Brain Death, Organ Donation, and Transplantation

Brain Death, Organ Donation, and Transplantation

The Precious Gift of Restoring Life

Edited by

ANNA TERESA MAZZEO
AND DEEPAK GUPTA

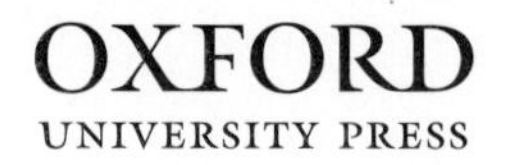

OXFORD
UNIVERSITY PRESS

Great Clarendon Street, Oxford, OX2 6DP,
United Kingdom

Oxford University Press is a department of the University of Oxford.
It furthers the University's objective of excellence in research, scholarship,
and education by publishing worldwide. Oxford is a registered trade mark of
Oxford University Press in the UK and in certain other countries

Published in India by
Oxford University Press
22 Workspace, 2nd Floor, 1/22 Asaf Ali Road, New Delhi 110 002, India

© Oxford University Press India 2022

The moral rights of the authors have been asserted

First Edition published in 2022

All rights reserved. No part of this publication may be reproduced, stored in
a retrieval system, or transmitted, in any form or by any means, without the
prior permission in writing of Oxford University Press, or as expressly permitted
by law, by licence or under terms agreed with the appropriate reprographics
rights organization. Enquiries concerning reproduction outside the scope of the
above should be sent to the Rights Department, Oxford University Press, at the
address above

You must not circulate this work in any other form
and you must impose this same condition on any acquirer

ISBN-13 (print edition): 978-0-19-013269-9
ISBN-10 (print edition): 0-19-013269-8

DOI: 10.1093/actrade/9780190132699.001.0001

Typeset in Minion Pro 10.5/14
by Newgen KnowledgeWorks Pvt. Ltd., Chennai, India

Printed in India by Rakmo Press Pvt. Ltd.

Cover art: Anna Teresa Mazzeo, *The Thousand Challenges of
the Anesthesiologist*, 1991, oil on canvas.

Dedicated to

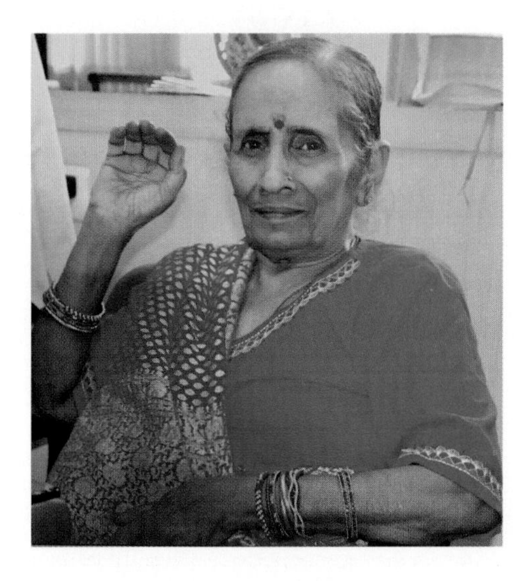

Amma

My mother for her omnipresent guiding force and selfless sacrifices

Deepak Gupta

To my Parents Angelo and Germana
bright guides illuminating my life
for their love, teaching, sacrifices, and exemplary dedication to Family

To the memory of my Grandparents Carmelo and Anna, Marco and Teresa
for teaching me honesty, humility, and justice

To my Patients and their Families
for sharing with me victories and defeats

Anna Teresa Mazzeo

To all the invisible Donors and their Families worldwide
for their precious gift of restoring life

To all Colleagues dedicated to organ donation and transplantation
for making the gift of life a dream that becomes reality

Anna Teresa Mazzeo and Deepak Gupta

Preface

Humanity facing one of the most dramatic pandemics of this century found itself weak and unprepared in front of invisible lethal threat—novel corona virus disease 2019 (COVID-19). It is in this actual and on-going scenario that I have been asked to write preface of this book 'Brain death, organ donation, and transplantation. *The precious gift of restoring life*'.

I felt especially proud of this commitment in my position as President of the World Federation of Neurosurgical Societies (WFNS). The mission of the WFNS is to work together to improve worldwide neurosurgical care, training, and research to benefit our patients.

I find a *similitude between global COVID-19 challenge and organ donation and transplantation need. Currently,* thousands of people are dying because of the virus and even the most organized and advanced healthcare systems are sometimes finding themselves inadequate to face such a challenge. *Similarly,* thousands of people are dying daily while waiting for a transplant as a more silent epidemic. Transplantation is a life-saving therapy for patients with end-stage organ failure, but donor shortage is still a significant problem in the clinical practice and a huge proportion of patients continue to die while on waiting list for a transplant.

World Health Organization and organizations from all over the world are nowadays working incessantly to stop the pandemic, to find resources, and to reduce the number of deaths. In the same way, transplant organizations are engaged in an endless activity to promote organ donation and transplantation all over the world.

Endless effort of healthcare providers and strategically work of several international organizations and professional societies represents nowadays the most important response to epidemic, while looking for future therapies.

Similarly, exchange of knowledge between countries, educational and training activities, national and international initiatives, are constantly playing an active role in the field of organ donation and transplantation all over the world.

Even if several countries are experiencing a tangible increase in numbers of donation and transplantation during recent years, nevertheless, the entire world is still facing the emergency, daily struggling against organ shortage and assisting to thousands of potentially avoidable deaths.

This book is expected to reach the international audience in a difficult moment for the humanity, a period in which we are all discovering to be united while fighting against a common enemy (COVID-19). The entire world stands united to find the best solution to control a threat towards which nobody was prepared. Solidarity, gratitude, generosity, sharing of knowledge and of research, are all themes of extraordinary actuality and are inherent characteristics of organ donation activity as well.

This book opera 'Brain death, organ donation, and transplantation. *The precious gift of restoring life*' is a well-balanced combination of different issues related to brain death diagnosis, organ donation (criteria for heart beating and non-heart beating death), organ donor management, and management of transplantation (patients, techniques, organization procedures). The ethical aspects are also covered in great detail. All these issues are discussed at a multidisciplinary level (clinicians and scientists, surgeons, internists, anaesthesiologists, psychologists, immunologists, etc.), at an international level, at a multi-cultural, religious level.

I wish that this book may help clinicians, students, institutions, organizations, politicians, in spreading the opportunities of organ donation and transplantation all over the world to give the immense gift of new lives to millions of patients who need transplant of organs or tissues.

Franco Servadei

President World Federation of Neurosurgical Societies (2017–2021)

Contents

About the Editors

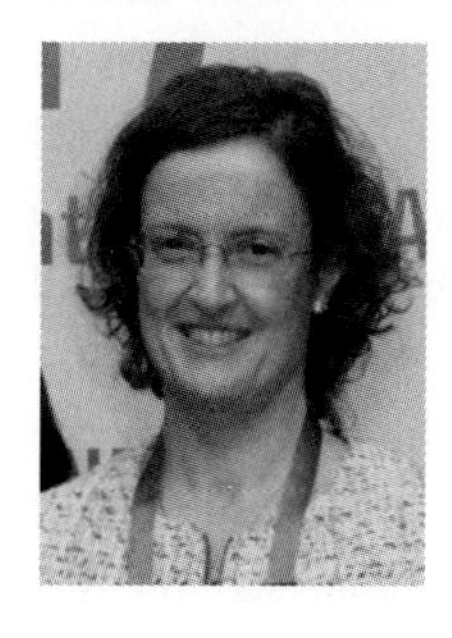

Anna Teresa Mazzeo is Associate Professor of Anesthesia and Intensive care at University of Messina, Italy. She previously served at University of Torino, A.O.U. Citta' della Salute e della Scienza di Torino, Molinette Hospital, which is one of the main transplantation centers in Europe.

She got trained as Research Fellow in 'Neurological Surgery and Neurointensive Care Monitoring' at Neuroscience ICU of Virginia Commonwealth University in Richmond, Virginia, USA. As part of her training she further completed several university stages in Europe and USA. Since 1996 she has been working as anesthesiologist and intensivist at University Hospitals and collaborating with international research groups.

Her main areas of interest are neurointensive care, neuroanesthesia, neuromonitoring, brain death and organ donor management, acute respiratory distress syndrome, extracorporeal membrane oxygenation, metabolic assessment during ex-vivo lung and liver perfusion, critical care management of severe COVID patients.

She has dedicated a significant part of her clinical and academic activity to the care of the acute brain injury patients, the critical care management of the potential organ donors, and, more recently, microdialysis monitoring of harvested organs requiring reconditioning procedures before transplantation.

She is highly interested and committed in residents and medical student education and training. Art-work and painting are her favorite hobbies.

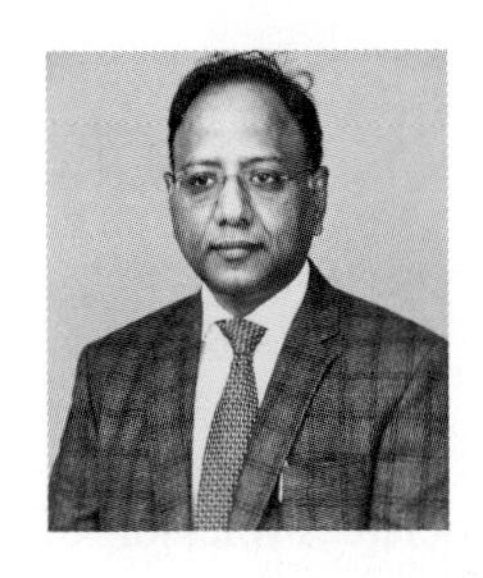

Deepak Gupta is a Professor of Neurosurgery at the All India Institute of Medical Sciences, New Delhi, India. He has over 20 years of experience in Neurosurgery, did his PhD on development of indigenous Finite Element Model of Craniovertebral junction in a joint collaboration with Indian Institute of Technology, Delhi. His key areas of interest include—Advanced Head and Spinal trauma care, Pediatric Craniofacial deformities, and Pediatric Neuro oncology. He is actively involved in looking after Organ donation and Transplantation services.

He has played a pivotal role in establishing a model head injury service at the Jai Prakash Narain Apex Trauma Centre, Delhi. He has significant contribution to head injury research—cerebral microdialysis and ICP monitoring. He is also involved in various guidelines on head trauma and pediatric neurosurgery diseases for India/globally (STF-ICMR for Head trauma, IndSPN society for hydrocephalus and meningomyelocele, NTSI national neurotrauma guidelines for head injury, ADAPT and Centre TBI for Head trauma studies).

He represents India as a member of neurotrauma section of World Federation of Neurological surgery (WFNS International). He is on the editorial boards of such journals as Child's Nervous System and Pediatric Neurosurgery. He is recipient of number of national and international awards.

He led the Craniopagus team of 125 doctors and paramedics leading to first successful separation surgery on Craniopagus conjoined twins of India in 2017. He has authored various books and has over 300 publications to his credit.

Contributors

Aadil Ali, BSc
Latner Thoracic Surgery Research Laboratories
University Health Network
Toronto, ON

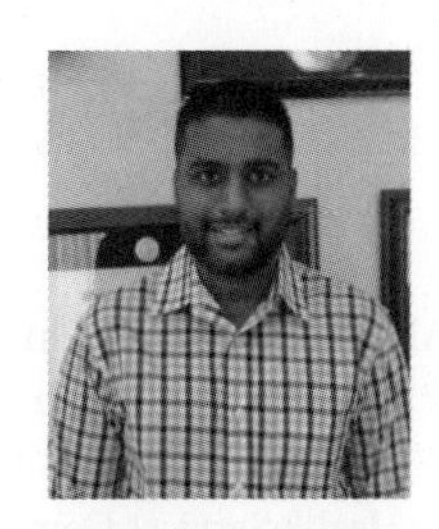

Ibrahim Asma Al Mannaei, MBBS and MPH
Executive Director, Research and
Innovation Center
Department of Health
Abu Dhabi, United Arab Emirates

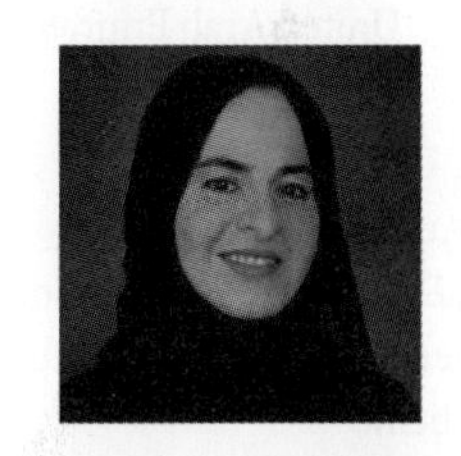

Abdulla A Al Sayyari, MD
Professor of Medicine, King Saudi Bin Abdulaziz
University for Health Sciences
Riyadh, Saudi Arabia

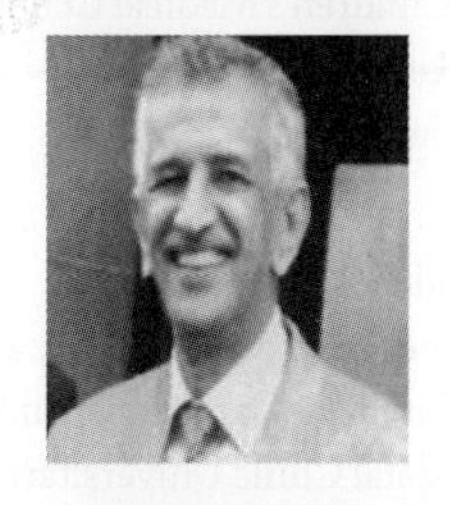

Fayez Alshamsi, MBBS, DABIM, FRCPC
Assistant Professor and Consultant in Internal and
Critical Care Medicine
Department of Internal Medicine, College
of Medicine & Health Sciences. United Arab
Emirates University
Al Ain, United Arab Emirates

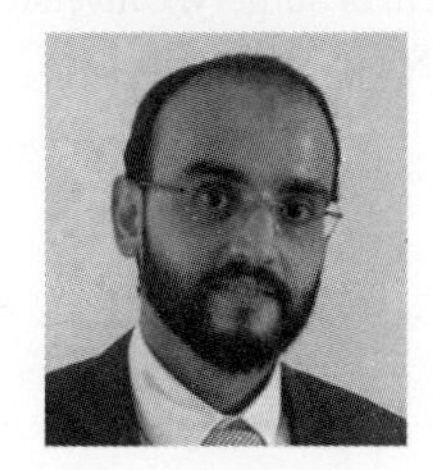

Juglans Alvarez, MD
Toronto General Hospital, University Health Network, Toronto, Division of Cardiac Surgery, University of Toronto
Toronto, ON, Canada

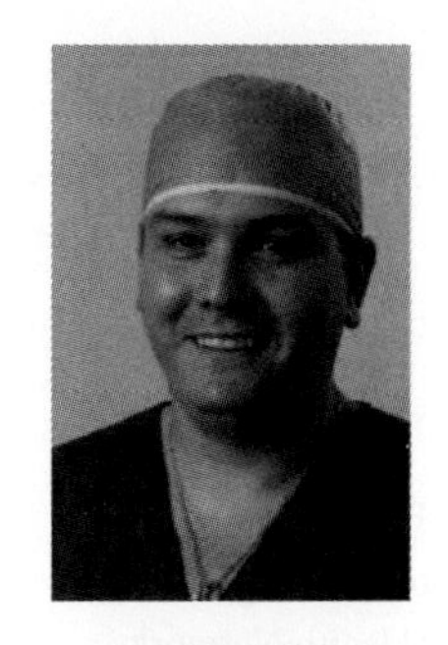

Zain Ali Al Yafei, BSc, M.Sc., PhD
Pharmacy and Allied Health Director
Corporate Medical & Clinical Affairs
Abu Dhabi Health Services Company – SEHA
Abu Dhabi, United Arab Emirates

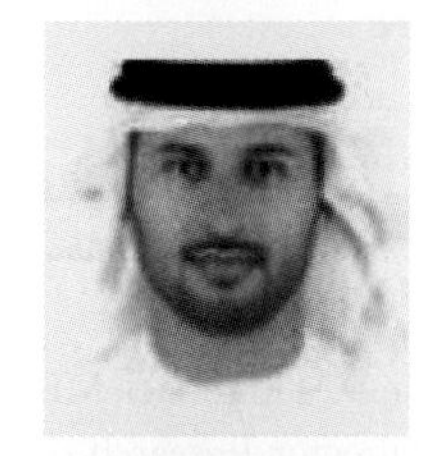

Takashi Araki, MD, PhD
Director, Division of Traumatology,
Department of Emergency, Trauma and Critical Care Medicine
Saitama Children's Medical Center, Saitama Medical University
Saitama, Japan

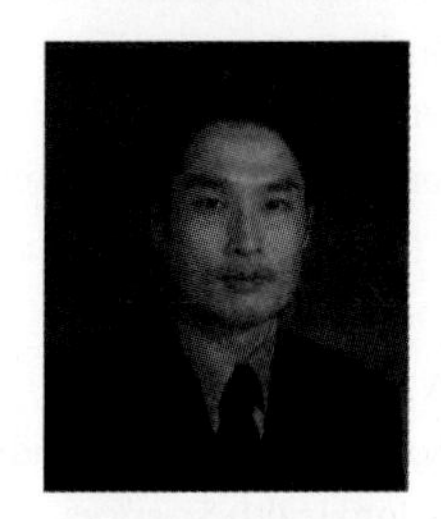

Rafael Badenes, MD
Department of Anaesthesiology and Surgical-Trauma Intensive Care Transplant Coordination Unit. Hospital Clinic Universitari de Valencia
Department of Surgery, University of Valencia
Valencia, Spain

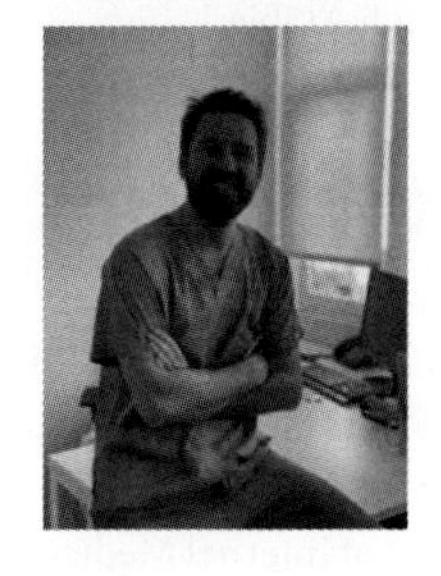

Chloë Ballesté Delpierre, MD
International Cooperation and Development
Director, DTI Foundation
Researcher, Transplantation Advisory Unit,
Hospital Clínic de Barcelona
Associate Professor, Department of Surgery and
Surgical Specialties, Universitat de Barcelona
European Society for Transplantation (ESOT)
Councilor
Barcelona, Spain

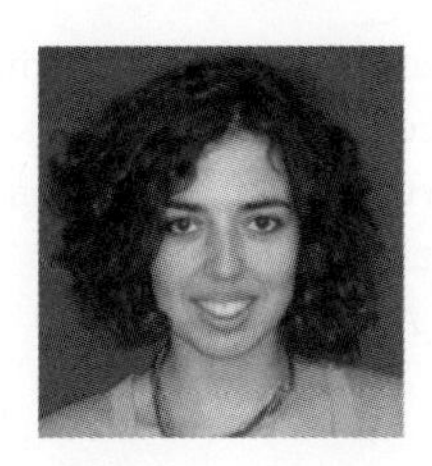

Ajit Kumar Banerji, MD
Emeritus Professor and Former Chief
Neurosciences Centre
All India Institute of Medical Science (AIIMS)
New Delhi, India

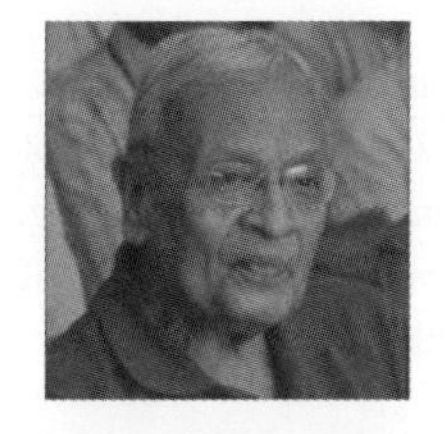

Cristina Barbero, MD, PhD
Heart and Lung Transplant Center, Cardiac
Surgery Division, Surgical Sciences Department,
Città della Salute e della Scienza,
University of Torino
Torino, Italy

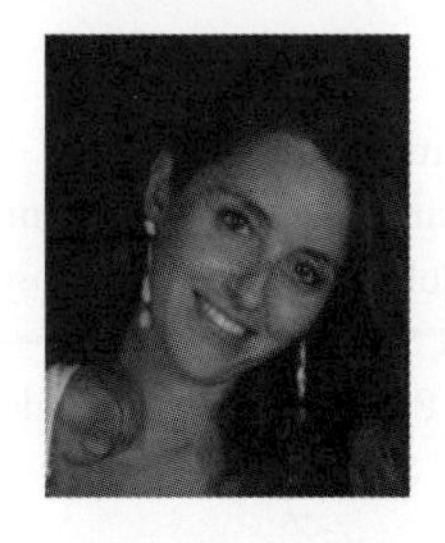

Stefania Barbieri, MD
Anesthesiology and Intensive Care, Department
of Medicine
University of Padova
Padova, Italy

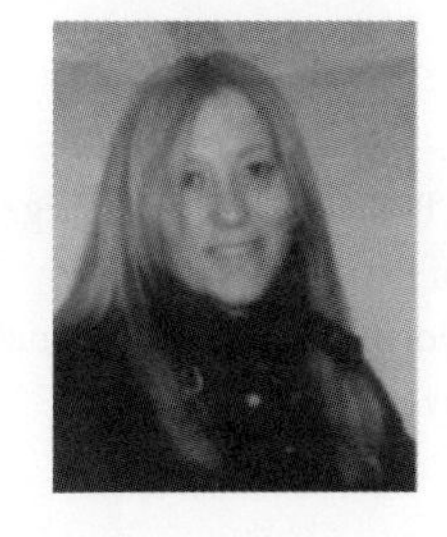

Lucinda Barry, RN, GradDip (Emerg)
Chief Executive Officer
Australian Organ and Tissue Donation and
Transplantation Authority
Canberra, Australia

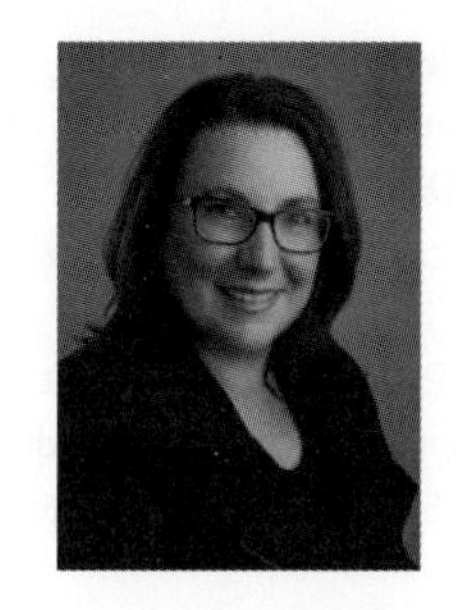

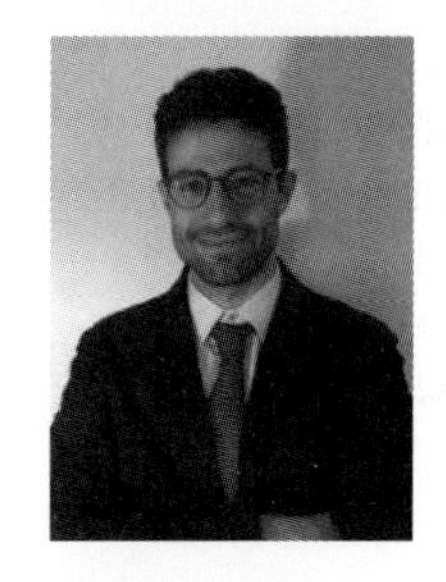

Michele Bartoletti, MD
Infectious Diseases Unit, S. Orsola Hospital,
Department of Medical and Surgical Sciences,
Alma Mater Studiorum University of Bologna
Bologna, Italy

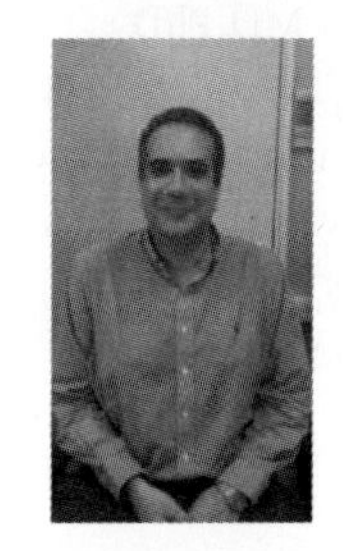

Adalia Ramon Bartolomé, MD
Head of Surgical Critical Care Unit.
Anesthesiology Department. Hospital del Mar.
Barcelona, Spain.
Associate Professor, Universitat de Barcelona
Barcelona, Spain

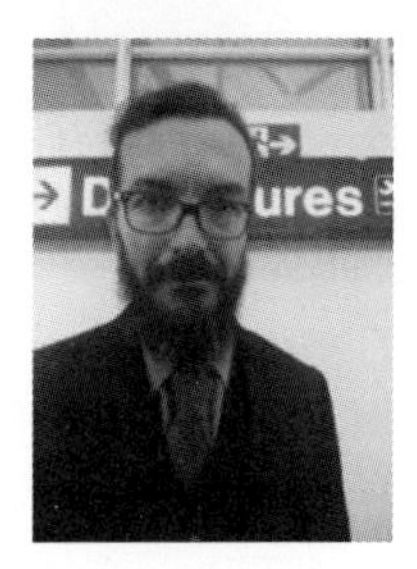

Tommaso Bellandi, PhD, Eur. Erg.
Director of Patient Safety Unit,
Tuscany Northwest Trust, Regional Health Service
Lucca, Italy

Gabriella Biffa, PsyD
Clinical Psychology Unit
IRCCS Ospedale Policlinico San Martino
Genoa, Italy

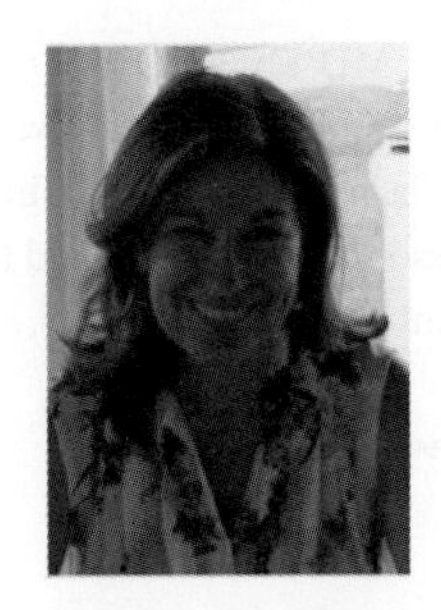

Carmen Blanco
DTI Foundation
TPM Courses coordinator
Barcelona, Spain

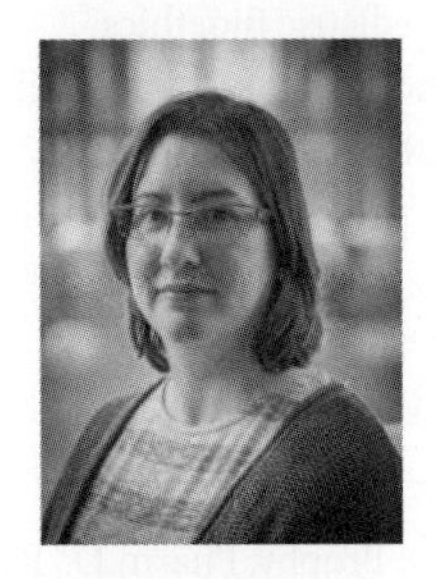

Massimo Boffini, MD
Associate Professor Heart and Lung Transplant Center, Cardiac Surgery Division, Surgical Sciences Department, Città della Salute e della Scienza, University of Torino
Turin, Italy

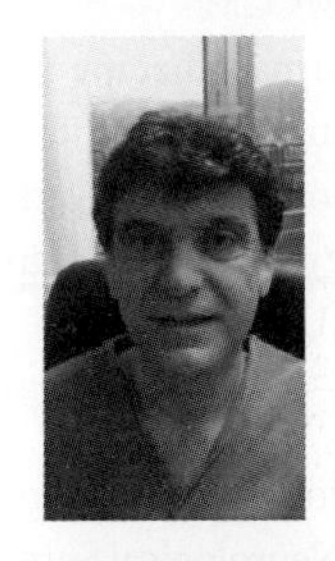

Deeplaxmi Borle, MD
Duke University School of Medicine
Department of Surgery, Division of Abdominal Transplant Surgery
Durham, NC, USA

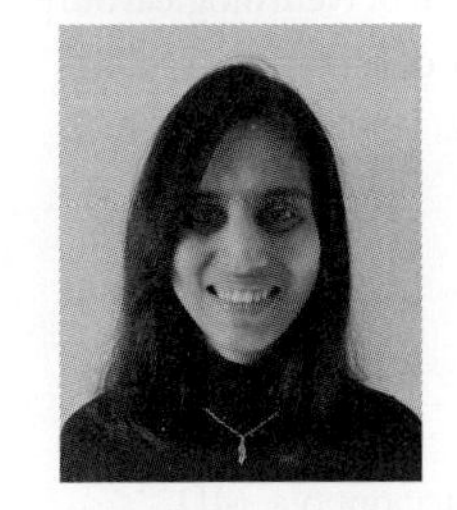

Luca Brazzi, MD, PhD
Director Anesthesia and Intensive Care, Città della Salute e della Scienza Hospital, Turin, Italy
Full Professor in Anaesthesia and Intensive Care, Department of Surgical Sciences, University of Turin
Turin, Italy

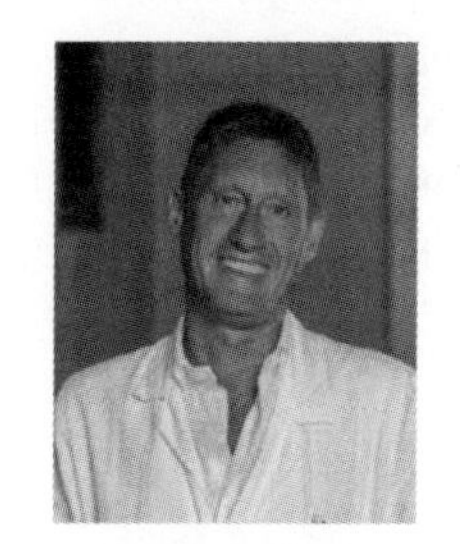

Joe Brierley, MBChB, FRCPCH, FFICM, MA
PICU & Paediatric Bioethics
Great Ormond St for Children NHS trust
London, UK

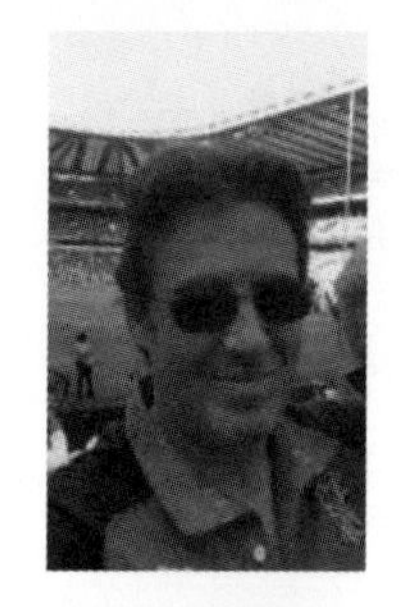

Gretchen M Brophy, Pharm.D., BCPS, FCCP, FCCM, FNCS, MCCM
Professor of Pharmacotherapy & Outcomes Science and Neurosurgery
Virginia Commonwealth University
Medical College of Virginia Campus
Richmond, VA, USA

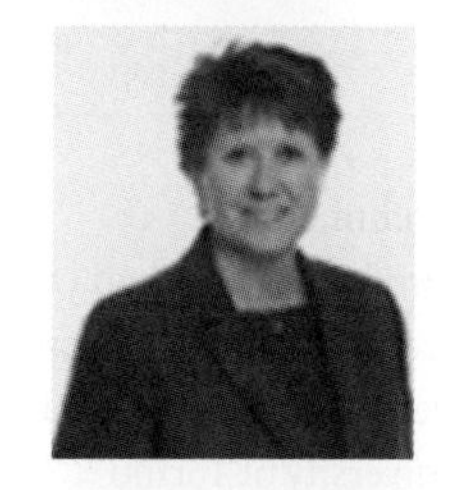

M Ross Bullock, MD, PhD
Professor Emeritus of Neurosurgery
Department of Neurological Surgery
University of Miami
Miami, FL, USA

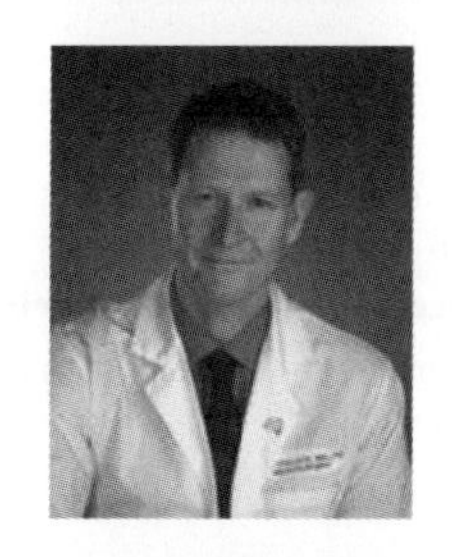

Alessio Caccioppola, MD
General Intensive Care Unit, Department of Anesthesia and Critical Care
Fondazione IRCCS Cà Granda-Ospedale Maggiore Policlinico
Milan, Italy

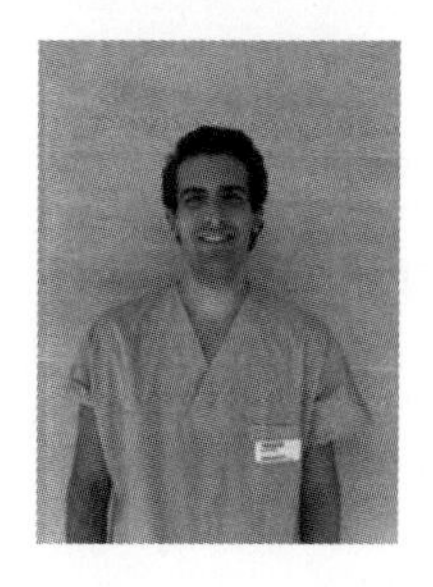

Adrian Caceres, MD
Pediatric Neurosurgery National Children's
Hospital of Costa Rica
Associated Professor University of Costa Rica
San Jose, Costa Rica

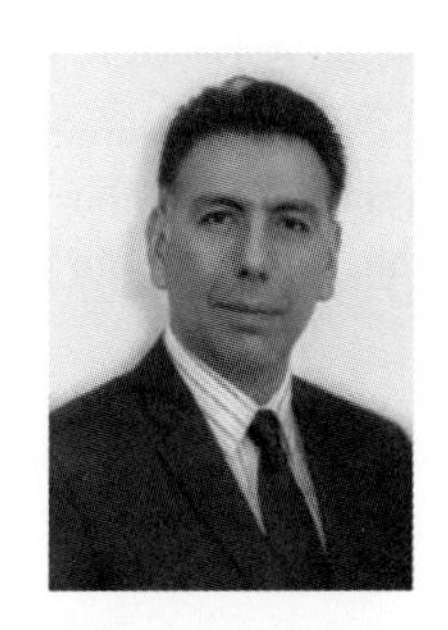

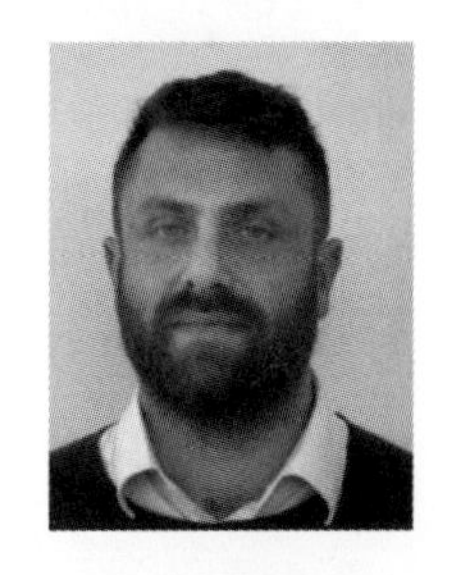

Marco Carbonara, MD
Neuroscience Intensive Care Unit, Department of
Anesthesia and Critical Care. Fondazione IRCCS
Cà Granda-Ospedale Maggiore Policlinico
Milan, Italy

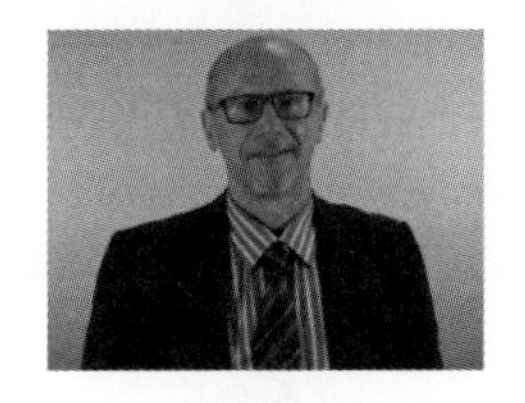

Massimo Cardillo, MD
Director Italian National Transplant Centre,
Italian National Institute of Health
Rome, Italy

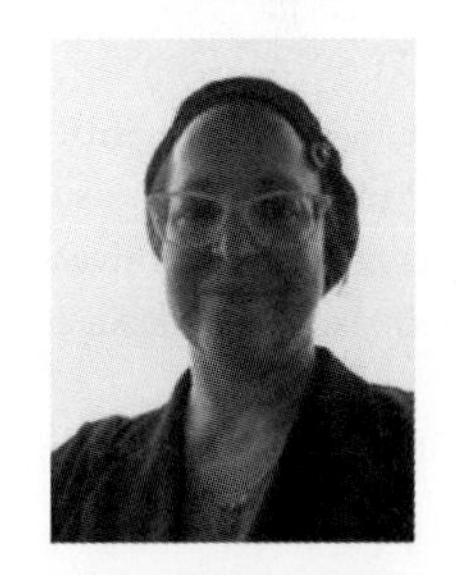

Cristiana Carollo, MD
Anesthesiology and Intensive Care, Department of
Medicine, University of Padova
Padova, Italy

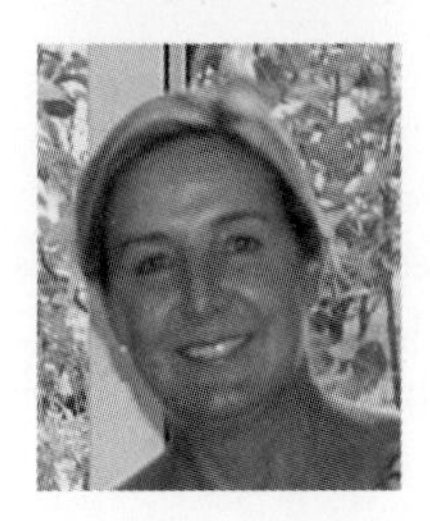

Carlotta Castagnoli, MD
Qualified Person, Turin Skin Bank Tissue and Cell
Factory, CTO, Città della Salute e della Scienza
Turin, Italy

Giuseppe Citerio, MD
Professor and Director Neurointensive Care, San Gerardo Hospital, ASST, Monza
Editor in Chief Intensive Care Medicine
Monza, Italy

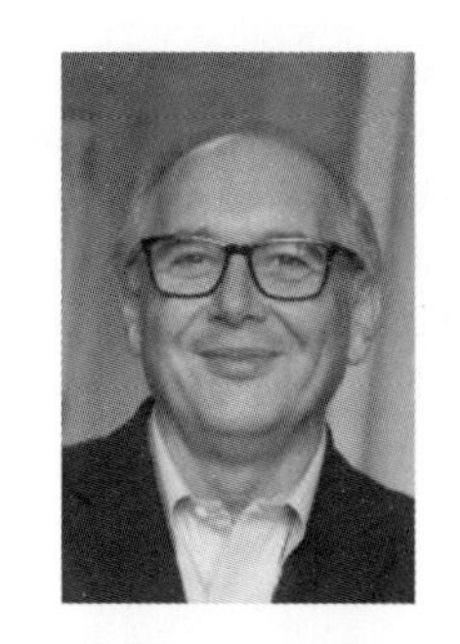

Liesl N Close, MD
Resident Physician, Department of Neurosurgery
University of Iowa Hospitals and Clinics
Iowa City, IA, USA

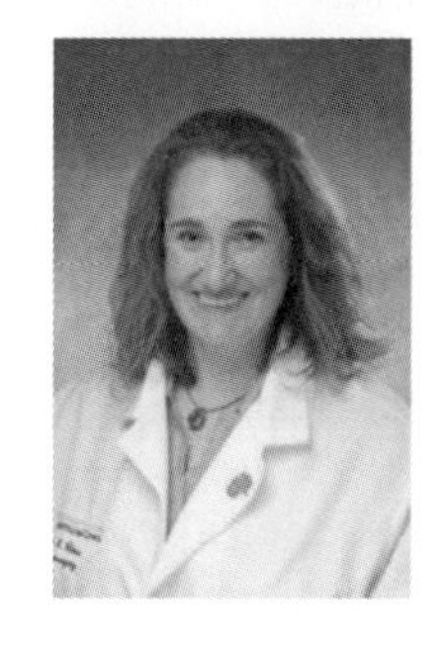

Alba Coll, PhD
DTI Foundation
Master and blended courses coordinator
Barcelona, Spain

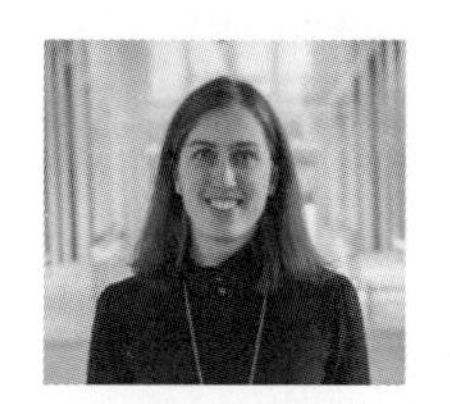

Alfredo Conti, MD, PhD, FEBNS
Associate Professor of Neurosurgery
Alma Mater Studiorum University of Bologna
IRCCS ISNB-Istituto delle Scienze Neurologiche Bellaria
Bologna, Italy

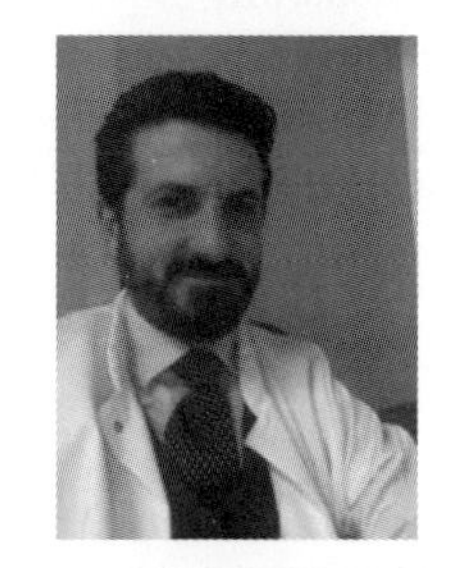

Silvia Corcione, MD
Department of Medical Sciences, Infectious Diseases, University of Turin
Turin, Italy

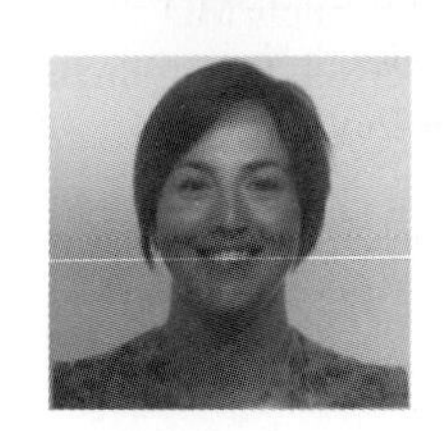

Joseph Costa, DHSc., PA-C
Instructor of Clinical Surgical Sciences in Surgery
Columbia University College of Physicians and Surgeons
Columbia University Medical Center
New York, NY, USA

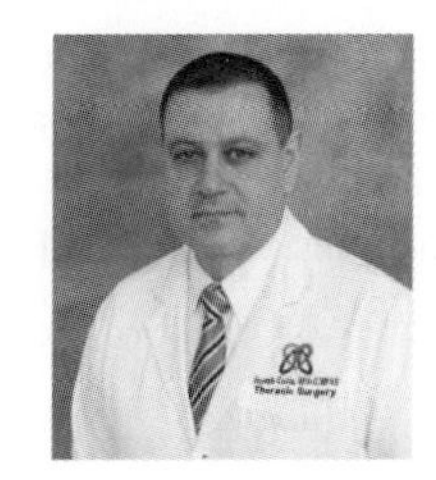

Paolo Costa, MD
Section of Clinical Neurophysiology, CTO Hospital
Città della Salute e della Scienza di Torino
Turin, Italy

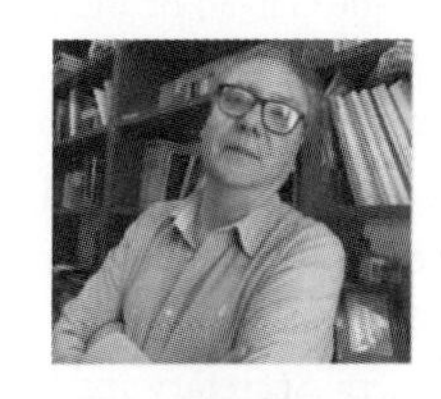

Andrea Costamagna, MD
Department of Anaesthesia and Critical Care,
Città della Salute e della Scienza di Torino,
Molinette Hospital
Turin, Italy

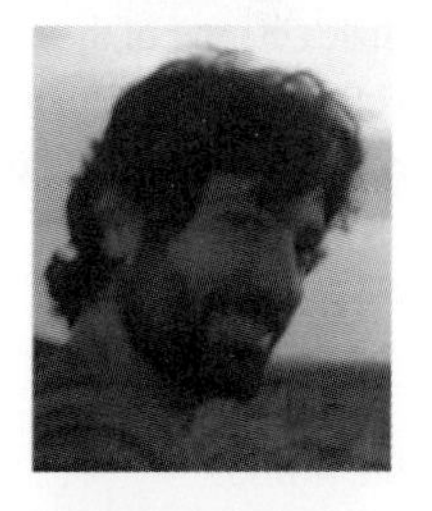

Colin Coulter, B.A. (Hons) MBChB
Anaesthetic Trainee
Barts Health NHS Trust
London, UK

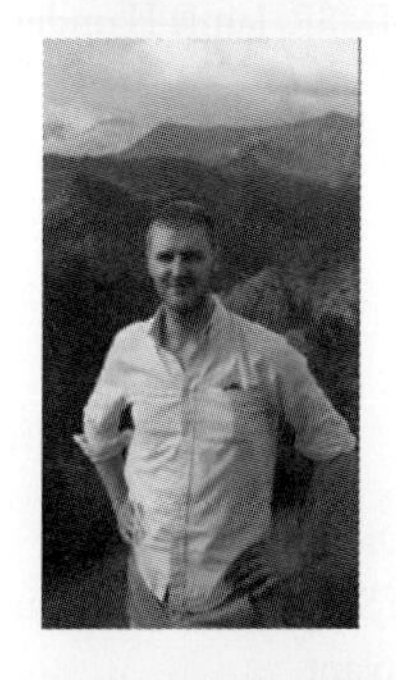

Marcelo Cypel, MD, MSc
Latner Thoracic Surgery Research Laboratories,
University Health Network
Division of Thoracic Surgery, University Health Network
Toronto, ON, Canada

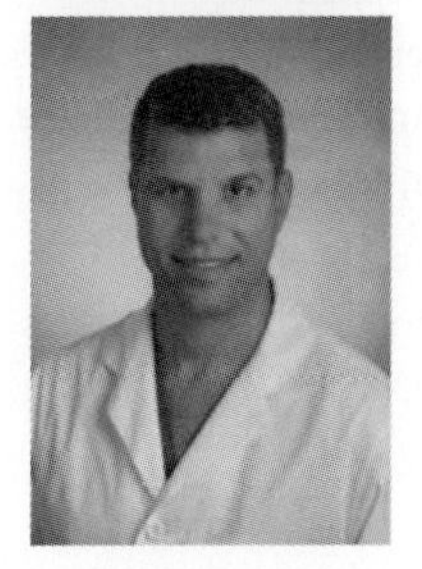

Tereza Eickmann Bruno Da Cunha
Journalist and researcher in the area of human rights
Teacher and translator English-Portuguese
Recife, Brazil

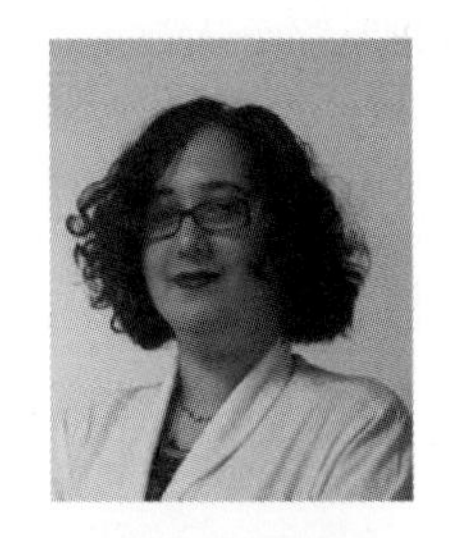

Artur Henrique Galvão Bruno Da Cunha, MD
Pediatric Neurosurgeon. President elected of GLEN 2021/2023
Chairman of the Board of KAAD in Recife.
Former President of the Brazilian Society of Pediatric Neurosurgery
Former General Secretary and former President of the Pediatric Chapter of the Latin American Federation of Neurosurgical Society. Member of the International Society of Pediatric Neurosurgery
Recife, Brazil

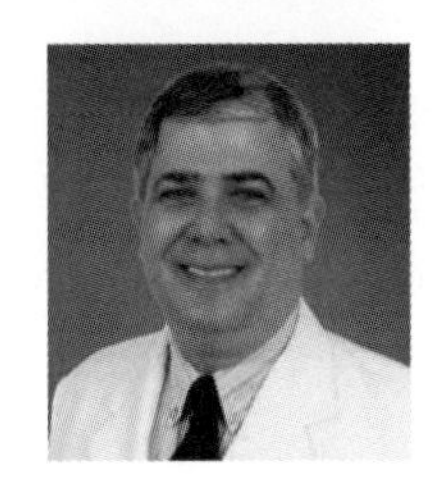

Tanshi Daljit, MBBS
Internist, HIMSR, Jamia Hamdard
Delhi, India

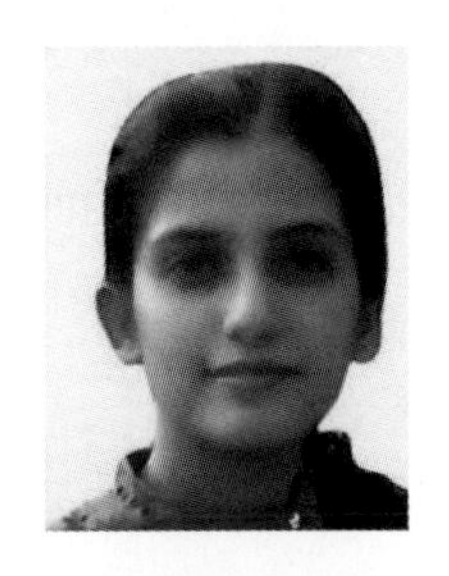

Richard C Daly, MD
Professor of Surgery, Surgical Director Heart and Lung Transplant
Department of Cardiovascular Surgery
Mayo Clinic School of Medicine, Mayo Clinic
Rochester, MN, USA

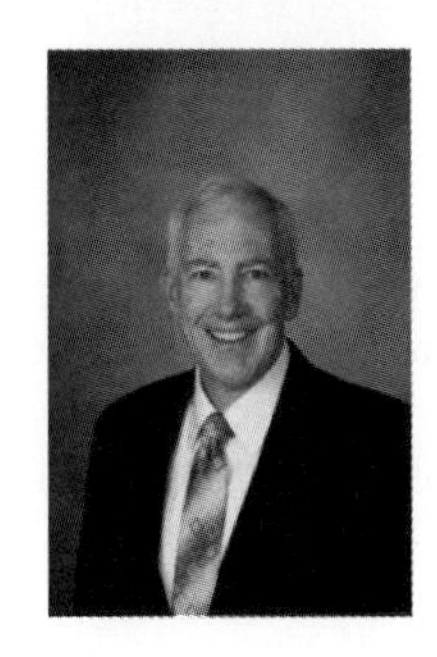

Valentina Della Torre, MD
Department of Surgery. University of Valencia. Spain. Department of Intensive Care, St Mary's Hospital Imperial College Healthcare NHS Trust, St Mary's Hospital
London, UK

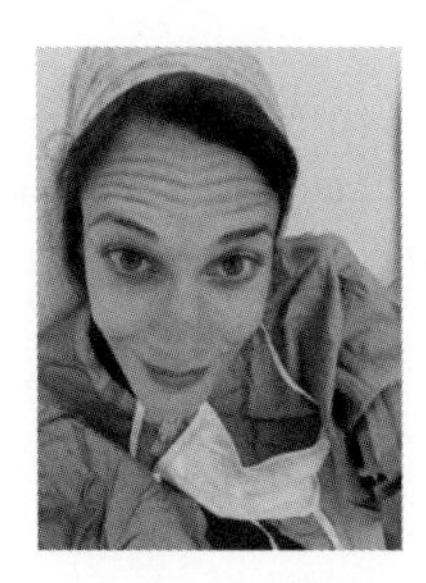

Lorenzo Del Sorbo, MD
Toronto General Hospital, University Health Network, Toronto
Interdepartmental Division of Critical Care Medicine University of Toronto
Toronto, ON, Canada

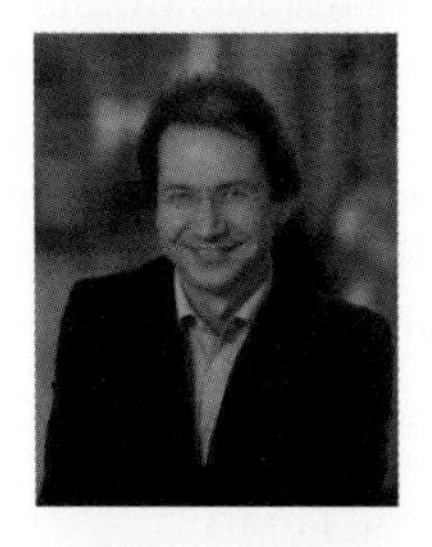

Francesco Giuseppe De Rosa, MD
Associate Professor, Department of Medical Sciences, University of Turin
Director, Infectious Diseases
City of Health & Science
Turin & Asti, Italy

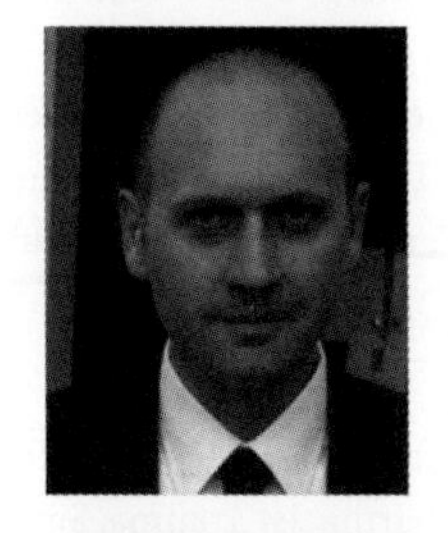

Antonia D'Errico, MD
Professor Pathology Unit, S.Orsola-Malpighi University Hospital
Bologna, Italy

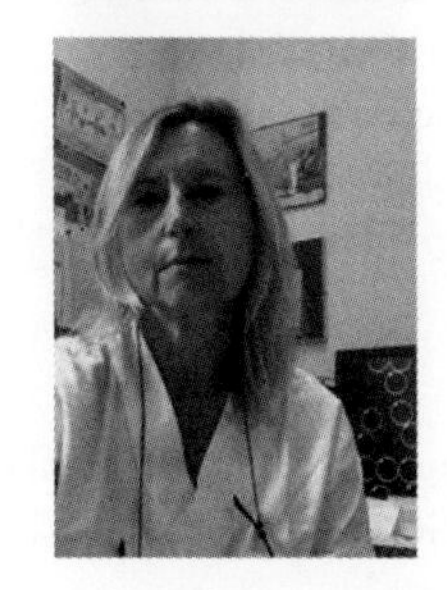

Paola Di Ciaccio, MD
Italian National Transplant Centre, Italian National Institute of Health, Rome
Rome, Italy

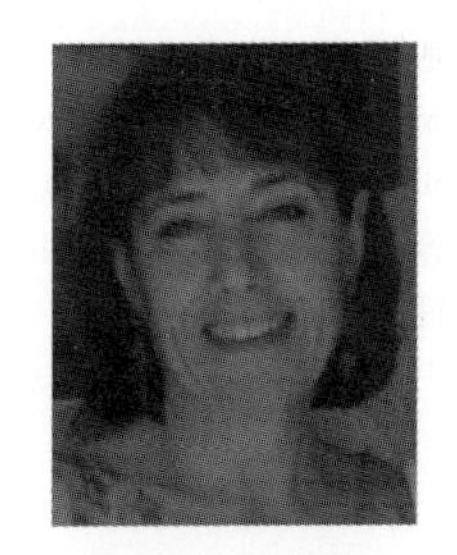

Carlo Di Giambattista, MD, PhD
President SSHM Scientific Society for Human Medicine
Medical Coordinator Isenior Group - elderly care
CEO Health International srl
Torino, Italy

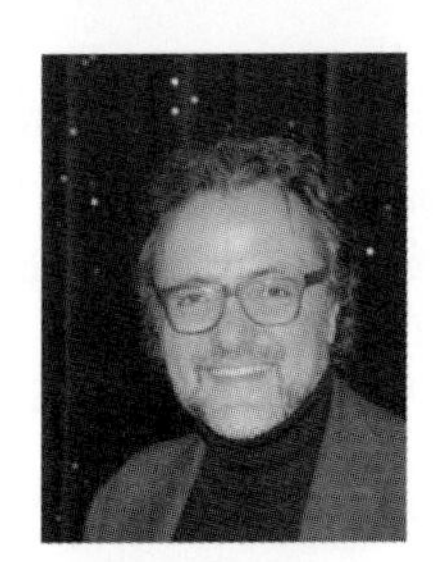

Matteo Di Nardo, MD
Pediatric Intensive Care Unit, Children`s Hospital Bambino Gesù, Rome, Italy
Toronto General Hospital, University Health Network, Toronto, Interdepartmental Division of Critical Care Medicine, University of Toronto
Toronto, ON, Canada

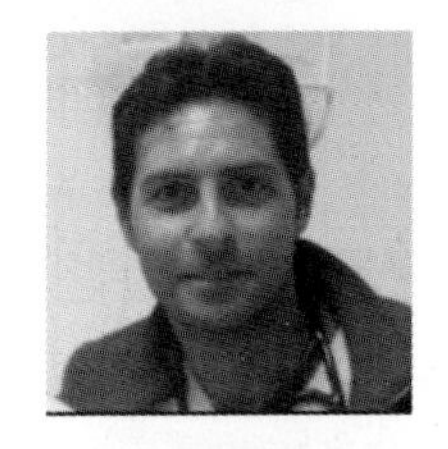

Russell Dixon, PharmD, BCCCP
Clinical Pharmacist Trauma, Surgical, and Neurologic Critical Care
St. John Medical Center
Tulsa, OK, USA

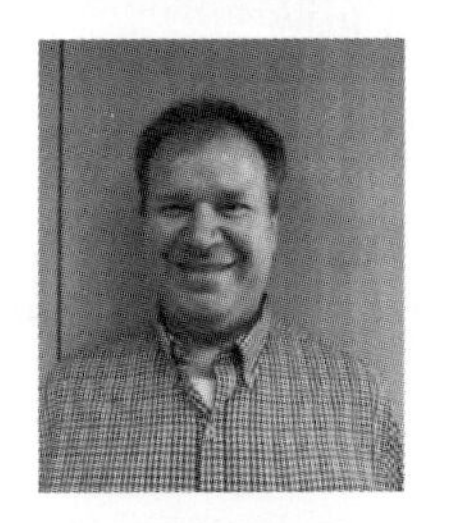

Beatriz Domínguez-Gil, MD, PhD
Director General, Organización Nacional de Trasplantes
Madrid, Spain

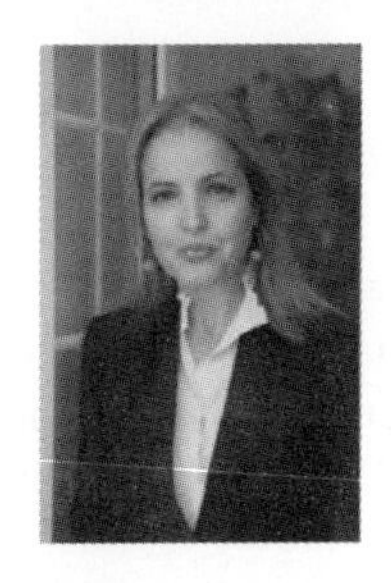

Frank D'Ovidio, MD, PhD
Associate Professor of Surgery
Surgical Director, Lung Transplant Program
Director, Ex-Vivo Lung Perfusion Program
Columbia University College of Physicians and Surgeons
Columbia University Medical Center
New York, NY, USA

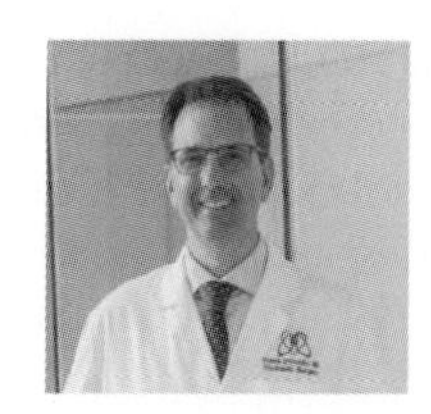

Tinus Du Toit, MD
Transplant surgeon, Department of Surgery,
Groote Schuur Hospital, University of Cape Town
Cape Town, South Africa

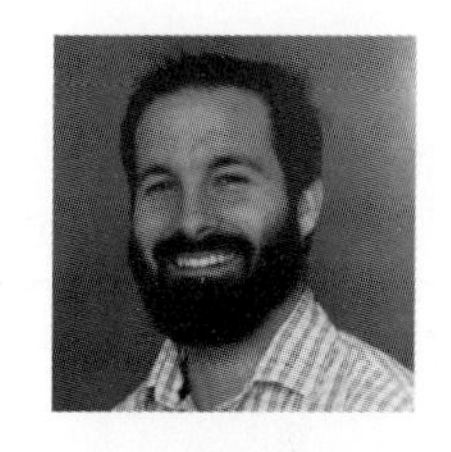

Deniz Dzhiner, MD
First Moscow State Medical University named after I.M. Sechenov Moscow, Russia

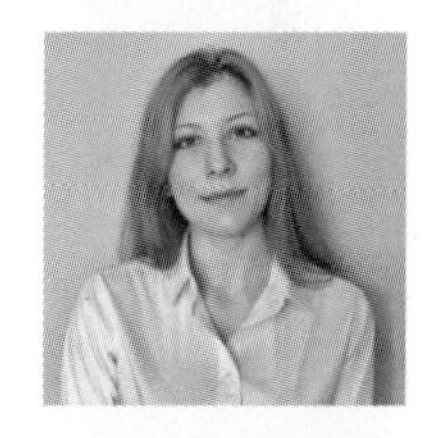

Albino Eccher, MD, PhD
Pathology Unit, Department of Pathology and Diagnostics, University and Hospital Trust of Verona
Verona, Italy

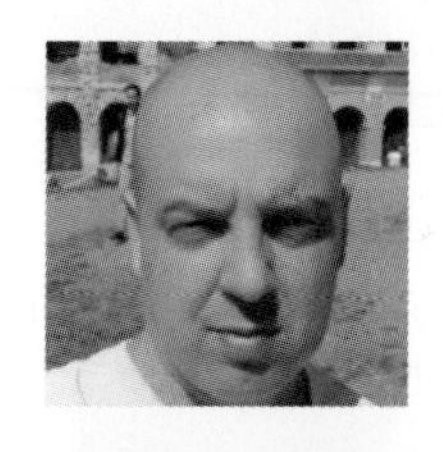

Hiroto Egawa, MD, PhD
Department of Surgery, Tokyo Women's Medical University,
Tokyo, Japan

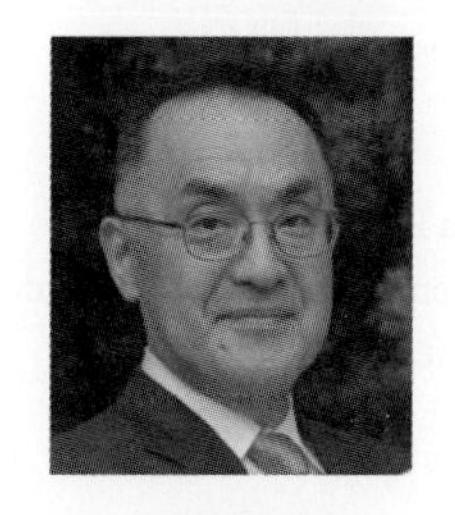

Gehad ElGhazali, MD, PhD
Professor Clinical Immunology
Consultant and Service Lead Immunologist
Sheikh Khalifa Medical City, Abu Dhabi, UAE

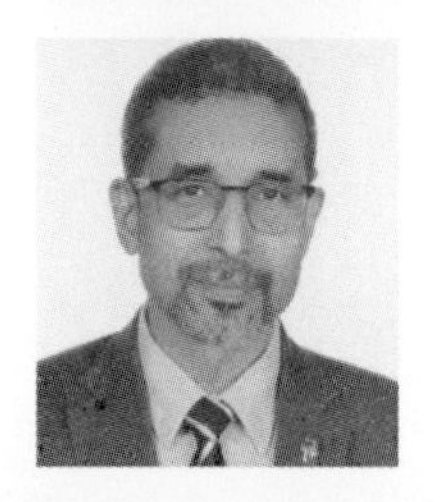

Vito Fanelli, MD, PhD
Associate professor of Anaesthesia and Critical Care, Città della Salute e della Scienza di Torino, Molinette Hospital
Department of Surgical Sciences, University of Torino
Turin, Italy

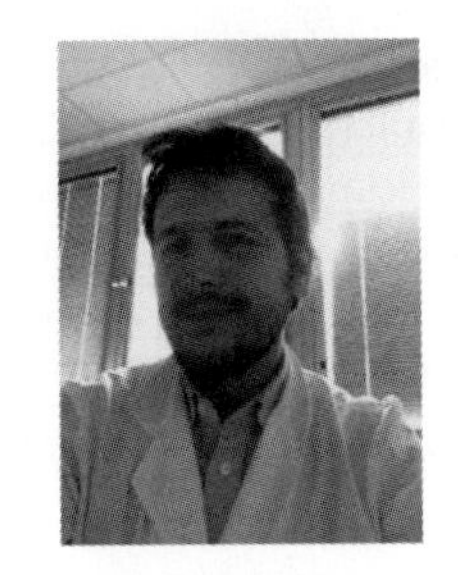

Ding-Yu Fei, PhD
Professor, Department of Biomedical Engineering
Virginia Commonwealth University
Richmond, VA, USA

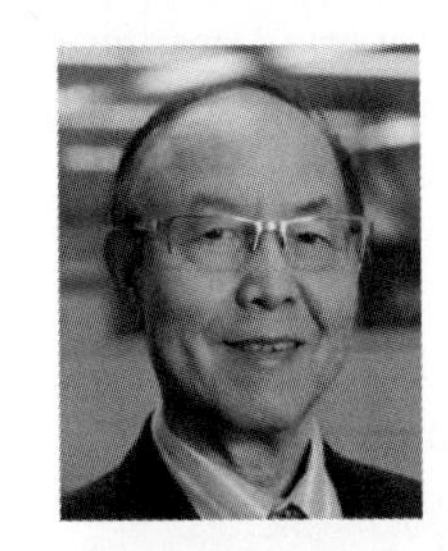

Paolo Feltracco, MD
Anesthesiology and Intensive Care, Department of Medicine
University of Padova
Padova, Italy

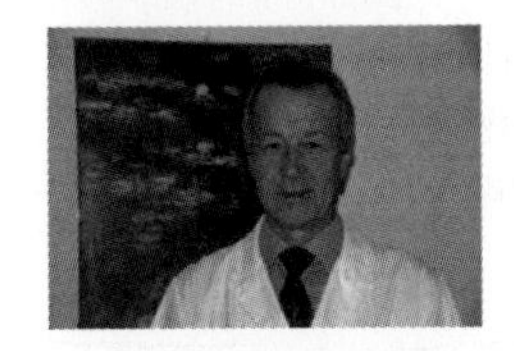

Stefano Ferrari, PhD
The Veneto Eye Bank Foundation
Venice, Italy

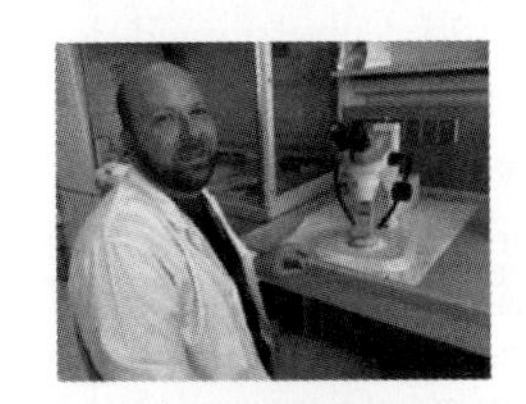

Francesca Fossi, MD
Neurointensive Care Unit, Grande Ospedale Metropolitano Niguarda
Milan, Italy

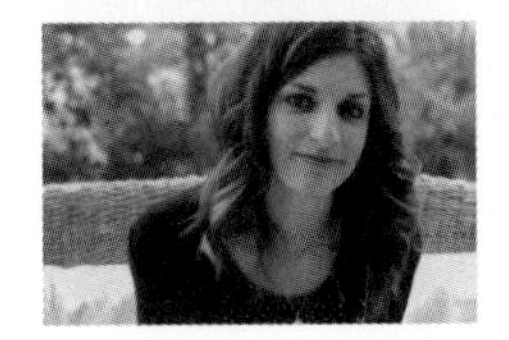

Paola Franco, MD
Paediatric Surgery, OIRM, Città della Salute e della Scienza
Turin, Italy

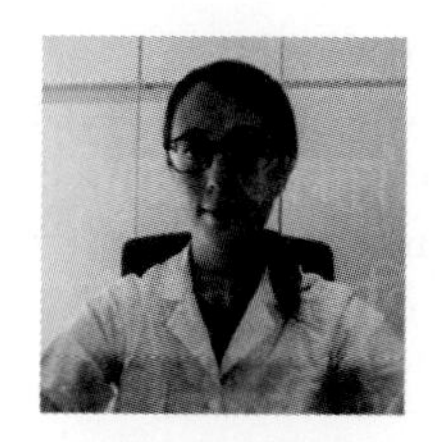

Alessandra Galeone, MD
University Hospital of Bari, Bari, Italy
The Veneto Eye Bank Foundation
Venice, Italy

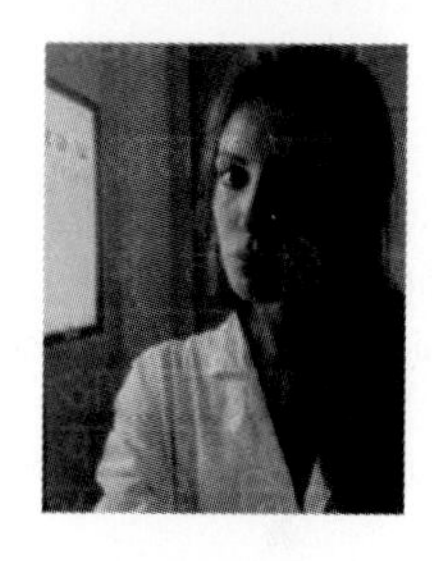

Domenica Garabello, MD
Radiology Consultant. Department of Radiology.
Citta' della Salute e della Scienza di Torino,
Molinette Hospital
Turin, Italy

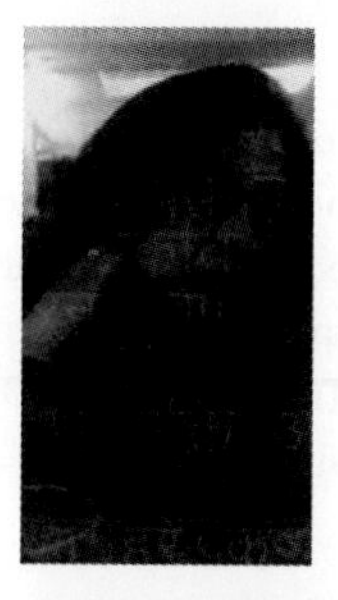

Sergey V Gautier, MD, PhD
Director of National Medical Research Center of Transplantology and Artificial Organs named after academician V.I. Shumakov, Moscow, Russia.
Head of Chair of Transplantology and Artificial Organs of I.M.Sechenov First Moscow State Medical University (Sechenov University)
Moscow, Russia

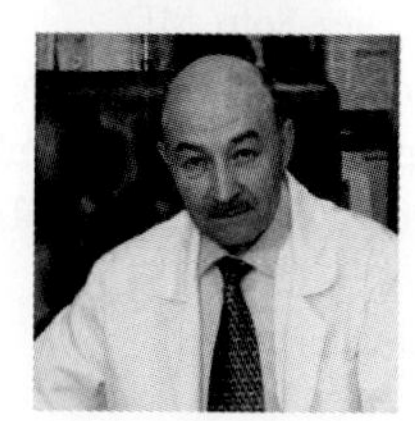

Federico Genzano Besso, MD, PHD
Piedmont Regional Transplant Agency
Tissue Banks and Biorepository, Department of Laboratory Medicine
Città della Salute e della Scienza di Torino
Turin, Italy

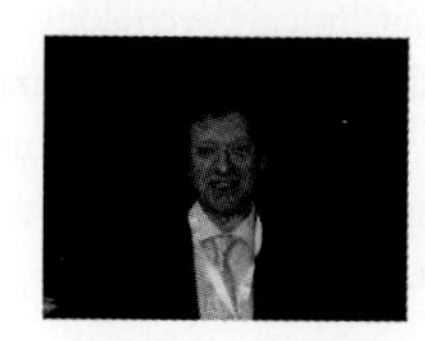

Nicola, Girtler, PsyD
Clinical Psychology Unit, IRCCS Ospedale Policlinico San Martino
Department of Neuroscience (DiNOGMI), University of Genoa
Genoa, Italy

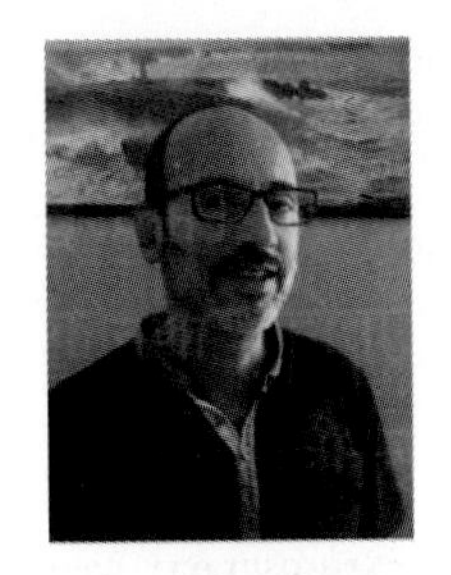

Lucia Golfieri, PsyD, PhD
UOC Medicina Interna Gravi Insufficienze d'organo
IRCCS - Azienda Ospedaliero Universitaria di Bologna
Bologna, Italy

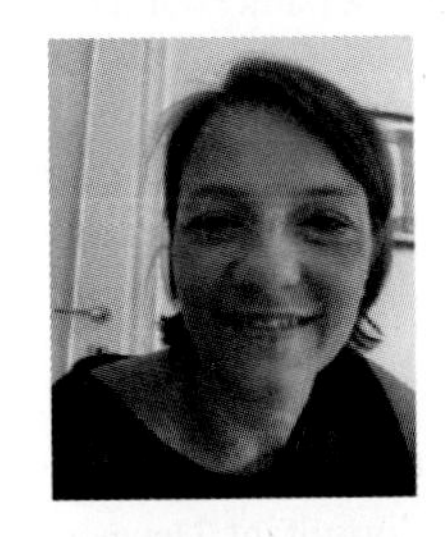

Maria Paula Gómez, MD
Transplant Procurement Manager
Executive Director, DTI Foundation. Medical Coordinator, International Registry in Organ Donation for Transplant—IRODaT
Barcelona, Spain

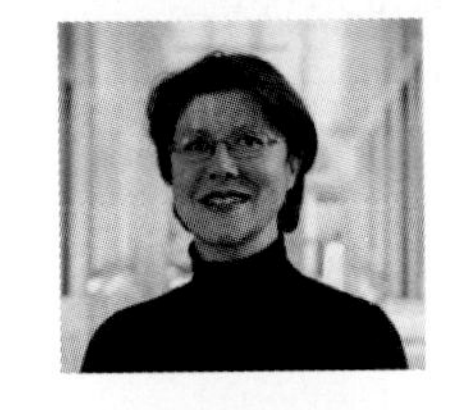

José A González-Soto, MD
Neurotrauma Research Group, MEDITECH Foundation, Bogotá/Cali (Colombia)
Neurosurgery Resident, Hospital Central de Maracay
Aragua State, Venezuela

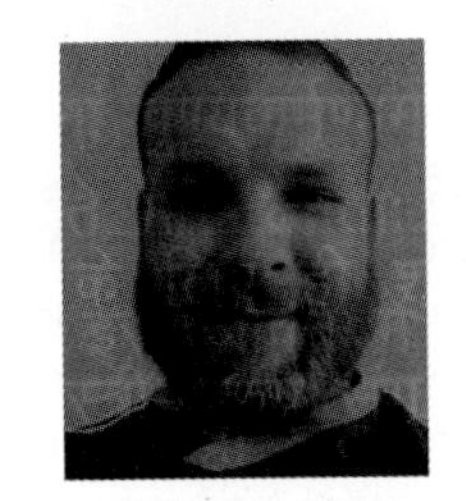

Silvana Grandi, MD
Professor of Clinical Psychology
Director Clinical and Psychosomatic Psychology Service for Organ Transplantation
Department of Psychology, University of Bologna
Bologna, Italy

Reginald Green
President
The Nicholas Green Foundation
USA

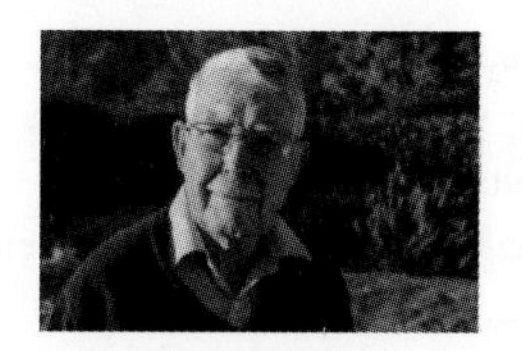

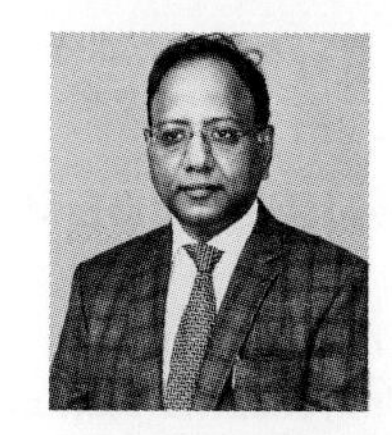

Deepak Gupta, MBBS, MS, MCH, PhD, FRCS
Professor of Neurosurgery. Department of Neurosurgery, All India Institute of Medical Sciences and Associated JPN Apex Trauma Centre
New Delhi, India

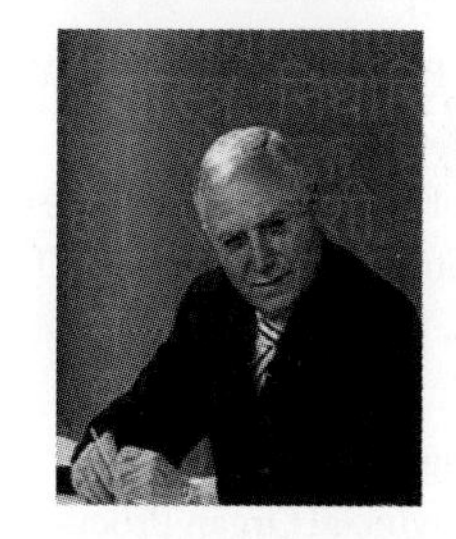

Mehmet Haberal, MD, FACS (Hon), FICS (Hon), FASA (Hon), FIMSA (Hon), Hon FRCS (Glasg)
Founder and Founder President, Baskent University
President of the Executive Supreme Board, Baskent University
Chair, Baskent University Division of Transplantation and Burns
Immediate Past-President, The Transplantation Society
Past-President, International Society for Burn Injuries
Member of the Board of Trustees, International Medical Sciences Academy
Distinguished Fellow, Royal Society of Medicine
Founder and Past President, Middle East Society for Organ Transplantation
Founder and President, Turkish Transplantation Society
Founder and President, Turkic World Transplantation Society
Editor-in-Chief, Experimental and Clinical Transplantation
Editor-in-Chief, Burn Care and Prevention
Ankara, Turkey

Farrokh Habibzadeh, MD
Shiraz Organ Transplant Center, Avicenna Hospital
Shiraz University of Medical Sciences
Shiraz, Iran

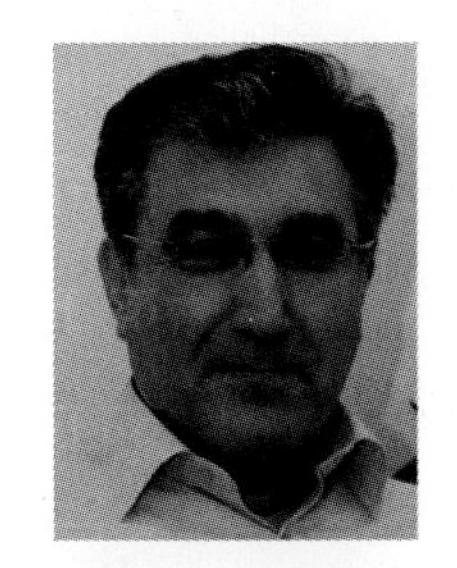

Ahmed Halawa, MD MSc MD MEd FRCS FRCS (Gen)
Consultant Transplant Surgeon
Transplant Unit, Sheffield Teaching Hospitals, Sheffield, UK.
Associate Professor, University of Liverpool, Programme.
Director of Master Degree Courses in Transplantation at University of Liverpool
Liverpool, UK

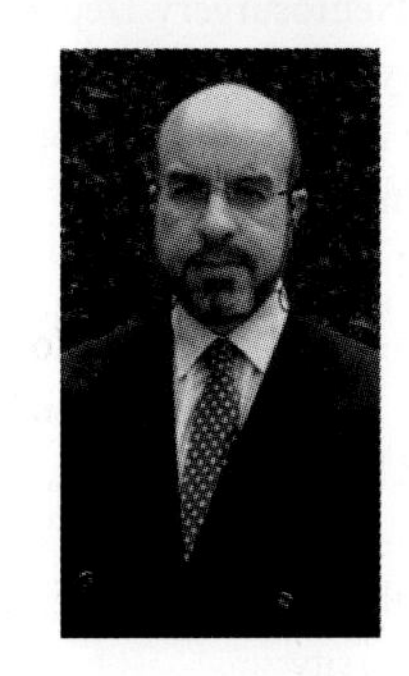

Xiangxiang He, MSc
Shanxi Provincial Organ Procurement And Allocation Center
Intelligence Sharing for Life Science Research Institute
Taiyuan, China

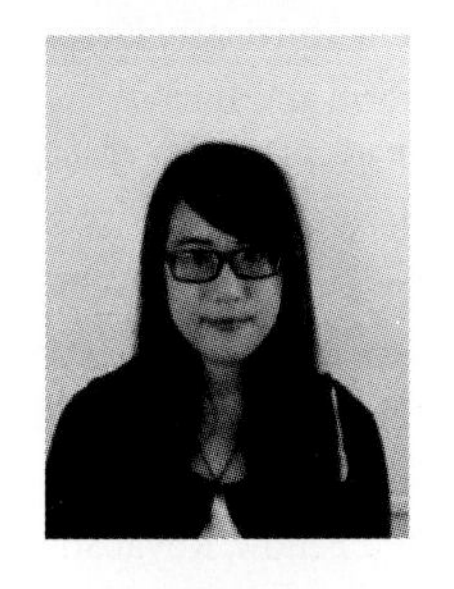

Ayman Ibrahim, BSc
Corporate Senior Medical Education Officer
Corporate Academic Affairs Abu Dhabi Health Services Company—SEHA
Abu Dhabi, United Arab Emirates

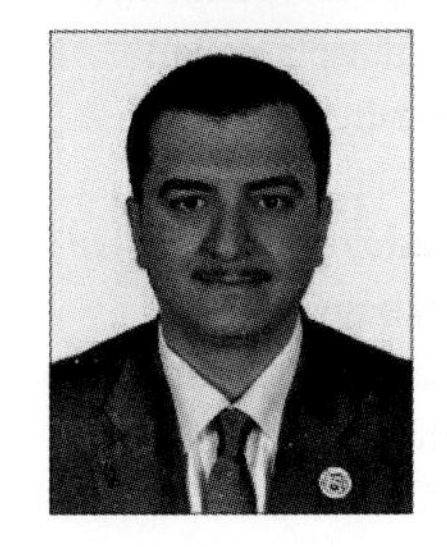

Wenshi Jiang, MSc
Shanxi Provincial Organ Procurement And Allocation Center
Intelligence Sharing for Life Science Research Institute
Taiyuan, China

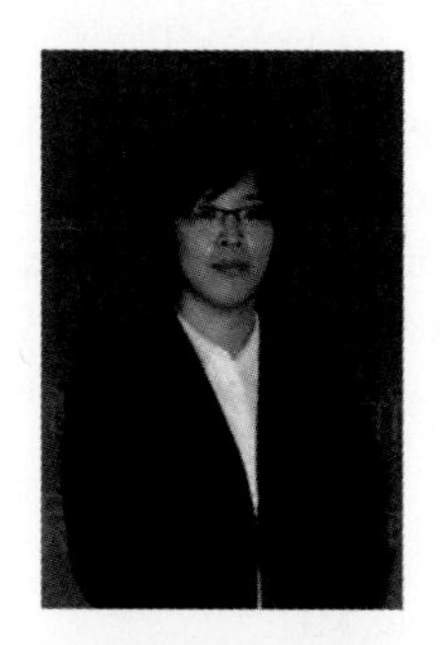

Shashank Sharad Kale, MD
Professor and Head, Department of Neurosurgery
All India Institute of Medical Science (AIIMS)
New Delhi, India

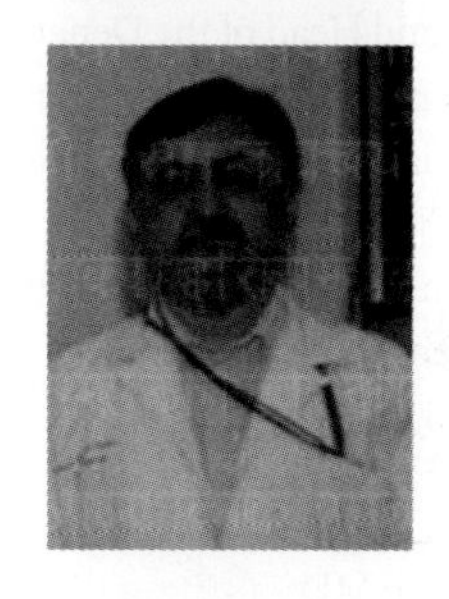

Samuel J Kesseli, MD
Duke University School of Medicine
Department of Surgery
Durham, NC, USA

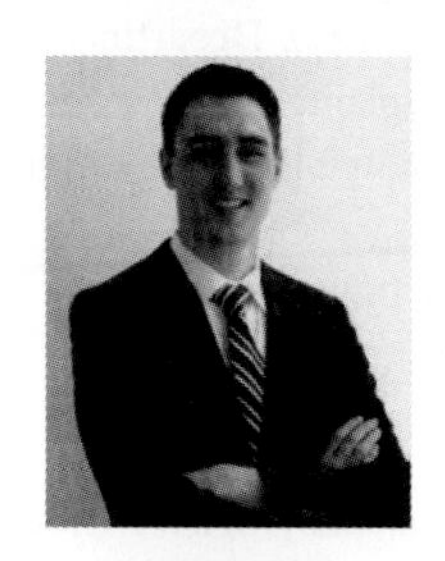

Sergey Khomyakov, MD, PhD
Deputy Director, Head of the Methodical Center in Transplantology of National Medical Research Center of Transplantology and Artificial Organs named after academician V.I. Shumakov
Moscow, Russia

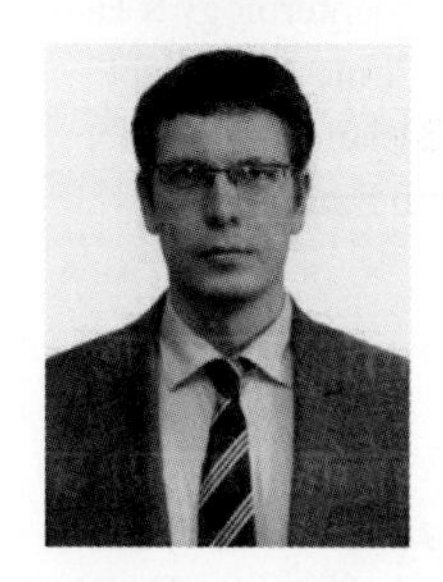

Vishal Khullar, MBBS
Assistant Professor of Surgery, Department of Cardiovascular Surgery
Mayo Clinic School of Medicine, Mayo Clinic
Rochester, MN, USA

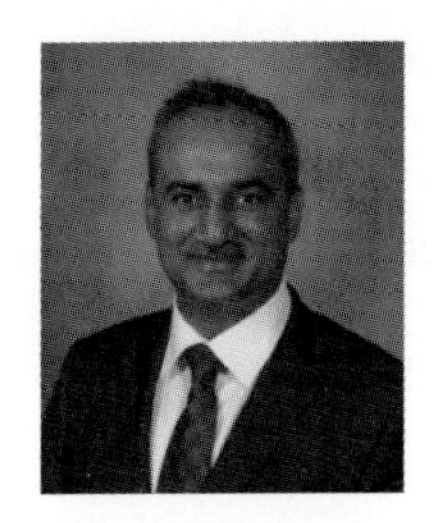

Anup Kumar, MD
Professor and Head of the Department.
Department of Urology and Renal Transplant.
Superspeciality Block, VMMC and Safdarjang Hospital
Expert panel member of Apex technical Committee to NOTTO
New Delhi, India

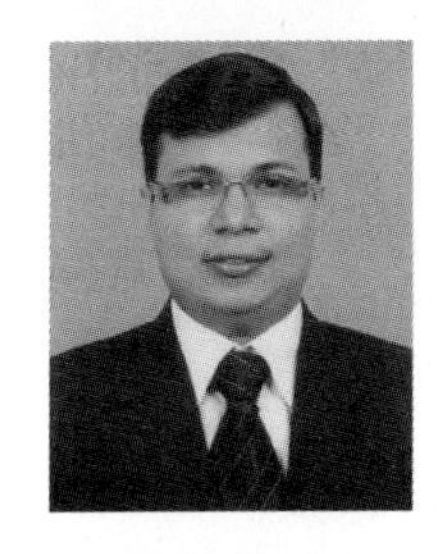

Niraj Kumar, MD
Assistant Professor Department of Urology and Renal Transplant,
Superspeciality Block, VMMC and Safdarjang Hospital
New Delhi, India

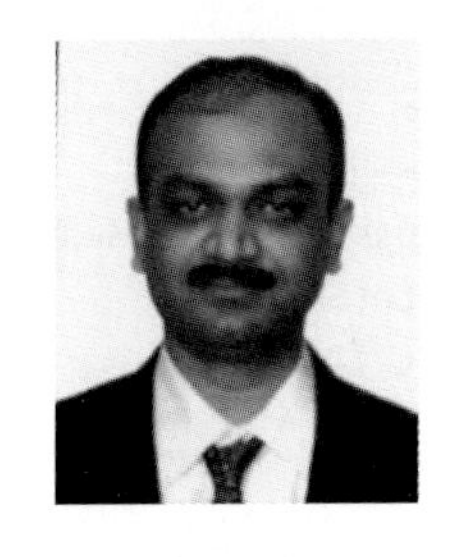

Shiva Kumar, MD, MHA, FAASLD
Chair, Gastroenterology & Hepatology
Cleveland Clinic Abu Dhabi
Al Maryah Island, Abu Dhabi
United Arab Emirates

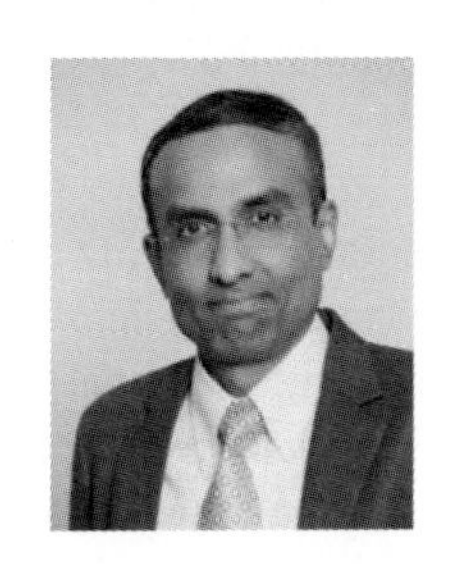

Kaori Kuramitsu, MD, PhD
Department of Surgery, Division of Hepato-biliary and Pancreatic Surgery, Kobe University
Kobe, Japan

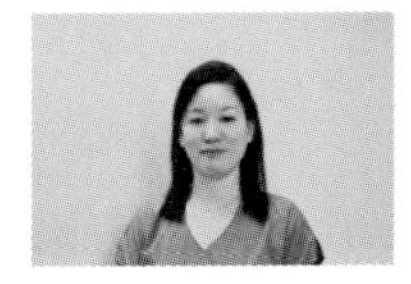

Sanjeev Lalwani, MD
Professor, Department of Forensic Medicine,
JPNATC,
All India Institute of medical Science, AIIMS
New Delhi, India

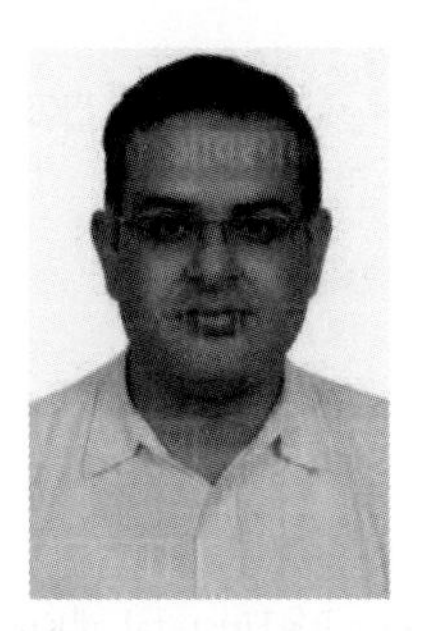

Stephen Ralph Large, MS, MA, FRCP, FRCS,
FETCS, ILTM, MBA
Consultant Cardiothoracic surgeon.
The Surgical Unit, Royal Papworth Hospital
Cambridge, UK

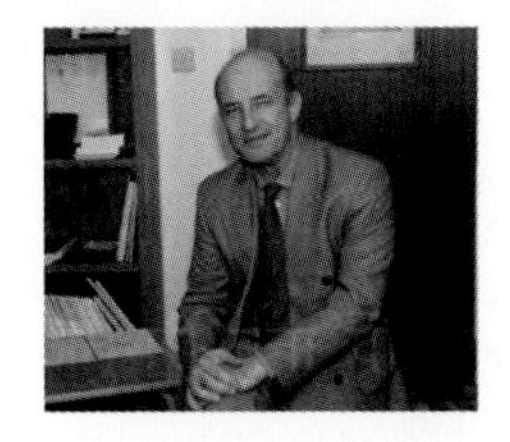

Chiara Lazzeri, MD
Intensive Care Unit and Regional ECMO
Referral Centre
Azienda Ospedaliero-Universitaria Careggi
Florence, Italy

Brian Le, MD
Assistant Professor, Department of Surgery,
Division of Plastic and Reconstructive Surgery
Virginia Commonwealth University
Richmond, VA, USA

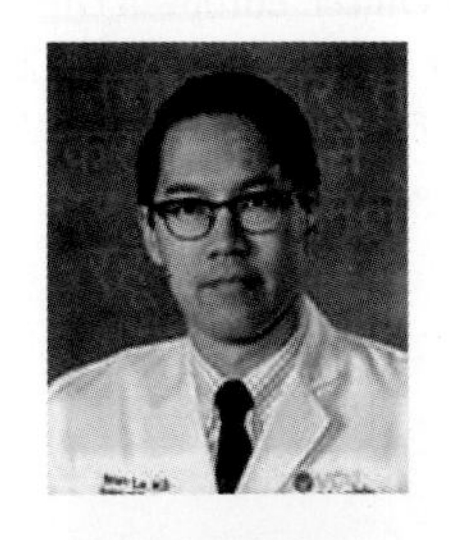

Bronwyn Levvey, RN B Ed Stud
Associate Professor, Lung Transplant Service,
Alfred Hospital and Monash University
Melbourne, Australia

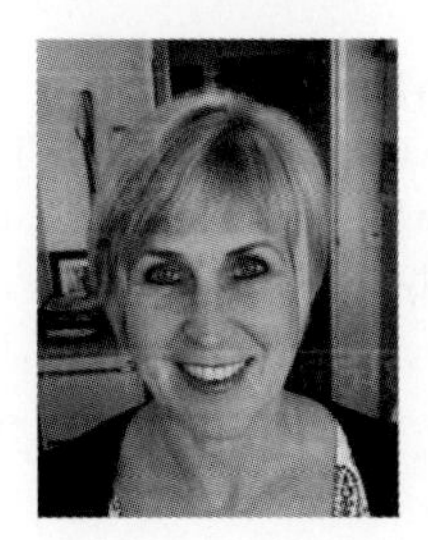

Chao Li, MD
The First People's Hospital of Kunming
Kunming, China

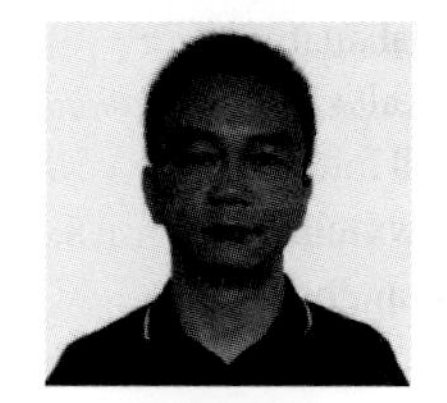

Li Li, MD
The First People's Hospital of Kunming
Kunming, China

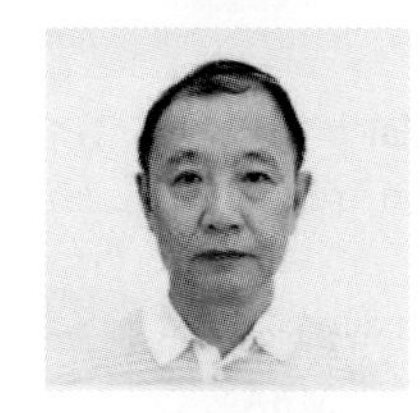

Letizia Lombardini, MD
Italian National Transplant Centre, Italian
National Institute of Health, Rome
Rome, Italy

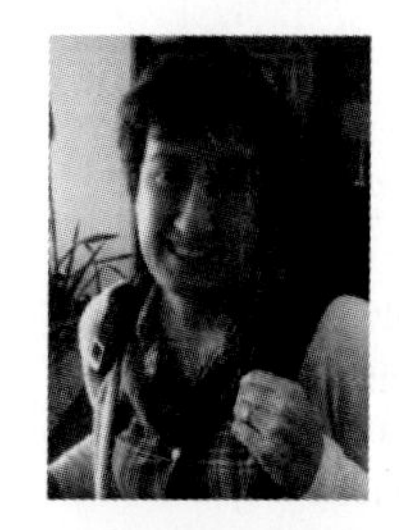

Marta López-Fraga, PhD
Scientific Officer, European Directorate for the
Quality of Medicines & HealthCare (EDQM)
Council of Europe
Strasbourg, France

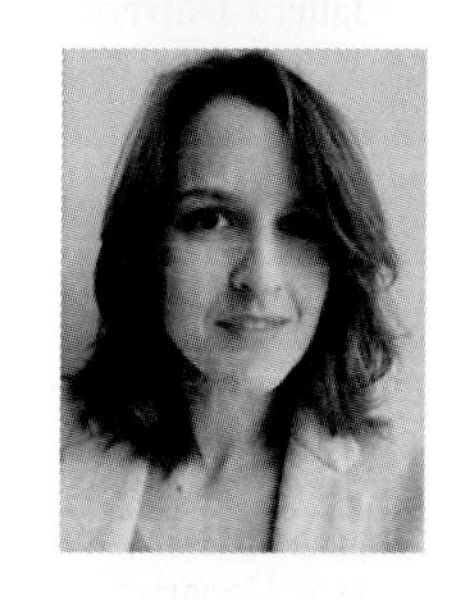

Francesco Lupo, MD, PhD
Chirurgia Generale 2U— Liver Transplant Centre
Cittá della Salute e della Scienza di Torino
Turin, Italy

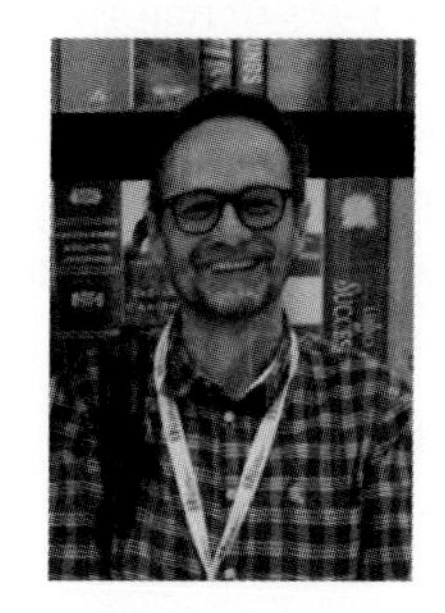

Ashok K Mahapatra, MCH
Director Health Programme SOA and Former Director, All India Institute of Medical Sciences, AIIMS, New Delhi, India
Bhubaneswar, India

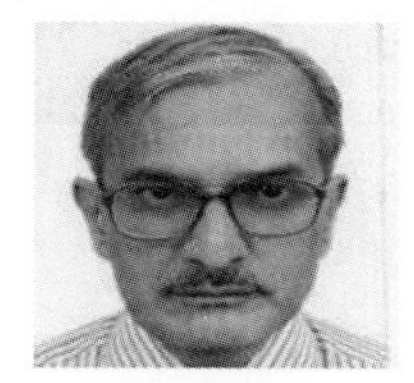

Seyed Ali Malek-Hosseini, MD, FACS (Hon)
Shiraz Organ Transplant Center, Avicenna Hospital
Shiraz University of Medical Sciences
Shiraz, Iran

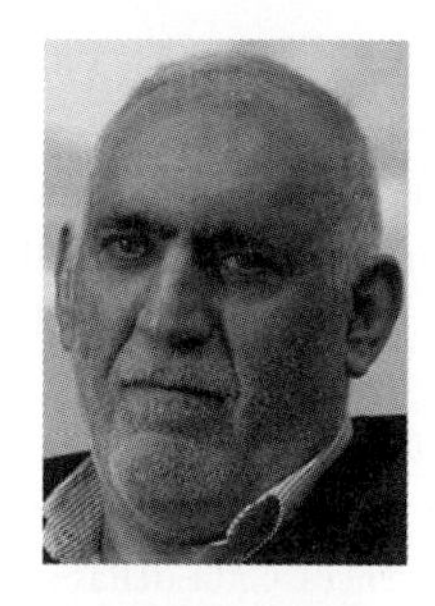

Deborah Malvi, MD
Pathology Unit, S.Orsola-Malpighi University Hospital
Bologna, Italy

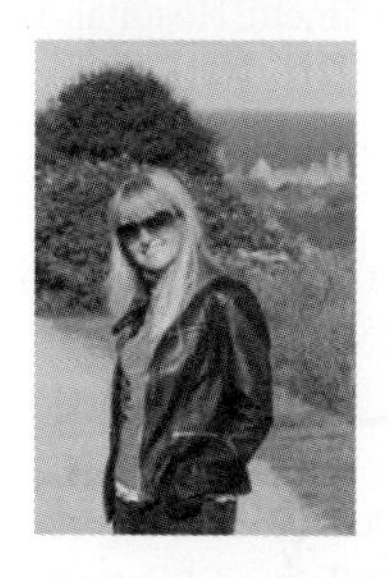

Marti Manyalich, MD, PhD
Transplant Procurement Manager
Head of the Transplantation Advisory Unit, Hospital Clínic de Barcelona
Associate Professor, Department of Surgery and Surgical Specialties, Universitat de Barcelona
President, DTI Foundation
Barcelona, Spain

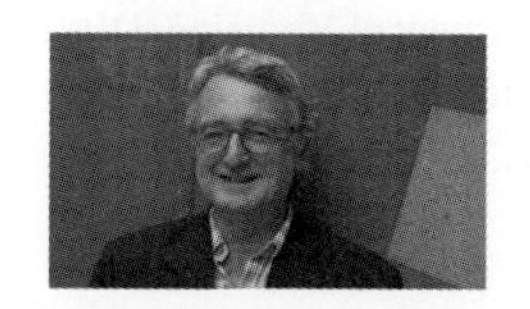

Luciana Mascia, MD, PhD
Associate Professor of Anesthesia and Intensive Care
Department of Biomedic and Neuromotor Sciences
University of Bologna
Bologna, Italy

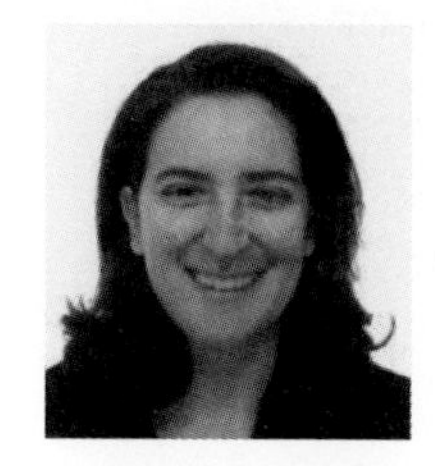

Marco Mazzeo, J.D.
Judge, Inspector General, Ministry of Justice, Italy
Rome, Italy

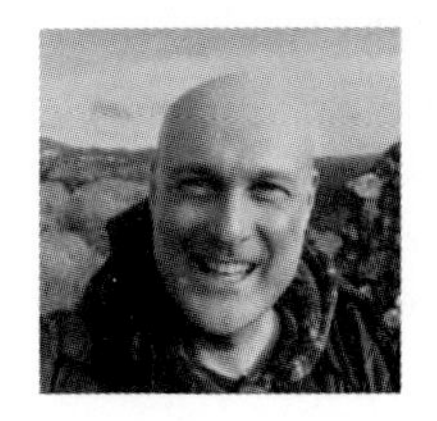

Anna Teresa Mazzeo, MD
Associate Professor of Anesthesia and Intensive care. Department of Human Pathology G. Barresi. University of Messina. AOU Policlinico Gaetano Martino.
Messina, Italy
Previously at University of Torino. Department of Surgical Sciences. Citta' della Salute e della Scienza di Torino, Molinette Hospital. Torino, Italy

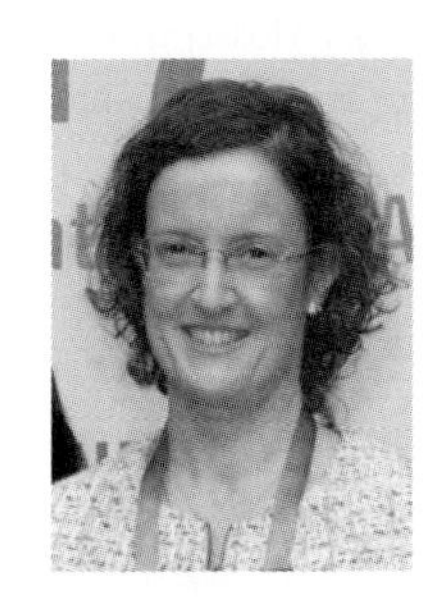

Brittny Medenwald, PharmD
Critical Care Pharmacist
University of Tennessee Medical Center
Knoxville, TN (USA)

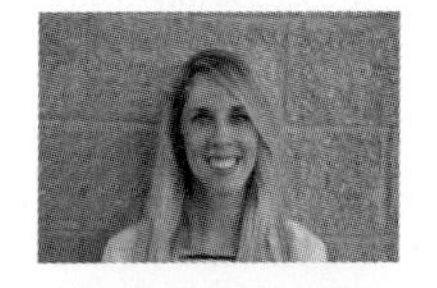

Claudia Mescoli, MD, PhD
Surgical Pathology and Cytopathology Unit, Department of Medicine (DIMED), University of Padua
Padua, Italy

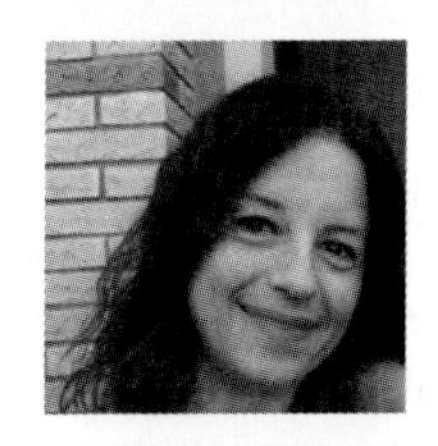

Simon Messer, PhD, MBChB
Cardiothoracic Transplant Registrar, Royal Papworth Hospital
Cambridge, UK

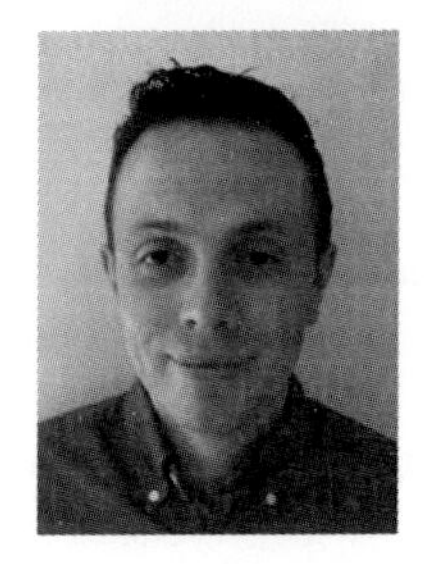

Pratick Metha, MD
Simmons Transplant Institute, Baylor University Medical Center
Dallas, Texas, USA

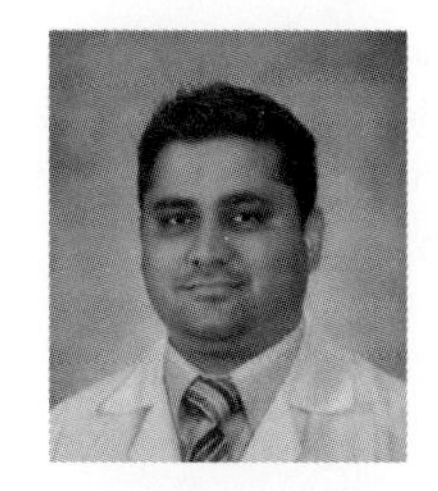

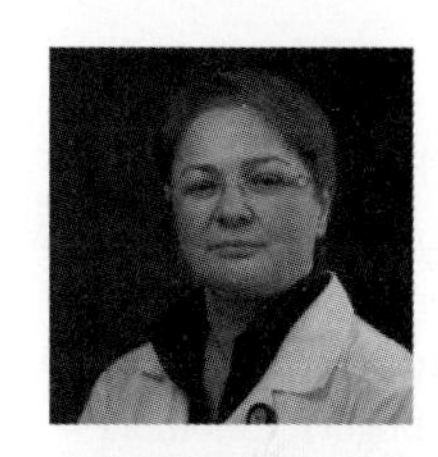

Marina G Minina, MD, PhD
Head of Moscow coordinating centre of organ donation.
Municipal hospital named after S.P.Botkin
Moscow, Russia

Artem Monakhov, MD
Chief of Surgical Department #2 (Liver Transplantation)
National Medical Research Center of Transplantology and Artificial Organs named after academician V.I. Shumakov, Moscow, Russia
Assistant Professor at Chair of transplantation and artificial organs of I.M. Sechenov First Moscow State Medical University (Sechenov University)
Moscow, Russia

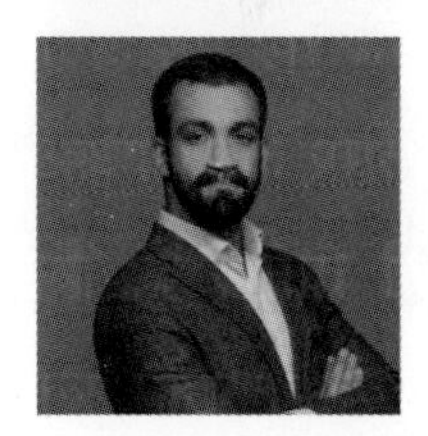

Elisa Montalenti, MD
Clinical Neurology, Transplant coordinator Città della Salute e della Scienza di Torino, Molinette Hospital
Turin, Italy

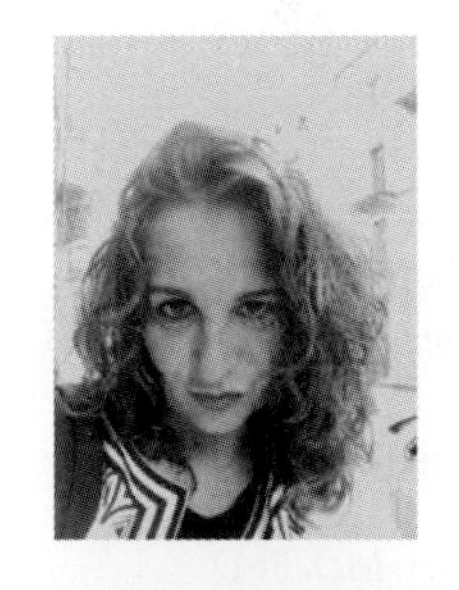

Juan S Montealegre, MS
Neurotrauma Research Group, MEDITECH Foundation, Bogotá/Cali
Medical Student, Universidad Nacional de Colombia
Bogotá, Colombia

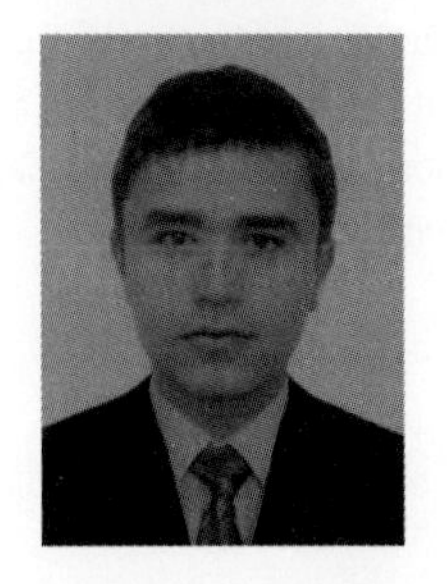

Antonino Montemurro
Nurse, Italian National Transplant Centre, Italian National Institute of Health
Rome, Italy

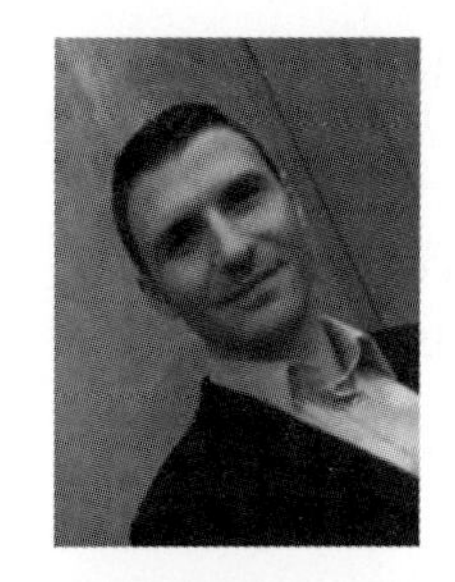

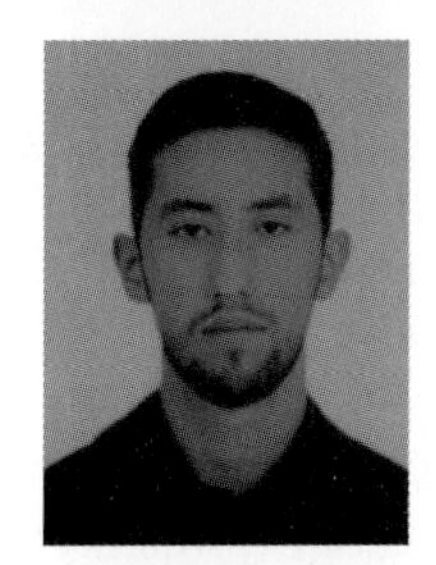

Killiam D Mora, MS
Neurotrauma Research Group, MEDITECH Foundation, Bogotá/Cali
Medical Student, Universidad Nacional de Colombia Bogotá, Colombia

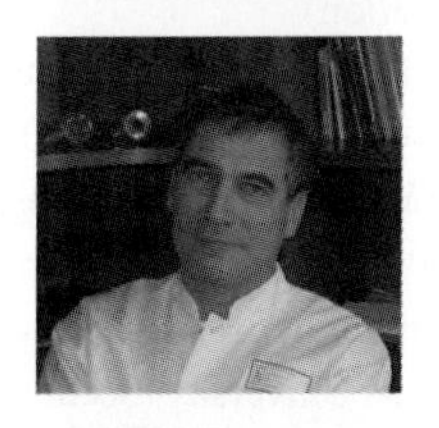

Emmanuel Morelon, MD
Department of Transplantation, Hopital Edouard Herriot
Lyon, France

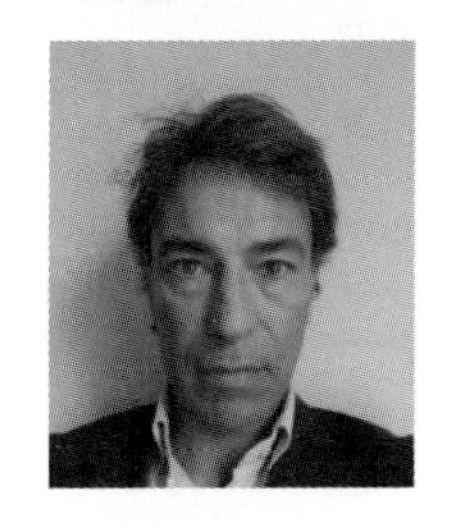

Paolo Muiesan, MD, FRCS, FEBS
Professor of HPB Surgery and Liver Transplantation
Liver Unit, Queen Elizabeth Hospital Birmingham and Birmingham Childrens' Hospital
Birmingham, UK
HPB Surgery Unit, University of Florence, Careggi Hospital
Florence, Italy

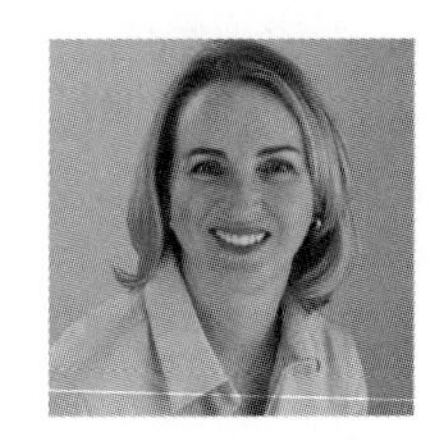

Elmi Muller, MD, PhD
Head of Division of General Surgery, Head of Transplant Unit, Department of Surgery, Groote Schuur Hospital, University of Cape Town
Cape Town, South Africa

Marina Munari, MD
Neurointensive Care Unit, UO Anesthesia and Intensive Care
University of Padua
Padua, Italy

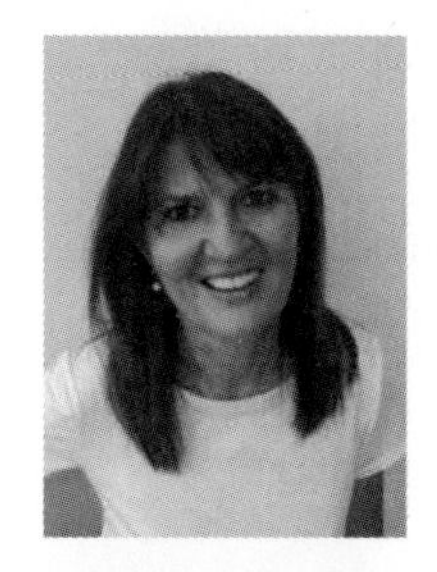

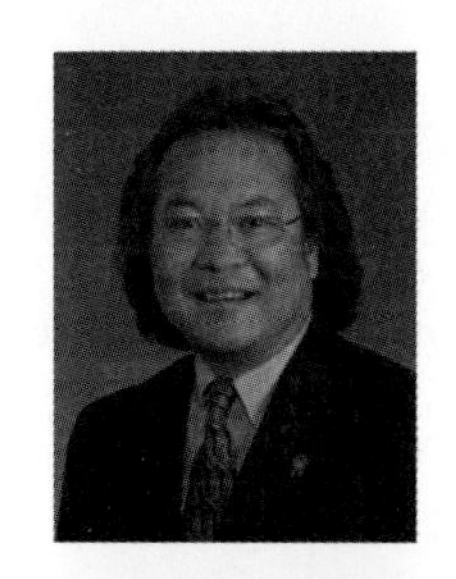

Thomas A Nakagawa, MD, FAAP, FCCM
Professor, Department of Pediatrics, Division of Critical Care Medicine
University of Florida College of Medicine
Medical Director, Pediatric Intensive Care
Wolfson Children's Hospital
Jacksonville, FL, USA

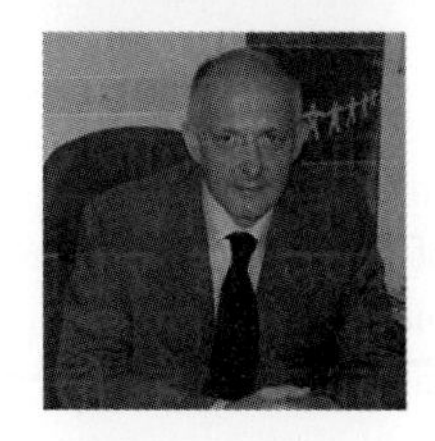

Alessandro Nanni Costa, MD
Past-Director Italian National Transplant Centre,
Italian National Institute of Health
Rome, Italy

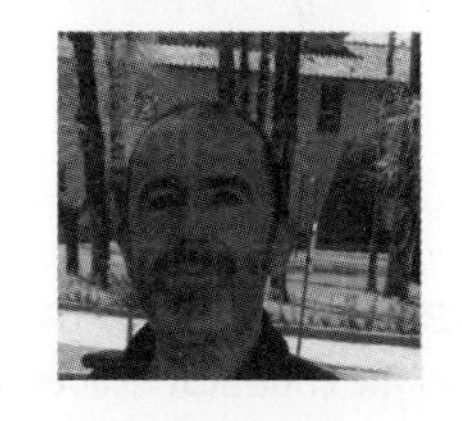

Luca Novelli, MD, PhD
Institute of Histopathology and Molecular Diagnosis
Careggi University Hospital
Florence, Italy

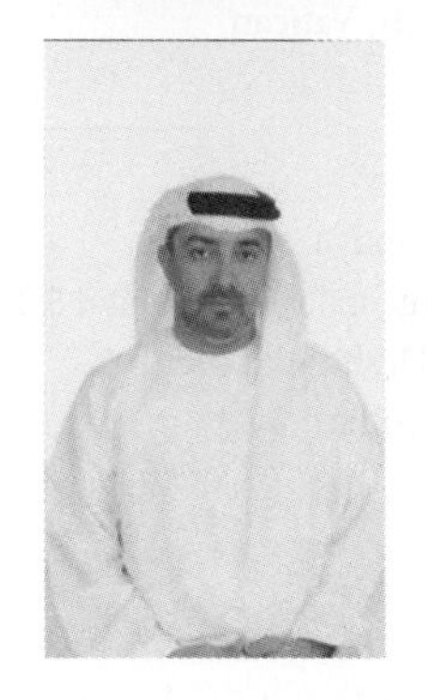

AI Ali Obaidli, MB, B.Ch. B.A.O, MPH
Group Chief Academic Affairs Officer
Corporate Academic Affairs Abu Dhabi Health Services Company—SEHA
Abu Dhabi

Helen Opdam, MD, MBBS, FRACP, FCICM
National Medical Director
Australian Organ and Tissue Donation and
Transplantation Authority
Canberra, Australia

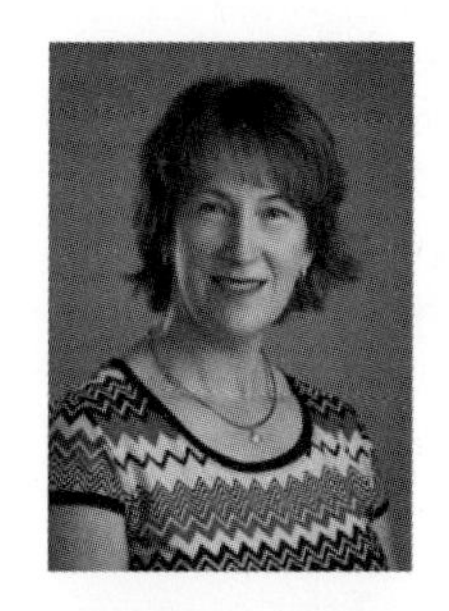

Kristine O'Phelan, MD
Professor of Clinical Neurology. Chief of
Neurocritical Care
Department of Neurology, University of Miami
Miami, FL, USA

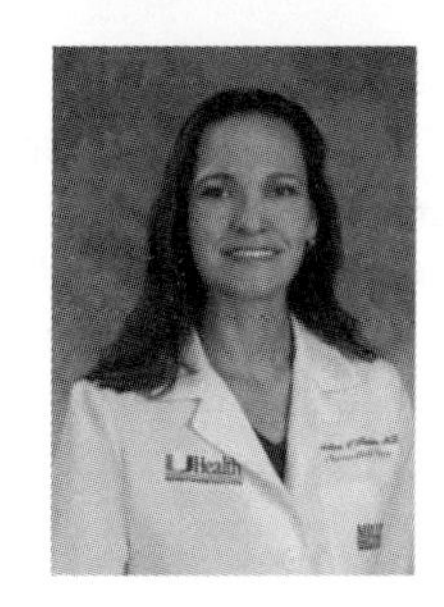

Alessandro Pacini, MD
Director of Donation and Organ S.O.S.D. of Local
Health Unit Toscana Centro
Firenze, Italy

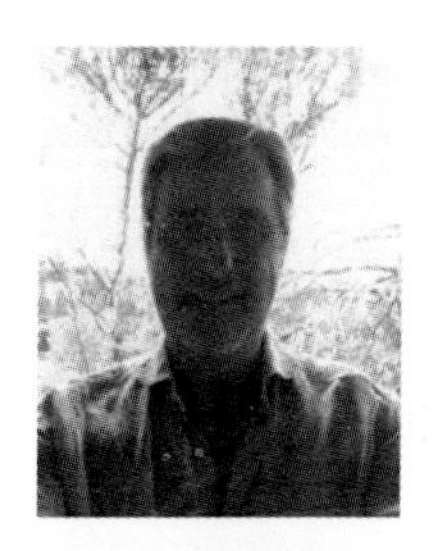

Vincenzo Paglia, STD, PhM, MPd
President of the Pontifical Academy for Life
Vatican City, Vatican

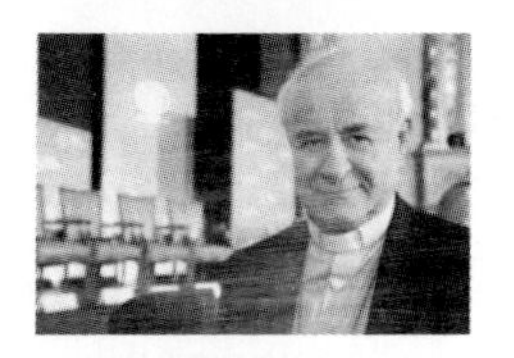

Sunil K. Pandya, M.S.
Neurosurgeon Jaslok Hospital & Research Centre
Dr. G. V. Deshmukh Marg
Mumbai, India

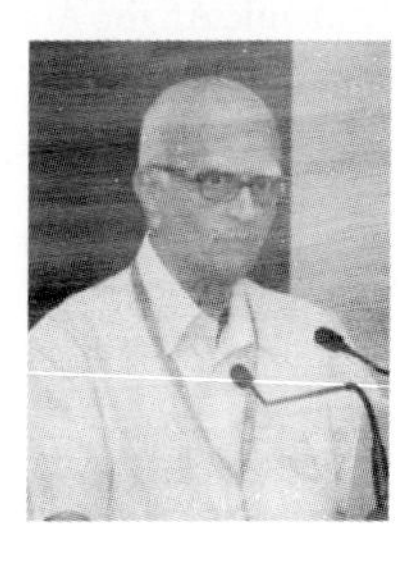

Laura Pastor, MD Neurotrauma Research Group, MEDITECH Foundation, Bogotá/Cali (Colombia)
Neurosurgery Resident, Hospital Universitario de Gran Canaria Doctor Negrín
Las Palmas de Gran Canaria, Spain

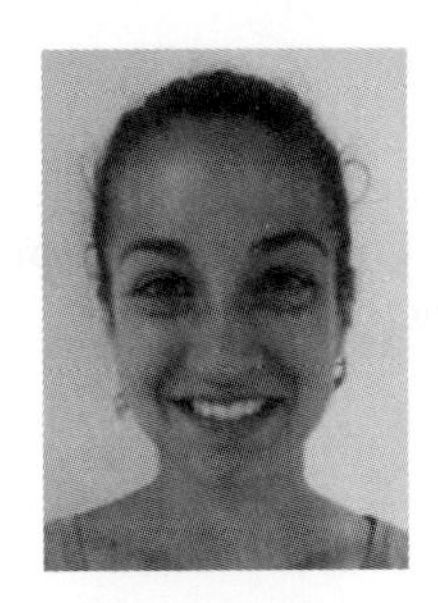

Damiano Patrono, MD, PhD
General Surgery 2U, Liver Transplant Unit, A.O.U. Città della Salute e della Scienza di Torino, University of Turin
Turin, Italy

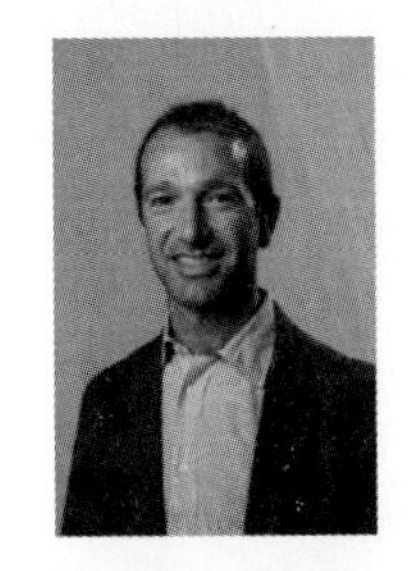

Jogi V Pattisapu, MD, FAAP, FACS, FAANS (L)
Professor, Pediatric Neurosurgery
University of Central Florida College of Medicine
Orlando, FL, USA

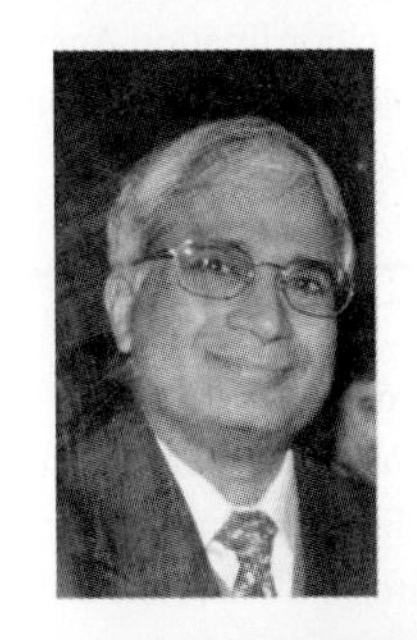

Alicia Pérez Blanco, MD, PhD
Intensive Care Medicine
MD Bioethics Organización Nacional de Trasplantes
Madrid, Spain

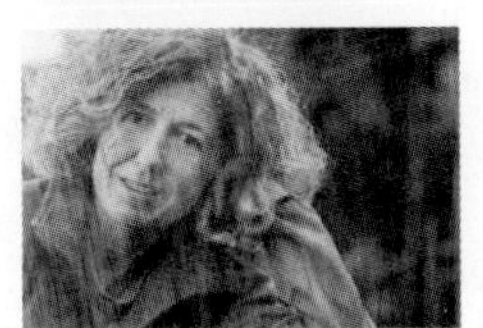

Palmina Petruzzo, MD
Department of Surgery, University of Cagliari, Italy
Department of Transplantation, Hopital Edouard Herriot, Hospices Civils de Lyon
Lyon, France

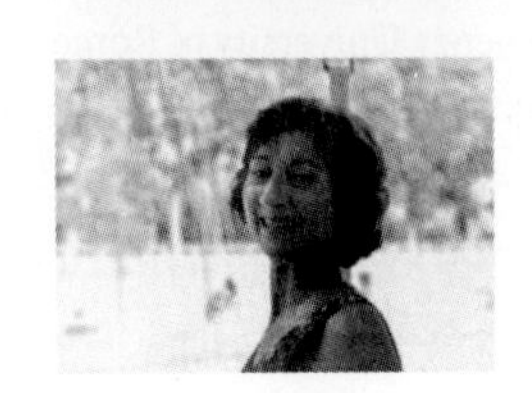

Edoardo Piervincenzi, MD
Department of Emergency, Intensive Care
Medicine and Anesthesiology, Fondazione
Policlinico Universitario "A. Gemelli" IRCCS
Rome, Italy

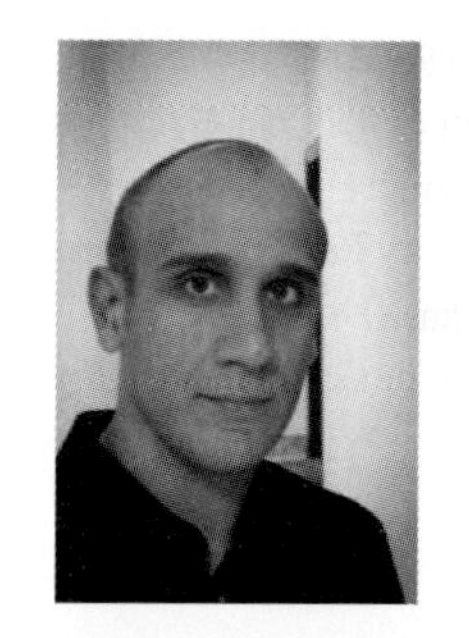

Diego Ponzin, MD
The Veneto Eye Bank Foundation
Venice, Italy

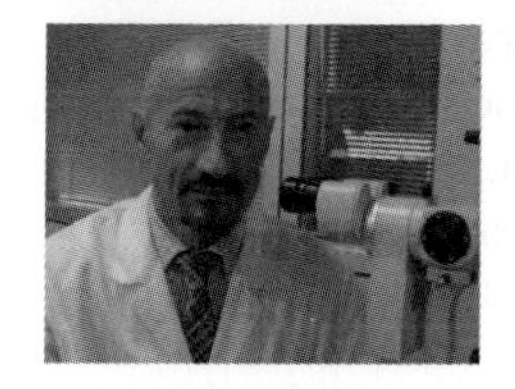

Raffaele Potenza, MD
Piedmont Regional Tissue and Organ
Procurement Coordination Agency
Città della Salute e della Scienza di Torino,
Molinette Hospital
Turin, Italy

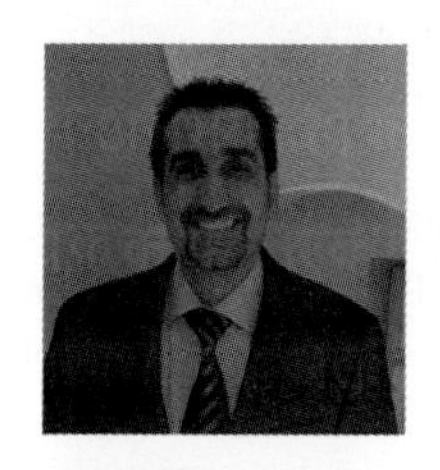

Francesco Procaccio, MD
Italian National Transplant Centre, Italian National
Institute of Health, Rome, Italy
Former Neuro ICU Director, University City
Hospital
Verona, Italy

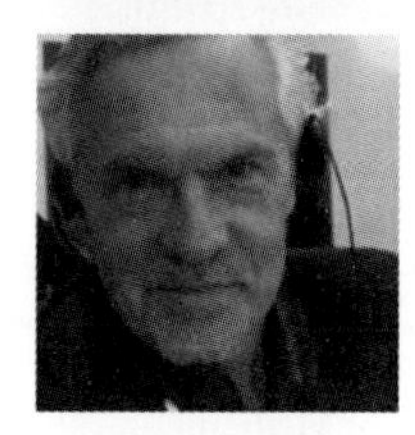

Francesco Pugliese, MD
Anesthesia and Intensive Care Medicine
La Sapienza University of Rome
Rome, Italy

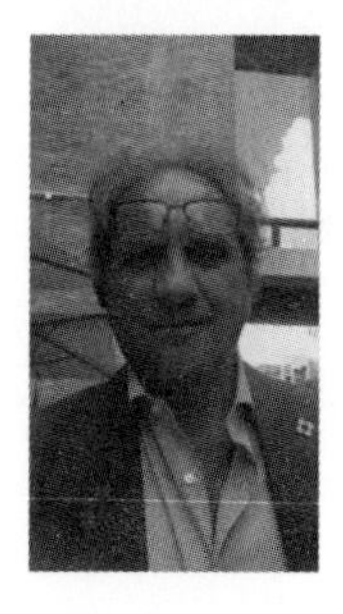

Francesco Puliatti, MD
Transplant Coordinator. Anesthesia and Intensive care Department. AOU Policlinico Gaetano Martino
Messina, Italy

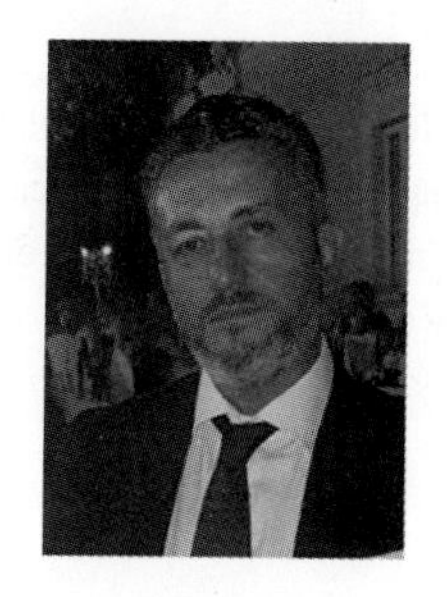

Arantxa Quiralte
DTI Foundation
Nursing and Practice Innovation
Barcelona, Spain

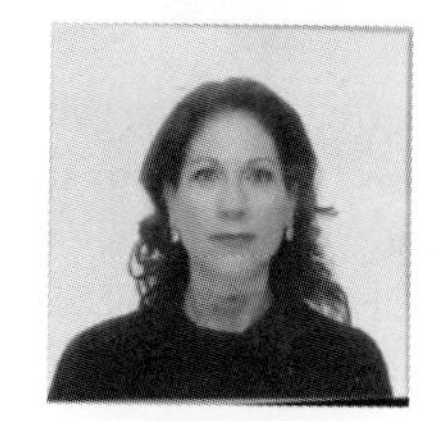

Azhar Rafiq, MD, MBA, MEd
Associate Professor, Department of Surgery
Virginia Commonwealth University
Richmond, VA, USA

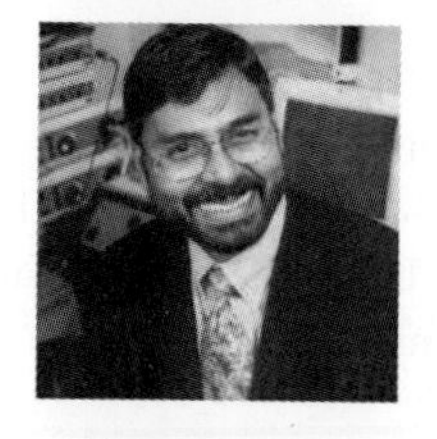

Kadiyala V Ravindra, MBBS
Duke University School of Medicine
Department of Surgery, Division of Abdominal Transplant Surgery
Durham, NC, USA

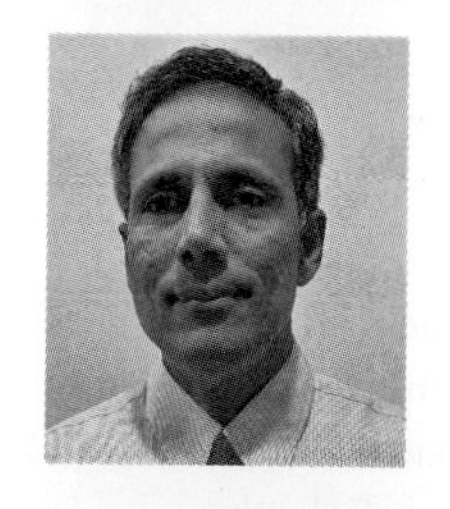

Davide Ricci, MD
Heart and Lung Transplant Center, Cardiac Surgery Division
Surgical Sciences Department, Città della Salute e della Scienza, University of Torino
Turin, Italy

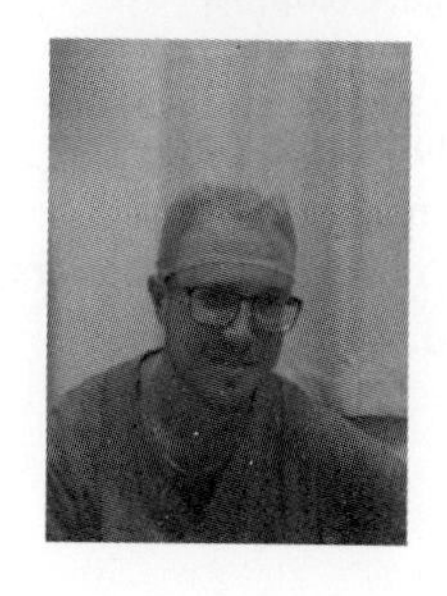

Mauro Rinaldi, MD
Director Heart and Lung Transplant Center,
Cardiac Surgery Division. Surgical Sciences
Department, Città della Salute e della Scienza,
University of Torino
Turin, Italy

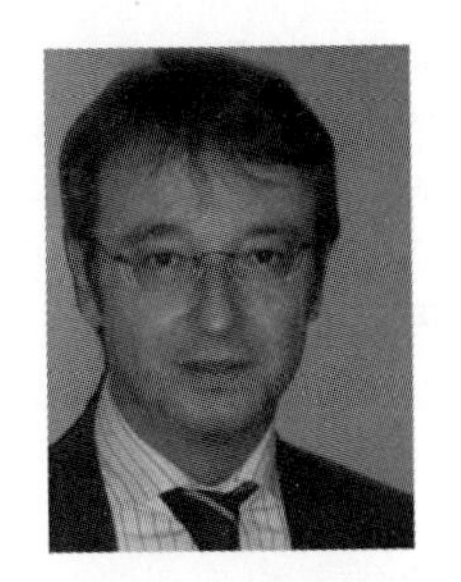

Lucia Rizzato
Head Nurse, UOC Chirurgia dei Trapianti di
Rene Pancreas - Azienda Ospedale-Università
Padova, Italy
Head Nurse, Italian National Transplant Centre,
Italian National Institute of Health
Rome, Italy

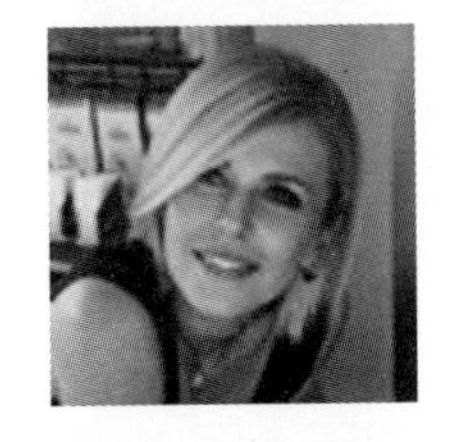

Renato Romagnoli, MD
Director General Surgery 2U - Liver Transplant
Unit, A.O.U. Città della Salute e della Scienza di
Torino, University of Turin
Turin, Italy

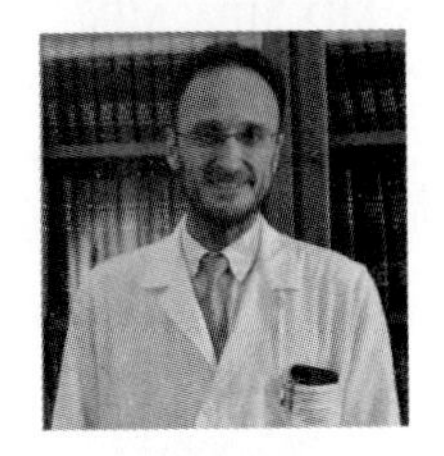

Andrés M Rubiano, MD, PhD
Neurotrauma Research Group, MEDITECH
Foundation, Bogotá/Cali
Trauma and Critical Care Neurosurgeon,
Neurosciences and Neurosurgery Professor,
Universidad El Bosque, MEDITECH Foundation
Bogotá/Cali, Colombia

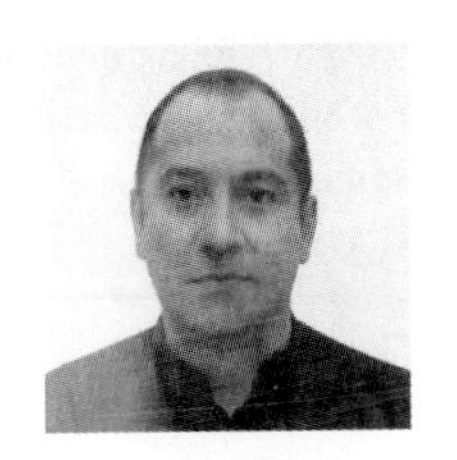

Brianna Ruch, MD
Department of Surgery
Virginia Commonwealth University
Richmond, VA, USA

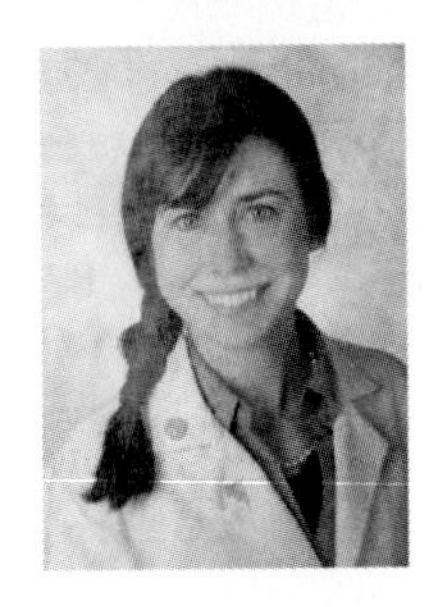

Iolanda Russo Menna, MD, PhD, MED, DABA
Associate Professor of Anesthesiology Clinical
Attending of Children's Hospital of Richmond
Faculty at Center for Human Simulation &
Patient Safety
Virginia Commonwealth University
Richmond, VA, USA

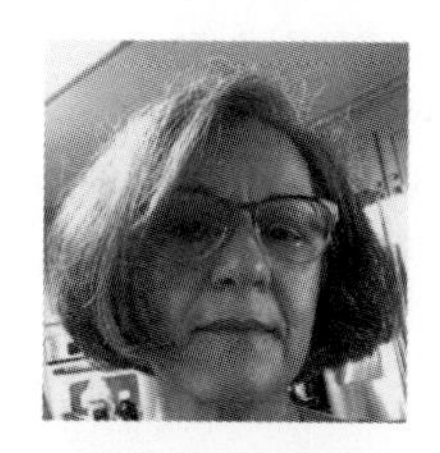

Sahar Saddoughi, MD, PhD
Senior Associate Consultant. Instructor in
Surgery, Department of Surgery
Division of Thoracic Surgery. Division of
Transplant Surgery,
Transplant Center. Mayo Clinic
Rochester, MN, USA

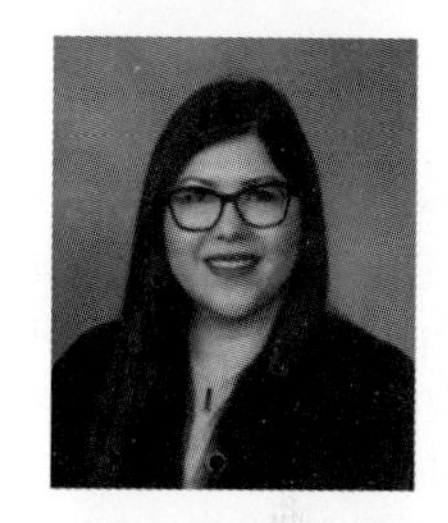

Mauro Salizzoni, MD
Former Director Liver Transplant Unit, AOU Città
della Salute e della Scienza di Torino. University
of Turin
Turin, Italy

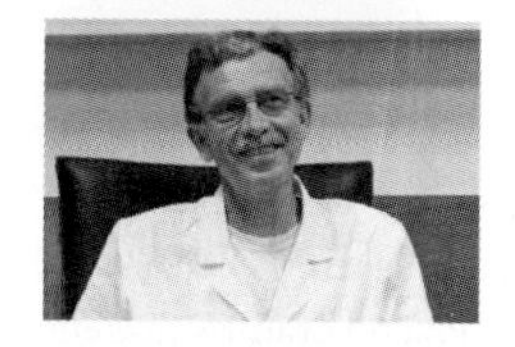

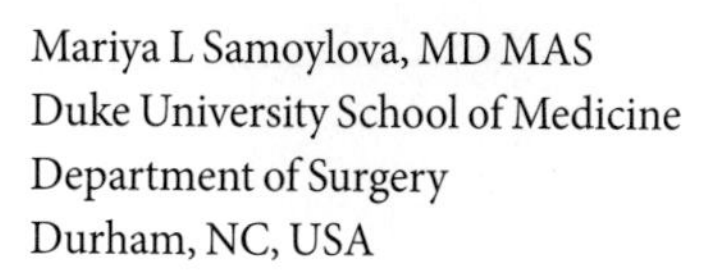

Mariya L Samoylova, MD MAS
Duke University School of Medicine
Department of Surgery
Durham, NC, USA

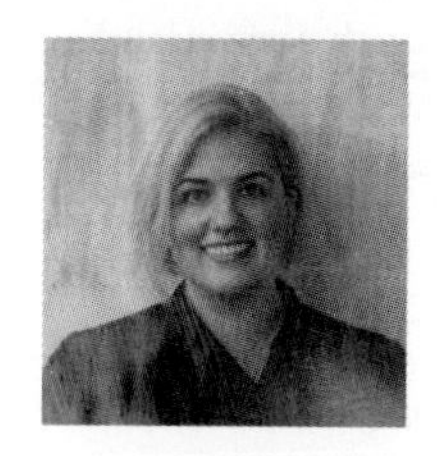

Bashir Sankari, MD, FACS
Chair, Surgical Subspecialties Institute
Cleveland Clinic Abu Dhabi
Abu Dhabi, United Arab Emirates

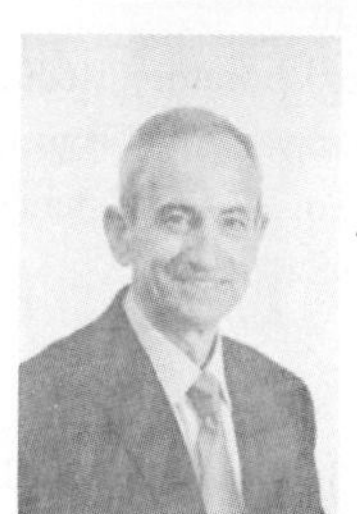

Vincenzo Sarnicola, MD
Sarnicola Eye Clinic
Grosseto, Italy

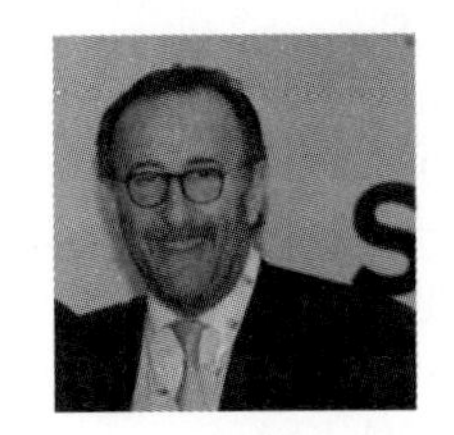

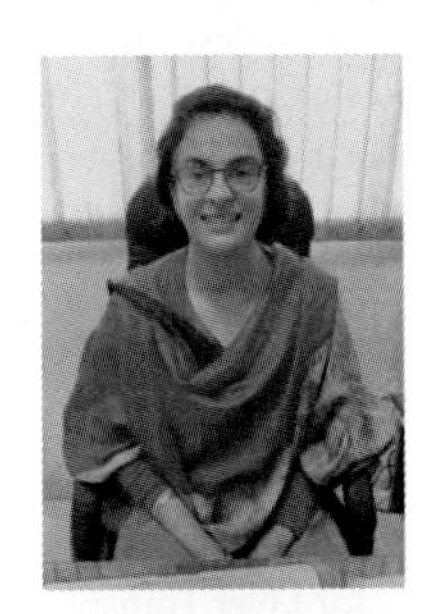

Chhavi Sawhney, MD
Professor, Department of Anesthesia, Jai Prakash Narayan Apex Trauma Centre (JPNATC), All India Institute of Medical Science (AIIMS)
New Delhi, India

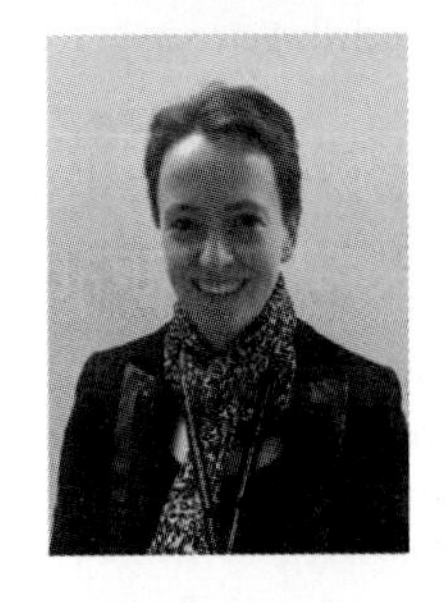

Andrea Schlegel, MD, MBA, FEBS
Swiss HPB and Transplant Center, Department of Visceral Surgery and Transplantation, University Hospital Zurich, Switzerland
Hepatobiliary Unit, Careggi University Hospital, University of Florence, Italy

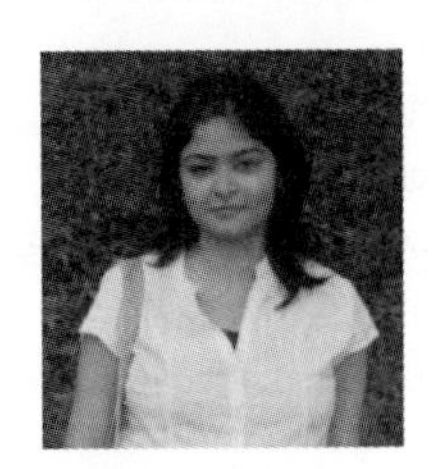

Kangana Sengar, MBBS, DCP, DNB
Senior Resident
Department of laboratory Medicine
Jai Prakash Narayan Apex Trauma Centre, All India Institute of Medical Science (AIIMS)
New Delhi, India

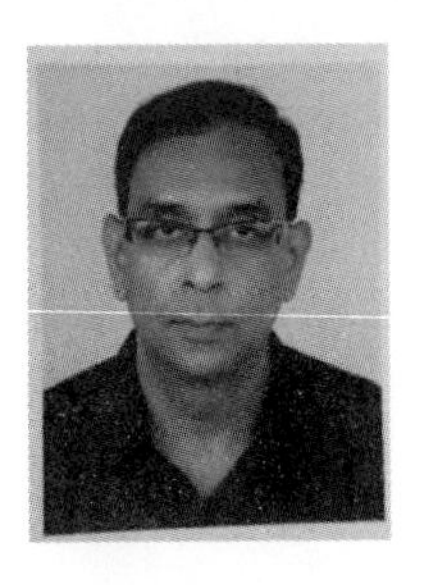

Manikandan Sethuraman, MD, PDCC
Professor and Head Division of Neuroanesthesia and Neurocritical Care. Department of Anesthesiology
See Chitra Tirunal Institute for Medical Sciences and Technology
Thiruvananthapuram, India

Faissal AM Shaheen, MD
Head of Nephrology and Senior Consultant
Physician and Nephrologist, Suleiman Fakeeh
Hospital
Jeddah, Saudi Arabia

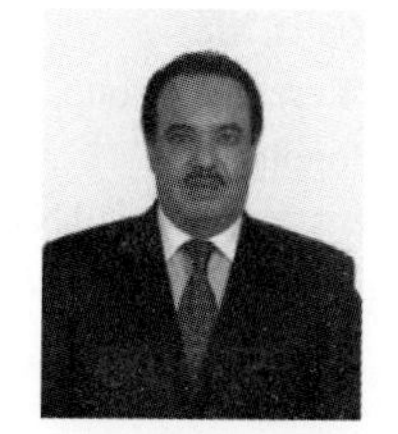

Mohamed F Shaheen, MD, MSc, FRCSC, DABS
Assistant Professor of Surgery and Abdominal
Multiorgan Transplantation Surgery Consultant.
Organ Transplant Center and Hepatobiliary
Sciences Department, King Saud Bin Abdulaziz
University for Health Sciences and King Abdullah
International Medical Research Center.
King Abdulaziz Medical City
Riyadh, Saudi Arabia

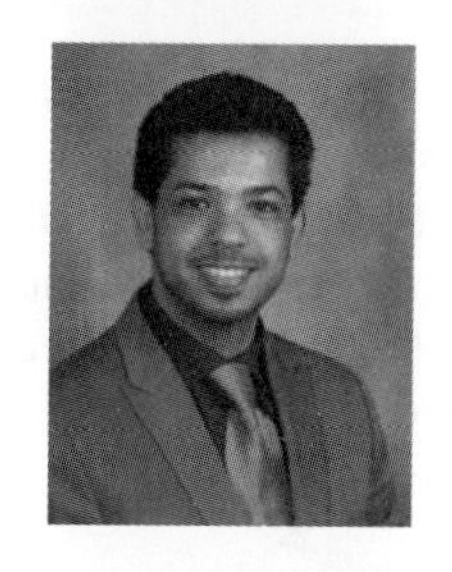

Amit Sharma, MD, MPhil, FACS
Associate Professor of Surgery
Division of Transplantation Surgery, Hume-Lee
Transplant Center
Virginia Commonwealth University
Richmond, Virginia, USA

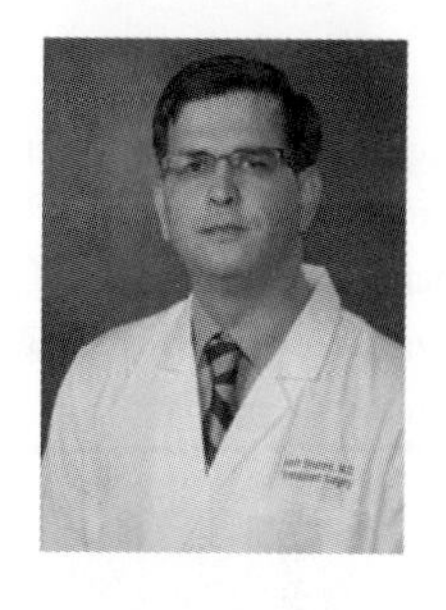

Kumar Ajay Sharma, MD
Consultant Surgeon in Transplantation and
Emergency Surgery
Transplant Unit, Royal Liverpool University Hospital
Deputy Director of Master Courses in
Transplantation at University of Liverpool
Senior Lecturer (Hon), University of Liverpool
Liverpool, UK

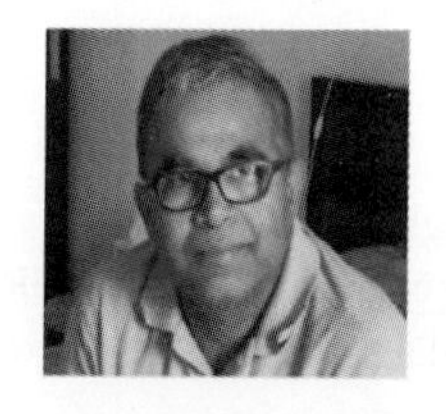

Anita Siletto
Recipient of transplant at Città della Salute e della
Scienza di Torino, Molinette Hospital.
Primary School Teacher
Volunteer of AITF - Associazione Italiana
Trapiantati di Fegato
Turin, Italy

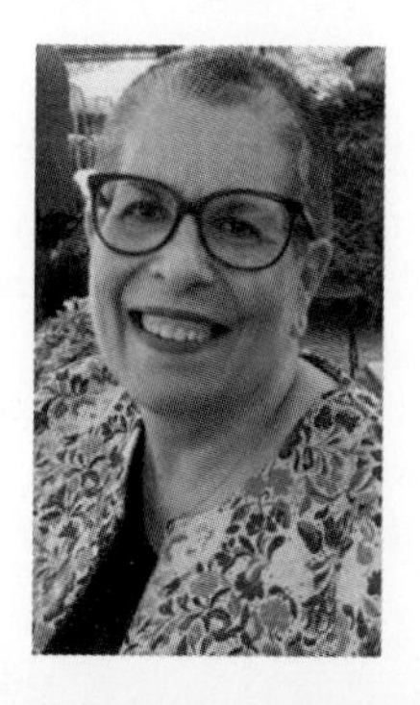

Nicolle Simmonds, MS
Neurotrauma Research Group, MEDITECH Foundation, Bogotá/Cali
Medical Student, Universidad Nacional de ColombiaBogotá, Colombia

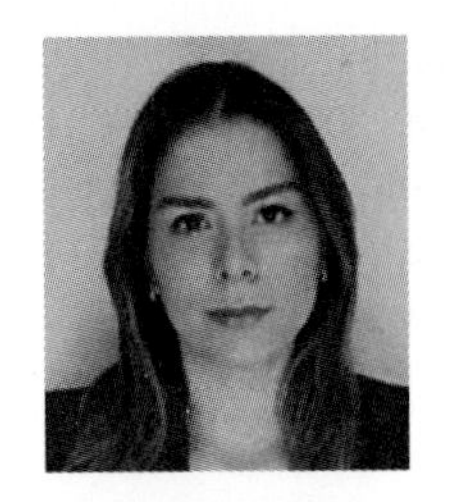

Erika Simonato, MD
Heart and Lung Transplant Center, Cardiac Surgery Division, Surgical Sciences Department, Città della Salute e della Scienza di Torino, University of Torino
Turin, Italy

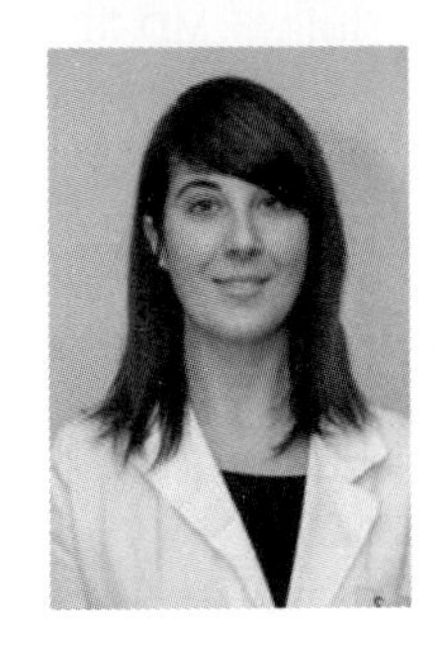

Abhay Singh, DNB (Neurosurgery)
Senior Resident, Department of Neurosurgery, Jai Prakash Narayan Apex Trauma Centre (JPNATC), All India Institute of Medical Science (AIIMS)
New Delhi, India

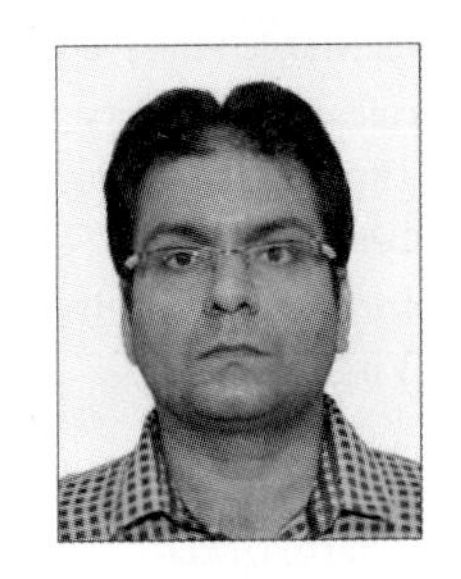

Daljit Singh, MS MCh
Professor Neurosurgery GIPMER
Delhi, India

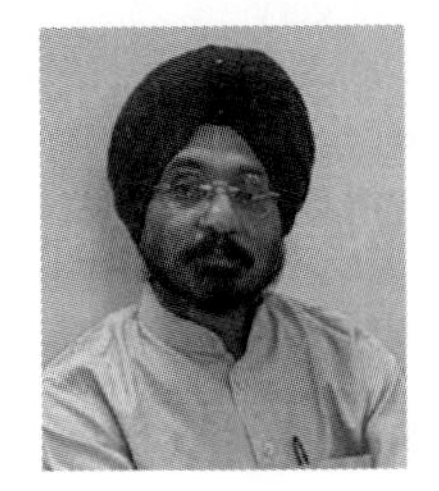

Gregory Snell, MBBS, FRACP, MD, OAM
Professor and Medical Head, Lung Transplant Service, Alfred Hospital and Monash University
Melbourne, Australia

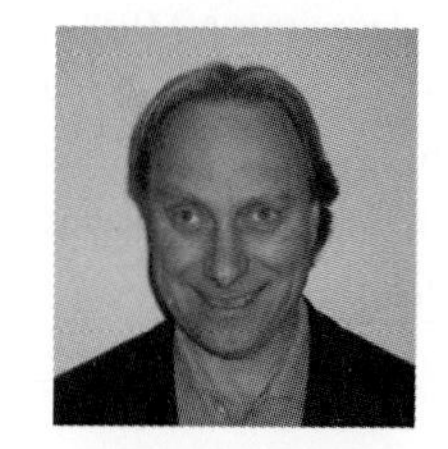

Maurizio Stella, MD
Director, Burn Centre and Turin Skin Bank Tissue and Cell Factory, CTO, Città della Salute e della Scienza di Torino
Turin, Italy

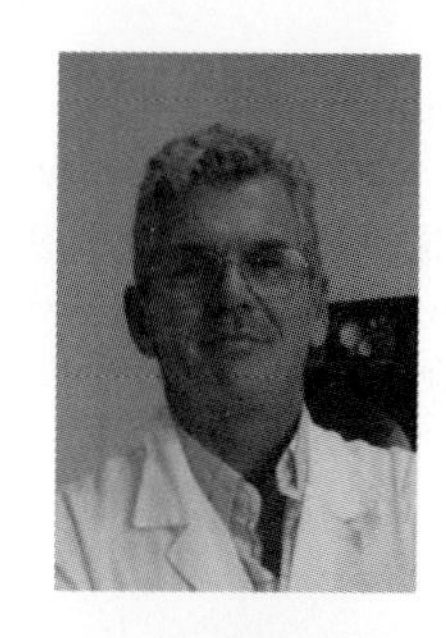

Nino Stocchetti, MD
Professor, Neuroscience Intensive Care Unit, Department of Anesthesia and Critical Care.
Fondazione IRCCS Cà Granda-Ospedale Maggiore Policlinico
Department of Pathophysiology and Transplantation, University of Milan
Milan, Italy

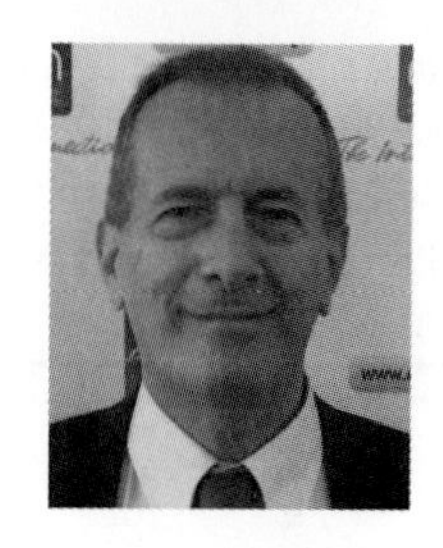

María N Suarez, MS
Neurotrauma Research Group, MEDITECH Foundation, Bogotá/Cali
Medical Intern, Universidad Surcolombiana
Neiva, Colombia

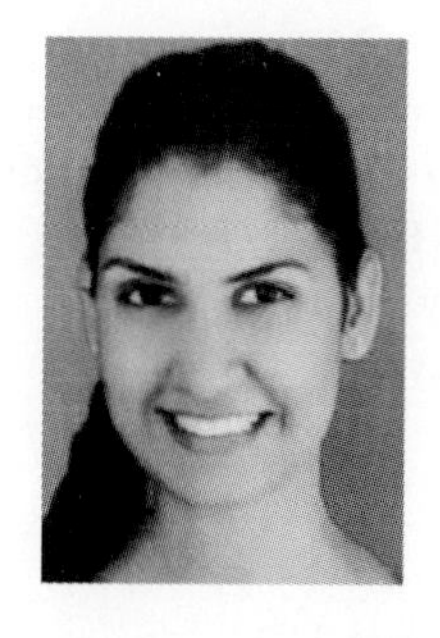

Arulselvi Subramanian, MBBS, MD
Professor Department of laboratory Medicine
Jai Prakash Narayan Apex Trauma Centre, All
India Institute of Medical Science (AIIMS)
New Delhi, India

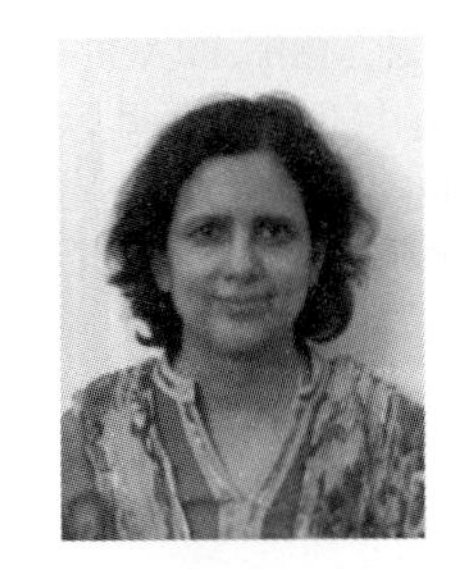

Francesco Tandoi, MD, PhD
Liver Transplant Unit. AOU Città della Salute e
della Scienza di Torino. University of Turin
Turin, Italy

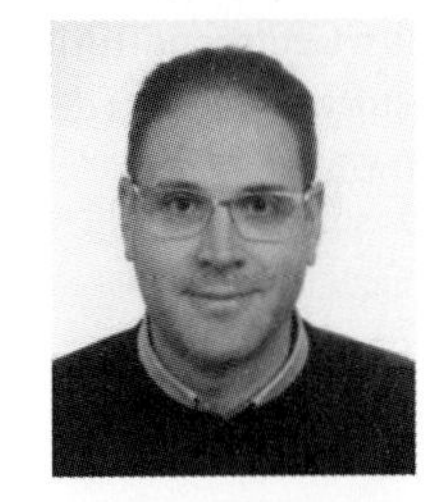

Prakash Narain Tandon, M.S., FRCS, D.Sc,
FAMS, FNA, FNASc, FASc, FTWAS, FRSM
National Research Professor
Emeritus Professor, All India Institute of Medical
Sciences, AIIMS
New Delhi, India

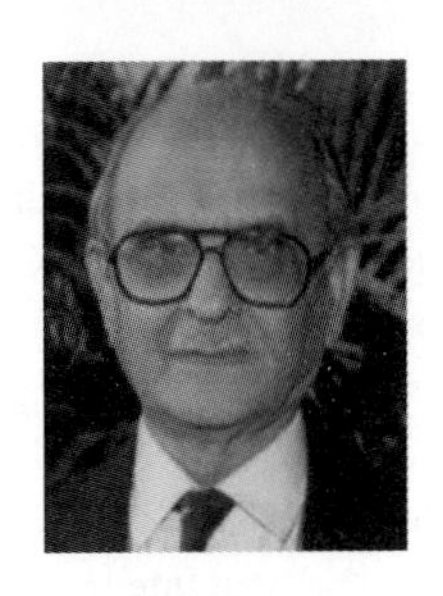

Sara Tardivo, MD
Department of Anesthesia and Intensive Care.
Città della salute e della scienza di Torino.
Molinette Hospital
University of Torino
Turin, Italy

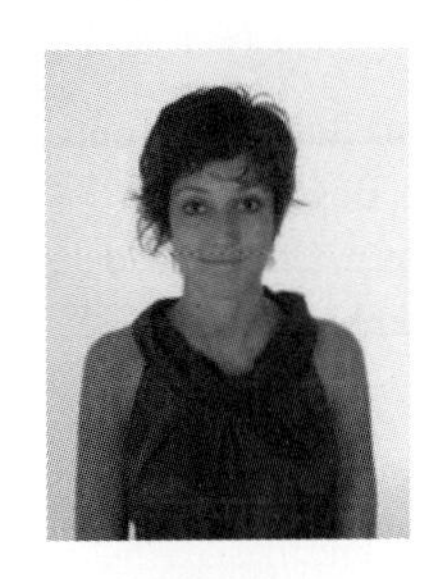

Giuliano Testa, MD
Simmons Transplant Institute, Baylor University
Medical Center
Dallas, Texas, USA

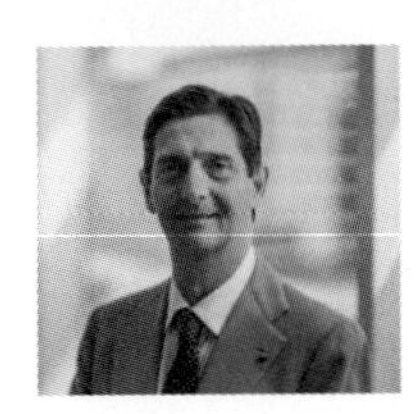

David Thomson, MD, Cert Critical Care (SA)
Critical Care Specialist and Transplant Surgeon,
Department of Surgery, Groote Schuur Hospital,
University of Cape Town
Cape Town, South Africa

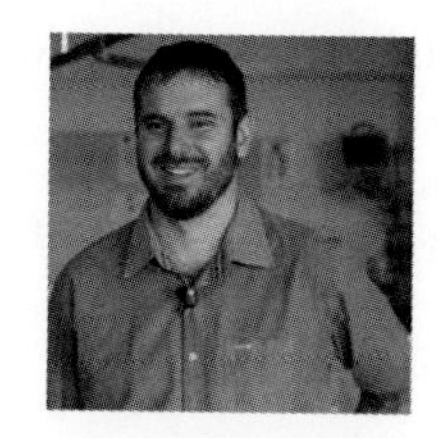

Olga M Tsiroulnikova, MD, PhD
Professor at Chair of transplantation and Artificial
organs of I.M.Sechenov First Moscow State
Medical University (Sechenov University)
Lead hepatologist of National Medical Research
Center of Transplantology and Artificial Organs
named after academician V.I. Shumakov
Moscow, Russia

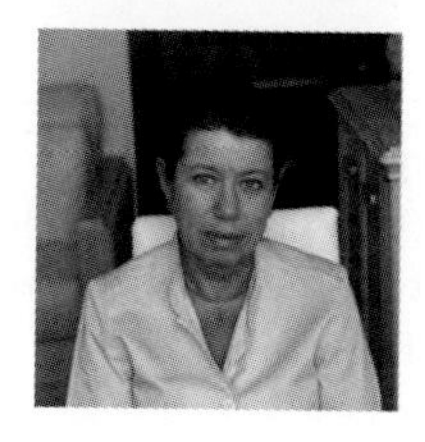

Steven Tsui, MD
Consultant Cardiothoracic Surgeon
Royal Papworth Hospital NHS Foundation Trust,
Papworth Everard, Cambridge, UK

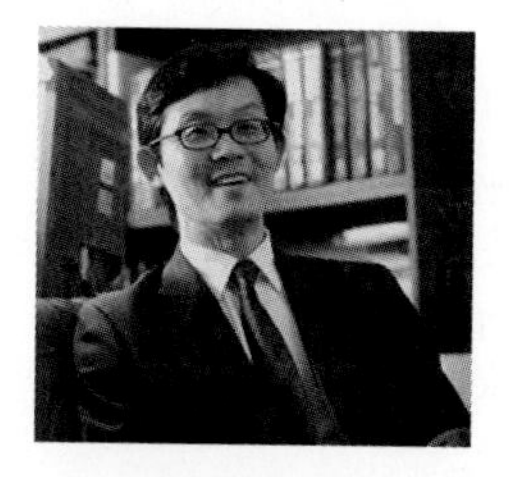

Rosario Urbino, MD
Medical Coordinator of Intensive Care Unit.
Department of Anesthesia and Intensive care.
Member of Transplant Coordination Team. Città
della Salute e della Scienza di Torino, Molinette
Hospital
Turin, Italy

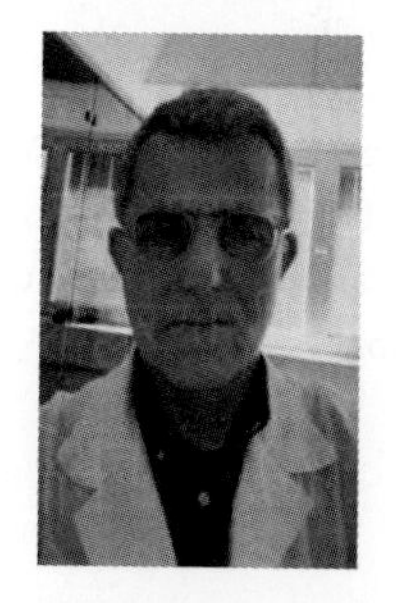

Ricard Valero, MD, PhD
Head of neuroanesthesia, Anesthesiology
Department, Hospital Clínic de Barcelona
Professor, Department of Surgery and Surgical
Specialties,
Universitat de Barcelona. Research Director, DTI
Foundation
DIBAPS, CIBER-SAM
Barcelona, Spain

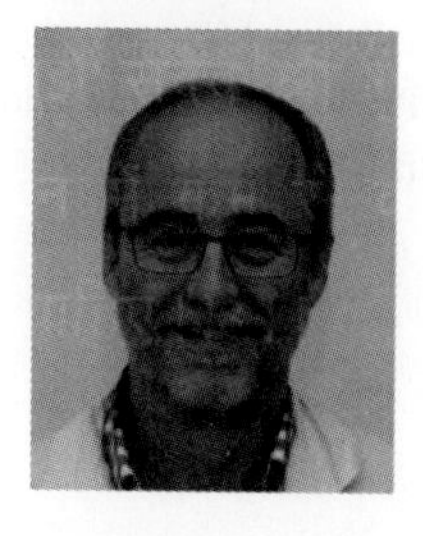

Murugusundaram Veeramani, MD
Radiologist, ER Division
Henry Ford Hospital
Detroit, MI 48202

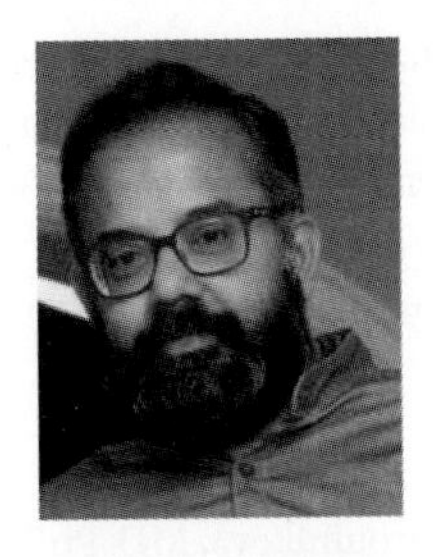

Simona Veglia, MD
Radiology Consultant. Department of Radiology.
Citta' della Salute e della Scienza di Torino,
Molinette Hospital
Turin, Italy

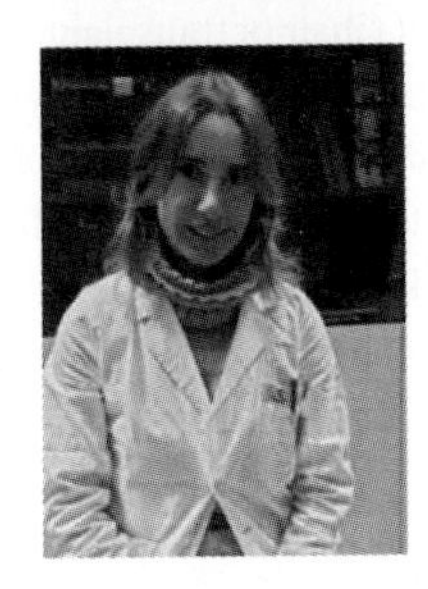

Elisa Vera
DTI Foundation
Project coordinator
Barcelona, Spain

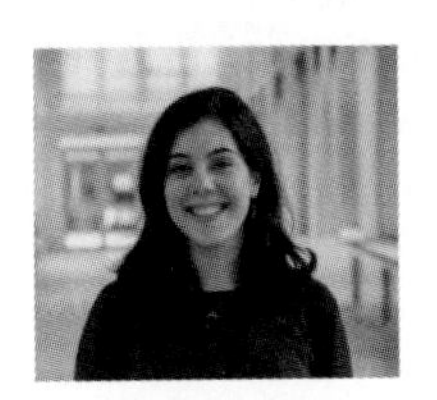

David S Vera, MD
Neurotrauma Research Group, MEDITECH
Foundation, Bogotá/Cali (Colombia)
Medical Researcher, Meditech Foundation
Cali, Colombia

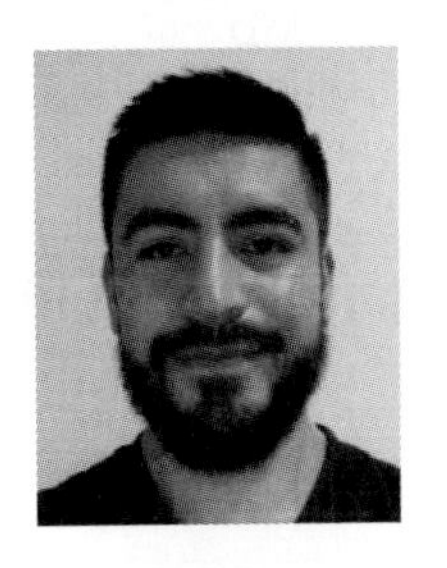

Rachna Wadhawa, MD
Associate Professor anaesthesiology GIPMER
Delhi, India

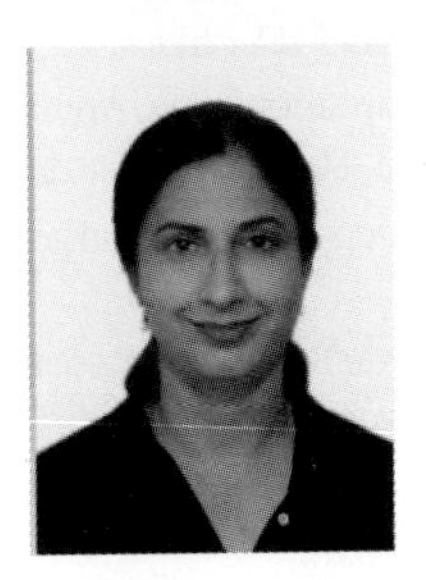

Walid Zaher, MD, MSc, PhD, MHPE
Group Clinical Research & Development Director
Corporate Academic AffairsAbu Dhabi Health
Services Company—SEHA
Abu Dhabi, United Arab Emirates

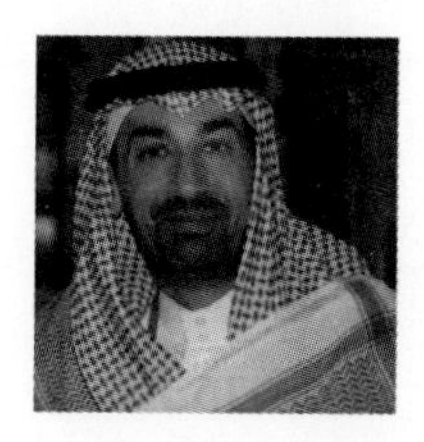

Marinella Zanierato, MD
Department of Anesthesia and Intensive Care,
Città della salute e della scienza di Torino,
Molinette Hospital
Turin, Italy

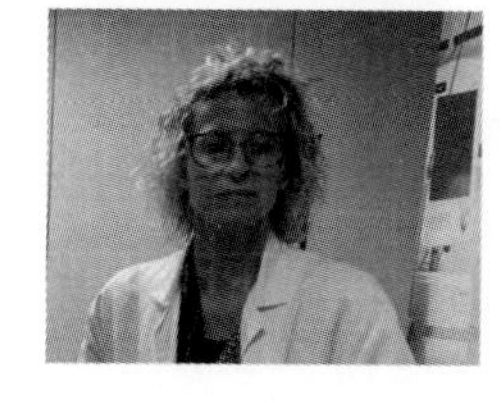

The Book aims at navigating the reader from the moment of diagnosis of death by neurologic criteria, to the entire process of organ donation and transplantation. A long-awaited comprehensive international book to share new science, to learn the best clinical practice, to debate controversies, to make an extraordinary gift of new lives happen.

Prof. PN Tandon, Emeritus Professor, All India Institute of Medical Sciences, National Research Professor New Delhi, India

For the first time all issues related to brain death, organ donation, and transplantation (criteria for diagnosis, donor identification and management, effective organization, and surgical pearls) are presented in a single book. All these issues are discussed at a multidisciplinary, international, and multicultural level. All these aspects make this book unique and a 'must have' on the desk of all professionals (healthcare personal, students, administrators, ethicists, politicians, transplant organizations) involved with transplant medicine.

Prof. V. Marco Ranieri, Chair Anesthesia and Intensive Care Medicine- Alma Mater Studiorum University of Bologna, Italy

This Book has extensive content germane to organ donation and transplant professionals of all disciplines, from around the world. It can promote education and training in the field of organ donation and transplantation that spark innovation, fuel research, and improve patient care.

Truly international and interdisciplinary.

Prof. Franco Servadei, President World Federation of Neurosurgical Societies

Introduction

The idea for this book was conceived in India during an international conference in Delhi while discussing the worldwide challenges posed by organ donation and transplantation with colleagues from different countries, cultures, religions, and specialties. Being aware of the variability in the approach to the diagnosis of brain death and contrasts in the numbers of organ donations and transplants in different parts of the world, we started to collect experiences from our international colleagues to analyse possible factors behind these differences. Significant contributions to this book came from the passionate work of transplant surgeons at the Citta' della Salute e della Scienza di Torino, Molinette Hospital, [Torino, Italy], and at All India Institute of Medical Sciences [New Delhi, India], where we had the opportunity to work as clinicians and researchers.

When the chapters for the book were almost ready, the world was hit by SARS-CoV2 pandemic. However, with the help of all the generous contributors and the OUP editorial office, the book moved forward despite the pandemic. Although the virus has inflicted abrupt and immense suffering around the world—including an impact on transplantation rates—it represented an opportunity to rethink and redefine priorities in our lives.

We are hopeful that the world will emerge from the pandemic in a better and more generous condition, and we hope this book will contribute to exchanging knowledge and promoting further achievements in the field of organ donation and transplantation. We designed this book to include experiences from several countries worldwide, and we regret not being able to include them all. Our critical objectives are to promote education and training, and to increase awareness in the field of organ donation and transplantation. We hope this book will serve as a multidisciplinary, international, and multicultural effort to help countries globally progress towards self-sufficiency in organ donation and transplantation.

Our patients on waiting lists to receive a transplant, regardless of their country of origin, may hope for the opportunity of restored life thanks to the precious gift of a donated organ. Moreover, we should offer to all patients who wish, the opportunity of organ donation after death. The gift of a new life for patients with end-stage organ failure is possible, and science and its advancement have made this a certainty. As physicians, researchers, and scientists we need to continue our mission of collaborating globally to help patients see a bright light waiting at the end of a tight and dark tunnel.

Anna Teresa Mazzeo and Deepak Gupta

Earthquake: *The gift of life may raise from brain death*

Coming from an earthquake area of Sicily, I have become accustomed to dealing with adversities since my childhood. Messina was destroyed twice in the recent centuries by disastrous earthquakes. The latest one, in 1908, was the most powerful and devastating, and I have always sought out photos of the terrible destruction it caused. The black-and-white pictures accentuate the grey and dust that was everywhere. They show crumbling buildings, pulverized roads, the absence of people in the streets, and nature crying for the sun, all witness of such destruction.

In these days, as an adult, I see my city so alive and energized that it seems almost impossible to imagine that people were able to achieve such full reconstruction. Life came back again after this apparent death of my city, palaces were rebuilt, old churches restored, trees and flowers planted, and new generations again are walking freely and confidently in the streets.

Brain death is like a terrible earthquake destroying what is the most precious in a human body. Moreover, it is also an earthquake for the families of the affected patients. A tsunami of emotions wipes away all the fervent hopes that relatives held onto while waiting in the intensive care unit for good news which doesn't arrive. The patient has died. No hope anymore. Then, in the blackest darkness, a tiny light is seen. A doctor comments that the person who died can offer life to someone else. They don't know them; they only know they can give a new smile to someone, also waiting somewhere with their families—the gift of a restored life. After an earthquake even so devastating, life can come back with the same strength as the pain of the loss. In a beautiful green garden, new flowers will grow.

Life can be donated through the generosity in death, and the pain of sorrowful families can be transformed to optimism and gratitude through the life of recipient patients.

This book is dedicated to all world donors and their families for their generosity.

Anna Teresa Mazzeo

Documented thoughts and current understanding on various aspects of brain death and organ transplantation by pioneers and exemplars in the medical sciences are scarce. The creation of this publication to inspire young minds while overcoming formidable odds imposed by Covid-19 pandemic is the raison d'etre for this book.

Some years ago, timidly but passionately, Anna Teresa asked me to consider jointly writing a book on Brain death and Organ Transplantation. Alone, I had neither the time nor energy for such a task. The book you hold in your hands follows innumerable hours of hard work and years of sleepless nights deliberating with masters in the field of brain death and organ donation programmes from various parts of the world. I do hope that you will learn much and emerge the richer for your understanding of current concepts on brain death and organ donation and transplantation as you turn the book's final page.

Deepak Gupta

SECTION 1.

THE DIAGNOSIS OF BRAIN DEATH

1

Harbingers of brain death

Prakash Narain Tandon

Introduction

Irreversible coma described as early as 1959,[1] later recognized as brain death was generally introduced in medical lexicon in 1965.[2] It was formally defined by the Ad Hoc Committee of the Harvard Medical School in 1968,[3] and first pronounced by the British Medical Establishment in 1976. It has, over the years, been globally accepted as equivalent to death of a human being.

Brain death implies irreversible loss of all functions of the brainstem, characterized by coma, pupillary abnormalities, absence of corneal reflex, arrest of respiration, and disturbance in thermoregulation and muscle tone. This was generally accepted by neurologists and neurosurgeons of that time. To avoid pit-falls of misdiagnosis, it is important to be aware of the confounding factors like drug intoxication, poisoning, or neuromuscular blocking agents, severe electrolytes, acid-base or endocrine disturbances, severe hypotension or hypothermia. Ancillary tests like EEG, Cerebral angiography, CT, MRI, Transcranial Doppler, or ICP monitoring are no longer considered mandatory for diagnosis of brain death but may be useful under certain circumstances specially as indicators of impending brain death.

Already in 1971, Mohandas and Chou,[4] on the basis of their clinicopathological studies on twenty-five patients with brain death, described damage to the brainstem as a critical component of severe brain damage resulting in death. It is worth mentioning that similar observations were described as early as 1960s.[5–7]

The declaration of brain death requires not only a series of careful neurological tests, but also the establishment of the cause of coma, the ascertainment of irreversibility, the resolution of any misleading clinical neurologic signs, and the recognition of possible confounding factors.[8] Notwithstanding reservations on the part of some critics, it is now generally accepted to equate brain death with death and that sufficient component of brain death is the brainstem.[9]

Currently, clinical neurological examination remains the standard for the determination of brain death and has been adopted by most countries (including India).[2,8,9]

An autopsy study reported by Tandon on 132 fatal head injury patients revealed brainstem haemorrhage in 49 (37%), while the remaining (83 cases) did not have any macroscopic abnormality in the brainstem.[1] Clinically these patients presented the commonly accepted signs of brainstem dysfunction—coma, papillary abnormality, disturbance of respiration, thermoregulation, and muscle tone. Comparison of the clinical features of the two groups (with and without structural damage to the brainstem) revealed no difference. More importantly, similar clinical features were also observed in some of the patients who survived.[1] Similarly, at least three out of twenty-five brains studied by Mohandas and Chou did not show any obvious structural damage of the brainstem.[4]

In October 1976, the Conference of Royal Colleges and their Faculties (UK) published a report expressing the opinion that 'brain death', when it had occurred, could be diagnosed with certainty with the Ad Hoc committee criteria.[3,10,11] This is now generally accepted. However, in a paper further elaborating the deliberations of this conference, an important concept was enunciated—'death is not an event but a process'. It was pointed out that, 'Exceptionally, as a result of massive trauma, death occurs instantaneously. Far more commonly death is not an event: it is a process, the various organs and systems supporting the continuation of life failing and eventually ceasing altogether to function, successively and at different times.'[11]

This concept has been further elaborated by Wijdicks, 'As brain death occurs, patients lose their reflexes in rostral—to caudal direction, and the medulla oblongata is the last part of the brain to cease to function. Several hours may be required for this destruction of the brainstem to be complete, and during that period there may still be medullary function.'[8] Prompt therapeutic intervention during this time may prevent brain death.

Premonitory signs of brain death

Tandon and Kristiansen elucidated the most significant fact to be learnt from the autopsy reported by Tandon as 'it is not possible on the basis of the clinical picture alone to predict whether the signs and symptoms of brainstem disturbances are reversible or irreversible'. Prompt actions resulted in saving twenty-one patients with evidence of severe brainstem dysfunction. To prevent brain death, it is important to detect these signs before they become irreversible. It is, therefore, essential to recognize the premonitory signs which are reversible.[7]

The prognostic values of individual clinical features as harbinger/premonitory signs of impending brain death are presented as follows.

Loss of consciousness

It is obvious that as long as consciousness is retained the brainstem functions are not impaired. However, there are a number of ominous signs which indicate impending risks to life. Loss of consciousness is conditio sine qua none of head injury. As a rule it starts to progressively recover spontaneously. However, failure to recover, persistence beyond a reasonable time, or deterioration following improvement, with or without a lucid interval should be a warning about impending brainstem dysfunction. Usually it is due to progressively increasing intracranial pressure (ICP) secondary to accumulating intracranial haematoma and/or progressing brain oedema associated with brain contusion, resulting in tentorial herniation. If not promptly relieved, it could result in brainstem damage and irreversible loss of brainstem function. Thus it is mandatory to carefully watch (and record) the state of consciousness at regular intervals and undertake prompt action to deal with the causative factor. The current routine use of the so-called aggressive treatment consisting of intubation, artificial ventilation, and use of sedatives soon after the arrival of the patient in the emergency room prevents repeated observations of the state of consciousness. Under these circumstances one has to rely on other indicators of risk to life. It must be pointed out that coma per se is not life threatening unless associated with loss of other vital functions. On the other hand, impairment of consciousness may be preceded by other symptoms and signs like increasing headache unresponsive to common analgesics, vomiting, and unexplained motor irritability. These symptoms are a harbinger of a more serious condition.

Pupillary reflex

Pupillary reflex to light is a sensitive test to detect brainstem compression. An increasing supratentorial mass results in tentorial herniation and compression of the brainstem. It is manifested initially as unilateral dilation of pupil. In case this is not relieved promptly it leads to bilateral dilation of pupil and loss of pupillary reflex to light which is a harbinger of brain death. A study of 164 cases of head injury revealed that patient with intracranial haematoma stands a much better chance of survival if the haematoma is evacuated before the pupil starts to dilate. Once one pupil is dilated and fixed the mortality rate goes up to 60–70%. Bilateral dilated and fixed pupils are one of the diagnostics criteria of brain death. Bilateral pin-point, non-reacting pupils, though much less frequently seen, also have a grave prognostic significance.[12]

Corneal reflex

This is one of the last brainstem reflexes to disappear and hence its bilateral absence is a grave sign. It is included among the criteria of brain death.

Vestibulo-Ocular Reflex (VOR)

VOR elicited by a cold caloric test is a reliable bed-side test to establish the integrity of the brainstem function. In a detailed prospective study of seventy-five patients with altered consciousness, Jadhav et al. reported a predictable relationship between the stage of unconsciousness and the pattern of VOR. We found that abnormality of VOR indicates the existence of a functional disturbance in the neuronal transmission at the ponto-mesencephalic level of the brainstem, before these functional changes have progressed to the stage of irreparable damage. An absent VOR is one of the important criteria of brain death.(13)

Based on the study of necroscopy on nine comatose patients submitted to the repeated neurological examination and the eliciting pattern of VOR, it has been revealed that abnormal VOR was observed sometime prior to death in all cases included in the study.(14) It may be pointed out that no patient with absent VOR survived while a number of patients with abnormal VOR recovered fully. Mahapatra and Tandon compared VOR with brainstem auditory evoked potentials (BAEP) and found the former to be as good or even better than BAEP in predicting outcome in severe head-injury patients.(15)

Decerebrate rigidity

While the total absence of motor activity following conventional sensory stimulation is one of the criteria for diagnosis of brain death, decerebration is an ominous sign of brainstem dysfunction. The underlying aetiology—intracranial space-occupying lesion, tentorial herniation, severe brain injury, brain oedema—if not urgently attended to may result in irreversible brainstem damage or brainstem death. However, as a life-threatening sign, it is not always a prelude to brain death even though it may be associated with other signs of brainstem dysfunction, for example, unconsciousness, papillary abnormality, and deranged VOR. Among sixty-two patients with severe head injury in Glasgow Coma Score (GCS) 4 with bilateral decerebration, twenty (33%) patients survived and half of them made a good recovery. While none of the eight with absent VOR survived, seven out of ten with abnormal VOR survived.(16)

Cushing reflex

In an experimental study on dogs, Cushing observed that rising ICP produces rising systolic pressure and slowing pulse rate. However, in clinical practice this has not proved to be a reliable sign.

Respiration

After establishing a free airway and excluding any significant chest injury or associated metabolic disturbances, a patient manifesting respiratory abnormality—hypo or hyper ventilation, Cheyne Stoke's or apneustic breathing—indicates an impending brainstem death. This is associated with depressed cough or gag reflex. Absence of respiration is a cardinal sign of brain death. To establish the irreversibility of the respiratory arrest the Apnoea Test is mandatory before diagnosing brain death.

Confirmatory tests for determination of brain death

It is now generally agreed that for diagnosis of brain death, clinical neurological examination along with apnoea test is all that is required. However, under exceptional circumstances ancillary confirmatory test may be desirable. Some of these tests are valuable in detecting premonitory signs of impending brain death. In any case, some of these tests are part of the standard management regime for a severe head injury patient.

ICP monitoring

Lundberg (1960) published his classic study on continuous recording of ICP using an indwelling intraventricular catheter in a series of 130 neurosurgical patients. He described three waveforms—A, B, and C. He found A—waves as pathological which were observed in the background of raised ICP. These were early indicators of neurological deterioration.[17] Ever since ICP monitoring started, using a variety of improved devices has been adopted as a routine component of management of severe head-injured patients.[18–20]

Increased ICP has been defined as pressure of more than 20 mm of Hg for more than 5 minutes. An ICP greater than 40mm of Hg suggests life-threatening intracranial hypertension and is associated with high mortality and morbidity.[21] Rising ICP adversely affects brain function by impairing cerebral perfusion pressure and on the other hand, it results in foraminal herniation leading to brainstem compression, a harbinger of brain death. While in initial stages raised ICP is amenable to medical or surgical therapy, it is not an uncommon experience that in some patients it becomes refractory to all treatment. Such patients have a fatal outcome.[22] Recent recommendations of the Lancet Neurology Commission in this regard are worth keeping in mind, 'Although population based targets for ICP and CPP management provide a useful initial basis for care, required target values or ranges differ between patients depending on the specific pathology.' Notwithstanding these limitations, the importance of ICP monitoring in patients with severe head injury cannot be underestimated. Persistent high ICP is a harbinger of a chain of events which lead to brainstem death. Lele et al studied 200 patients with head injury of which 126 (63%) had ICP monitoring; they concluded that ICP monitor placement was associated with lower hospital mortality than patients without ICP monitoring.[23]

Transcranial doppler ultrasonography

This is a non-invasive technique which could easily be utilized at the patient's bedside to evaluate the intracranial blood flow in the major vessels. Measuring blood flow velocity (BFV) and the pulsatile index (PI) provided valuable information about the existence of vasospasm, which accompanies severe rise in ICP.[24] Detecting it prior to complete cerebral circulatory arrest which indicates brain death may provide a therapeutic window to prevent fatal outcome.[25,26]

Cerebral angiography

In earlier years, cerebral angiography was the most common investigation for diagnosing brain pathology. Cerebral vasospasm could be easily visualized.[27–29] This vasospasm affecting the main arteries at the point of their entrance in the skull is a prelude to total cerebral vascular arrest, which was included as one of the essential criteria of brain death. However, except in rare circumstances, especially in children, this is no more required.[30] In place of angiography, cerebral scintigraphy using Tc 99m has also been used for this purpose.

Computerized axial tomography

A computerized axial tomography (CT) scan is for all practical purposes a routine investigation for all seriously ill neurological patients. It is essential for determining the cause of death. It helps in demonstrating a space-occupying lesion with brain oedema or brain swelling alone. While the CT scan may be normal in the early period of cardiorespiratory arrest, the findings including obliteration of basal cisterns, shift of the midline, and compressed ventricles should forewarn an imminent brainstem compression and impending death. A repeat CT scan, even if initially normal, is necessary if the patient's clinical state deteriorates or fails to improve. Agarwal et al, in 2016, have published their experience on bedside CT scans in traumatic brain injury. Based on their evaluation of the first 1000 patients they concluded that, 'Inclusion of a mobile CT scanner in the armamentarium of a neurosurgeon as a bed side tool' can dramatically change decision-making and the response time.[31]

Continuous Electroencephalographic (EEG) monitoring

In earlier years absence of all electrical activity in the EEG was included as one of the criteria of brain death. Besides this, it demonstrated a lack of reactivity to intense somato-sensory or audio-visual stimuli. However, it is no more as an essential requirement and in any case, it does not provide reliable evidence of premonitory signs of impending brain death.

Conclusion

Brain death is an irreversible loss of all functions of the brainstem. It is now generally recognized that death is not an event but a process.[11] This implies that there may be a 'time window' where the loss of brainstem function may be reversible.[7] To successfully utilize the time window for preventing brain death, it is important to carefully look for the premonitory signs of brain death. The evolution of the clinical signs of brain death before these becomes irreversible can be predicted by these premonitory signs described in this chapter. While it is now generally accepted that clinical neurological examination is enough to diagnose brain death, as a rule, it does not require ancillary investigations. Such investigations like ICP monitoring, Transcranial Doppler study for cerebral blood flow assessment, CT scan can provide an early warning of an impending brainstem dysfunction. It needs to be emphasized that brainstem death can occur in the absence of structural damage. On the other hand, useful survival is well known for patients with such structural damage, as brainstem haemorrhage as has been confirmed by imaging.[4,6] All efforts must, therefore, be made to detect the brainstem dysfunction when it is still reversible.

Highlights

- Death = brain death = brainstem death; Brainstem death is usually not an instantaneous event but a process.
- Death is the irreversible loss of brainstem functions.
- Irreversible brainstem function can occur in the absence of observable structural damage.
- The diagnosis of brain death can be established on the basis of clinical neurological examination specially, brainstem reflexes. Ancillary tests can be supportive.
- For irreversibility of the clinical state, it is necessary that all brainstem reflexes are lost. Loss of individual reflex, while indicative of the gravity of the clinical condition does not herald brain death.
- Harbingers or premonitory signs of impending brain death can be identified during the 'time window' where the loss of function may be reversible.

- Therapeutic steps instituted prior to irreversibility of the signs of brain death can save life.

References

1. Mollaret P, Goulan M. Le coma depasse (memoir preliminaire). Rev Neurol (Paris) 101, 3–5, 1959.
2. Kerridge IH, Saul P, Lowe M, MePhee J, Williams D. Death, dying and donation: Organ transplantation and the diagnosis of death. J Med Ethics 28, 89–94, 2002.
3. Ad Hoc Committee of the Harvard Medical School: A definition of irreversible coma. J. Amer Med Assoc 205, 337–340, 1968.
4. Mohandas A, Chou SN. Brain death: A clinical and pathological study. J Neurosurg 35, 211–218, 1971.
5. Kristiansen K, Tandon PN. Diagnosis and surgical treatment of severe head injury. J Oslo City Hospital (Supplement) 10, 107--213, 1960.
6. Tandon PN. Brainstem haemorrhages in cranio-cerebral trauma: Acta Neurol Scandinav 40, 375–385, 1964.
7. Tandon PN, Kristianen K. Clinico-pathological observations on brainstem dysfunction in cranio-cerebral injuries. Excerpta Medica International Congress Series 110, 23–28, 1965.
8. Wijdicks EFM. The diagnosis of brain death. N Eng J Med 344, 1215–1221, 2001.
9. Pallis C. ABC of brain stem death: Reappraising death. Brit Med J 285, 1409–1412, 1982.
10. Conference of the Medical Royal Colleges: Diagnosis of brain death. Brit Med J ii, 1187–1188, 1976.
11. Diagnosis of death. Memorandum issued by the honorary secretary of the conference of Medical Royal Colleges and their faculties in the United Kingdom on 15th January 1979. Brit Med J 1 (6150) 332, 1979.
12. Tandon PN. Pupillary signs in intracranial haematomas. Indian J Surg 26, 890, 895, 1964.
13. Jadhav, WR, Sinha A, Tandon PN, Kacker SK, Banerji AK. Cold caloric test in altered states of consciousness. Laryngoscope 81, 391–402, 1971.
14. Tandon PN., Bhatia R, Banerji AK. Vestibulo-ocular reflex and brainstem. Neurology (India) 21, 193, 1973.
15. Mahapatra AK, Tandon PN. Brainstem auditory evoked reflexes and vestibulo-ocular reflex in severe head injured patients: A prospective study of 60 cases. Acta Neurochir (Wien) 87, 40, 1987.
16. Mahapatra AK, Tandon PN., Bhatia R, Baneji AK. Bilateral decerebration in head injury patients. An analysis of 62 cases. Surg. Neurol 23, 36–40, 1985.
17. Lundberg N. Continuous recording and control of ventricular fluid pressure in neurosurgical practice. Acta Psychiat Neurol Scand (Suppl), 36, 1–93, 1960.
18. Lundberg N, Troupp H, Lorin H. Continuous recording of ventricular fluid press in patients with severe acute traumatic brain injury. J. Neurosurg 22, 581–590, 1965.

19. Becker DP, Miller JD, Greenberg R et al. The outcome from severe head injury with early diagnosis and intensive management. Neurosurg 47, 491–502, 1977.
20. Marshall LF, Smith RW, Shapiro HM. The outcome with aggressive treatment in severe head injury: The significance of intracranial pressure monitoring. Neurosurg 50, 20–25, 1979.
21. Marshall LF, Gautille HE Jr, Klauber MR et al. The outcome of severe closed head injury. J Neurosurg 75, 528–536, 1991.
22. Tandon PN. Head injury management: Future trends. In *Textbook of Neurosurgery*. 2nd edition (eds) Ramamurthi B, Tandon PN. B.I Churchill Livigston Pvt Ltd., New Delhi. Chapter 21, pp. 337–338, 1996.
23. Lele A, Kannan N, Vavilala MS, Sharma D, Mossa-Basha M, Agyem K, Mock C, Pandey RM, Dash HH, Mahapatra A, Gupta D. Patients who benefit from intracranial pressure monitoring without cerebrospinal fluid drainage after severe traumatic brain injury. Neurosurgery 2019 Aug 1;85(2):231–239.
24. Grolimund P, Weber M, Seiler RW et al. Time course of severe vasospasm after severe head injury. Lancet 1, 1173, 1988.
25. Petty GW, Mohr JP, Pedley TA et al. The role of Transcranial Doppler in confirming brain death: Sensitivity, specificity and suggestions for performance and interpretation. Neurology (Minneap) 40, 300, 1990.
26. Marin NA, Doberstein C, Zane C et al. Post traumatic cerebral arterial spasm: Transcranial Doppler Ultrasound cerebral blood flow and angiographic findings. J Neurosurg 77, 575–583, 1992.
27. Tandon PN, Prakash B, Banerji AK. Temporal lobe lesions in head injury. Acta Neurochirug 41, 205–221, 1978.
28. Brade GB, Simon BS. Angiography in brain death. Neuroradiol 7, 25–28, 1974.
29. Lindegaard KF, Nornes H, Bakke SJ, et al. Cerebral vasospasm diagnosed by means of angiography and blood velocity measurements. Acta Neurochir (Wien) 100, 12–24, 1989.
30. Ashwal S: Brain death in newborn: Current perspectives. Clin PErinatal 24, 859–882, 1997.
31. Agarwal D, Saini R, Singh PK et al. Bedside computed tomography in traumatic brain injury: Experience of 10,000 consecutive cases in neurosurgery at a level 1 trauma centre in India. Neurol India 64, 62–5, 2016.

2

Brain death: History of the concept and implications for organ donation

Sunil K. Pandya

Introduction

The *Oxford English Dictionary* had not yet been completed in the 1890s. The standard work of reference for legal definitions was *Black's Law Dictionary* (1891).(1) Its first edition had the entry under 'death' as 'The extinction of life; the departure of the soul from the body the ceasing to exist; deemed by physicians as a total stoppage of the circulation of the blood and a cessation of the animal and vital functions consequent thereupon, such as respiration, pulsation, etc.'(1)

The entry was modified in 1999 to read: 'Death—The ending of life; the cessation of all vital functions and signs. Brain death.—The bodily condition of showing no response to external stimuli, no spontaneous movements, no breathing, no reflexes and a flat reading (usu. for a full day) on a machine that measures the brain's electrical activity.—Also termed *legal death*.'(2)

Death has been looked upon with trepidation by most individuals throughout history. On the other hand, philosophers, especially in India, have considered it the gateway to rebirth with a succession of births and deaths till the individual reached the state of *nirvana* when the cycle ended and the atman (soul) of the individual merged with Brahma, the universal spirit.

The Venerable Bede (673–735 A.D.), the English Benedictine monk in Northumbria, enunciated the views of most thinkers when he pointed out that we are utterly ignorant of what precedes birth and follows death.(3)

As is often the case, Shakespeare (1564–1616) most elegantly describes the diagnosis of death(4) before Harvey's discovery of the circulation of blood(5):

Prince Henry (watching by the King): 'By his gates of breath there lies a downy feather, which stirs not. Did he suspire, that light and weightless down perforce must move.' (King Henry IV: IV, v)

Another example is found in King Lear's statement when he holds Cordelia in his arms: 'I know when one is dead and when one lives; she's dead as earth—lend me a looking glass; if that her breath will mist or stain the stone, why then she lives' (King Lear V, iii).

William Harvey (1578–1657) published '*An anatomical disquisition on the motion of the heart and blood in animals*'[5] in 1628 and in doing so, provided another criterion for the diagnosis of death—permanent cessation of the action of the heart manifested by an absence of arterial pulses and heart sounds.

Over the next 350 years or so, the diagnosis of death rested on the stoppage of the action of the heart and of breathing.

The advent and use of the ventilator disabled the use of stoppage of breathing in identifying death. Were we to carry on with the therapy on the basis that the heart continues to pump blood, when the brain is irreversibly damaged, survival would be prolonged. Such an individual, however, would never have a meaningful life. Inevitably, under this circumstance, death will follow in hours or days.

Brain death

Increasing awareness of the need for an intact brain, especially the deep cerebrum and brainstem, to sustain life led to the development of criteria that could identify their permanent and irrevocable destruction.

Addressing an International Congress of Anaesthesiologists in 1957, Pope Pius XII[6] asked, 'Can the doctor remove the artificial respiration apparatus before the blood circulation has come to a complete stop?' He then provided the answer in the affirmative 'when death has already occurred after grave trauma of the brain, which has provoked deep unconsciousness and central breathing paralysis, the fatal consequences of which have nevertheless been retarded by artificial respiration.'

In 1959, Mollaret and Goulon[7] described twenty-three patients with 'total and definitive abolition of vegetative functions with abolition of the functions of relation'. It was only possible to observe this state in patients with damaged brains who were being treated with artificial ventilation. Terming this condition *coma dépassé*, they suggested the need for a new means for assessing the frontier between life and death as patients in this state could take hours or even days before organs other than the brain, which was already dead, would cease to function even on being artificially maintained. Modern dictionaries translate *coma dépassé* as 'brain death'.

The importance of the EEG

Beecher et al, constituting the *Ad Hoc Committee of the Harvard Medical School* to examine brain death, defined irreversible coma in 1968.[8] In their opening paragraph they explained the need for such definition on two grounds: (1) To avoid burdening the families of those who suffer permanent loss of intellect consequent to irreversible damage to the brain and on hospitals in which they were being treated. (2) Revise obsolete criteria for the definition of death that led to controversy in obtaining organs for transplantation. They realized that moral, ethical, religious, and legal issues accompanied the medical problems involved in the process. They listed the characteristics of a permanently non-functioning brain, including a flat electroencephalogram (EEG) recorded over at least 10 but preferably 20 minutes. Tests were to be performed to identify these in the patient after excluding hypothermia (below 90 degrees F) and presence of central nervous system depressants such as barbiturates in the patient. All tests were to be repeated after 24 hours. Once the patient was declared dead and the family was informed of this event, the respirator was to be turned off. All decisions were to be made by the physician-in-charge in consultation with other physicians directly involved in the care of the patient. The Committee concluded that responsible medical opinion was ready to adopt the new criteria for pronouncing death and that no change in law was required since 'the cessation of life: the ceasing to exist' was to be defined by physicians. The Committee clarified that judgement on these criteria was solely a medical issue.

The emphasis on EEG findings was challenged in the USA in 1972 by the Task Force on Death and Dying of the Institute of Society, Ethics and Life Sciences.[9] It concluded: 'We urge that the clinical and more comprehensive criteria of the Harvard Report be adopted. We are supported in this conclusion by the report that a majority of neurologists have rejected the proposition that EEG determinations are sufficient as the sole basis for a determination of death.'

Professor Bryan Jennett in Glasgow described his dilemma and, in doing so, coined the term *brain death* in the English medical literature.[10] Worried by the need to decide how long life-supporting measures were to be continued when brain death was evident and the need to provide much-needed organs for transplantation, he discussed medical, philosophical, and legislative issues. As the first step, he emphasized the need for defining brain death, irrespective of organ transplantation. He defined circumstances under which brain death might be considered and the criteria to establish the diagnosis. He focused on death of the brainstem. He pointed out that EEG was available in few British hospitals and that the standard of recording it was variable. He felt that EEG records were not required. He did not advocate cerebral angiography as 'it is possible to have brain death with the circulation still intact'. He described sources of error in the diagnosis of brain death and discussed briefly the persistent vegetative state, locked-in syndrome, and peripheral paralysis, and emphasized that spinal cord function with reflex movements may persist after brain death. He did not use the term *brainstem death* anywhere in his paper.

Brainstem death: A historical overview

The term brainstem death was encountered in the conference of the Medical Royal Colleges of the United Kingdom on 11 October 1976.[11] It was reported, 'it is agreed that permanent functional death of the brainstem constitutes brain death and that once this has occurred further artificial support is fruitless and should be withdrawn.'

A committee appointed by the president of the United States of America in 1981[12] differed with regards to one of the conclusions reached by the Ad Hoc Committee of the Harvard Medical School. It concluded that a statute was needed to provide a clear and socially accepted basis for making determinations of death. It provided a draft for such a statute: 'An individual who has sustained either (1) irreversible cessation of circulatory and respiratory functions, or (2) irreversible cessation of all functions of the entire brain, including the brainstem, is dead.' It approved the Harvard criteria referred to above and drew on several other documents. In addition to EEG, it also approved of tests to ensure that there was no arterial flow to the brain. It validated the American emphasis on ensuring cessation functions of the entire brain rather than the British focus of death of the brainstem alone as the latter was 'closer to a prognostic return (that a *point of no return* has been reached in the process of dying), while the American approach is more diagnostic in seeking to determine that all functions of the brain have irreversibly ceased at the time of the declaration of death.'

Shemie (2012)[13] highlighted difficulties in gaining acceptance of the concept of brain death. 'As with most discussions about death, the challenges are complex due to:

- Philosophical, religious, and cultural differences in the concept and definitions of death.
- The difficulties in performing research in this field and the resultant deficits in information and evidence on a number of aspects of the dying process.
- Controversies regarding the validity of death determination practices.
- Lack of understanding and/or awareness by the public and health professionals.
- The emotionally charged nature of the subject matter.'

Burkle et al (2014)[14] provided an unequivocal response and emphasized that 'neurologic determinations of death and state laws concerning these matters are clear and unambiguous ... A strong and well-established consensus regarding brain death has been forged from decades of sustained discussions in medicine, law, and ethics ... An informed public is the best defense against unanticipated outcry ... and thus we encourage our colleagues in critical care, neurosciences, and biomedical ethics to engage patients and local communities about matters related to brain death.'

Dhanwale (2014)[15] has provided a review of the Indian policy where irreversible and extensive damage to the brainstem forms the basis for the diagnosis of death. He has described the tests prescribed for the purpose of making this diagnosis, with emphasis on the apnoea and other newer ancillary tests.

Vrselja et al (2019)[16] have recently published their report on the restoration and maintenance of microcirculation, molecular, and cellular functions of the intact pig brain up to 4 hours post-mortem. They concluded that 'These findings demonstrate that under appropriate conditions the isolated, intact large mammalian brain possesses an underappreciated capacity for restoration of microcirculation and molecular and cellular activity after a prolonged post-mortem interval.' While debates are already underway on the ethical implications of these findings, it is evident that these findings need to be confirmed by other researchers and further studies will be needed to assess the functional capabilities of these neurons and their connections over the long term.

Implications regarding organ transplants

A common criticism against the use of the concept of brain death has been that it was devised to enable organ transplants. As we have seen in Mollaret and Goulon,[7] once the concept evolved, it became evident that it could be used to benefit those in need of life-saving organ transplants.

The prime purpose, however, was to spare the family prolongation of the process of death of their loved one and to ensure that scarce utilities in the form of intensive care beds were made available to those whose illnesses could be cured and meaningful lives prolonged.

Machado et al (2007)[17] showed that while transplantation developed as a consequence of advances in surgery and immunosuppressive treatment, brain death owed its origin to the need to optimize intensive care.

Discussing law and ethics in organ transplantation, Woodcock and Wheeler (2010)[18] pointed out that the ideal organ donor is the one who cannot be harmed by donation. This makes the dead most acceptable as donors. Expanding the definition of death to include brain dead persons provides 'a pool of heart-beating donors'.

Machado (2005)[19] described the first organ transplant from a brain-dead donor. 'Five years before the Harvard criteria appeared, Guy Alexandre, a Belgian surgeon ... introduced a set of brain death criteria based on the description of *coma dépassé* and carried out the first transplant in his country.' It is learned that Alexandre and his team did not discontinue mechanical ventilation and wait for the donor's heart to stop. 'Theirs was the first transplantation ever to make use of a heart-beating, brain dead donor.' Machado provided details of the kidney transplant in June 1963. The transplanted kidney functioned well till the recipient died of sepsis eighty-seven days after surgery. At the CIBA Symposium on Transplantation, Alexandre described nine patients with severe craniocerebral injuries who had served as organ donors. The criteria used by him to diagnose brain death included complete, bilateral mydriasis, complete absence of reflexes and of breathing even after stopping mechanical respiration for 5 minutes, a progressive fall in blood pressure and persistently flat EEG.

This paper deserves study for the details it provides not only on Alexandre's pioneering operation but also for some of the discussion that followed his presentation at the symposium.

For instance, Hamburger's publication in 1959[(19)] describes a patient in whom breathing and the circulation of blood were maintained artificially. The professor of neurology, when consulted, opined that the patient had been dead for several days.

As quoted by Machado,[(19)] Thomas Starzl, and Roy Calne, then the world leaders in organ transplantation, did not accept the clear and logical presentation of Alexandre's criteria for the diagnosis of brain death. Starzl concluded his discussion by asking, 'Would any physician be willing to remove an unpaired organ before circulation had stopped?' Calne agreed with Starzl. 'Although Dr. Alexandre's criteria are medically persuasive, according to traditional definitions of death, he is in fact removing kidneys from live donors. I feel that if a patient has a heartbeat, he cannot be regarded as a cadaver.' Calne later admitted that his fears were unfounded and credited Alexandre with an important medical advancement.

Conclusion

Reviewing the Harvard Report on brain death fifty years after it was issued, Truog et al (2018)[(20,21)] noted that the recommendations in it had no legal force. Kansas adopted a variation of the Harvard criteria into its law two years after the report had been issued. The Uniform Determination of Death Act was passed in 2008 but four American states permit families to assert various degrees of conscientious objection.[20] They concluded their review thus[20]:

'History is full of ironies, and the 50-year legacy of the Harvard report is no exception. From one perspective, the report laid the foundation for laws that have both saved and improved the lives of hundreds of thousands of patients through organ and tissue donation. Conversely, decades of attempts to find a conceptual justification for linking this diagnosis to the death of the patient remain incomplete.

The significance of brain death may diminish in the near future. If new genetic technologies render xenotransplantation safe, there could be a supply of transplantable organs without resorting to human donors (although the approach would raise its own ethical concerns). Tissue engineering and 3-dimensional printing might yield synthetic organs. Such developments would make the diagnosis of brain death irrelevant for organ procurement. Until then, however, one warning remains apt—Capron, one of the architects of the UDDA, summarized the situation well in 2001 when he described efforts to determine when death has occurred as both well settled, yet still unresolved.'

Highlights

- The criteria for making the diagnosis of death has changed over the centuries from permanent cessation of breathing to permanent cessation of breathing, and heart beat and, more recently, to irreparable and permanent damage to the brainstem.
- The use of irreparable and permanent damage to the brainstem as the sole criterion for the diagnosis of death spares the family the agony and expense of futile 'treatment' in the intensive care unit over days, weeks, or more.
- It also enables retrieval of organs for transplantation while they are continuing to be perfused by oxygenated arterial blood.
- New genetic technologies may render xenotransplantation safe. It may also be possible to create synthetic organs. In that future, organ retrieval from beating-heart cadavers will be rendered unnecessary.

Acknowledgements

I am grateful to Dr Bindu T. Desai (USA) and Dr Reeta Mani (Bengaluru, India) for providing me with the full texts of papers I could not access locally.

References

1. Black Henry Campbell. *A dictionary of law. Definitions of the terms and phrases of American and English jurisprudence, ancient and modern.* St. Paul, MN: West Publishing Co. 1891, 334–335
2. Garner Bryan A (Editor-in-chief): *Black's Law Dictionary. Seventh Edition.* St. Paul, MN: West Publishing Co. 1999
3. San Filippo David. Historical perspectives on attitudes concerning death and dying. (2006). Faculty Publications 2006; 29:1–16 https://digitalcommons.nl.edu/faculty_publications/29 Accessed on 13 March 2019
4. Turner TJ. The signs of approaching death illustrated from Shakespeare. Shakespeariana 1884;1:274–276
5. Harvey William. *An anatomical disquisition on the motion of the heart and blood in animals.* In Willis Robert (Ed.): *The works of William Harvey M.D. Physician to the King, Professor of Anatomy and Surgery to the College of Physicians. Translated from the Latin with A Life of the Author.* London: Printed for the Sydenham Society. 1847, 3–86
6. Pope Pius XII. Address to an international congress of anesthesiologists. 25–26 November 1957. http://lifeissues.net/writers/doc/doc_31resuscitation.html Accessed on 3 April 2019
7. Mollaret P, Goulon M. Le coma dépassé. Rev Neurol (Paris) 1959;101:3–15
8. Beecher Henry K, Adams Raymond D, Barger Clifford A et al. (Constituting the Ad Hoc Committee of the Harvard Medical School to examine the definition of brain death): A definition of irreversible coma. JAMA 1968;205:85–88
9. Eric, Kass Leon R (co-chairmen). Task force on death and dying of the institute of society, ethics and life sciences: Refinements in criteria for the determination of death: An appraisal. *JAMA* 1972;221:48–53
10. Jennett Bryan. The donor doctor's dilemma: Observations on the recognition and management of brain death. *Journal of Medical Ethics* 1975;1:63–66
11. Honorary Secretary of the Conference of Medical Royal Colleges and their Faculties in the United Kingdom: Diagnosis of brain death. *British Medical Journal* 1976;2:1187–1188
12. President's Commission for the Study of Ethical Problems in Medicine and Biomedical and Behavioural Research (Chairman: Morris B. Abram): *Defining death. A report on the medical, legal and ethical issues in the determination of death.* Washington D.C.: U. S. Government Printing Office. July 1981;1–166
13. Shemie Sam (Forum Chair). *International guidelines for the determination of death—Phase 1* Ottawa: Canadian Blood Services 2012;1–49

14. Burkle Christopher M, Sharp Richard R, Wijdicks Eelco F. Why brain death is considered death and why there should be no confusion. *Neurology* 2014;783:1464–1469
15. Dhanwale Anant Dattatray. Brainstem death: A comprehensive review in Indian perspective. *Indian Journal of Critical Care* 2014;18:596–605
16. Vrselja Zvonimir, Daniele Stefano G, Silbereis, Talpo Francesca et al. Restoration of brain circulation and cellular functions hours post-mortem. *Nature* 2019;568:336–343
17. Machado Calixto, Korein Julius, Ferrer Yazmina et al. The concept of brain death did not evolve to benefit organ transplants. *Journal of Medical Ethics* 2007;33:197–200
18. Woodcock Tom, Wheeler Robert. Law and ethics in organ transplantation surgery. *Annals of the Royal College of Surgeons of England* 2010;92:282–285
19. Machado Calixto. The first organ transplant from a brain-dead donor. *Neurology* 2005;64:1938–1942
20. Truog Robert D, Pope Thaddeus Mason, Jones David S. The 50-year legacy of the Harvard report on brain death. *JAMA* 2018;320:335–336
21. Truog Robert D, Berlinger Nancy, Zacharias Rachel L, Solomon Mildred Z. Brain death at fifty: Exploring consensus, controversy and contexts. *Hastings Center Report* 2018;48:S2–S5

3

Determination of death by neurological criteria (brain death)

Francesco Procaccio and Marina Munari

Introduction

What is death? Taking into account the continuous intense discussion among experts regarding the concept of death, this question may prove difficult to answer.[1–3] Nevertheless, using a pragmatic medical approach, a simple point can be affirmed and endorsed: death is 'brain death' (BD). According to Uniform Determination of Death Act (UDDA),[2] death of a person is 'the irreversible loss of all functions of the brain, including the brainstem'. In fact, BD is the only death, regardless of the mechanisms that cause total irreversible damage of the brain (a respiratory and circulatory arrest or a direct devastating cerebral lesion).[4,5]

Unfortunately, from 1960s onwards, BD has been strictly connected with the increasing new organ transplant possibilities, sometimes culminating in the suspect of a legal fiction established to facilitate organ transplantation.[6–8] Moreover, several criticisms have been made regarding the concept of death and accuracy of related criteria in the scientific community.[3–9]

The *whole BD* is the most accepted concept worldwide.[10,11] But many Anglo-Saxon medical schools utilize the *brainstem death* as the focal point to the BD concept. Based on the pathophysiological and clinical evidence, the brainstem, easily testable with the examination of cranial nerve reflexes, is the fundamental centre of brain functions.[12] The two essential components of human life, the capacity for consciousness and the capacity to breathe, depend on the integrity of these few cubic centimetres of (brainstem) tissue.[13] It should be underlined that the irreversible cessation of brainstem function implies death of the brain as a whole, even if it does not necessarily imply the immediate death of every cell in the brain. There is no difference between the two BD concepts when performing a clinical neurological examination. Nevertheless, the *whole BD* concept would require the complete absence of hemispheric functions, not clinically verifiable in comatose patients.

The diagnosis of BD should be based on a complete clinical examination performed by trained physicians, such as ICU personnel and neurologists, with documented experience, who meticulously follow international and national criteria, the knowledge of which should be part of the medical university curriculum.[14]

The purpose of this chapter is to discuss critical aspects related to the BD concept and detail the prerequisites and clinical criteria to establish a BD diagnosis.

Critical aspects of BD concept and diagnosis

BD is and must be a clinical diagnosis; despite this it is evident that clinical tests used for BD diagnosis cannot examine the whole brain or all the brainstem neurons. Thus some hidden unspecified cerebral functions might go undetected; likewise some basic hormonal or autonomic and neurophysiological functions, reasonably linked to still active neurons somewhere in the brain, are seen in subjects in whom BD has been correctly determined.[15]

For example, despite the absence of intracranial blood flow, in a number of BD patients the hypothalamic-hypophyseal axis can secrete antidiuretic hormone and prevent neurogenic diabetes insipidus.[16] Moreover, circulatory and other homeostatic functions of the brain, including temperature modulation, are excluded from BD diagnostic criteria. The loss of blood pressure and heart variability and baroflex sensitivity after BD are specific BD signs, but are rarely used in addition to the classical neurological standard.[17]

Thus, the absence of testable brainstem reflexes included in the BD neurological standard is the only best, clinically achievable *proxy* of a complete brainstem destruction. Moreover, the timing and the clinical insight based on the neurological examination cannot define the loss of cerebral functions 'irreversible', but precisely 'permanent' during the time of clinical observation.[18,19] The real clinical state enhanced by the BD neurological standard might consequently be defined as 'permanent apnoeic unconsciousness' under artificial ventilatory support.[20]

Since Harvard criteria in 1968[21] and the UDDA[22] in 1981, intensive care has greatly improved and the clinical experience of BD patients has grown immensely. The concept commonly accepted in the 1980s was that BD is death because it is the permanent cessation of essential integrative and modulating functions necessary for maintaining the organism as a whole[23–26] and preventing a rapid deterioration of the homeostatic milieu leading to circulatory arrest despite any extraordinary medical support. With our current knowledge, this concept is hardly acceptable from a strict biological point of view.

Severe cardiovascular instability caused by brain coning, autonomic storm, and hypothalamic-brainstem infarct, rapidly leading to a circulatory arrest in the 1970s, may presently recover if appropriate treatment is implemented in a timely fashion and continued in ICU. Other acute disorders, including heart function,[27] may self-resolve within few days or more[28] and 'chronic' BD clinical stabilization may occur if ventilator support is not withdrawn and quality intensive care is offered. The assumption that the body without brain function will rapidly disintegrate and cardiocirculatory arrest will be soon unavoidable is definitely false.[29]

All these facts would contradict the BD definition (*irreversible* loss of *all* the cerebral functions) literally taken and its biological justification (loss of integrative functions and unavoidable body disintegration). Consequently, it might be reasonable to say that equating BD with death involves some levels of incoherence between concept and criterion, criterion and tests, and tests and concept.[30] It is mandatory to say that the patient must be *dead* and not *almost* dead when his or her death is declared.[31] This may depend on the acceptance of unique or variable concepts of death.[11]

Nevertheless, the core significance of a human being death deserves a deeper medical insight. The survival of several parts and functions of a BD human body are fully compatible with the death of that organism, i.e., of that person. In fact, organs and functions contribute to achieving the finality of maintaining the organism as a whole, which does not only mean to preserve the physiological milieu of the body but principally to sustain the unique *emergent* function of mammals that is *conscious awareness*. This essential function, i.e., the most important mystery of human life, is unique among biological phenomena and is the prodigious result of encephalic integrative actions; to date, it is completely irreplaceable by any technological process and support.(32) Thus, the loss of this emergent function can be considered as the most acceptable and concrete border between human life and death. If the residual activity of some neurons is philosophically disturbing and not coherent with BD definition, clinical tests could be improved and tightened(33) and procedures could be modified to better assure 'irreversibility'.

Clinically, a strict observance of the complete examination and a careful exclusion of any possible confounding factor are the most important requisites to eliminate the possibility of misdiagnosis and quell any doubts. In the real world of ICUs, BD diagnosis maintains and respects the dignity of all the patients who die in the secure awareness that there is no possible chance of any recovery despite extreme medical care.

Three working traits for a feasible concept of death could be: (1) a simple, uniform concept defined as a single phenomenon; (2) death of the *organism as a whole* (not of the whole organism); and (3) relevant to most prevalent situations and practices, including the new clinical and technological scenarios.(34)

Death determination by neurological criteria

Early suspicion that a patient with devastating untreatable cerebral lesion is deteriorating to BD should be always and promptly raised in ICU,(35) even under sedation, when coma combines with no response to painful stimulation and absence of normally monitored brainstem reflexes during ICU nursing and treatment (bilateral areflexic pupillary mydriasis, loss of gag, cough reflexes to suction, etc.).(36)

BD prediction in neurocritical patients

BD can be expected during neurocritical care if diagnostic imaging and advanced neuromonitoring, including ICP, TCD, EEG, EvPot, etc., concurrently show a deterioration towards failing cerebral blood flow and irrecoverable global cerebral dysfunction.

Correct and timely prevision of BD deterioration in ICU facilitates the prevention of severe circulatory instability due to brain coning leading to spinal shock that may impede a reliable and prompt BD diagnosis.

A clinical evaluation for BD diagnosis should be routinely considered in patients with massive untreatable and irreversible brain injury of identifiable aetiology but, nowadays, BD testing is not undertaken when this is a likely diagnosis in up to 21% of cases in European hospitals.(37)

Prerequisites and key factors for BD diagnosis

The three essential findings in BD are unconsciousness (coma), absence of brainstem reflexes, and spontaneous respiratory drive (apnoea). Careful adherence to three main recommendations is obligatory(38,39):

1. The precise diagnosis of the devastating cerebral lesion aetiology and definition of the pathogenesis possibly leading to BD are essential *sine qua non*-prerequisites for clinically diagnosing BD and zeroing any pitfall and mistake.(40,41) Consequently, investigations and imaging aimed at a precise definition of the aetiology and the evaluation of the severity of the brain damage and its consistency with the development of BD should always be performed and clearly requested by any national guidelines.

   Neuroimaging and laboratory tests (meningitis, encephalitis, poisoning, etc.) should be used and repeated as needed at the best quality possible. BD can be diagnosed in comatose patients of unknown aetiology only if the pathogenesis of the devastating cerebral injury is clear, and eventually confirmed by ancillary tests.

   The exclusion of any disease and clinical situation that can mimic BD is imperative and must be performed using the tools available, such as an accurate patient history and proper diagnostic testing.

Such conditions include brainstem encephalitis, Guillain-Barré syndrome involving all peripheral, and cranial nerves (Miller-Fisher syndrome), demyelinating conditions, endocrine crisis, subclinical status epilepticus, snake bite, and poisoning as baclofen overdose (potentially reversible situations). Chronic or sub-acute states as Locked-in syndrome, vegetative or minimally conscious state should be carefully investigated and diagnosed.

Any possible consequence of a transient brain 'penumbra', i.e., a recoverable loss of cerebral functions, on exam reliability should be excluded in particular when a severe diffuse ischemic or anoxic insult is probable (waiting at least 24 hours).

2. Clinical BD diagnosis cannot be reliable and should not be performed if any confounding factor has not been excluded or reversed. This is a golden rule and a 'clinical must' for avoiding any possible pitfalls and mistakes. Factors like hypotension, hypoxia, hypothermia, etc. that can interfere with the neurological examination, possibly masking residual cerebral functions and being potentially reversible, must be excluded. If a potential confounding factor cannot be reversed or excluded, BD diagnosis must be completed with proper confirmatory ancillary tests. General clinical principles of good medicine or existing detailed guidelines can be followed as well.

No severe derangement in circulatory, metabolic, and respiratory functions can be underestimated or neglected. Thus, some preconditions before neurological examination must be strictly fulfilled and a step-by-step procedure should invariably be followed:

- The long-term and recent clinical history of the patient must be well known and, as needed, investigated. All acute therapies should be recorded and analysed. Previous diseases and treatments should be considered. The drug history should be reviewed and a toxicological screening obtained, if necessary.
- Core temperature >35°C is a fundamental prerequisite. The response to light is lost between 28°C and 32°C and brainstem reflexes may disappear below 28°C. Long-term therapeutic hypothermia (i.e., 32°C to 34°C in anoxic brain injury), particularly if associated with sedation and metabolic alterations, requests more time after rewarming to completely reverse and avoid any possible pitfall.[42,43]

- Mean arterial blood pressure >65 mmHg (>8.7 kPa) in normotensive subjects and hemodynamic stability with adequate oxygenation and volemia must be ensured.
- Severe derangement in electrolytes (particularly sodium, calcium, and magnesium), glucose, acid-base, or endocrine function (hypothyroidism, adrenal dysfunction, hypo-hyperglycaemia) should be excluded or reversed (cortisol, T3–T4 blood levels). Uraemia and hepatic failure can affect the level of consciousness and arousal response.
- Any possible effect of CNS-depressant drugs and neuromuscular blocking agents should be carefully evaluated and excluded (barbiturates, opioids, benzodiazepines, tricyclic anti-depressants, etc.).[44]. Blood screening tests may be helpful, but not definitive in some cases. The neuronal level of drugs cannot be clinically investigated and associated actions of drugs and toxics may not be detectable by routine assessments. Pharmacokinetic data and blood level references for common anaesthetic drugs exist but only a careful clinical judgement, including the evaluation of kidney and liver functions, possible active metabolites, temperature and preexisting cerebral metabolic damage can guide clinicians to reliable conclusions. If there is any doubt regarding the timing of some pharmacological agents, withholding the BD neurological examination for hours or days (at least four times the clearance half-life of the substance) can be considered, but, preferably, ancillary test should be considered and utilized.[45,46] In this instance, electroencephalogram is not the preferable test as CNS-depressant drugs easily affect it.

In chronic use of antiepileptic drugs, levels below or in the therapeutic range cannot interfere with BD diagnosis. Specific drug antagonists may be used if appropriate (naloxone or flumazenil). Drug evaluation in patients under non-pulsatile, continuous-flow mechanical circulatory support devices must be done with extreme caution. A peripheral nerve stimulator can be used to confirm intact neuromuscular conduction.

3. If the prerequisites for clinical diagnosis of BD cannot be fully satisfied, an objective demonstration of the absence of intracranial blood flow is required.

Clinical neurological examination

The clinical examination must be complete, rigorous, and reliable (Box 3.1). Self-fulfilling prophecy may lead to an incomplete examination of bilateral brainstem reflexes; possible pitfalls may also depend on facial, ocular, or high cervical trauma, pre-existing pupillary abnormalities and peripheral cranial or spinal nerve lesions. Severe chronic respiratory dysfunction, severe circulatory reaction to acute hypercapnia and acidosis

Box 3.1 Clinical diagnosis of death by neurological criteria (brain death)

Prerequisites for clinical determination of death by neurological criteria (brain death)

- Knowledge of patient's clinical history, brain injury aetiology, and/or pathogenesis of untreatable cerebral damage
- Cerebral diagnostic imaging
- Irreversible devastating Cerebral lesion
- Exclusion of any possible confounding factors that may make the clinical examination unreliable:
  - Hypothermia (core temperature < 35°C)
    Hypotension, hypoxia, severe hypercapnia, severe electrolytes, acid-base, or endocrine disturbances
  - Central nervous system-depressant drugs and poisoning
  - Neuromuscular blocking agents and dilating pupil agents
  - Acute/chronic neuromuscular and demyelinating diseases
  - Brainstem encephalitis, Guillain-Barré syndrome, subclinical status epilepticus
- At least 24 hours after a severe anoxic insult
- Experienced physicians

Box 3.1 Continued

Clinical neurological examination

Complete and rigorous neurological examination to diagnose the permanent absence of:

(1) Any sign of arousal and consciousness (hypotonic coma [GCS 3]—no arousal response to painful stimuli, no seizures, no myoclonic jerks, no ventilator drive)
(2) Brainstem reflexes (Standardized methodology of brainstem reflexes testing is mandatory) [see text]
(3) Spontaneous respiratory drive at the maximal hypercapnic stimulation (apnoea test) [see text]

Irrefutable results of brainstem reflexes testing:

–Bilateral complete absence of any motor or autonomic response to:

(1) Oculomotor reflex
(2) Corneal reflex
(3) Oculocephalic reflex
(4) Painful stimulation of the trigeminal area
(5) Pharyngeal (gag) reflex
(6) Carinal (tracheal) reflex
(7) High dose (0.04 mg/kg) atropine i.v. administration

Irrefutable result of the apnoea test *(see text for the recommended methodology):*

–Complete continuous absence of any respiratory drive and ventilator movement with documented (blood gas analysis) $PaCO_2 \geq 60$ mmHg ($\geq$8 kPa)

Spinal reflexes

Meticulous evaluation of any spontaneous or provoked movements of the trunk, arms, or legs and autonomic response to stimuli:

–Confirmation of the spinal origin (motor and viscera-visceral spinal reflexes) [see text]

Recourse to confirmatory ancillary tests if complete testing is not possible or even a minimal doubt about cerebral pathogenesis or clinical examination remains.

Percentage of misdiagnosis or mistake must be zero.

If all the brain death criteria are fulfilled, death declaration by neurological criteria should always be performed regardless the possibility of organ donation.

and technical problems under extracorporeal membrane oxygenation (ECMO) may make the apnoea test unreliable. In all these conditions of incomplete examination, an ancillary test is recommended.[45,46]

Clinical testing should be performed under stable physiologic conditions in an adequate and quiet environment; the presence of at least two physicians and ICU nurses is recommended. It is advisable to use a proper checklist form in which all the preconditions, the clinical parameters, the detailed neurological examination, and the apnoea test are listed. Ethically, the clinical examination in a patient still hypothetically alive should be performed from the less detrimental to the most potentially dangerous test, i.e., the apnoea test. For this reason, in some countries, the apnoea test can be performed only at the end of the second and final examination for BD declaration.

Optimal oxygenation and normocapnia, proved by arterial blood gas analysis, and continuous heart rate and blood pressure monitoring are recommended before starting and during the examination. In trauma patients, any bleeding or cerebrospinal fluid (CSF) leakage from tympanic regions and possible facial and temporal bone fractures and swelling should be detected, to evaluate and exclude possible cranial nerve peripheral lesions that could prevent a reliable testing of brainstem reflexes. Clinical progression of brainstem reflexes should be known in order to investigate possible infrequent, multiple traumatic cranial nerve lesions, i.e., oculomotor, abducens, vestibular, and facial nerves.

Evidence-based data regarding clinical criteria for BD diagnosis do not exist and such prospective and controlled studies can be hardly imagined; nevertheless, no recovery of neurologic functions has ever been reported in patients in which the correct and complete neurological standard, produced 50 years ago by the Harvard Ad Hoc committee, had been applied.[46]

The clinical neurological standard for BD diagnosis is as follows[45–48]:

Unconsciousness

As part of initial clinical assessment, unconsciousness and deep coma must be confirmed; any spontaneous movement, blood pressure, and heart rate variations should all be detected and documented. If seizures, myoclonus, posturing, or eyes blinking are observed, BD can be excluded. Not purposeful movements of the arms, provoked or spontaneous, can be present or reported but it is usually very difficult to confirm their cerebral or spinal origin before performing a complete and specific neurological examination.

Brainstem reflexes

The brainstem sensory nuclei can be bilaterally stimulated in a rostro-caudal sequence from midbrain to pons and medulla oblongata and any reaction coming from the motor nerves must be excluded.

Pupillary reflex to light: Photomotor reflex (afferent II cranial nerve, efferent III)
Dilated (8–9 mm) or mid-position (4–6 mm) fixed pupils should not react to direct intense light stimulation in semi-darkness; sometimes, fixed anisocoric pupils may occur, particularly if BD results from initial ipsilateral brain herniation. When uncertainty exists, a magnifying glass or a pupillometer should be used. Rarely, irregular pupillary margins or hippus, i.e., automatic spasmodic dilating and contracting pupillary movements, can be observed. The presence of glass eyeball should be excluded. No blinking reflex should be noted upon stimulation.

Corneal reflexes (afferent V cranial nerve, efferent VII)
Corneal stimulation by a cotton swab or a drop of saline should be performed and no blinking, tearing, reddening, or increase in heart rate should be obtained.

Oculovestibular and Oculocephalic reflexes (afferent VIII cranial nerve, efferent III and VI)

- *Oculovestibular reflex*: After inspection of tympanic membranes, the auditory canal has to be slowly irrigated with 50 cc icy (4°C) saline with both eyes open. Any deviation or even minimal movement of eyeballs and any autonomic response must be excluded within a timeframe of 1–2 minutes. Typically, the contralateral side should be tested after around 5 minutes in order to balance vestibular temperature.

- *Oculocephalic reflex (Doll's eye reflex)*: When the head is turned abruptly from side to side with open eyes, no change in the axis of eyeballs must be detected in BD while delayed movement following head turning can occur when the reflex is present. This reflex investigates the same brainstem regions activated by the oculocephalic reflex but may be dangerous for patients with cervical instability or trauma. For these reasons, several guidelines do not include the 'Doll's eyes reflex' in the brainstem testing.

Pharyngeal (gag) and carinal reflexes (afferent IX cranial nerve, efferent X)

No movement or autonomic response to posterior pharynx stimulation with a tongue blade and no response to carinal stimulation during tracheo-bronchial suctioning must be observed.

Trigeminal stimulation by noxious stimuli (afferent V cranial nerve, efferent VII) and painful stimulation of the body (afferent spinal nerves, efferent VII cranial nerve)

No response, including any movement or change in blood pressure and heart rate, to bilateral intense painful stimulation of the trigeminal area (i.e., at the supraorbital ridges) must be observed. No movements or grimacing must be observed in the facial areas following painful stimuli to body areas not innervated by the cranial nerves (neck, thorax, limbs, or abdomen). If any movement is recorded or elicited outside the facial territory, the possible concurrent presence of spinal reflexes must be deeply investigated and confirmed before declaring BD. Any spontaneous or provoked arousal reaction is not compatible with BD.

Apnoea testing

Complete loss of any capacity of spontaneous ventilation due to irreversible damage of the lower brainstem neurons producing the respiratory drive must be proved.[49] It is an invasive test that may worsen the cerebral compliance increasing the intracranial pressure in still living patients with residual cerebral blood flow.[50] For this reason, it should be performed as the last test when all the other criteria have been already fulfilled. Moreover, the acute respiratory acidosis may be detrimental in hypovolemic states causing severe hypotension and arrhythmias, preventing the completion of the test. Thus, before starting, adequate oxygenation and volemia, as well as normocapnia around 35–45 mmHg (4.7–5.9 kPa) and pH of approximately 7.40, should be ensured. Measures to optimize compliance to the apnoea test include pre-oxygenation of the patient with at least 10 minutes of 100% concentration of inspired oxygen as well as modulation of mechanical ventilation and volemic optimization. Prevention of hypoxia and circulatory instability during the apnoea test is a key factor in BD declaration. Baseline gas analysis is mandatory before disconnecting the patient from the ventilator in order to monitor the increase of $PaCO_2$ (it may be useful to support oxygenation during the procedure through apnoeic O_2 diffusion using an inflated soft balloon or a catheter inside the tracheal tube).[51] Modern ventilators with continuous positive airway pressure (CPAP) may avoid disconnection from the ventilator after the exclusion of automatic insufflation and that of the backup drive. The target of the test is to obtain a maximal stimulation of respiratory neurons reaching a $PaCO_2 \geq 60$ mmHg (≥8.0kPa) with a concomitant decrease of the pH in the acidity range. When pre-existing hypercapnia is reported an increase of around 20 mmHg (2.7 kPa) over the baseline is requested in most guidelines. Any ventilator movement or any respiratory drive must be excluded by careful observation of the chest and/or continuous capnographic monitoring. A flat $EtCO_2$ line should be recorded, even if rapid comb waves, with the same frequency of the heart rate, may be caused by aorta elastic widening in thin subjects. Ventilator self-cycling should be avoided and not confused with cerebral-mediated drive.[52] At the end of the test, a second arterial blood gas sample is obtained to document that the target CO_2 and pH have been achieved.

If a lung donation is possible, atelectasis and oedema should be better prevented during the apnoea test with continuous CPAP and final recruitment manoeuvres.[53]

The apnoea test can be performed under ECMO modulating the artificial gas support without changing the target.[54,55]

Atropine test (afferent X cranial nerve root receptors, efferent X cranial nerve)
The intravenous administration of 0.04mg/kg atropine will cause a dramatic increase in heart rate in non-BD patients, stimulating the nucleus of the vagus nerve in the lower brainstem medulla. No reaction or less than 10% increase due to direct heart stimulation must be recorded in BD. Atropine test is not dangerous and is capable of investigating the same crucial part of the brainstem in a different way from hypercapnia during the apnoea test.[56] Nevertheless, it is an additional test included in only a few guidelines and cannot replace the mandatory apnoea test.

Spinal reflexes

Since spinal blood flow may be totally preserved in BD, neurologic and autonomic activities depending on spinal cord neurons may cause both somatic movements and changes in cardiocirculatory state that can become evident either clinically or with neurophysiological tests. After a variable period of 'spinal shock' due to acute loss of the cerebral activation input, the simple diastaltic arch activity of spinal neurons may cause spontaneous or provoked movements with exclusion of the facial area. Without any encephalic control, the spinal neurons may easily react to even minimal stimuli (i.e., body touching, respiratory acidosis during the apnoea test, or any painful stimulation). These reflexes can become extremely active with gross movements of the arms (triple leg flexion) and the trunk (opisthotonus posturing till the Lazarus sign, not rarely observed during apnoea test in children). A huge variety of spinal reflexes have been described and studied.[57,58] Normal or increased tendon reflexes can be elicited after a variable period of spinal shock.

A clear distinction from the movement of cerebral origin can be easily achieved in most of the cases; spinal movements are usually gross and rough, cannot localize or remove the stimuli, and hardly affect the contralateral side. Slow turning of the head may be caused by cervical area stimulation. Sometimes, posturing-like movements may create doubts that need a confirmatory ancillary test. Post-anoxic myoclonus is not a spinal reflex and has origin in cortical/subcortical encephalic structures and maybe only variably associated with EEG spike and waves. Severe hypertension and tachycardia are easily caused by painful stimulation of the trunk or visceral tractions. These viscero-somatic and viscero-visceral reflexes[59] can be attenuated or abolished by spinal neurons anaesthesia. The spinal origin of these reflexes should be explained to all the professionals dealing with BD patients (see Chapters 41–43).

In BD, subjects kept under ventilation in ICU for weeks and months (e.g., when waiting for foetus maturation in pregnant women,[60] in countries where BD law does not exist, yet, when family opposition to BD declaration is possible or in cases where withdrawal of ventilatory support is allowed only for organ recovery) a quite stable circulatory function is maintained by spinal neurons without any pharmacological support. Somatic growth, sweating, immune response, inflammatory responses, wound healing, and pregnancy in the dead person do not depend on cerebral function and are all compatible with 'chronic BD' as well.[61]

Irreversibility

Irreversibility of the clinical situation of BD is the key factor for death declaration using both neurological and circulatory criteria. Certainty depends on (1) careful evaluation of congruent severity of the cerebral lesion and coherent clinical progression, (2) exclusion of any possibilities of medical or surgical treatment, (3) exclusion of any potential confounding factor, and (4) absence of any clinical variation during a specific observational time. This interval after the onset of coma or initial clinical observation and between at least two clinical examinations may vary as per patient age and among countries, depending on national guidelines. Voluntary or accidental failure to comply with these strict recommendations may lead to single or incomplete examination[62,63] and cause a BD misdiagnosis or a near-miss clinical disaster, particularly in post-anoxic patients and in the presence of cerebral penumbra. It is reasonable to monitor all the clinical signs over a period of time before confirming BD, particularly in post-anoxic patients. At least 24 hours should be the interval between the anoxic insult and a reliable neurological examination. When therapeutic hypothermia has been used, this interval should be extended to 72 hours.[43]

BD declaration

BD declaration is the pronouncement that the patient is medically and legally dead. In most countries an adherence to strict procedures is mandatory to give legal and social validity to the clinical diagnosis. A national protocol for BD diagnosis is strongly recommended[64] to preserve the quality and safety of clinical examinations and protect both the health professionals and the patients.[65] The final target is a 'zero mistake' practice of death determination. A clear transparency in rules and procedures can increase the public trust in BD declaration, increasing at the same time the social acceptance of BD diagnosis and the positive attitude towards organ donation.

Unfortunately, the wide variability among countries[66,67] in legal procedures for BD declaration may create doubts and unsolved criticisms, despite the clinical standard remains the same worldwide.

Conclusion

The death of a human being should be based on a simple and unique concept, i.e., the irreversible loss of cerebral functions commonly named BD, regardless of the pathophysiological circulatory or neurological mechanism leading to death. Furthermore, it is advisable to abandon the colloquial wording BD in favour of 'death determined by neurological or circulatory criteria'.

No differences exist if death occurs under extracorporeal life support treatment and both circulatory and neurological criteria can be used as indicated. The concept that death occurs after circulatory arrest only when BD takes place, and not before, has been and still is one of the most critical points in developing and accepting donation after circulatory death (DCD).[68] Definitely, BD could be the unique concept of the death of a human being in the foreseeable future of medicine and technology.

Specific wide information regarding the concept of death, the different mechanisms for dying, and the different criteria for diagnosing death are mandatory for both professionals and citizens.

BD diagnosis is simple and reliable if complete and rigorous. Standardization and documented proficiency should be ensured by every physician performing the BD clinical examination[45,46] Physicians and nurses should receive specific education, including simulation sessions,[69] about the ethical, legal, and clinical aspects of death diagnosis, in both the devastating cerebral injury and circulatory arrest scenarios.

Unambiguous and homogeneous national procedures based on international standards regarding all the possible implications of death declaration by neurological criteria and a clear indication about the time of death are desirable, thus facilitating the delicate relationship between medical practice and families and increasing social acceptance of death declaration.[70] Social confidence and family trust in the dead donor rule[71] would benefit from BD declaration in all subjects who fulfil BD criteria. This medical practice could support the fundamental idea that there is no difference in timing and modality of death between potential donors and other patients.

Timely death diagnosis and organ donation are essential parts of neurocritical care and greatly depend on the quality of treatment in ICU.[28] To date, despite speculative criticisms, (brain) death determination by neurological criteria appears as the most reliable, wise, usable, pragmatic, acceptable, and useful way to ensure death declaration in acute patients with direct or secondary diffuse cerebral damage.[72]

Highlights

- BD is the irreversible loss of capacity for consciousness, all brainstem functions, and capacity to breathe.
- BD diagnosis is an essential part of neurocritical care; only mechanically ventilated patients with acute devastating cerebral injury may deteriorate to BD.
- Despite different procedures for BD declaration worldwide, only one clinical standard is used.
- BD should be declared regardless of the possibility of organ donation when all BD criteria are fulfilled and indicates a clear point for withdrawal of any artificial support.
- A complete clinical examination must be performed by trained physicians who follow international criteria and national procedures.
- BD is coherent with the ethical possibility of recovering organs for transplantation.

References

1. Bernat JL, Culver CM, Gert B. On the definition and criterion of death. Ann Int Med. 1981;94:389–394.
2. President's Commission for the Study of Ethical Problems in Medicine and Biomedical and Behavioral Research. Defining Death: A Report on the Medical, Legal and Ethical Issues in the Determination of Death. Washington: Government Printing Office; 1981. 3–166. Accessed July 2019. Available at https://repository.library.georgetown.edu/bitstream/handle/10822/559345/defining_death.pdf?sequence=1
3. The President's Council on Bioethics. Controversies in the Determination of Death: A White Paper by the President's Council on Bioethics; 2008. 1–144. Accessed July 2019. Available at: https://www.google.it/url?sa=t&rct=j&q=&esrc=s&source=web&cd=6&cad=rja&uact=8&ved=2ahUKEwiZ4JPViuHjAhVNmIsKHRuxCd8QFjAFegQIBhAC&url=https%3A%2F%2Fwww.thenewatlantis.com%2FdocLib%2F20091130_determination_of_death.pdf&usg=AOvVaw03QrFZ9uiJFVFymnekF9ew
4. Shemie SD, Hornby L, Baker A, et al. International guideline development for the determination of death. Intensive Care Med. 2014;40:788–797.
5. Manara AR. All human death is brain death: The legacy of the Harvard criteria. Resuscitation. 2019;138:210–212. Epub 2019 Mar 15.
6. Truog RD. Is it time to abandon brain death? Hastings Cent Rep. 1997;27:29–37.
7. Veatch RM. Killing by organ procurement: Brain-based death and legal fictions. J Med Philos. 2015;40:289–311. Epub 2015 Apr 18.
8. Truog RD, Berlinger N, Zacharias RL, Solomon MZ. Brain death at fifty: Exploring consensus, controversy, and contexts. Hastings Cent Rep. 2018;48(Suppl 4):S2–S5.
9. Veatch RM. Would a reasonable person now accept the 1968 Harvard brain death report? A short history of brain death. Hastings Cent Rep. 2018 Nov;48(Suppl 4):S6–S9.
10. Bernat JL. The biophilosophical basis of whole-brain death. Soc Philos Policy. 2002;19:324–342.
11. Bernat JL. Contemporary controversies in the definition of death. Prog Brain Res. 2009;177:21–31.
12. Diagnosis of brain death: Statement issued by the honorary secretary of the conference of Medical Royal Colleges and their faculties in the United Kingdom on 11 October 1976. Br Med J. 1976; 2:1187–1188.
13. Pallis C, Harley DH. *ABC of Brainstem Death*. 2nd ed. London: BMJ Publishing Group; 1996.
14. Wijdicks EFM. Clinical diagnosis and confirmatory testing of brain death. In: Wijdicks EFM, ed. *Brain Death*. Philadelphia: Lippincott Williams & Wilkins; 2001, pp. 61–69. ISBN 0-7817-3020-1
15. Bernat JL. How much of the brain must die in brain death? J Clin Ethics. 1992;3:21–26.
16. Collins M, Northrup J, Olcese J. Hypothalamic-pituitary function in brain death: A review. J Intensive Care Med. 2014;31:41–50.
17. Conci F, Di Rienzo M, Castiglioni P. Blood pressure and heart rate variability and baroreflex sensitivity before and after brain death. J Neurol Neurosurg Psychiatry. 2001;71:621–631.

18. Bernat JL. On irreversibility as a prerequisite for brain death determination. Adv Exper Med Biol. 2004;550,161–167.
19. Bernat JL. How the distinction between 'irreversible' and 'permanent' illuminates circulatory–respiratory death determination. J Med Philos. 2010;35:242–255.
20. Zamperetti N, Bellomo R, Defanti CA, Latronico N. Irreversible apnoeic coma 35 years later. Towards a more rigorous definition of brain death? Intensive Care Med. 2004;30:1715–1722.
21. Ad Hoc Committee. A definition of irreversible coma: Report of the ad hoc committee of the Harvard medical school to examine the definition of brain death. JAMA. 1968;205:337–340.
22. National Conference of Commissioners on Uniform State Laws: Uniform Determination of death Act (UDDA). Annual Conference Meeting on its eighty-ninth year on Kauai, Hawaii July 26—1 August 1980. Accessed July 2019. Available at: http://www.lchc.ucsd.edu/cogn_150/Readings/death_act.pdf
23. Loeb J. *The Organism as a Whole: From a Physicochemical Viewpoint.* New York: G. P. Putnam's Sons; 1916.
24. Bonelli RM, Prat EH, Bonelli J. Philosophical considerations on brain death and the concept of the organism as a whole. Psychiatr Danub. 2009;21:3–8.
25. Bernat JL, Culver CM, Gert B. On the definition and criterion of death. Ann Intern Med. 1981;94:389–394.
26. Bernat JL. A defense of the whole-brain concept of death. Hastings Cent Rep. 1998;28:14–23.
27. Casartelli M, Bombardini T, Simion D, Gaspari MG, Procaccio F. Wait, treat and see: Echocardiographic monitoring of brain-dead potential donors with stunned heart. Cardiovasc Ultrasound. 2012;10:25.
28. Martin-Loeches I, Sandiumenge A, Charpentier J, et al. Management of donation after brain death (DBD) in theICU: The potential donor is identified, what's next? Intensive Care Med. 2019;45:322–330. Epub 2019 Feb 28. Review.
29. Shewmon AD. The brain and somatic integration: Insights into the standardbiological rationale for equating 'brain death' with death. J Med Philos. 2001;26:457–478.
30. Shewmon DA. Brain death: A conclusion in search of a justification. Hastings Cent Rep. 2018;48(Suppl 4):S22–S25.
31. Shewmon DA. Brain death or brain dying? J Child Neurol. 2012;27:4–6.
32. Bernat JL. A conceptual justification for brain death. Hastings Cent Rep. 2018;48(Suppl 4):S19–S21.
33. Dalle Ave AL, Bernat JL. Inconsistencies between the criterion and tests for brain death. J Intensive Care Med. 2020;35:772–780. Epub 2018 Jan 1
34. International Guidelines for the Determination of Death—Phase I, May 2012 Forum Report 2012 Canadian Blood Services, pp. 7–8. Accessed July 2019. Available at: https://www.who.int/patientsafety/montreal-forum-report.pdf
35. Manara AR, Thomas I, Harding R. A case for stopping the early withdrawal of life sustaining therapies in patients with devastating brain injuries. J Intensive Care Soc. 2016;17:295–301. Epub 2016 May 5.
36. de Groot Y, Jansen N, Bakker J, et al. Imminent brain death: Point of departure for potential heart-beating organ donor recognition. Intensive Care Med. 2010;36:1488–1494.

37. Domínguez-Gil B, Murphy P, Procaccio F. Ten changes that could improve organ donation in the intensive care unit. Intensive Care Med. 2016;42:264–267. Epub 2015 May 19.
38. Guidelines for the diagnosis of brain death. Canadian Neurocritical Care Group. Can J Neurol Sci. 1999;26:64–66.
39. Practice parameters for determining brain death in adults (summary statement). The Quality Standards Subcommittee of the American Academy of Neurology. Neurology. 1995;45:1012–1014.
40. Busl KM, Greer DM. Pitfalls in the diagnosis of brain death. Neurocrit Care. 2009;11:276–287. Epub 2009 May 15.
41. Wijdicks EF. Pitfalls and slip-ups in brain death determination. Neurol Res. 2013;35:169–173. Review.
42. Webb AC, Samuels OB. Reversible brain death after cardiopulmonary arrest and induced hypothermia. Crit Care Med. 2011;39:1538–1542.
43. Rossetti AO, Oddo M, Logroscino G, et al. Prognostication after cardiac arrest and hypothermia: A prospective study. Ann Neurol. 2010;67:301–307.
44. Molina DK, McCutcheon JR, Rulon JJ. Head injuries, pentobarbital, and the determination of death. Am J Forensic Med Pathol. 2009;30:75–77.
45. Wijdicks EF. The diagnosis of brain death. N Engl J Med. 2001;344:1215–1221.
46. Wijdicks EF, Varelas PN, Gronseth GS, et al. Evidence-based guideline update: Determining brain death in adults: Report of the quality standards subcommittee of the American Academy of Neurology. Neurology. 2010;74:1911–1918.
47. Wijdicks EF. Brain death guidelines explained. Semin Neurol. 2015;35:105–115. Epub 2015 Apr 3. Review.
48. Wijdicks EFM. Critical synopsis and key questions in brain death determination. Intensive Care Med. 2019;45:306–309. Epub 2019 Feb 6.
49. Scott JB, Gentile MA, Bennett SN, Couture M, MacIntyre NR. Apnea testing during brain death assessment: A review of clinical practice and published literature. Respir Care. 2013 Mar;58(3):532–538. Review.
50. Goudreau JL, Wijdicks EF, Emery SF. Complications during apnea testing in the determination of brain death: Predisposing factors. Neurology. 2000;55:1045–1048.
51. Daneshmand A, Rabinstein AA, Wijdicks EFM. The apnea test in brain death determination using oxygen diffusion method remains safe. Neurology. 2019;92:386–387. Epub 2019 Jan 11.
52. Schwarz G, Errath M, Arguelles Delgado P, Schöpfer A, Cavic T. Ventilator autotriggering: An underestimated phenomenon in the determination of brain death. Anaesthesist. 2019;68:171–176.
53. Paries M, Boccheciampe N, Raux M, et al. Benefit of a single recruitment maneuver after an apnea test for the diagnosis of brain death. Crit Care. 2012;16:R116.
54. Giani M, Scaravilli V, Colombo SM, et al. Apnea test during brain death assessment in mechanically ventilated and ECMO patients. Intensive Care Med. 2016;42:72–81. Epub 2015 Nov 10.
55. Lie SA, Hwang NC. Challenges of brain death and apnea testing in adult patients on extracorporeal membrane oxygenation—A review. J Cardiothorac Vasc Anesth. 2019;33:2266–2272. Epub 2019 Jan 17. Review.

56. Domínguez-Roldán JM, Procaccio F, Villar-Gallardo J, et al. Diagnosis of death by neurologic criteria (brain death). In: Valero R, ed. *Transplant Coordination Manual.* Barcelona: DTI Foundation Editor; 2014, pp. 155–180.
57. Jorgensen EO. Spinal man after brain death. The unilateral extension-pronation reflex of the upper limb as an indication of brain death. Acta Neurochirurgica. 1973;28:259–273.
58. Saposnik G, Bueri JA, Mauriño J, Saizar R, Garretto NS. Spontaneous and reflex movements in brain death. Neurology. 2000;54:221–223.
59. Conci F, Procaccio F, Arosio M, Boselli L. Viscero-somatic and viscero-visceral reflexes in brain death. J Neurol Neurosurg Psychiatry. 1986;49:695–698.
60. Lane A, Westbrook A, Grady D, et al. Maternal brain death: Medical, ethical and legal issues. Intensive Care Med. 2004;30:1484–1486.
61. Shewmon DA. Chronic 'brain death': Meta-analysis and conceptual consequences. Neurology. 1998;51:1538–1545.
62. Wang MY, Wallace P, Gruen JP. Brain death documentation: Analysis and issues. Neurosurgery. 2002;51:731–736.
63. Braksick SA, Robinson CP, Gronseth GS, et al. Variability in reported physician practices for brain death determination. Neurology. 2019;92:e888–e894. Epub 2019 Jan 25.
64. Choi EK, Fredland V, Zachodni C, et al. Brain death revisited: The case for a national standard. J Law Med Ethics. 2008;36:824–836. Review.
65. Bernat JL, Brust JCM. Strategies to improve uniformity in brain death determination. Neurology. 2019;92:401–402. Epub 2019 Jan 25.
66. Wahlster S, Wijdicks EF, Patel PV, et al. Brain death declaration: Practices and perceptions worldwide. Neurology. 2015;84:1870–1879. Epub 2015 Apr 8.
67. Greer DM, Wang HH, Robinson JD, et al. Variability of brain death policies in the United States. JAMA Neurol. 2016;73:213–218.
68. Dalle Ave AL, Bernat JL. Donation after brain circulation determination of death. BMC Med Ethics. 2017;18:15.
69. Hocker S, Wijdicks EF. Simulation training in brain death determination. Semin Neurol. 2015;35:180–187. Epub 2015 Apr 3. Review.
70. Smith M. Brain death: Time for an international consensus. Br J Anaesth. 2012;108(Suppl 1):i6–i9.
71. Dalle Ave AL, Sulmasy DP, Bernat JL. The ethical obligation of the dead donor rule. Med Health Care Philos. 2020;23:43–50. Epub 2019 May 13
72. Greer DM, Shemie SD, Lewis A et al. Determination of brain death/death by neurologic criteria: The World Brain Death Project. JAMA 2020;15:1078–1097.

4

Facing brain death: Prelude to brain death diagnosis and testing

Liesl N. Close, Kristine O'Phelan, M. Ross Bullock

Transition between severe brain injury and brain death

For many clinicians who work in acute neuroscience, there is a 'grey area' between an unsalvageable, very severely brain-injured patient and a salvageable one. This holds true regardless of the aetiology of the acute injury and is especially true in the early years of practice. No two patients are the same and there are few guidelines or rule books other than the criteria for brain death. This is compounded by the desperate need for reassurance and 'need for decisive action' that most families bring to such situations. The cardinal rule in such situations is to allow the passage of time. This serves two purposes, first it may provide time for some recovery of function to take place. Anticipating the transition to brain death in a patient with a severe brain injury must take into account the aetiology and its unique natural history of recovery for the specific type of brain injury. For example, acute intoxications may recover over a shorter time span of days, while traumatic brain injury (TBI) or intracranial haemorrhage may take much longer to 'declare' their trajectory towards deterioration or recovery. Unfortunately, many of these mechanisms may be present and overlap in the same patient. For example, in TBI with hematoma removal there may be hypoxic-ischemic injury, brain herniation, and the effect of high intracranial pressure. The patient's age is the second most important factor in formulating a picture of the likely outcome. In elderly patients over seventy years with prolonged coma after severe brain injury meaningful recovery is very unusual.[1]

The neurologic exam and imaging studies can be helpful. However, the neurological exam may be clouded by medications and physiological factors, as discussed below. Reviewing the brain imaging is important when advising families about prognosis, for example, if a large brainstem haemorrhage is seen on the Computed Tomography (CT) or if the Magnetic Resonance Imaging (MRI) shows severe brainstem ischemia. Over the course of several days the clinician is often able to establish the anticipated course the patient will take. This course may be some degree of expected recovery, progression to a vegetative state, or deterioration to brain death. However, no single clinician is infallible or even completely accurate in making these difficult assessments. Therefore, consultation with senior colleagues and other disciplines such as Neurology or Intensive care teams is always helpful. Several days or even a week (when the situation is more uncertain) should be allowed to pass before such prognostic decisions are made and acted upon. This allows the family to come to terms with the situation, to see that all possible care is being given, and to allow time for any possible improvement to declare itself. While care is aimed at maximizing neurologic recovery, an experienced clinician can often identify those patients who will progress to brain death. Clinicians should resist the temptation to tell families that recovery is completely impossible during the first few days after injury. In many cases patients who display no brainstem function early after a catastrophic brain event such as TBI or subarachnoid haemorrhage (SAH) can show some recovery over several days. This is especially true in children and infants, hence the different brain death criteria used for children in many countries. It is far preferable to communicate to the family that the outcome is initially uncertain and that time is needed for any possible improvement to declare itself.

Role of computerized prediction algorithms

Prognostic calculators exist for estimating expected outcome after TBI and cardiac arrest. Prognostic tools should be applied after at least 24 hours for stabilization. They are not infallible and should only be used to support the clinical impression, not to define it. An excellent role for these computerized prediction tools has been as an adjunct to family meetings to support the decision of transition to comfort measures, often after many days of aggressive support have failed to produce improvement and when death or vegetative survival seems the likely outcome. Ideally, such meetings can be timed to occur before tracheostomy and gastrostomy tube placement in patients with very severe brain damage.

Organ recovery agency factors

In the USA, most countries in Europe, and the UK, organ recovery is under the control of organizations such as the association of organ procurement organizations (AOPO) and the united network for organ sharing (UNOS) in the USA. These, in turn, work with regional and local organ procurement agencies in each major accredited hospital and city to request consent for organ donation from the families of patients with irreversible major brain injury. Recovered organs are nationally matched and allocated to optimize lifesaving transplants. In order to achieve this, all accredited hospitals are required to ensure that local organ recovery agencies (OPO) are informed whenever a patient with a Glasgow Coma Scale score of 5 or below is admitted to the emergency department or intensive care unit. The OPO then follows the case to determine eligibility for organ donation. The relationship between the treating team and the OPO must remain transparent to avoid real or perceived conflicts of interest. The OPO will remain advised on the clinical course of a particular case but cannot become actively involved with the patient until brain death is determined or the decision to withdraw mechanical ventilation in the setting of comfort care is reached. Furthermore, the treating team, OPO, and the transplant team remain separate in their management and relationships with the patient and their family. This 'decoupling' helps to minimize conflicts of interest.[2]

Progression of brainstem injury

As the transition occurs from severe injury to the irreversible loss of all brain function, the neurologic exam will change in characteristic ways. The motor component of the neurologic exam deteriorates in a sequential fashion, from a flexion response to central noxious stimulus, to decorticate posturing, decerebrate posturing, and finally loss of motor function with the exception of spinal reflexes. Progressive loss of brainstem reflexes occurs with ongoing injury to the brainstem. Pupils may dilate unilaterally from compression of the third cranial nerve, or bilaterally with an injury at the level of the tectum. With caudal progression of injury, pupils may become pinpoint at the level of the pons, and finally come to rest in mid-position. There is concurrent loss of the pupillary light reflex with injury to the oculomotor nerve or midbrain. The oculovestibular and corneal reflexes are lost with injury to the pons. Finally, there is loss of the cough and gag reflexes when injury progresses to the level of the medulla. It is often useful at this stage to consider using the oculocephalic and cold caloric tests as well as the pupillary and ocular movements as a diagnostic tool to assess brainstem function.[3]

In addition to the changes in the neurologic exam that occur with the progression to brain death, other physiologic changes arise, which can provide an indication that the brainstem has been critically injured. Changes in blood pressure, urine output, and respiration are seen as areas of the brain that are progressively injured from rostral to caudal. When a craniotomy has already been performed, such a 'classic' progression towards herniation may not occur. However, diabetes insipidus, a sign of hypothalamic ischemia or infarction, is almost always a harbinger of progression towards brainstem death. These changes may be rapid in onset; they should always be treated aggressively with vigorous volume resuscitation, vasopressin infusion, or intravenous deamino D-arginine vasopressin (DDAVP) to reverse diabetes insipidus, and pressor agents as needed to maintain mean arterial pressure. Close attention to adjusting mechanical ventilation for adequate oxygenation and ventilation should be continued. During this phase of care the family has time to process and adjust to the large amount of information they will be given. Additionally, ongoing aggressive support will allow patients who do progress to brain death to be appropriately evaluated for eligibility for organ donation. A nihilistic approach with early de-escalation is inappropriate as it precludes eligibility for organ donation.

Factors clouding the determination of brain death

In order to avoid a potentially disastrous misdiagnosis, it is important to be able to recognize states which may mimic brain death. These include intoxication with medications or drugs of abuse taken before the catastrophic brain event, or medications given during early clinical care in the intensive care unit or emergency department. Specifically, benzodiazepines, barbiturates and opiates, electrolyte abnormalities (hyponatremia Na<120 mEq/L, Hypernatremia Na>160 mEq/L, hyperglycaemia>300mg/dL, severe hypocalcaemia), hypothermia <36° C, and locked-in syndrome must be identified and reversed before brain death testing can occur.

Paediatric considerations

Severe brain damage in infants and children is especially difficult to diagnose and manage, because of the more labile physiology, the need to address the needs of the family as well as the child, and most importantly, the remarkable ability for children and infants to recover from severe brain injury. This is especially evident in ice water drowning victims, and in cases where children have recovered after long periods of circulatory and respiratory arrest. For these reasons, the criteria for brain death determination in children require longer time intervals before the initial testing is done and require waiting for a specific time interval between sequential clinical examinations.[4]

Management in the prelude to brain death testing

Caring for a patient with a severe brain injury is multidisciplinary and multifaceted. Care during this period often involves collaboration between neurocritical care, neurosurgery, or neurology and a social worker or hospital chaplain. Benefits of this approach include increasing time providers spend with the family to explain the diagnosis and prognosis and to answer questions. The additional time also allows for evaluation of the family's need for emotional support. It is crucial that families are given the chance to process the information they obtain and perceive the depth of medical support their loved one is receiving.

Initial resuscitation and stabilization following an insult to the brain primarily involve re-establishing and maintaining normal physiologic parameters. Initially efforts should focus on supporting the possibility of neurological recovery until the prognosis becomes clearer. This includes treatment of intracranial hypertension and supporting cerebral perfusion pressure. If progression to brain death is anticipated, then the focus shifts to achieving the strictly defined parameters necessary for performing a brain death examination. After brain death has been determined, attention is shifted to optimizing the patient for potential organ donation. Luckily there is overlap in the therapies used for these two goals as both focus on normalization of physiologic parameters and optimizing organ perfusion and function. Hemodynamic support, respiratory support with adequate oxygenation and ventilation and correction of deranged fluid status and electrolytes are crucial. Once the patient is normothermic, normo-natremic with adequate oxygenation and without hypotension brain death testing may proceed.

Temperature

Temperature management is a vital part of caring for any patient with acute brain injury. The specific target temperature varies depending on the type of injury. Patients with a traumatic injury, who are found down, may be hypothermic due to exposure to the elements. These patients should be rewarmed to normothermia as part of the resuscitation and stabilization efforts. If a patient's core temperature is low due to exposure, slow rewarming is used in order to avoid complications associated with cooling such as coagulopathy and arrhythmias. When targeted temperature management is used, slow rewarming avoids precipitating rebound brain oedema which can occur with rapid rewarming. A definitive neurologic exam should not be performed until the patient has a core temperature of at least 36° C, as hypothermia can cause diminished brainstem reflexes. Additionally, hypothermia will affect the metabolism of any medications that are given. Therefore, enough time must pass after normothermia is achieved to allow for the clearance of sedating medications.

Sedation and neuromuscular blockade

Sedation plays an important role in caring for critically ill patients with neurologic injuries. Although the effects of sedation can cloud or obscure an accurate neurologic exam, sedation can also be protective against pain, agitation, and secondary injury related to increases in intracranial pressure. However, when barbiturates are used patients need to be fully weaned off for a period of time that allows the barbiturate levels to dissipate before brain death testing is performed. This may require several days and verification by testing blood levels to allow for a valid neurologic exam. Paralytics can sometimes be used to manage refractory intracranial hypertension. In order to obtain an accurate neurologic examination, it is important to ensure that there are no residual effects of neuromuscular blocking agents. This is easily achieved by using a 'train of 4' nerve stimulator which will show 4 responses when 4 shocks are delivered to demonstrate lack of pharmacological paralysis. Train of 4 testing is carried out before brain death testing in any patient who has received neuromuscular blockade.[(5)]

Drug intoxication must be ruled out as this is one of the most common mimics of brain death. This is specifically important in patients without catastrophic injury on brain imaging. Intentional or accidental overdoses of medications, illicit drugs, and alcohol can all contribute to a state of coma. The current recommendation is to wait 4–5 times the drug's half-life, to ensure adequate metabolism. Clinicians must be aware of the possibility of delayed drug metabolism, such as in the case of renal or hepatic dysfunction, or following hypothermia therapy.

Adjunctive testing and their limitations

Confirmatory brain death testing should be used when an apnoea test cannot be safely performed. In these cases, a full neurological exam is performed and a confirmatory test is ordered in addition. Confirmatory testing may include the following: nuclear medicine blood flow studies, cerebral angiography, electroencephalography, or transcranial Doppler studies. Each test has its own benefits and liabilities which are used to choose the best confirmatory test for any specific patient. Cerebral angiograms are definitive, yet use significant human and facility resources which may not be available or may take some time to assemble. Electroencephalography is portable so can be used on the most unstable patients; however, the studies are highly prone to electrical artefacts which are common in the intensive care unit. Nuclear medicine studies may not be broadly available and require the patient to move to the radiology department. Transcranial Doppler studies are portable and not expensive; however, the results are highly dependent on the skill of the technician and so they may not always be reliable. The best confirmatory test to use should be decided based on the needs of the patient and local hospital factors.[4] For the role of confirmatory/ancillary tests to document absent cerebral blood flow, refer to Chapter 9 of this book.

Brain death within the continuum of severe brain damage

Histopathological analysis of the brain in those who are pronounced brain dead seldom occurs until days have elapsed between the brain death determination and the autopsy. Nevertheless, the studies which have been reported show that some populations of neurons and the majority of astrocytes remain grossly intact after brain death is determined. Recently, a case report on McMath was published documenting 4.5 years of survival after brain death was declared. The case has caused legal and ethical introspection and discussion, and since this case, several families have refused to accept the diagnosis of brain death. What is truly clear from the McMath case is that the level of neurologic function this patient exhibited was minimal and insufficient to communicate with her environment.[5] Clinicians need to be absolutely certain that the strict preconditions and details of the brain death testing are observed and fully documented each time brain death is determined. Local hospitals must decide how they will respond to such cases if they arise. Despite improvements in MRI imaging, electrophysiology, and improved understanding of brain and neuronal pathomechanisms, clinical brain death testing with an apnoea test is the best means available to diagnose brain death.[6] Once brain death is declared, we know that independent, sentient, fully human recovery of the brain will not occur by medical care currently available.

Futile care in the face of brain death

In many cases, especially when older patients sustain major brain damage, the treating physician becomes aware that functional recovery is unlikely. In these cases the team must explain the likely outcome scenarios with the family. After the family has had time to process this information a conversation to establish goals of care for the patient should be arranged. Goals of care discussions should include a clear picture of what the range of possible disabled survival scenarios may look like, including the need for tracheostomy, tube feeding, nursing home care, or full-time in-home caregivers. Few patients over seventy who are in coma for a week or more due to a catastrophic brain injury will survive, and very few will recover to be independent. Ideally, an advance directive will help the family and caregivers clearly understand the wishes of the injured patient. This often allows families to transition to comfort measures more easily sparing the patient unnecessary procedures and non-beneficial care. Such patients may still be evaluated for organ donation after cardiac death and should be reported to the local OPO when the decision to pursue comfort measures only is made. As always, discussions surrounding organ donation should be initiated and led by the organ recovery agency.

Critical injury or illness of a loved one is a stressful event. Some patients have made very clear their wishes to family in the event of critical illness or injury, while others have not or are estranged from those who can help with decision making at the end of life. In these difficult cases consultation with an ethics team can be helpful. If the family is available and having trouble reaching a decision the ethics team can guide them often calling on clergy or additional friends and family for support. If there is no family available the ethics teams may serve as a surrogate decision-maker. For those family members who are hesitant to carry out their loved ones wishes, a clear conversation between the care team and the family should be held. It is helpful to frame the conversation and highlight that the role of the surrogate decision-maker is to act as the voice of the patient rather than report their own wishes. Compassion is critical during these conversations as this can be a difficult task for grief-stricken families who are not emotionally ready to accept that their loved one has suffered a non-survivable brain injury.

Strategies for managing the family in the face of brain death

Almost all families will accept the veracity of a diagnosis of brain death if sufficient time has been taken for effective discussion and for them to see that their loved one shows no sign of recovery. When discussing brain injury and brain death with families, it is important to use non-medical language as much as possible. This will help them understand the injuries that the patient has suffered and the consequences of such injuries. For example, when brain death is determined, the family should be told in plain terms that the patient has died. When explaining brain death, discussing residual reflexes that could be misinterpreted as brain function is important. Families should be informed that these movements can come from the spinal cord rather than reflecting preserved brain activity. This prevents the family from holding on to false hope in the face of clinical evidence. Some families appreciate the offer of being shown CT or MRI scans with a clear explanation of the findings. Finally, when engaging in these difficult discussions with families, it is important to show empathy and compassion. By establishing a rapport with the family through several discussions each day they may be able to take comfort knowing that their loved one received the best care possible.

Specific policies should be established in each hospital to guide the management of those very few families who refuse to accept the diagnosis of brain death, and who are given sufficient time to come to terms with the death. In general, the law supports withdrawal of pressor and ventilator support once death is declared. However, many hospitals will be sensitive to the potential for negative publicity and will want to manage these cases in a non-confrontational manner.

Highlights

- In the early period following brain injury, it is often difficult to discern the clinical course the patient will take. Time must be allowed for any possible recovery to occur.
- Care of a severely brain-injured patient is multidisciplinary.
- There is significant overlap in the goals of management of a patient with a severe brain injury, parameters necessary for diagnosing brain death, and optimizing a patient for organ donation.
- Mimics of brain death must be ruled out.
- Frequent communication with families and compassionate, empathetic care are important factors in the care of a brain-injured patient.

References

1) Maiden MJ, Cameron PA, Rosenfeld JV et al. Long-term outcomes after severe traumatic brain injury in older adults. A registry-based Cohort study. Am J Respir Crit Care Med 201, 2, 167–177. 15 Jan2020.
2) Shemie, SD, Robertson A, Beitel J, Chandler J et al. End of life conversations with families of potential donors. Transplantation May 2017, 101, 5s;S17–S26.
3) Posner JB, Saper CB, Schiff ND, Plum F. Diagnosis of stupor and coma, Fourth edition. Oxford University Press. 2007.
4) Wijdicks, EFM. Determining brain death. Continuum 2015; 21(5): 1411–1424.
5) Leweis, A. Reconciling the case of Jahi McMath. Neurocrit Care 2018 Aug;29(1):20–22.
6) Wijdicks EF, Varelas PN, Gronseth GS, Greer DM. American Academy of N. Evidence-based guideline update: Determining brain death in adults: Report of the Quality Standards Subcommittee of the American Academy of Neurology. Neurology 2010;74(23):1911–1918.

5

Pathophysiology and mechanisms of brain death in adults

Marco Carbonara, Alessio Caccioppola, Nino Stocchetti

Introduction

Death was always historically defined as the permanent loss of all vital bodily functions,[1] with the cessation of cardiopulmonary function. However, due to major technical improvements, such as mechanical ventilation and cardiopulmonary resuscitation, around the middle of the 20th-century reports appeared describing patients in deep coma and without respiratory drive, whose central nervous system was unreactive but whose circulatory system was still functioning, with artificial support. Mollaret and Goulon[2] introduced the term *coma dépassé* to describe twenty-three patients without consciousness, no brainstem reflexes, and total absence of cerebral electrical activity in an electroencephalogram. This clinical syndrome was further characterized by the Harvard Medical School Committee, which in 1968 introduced more stringent criteria for the diagnosis of irreversible coma, now referred to as brain death, defined as the lack of motor response, respiratory activity, and brainstem reflexes in a 'beating-heart corpse'.[3] Since then, national legislations across the world have introduced different criteria to establish brain death. While these always include clinical criteria (coma and absence of brainstem reflexes), as proposed by the American Academy of Neurology,[4] there is wide variation among countries regarding ancillary testing, such as apnoea tests or electroencephalography.[5] This chapter focuses on adults, since the pathophysiology of brain death in infants and children may be different.

From the insult to death: Aetiology of brain death

Brain death is a condition of irreversible loss of all functions of the entire brain, including the brainstem, coupled with cessation of circulation in the structures cranial to the foramen magnum. Different countries apply different criteria and laws to define patients as brain-dead. A few countries (among others, the United Kingdom) use different definitions/terminology for brainstem death, highlighting the brainstem's central role in consciousness and respiratory control.[6] Such definitions leave out functions attributed to the supratentorial central nervous system, but includes core features of brain death, i.e. loss of consciousness and respiratory drive.

In adults, the events most frequently associated with brain death are traumatic brain injury and cerebral haemorrhage[7]; other significant causes are anoxic brain injury, hydrocephalus, ischemic stroke, neoplasms, brain abscesses, and central nervous system infective diseases like encephalitis and meningitis. Less frequently, brain death can result from direct damage to the brainstem, generally due to trauma, ischemic, or haemorrhagic stroke, and neoplasms. A more recent report by Kramer[8] on a cohort of Canadian brain-dead patients, published in 2008, corroborates these findings, confirming the main contributing elements while illustrating the reduction in the proportion of brain death diagnosis among critically ill patients.

Originating from different central nervous system pathologies, brain death can be considered a syndrome—a collection of signs rather than a single clinical entity. Its unifying factor is a catastrophic, irreversible brain injury driving acute ischemia of the main intracranial portions of the central nervous system.

To simplify, causes of brain death can be classified as either extracranial or intracranial (see Figure 5.1). The most frequent extracranial event causing brain death is cardiopulmonary arrest followed by delayed or inadequate cardiopulmonary resuscitation, causing prolonged, severe impairment of the blood supply to the brain. The subsequent hypoxia and ischemia cause perturbations in cellular osmoregulation, leading to brain oedema. Since the brain is held inside a rigid skull, this swelling will ultimately cause blood flow disturbances and induce further ischemia/

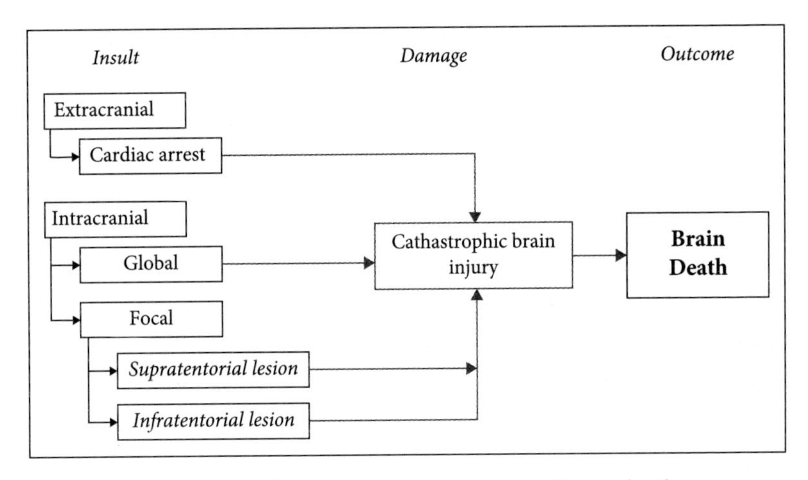

Figure 5.1. Summary of the most common causes of brain death

hypoxia in a vicious, self-sustaining cycle. The detrimental consequence of this continuing fluid accumulation in the brain is an extreme rise in intracranial pressure (ICP), leading to compression of the entire brain and brainstem; this high intracranial hypertension (HICP) causes either herniation or complete cessation of cerebral circulation, leading to aseptic necrosis of brain tissue.

The most common intracranial causes of brain death in adults are traumatic brain injury and subarachnoid haemorrhage, while in children abuse is more common than motor vehicle accidents or asphyxia. From an anatomical point of view, intracranial causes can be further divided into global—such as central nervous system infections and hydrocephalus, and localized/focal—such as supratentorial, which make up the majority, or infratentorial (see Figure 5.1). Focal disorders of the supratentorial brain most frequently linked to brain death are traumatic brain injury, ischemic, or haemorrhagic strokes. When lesions are large enough or localized in or next to vital areas, they will cause HICP; at extreme levels HICP may result in herniation, with descent of the supratentorial portion of the brain (usually the uncus, the medial part of the temporal lobe), transferring HICP to infratentorial structures. A second effect of HICP is complete global ischemia when cerebral perfusion pressure (CPP) drops close to zero. Localized infratentorial lesions, on the other hand, have a different pathophysiological pathway. In these cases, the definition of brainstem death is more appropriate as these are terminal events of extensive disruptions of the brainstem, such as haemorrhage, trauma, or tumour.

Pathophysiological pathways to brain death

As outlined earlier, different aetiologies underlie the mechanisms causing brain death. There are two main pathophysiological pathways: (1) alteration of cerebral hemodynamics resulting in global ischemia, which is the most common pathway, or (2) direct lesion of the brainstem, less frequently.

The mechanism common to extracranial, global intracranial, and supratentorial intracranial causes of brain death is global ischemia, either from cardiac arrest or due to ICP rising to a point beyond the mean arterial pressure, resulting in cessation of cerebral blood flow (CBF) and leading to permanent cytotoxic injury of the intracranial neuronal tissue.[9] The mechanism linking cerebral ischemia to cardiac arrest is self-evident.

Cerebral hemodynamics

The role of ICP in CBF is briefly reviewed with basic cerebral hemodynamics.[10] The force driving CBF, just like in any organ, is the difference between mean arterial and venous pressures. Since measuring intracranial venous pressure is problematic, ICP is employed as a surrogate, as cerebral venous pressure must be slightly higher than ICP to prevent venous collapse.[10] When ICP is higher than mean arterial pressure, CPP is equal to (or less than) zero, and blood flow ceases.

Hypoperfusion leads to cerebral ischemia as CPP drops towards the lower limit of autoregulation (approximately 50 mmHg), arteriolar resistance vessels dilate and cerebral blood volume increases. Beyond this point, the capacity for vasodilation is exhausted, the circulation cannot reduce resistance any further to maintain flow, and CBF begins to decline passively as CPP falls further. At first, an increase in oxygen extraction can compensate for the passive decline in CBF but when oxygen extraction reaches maximum the cerebral metabolic rate of oxygen begins to diminish. Accordingly, synaptic transmission becomes impaired and eventually fails completely, as manifested by an isoelectric EEG. At this point, sufficient energy is available to keep the neurons alive, but synaptic work is abolished. Even lower flow levels result in membrane failure (Na^+, Ca^{2+}, and water enter, and K^+ exits the cell: i.e. cytotoxic oedema). These reductions in CBF are in the lethal range and result in infarction if not corrected (see Figure 5.2). The development of cerebral infarction depends on both the degree of flow reduction and its duration.

Zero CPP (corresponding to interruption of CBF) has been postulated in the majority of cases of brain death.[4,11] With ICP exceeding mean arterial pressure, there is no positive CPP. In contrast to these theoretical

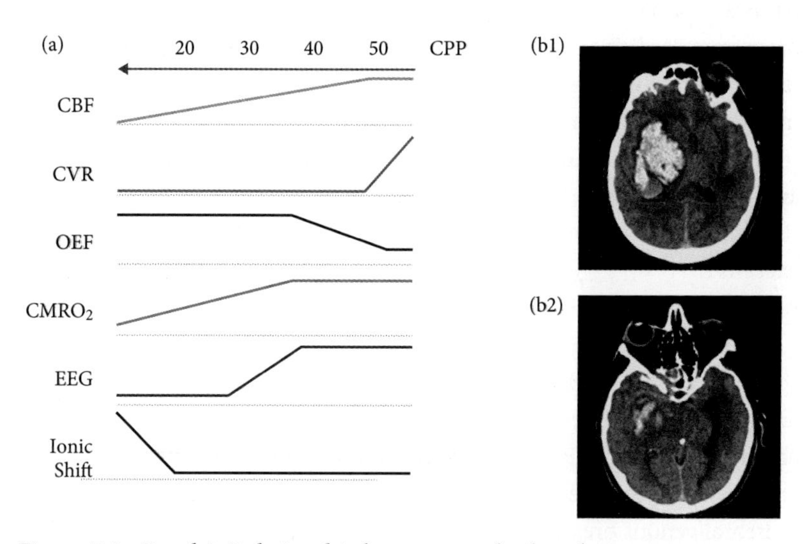

Figure 5.2. Panel A. Relationship between cerebral perfusion pressure (CPP) and cerebral blood flow (CBF): below a certain CPP threshold (usually 50 mm Hg), cerebral vascular resistance (CVR) can fall no further so blood flow will decrease. Oxygen extraction fraction (OEF) will be maximized until synaptic activity (expressed here as EEG) begins to drop. Eventually, further CBF reduction will lead to impairment of ionic pumps, causing cell death. Adapted from Young[10]

Panel B. Two slices from a single patient's brain CT scan of a devastating cerebral hemorrhage, showing signs of intracranial hypertension with ongoing cerebral transfalcine (B1) and uncal (B2) herniation considerations, however, clinical data has revealed patients with slightly positive CPP during brain death. Pathological ICP, incompatible with adequate CPP, was measured in twenty-eight patients by Salih.[12] CPP was negative in the majority of cases; in a few patients, however, a residual—though minimal—positive CPP was detectable.

To explain these contradictory findings, with other mechanisms leading to global ischemia preserved, minimal CPP was hypothesized: the collapse of cerebral veins was proposed as leading to blood flow stasis, with further increases in ICP.[13] This mechanism might also lead to cerebral circulation arrest due to secondary brain oedema. Some authors prefer the hypothesis of critical closing pressure, defined as the arterial pressure threshold below which arteries collapse.[12]

Few experimental studies have directly observed the pathophysiologic pathway leading to brain death but, as far as we know, all of them are based on perturbations of cerebral hemodynamics, after ligation of arteries that supply blood to the brain or progressive but critical increases in ICP.

A brain death model in pigs showed that a progressive increase of ICP and consequent drop in CPP could lead to a marked decrease in brain tissue oxygenation and increase in the lactate: pyruvate ratio. If the insult exceeds the threshold for cerebral ischemia the damage is irreversible and results in brain death.[14]

Valenza et al.[15] also used a pig model to show how the complete absence of CBF is the pathophysiological process leading to brain death. They raised the ICP over the mean arterial pressure for more than 60 min, and confirmed brain death on the basis of clinical signs, apnoea test and electroencephalogram (see Figure 5.3).

In a clinical study, Roth[16] (2019) recently thoroughly described how all patients experienced very high ICP, reaching ≥96 mmHg during the total observation period, with a median CPP of -2.5 mmHg at brain death determination, suggesting the arrest of cerebral circulation. This pathological situation triggers processes of apoptosis and neuronal necrosis that lead to irreversible loss of activity of the whole brain and, therefore, to a condition incompatible with life. The main explanation is the progressive and sustained decrease in CBF to below the threshold for cerebral ischemia and the consequent irreversible neuronal metabolic failure and death.

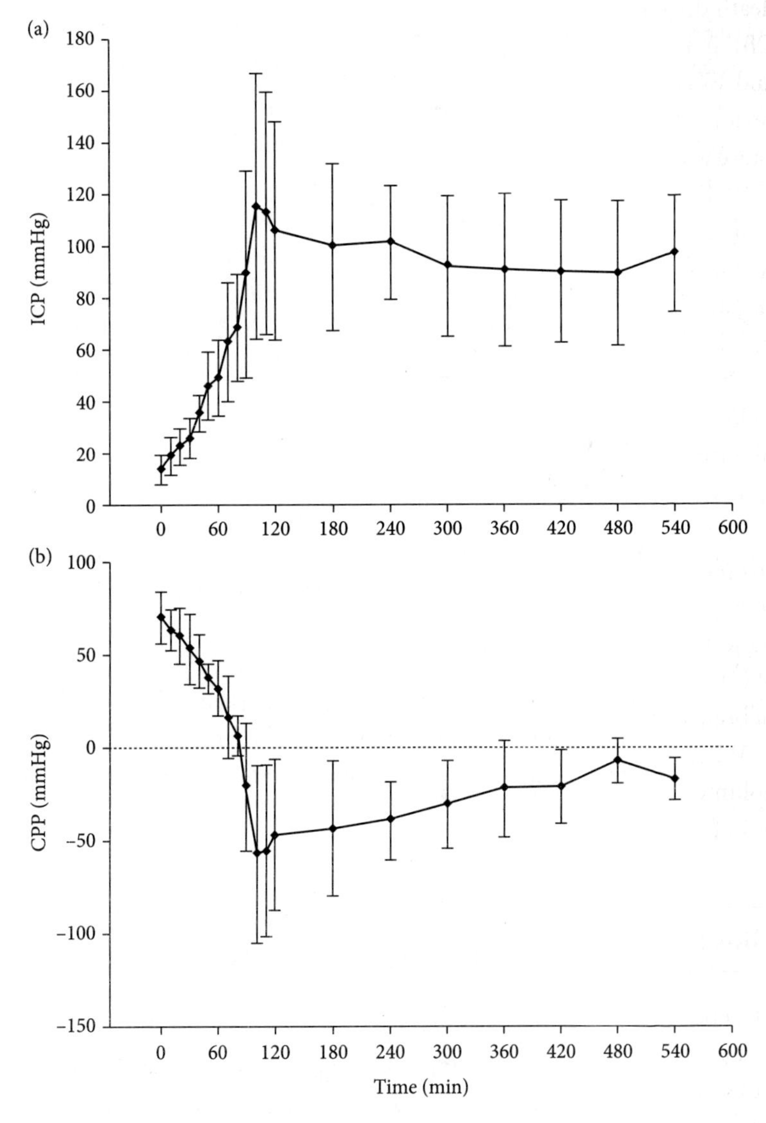

Figure 5.3. Induction and maintenance of intracranial hypertension to reach zero or negative cerebral perfusion pressure is the most common method of inducing brain death in pigs (reproduced with permission from Valenza [15])

The 'no blood flow' theory is certainly not bullet-proof, since it does not encompass every case of brain death and it comes mainly from case series and anecdotal reports, but it seems to explain most cases. In fact, there are several anecdotal cases in which CBF was still detectable at brain death diagnosis, well summarized by Flowers,[17] who reported residual CBF in two patients (out of 219, less than 1%) whose clinical diagnosis and EEG findings suggested brain death. This prompted a thoughtful review of all possible causes of persistent CBF in brain death. The main cause was identified in cases where HICP was not yet high enough to stop CBF. There is a possibility, suggested more recently by Ala[18] (2006) that CBF might have been tested too early, before a complete circulatory stop was reached in the brain. Also, in Roth's paper[16] half the patients had slightly positive CPP at brain death. Their ICP and CPP varied during the development of brain death and even after confirmation.

The time of determination of brain death is set free and might even be influenced by the availability of clinicians to do the tests. The presence of positive CPP during or after brain death therefore may depend on the time when brain death is determined.

The other plausible pathophysiology is a direct lesion causing catastrophic damage to the brainstem. Even though these cases are a minority they are challenging since a major requirement for brain death determination in a number of legislations, CBF, is absent. CBF may still be detectable in these patients; even so, they may present the clinical core features of brain death: deep coma, apnoea, and absent brainstem reflexes.

When the brain is no longer enclosed in a rigid envelope (i.e. skull), volume increase does not, generally, correspond to increase in pressure, as in Decompressive Craniectomy (see Box 5.1).

Box 5.1: Special case: Decompressive craniectomy

Decompressive craniectomy (DC) is a treatment for refractory HICP, since freeing the brain from part of its rigid envelope should prevent the pressure rise. Patients submitted to DC usually do not reach the extreme level of HICP that leads to the abolition of CPP. Therefore, they rarely evolve towards brain death. However, there are exceptions to this general rule, with two studies reporting DC patients who developed refractory HICP leading to brain death, through the same mechanisms described above of critical reduction of CPP due to extreme ICP[19,20]

Mimicking conditions

Some conditions mimic brain death, with very similar clinical presentation but their pathophysiology is very different, and the CBF is not low like in brain death. It is important to exclude the following conditions when evaluating a patient for diagnosis of brain death.

Locked-in syndrome

In 1966, Plum and Posner[21] introduced the term 'locked-in syndrome' to define a neurological condition associated with infarction of the ventral pons commonly resulting from an infarct, haemorrhage, or trauma. It is most often caused by a stroke in the basilar artery territory. The syndrome was described as causing quadriplegia, lower cranial nerve paralysis, and mutism with preservation of only vertical gaze and upper eyelid movement. Consciousness remains intact, and the patient is able to communicate intelligibly by eye blinking. The patient with 'locked-in syndrome' is literally locked inside his body, aware of his environment but with severely limited ability to interact with it. Consciousness persists because the tegmentum, with the reticular formation, is not affected.

Hypothermia

Hypothermia is defined as a body temperature lower than 35°C and may be accidental or therapeutic—for instance, for refractory HICP or after cardiac arrest. Hypothermia causes a downward spiral of loss of brainstem reflexes and pupillary dilatation, and also slows drug metabolism, making the neurological assessment of brain death problematic. The response to light is lost at core temperatures of 28–32°C, and brainstem reflexes disappear when the core temperature drops below 28°C. These deficits are all potentially reversible, even after extreme hypothermia. In therapeutic hypothermia as well as in accidental environmental exposure cases, the confounders are so significant that diagnosis of brain death should not even be attempted.[7]

Drug intoxication

Various drugs and/or their metabolites, including narcotics, benzodiazepines, tricyclic antidepressants, anticholinergics, and barbiturates, can closely mimic brain death. Cases of tricyclic or barbiturate overdose presenting the clinical features resembling brain death have been reported[22,23] This is why guidelines recommend excluding the effects of depressant drugs on the central nervous system, on the basis of history, drug screening, and calculation of clearance using five times the drug's half-life (assuming normal hepatic and renal function) or, if available, drug plasma levels below the therapeutic range.[7]

Conclusion

Despite their clinical and ethical importance, the mechanisms of brain death are still not completely clear. Brain death is not a single clinical entity, but can be considered a syndrome, which has been labelled 'brain death' or 'brainstem death' with different definitions across different countries. Therefore, it is not possible to group brain death in any single pathophysiological theory. Two distinct pathways are proposed for brain death, bearing in mind that the *primum movens* is always a catastrophic, irreversible injury:

- The first, which covers the majority of cases, is the 'no flow theory'. From extracranial or intracranial causes, CBF is abolished or severely impaired focally in the brainstem or globally. Through a self-sustaining mechanism, ischemia causes cytotoxic oedema, resulting in HICP and a consequent further reduction or abolition of CBF. The increasing oedema will eventually lead to supratentorial herniation and compression of the brainstem, which is the final stage of brain death.
- The second covers the remaining brain death patients. Direct lesion of the brainstem by conditions such as neoplasm, ischemia, or haemorrhage can trigger its own death. Such cases are still a minority, and some consider them anecdotal.

The conditions causing brain death are normally considered catastrophic and irreversible since the central nervous system is highly vulnerable to hypoxemia/ischemia, not replaceable and not repairable. This is our current state of knowledge, but scientific progress may change it. In a recently published, elegant paper by Vrselija and colleagues,[(24)] pig brains were perfused *ex-vivo* 4 hours after disembodiment: the authors succeeded in restoring some cellular and tissue functions and even synaptic activity. Future research may interrupt the vicious cycle of events that leads to brain death and may even recover the entire brain and its functions, making the whole concept of brain death outdated.

Highlights

- Brain death is a condition of irreversible loss of all functions of the entire brain: brain-dead patients are in deep coma, apnoeic and have no brainstem reflex.
- The main causes of brain death are exemplified by cardiac arrest for extracranial conditions, and traumatic brain injury and haemorrhagic stroke for intracranial ones.
- Different aetiologies and different characterization in national legislation mean that brain death can be considered a syndrome, differing in its plausible pathophysiology, but the ultimate outcome is always an irreversible, catastrophic brain injury.
- The most common pathophysiological pathway is global cerebral ischemia, caused either by cardiac arrest or extreme HICP that abolishes CPP.
- Less frequently, brain death may evolve from direct lesions to the brainstem.

References

1. Powner DJ, Ackerman BM, Grenvik A. Medical diagnosis of death in adults: Historical contributions to current controversies. Lancet. 1996 Nov 2;348(9036):1219–1223.
2. Mollaret P, Goulon M. The depassed coma (preliminary memoire). Rev Neurol (Paris). 1959 Jul;101:3–15.

3. Report of the Ad Hoc Committee of the Harvard Medical School to examine the definition of brain death. A definition of irreversible coma. JAMA. 1968 Aug 5;205(6):337–340.
4. Wijdicks EF, Varelas PN, Gronseth GS, Greer DM. American Academy of Neurology. Evidence-based guideline update: Determining brain death in adults: Report of the Quality Standards Subcommittee of the American Academy of Neurology. Neurology 2010;74:1911–1918.
5. Wahlster S, Wijdicks EF, Patel PV, Greer DM, Hemphill JC 3rd, Carone M, Mateen FJ. Brain death declaration: Practices and perceptions worldwide. Neurology. 2015 May 5;84(18):1870–1879.
6. Smith M. Brain death: The United Kingdom perspective. Semin Neurol. 2015 Apr;35(2):145–151.
7. Wijdicks EF, Varelas PN, Gronseth GS, Greer DM. American Academy of Neurology. Evidence-based guideline update: Determining brain death in adults: Report of the Quality Standards Subcommittee of the American Academy of Neurology. Neurology. 2010 Jun 8;74(23):1911–1918.
8. Kramer AH, Zygun DA, Doig CJ, Zuege DJ. Incidence of neurologic death among patients with brain injury: A cohort study in a Canadian health region. CMAJ. 2013 Dec 10;185(18): E838–E845.
9. Spinello IM. Brain death determination. J Intensive Care Med. 2015 Sep;30(6):326–337.
10. Joshi S, Ornstein E, Young W. Cerebral and spinal cord blood flow. In Cottrell J Young W, eds. *Cottrell and Young's Neuroanesthesia*. Philadelphia: Mosby Elsevier, 2010; 17–59.
11. Welschehold S, Kerz T, Boor S, et al. Detection of intracranial circulatory arrest in brain death using cranial CT-angiography. Eur J Neurol. 2013 Jan;20(1):173–179.
12. Salih F, Holtkamp M, Brandt SA, et al. Intracranial pressure and cerebral perfusion pressure in patients developing brain death. J Crit Care. 2016 Aug; 34:1–6.
13. Yu Y, Chen J, Si Z, et al. The hemodynamic response of the cerebral bridging veins to changes in ICP. Neurocrit Care. 2010 Feb;12(1):117–123.
14. Purins K, Enblad P, Wiklund L, Lewén A. Brain tissue oxygenation and cerebral perfusion pressure thresholds of ischemia in a standardized pig brain death model. Neurocrit Care. 2012 Jun;16(3):462–469.
15. Valenza F, Coppola S, Froio S, et al. A standardized model of brain death, donor treatment, and lung transplantation for studies on organ preservation and reconditioning. Intensive Care Med Exp. 2014 Dec;2(1):12.
16. Roth C, Ferbert A, Matthaei J, Kaestner S, Engel H, Gehling M. Progress of intracranial pressure and cerebral perfusion pressure in patients during the development of brain death. J Neurol Sci. 2019 Mar 15; 398:171–175.
17. Flowers WM, Patel BR. Persistence of cerebral blood flow after brain death. South Med J. 2000 Apr;93(4):364–370.
18. Ala TA, Kuhn MJ, Johnson AJ. A case meeting clinical brain death criteria with residual cerebral perfusion. AJNR Am J Neuroradiol. 2006 Oct;27(9):1805–1806.
19. Pereyra C, Benito Mori L, Schoon P, et al. Decompressive craniectomy and brain death prevalence and mortality: 8-year retrospective review. Transplant Proc. 2012 Sep;44(7):2181–2184.

20. Salih F, Finger T, Vajkoczy P, Wolf S. Brain death after decompressive craniectomy: Incidence and pathophysiological mechanisms. J Crit Care. 2017 Jun; 39:205–208.
21. Plum F, Posner JB. The diagnosis of stupor and coma. FA Davis, Philadelphia, PA (1966)
22. Grattan-Smith PJ, Butt W. Suppression of brainstem reflexes in barbiturate coma. Arch Dis Child. 1993 Jul;69(1):151–152.
23. Yang KL, Dantzker DR. Reversible brain death. A manifestation of amitriptyline overdose. Chest. 1991 Apr;99(4):1037–1038.
24. Vrselja Z, Daniele SG, Silbereis J et al. Restoration of brain circulation and cellular functions hours post-mortem. *Nature.* 2019 Apr;568(7752):336–343.

6
Histology and pathology of brain death

Kangana Sengar, Arulselvi Subramanian

Introduction

According to American Academy of Neurology (AAN) Practice Parameters,[1] brain death (BD) is a precisely defined clinical diagnosis caused by a catastrophic injury leading to irreversible loss of function of the entire brain including brainstem, absent brainstem reflexes, and apnoea along with presence of clinical or neuro-imaging evidence of acute Central Nervous System (CNS) catastrophe severe enough to explain the condition, core temperature greater than 32°C (90°F), no drug intoxication or poisoning, and absence of confounding medical conditions such as severe electrolyte, acid-base, or endocrine disturbances.[1,2] There is no recovery from BD by any mechanism. The body may be supported by artificial means for a limited period of time but most often the organs will fail over time despite artificial support.

In contrast to BD, coma refers to a severely depressed level of consciousness, with complete unresponsiveness but presence of spontaneous breathing.[3–5] In vegetative state, brainstem functions are preserved thus breathing and involuntary movements remain intact. However, such patients lack any awareness or meaningful interaction with their environment.[5] There are many causes of BD such as haemorrhagic/ischemic stroke, traumatic brain injury (TBI), cardiac arrest, brain infections, hypoxic encephalopathy, and so on.[3,6] Differential diagnosis of BD such as barbiturate overdose, alcohol intoxication, sedative overdose, hypothermia, hypoglycaemia, coma, and chronic vegetative state must be ruled out clinically as well as neuro-pathologically.[3,6]

Historical overview

Perhaps no subject has generated more debate in medicine than the diagnosis of BD. Concept of BD did not exist before the advent of technology to provide artificial support to organs, as patients succumbed to brain injuries that were severe enough to affect breathing and heart function. However, after the invention of ventilators, declaration of death by neurological criteria became necessary. Since the late 1950s and 1960s strict policies are being adopted to ensure correct determination of BD, and in accordance with medical standards and state laws.[7–10]

BD has been synonymously used with the terms like *coma depasse*, dissociated BD, BD syndrome, and respirator brain.[3]

Maintenance of hemodynamics by using vasopressors and oxygenation by mechanical ventilation can support somatic organs and allow ongoing brain necrosis. In the 1970s neuropathologists coined the term 'respirator brain' to describe the typical features of total brain necrosis found at autopsy in brain-dead cases kept on life support, and hence it was considered a BD pathologic hallmark.[7–10] The typical features of a respirator brain (total brain necrosis) are dusky, congested, and discoloured brain containing liquid portions and brain fragmentations.[11] However now, due to organ transplant protocols, the time to brain fixation has been shortened. As a result, respirator brain is rarely observed in modern transplant era and neuropathological findings may be different than described in the past.

Autopsy studies in patients who have been declared brain dead are limited resulting in paucity of literature. The largest study on neuropathology in BD was done by the Collaborative Study of Cerebral Death directed by Walker et al. on 226 brains.[4] Larger number of autopsy studies in BD will be helpful for the growing demand of biospecimen in the new and innovative research field of brain biobanks. In India, Human brain bank is at National Institute of Mental Health and Neurosciences (NIMHANS), Bangalore, which is functional since fifteen years.[12]

Histology of brain

When brain is sectioned, two major areas of brain tissue are seen according to their colour in fixed, unstained tissue.

- Grey matter comprising Neuron cell bodies, glial cells, dendrites, and synapses
- White matter comprising Axons (myelinated and unmyelinated) and glial cells

Brain tissue consists of two major cell types: Neurons or nerve cells and supporting or non-neuronal cells.[13–15]

Neurons/nerve cells

Neurons perform conduction, propagation, and reception of nerve impulses. Neuron consists of three parts, namely cell body, dendrites, and axon. Cell body has nucleus and abundance of rough endoplasmic reticulum (RER) and polyribosomes forming clumps called Nissl bodies. Processes called dendrites extend from cell body which receives input from other neurons or receptors. Axon is the extension of the cell body that is specialized for conducting electrical impulses/action potentials. Axon lacks Nissl bodies and does not stain with routine histological stains. They are either myelinated (surrounded by fatty insulating sheath that speeds conduction of the electrical impulse) or non-myelinated (lacking myelin sheath and thus conduct impulses slowly).

Supporting cells (non-neuronal cells/glial cells/neuroglia cells)

As their name suggests, these cells provide support in the form of nutrition, insulation, and protection to the neurons and outnumber them in the ratio of 10:1. They are generally situated among the neurons and are smaller with no axon or dendrites in contrast to neurons. In routine sections stained with Haematoxylin & Eosin (H

& E) usually only the glial cell nuclei are seen. Special staining techniques are necessary if they are to be easily differentiated from surrounding cells.

- **Astrocytes:** These star-shaped cells play critical roles in various supportive functions such as recycling neurotransmitters, secreting neurotrophic factors like neural growth factors for growth and maintenance of neurons, dictating and modulating synapses, and maintaining appropriate ionic composition of extracellular fluid surrounding neurons. Astrocytes are analogous to fibroblasts elsewhere in the body, and in reaction to injury form intracytoplasmic glial filaments (scar tissue). Normally, cytoplasm of astrocyte is inconspicuous. However, in brain injury astrocyte secretes a large amount of perinuclear cytoplasm and synthesizes glial filaments and forms reactive/hypertrophic/gemistocytic astrocytes. Reactive astrocytosis/gliosis becomes evident histologically in four days, well established in seven to ten days, and maximal at two to three weeks. Immunostain for glial filaments is glial fibrillary acidic protein (GFAP) which highlight the star-shaped astrocytes (see **Figure 6.1**), vimentin, and S100.[16]
- **Oligodendrocytes:** Analogous to the Schwann cell of the peripheral nervous system (PNS), these cells myelinate axons in grey as well as white matter. Injury to oligodendrocytes with preservation of underlying axon may result in myelin breakdown called as demyelination. Immunostain for oligodendrocyte is myelin basic protein (MBP).[16]
- **Microglial cells:** These are the smallest glial cells and are responsible for the underlying inflammatory response that occurs following damage to the CNS and the invasion of microorganisms. The brain contains several different macrophages/monocytes populations, including resident brain macrophages (microglia) and perivascular macrophages. All of these macrophages/monocyte cells are of bone marrow origin and have roles in phagocytosis of debris and immune surveillance. The resident microglia clean-up the minor debris, but the clean-up of larger amounts of necrotic debris requires the recruitment of blood-borne monocytes/macrophages to the area. Activated macrophages within the brain typically have spindle-shaped nuclei

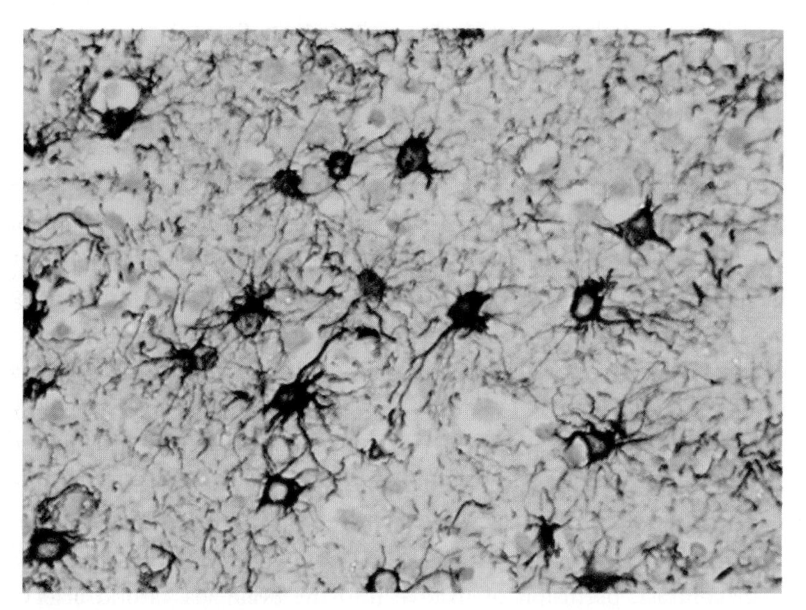

Figure 6.1. GFAP positive Astrocytes (brown staining) and oligodendrocytes (blue stained nucleus) with perinuclear halos (IHC, 400X)

(rod cells). As the macrophages ingest debris, they become the lipid-filled macrophages (foam cells) and are found around areas of brain necrosis. Microglia can be highlighted by Immunomarker Iba1 and CD68.[16]

- **Ependymal cells/Ependymocytes:** These cells form ciliated simple columnar epithelium that line ventricles of the brain and central canal of the spinal cord. Ependymal cells do not proliferate in response to a brain injury, unlike astrocytes.
- **Epithelial cells of choroid plexus:** These cells closely resemble ependymal cells and line fibro-vascular papillae of the choroid plexus found in lateral, third, and fourth ventricles and produces cerebrospinal fluid (CSF).
- **Schwann cells/Lemmocytes:** These cells wrap around the segments of axon and form myelin sheath along the axon. This myelin sheath is composed primarily of lipids which serve as an insulator and thus increase the transmission rate of action potentials along the axon.

Neuropathological techniques

A good fixation of brain is an essential prerequisite for histopathologic examinations. The fixation is done in neutral and buffered, 10% formalin concentration, in ten times of the volume of brain suspended in it.[17–19] Two types of techniques can be used namely, immersion and perfusion fixation.

With immersion fixation, a fixation time of at least two weeks is recommended for a larger brain. Also, precaution should be taken for fixation not to exceed four weeks (as formalin becomes acidic), and the formalin should be changed after 24 hours and at the end of the first week. However, immersion fixation of brain leads to unavoidable mechanical damage and the development of artefacts, but any intravascular pathology is not disturbed. Also, immersion fixation with formalin may increase the weight of the brain by up to 10%, which usually returns to its fresh state weight after three weeks of fixation.

In contrast, perfusion of fixative into the brain via carotid artery stumps fixes neural tissue *in-situ* in about 2–3 hours and minimizes mechanical artefacts. After perfusion, the brain should remain *in situ* for at least 2 hours and upto 24 hours with large brains, to permit adequate penetration of the fixative. However, perfusion fixation is often impractical, and the lengthy death-to-autopsy interval very frequently encountered in forensic cases means that perfusion will be incomplete and inconsistent. Artefactual brain shrinkage may be caused by unduly high osmolality (>0.1 mol/l) of the perfusate.[17–20]

After adequate fixation, the entire brain is sectioned in a transverse plane at about 0.5-1cm intervals. It should be noted that the high lipid and water content of the brain requires longer dehydration times during processing.[17–20] Adequate sampling from different areas of brain is done by taking sections from the frontal lobe including right or left superior medial frontal gyrus, temporal lobe, thalami, basal ganglia, hippocampi, and cerebellum including cortex and dentate nuclei.[15] Immunohistochemistry has now replaced many traditional special neuropathology stains. Antibodies for use in formalin-fixed, paraffin-embedded material are now widely available. However, care must be taken of appropriate fixation times and antigen retrieval methods, correct antibody dilutions, and positive and negative controls.[15,16]

Neuropathology of BD in the transplant era

BD is caused by catastrophic and diffuse insult like ischemic brain injury caused by insufficient blood supply, vascular injury caused by haemorrhage, brain oedema, and diffuse axonal injury (DAI) leading to intracranial circulatory arrest and ischemic total cerebral infarction.[21] Lack of perfusion accompanies secondary cerebral swelling and intravital autolysis of the brain. Maintenance of hemodynamics and oxygenation (using ventilator) can support somatic organs for a period of time, while brain necrosis continues.[10] Therefore, the pathological sequelae depend on various factors such as duration of cerebral anoxia, time on ventilator, age of patient, primary cause of hypoxic damage, and secondary neurochemical injury causing additional neuronal damage.[3,10] Flow arrest caused by asphyxiation is more injurious to the brain than the same period of normovolemic ventricular fibrillation arrest, while that caused by exsanguination may be less injurious.[3]

Gross examination

Since the primary pathological lesions in BD are so varied, more generalized changes are discussed. Depending upon the time on respirator and primary cause of brain damage, the brain may be well-preserved or may exhibit oedema resulting in flattened convolutions and narrowed sulci or softening of brain into a non-descript mushy mass. Brain weight is increased with duration on respirator. Cerebral hemispheres may be swollen and congested having a dusky hue and the leptomeninges often show a quantitatively variable extent of congestion indicating reflow phenomenon. Transtentorial herniations are commonly seen and the brainstem is often distorted by local oedema or torn and fragmented. Cerebellum shows swelling and congestion along with softening and fragmentation of herniated cerebellar tonsils. The cut sections may appear normal or oedematous and soft. Weight gain after 24 hours on respirator, softening, and swelling are the most common changes.[3,7,10,19]

Microscopic examination

The microscopic features are highly variable because brain is not uniformly affected and all neuroanatomical regions are selectively vulnerable. Apart from the cause of injury, the cerebral cortex is diffusely congested and oedematous. Areas of ischemic infarcts and haemorrhagic infarcts are seen due to occlusion of cerebral arteries.[10] The cortical neurons show cloudy swelling, loss of basophilia, red cell change (neuronal ischemic change), and loss of neuronal cells.[22] White matter shows perivascular haemorrhages and axonal swellings, varicosities, and retraction bulbs.[10,22,23] The brainstem shows pericellular oedema, haemorrhage, infarction, necrosis, and neuronal loss. Autolysis of the granular layer of the cerebellar cortex is particularly common.[24] No glial reaction is seen. If patients with any insult to the brain that may lead to BD survive for few days, laminar necrosis, pituitary gland infarction, and perivascular haemorrhages are seen in the white matter. Histopathological findings are usually less impressive than gross appearance may suggest. This may be due to cessation of the arterial circulation, which thereby does not allow the influx of inflammatory cells.[2,10,24] The capillaries do not show endothelial proliferation or neovascularization.[2,10]

Changes in axons

Axonal changes are identifiable in the white matter or in large fibre bundles (corpus callosum, internal capsule, or corticospinal fibres of the brainstem).[25,26]

- **Axonal swellings (spheroids):** Axonal swellings are the ovoid enlargements found in injured axons and are observed within several hours in case of TB1. Since there is a constant antero- and retrograde movement of various cargoes in axons, they react to any transport disruption by swelling and forming spheroids. The number and size of axonal spheroids increase over the ensuing 24 hours[10,17,18,25,27] (see **Figure 6.2**).
- **Axonal varicosities:** Axonal varicosities are caused by axonal elongation without rupture. These are characterized by a periodic arrangement of enlargements separated by shrunken areas and become swollen, beaded, and varicose[10,25,28] (see **Figures 6.3 & 6.4**).

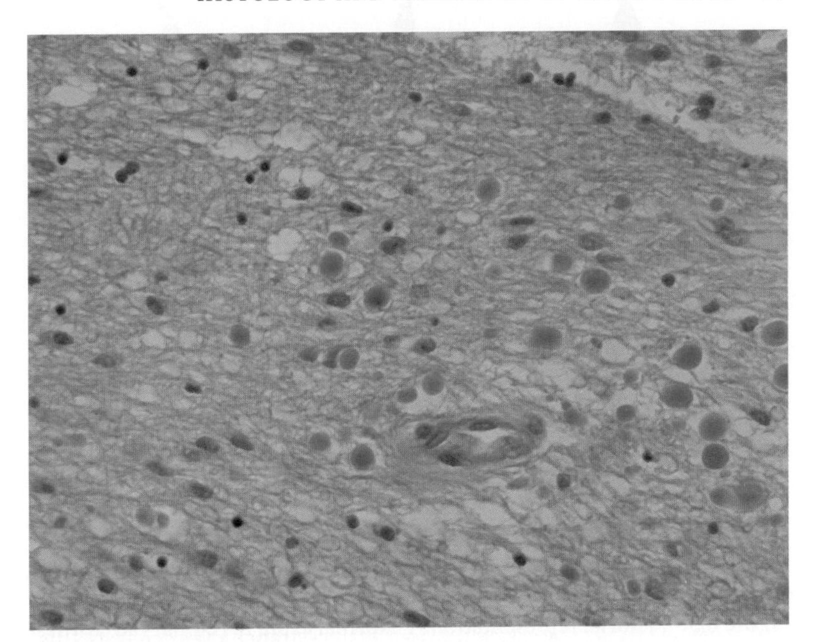

Figure 6.2. Axonal swellings in cerebral white matter (H&E, 400X)

- **Retraction balls:** Retraction balls (club) are caused by rupture of axonal fibre. The proximal stub forming a mass of axoplasm identifiable as round or elliptical eosinophilic masses, with varying sizes from 5 to 40 microns, and are seen as early as 2 hours after the initial injury(10,25,30–32) (see **Figures 6.3 & 6.4**).

Changes in neurons

- **Red neurons**: Red neurons are characterized by shrinkage of cell body, intense eosinophilic cytoplasm devoid of Nissl granules and shrunken pyknotic nucleus (see **Figure 6.5**). These may appear as early as within 2 hours, sometimes in asynchronous waves and more rapidly in smaller neurons than larger neurons.(10,17) These eosinophilic neurons (red neurons) reaching a moderate/severe degree are present in 34% to 68% of the cases in different regions.(10) However, red neurons are not pathognomonic in BD.(3,10,17)

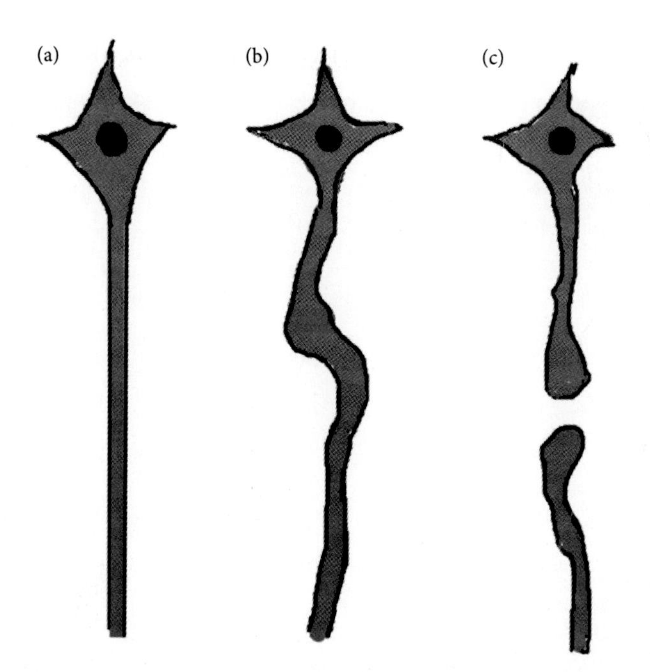

Figure 6.3. Pictorial representation A. Normal axon; B. Axonal varicosities; C. Retraction bulb

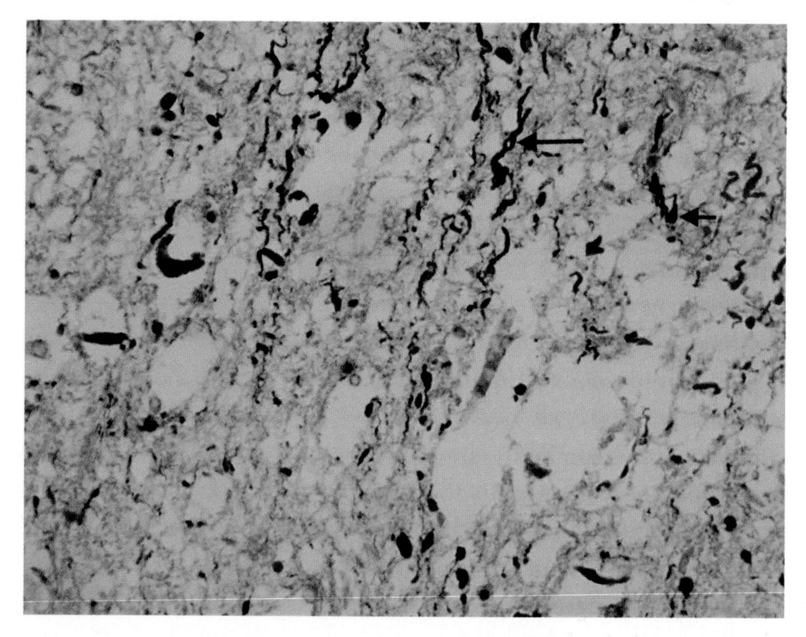

Figure 6.4. Axonal retractions (short arrow) and varicosities (long arrow) in a case of traumatic brain injury (IHC- β-APP, 400X)

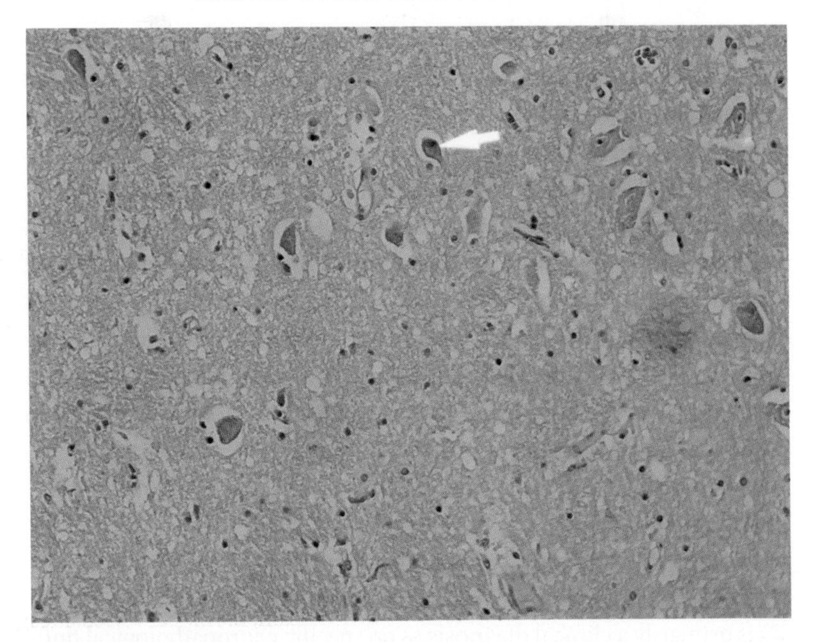

Figure 6.5. Red neurons, with hypereosinophilic cytoplasm and nuclear changes (H&E, 400X)

DAI and multiple contusions are seen in patients after TBI. Destructive haemorrhagic stroke and ischemic stroke with mass effect show various degrees of neuronal ischemic changes in different areas of brain. Patients with anoxic-ischemic injury have severe neuronal necrosis in all hemispheric samples, but moderate neuronal ischemic changes in the brainstem.

Respirator brain

The typical respirator brain is the extreme end of spectrum and is typically seen in patients with more than 72 hours on ventilator after BD. Features are dusky congestion, oedema, and softening and fragmentation of entire brain, necrotic and sloughing tonsillar herniation and mass effect.[3,6,10,33] Microscopic changes are characterized by diffuse neuronal ischemic changes, autolysis of cerebellar structures and pallor of myelin. However, respirator brains are rarely observed nowadays when fixation occurred within 12 hours.[10] Classically, neuronal and axonal changes were identified using H & E or silver stains. However, some of the changes are difficult to identify as well as underestimated using H & E stains. Silver stains are more sensitive than H & E. However, they positively label all axons, occasionally making it difficult to interpret the presence of axonal diameter irregularities.[25,32] In silver stains, identifiable enlarged neurons are seen at 2 hours post-injury which become more apparent with time. Axonal features can be best appreciated by Immunohistochemistry stain—β-APP in TBI.[32,34] By electron microscopy, these neurons show irreversible changes such as the breaks in the nuclear and cell membranes and dense deposits in mitochondria characteristic of necrosis, rather than apoptosis.[29]

Conclusion

BD is primarily a clinical diagnosis as no specific neuropathological findings in BD is identified and also, autopsy findings in BD lack distinction from other comatose states such as persistent vegetative state or minimally conscious state. However, autopsy studies remain the best method to confirm the direct cause of death leading to irreversible destruction of brain and to correlate clinical findings. In the majority of studies done till date, the cause of BD was TBI, perhaps accurately representing the 'neuropathology of BD after trauma' rather than the neuropathology of BD. However, we still don't have clear answers for queries like: Is the absence of perfusion essential for confirming BD? Degree of damage to diagnose a 'dead brain' or BD? Larger studies with the predetermined criteria for BD as defined by AAN, short intervals between BD and cardiac arrest and standardized brain pathology protocol are required to be done in order to provide an analysis of the neuropathological features that correlate diagnosis of BD. Also, it will provide biospecimen for the new and innovative research field of brain biobanks.

Highlights

1. BD is primarily a clinical diagnosis as no specific neuropathological features are recognized.

2. In majority of studies done till date, the cause of BD was TBI, perhaps accurately representing the 'neuropathology of BD after trauma' rather than the neuropathology of BD.
3. The relatively short time on life support does not result in development of typical respirator brain that was reported in earlier literature when transplantation was not an issue.
4. The pathological sequelae depend on various factors such as duration of cerebral anoxia, time on ventilator, age of patient, primary cause of hypoxic damage, and secondary neurochemical injury.
5. Microscopically changes seen in BD are axonal swellings, varicosities, retraction bulbs, red neurons (neuronal ischemic change), and neuronal loss.
6. Larger studies with the predetermined criteria for BD as defined by AAN and standardized brain pathology protocol are required to be done to analyse neuro-pathologic features.

References

1. Practice parameters for determining brain death in adults (summary statement). The quality standards subcommittee of the American Academy of Neurology. Neurology 1995;45(5):1012–1014.
2. Editorial, Saponsik G, Munoz DG. Dissecting brain death Time for a new look, Neurology® 2008;70:1230–1231.
3. Oehmichen M. Brain death: neuropathological findings and forensic implications. Forensic Science International 69(1994) 205–219.
4. Korein J. Terminology, definitions, and usage. Annals of the New York Academy of Sciences 1978 Nov 1;315(1):6–10.
5. Laureys S, Owen AM, Schiff ND. Brain function in coma, vegetative state, and related disorders. The Lancet Neurology 2004 Sep 1;3(9):537–546.
6. Walker AE. Cerebral death.3rd ed. Baltimore: Urban and Schwarzenberg 1985; 1–198.
7. Walker A, Diamond E, Moseley J. The neuropathological findings in irreversible coma. A critique of the 'respirator.' J Neuropathol Exp Neurol 1975;34:295–323.
8. Towbin A. The respirator brain death syndrome. Hum Path 1973;4:583–594.
9. Adams RD, Jequier M. The brain death syndrome-hypoxemic panencephalopathy. Schweiz Med Wochenschr 1969;99:65–73.
10. Wijdicks EF, Pfeifer EA. Neuropathology of brain death in the modern transplant era. Neurology. 2008 Apr 8;70(15):1234–1237.
11. Walker A. Pathology of brain death. Ann NY acad Ci 1978;315:272–280.
12. Netravathi M, Kamble N, Satishchandra P, Gourie-Devi M, Pal PK. Six decades of Neurology at NIMHANS: A historical perspective. Neurology India. 2018;66(2):459.

13. Young B, Woodford P, O'Dowd G. Wheater's functional histology e-book: A text and colour atlas. 6th ed. Elsevier Health Sciences; 2013; Chapter 20, Central nervous system: 384–401.
14. Garman RH. Histology of the central nervous system. Toxicologic pathology. 2011 Jan;39(1):22–35.
15. Rosai J. Rosai and Ackerman's surgical pathology e-book. 11th ed. Elsevier Health Sciences; 2011; Chapter 43, Central nervous system: 2308–2309.
16. Dabbs DJ. Diagnostic Immunohistochemistry. Philadelphia, PA: Saunders Elsevier; 2010.
17. Finnie JW. Forensic pathology of traumatic brain injury. Veterinary pathology 2016 Sep;53(5):962–978.
18. Itabashi HH, Andrews JM, Tomiyasu U, Erlich SS, Sathyavagiswaran L. Forensic neuropathology: A practical review of the fundamentals. Academic Press; 2011 Aug 29.
19. Oemichen M, Auer RN, Konig HG. Forensic Neuropathology and Associated Neurology. Berlin, Germany: Springer; 2006.
20. Kalimo H, Saukko P, Graham D. Neuropathological examination in forensic context. Forensic Sci Int 2004;146:73–81.
21. Perez-Nellar J, Machado C, Scherle C, Alvarez R, Areu A. Clinical and neuropathologic study of a series of brain-dead patients from a tertiary hospital in Cuba. Functional Neurology, Rehabilitation, and Ergonomics 2011;1(1):25.
22. Leestma JE, Hughes JR, Diamond ER. Temporal correlates in brain death: EEG and clinical relationships to the respirator brain. Archives of neurology 1984 Feb 1;41(2):147–152.
23. Graham DI, Adams JH, Murray LS, Jennett B. Neuropathology of the vegetative state after head injury. Neuropsychological rehabilitation 2005 Jul 1;15(3–4):198–213
24. Auer R, Benveniste H. In Grahan DI, Lantos PL, eds. Hypoxia and Related Conditions. London: 1977.
25. Hostiuc S, Pirici D, Negoi I, Ion DA, Ceausu M. Detection of diffuse axonal injury in forensic pathology. Rom J Leg Med 2014 Sep1;22:145–152.
26. Imajo T, Challener RC, Roessmann U. Diffuse axonal injury by assault. The American journal of forensic medicine and pathology 1987;8:217–219.
27. Oemichen M, Meissner C, Schmidt V, et al. Axonal injury—a diagnostic tool in forensic neuropathology? A review. Forensic Sci Int 1998;95: 67–83.
28. Johnson VE, Stewart W, Smith DH. Axonal pathology in traumatic brain injury. Experimental neurology.2013;246:35–43.
29. Colbourne F, Sutherland GR, Auer RN. Electron microscopic evidence against apoptosis as the mechanism of neuronal death in global ischemia. J Neurosci 1999; 19:4200–4210.
30. Peerless SJ, Rewcastl, Nb. Shear injuries of brain. Can Med Assoc J. 1967;96:577.
31. Cajal SR. Degeneration & regeneration of the nervous system: Oxford University Press, Humphrey Milford; 1928.
32. Gleckman AM, Bell MD, Evans RJ, Smith TW. Diffuse axonal injury in infants with nonaccidental craniocerebral trauma: Enhanced detection by β-amyloid precursor protein immunohistochemical staining. Archives of Pathology and Laboratory Medicine 1999 Feb;123(2):146–151.

33. Schneider H, Masshoff W, Neuhaus GA. Klinische und morphologische Aspekte des Hirntodes. Klinische Wochenschrift 1969 Aug 1;47(16):844–859.
34. Hortobágyi T, Wise S, Hunt N, Cary N, Djurovic V, Fegan-Earl A, et al. Traumatic axonal damage in the brain can be detected using beta-APP immunohistochemistry within 35 min after head injury to human adults. Neuropathol Appl Neurobiol. 2007 Apr;33(2):226–237.

7

Neuroimaging of brain death

Murugusundaram Veeramani

Introduction

Brain death (BD) is clinically determined. Ancillary tests including neuroimaging are used when clinical tests cannot be performed conclusively. Neuroimaging tests recommended by the American Association of Neurology (AAN) include cerebral angiography (CA), TCD (transcranial doppler) ultrasound, nuclear medicine cerebral scintigraphy with technetium Tc 99m Hexamethyl-propyleneamine oxime (^{99m}Tc HMPAO).[1] Some countries including France and Netherlands also require the clinical diagnosis to be confirmed with demonstration of lack of brain function or cerebral circulatory arrest.[2] There is insufficient evidence to determine if newer ancillary tests accurately confirm the cessation of function of the entire brain. In neuroimaging, these tests include CTA (Computed tomography angiography), CT Perfusion, MRI (magnetic resonance imaging), MRA (magnetic resonance angiography), and MR Perfusion.

Diagnosis of cause

In the USA, after the Uniform Declaration of Death Act, a practice parameter was published by AAN in 1995 to outline the medical standards for the definition of brain death.[2] Coma with a known cause is one of the clinical findings necessary to confirm the irreversible cessation of the entire brain functions present with brain death. Neuroimaging performed to evaluate the cause of coma has been included by AAN as one of the prerequisites to be checked before the determination of BD. Computed tomography (CT) and MRI may help to establish the cause of coma. A relatively normal-appearing brain on imaging should prompt an alternative diagnosis and a search for conditions that can mimic BD.[2] Causes for BD would include intracranial haemorrhage including extra and intra-axial haemorrhages, brain infarcts including brainstem infarcts, diffuse brain oedema, midline shift, and brain herniation (see Figures 7.1, 7.2, and 7.3). The end result of all causes would be death of neuronal and glial cells. CT and MRI would help to work up the underlying causes for BD. CT would show diffuse brain oedema with loss of grey white matter differentiation, effacement of sulci and ventricles, and trans-compartmental herniations. MRI may additionally show changes of restricted diffusion and loss of flow voids in the major intracranial vessels related to loss of intracranial blood flow as well.[2]

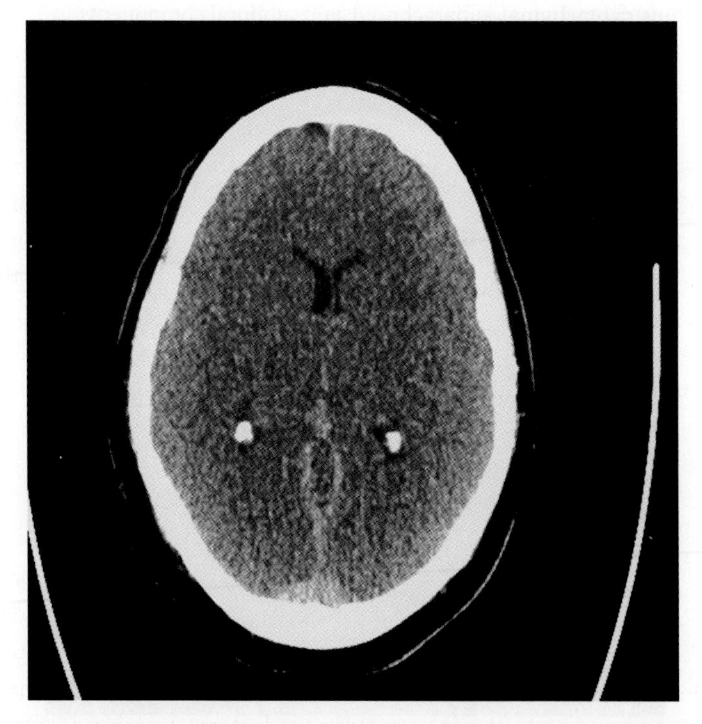

Figure 7.1. 65-year-old male found with unknown down time. Diffuse brain oedema seen with loss of grey white matter differentiation and with effacement of sulci and ventricles

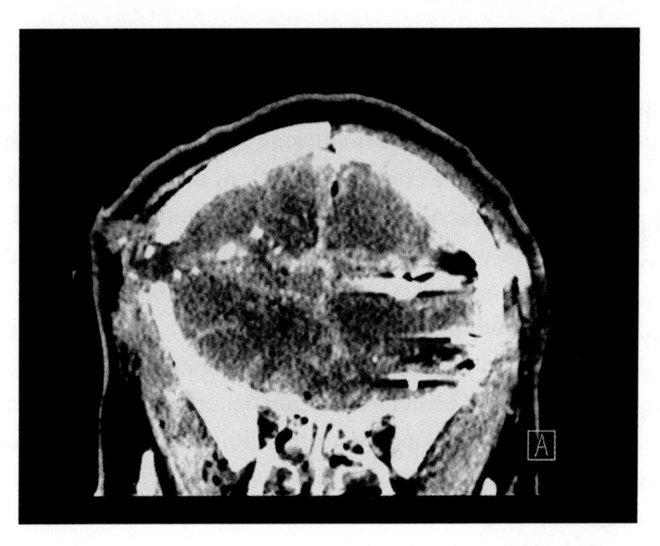

Figure 7.2. 18-year-old male with GSW (gunshot wound) in the head—CT shows intracranial bullet and skull fragments with extensive haemorrhage including parenchymal, subarachnoid, and subdural components

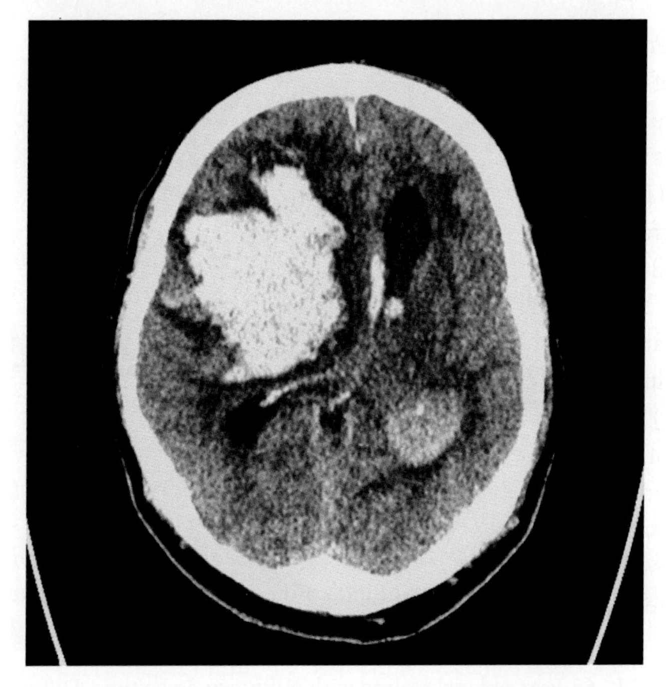

Figure 7.3. 73-year-old who presented unresponsive with high blood pressure. Head CT shows extensive right sided parenchymal brain haemorrhage centred in the basal ganglia with ventricular extension. There is associated midline shift to the left and hydrocephalus. Despite emergent hematoma evacuation, the patient did not improve and was declared brain dead

There is limited space within the closed cranial cavity. Pathologies resulting in irreversible coma can cause increase in intracranial pressure. This could be due to substances such as blood from haemorrhage or fluid from oedema of either vasogenic or cytotoxic types. The build-up of pressure eventually exceeds the pressure of blood in the arterial system which prevents inflow of fresh oxygenated blood into the cranial cavity. It is axiomatic that cessation of all blood flow to the brain for a reasonable amount of time results in irreversible cell death intracranially. This eventually leads to BD which can be demonstrated clinically with neurological testing. When the results of the clinical tests are not clear or the tests are difficult to perform, ancillary tests may be necessary. The imaging studies used demonstrate cessation of blood flow to the brain.

Cerebral angiography

Conventional CA is considered the reference standard in demonstrating lack of cerebral circulation. It is performed by injecting iodinated contrast material into the aortic arch under pressure or selectively in the neck vessels arising from the aorta. Imaging is obtained in anteroposterior and lateral projections using a biplane angiographic system. Normally there is intracranial blood flow to the brain via bilateral internal carotid arteries and bilateral vertebral arteries. In BD, there is no flow or little meaningful blood flow to the brain. Non-visualization of intracranial internal carotid arteries beyond the petrous segment, vertebral arteries beyond the intradural segment with normal visualization of external carotid arteries (ECA) and non-visualization of the internal cerebral veins (ICV), and vein of Galen is considered positive for BD diagnosis. Stasis filling with delayed, weak, and persistent opacification of the proximal cerebral arterial segments without opacification of the cortical branches or venous outflow can also be seen with BD.[3] Delayed opacification may be seen in the superior longitudinal sinus.

Computed tomography angiography

The CTA is done more frequently than CA. Iodinated contrast is injected into the peripheral or central venous system through an intravenous line and imaging is done in a CT scanner over the head and neck region. It is much faster, easily accessible, safer, and less operator dependent. However, this is not considered equivalent to CA in diagnosing BD in several countries, including the USA. In France and Canada, CTA is accepted with established criteria.[4–6] It is based on a 7-point scoring system with 2 points each for non-opacification of pericallosal branches of the anterior cerebral arteries (ACA), middle cerebral artery (MCA) branches in Sylvian fissure, ICV and 1 point for great cerebral vein (GCV). Four-point evaluation with bilateral cortical MCA branches and ICVs have been shown to be more sensitive.[3] Studies have shown the ICV to be the most sensitive and specific of these criteria.[4,7,8] Some studies have shown the findings on CTA to be falsely negative or falsely positive.[9,5]

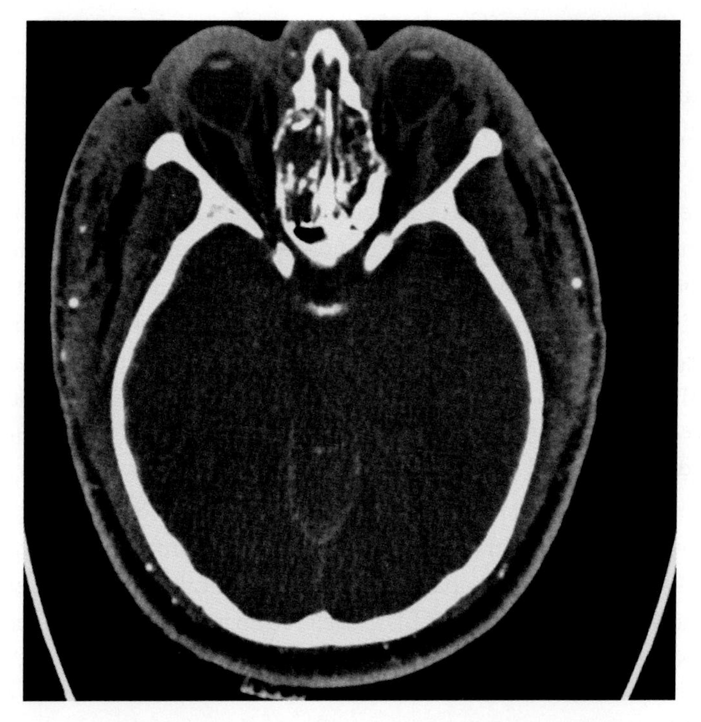

Figure 7.4. CTA in 18-year-old male with GSW. There is normal visualization of the Superficial temporal arteries (STA) on both sides. There is no visualization of any of the blood vessels at the Circle of Willis or of the ICV or Great cerebral vein consistent with the clinical picture of BD

This is partly related to nonuniform criteria used in diagnosis of BD with CTA and comparing them to other ancillary tests which themselves have been shown to have varying sensitivities and specificities.[5] False negative findings can be seen with craniotomy which releases the intracranial pressure. Blood flow and hence opacification are seen in the neck vessels and branches of the ECAs including the superficial temporal arteries (see Figure 7.4). Criteria have included no flow being seen in the ICAs at the siphon and distally, and in the vertebral arteries in their intradural course[10] though there may be some filling of the proximal V4 vertebral artery segments. No venous return should be seen as well.

There is growing medical literature to support the inclusion of CTA in the diagnosis of BD.[3,5,7] The accuracy of CTA depends on the criteria used.[11] The meta-analysis of 337 patients, demonstrated a sensitivity of 84–85% and suggested that, although the available evidence cannot support the use of CTA as a complete replacement for neurological testing for diagnosis of brain death, it may be useful as a confirmatory test.[10,12] Iodinated contrast used in conventional CA and CTA can contribute to renal damage.

Nuclear medicine BD scan

The scan involves dynamic imaging of the cerebral perfusion and delayed static Single-photon emission computed tomography (SPECT) images by injecting ^{99m}Tc Hexamethyl-propyleneamine oxime (HMPAO) intravenously. This is a lipophilic compound and the distribution corresponds to the blood flow. It crosses the blood brain barrier and is taken up by the brain parenchyma. In BD, the angiographic phase shows blood flow in the bilateral common carotid arteries (CCAs), ECA systems, and extracranial vertebral arteries. The radionuclide activity is seen in the soft tissue of the neck and scalp with no activity in the brain within the cranial cavity (light bulb appearance). There is 'hot nose' appearance due to relatively increased activity in the nasal tissues supplied by branches of the ECA (see Figures 7.5a and 7.5b). There may be delayed activity seen in the superior sagittal sinus, but this is not a certain sign compatible with brain life. SPECT images help to evaluate the brainstem and posterior fossa structures better.[13]

(a)

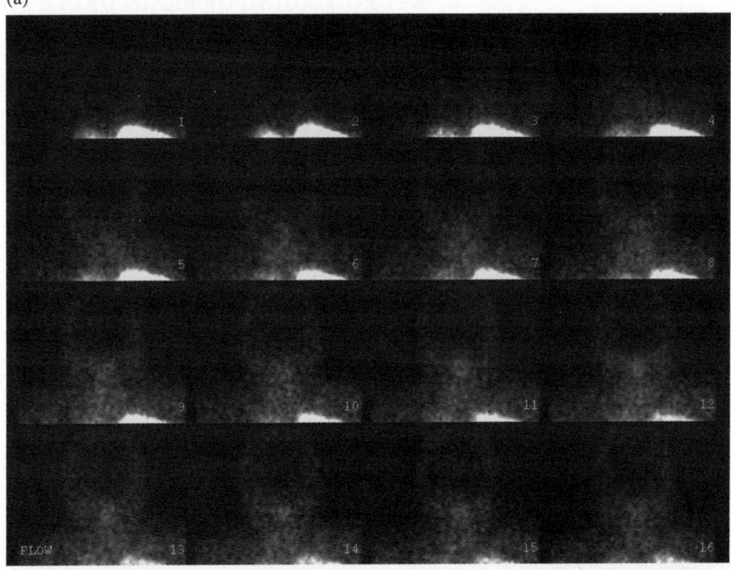

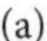

(b)

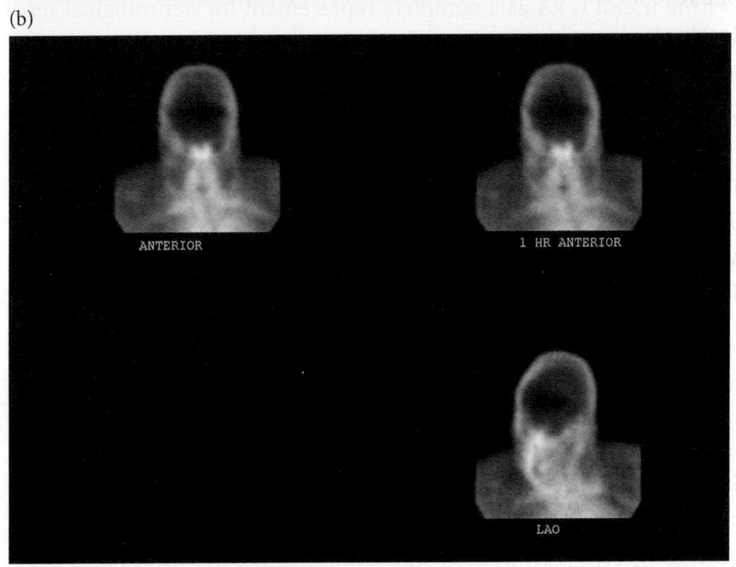

Figure 7.5a and 7.5b. Tc 99m DTPA dynamic injection phase on 7.5a shows normal flow related activity in the region of extracranial blood vessels in the neck and the ECA branches supplying the scalp with no blood flow being shown intracranially. The blood pool and 1 hour delayed images on 7.5b show 'hot nose' sign from increased activity in the nasal mucosa supplied by ECA branches with no activity seen in the ICA or vertebral artery territories intracranially. These are consistent with clinical BD in a 33-year-old male overdosed on cocaine with multiple brain infarcts including that of the brain stem

Alternate lipophilic radionuclide used for brain perfusion imaging is ^{99m}Tc ECD (ethyl cysteinate dimer). ^{99m}Tc DTPA (diethylenetriaminepentaacetic acid) does not cross the blood brain barrier and hence does not bind to the brain. Angiographic phase alone is performed and there is no delayed parenchymal phase.(14)

Transcranial Doppler ultrasound evaluation

Ultrasound beams are used to evaluate intracranial blood flow. The flow in the intracranial ICAs, MCAs, ACAs, vertebral arteries, and basilar artery is evaluated.(15) The patterns seen with the diagnosis of brain death are brief systolic forward flow or systolic spikes and diastolic reversed flow, brief systolic forward flow or systolic spikes and no diastolic flow, or no demonstrable flow in a patient in whom flow had been clearly documented in a previous TCD examination. Abnormal flow needs to be demonstrated bilaterally or in at least three vessels for 3 minutes during the same exam.(16) Oscillating or reverberating flow has been described.(17,18) TCD may be exceedingly difficult or impossible in a brain-dead patient with intubation with no insonation window. Operator expertise is also necessary for performing these studies. A meta-analysis of 684 patients showed a sensitivity of 89% with a specificity of 99%.(18)

MRA, CT perfusion, and MR perfusion

The MRA done with Time of Flow technique demonstrates a lack of normal flow-related enhancement signal in the intracranial supraclinoid portions of the internal carotid arteries and the vertebral arteries.(19) It does not usually require the injection of contrast. It also appears to be unaffected by the stasis filling finding in the CTA. High sensitivity and specificity of up to 100% have been described with these studies.(20) However, performing an MR study is much more difficult in a critical care patient on life support and this may result in artefacts as well.

CT perfusion and MR perfusion studies demonstrate lack of perfusion to both supratentorial and infratentorial compartments of the brain. These are considered functional studies. Both need intravenous contrast injection. The MR perfusion may also show an MRI equivalent of the 'hot nose' sign.[21] These two techniques are still considered experimental.

Conclusion

BD remains a clinical diagnosis. Ancillary tests including the accepted neuroimaging tests may have geographic variations to their order of preferences. Some places do not require these tests to make the diagnosis of BD arrived by clinical criteria while others need confirmation by a test. They may also help to shorten the time of observation in some cases which is also valuable, including for organ procurement.

Highlights

- Neuroimaging helps to identify the cause of irreversible coma, a criterion for BD.
- BD is a clinical diagnosis. Neuroimaging studies are ancillary tests to confirm BD.
- CA is considered the standard in imaging confirmation of BD.
- CTA has been accepted as an alternative to conventional angiography in the diagnosis of BD in some countries.
- Nuclear medicine BD scans are an accepted imaging study to diagnose BD.
- TCD evaluation is another well-established modality to establish the diagnosis.

References

1. Wijdicks EFM, Varelas PN, Gronseth GS, Greer DM. Evidence-based guideline update: Determining brain death in adults. Report of the Quality Standards Subcommittee of the American Academy of Neurology, 2010.
2. Rizvi T, Batchala P, Mukherjee S. Brain death: Diagnosis and imaging techniques. Semin Ultrasound CT MR. 2018 Oct; 39(5):515–529.

3. Sawicki M, Bohatyrewicz R, Safranow K, Walecka A, Walecki J, Rowinski O et al. Computed tomographic angiography criteria in the diagnosis of brain death-comparison of sensitivity and interobserver reliability of different evaluation scales. Neuroradiology. 2014 56:609–620.
4. Frampas E, Videcoq M, de Kerviler E, Ricolfi F, Kuoch V, Mourey F, et al. CT angiography for brain death diagnosis. AJNR Am J Neuroradiol. 2009;30:1566–1570.
5. Garrett MP, Williamson RW, Bohl MA, Bird CR, Theodore N. Computed tomography angiography as a confirmatory test for the diagnosis of brain death. J Neurosurg. 2018 Feb;128(2):639–644.
6. Chakraborty S, Dhanani S. Guidelines for use of computed tomography angiogram as an ancillary test for diagnosis of suspected brain death. Can Assoc Radiol J. 2017;68:224–228.
7. Sawicki M, Bohatyrewicz R, Walecka A, Solek-Pastuszka J, Rowinski O, Walecki J. CT angiography in the diagnosis of brain death. Pol J Radiol. 2014;79:417–421.
8. Marchand AJ, Seguin P, Malledant Y, Taleb M, Raoult H, Gauvrit JY. Revised CT angiography venous score with consideration of infratentorial circulation value for diagnosing brain death. Ann. Intensive Care. 2016; 6:88.
9. Quesnel C, Fulgencio JP, Adrie C, Marro B, Payen L, Lembert N, et al. Limitations of computed tomographic angiography in the diagnosis of brain death. Intensive Care Med. 2007;33:2129–2135.
10. Sadeghian H, Raeisi M, Dolati P, Motiei-Langroudi R. Brain computed tomography angiography as an ancillary test in the confirmation of brain death. Cureus. 2017;9(7): e1491. DOI 10.7759/cureus.1491
11. Lugt A. Imaging tests in determination of brain death. Neuroradiology. 2010;52:945–947.
12. Taylor T, Dineen RA, Gardiner DC, Buss CH, Howatson A, Pace NL. Computed tomography (CT) angiography for confirmation of the clinical diagnosis of brain death. Cochrane Database Syst Rev. 2014;3:CD009694.
13. Donohoe KJ, Agrawal G, Frey KA, et al. SNM practice guideline for brain death scintigraphy 2.0. J Nucl Med Technol. 2012;40:198–203.
14. Zuckier LS. Radionuclide evaluation of brain death in the post-McMath era. J Nucl Med. 2016 Oct;57(10):1560–1568.
15. Walter U, Schreiber SJ, Kaps M. Doppler and Duplex sonography for the diagnosis of the irreversible cessation of brain function ('brain death'): Current guidelines in Germany and neighboring countries. Ultraschall Med. 2016 Dec;37(6):558–578.
16. Poularas J, Karakitsos D, Kouraklis G, Kostakis A, De Groot E, Kalogeromitros A, et al. Comparison between transcranial color Doppler ultrasonography and angiography in the confirmation of brain death. Transplant Proc. 2006 Jun;38(5):1213–1217.
17. Lupetin AR, Davis DA, Beckman I, Dash N. Transcranial Doppler sonography. Part 2. Evaluation of intracranial and extracranial abnormalities and procedural monitoring. Radiographics. 1995 Jan;15(1):193–209.
18. Monteiro LM, Bollen CW, van Huffelen AC, Ackerstaff RG, Jansen NJ, van Vught AJ. Transcranial Doppler ultrasonography to confirm brain death: A meta-analysis. Intensive Care Med. 2006 Dec;32(12):1937–1944.

19. Ishii K, Onuma T, Kinoshita T, et al. Brain death: MR and MR angiography. AJNR Am J Neuroradiol. 1996 Apr;17: 731–735.
20. Sohn CH, Lee HP, Park JB, et al. Imaging findings of brain death on 3-tesla MRI. Korean J Radiol. 2012 Sep/Oct; 13(5): 541–921.
21. Orrison WW, Champlin AM, Kesterson OL, Hartshorne MF, King JN. MR 'hot nose sign' and 'intravascular enhancement sign' in brain death. AJNR Am J Neuroradiol. 1994 May;15(5): 913–916.

8

The role of neurophysiology

Elisa Montalenti, Paolo Costa

Historical overview

Early definitions of brain death (BD)[1–3] included, in addition to the clinical triad (unresponsiveness, absence of cephalic reflexes and apnoea), cerebral electrical inactivity documented by Electroencephalography (EEG), at that time the most sophisticated technological methodology to test brain function.

In a couple of studies in 1975 and 1976, few years after the original description by Jewett and Williston,[4] Starr and Achor studied short-latency brainstem auditory evoked potentials (BAEPs) in patients with consciousness disorder as a test to assess brainstem function and describe the specific alterations of BD.[5,6]

In 1980, Anziska and Cracco,[7] using extra-cephalic reference, demonstrated the absence of cortical components of median nerve somatosensory evoked potentials (mn-SEPs) in subjects fulfilling clinical criteria of BD. In 1981, Goldie et al.[8] studied mn-SEPs with simultaneous recording at different levels of somatosensory pathway and clearly defined the pattern of cerebral death.

A further step forward was the study of Sonoo et al.,[9] who showed that N18 far-field is preserved in non-brain-dead comatose patients, whereas it is not recordable in patients judged to be brain dead.

Rationale for the use of Clinical Neurophysiology Techniques in Intensive Care Unit

The clinical examination of Intensive Care Unit (ICU) patients is typically limited by structural damage and/or administered therapies. Conversely, due to their intrinsic nature (type of signal, presence or absence of components, latency, repeatability) Clinical Neurophysiology Techniques (CNTs) allow a quantitative assessment of nervous system that is often not possible only on clinical grounds.[10,11] Therefore, CNTs are widely used in ICU for many technical and practical reasons: they are related to cerebral metabolism, are sensitive to the most common causes of brain damage, correlate with brain topography and are able to identify neuronal dysfunction in a reversible phase.[12] CNTs are non-invasive, commonly available bedside, economical, and easy to interpret by qualified personnel. Finally, CNTs, in particular EEG, consent a fast diagnosis and are still the most used confirmatory tests for BD.

The EEG is generated by spatio-temporal summation of excitatory and inhibitory postsynaptic potentials of cortical neurons, in turn influenced by thalamus-cortical projections.[12] Many cortical neurons need to sum their activity in order to produce a detectable signal from the scalp. EEG reflects the synchronous firing of pyramidal cells of layers 3 and 5; this activity is an epiphenomenon of cellular metabolic activity.[12, 13] The EEG therefore alters in the case of metabolic suffering of the generators; in this sense is a robust, although often aspecific, indicator of brain sufferance.[13] Evoked Potentials (EPs) are generated in the peripheral and in central nervous system at subcortical/cortical levels: any structural damage causes the disappearing of responses generated at that level. Contrary to EEG, they are resistant to metabolic disturbances and medications effects.[14]

The CNTs strictly correlate with cerebral blood flow (CBF). In 1981 Astrup et al.[15] demonstrated that EEG abnormalities begin when CBF fell down from normal values (50–70 ml/100 g/min) to 25–30 ml/100 g/min. Progressive modifications in EEG parameters (morphology, amplitude, and frequency) correlate with the severity and size of cerebral ischemia.[16,17] The EEG picture of brain bioelectric inactivity represents the electrical epiphenomenon of cellular energy failure and loss of cell membrane integrity (i.e. cell death).

Electroencephalography in the diagnosis of BD

As previously mentioned, the EEG was included in the original descriptions of BD. This is probably the reason why, both in countries where

Table 8.1 Countries where Confirmatory Tests are optional or mandatory

Confirmatory Tests	Optional	Mandatory
North America	United States, Canada	—
Caribbean	Barbados, Cuba, Trinidad e Tobago	Jamaica
Central and South America	Brazil, Columbia, Costa Rica, Ecuador, Paraguay, Uruguay Venezuela	Argentina, Chile, El Salvador, Mexico
Africa	South Africa, Tunisia	Tanzania
Middle East	Oman, United Arab Emirates	Iran, Israel, Jordan, Lebanon, Qatar, Saudi Arabia
Asi	Armenia, Bangladesh, China, Hong Kong, Indonesia, South Korea, Philippines, Singapore, Taiwan, Thailand, Vietnam	Georgia, India, Japan, Malaysia
Oceania	Australia, New Zealand	
Europe	Austria, Bulgaria, Cyprus, Estonia, Finland, Greece, Ireland, Poland, Portugal, Russia, Spain, Sweden, Switzerland, UK	Belgium, Bosnia, Croatia, Denmark, France, Germany, Hungary, Italy, Lithuania, Netherlands, Norway, Romania, Slovenia, Turkey

confirmatory tests are mandatory, as well as in those where they are optional (Table 8.1), it is the most used confirmatory test.

The EEG pattern identifying BD is electrocerebral inactivity (ECI) or electrocerebral silence (ECS). Since 1970, these terms have replaced other non-physiologic descriptions as 'isoelectric', 'linear', or 'flat' EEG.[18]

The ECI is defined as no EEG activity over 2 uV when recording from scalp electrode pairs, 10 or more cm apart, with interelectrode impedances under 10,000 Ohms (10 KOhms), but over 100 Ohms.[18, 19] This pattern is maintained even when auditory and nociceptive stimuli are performed in a bilateral manner. However, the EEG is extremely sensible to CNS-depressant drugs; therefore, the absence of any possible pharmacological interference has to be ruled out before recording. In particular the presence of barbiturates, propofol, and benzodiazepines should be excluded by history, drug screen, or drug plasma levels over the therapeutic range. If an effect of sedative drugs cannot be excluded, French guidelines[20] recommend techniques based on the study of intracerebral blood flow.

According to Italian Law,[21] in case of concomitant factors (depressive drugs of the central nervous system or muscle relaxants, hypothermia, endocrine-metabolic alterations, previous systemic hypotension) cerebral flow techniques have to be used; alternatively, it is possible to wait for a reasonable period of time to correct or eliminate these factors. According to Italian Law[21] and French Guidelines,[20] the patient's body temperature has to be maintained respectively above 34°C and 35°C.

American Clinical Neurophysiology Society (ACNS) guidelines[19] recommended to record blood pressure and oxygen saturation.

There are several technical issues to be kept in mind in order to use EEG as a confirmatory test in BD diagnosis. In order to cover all the regions of the scalp a minimum of 8[20, 21] or 16[19] EEG scalp electrodes are required. French Guidelines[20] and Italian Law[21] recommend placement of electrodes at FP2, C4, O2, T4, FP1, C3, O1, T3 of the 10–20 International System, with one-channel ECG and one-channel non-cephalic recording. ACNS guidelines[19] suggest including midline electrodes (Fz, Cz, Pz) because of their sensitivity to detect the residual low-voltage physiologic activity. A sampling rate of 128[21]–256[20] Hz is recommended. The sensitivity must be increased to a maximum of 2 μV/mm. The calibration voltage should be 2 μV; impedance for each electrode must be between 100 and 10,000W. Integrity of the system should be tested by touching each electrode with a cotton swab to voluntarily create an artefact potential. The recording has to be at least of 30' and auditory and somatosensory stimuli (touch and pain) should be repeatedly performed.

According to ACNS[19] high-frequency filters should not be set below 30 Hz, and low-frequency (high pass) filters should not be set above 1Hz; French Guidelines[20] suggest a bandwidth of 0.53–70 Hz.

The 50/60 Hz notch filter can be used with care, but there should be segments of EEG that are recorded without this filter for comparison.[19]

The relevance of technologists in recording electrophysiological confirmatory tests is agreed by many guidelines.[19, 21] The role of technologist is to guarantee a technically correct recording, by identifying and eliminating artefacts, implementing the required settings, performing standard activation procedures, and documenting all relevant data in the recording. According to Italian Law[21] recording is made by a qualified technician under medical supervision. Traces have to be interpreted by a qualified electroencephalographist.

Role of evoked potentials in BD diagnosis

Evoked potentials are responses generated in central or peripheral nervous system following a sensitive/sensorial stimulation. EPs consist of a series of positive or negative deflections, with specific latency amplitude, and polarity. The stimulation modalities are the auditory (AEPs: auditory evoked potentials), visual (VEPs: visual evoked potentials), somatosensorial (SEPs: somatosensory evoked potentials), and the stimulation of the motor pathways (MEPs: motor evoked potentials). The events to be recorded are generally low voltage and are therefore in some way 'obscured' by chaotic electrical activity (EEG, EMG), unrelated to the stimulus. It is therefore necessary to average many events to allow EPs to stand out from the underlying activity. Cortical potentials are largely determined by the temporal summation of excitatory and inhibitory postsynaptic potentials generated in the cellular soma and dendrites in response to stimulus.

Subcortical potentials are probably made up of two types of components: (1) postsynaptic potentials generated near subcortical nuclei and (2) axon action potentials. The first component, due to stationary generators, is probably the basis of potentials that are widely recorded with stable latencies (e.g. the N13 of the median SEPs). The second component, by the waves propagated by the afferent volley, generates potentials whose latency varies by a few milliseconds depending on the recording site.

The term near-field potential (NFP) means that the signal is located immediately below the recording electrode. Therefore, the electrode records the variation in potential that occurs between the depolarization area and the repolarization area. As a result, the localization of the electrode is very important, since the amplitude of the signal is attenuated by the bony and cutaneous structures interposed between the generator and the electrode.

Far-field potentials (FFPs) are also generated by the depolarization of the cell membrane. The electrode (located away from the generator) does not 'see' the variation in potential between areas of depolarization and repolarization, but rather the polarization front; they are therefore widely distributed. FFPs account for a large percentage of registered PE, because generators are often located deeply in the nervous system. FFPs (whose morphology consists of a simple positive deflection) are of low voltage and sometimes difficult to record, due to the distance between the generator and the electrode; their amplitude is however less attenuated by bone and cutaneous structures.

The EPs consist of a series of waves or peaks generated in response to a particular stimulus. Each component can be defined on the basis of the following characteristics: polarity (positive or negative), sequential numbering, latency, amplitude, morphology.

Traces are examined by evaluating the presence or absence of the components present in normal subjects, the absolute or interpeak latencies and, in some cases, the amplitude ratios. The complete absence of an EP component is indicative of a complete interruption of the conduction generated by a pathological process whose lesion level is placed caudally to the generator of the first expected component. The absence of components can be considered as the maximum level of severity of a lesion which, in a milder form, produces a reduction in amplitude, an increase in latency or both anomalies. A detailed description of EPs goes beyond the purposes of this chapter; therefore the attention will be focused on the short-latency BAEPs and the mn-SEPs, the most used EPs in ICU.

Brainstem Auditory Evoked Potentials

The BAEPs are electrical events recordable in the first 10 milliseconds (ms) after an acoustic stimulus; they are FPPs consisting of 5 waves expressed in Roman numerals, of which 3 (I, III, and V) are recordable in 100% of normal subjects. The path explored goes from the VIII nerve to the midbrain. BAEPs are not modified by the majority of sedative/hypnotic drugs[22] and by anaesthetics, even at doses that flatten the EEG.[23]

Waveforms and generators

Wave I: This is the component of BAEPs whose generator is better known; in fact, it is generated by the Nerve VIII, probably at the proximal level and corresponds to the N1 of the electrocochlearogram.[24]

Wave II: For many years it was thought to be generated by the ipsilateral cochlear nucleus. But intraoperative recording[24–26] and the recordability of the II wave in brain-dead subjects[27] clarified that the intracranial portion of VIII nerve, very close to the brainstem, may at least partly contribute to the genesis of wave II.

Wave III: The III wave generator is located in the caudal pons; in fact this wave is abolished by the lesion or anesthetization of the trapezoid body[28, 29] and from lesions of the medial part of the contralateral superior olive complex.[29] Probably it is the correlate of the contralateral trapezoid body activation[30] or of the outflow from the superior olivary complex lateral to the lateral lemniscus.[31]

Wave IV and V: The generators hypothesized for the IV–V wave complex are located at high pontine/low mesencephalic level. The structures of the brainstem that give the greatest contribution to the V wave are the lateral lemniscus and / or the inferior colliculus ipsi and contralateral lemniscus on the stimulated side.[32–34]

As mentioned earlier, waves I, III, and V are present in all normal subjects. Thus, the absence of wave V is an expression of lesion of the mesencephalic level, the absence of wave III indicates lesion at the level of the caudal pons.

BAEPs finding in BD

Patients who meet the clinical and EEG criteria of BD have 2 characteristic patterns[27]:

1. In 75% of cases no component of the BAEPs (including wave I) is recordable, even at the maximum stimulation intensity.
2. In the remaining cases, wave I or waves I and II (generated by the VIII nerve and the cochlear nucleus) are recordable and repeatable (Figure 8.1 B); this condition is certainly indicative of BD (that is of the brainstem).

However, the most frequent situation, in which no component of BAEPs is recognizable, does not allow to exclude a serious damage of

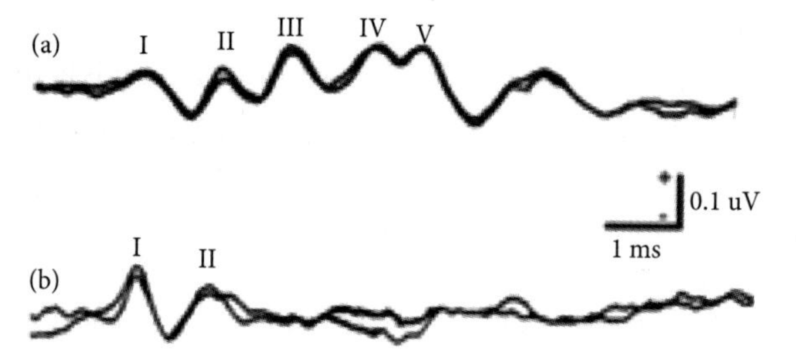

Figure 8.1. (A) Normal BAEPs in a healthy subject. (B) Loss of components following wave II in a brain death patient.

the peripheral portion of acoustic pathway, either acquired (i.e. cochlear damage due to a transverse fracture of the temporal bone) or pre-existing.

The absence of all BAEP waves in BD is probably due to due to cochlear ischaemia from arrest of the cerebral circulation. This is the reason why the BAEPs cannot be the only method for evaluating the brainstem, though they are generally used in association with the SEPs.[35]

Median nerve somatosensory evoked potentials

The mn-SEPs are electrical potentials generated by various portions of the ascending sensory pathways. They are widely used in the ICU in the evaluation of coma and BD because the amplitude of the signal is robust even in sedated and curarized patient.

The mn-SEPs consent the recording of the ascending volley from brachial plexus to spinal cord, to brainstem up to the cerebral cortex. The generators of waves used for clinical diagnostics (particularly in ICU) will be described below.

Waveforms and generators

N9: The first event from the ipsilateral Erb point to the stimulated side is a negative-positive-negative complex, with a latency of about 9 ms, called N9. This NFP is not detectable from the contralateral neck to the stimulated side and is attributed to the passage of the afferent volley through the brachial plexus and the cervical roots proximal to the Erb point.[36]

N13: This is an NFP with a phase-reversal, becoming positive (P13) with both oesophageal and surface recording.[36–38] The N13 is thought to be generated by excitatory postsynaptic potentials in the interneurons of the IV-V laminae of the posterior horns of the spinal cord, being the axis of the dipole equivalent horizontally from the back to the front.[39]

P14: It is an FFP that is thought to be generated by the caudal portion of the medial lemniscus[38, 40] and which represents the electrical correlate of the afferent volley in the medial lemniscus.

N18: This is a widespread negativity with the characteristics of the FFP. It has been hypothesized that it is the correlative of excitatory post-synaptic potentials in the soma or in the dendrites of the cuneate nucleus and / or in the nuclei of the brainstem that receive afferents from the cuneate nucleus.[41] According to another, more revolutionary hypothesis, the N18 could represent the electrical correlate of the volley afferent to the cuneate nucleus and have, therefore, more caudal generators than those of the P14.[42, 43]

N20: This is the first NFP recordable by the scalp. It is recordable only from the contralateral parietal regions to the stimulated side where it is superimposed to the N18. A majority of authors consider the N20 as the electrical correlate of the initial response of the sensory cortex to the arrival of the afferent volley.[44–48]

Therefore, by stimulating the median nerve we can record responses generated by the brachial plexus, cervical cord, brainstem, and cortex (Figure 8.2). This is extremely important to assess the functionality of the

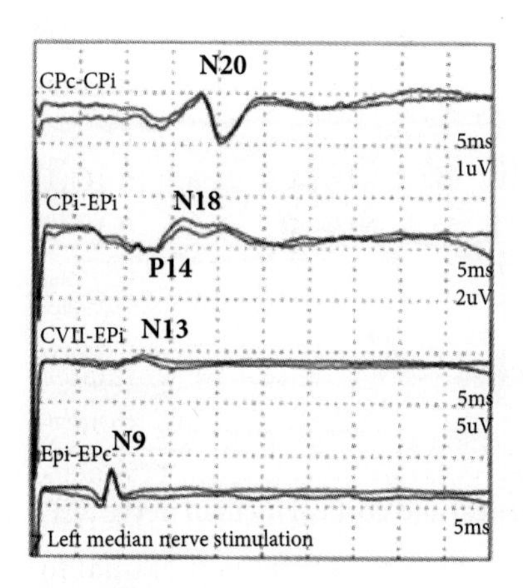

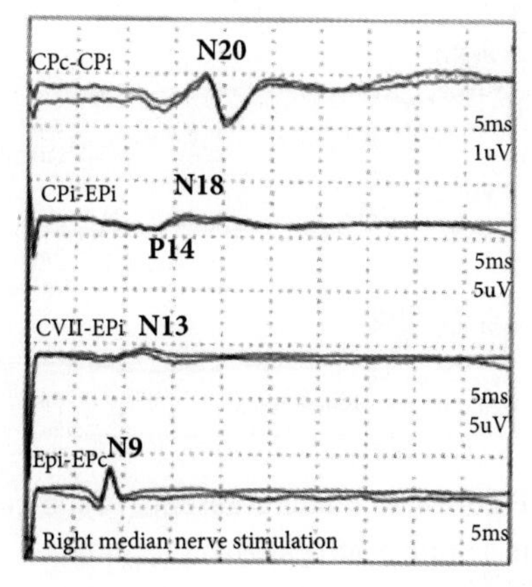

Figure 8.2. Bilateral normal median nerve SEPs in a healthy subject.

nervous system in subjects with consciousness disorder and to confirm the diagnosis of BD.

mn-SEPs finding in BD

The characteristic finding of BD is constituted by the recording of plexual N9 and cervical N13, in the absence of the other components (subcortical and cortical—Figure 8.3). The pathophysiological significance of this finding fits well with BD, indicating conduction block at bulbar level, with preservation of the sensory input. The recordability of P14 can explain some residual respiratory function in subjects who also meet all the criteria for the diagnosis of BD.[49] Wagner et al.[50, 51] showed that nasopharyngeal recordings of P14 could correctly differentiate between non-brain-dead coma and BD, but the technical difficulty may prevent its routine application.

Sonoo et al.[9] showed that N18 far-field is preserved in non-brain-dead comatose patients, whereas it is not recordable in patients judged to be brain dead. The combined use of BAEPs and mn-SEPs have demonstrated to improve the reliability of diagnosis.[52]

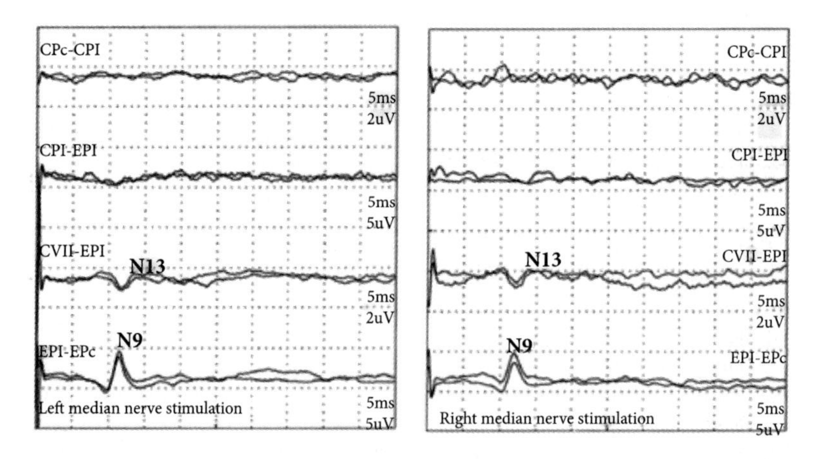

Figure 8.3. Bilateral absence of sub-cortical and cortical median nerve SEPs in a brain death patient.

Conclusion

When confounding factors are excluded, CNTs consent a fast diagnosis of BD. The combined recording of EEG, BAEPs, and mn-SEPs consent a quick and sensitive evaluation of brainstem and cortical functions. CNTs are widely used in ICU for many technical and practical reasons; they are related to cerebral metabolism, are sensitive to the most common causes of brain damage, correlate with brain topography and are able to identify neuronal dysfunction in a reversible phase.[12] Finally, CNTs, in particular EEG consent a fast diagnosis and are still the most used confirmatory tests for BD.

Highlights

- CNTs, in particular EEG, are the most used confirmatory test for BD.
- When confounding factors are excluded the pattern of BD is clear and easy to interpret by expert personnel.
- The combined use of EEG and multimodal EPs may improve the reliability of diagnosis.

References

1. Mollaret P, Goulon M. Le coma dépassé. Rev Neurol (Paris) 1959;101:3–15.
2. Wertheimer P, Jouvet M, Descotes J. Diagnosis of death of the nervous system in comas with respiratory arrest treated by artificial respiration. Presse Med. 1959; 67:87–88.
3. A definition of irreversible coma: Report of the Ad Hoc Committee of the Harvard Medical School to examine the definition of brain death. JAMA 1968; 205:337–340.
4. Jewett, DL Williston, JS. Auditory evoked far-fields averaged from the scalp of humans. Brain, 1971; 94: 681–696.
5. Starr A, Achor J. Auditory brain stem responses in neurological disease. Arch Neurol. 1975 Nov;32(11):761–768.
6. Starr A. Auditory brain-stem responses in brain death. Brain, 1976; 99: 543–554.
7. Anziska BJ, Cracco RQ. Short latency somatosensory evoked potentials in brain dead patients. Arch Neurol, 1980; 37:222–225.

8. Goldie WD, Chiappa KH, Young RR, Brooks EB. Brainstem auditory and short-latency somatosensory evoked responses in brain death. Neurology. 1981 Mar;31(3):248–256.
9. Sonoo M, Tsai-Shozawa Y, Aoki M, et al., N18 in median somatosensory evoked potentials: A new indicator of medullary function useful for the diagnosis of brain death. J Neurol Neurosurg Psychiatry. 1999 Sep;67(3):374–378.
10. Amantini A, Carrai R, Lori S et al. Neurophysiological monitoring in adult and pediatric intensive care. Minerva Anestesiol. 2012;78:1067–1075.
11. Guérit JM, Amantini A, Amodio P et al. Consensus on the use of neurophysiological tests in the intensive care unit (ICU): electroencephalogram (EEG), evoked potentials (EP), and electroneuromyography (ENMG). Neurophysiol Clin. 2009;39(2):71–83.
12. Jordan KG. Continuous EEG monitoring in the neuroscience intensive care unit and emergency department. J Clin Neurophysiol, 1999;16:14–39.
13. Jordan KG. Continuous EEG and evoked potential monitoring in the neuroscience intensive care unit. J Clin Neurophysiol 1993;10:445–475.
14. Sloan TB, Jäntti V. Anesthetic effects on evoked potentials. In Nuwer MR (ed.), Intraoperative monitoring of neural function. Handbook of clinical neurophysiology, 8. Amsterdam, Elsevier; 2008: 94–126.
15. Astrup J, Simon L, Siesjo BK, et al. Thresholds in cerebral ischemias—the ischemic penumbra. Stroke 1981; 2:723–725.
16. Sharbrough FW, Messick JM, Sundt TM. Correlation of continuous electroencephalograms with cerebral blood flow measurements during carotid endarterectomy. Stroke 1973; 4:674–683.
17. Sundt TM Jr, Sharbrough FW, Piepgras DG et al. Correlation of cerebral blood flow and electroencephalographic changes during carotid endarterectomy with results of surgery and hemodynamics of cerebral ischemia. Mayo Clin Proc 1981; 56:533–543.
18. Chatrian GE, Bergamini L, Dondey M, Klass DW, Lennox-Buchthal M, Peterson I. A glossary of terms most commonly used by clinical electroencephalographers. Electroencephalogr Clin Neurophysiol 1974;37:538–548.
19. Stecker MM, Sabau D, Sullivan L, Das RR, Selioutski O, Drislane FW et al. American Clinical Neurophysiology Society Guideline 6: Minimum technical standards for EEG recording in suspected cerebral death. J Clin Neurophysiol 2016;33:324–327.
20. Szurhaj W, Lamblin MD, Kaminska A, Sediri H. Société de Neurophysiologie Clinique de Langue Française. EEG guidelines in the diagnosis of brain death. Neurophysiol Clin. 2015 Mar;45(1):97–104.
21. Law no. 578 dated 29/12/1993; The Ministerial Decree relating to the modalities of ascertaining and certifying death, no. 582 dated 22/09/1994, updated on 20/02/2009.
22. Stockard JJ, Rossiter VS, Jones TA, Sharbrough FW. Effects of centrally acting drug on brainstem auditory responses. Electroencephalogr Clin Neurophysiol 1977; 43: 550–551.
23. Markand ON. Brainstem auditory evoked potentials. J Clin Neurophysiol 1994; 11 (3): 319–342.
24. Moller AR, Jannetta PJ, Moller MB. Neural generators of brainstem auditory evoked potentials. Results from human intracranial recordings. Ann Otol Rhinol Laryngol 1981; 90: 591–596.

25. Hashimoto I, Ishiyama Y, Yoshimoto Y, Nemoto S. Brainstem auditory evoked potentials recorded directly from human brainstem and thalamus. Brain 1981; 104: 841–859.
26. Jannetta PJ, Moller MB. Neural generators of brainstem auditory evoked potentials. Results from human intracranial recordings. Ann Otol Rhinol Laryngol 1981; 90: 591–596.
27. Goldie WD, Chiappa JH, Young RR, Brooks EG. Brainstem auditory and short-latency somatosensory evoked responses in brain death. Neurology 1981; 31: 248–256.
28. Brown RH, Chiappa KH, Brooks EB. Brainstem auditory evoked responses in 22 patients with intrinsic brainstem lesions. Electroencephalogr Clin Neurophysiol 1981; 51: 38P.
29. Wada SI, Starr A. Generation of brainstem auditory evoked responses (ABRs) II Effects of surgical section of the trapezoidal body on the ABR of guinea pigs and cats Electroencephalogr Clin Neurophysiol, 1983, 56: 340–351.
30. Buchwald JS. Generators. In Moore EJ (ed.) *Basis of auditory brainstem responses.* New York, Grune & Stratton, 1983: 157–195.
31. Krumholz A, Felix JK, Goldstein PJ, et al. Maturation of the brainstem auditory evoked potential in premature infants. Electroencephalogr Clin Neurophysiol 1985; 62: 124–134.
32. Hashimoto I, Ishiyama Y, Tozuka G. Bilaterally recorded brainstem auditory evoked responses, their asymmetric abnormalities and lesions of the brainstem. Arch Neurol 1979; 36: 161–167.
33. Oh SJ, Kuba T, Soyer A, Choi S, Bonikowski FP, Vtek J. Lateralization of brainstem lesions by brainstem auditory evoked potentials. Neurology 1981; 31: 14–18.
34. Starr A, Achor J. Auditory brainstem responses in neurological disease. Arch Neurol 1975; 32: 761–768.
35. Facco E, Munari M, Gallo F, Volpin SM, Behr AU, Baratto F, Giron GP. Role of short latency evoked potentials in the diagnosis of brain death. Clin Neurophysiol 2002;113:1855–1866.
36. Emerson RG, Seyal M, Pedley TA. Somatosensory evoked potentials following median nerve stimulation. I. Cervical components. Brain 1984; 107: 169–182.
37. Desmedt JE. Non invasive analysis of the spinal cord generators activated by somatosensory input in man: near field and far-field potentials. Exp Brain Res 1984; 9: 45–62.
38. Seyal M, Gabor AJ. Generators of human spinal somatosensory evoked potentials. J Clin Neurophysiol 1987;4: 177–187.
39. Desmedt JE, Nguyen TH. Bit mapped colour imaging of the potentials fields of propagated and segmental subcortical components of somatosensory evoked potentials in man. Electroencephalogr Clin Neurophysiol 1984; 59: 481–497.
40. Kaji R, Ritsuho T, Kawaguchi S, MsCormick F, Kameyama M. Origin of short-latency somatosensory evoked potentials to median nerve stimulation in the cat. Comparison of the recordings montages and effect of laminectomy. Brain 1986; 109: 443–468.
41. Desmedt JE. Neuromonitoring in surgery (Clinical Neurophysiology Updates vol I). Elsevier, Amsterdam,1989.

42. Noel P, Ozaki I, Desmedt JE. Origin of N18 and P14 far-fields of median nerve somatosensory evoked potentials studied in patients with a brain-stem lesion. Electroencephalogr Clin Neurophysiol 1996; 98: 167–170.
43. Sonoo M, Tsai-Shozawa Y, Aoki M, et al., N18 in median somatosensory evoked potentials: a new indicator of medullary function useful for the diagnosis of brain death. J Neurol Neurosurg Psychiatry 1999;67:374–378.
44. Allison T, Goff WR, Williamson PD, van Gilder JC. On the neural origin of early components of the human somato-sensory evoked potential. In JE Desmedt (ed.): *Clinical uses of cerebral, brainstem and spinal somatosensory evoked potentials*. Karger, Basel, 1980: 51–68.
45. Allison T, Hume AL. A comparative analysis of short-latency somatosensory evoked potentials in man, monkey, cat, rat. Exp Neurol 1981;72:592:611.
46. Desmedt JE, Cheron G. Prevertebral (oesophageal) recording of subcortical somatosensory evoked potentials in man: The spinal N13 component and the dual nature of the spinal generators. Electroencephalogr Clin Neurophysiol 1981; 52: 257–275.
47. Hume AL, Cant BR. Conduction time in central somatosensory pathways in man. Electroencephalogr Clin Neurophysiol 1978; 45: 361–375.
48. Mauguiére F, Desmedt JE, Courion J. Astereognosis and dissociated loss of frontal or parietal components of somatosensory evoked potentials in hemispheric lesions. Brain 1983;106: 271–311.
49. Chiappa KH, Hill AR. Short-latency somatosensory evoked potentials: Interpretation. In Chiappa KH (ed.) Evoked potentials in clinical medicine [3th. Edition]. Lippicott-Raven Publishers. 1997: 341–400.
50. Wagner W. SEP testing in deeply comatose and brain dead patients: The role of nasopharyngeal, scalp and earlobe derivations in recording the P14 potential. Electroencephalogr Clin Neurophysiol 1991;80:352–363.
51. Wagner W. Scalp, earlobe and nasopharyngeal recordings of the median nerve somatosensory evoked P14 potential in coma and brain death: Detailed latency and amplitude analysis in 181 patients. Brain 1996;119:1507–1521.
52. Facco E, Munari M, Gallo F et al. Role of short latency evoked potentials in the diagnosis of brain death. Clin Neurophysiol 2002;113:1855–1866.

9

The role of cerebral blood flow studies

Anna Teresa Mazzeo, Simona Veglia, Domenica Garabello, Deepak Gupta

Introduction

The diagnosis of brain death (BD) is essentially a clinical diagnosis, which should be systematic, rigorous, and complete. Documentation of each component of the clinical examination performed for the diagnosis of BD is essential. Determination of BD with clinical examination is possible in the majority of cases, in the clinical practice.

However, there are specific situations in which neurologic clinical examination cannot be complete, or the eventuality of confounding factors cannot be excluded, where the use of ancillary tests become an essential component of the diagnosis of BD. These tests originally referred to as 'confirmatory tests' have been more recently termed 'ancillary tests', as the latter term appears more appropriate to describe their role in assisting the clinician in the diagnosis of BD. In any case, ancillary tests can never be used to replace neurological clinical examination which remains the cornerstone of the diagnosis.

Rationale for the use of cerebral blood flow studies

The key role of cerebral blood flow (CBF) studies as ancillary tests in the diagnosis of BD can be appreciated only if the underlying pathophysiological mechanisms of BD are understood. CBF is normally maintained within a range of 45–60 mL/100 g of brain tissue/min. The occurrence of a catastrophic acute brain injury results in cerebral oedema due to numerous event cascades which further develops intracranial hypertension with consequent reduced cerebral perfusion pressure (CPP) and eventually reduced CBF. A CBF below 35 mL/100g/min will determine a cessation of neuronal protein synthesis and below 15–20 mL/100g/min, 'electric failure' with modification of synaptic transmission and isoelectric EEG will occur. The flow threshold for 'ion pump failure', irreversible damage and neuronal death occurs at 10 to 12 mL/100 g/min.[1]

This progressive acute ischemic damage will spread involving the whole brain as well as the intracranial vessels which will become compressed, further extending infarction, and leading to necrosis. When intracranial pressure (ICP) overcomes systolic arterial pressure (SAP), cerebral perfusion will cease and BD will occur. The arrest of cerebral circulation is a gradual phenomenon rather than an on and off effect, which will primarily affect the deep cerebral veins and capillaries, and then large arteries.[2,3] Furthermore, it should be remembered that a rostro-caudal progression of cerebral circulatory arrest is usually observed, with an increase in ICP first in supratentorial region than in infratentorial region, due to an initial protective function of the cerebellar tentorium. Therefore, as an adequate CBF is essential to maintain cerebral function, the arrest of cerebral circulation is the anatomopathological substrate of irreversibility of BD. To be consistent with the concept of BD, CBF studies have to document the absent blood flow in the anterior circulation as well as in the posterior circulation.[4]

Tests demonstrating absence of CBF represent the ideal ancillary tests for the diagnosis of BD, as they are not affected by metabolic disturbances, by residual effect of sedatives, hypothermia, or by other factors potentially affecting neurological clinical examination.

Indications for CBF studies

Before starting neurological clinical examination for the diagnosis of BD, it is imperative for the clinician to document essential prerequisites which are the certainty of aetiology and the exclusion of confounding factors. Neuroimaging should demonstrate a catastrophic brain damage consistent with the clinical picture. The exclusion of confounding factors which may interfere with the clinical examination is of paramount importance and must always precede the clinical examination. Clinicians should take enough time to exclude any factor which may mimic BD or affect the neurological examination. The confirmation of the absence of residual effects of analgesics or sedative drugs that could interfere with the clinical picture is essential. If reversible alterations in thermal, metabolic, and hemodynamic homeostasis are identified, these should be treated and corrected whenever possible. When reliability on some part of clinical examination is not certain, or if some component of the clinical examination cannot be completed, then clinicians should order a CBF test to confirm the clinical diagnosis. The indications to the use of CBF studies as ancillary tests in the diagnosis of BD are presented in Box 9.1.

For the purpose of BD diagnosis, the ideal CBF study should be a safe, bedside procedure that is not invasive or minimally invasive, readily available, and operator independent. Furthermore, it should provide 100% specificity, meaning that no false-positive results are allowed. A false-positive result is defined when a test detects no CBF but the patient is not clinically dead. Indeed, when used to confirm BD diagnosis, high specificity is of paramount importance and is more important than

Box 9.1 Indications for cerebral blood flow studies to confirm the diagnosis of brain death

- When even a single component of clinical diagnosis cannot be reliably performed (i.e. severe maxillofacial trauma precluding elicitation of some brainstem reflexes, fracture of rocca petrosa precluding oculovestibular reflex etc.)
- In presence of mimicking medical conditions or confounding factors, such as severe alterations in thermal, metabolic, hemodynamic, and endocrine homeostasis, that could interfere with the clinical picture (i.e hypothermia, severe sodium alterations etc.)
- High cervical spinal cord injury (which may affect apnea test or neurological clinical examination)
- When it is not possible to exclude the effect of sedative or analgesic drugs, or in the presence of organ dysfunction interfering with drug pharmacokinetics.
- Impossibility to complete apnea test for physiological instability
- Children less than one year of age
- If required by specific national laws

high sensitivity.[5,6] None of the tests, in fact, should demonstrate signs of BD when the patient is not clinically BD.

While all tests used in the clinical practice to document absence of CBF provide 100% specificity, they differ in their sensitivity and negative predictive value.[7] Maximizing sensitivity will reduce false-negative classifications. A false-negative result occurs when a test still detects residual CBF but the patient is already clinically BD. This will require a repetition of the test after some hours and will postpone the determination of death. False-negative results are described in the presence of a skull defect, as in the case of an extensive fracture, when decompressive craniectomy has been performed, if ventricular drain has been placed, or in some specific circumstances such as open fontanelles and expansible skulls in infants (events that may all limit the effects of an increased ICP).

Several CBF studies are used worldwide to confirm the clinical diagnosis of BD and are approved by respective national guidelines for this purpose.[8–12] The choice of the test depends on local availability and preferences, different invasiveness, and costs. A rich literature has been growing during the last decades to confirm their role for the purpose of this diagnosis. In this chapter we will describe the role of cerebral angiography, computed tomography angiography (CTA), nuclear medicine, and magnetic resonance (MR) angiography as CBF studies to confirm clinical diagnosis of BD. The role of transcranial doppler for this purpose will be addressed in Chapter 10 of this book.

Four-vessel contrast intra-arterial cerebral angiogram

Cerebral angiography has been considered the gold standard of CBF studies to which all the other tests have been compared. After selective injection of contrast media in carotids and vertebral arteries, criteria for BD confirmation in conventional angiography are: documentation of non-filling of intracranial arteries at the entry to the skull in both anterior and posterior circulation; arrest of the contrast at the petrosal portion of the internal carotid arteries and at the foramen magnum in the vertebral arteries; normal flow in external carotid arteries which remain patent and fills rapidly and early; and non-visualization of the internal cerebral veins and vein of Galen. Longitudinal sagittal sinus or lateral sinus contrast may occur in the presence of shunt through emissary vein from the external carotid circulation.[3,4,13,14]

In the clinical practice, cerebral angiography is the least used among other CBF examinations to confirm BD, due to its invasiveness, need of large quantity of contrast medium, need to access angiographic suite which may not be readily available in many peripheral hospitals and greater technical complexity than other more widely available tests. In Figure 9.1 cerebral angiography documenting absence of CBF is illustrated.

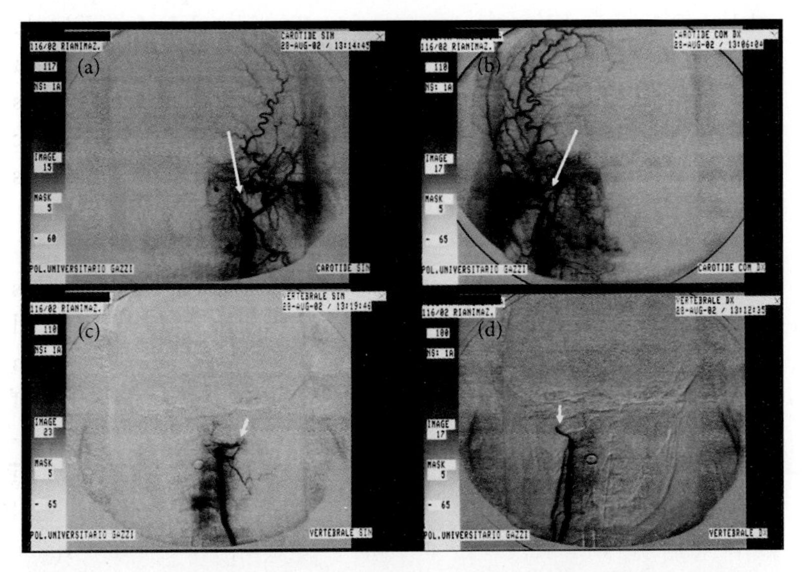

Figure 9.1. Catheter angiogram after aortic arch injection shows lack of contrast in intracranial segments of internal carotid and vertebral arteries and with contrast in external carotid artery branches. The white arrows indicate the stop of CBF at the level of right and left internal carotid arteries at skull base for the anterior circulation, and at the level of the two vertebral arteries at foramen magnum for the posterior circulation

Computed tomography angiography

Among CBF studies which can be used to confirm cerebral circulatory arrest, CTA is easily available 24 hours per day in most hospitals; it is rapid, non-invasive, inexpensive, and non-operator dependent.[5] It was first proposed by Dupas in 1998[15] as a reliable tool to confirm BD. Since then CTA has been widely investigated in literature and several national guidelines have included it among CBF studies for confirming BD.[8,10–12,16–18]

When CTA is used to confirm cerebral circulatory arrest, a complete assessment of the cerebral vasculature is required, including both anterior and posterior circulation, and the exam will be positive if it will document the absence of filling of intracranial arteries at the level of intracranial entrance. For a correct exam, external carotid arteries should be normally visualized, which will confirm the successful intravenous contrast injection and will rule out hemodynamic compromise causing a delay of contrast delivery to vessels of neck and head. In fact a severe hypotension could affect the result of the exam and needs to be excluded.

In Figure 9.2, CTA showing the absence of filling of intracranial arteries at the level of intracranial entrance is presented.

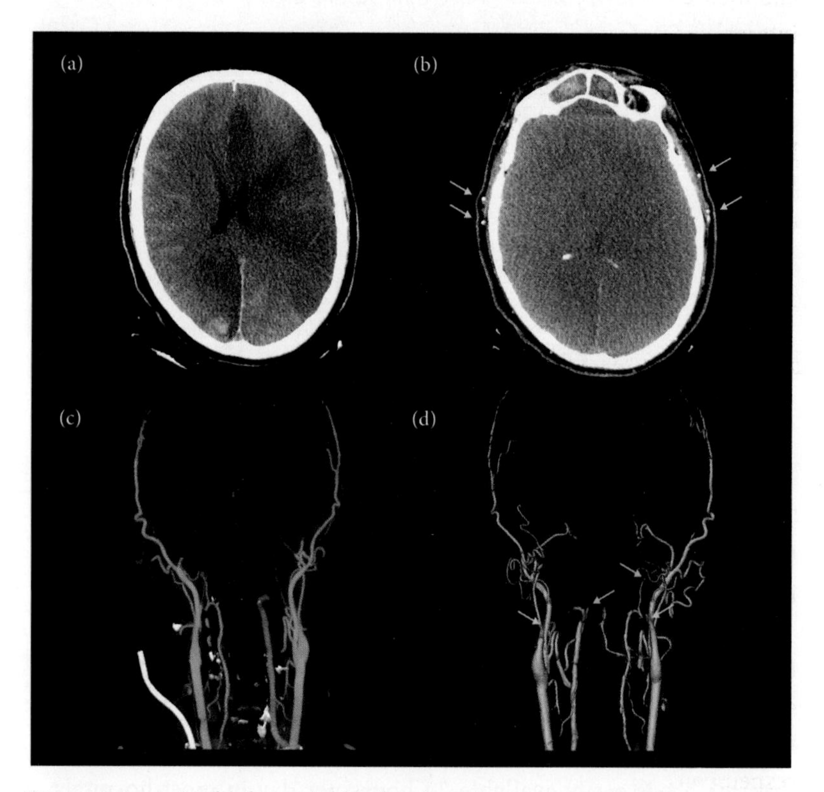

Figure 9.2. A. Multiple cerebral infarctions associated with right occipital intracerebral haemorrhage. B. CT-Angiography, axial plane: Regular extracranial vessels opacification (arrows). C and D: MIP and Volume-Rendering: Absence of carotid (yellow arrows) and vertebral arteries (green arrows) before intracranial entrance

Several protocols of CTA have been described in literature, explaining the difficulties in comparing results between different studies.[4,10] A summary of the CTA protocol revised in 2014 by the Italian Council of the National Transplant Center (Consulta tecnica nazionale per i trapianti)[11] regarding the application of CBF in the determination of BD is presented in Box 9.2.

According to published literature,[15,19,20] for the diagnosis of BD, opacification of the following vessels is recorded: Superficial temporal arteries (STA), the right and left anterior cerebral arteries and their pericallosal segments (ACA-A3), the right and left middle cerebral arteries and their cortical segments (MCA-M4), the right and left posterior cerebral arteries and their cortical segments (PCA-P2), basilar artery (BA), right and left internal cerebral veins (ICV), and the great cerebral vein (GCV)—the vein of Galen.

Either 4-points or 7-points or 10-points measurements have been proposed as diagnostic criteria for BD confirmation in literature, with a diagnostic sensitivity differing depending on the adopted criteria.

10-point: • BA, • Right and left PCA-P2, • Right and left ACA-A3, • Right and left MCA-M4; • Right and left ICV; • GCV[19]

7-point: • Right and left ACA-A3; • Right and left MCA-M4; • Right and left ICV; • GCV[15]

4-point: • Right and left MCA-M4; • Right and left ICV[20]

The main critique of the use of the 4- and 7-point grading scales is that they do not fulfil the condition of the concept of whole BD, as they do not include posterior circulation.

In a study comparing sensitivity of these three scales to confirm the diagnosis of BD, Sawiski et al.[21] reported that in the 10-, 7-, and 4-point scales sensitivities were 67%, 74%, and 96%, respectively, with an inter-observer agreement percentage of 93%, 89%, and 95%, respectively.

In a meta-analysis on twelve studies involving 541 patients, Kramer et al[5] showed that CTA diagnostic accuracy is highly dependent on the methodology and specific criteria are used to confirm cessation of intracranial blood flow: if complete lack of opacification of

Box 9.2 Summary of the Computed Tomography Angiography protocol for the determination of absent cerebral blood flow to confirm brain death, by the Italian Council of the National Transplant Center (Consulta tecnica nazionale per i trapianti).

CH CTA exam phases:

1) First a non-enhanced spiral scanning (from C2 to vertex) is used as a reference, with 0.4–0.6 mm increments, and multiple planar reconstruction (MPR) images of 3–4 mm.
2) Administration of contrast medium (1ml/Kg body weight) in an antecubital vein or a central venous catheter with a power injector, followed by 30 ml (15 ml in children) of an isotonic saline solution (rate: 3.5 ml/s). Post contrast CT acquisition (from C6 to vertex, with 0.4–0.6 mm increments) will start 5 seconds after opacification of aortic arch. Multiple Intensity Reconstruction is used. Regular opacification of external carotid arteries and in particular, STA is used as an indicator of adequacy of the exam.
3) For the venous phase CTA a repeated acquisition will start after 40 sec after the end of arterial phase, with MPR images with 3–4 mm increments as in the first scanning.

CH Interpretation of the results:

- CTA indicates ***absent CBF*** if there is a stop of contrast medium at siphon level and foramen magnum with absence of opacification of intracranial arterial vessels.
- CTA indicates ***persistent CBF*** if opacification of distal tracts of middle cerebral artery (M3/M4) or anterior cerebral artery (A3/A4) or posterior cerebral artery (P2/P3) is present.
- If there is opacification of proximal tracts of middle cerebral artery (M1/M2) or of anterior cerebral artery (A1/A2) or of basilar artery (BA) or of posterior cerebral artery (P1), as expression of stasis filling, a venous phase is required:
  - if one or both internal cerebral veins are opacified, the exam indicates ***persistent CBF.***
  - if there is no opacification of both internal cerebral veins, the exam indicates ***absent CBF.***

intracranial vessels was the referral criterion, sensitivity was 84% (95% Confidence Interval (CI) 75–94%) for CTA performed during the arterial phase. If the CTA criterion for declaration of BD was absence of any opacification of blood vessels supplying the brain during the venous phase, then the sensitivity of CTA was 62% (95% CI 50–74%).[5] Using the 4-point criteria (absence of opacification of distal MCA branches and internal cerebral veins) improved the sensitivity of CTA in the venous phase to 85% (95% CI 77–93%,[5] while the sensitivity of the 7-point scale was 71% (95% CI 61–81%). In another meta-analysis with reportedly significant heterogeneity encountered while using CTA criteria for BD, Taylor and colleagues[22] reported a pooled sensitivity of 84% (95% CI 69–93%). More recently, in a study to assess CTA in diagnosing BD, CTA had a sensitivity of 75%, a specificity of 100%, a positive predictive value of 100%, and a negative predictive value of 33%.[23]

Stasis filling

The term stasis filling has been used to describe a delayed, weak, and persistent intracranial opacification of proximal segments of the cerebral arteries in patients with BD.[24,25,6] Its occurrence has been variably reported with an incidence of 5%,[26] 12.5%,[13] 28%,[3] and 43%[15] in angiographic studies, and even higher 43–59% in CTA.[15,4]

Stasis filling has been related to increased ICP, high cerebrovascular resistance, and altered cerebral autoregulation mechanisms which determine the cessation of capillary circulation while proximal arterial segments may remain patent.[6,25] The occurrence of stasis filling does not preclude the diagnosis of BD, as it does not indicate any residual brain perfusion but only ineffective propagation of contrast in cerebral vessels.[25,27] Nevertheless, to exclude any persistent CBF, several CTA protocols will include the venous phase.

Furthermore, Shankar et al.[28] demonstrated computed tomographic perfusion (CTP) parameters consistent with nonviable brainstem in patients with preserved filling of supratentorial vessels when using CTA, therefore confirming that stasis filling does not preclude BD diagnosis.[27] Indeed, CT perfusion has been evaluated as an ancillary test in the diagnosis of BD,[29] showing a sensitivity of 100%. CTP findings were interpreted as consistent with BD diagnosis if CBF and cerebral blood volume values were below the thresholds for neuronal necrosis (i.e. 10 mL/100 g/min and 1.0 mL/100 g, respectively). Therefore, it was suggested that performing CTP together with the commonly used CTA, especially if the CTA finding shows intracranial filling, could increase the sensitivity of CTA.[27]

In a systematic review to assesses the accuracy of CTA and CTP in confirming BD, including studies from 1998 to 2014 and involving 322 patients, a sensitivity of 87.5% was reported.[30] Figure 9.3 illustrates CTA appearance of stasis filling.

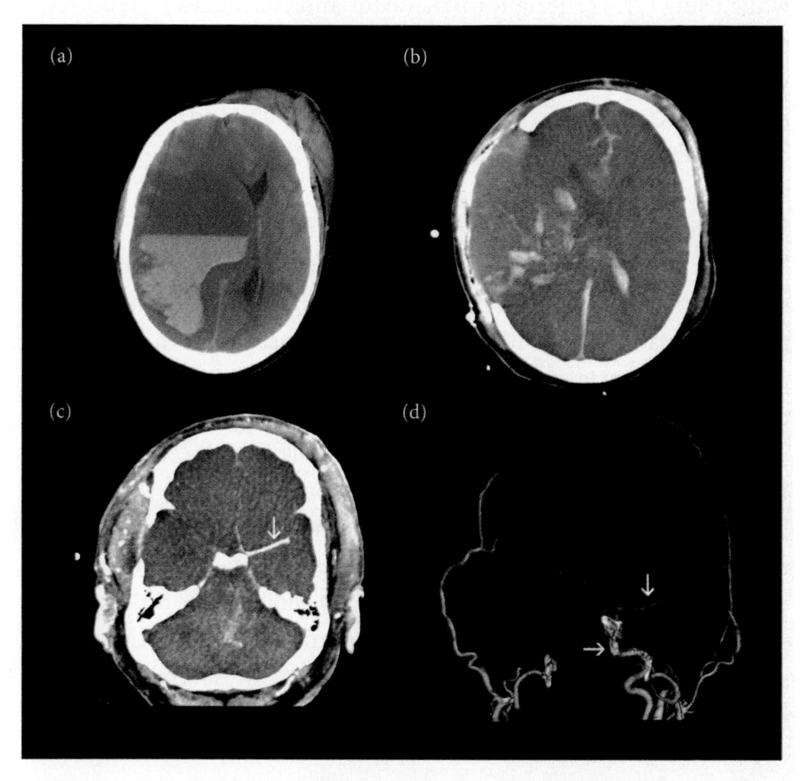

Figure 9.3. A. Large traumatic intracerebral haemorrhage, with subarachnoid haemorrhage. B. After decompressive craniectomy. C and D: CT-Angiography and Coronal 3D: Regular extracranial vessels opacification. Absence of opacification of intracranial arteries except for the left common carotid artery (yellow arrow). Partial opacification of left M1-M2 tracts (white arrows) due to 'stagnant' blood flow

Cerebral perfusion scintigraphy and SPECT

Cerebral perfusion scintigraphy is a simple, non-invasive tool which can be used to document absence of radionuclide detection in the brain, as an expression of cerebral circulatory arrest and absent brain function. Single-photon emission computer tomography (SPECT) uses

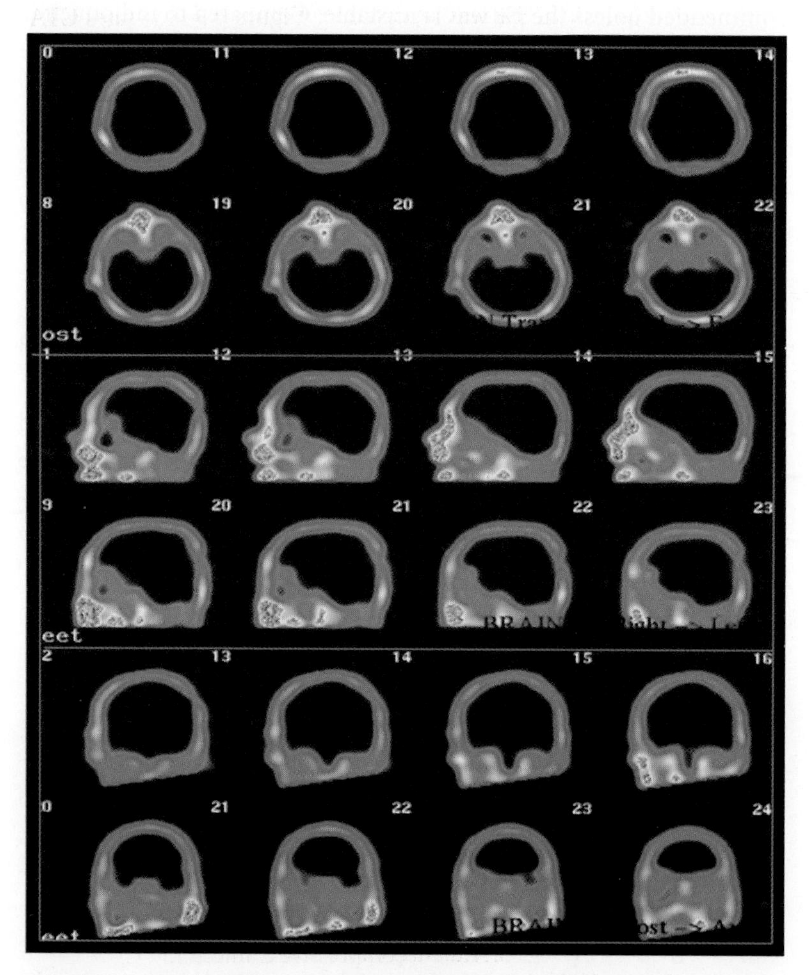

Figure 9.4. Axial, sagittal and coronal sections of HMPAO SPECT study to confirm absent cerebral blood flow in a case of brain death. There is no evidence of brain perfusion. The hot nose sign due to shunting of carotid blood flow to the maxillary branches is visualized

brain-specific agents, such as 99mTc-bicisate (ECD; ethyl cysteinate dimer) and 99mTc-exametazime (HMPAO; hexamethylpropylene amine oxime), which are lipophilic radiopharmaceuticals that cross the blood-brain barrier and enter normally perfused cerebral tissue, in proportion to regional perfusion. If the neuronal cells are not perfused and viable, the tracer is not taken up.[31,26] Lateral and posterior projection planar imaging are obtained as needed. SPECT imaging is recommended unless the patient is unstable. Compared to radionuclide angiography, SPECT allows better visualization of perfusion to the posterior fossa and brainstem structures.[31–33,26] For a SPECT study to be considered positive, there must be no perfusion to the brain. Expected activity can be seen in the scalp or projecting over the nose (known as the hot-nose sign) due to shunting of carotid blood flow to the maxillary branches. The sensitivity of planar imaging and SPECT with Tc99m HMPAO is very high (78% and 88%, respectively) while the specificity is 100%.[34,35]

In a study enrolling twenty BD patients, Munari et al[26] demonstrated a perfect agreement between angiography and SPECT results.

Guidelines with recommendations on how to perform, interpret, and report brain perfusion imaging as ancillary test in the diagnosis of BD are available in the literature.[33,36]

In Figure 9.4 SPECT showing absent cerebral perfusion in a case of BD is showed.

Magnetic Resonance Imaging (MRI) angiography

MRI and MRI angiography have been investigated as an accurate, non-invasive, and a reliable technique to demonstrate the absence of CBF, thus confirming BD diagnosis.[37–42] However, transportation, monitoring, and ventilation of an unstable BD patient inside the MRI suite poses several challenges and limit its use in the clinical setting.[43]

MRI signs of BD have been described in literature.[38,39,44,45] Absence of any cerebral vessels above the level of the supraclinoid portions of the ICA on MR angiograms, loss of flow void in the intracranial ICA, central and tonsillar herniation, and diffuse brain swelling on MR images are findings suggestive of BD described by Ishii et al.[38] Sohn et al[46] described absent intracranial vascular flow void in both conventional MRI and MRA, tonsillar herniation, diffuse cortical high signal intensity and swelling of the cerebral sulci on T2 weighted image, diffuse hemispheric hyperintensities on diffusion-weighted MRI and a drop in the apparent diffusion coefficient due to cytotoxic oedema, as conventional diagnostic criteria for BD on MRI. Recently, Sohn et al[46] in a smaller study found 3 Tesla MRA to be 100% sensitive and specific for the diagnosis of BD.

Transcranial doppler

Transcranial doppler is a non-invasive, inexpensive, portable, and efficient device for determining CBF and has become a widely used technique with diagnostic, therapeutic, and prognostic implications in the neuro intensive care unit. For the role of transcranial doppler as an ancillary test to document absent CBF, refer to Chapter 10 of this book.

Conclusions

In accordance with the concept that diagnosis of BD is essentially a clinical diagnosis, when reporting results of CBF studies, the neuroradiologist should avoid the terminology 'consistent with BD' and should only comment on the presence or absence of CBF.[8,33]

This chapter was aimed at describing why, when, and which CBF studies should be performed to confirm the clinical diagnosis of BD. **Why:** To demonstrate substratum of BD. **When:** If neurologic clinical examination cannot be complete or the eventuality of confounding factors cannot be excluded. **Which:** Depending on local availability and preferences, differences in invasiveness and costs, CT angiography, cerebral angiography, cerebral scintigraphy with SPECT, MRI angiography, and transcranial Doppler (refer Chapter 10) can demonstrate absence of CBF.

A worldwide consensus on the use, limitation and interpretation of ancillary tests for determination of BD would help to reduce actual variability around the world.[47]

Highlights

- If an adequate CBF is the physiologic requisite to sustain cerebral metabolism and function, cerebral circulatory arrest is the pathophysiological mechanism underlying the loss of all functions of the brain, including the brainstem, and is the essence of irreversibility of BD.
- CBF studies are required as ancillary tests if neurologic clinical examination cannot be complete or the eventuality of confounding factors cannot be excluded.
- CBF studies are complementary, and never a replacement, of the clinical diagnosis of BD.
- In the clinical practice the choice of CBF study depends on local availability and preferences, different invasiveness, and costs.
- When reporting results of CBF studies, the neuroradiologist should only describe the presence or absence of CBF, avoiding the terminology consistent with BD.

References

1. Branston NM, Symon L, Crockard HA, Pasztor E. Relationship between the cortical evoked potential and local cortical blood flow following acute middle cerebral artery occlusion in the baboon. Exp Neurol. 1974;45:195–208.
2. Sawicki M, Bohatyrewicz R, Walecka A, Sołek-Pastuszka J, Rowiński O, Walecki J. CT Angiography in the diagnosis of brain death. Pol J Radiol. 2014;79:417–421.
3. Savard M, Turgeon AF, Gariepy JL, Trottier F, Langevin S. Selective 4 vessels angiography in brain death: A retrospective study. Can J Neurol Sci 2010; 37:492–497.
4. Welschehold S, Kerz T, Boor S, et al. Detection of intracranial circulatory arrest in brain death using cranial CTangiography. Eur J Neurol 2013; 20:173–179.
5. Kramer AH, Roberts DJ: Computed tomography angiography in the diagnosis of brain death: A systematic review and meta-analysis. Neurocrit Care 2014; 21: 539–550.
6. Suarez-Kelly LP, Patel DA, Britt PM, et al. Dead or alive? New confirmatory test using quantitative analysis of computed tomographic angiography. J Trauma Acute Care Surg. 2015;79:995–1003.
7. MacDonald D, Stewart-Perrin B, Shankar JJS. The role of neuroimaging in the determination of brain death. J Neuroimaging. 2018;28:374–379.
8. Shemie SD, Lee D, Sharpe M, Tampieri D, Young B. Canadian Critical Care Society. Brain blood flow in the neurological determination of death: Canadian expert report. Can J Neurol Sci. 2008;35:140–145.

9. Wijdicks EF, Varelas PN, Gronseth GS, et al. Evidence-based guideline update: Determining brain death in adults: Report of the Quality Standards Subcommittee of the American Academy of Neurology. Neurology 2010;74:1911–1918.
10. Chakraborty S, Dhanani S. Guidelines for use of computed tomography angiogram as an ancillary test for diagnosis of suspected brain death. Can Assoc Radiol J. 2017;68:224–228.
11. Amendment to the national Guidelines of the Committee. 'Application of the cerebral Blood flow studies released on February 20th 2009. Italian National Transplant Center. Approved 2014. available online at: http://www.trapianti.salute.gov.it/imgs/C_17_cntPubblicazioni_38_allegato.pdf Emendamento alle Linee guida nazionali della Consulta Applicazione delle indagini strumentali di flusso ematico cerebrale' emanate il 20 febbraio 2009. Centro Nazionale Trapianti. Approved 2014. available online at: http://www.trapianti.salute.gov.it/imgs/C_17_cntPubblicazioni_38_allegato.pdf
12. Leclerc X. CT angiography for the diagnosis of brain death: Recommendations of the French Society of Neuroradiology (SFNR). J Neuroradiol. 2007;34:217–219.
13. Bradac GB, Simon RS. Angiography in brain death. Neuroradiology. 1974; 7: 25–28.
14. Nau R, Prange HW, Klingelhöfer J, Kukowski B, Sander D, Tchorsch R, Rittmeyer K. Results of four technical investigations in fifty clinically brain dead patients. Intensive Care Med. 1992;18:82–88.
15. Dupas B, Gayet-Delacroix M, Villers D, Antonioli D, Veccherini MF, Soulillou JP. Diagnosis of brain death using two-phase spiral CT. Am J Neuroradiol. 1998; 19: 641–647.
16. Société française de neuroradiologie. Société française de radiologie. Agence de la biomédecine. Recommandations sur les critères diagnostiques de la mort encéphalique par la technique d'angioscanner cerebral. Recommendations on diagnostic criteria of brain death by the technique of CT angiography. Journal of Neuroradiology 2011;38:36–39.
17. Swiss Academy of Medical Sciences. Determination of death with regard to organ transplantation and preparation for organ removal; approved by the Senate of the SAMS on 16 May 2017. Swiss Med Wkly. 2018 Oct 22; 148:w14524. doi: 10.4414/smw.2018.14524.
18. Health Council of the Netherlands. Brain Death Protocol. The Hague: Health Council of the Netherlands, 2006; 1–70. publication no. 2006/04E. ISBN: 978-90-5549-886-4
19. Combes JC, Chomel A, Ricolfi F, d'Athis P, Freysz M. Reliability of computed tomographic angiography in the diagnosis of brain death. Transplant Proc. 2007;39(1):16–20.
20. Frampas E, Videcoq M, de Kerviler E, Ricolfi F, Kuoch V, Mourey F, Tenaillon A, Dupas B. CT angiography for brain death diagnosis. AJNR Am J Neuroradiol. 2009;30:1566–1570.
21. Sawicki M, Bohatyrewicz R, Safranow K, et al. Computed tomographic angiography criteria in the diagnosis of brain death—comparison of sensitivity and interobserver reliability of different evaluation scales. Neuroradiology 2014;56:609–620.
22. Taylor T, Dineen RA, Gardiner DC, Buss CH, Howatson A, Pace NL. Computed tomography (CT) angiography for confirmation of the clinical diagnosis of

brain death. Cochrane Database of Systematic Reviews 2014, Issue 3. Art. No.: CD009694. DOI: 10.1002/14651858.CD009694.pub2.

23. Garrett MP, Williamson RW, Bohl MA, Bird CR, Theodore N. Computed tomography angiography as a confirmatory test for the diagnosis of brain death. J Neurosurg 2018; 128:639–644.
24. Kricheff II, Pinto RS, George AE, Braunstein P, Korein J. Angiographic findings in brain death. Ann N YAcad Sci 1978; 315:168–183.
25. Sawicki M, Bohatyrewicz R, Safranow K et al. Dynamic evaluation of stasis filling phenomenon with computed tomography in diagnosis of brain death. Neuroradiology, 2013; 55: 1061–1069.
26. Munari M, Zucchetta P, Carollo C, et al. Confirmatory tests in the diagnosis of brain death: Comparison between SPECT and contrast angiography. Crit Care Med 2005; 33:2068–2073.
27. Sawicki M, Sołek-Pastuszka J, Chamier-Ciemińska K, Walecka A, Walecki J, Bohatyrewicz R. Computed tomography perfusion is a useful adjunct to computed tomography angiography in the diagnosis of brain death. Clin Neuroradiol. 2019;29:101–108.
28. Shankar JJ, Vandorpe R: CT perfusion for confirmation of brain death. Am J Neuroradiol, 2013; 34: 1175–1179.
29. Sawicki M, Sołek-Pastuszka J, Chamier-Ciemińska K, Walecka A, Bohatyrewicz R. Accuracy of computed tomographic perfusion in diagnosis of brain death: A prospective cohort study. Med Sci Monit. 2018;24:2777–2285.
30. Brasil S, Bor-Seng-Shu E, de-Lima-Oliveira M, K Azevedo M, J Teixeira M, Bernardo L, M Bernardo W. Role of computed tomography angiography and perfusion tomography in diagnosing brain death: A systematic review. J Neuroradiol. 2016;43:133–140.
31. Keske. Tc-99m-HMPAO single photon emission computed tomography (SPECT) as an ancillary test in the diagnosis of brain death. Intensive Care Med 1998; 24:895–897.
32. Facco E, Zucchetta P, Munari M, et al. 99mTc-HMPAO SPECT in the diagnosis of brain death. Intensive Care Med 1998;24:911–917.
33. Donohoe KJ, Agrawal G, Frey KA, et al. SNM practice guideline for brain death scintigraphy 2.0. J Nucl Med Technol. 2012;40:198–203.
34. Joffe AR, Lequier L, Cave D. Specificity of radionuclide brain blood flow testing in brain death: Case report and review. J Intensive Care Med 2010;25:53–64.
35. Sinha P, Conrad GR. Scintigraphic confirmation of brain death. Semin Nucl Med 2012;42:27–32.
36. ACR–SPR Practice Parameter for the Performance of Single Photon Emission CT (SPECT) Brain Perfusion and Brain Death Examinations Res. 26 – 2016. Available at: www.acr.org/Quality-Safety/Standards-Guidelines/Practice-Guidelines-by-Modality.
37. Jones KM, Barnes PD. MR diagnosis of brain death. AJNR Am J Neuroradiol 1992;13:65–66.
38. Ishii K, Onuma T, Kinoshita T, Shiina G, Kameyama M, Shimosegawa Y. Brain death: MR and MR angiography. AJNR Am J Neuroradiol. 1996;17:731.

39. Karantanas AH, Hadjigeorgiou GM, Paterakis K, Sfiras D, Komnos A. Contribution of MRI and MR angiography in early diagnosis of brain death. Eur Radiol. 2002;12:2710.
40. Aichner F, Felber S, Birbamer G, Luz G, Judmaier W, Schmutzhard E. Magnetic resonance: A noninvasive approach to metabolism, circulation, and morphology in human brain death. Ann Neurol 1992;32:507–511.
41. Matsumura A, Meguro K, Tsurushima H, Komatsu Y, Kikuchi Y, Wada M, Nakata Y, Ohashi N, Nose T. Magnetic resonance imaging of brain death. Neurol Med Chir (Tokyo). 1996;36:166.
42. Lovblad KO, Bassetti C. Diffusion-weighted magnetic resonance imaging in brain death. Stroke 2000;31:539–542.
43. Luchtmann M, Bernarding J, Beuing O, Kohl J, Bondar I, Skalej M, Firsching R. Controversies of diffusion weighted imaging in the diagnosis of brain death. J Neuroimaging 2013;23:463–468.
44. Orrison WW, Champlin AM, Kesterson OL, Hartshorne MF, King JN. MR 'hot nose sign' and 'intravascular enhancement sign' in brain death. AJNR Am J Neuroradiol. 1994;15:913–916.
45. ECR G. Santacana-Laffitte, D. Loubriel-Torres, D. Del Prado; San Juan, Novel white matter and subependymal MRI findings in Brain Death. European Society of radiology 2013; doi 10.1594/ecr2013/C-2105
46. Sohn CH, Lee HP, Park JB, et al. Imaging findings of brain death on 3-tesla MRI. Korean J Radiol 2012; 13:541–549.
47. Lewis A, Liebman J, Kreiger-Benson E, Kumpfbeck A, Bakkar A, Shemie SD, Sung G, Torrance S, Greer D. Ancillary testing for determination of death by neurologic criteria around the world. Neurocrit Care. 2021;34:473–484.

10

The role of Transcranial Doppler

Alfredo Conti

Introduction

The state defined as 'brain death' (BD) is a neurologic condition engendered by technological advances of contemporary medicine that allow to maintain the integrity of the cardiopulmonary system in patients with the loss of every brain function.[1–6] In many countries, practice guidelines are available for the determination of BD.[2] The guidelines specify a prerequisite (a known cause of persistent, irreversible, and totally unresponsive comatose state), and comprises a differential diagnosis process to exclude states that may mimic BD (hypothermia, metabolic disorders, drugs, neurologic diseases). Clinical criteria include absent motor response, absent brainstem reflexes, and apnoea testing, using a PCO_2 target.[2–6]

Nevertheless, there are circumstances in which clinical criteria cannot be reliably applied, e.g., when cranial nerves cannot be adequately examined, in cases of neuromuscular paralysis or heavy sedation, or in some patients for whom the apnoea test is precluded (respiratory instability or high cervical spine injury). In these situations, ancillary tests may support the diagnosis.

Truly confirmatory ancillary tests for BD should meet the following criteria: (1) There should be no 'false positives', i.e., when the test confirms BD, there should be none who recover or who have the potential to recover. (2) The test should be sufficient on its own to establish that BD is or is not present. (3) The test should not be susceptible to 'confounders' such as drug effects or metabolic disturbances. (4) The test should be standardized in technology, technique, and classification of results. (5) The test should be available, safe, and readily applied.[7]

Though a laboratory study support to the clinical diagnosis can be valuable, a delay in the diagnosis of BD can affect the quality of organs, or make them unsuitable to be transplanted by permitting the occurrence of events such as multiple organ failure or cardiac arrest. For this reason, ancillary tests should meet another condition; they should not cause the delay of diagnosis.

Most national practice guidelines,[8] actually, mandate confirmatory testing in patients who meet the neurological standards. Those tests evaluate the electric activity of the brain, the cerebral metabolism, or the cerebral blood flow (CBF). Testing modalities which demonstrate the absence of blood flow to the brain meet the abovementioned criteria. Among those tests, four-vessel contrast angiography remains the most reliable, but the method is invasive, expensive, and requires transporting critically ill patients. Radioisotope techniques are equally costly and require the use of radiopharmaceutical agents and cumbersome equipment.

Ultrasounds represent a relatively simple, non-invasive diagnostic tool to repeatedly determine the status of cerebral circulation. In many countries, Transcranial Doppler (TCD) has been recommended by medical councils as one of the methods, which can shorten the waiting time for fulfilling the criteria for diagnosis of cerebral death.[9]

Basic principles of TCD sonography

TCD ultrasonography is based on the so-called Doppler effect, from the eponym of the inventor of ultrasounds emitting systems. The Doppler effect is based on the principle that there is a shift in the frequency between the emitted and reflected ultrasound waves when the reflecting object is moving and that this shift is proportional to the velocity of the reflecting objects.[10,11] In medical terms, the reflecting objects are represented by blood cells (see Figure 10.1). As these cells move in the vessels with a laminar movement (with lower resistance and higher speed in the centre and high resistance and slower speed close to the vessels walls), the Doppler signal will be a mixture of different Doppler frequency shifts forming a spectral display of the distribution of the velocities of individual blood cells. The spectral analysis (see Figure 10.2) can be used to measure the blood flow velocity (FV) and a few other characteristics of the CBF.

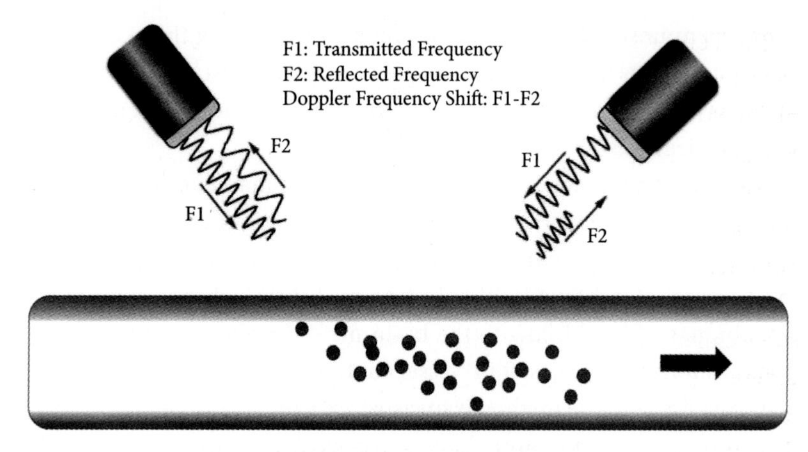

Figure 10.1. Graphic representation of the Doppler frequency shift

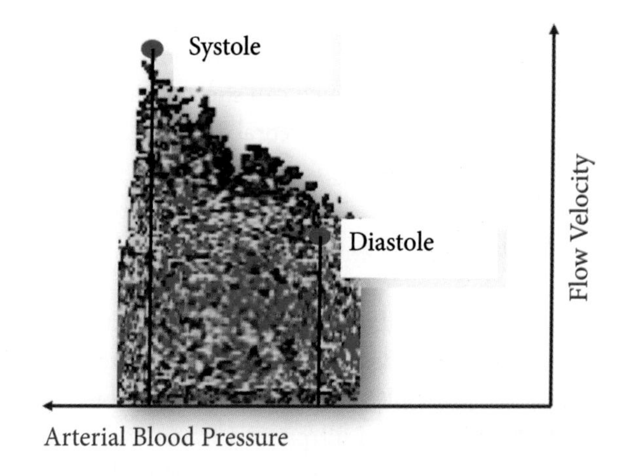

Figure 10.2. Spectral display of the distribution of the velocities of individual blood cells

The specific parameters obtained from this spectral analysis include peak systolic velocity (Vs), end diastolic velocity (Vd), systolic upstroke or acceleration time, pulsatility index (PI), and time-averaged mean maximum velocity (V_{mean}). The V_{mean} is a continuous trace of peak velocities as a function of time and in most TCD instruments, it is calculated and displayed automatically.[11]

The TCD examination is performed using a 2 MHz frequency ultrasound probe. Higher frequency probes are not applicable for intracranial measurements because they cannot adequately penetrate the skull. Furthermore, insonation of the cerebral arteries is possible only through specific areas of the skull, termed acoustic windows, where the skull is sufficiently thin to be penetrated by the ultrasounds (see Figure 10.3). Four acoustic windows are commonly used: (1) the temporal window, (2) the transorbital window, (3) the submandibular window, and (4) the suboccipital window. Although each window has unique advantages for different arteries and indications, a complete TCD examination should include measurements from all four windows and the course of blood flow at various depths within each major branch of the circle of Willis should be assessed. Specific arteries of the circle of Willis are identified

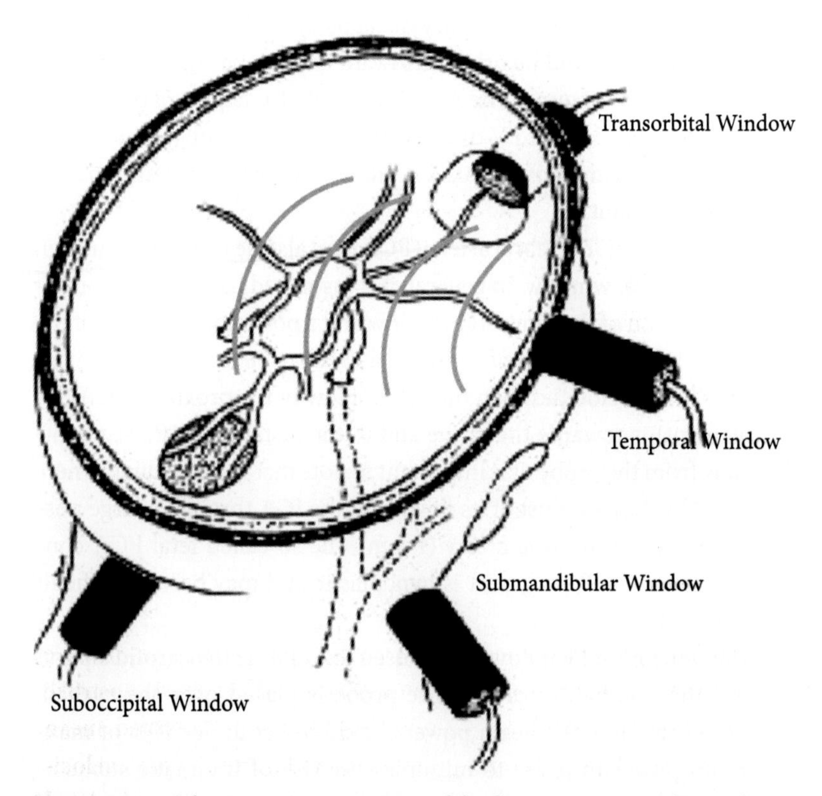

Figure 10.3. Schematic representation of the four acoustic windows of the skull

using the following criteria: (1) relative direction of the probe within a specific acoustic window, (2) direction of blood flow relative to the probe, (3) depth of insonation, and (4) in difficult cases when it is not possible to differentiate the anterior from the posterior circulation, the blood flow response to carotid compression or vibration.

- The temporal window allows the insonation of the intracranial carotid artery (ICA) bifurcation that can be identified at depths of 55 to 65 mm. It shows simultaneous flow towards and away from the probe as the ICA bifurcation terminates in the anterior (flow away from the probe) and middle (flow toward the probe) cerebral arteries (ACA and MCA). The ICA bifurcation (with the typical dual flow) is a convenient anatomic landmark to locate the vessels of the anterior circulation. The middle cerebral artery (MCA), is usually insonated at depths of 35 (very distal part) to 55 mm (origin). Flow in the MCA should be oriented towards the probe and it has a characteristic acute sound. The ACA is insonated at depths of 60–70 mm and often has a lower FV directed away from the probe. An agenesia of the A1 segment of the ACA represents a relatively common anatomical variant.

  The posterior cerebral artery (PCA) can also be insonated through the temporal window. In general, it is insonated using a more posterior portion of the temporal window and a posterior direction of the beam. It lies at a depth of approximately 60 to 70 mm and exhibit always lower velocities than the MCA. Flow in the proximal PCA (P1 segment) is towards the probe and in the distal PCA (P2 segment) away from the probe. It is important to note that in individuals where the PCA derives most of its flow from the ICA through a large posterior communicating artery (Pcom), the so-called fetal PCA configuration, the P1 segment is hypoplastic and may be very difficult to identify.
- The transorbital window can be used to examine the carotid siphon and the ophthalmic artery. The probe is placed over the eyeball. Before starting, the beam power should be set under 10% of maximum power in order to minimize the risk of traumatic subluxation of the crystalline lens. In addition to lowering the amount of

power, the time of insonation also needs to be kept to a minimum. The probe is directed towards the optic canal at a depth of 55 to 70 mm to insonate the carotid siphon. The flow is directed towards the probe in the infraclinoid siphon, it is bidirectional in the genu and away from the probe in the supraclinoid segment. The ophthalmic artery will be found at depths of 40 to 50 mm. The low flow of the ophthalmic artery is towards the probe, but it represents a collateral system between the external carotid artery and the anterior intracerebral circulation.

- The suboccipital window with the neck flexed, can be used to insonate the basilar and vertebral arteries. The basilar artery is typically found at depths of 70 to 80 mm and can sometimes be followed to depths up to 100 mm. Although the basilar artery is found with the probe directed medially, vertebral arteries are best insonated with the probe slightly shifted laterally, at a depth of 80 to 115 mm. Flow at the top of the basilar artery and in the vertebral arteries is typically away from the probe.[12–15]
- The submandibular window is at the angle of the jaw and can be used to locate the distal ICA in the neck at a depth of 40 to 60 mm. Flow at this point is usually away from the probe.

Patterns featuring BD

After a brain injury causes total neuronal death, the physiologic cerebral circulation is progressively transformed into a high resistance and low-flow system, a process that culminates with the arrest of the CBF. The TCD is a valuable diagnostic tool in detecting such changes, its application in this field dates back to the late 1980s, and the advantages of its use are widely recognized.[13,16–22]

The brain has the characteristics of being perfused during the whole cardiac cycle (see Figure 10.2). During the systole, the CBF is conducted by the systolic output of the heart. The elastic component of the basal arteries of the brain stores the potential energy through arterial wall dilatation during this stage of the cardiac cycle. This energy will be then released during the diastole. The diastolic forward flow is therefore due to the elastic impulse of the basal arteries of the brain. While the intracranial pressure (ICP) increases, the transmural pressure increases reducing the diastolic component of the cerebral flow. Therefore, an increase in ICP results in an increase in the 'pulsatility' of flow, that is in the difference between the systolic and diastolic components of flow velocities as displayed by the TCD spectral analysis. When the ICP equals the diastolic arterial pressure, the brain is perfused only in systole and with further increase of ICP over the systolic arterial pressure (see Figure 10.4A). This flow is characterized by the presence of 'systolic peaks' pattern, namely a systolic-only flow.

When the values of the ICP reach those of the systolic blood pressure (BP), the CBF progressively ceases. Due to elasticity of the arterial wall, the early stage of the cerebral circulatory arrest (CCA) is featured by Doppler evidence of oscillatory movement of blood in the large arteries of the base of the brain. In a nutshell, the blood can reach the capacitance arteries of the skull base. Nonetheless, there is no forward flow because the ICP has caused a collapse of bridging veins and arterioles. As a consequence, the flow reverberates backward so that the flow will be featured by a 'to and fro' movement. With increase of ICP that equals the systolic BP, reverberating flow with forward and reverse flow is nearly equal and cerebral perfusion ceases. Net flow is zero when there is equality among both the flow components and if the area under the envelope of the positive and negative deflection is the same (see Figure 10.4B).

With a further increase of ICP over the systolic BP, only systolic spikes can be registered, and their amplitudes decrease with time. Such systolic spikes, which represent simply oscillations of the arterial wall (see Figure 10.4C), have characteristic pattern of CCA, but may resemble high resistance pattern with reduction of diastolic flow, the phase before development of reverberating flow. Due to the usage of high pass filters for elimination of artefacts from wall movement, reverberating flow can be missed. Therefore, the filters must be set at its lowest level, being 50 Hz.

With further reduction of blood movement, the further decrease of amplitude can be registered until the complete cessation of signals. With time the oscillations decrease in amplitude of spectral spikes until no pulsations are detectable.

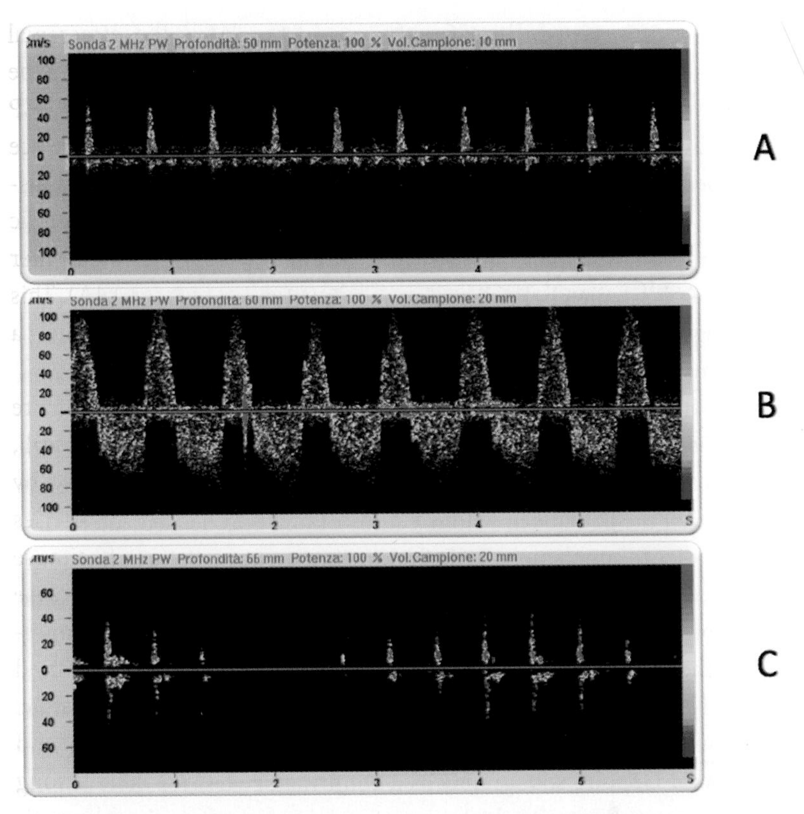

Figure 10.4A. The initial stage of cerebral circulation arrest has a typical pattern characterized by systolic peaks without diastolic spectrum.

Figure 10.4B. As intracranial pressure increases, the small vessels collapse. In such a situation, a small degree of antegrade blood flow during systole is allowed. However, since forward flow is negated, blood reverberates backward. This produces a characteristic oscillating flow velocity wave form on TCD evaluation described as 'To and Fro' movement.

Figure 10.4C. The following stage is represented by the appearance of the 'systolic spikes' characterized by sharp, narrow peaks at the beginning of the systole due to a short vibration of the vessel. Flow velocity during the rest of the cardiac cycle is zero. The systolic TCD spikes show a typical respiration-dependent fluctuation in amplitude.

Guidelines for the use of Doppler sonography in BD

According to the Italian guidelines[23] for the determination of BD, established in 1994, the study of CBF is compulsory in the following conditions: (1) infants below one year of age; (2) presence of factors that may interfere with the clinical picture (intoxication, hypothermia, neuromuscular paralysis, metabolic disorders not readily reversed); (3) uncertain aetiology, or clinical situations preventing from an adequate exploration of brainstem reflexes (orbital or middle and inner ears trauma, cranial neuropathies).

Precise criteria for the use of TCD were established in 2003 by a working group of the National Commission for Transplant.[24] Accordingly, up to 2003, in all the patients in whom a study of flow was needed, alternative flow studies to supplement TCD findings are performed, including four-vessel cerebral angiography, 99mTC HMPAO-Single Photon Emission Computed Tomography (SPECT); CT angiography (refer to Chapter 9 for further details on these cerebral blood flow studies).

The Neurosonology Research Group (NSRG) of the World Federation of Neurology (WFN) created a Task Force Group in order to evaluate the role of Doppler sonography as a confirmatory test for determining BD, and created criteria which are defined and guidelines for the use of Doppler sonography in this setting,[25] and these guidelines were adopted and endorsed by numerous national societies.[26–29] According to aforementioned findings, Task Force Group of the NSRG WFN[25] set guidelines for the use of Doppler sonography as a confirmatory test for CCA as follows:

1. *Circumstances*

Vascular testing can be used to confirm CCA thus confirming BD only if the following diagnostic prerequisites are fulfilled:

(i) The cause of coma is established and is sufficient to account for a permanent and irreversible loss of brain functions;
(ii) Other conditions such as intoxication, hypothermia, severe arterial hypotension, metabolic disorders have been excluded;

(iii) Clinical evidence of brain function loss was assessed by at least two experienced examiners.

2. *Clinical Prerequisites*

Clinical and instrumental criteria set by Italian medical college[24] to declare the death were: (a) absence of brainstem reflexes and oculovestibular responses; (b) absence of motor responses following painful stimuli in trigeminal areas; (c) absence of oropharyngeal and respiratory reflexes, and apnoea (with a Pa-CO_2 >60 mmHg); (d) flat EEG (three recordings, each lasting at least 30 min, at the beginning, in the middle, and at the end of the period of observation); (e) observation lasting 6 hours; (f) demonstration of CCA in infants below one year of age.

Criteria for determination of CCA by TCD

CCA can be confirmed if the following extra- and intracranial Doppler sonographic findings have been recorded and documented both intra- and extracranially, and bilaterally on two examinations at an interval of at least 30 min.[30]

1. Systolic spikes or oscillating flow recorded by bilateral transcranial insonation of the ICA and MCA, and posterior circulation. Oscillating flow is defined by signals with forward and reverse flow components in one cardiac cycle exhibiting almost the same area under the envelope of the waveform (to and fro movement). Systolic spikes are sharp unidirectional velocity signals in early systole of less than 200 milliseconds duration, less than 50 cm/s peaks systolic velocity, and without a flow signal during the remaining cardiac cycle. Transitory patterns between oscillating flow and systolic spikes may be seen. In order to enable visualization of the low signals, wall filter must be set at its lowest level (50 Hz).
2. The diagnosis established by the intracranial examination must be confirmed by the extracranial bilateral recording of the CCA, ICA, and VA.

3. The lack of signal during transcranial insonation of the basal cerebral arteries is not a reliable finding because this can be due to transmission problems. But the disappearance of intracranial flow signals in conjunction with typical extracranial signals can be accepted as a proof of circulatory arrest.
4. No ventricular drains or large openings of the skull, like in the case of decompressive craniectomy, should be present as they possibly interfere with the development of the ICP.

Diagnostic accuracy

Diagnostic accuracy of any diagnostic procedure or a test gives an answer to the following question: 'How well this test discriminates between certain two conditions of interest (i.e. health and disease)?' This discriminative ability can be quantified by the measures of diagnostic accuracy such as sensitivity and specificity, predictive values, likelihood ratios, the area under the ROC curve, Youden's index, and diagnostic odds ratio.

Specificity

As regards the specificity, in most series the TCD was 100% specific in diagnosing the CCA. Twelve false-positive results have been reported to date.[16–18,31–39] Specifically, Kirkham et al.[32] and Newell et al.[17] reported a preserved weak spontaneous respiration for a short period of time (1 h) in patients with TCD evidence of CCA. In neither of those studies, the cases were regarded as false positives by those authors, because the signs of circulatory arrest proved to be irreversible, and the patients soon became apnoeic. In fact, those and most of the other reported cases cannot be considered as true false positives when currently accepted criteria to define the CCA are applied. In only two of those twelve cases, actually, both the anterior and posterior circulation were studied.[30] In a study by Hadani e al.[31] a patient with CCA demonstrated weak respiration, but BD occurred a few hours later. Van Velthoven et al.[18] reported a clinically brain-dead patient with CCA, confirmed by angiography, in whom EEG became iso-electric only several hours later.

Furthermore, acutely raised ICP due to bleeding or rebleeding from an aneurysm has been observed with transient flow patterns similar to those in CCA.[35,37] A similar high resistance pattern can occur shortly after cardiac arrest during the 'no reflow phase'. Both conditions are transient and the flow abnormalities will reverse at least partially within less than 30 minutes.

Accordingly, to date none of the patients with TCD evidence of circulation arrest survived for a clinically relevant interval of time. Aortic insufficiency, especially in aortic dissection, may also pose problems for interpretation of the flow pattern. Nevertheless, reverse component, if present, is smaller than the forward component of the flow signals. In patients with both ICA distal occlusion, only systolic spikes in both ICAs would be detected. These patients would be mistaken if examination of the posterior circulation is not part of the protocol.

In conclusion, it is extremely important that the examination is performed according to guidelines including two separate examinations at an interval of at least 30 minutes and the exploration of both posterior and anterior circulation.

Sensitivity

Although TCD examination for detection of CCA is 100% specific, the sensitivity did not reach 100% in most series. [13,16–18,30,31,33,36,40–57] The sensitivity of TCD is limited by several factors, the failure of the temporal window to permit the insonation of cerebral arteries being the most frequent reason. This phenomenon is usually due to the coexistence of several factors: a weak sonographic signal due to low blood FV; a small window, which is more frequent in elderly patients; a surgical wound in the temporal region.

The other source of reduced sensitivity was represented by the presence of patients with persistent CBF, despite the clinical evidence of whole BD. Those cases, regarded as true false negatives, are commonly associated with the presence of large craniotomies, bone defects, such as decompressive craniectomies or skull fractures, or external ventricular drainages. These conditions, in fact, may interfere with the mechanism of ICP rising and fall of cerebral perfusion pressure that characterizes the

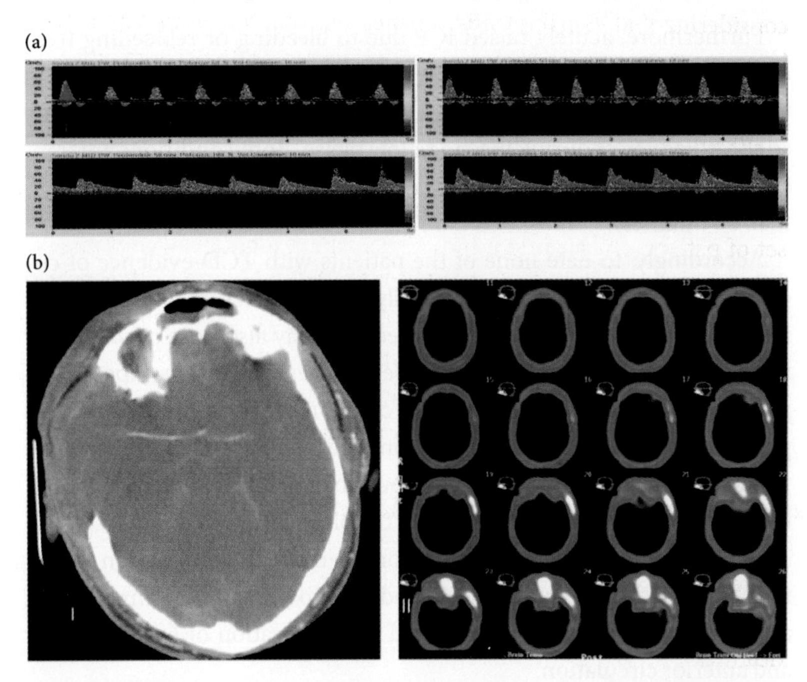

Figure 10.5A. *Upper*. Bilateral reverberating flow on MCA recorded before surgical treatment. *Lower*. After a fronto-temporal craniectomy, a new TCD examination was performed showing the recovery of diastolic flow

Figure 10.5B. Discrepancy between 'arteria circulation' and 'brain perfusion' as demonstrated by the discrepancy between the CT angiogram (I) showing persisting arterial filling and the 99mTc-HMPAO SPECT (II) showing an 'empty skull'. This can be explained considering that 99mTc-HMPAO penetrates into the brain parenchyma in proportion to regional blood flow, but its cerebral uptake requires the persistence of a viable brain

death of the brain, thus preventing the arrest of cerebral circulation. In this setting, it is also possible for a recovery from CCA without changes in the clinical status.[35,37,38]

Recovery from CCA is also possible, for instance after a decompressive craniectomy. An example is reported in Figure 10.5A. The case described is worthy of note also because a discrepancy was recorded between the TCD and the radioisotope study performed on the same day. In fact, TCD showed a persistent diastolic flow whereas the 99mTc-HMPAO SPECT showed an 'empty skull' (see Figure 10.5B). This can be explained considering that 99mTc-HMPAO penetrates into the brain parenchyma in proportion to regional blood flow, but its cerebral uptake requires the persistence of a viable brain.

Meanwhile, in particular circumstances, TCD may show the persistence of arterial circulation in brain dead patients, whereas 99mTc-HMPAO SPECT may demonstrate absence of brain perfusion in the same set of patients. Accordingly, in patients who underwent decompressive craniectomies or ventriculostomies, it is advisable to use other tests to confirm the clinical diagnosis of BD. This holds true also in infants below the age of one year who, because of immature skull, may present similar problems. In such infants, Key Doppler alterations, such as absent or retrograde flow during diastole, are not uniquely associated with the diagnosis of BD, particularly in the setting of congenital heart disease.(58)

Another cause of persistent flow in patients with the absence of any brainstem activity is the dissociation between the carotid and the vertebro-basilar circulation.(45) In patients with severe vascular accidents involving the posterior circulation only, a condition of brainstem death can be identified while the telencephalon is still perfused by the anterior circulation. Similar cases can be regarded as false negatives only if a brainstem formulation of death is applied.(59) In most Western countries, including Italy, a whole-brain formulation of BD is adopted, and death is defined by the irreversible cessation of all functions of the entire brain. The TCD may assist the differential diagnosis between whole BD and brainstem death.

Improving sensitivity

As mentioned, TCD is highly specific (100% when all prerequisites and criteria are respected), but not completely sensitive. The question thus arises whether there are technical strategies that may increase sensitivity of the examination. It has been demonstrated that the insonation of the ICA at the level of the siphon and at the extracranial level, through transorbital and cervical insonation, may show a sonographic pattern of circulatory arrest.(60,61) This gives evidence for the absence of flow in the whole anterior cerebral circulation, even in case of lack of temporal windows.

The inclusion of a transorbital and transcervical approach in our study protocol increased sensitivity from 82.1% to 88%[13] allowing the diagnosis of CCA in further eleven patients lacking the temporal ultrasonic window. Nevertheless, twenty-two patients (11.9%) had weak persistent diastolic flow. This finding agrees with those of others. In fact, ICA diastolic flow could be present in up to 20% of patients with clinical evidence of BD.[62] Extracranial ICA diastolic flow has also been reported in 10.7% of patients with the evidence of intracranial circulation arrest.[45]

It has been observed that changes of flow pattern in the extracranial segment of the ICA were similar to those recorded in the intracranial vessels, with progressive disappearance of the diastolic spectrum culminating in a reverberating flow. According to the angiographic observations of Hassler et al.,[63,64] the origin of the intracranial ICA remains patent during the early stage of intracranial circulation arrest. Persistent diastolic forward flow in the ICA is therefore compatible with early intracranial CCA, with the hypothesis that basal arteries are still patent, and blood shunts into the external carotids through collaterals, such as the ophthalmic arteries.

In such cases, the progressive passage towards a reverberating flow in the ICA could be recorded during serial examinations, with an earlier appearance on the side in which a greater ICP could be expected. This allowed to increase sensitivity from 88% to 95.6%. Of note, the presence of oscillating flow in the extracranial ICA corresponded in all cases to an intracranial circulation arrest demonstrating that the detection of circulation arrest on the extracranial ICA reliably reflects intracranial flow absence.

Conclusion

Ultrasounds represent a relatively simple, non-invasive diagnostic tool to repeatedly determine the status of the cerebral circulation. In many countries, TCD has been recommended by medical councils as one of the methods which can shorten the waiting time for fulfilling the criteria for diagnosis of cerebral death. If the study is performed correctly, according to the currently available guidelines, the false identification of positive cases is not possible. Thus, the specificity of TCD in the diagnosis of CCA is 100%.

This technique is, however, not completely sensitive. The sensitivity of TCD is limited by several factors, the failure of the temporal window to permit the insonation of cerebral arteries being the most frequent reason. The other source of reduced sensitivity is represented by the presence of patients with persistent CBF, despite the clinical evidence of whole BD. Those cases regarded as true false negatives are commonly associated with the presence of large craniotomies, bone defects, such as decompressive craniectomies or skull fractures, or external ventricular drainages.

In patients lacking the temporal window, the transcervical and transorbital study of the ICA may increase the sensitivity of the exam. Nevertheless, there is a quota of patients in which diastolic flow is still present on the ICA despite clinical evidence of BD. In those patients awaiting the later stages of CCA, when the process of CCA is completed, reverberating flow appears in the intra- and extracranial carotid artery which may further increase sensitivity.

Highlights

- TCD ultrasonography represents a relatively simple, non-invasive diagnostic tool to repeatedly determine the status of cerebral circulation.
- TCD has been adopted by many national Medical Councils as confirmatory testing in patients who meet the neurological standards for the diagnosis of BD.
- TCD is 100% specific if the examination is correctly conducted.
- TCD is not completely sensitive because of possible lack of sonographic windows or skull defects.
- The insonation of the proximal ICA and repeated examination may increase sensitivity of TCD up to 90%.

References

1. Beecher, Henry K, A definition of irreversible coma: Report of the Harvard Medical School Comm to examine the definition of brain death. Journal of the American Medical Association, 1968, 205:85–88.

2. Wahlster S, Wijdicks EF, Patel PV, Greer DM, Hemphill JC, 3rd, Carone M, et al. Brain death declaration: Practices and perceptions worldwide. Neurology. 2015;84(18):1870–1879.
3. Bernat JL, Culver CM, Gert B. On the definition and criterion of death. Ann Intern Med. 1981;94(3):389–394.
4. Diagnosis of brain death. Statement issued by the honorary secretary of the Conference of Medical Royal Colleges and their faculties in the United Kingdom on 11 October 1976. Br Med J. 1976;2(6045):1187–1188.
5. Wijdicks EF. The diagnosis of brain death. N Engl J Med. 2001;344(16):1215–1221.
6. Wijdicks EF. Brain death worldwide: Accepted fact but no global consensus in diagnostic criteria. Neurology. 2002;58(1):20–25.
7. Young GB, Lee D. A critique of ancillary tests for brain death. Neurocrit Care. 2004;1(4):499–508.
8. Eelco F.M. Wijdicks, Panayiotis N. Varelas, Gary S. Gronseth, David M. Greer. Evidence-based guideline update: Determining brain death in adults: Report of the Quality Standards Subcommittee of the American Academy of Neurology. Neurology 2010;74;1911–1918.
9. Haupt WF, Rudolf J. European brain death codes: A comparison of national guidelines. J Neurol. 1999;246(6):432-437. doi:10.1007/s004150050378
10. Considine GD (ed.) (2015). Doppler Effect. In *Van Nostrand's Scientific Encyclopedia*, doi:10.1002/0471743984.vse2663 Wiley-Interscience; 10th edition (2008); pp 1–5.
11. Naqvi J, Yap KH, Ahmad G, Ghosh J. Transcranial Doppler ultrasound: A review of the physical principles and major applications in critical care. Int J Vasc Med. 2013;2013:629378.
12. Conti A, Iacopino DG, Fodale V, Micalizzi S, Penna O, Santamaria LB. Cerebral haemodynamic changes during propofol-remifentanil or sevoflurane anaesthesia: Transcranial Doppler study under bispectral index monitoring. Br J Anaesth. 2006;97(3):333–339.
13. Conti A, Iacopino DG, Spada A, Cardali SM, Giusa M, La Torre D, et al. Transcranial Doppler ultrasonography in the assessment of cerebral circulation arrest: Improving sensitivity by transcervical and transorbital carotid insonation and serial examinations. Neurocrit Care. 2009;10(3):326–335.
14. Fodale V, Schifilliti D, Conti A, Lucanto T, Pino G, Santamaria LB. Transcranial Doppler and anesthetics. Acta Anaesthesiol Scand. 2007;51(7):839–847.
15. Iacopino DG, Conti A, Battaglia C, Siliotti C, Lucanto T, Santamaria LB, et al. Transcranial Doppler ultrasound study of the effects of nitrous oxide on cerebral autoregulation during neurosurgical anesthesia: A randomized controlled trial. J Neurosurg. 2003;99(1):58–64.
16. Ducrocq X, Braun M, Debouverie M, Junges C, Hummer M, Vespignani H. Brain death and transcranial Doppler: Experience in 130 cases of brain dead patients. J Neurol Sci. 1998;160(1):41–46.
17. Newell DW, Grady MS, Sirotta P, Winn HR. Evaluation of brain death using transcranial Doppler. Neurosurgery. 1989;24(4):509–513.
18. Van Velthoven V, Calliauw L. Diagnosis of brain death. Transcranial Doppler sonography as an additional method. Acta Neurochir (Wien). 1988;95(1–2):57–60.

19. Consensus Group on Transcranial Doppler in Diagnosis of Brain D. Latin American consensus on the use of transcranial Doppler in the diagnosis of brain death. Rev Bras Ter Intensiva. 2014;26(3):240–252.
20. Al-Jehani HM, Sheikh BY. Transcranial Doppler in brain death assessment. Perspective and implications in the Saudi Arabian health system. Neurosciences (Riyadh). 2013;18(2):122–125.
21. Orban JC, El-Mahjoub A, Rami L, Jambou P, Ichai C. Transcranial Doppler shortens the time between clinical brain death and angiographic confirmation: A randomized trial. Transplantation. 2012;94(6):585–588.
22. Sharma D, Souter MJ, Moore AE, Lam AM. Clinical experience with transcranial Doppler ultrasonography as a confirmatory test for brain death: A retrospective analysis. Neurocrit Care. 2011;14(3):370–376.
23. Linee guida relative all'applicazione delle indagini strumentali di flusso ematico cerebrale in situazioni particolari, ai fini della diagnosi di morte in soggetti affetti da lesioni encefaliche (Decreto Ministeriale 22 agosto, 1994, n° 582). https://www.societaitalianatrapiantidiorgano.com/wp-content/uploads/2018/06/LG-su-Metodiche-di-Flusso-aggiornate-al-20-febbraio-2009.pdf
24. Beltramello A, Ricciardi GK, Pizzini FB, Piovan E. Updates in the determination of brain death. Neuroradiol J. 2010;23:145–150.
25. Ducrocq X, Hassler W, Moritake K, et al. Consensus opinion on diagnosis of cerebral circulatory arrest using Doppler-sonography: Task Force Group on cerebral death of the Neurosonology Research Group of the World Federation of Neurology. *J Neurol Sci.* 1998;159(2):145–150. doi:10.1016/s0022-510x(98)00158-0
26. Segura T, Calleja S, Irimia P, Tembl JI. Spanish Society of N. Recommendations for the use of transcranial Doppler ultrasonography to determine the existence of cerebral circulatory arrest as diagnostic support for brain death. Rev Neurosci. 2009;20(3–4):251–259.
27. Calleja S, Tembl JI, Segura T, Sociedad Espanola de N. Recommendations of the use of transcranial Doppler to determine the existence of cerebral circulatory arrest as diagnostic support of brain death. Neurologia. 2007;22(7):441–447.
28. Marinoni M, Alari F, Mastronardi V, Peris A, Innocenti P. The relevance of early TCD monitoring in the intensive care units for the confirming of brain death diagnosis. Neurol Sci. 2011;32(1):73–77.
29. Alexandrov AV, Sloan MA, Tegeler CH, Newell DN, Lumsden A, Garami Z, et al. Practice standards for transcranial Doppler (TCD) ultrasound. Part II. Clinical indications and expected outcomes. J Neuroimaging. 2012;22(3):215–224.
30. Monteiro LM, Bollen CW, van Huffelen AC, Ackerstaff RG, Jansen NJ, van Vught AJ. Transcranial Doppler ultrasonography to confirm brain death: A meta-analysis. Intensive Care Med. 2006;32(12):1937–1944.
31. Hadani M, Bruk B, Ram Z, Knoller N, Spiegelmann R, Segal E. Application of transcranial doppler ultrasonography for the diagnosis of brain death. Intensive Care Med. 1999;25(8):822–828.
32. Kirkham FJ, Levin SD, Padayachee TS, Kyme MC, Neville BG, Gosling RG. Transcranial pulsed Doppler ultrasound findings in brain stem death. J Neurol Neurosurg Psychiatry. 1987;50(11):1504–1513.

33. Powers AD, Graeber MC, Smith RR. Transcranial Doppler ultrasonography in the determination of brain death. Neurosurgery. 1989;24(6):884–889.
34. Qian SY, Fan XM, Yin HH. Transcranial Doppler assessment of brain death in children. Singapore Med J. 1998;39(6):247–250.
35. Grote E, Hassler W. The critical first minutes after subarachnoid hemorrhage. Neurosurgery. 1988;22(4):654–661.
36. Paolin A, Manuali A, Di Paola F, Boccaletto F, Caputo P, Zanata R, et al. Reliability in diagnosis of brain death. Intensive Care Med. 1995;21(8):657–662.
37. Eng CC, Lam AM, Byrd S, Newell DW. The diagnosis and management of a perianesthetic cerebral aneurysmal rupture aided with transcranial Doppler ultrasonography. Anesthesiology. 1993;78(1):191–194.
38. Steinmetz H, Hassler W. Reversible intracranial circulatory arrest in acute subarachnoid haemorrhage. J Neurol Neurosurg Psychiatry. 1988;51(10):1355–1356.
39. Shiogai T, Sato E, Tokitsu M, Hara M, Takeuchi K. Transcranial Doppler monitoring in severe brain damage: Relationships between intracranial haemodynamics, brain dysfunction and outcome. Neurol Res. 1990;12(4):205–213.
40. Azevedo E, Teixeira J, Neves JC, Vaz R. Transcranial Doppler and brain death. Transplant Proc. 2000;32(8):2579–2581.
41. Davalos A, Rodriguez-Rago A, Mate G, Molins A, Genis D, Gonzalez JL, et al. Value of the transcranial Doppler examination in the diagnosis of brain death. Med Clin (Barc). 1993;100(7):249–252.
42. de Freitas GR, Andre C. Sensitivity of transcranial Doppler for confirming brain death: A prospective study of 270 cases. Acta Neurol Scand. 2006;113(6):426–432.
43. Dominguez-Roldan JM, Jimenez-Gonzalez PI, Garcia-Alfaro C, Rivera-Fernandez V, Hernandez-Hazanas F. Diagnosis of brain death by transcranial Doppler sonography: Solutions for cases of difficult sonic windows. Transplant Proc. 2004;36(10):2896–2897.
44. Dosemeci L, Dora B, Yilmaz M, Cengiz M, Balkan S, Ramazanoglu A. Utility of transcranial doppler ultrasonography for confirmatory diagnosis of brain death: Two sides of the coin. Transplantation. 2004;77(1):71–75.
45. Feri M, Ralli L, Felici M, Vanni D, Capria V. Transcranial Doppler and brain death diagnosis. Crit Care Med. 1994;22(7):1120–1126.
46. Kirkham FJ, Neville BG, Gosling RG. Diagnosis of brain death by transcranial Doppler sonography. Arch Dis Child. 1989;64(6):889–890.
47. Kuo JR, Chen CF, Chio CC, Chang CH, Wang CC, Yang CM, et al. Time dependent validity in the diagnosis of brain death using transcranial Doppler sonography. J Neurol Neurosurg Psychiatry. 2006;77(5):646–649.
48. Lampl Y, Gilad R, Eschel Y, Boaz M, Rapoport A, Sadeh M. Diagnosing brain death using the transcranial Doppler with a transorbital approach. Arch Neurol. 2002;59(1):58–60.
49. Nebra AC, Virgos B, Santos S, Tejero C, Larraga J, Araiz JJ, et al. Clinical diagnostic of brain death and transcranial Doppler, looking for middle cerebral arteries and intracranial vertebral arteries. Agreement with scintigraphic techniques. Rev Neurol. 2001;33(10):916–920.
50. Petty GW, Mohr JP, Pedley TA, Tatemichi TK, Lennihan L, Duterte DI, et al. The role of transcranial Doppler in confirming brain death: Sensitivity, specificity, and suggestions for performance and interpretation. Neurology. 1990;40(2):300–303.

51. Poularas J, Karakitsos D, Kouraklis G, Kostakis A, De Groot E, Kalogeromitros A, et al. Comparison between transcranial color Doppler ultrasonography and angiography in the confirmation of brain death. Transplant Proc. 2006;38(5):1213–1217.
52. Ropper AH, Kehne SM, Wechsler L. Transcranial Doppler in brain death. Neurology. 1987;37(11):1733–1735.
53. Zurynski Y, Dorsch N, Pearson I, Choong R. Transcranial Doppler ultrasound in brain death: Experience in 140 patients. Neurol Res. 1991;13(4):248–252.
54. Cestari M, Gobatto ALN, Hoshino M. Role and limitations of transcranial doppler and brain death of patients on Veno-Arterial Extracorporeal Membrane Oxygenation. ASAIO J. 2018;64(4):e78.
55. Li Y, Liu S, Xun F, Liu Z, Huang X. Use of transcranial doppler ultrasound for diagnosis of brain death in patients with severe cerebral injury. Med Sci Monit. 2016;22:1910–1915.
56. Hashemian SM, Delavarkasmaei H, Najafizadeh K, Mojtabae M, Ardehali SH, Kamranmanesh MR, et al. Role of transcranial doppler sonography in diagnosis of brain death: A single center study. Tanaffos. 2016;15(4):213–217.
57. Chang JJ, Tsivgoulis G, Katsanos AH, Malkoff MD, Alexandrov AV. Diagnostic accuracy of transcranial doppler for brain death confirmation: Systematic review and meta-analysis. AJNR Am J Neuroradiol. 2016;37(3):408–414.
58. Rodriguez RA, Cornel G, Alghofaili F, Hutchison J, Nathan HJ. Transcranial doppler during suspected brain death in children: Potential limitation in patients with cardiac 'shunt'. Pediatr Crit Care Med. 2002;3(2):153–157.
59. Pallis, C. From brain death to brain stem death, BMJ, 285, Nov 20;285(6353):1487–90.doi: 10.1136/bmj.285.6353.1487.
60. Nornes H, Angelsen B, Lindegaard KF. Precerebral arterial blood flow pattern in intracranial hypertension with cerebral blood flow arrest. Acta Neurochir (Wien). 1977;38(3-4):187–194.
61. Yoneda S, Nishimoto A, Nukada T, Kuriyama Y, Katsurada K. To-and-fro movement and external escape of carotid arterial blood in brain death cases. A Doppler ultrasonic study. Stroke. 1974;5(6):707–713.
62. Cabrer C, Dominguez-Roldan JM, Manyalich M, Trias E, Paredes D, Navarro A, et al. Persistence of intracranial diastolic flow in transcranial Doppler sonography exploration of patients in brain death. Transplant Proc. 2003;35(5):1642–1643.
63. Hassler W, Steinmetz H, Gawlowski J. Transcranial Doppler ultrasonography in raised intracranial pressure and in intracranial circulatory arrest. J Neurosurg. 1988;68(5):745–751.
64. Hassler W, Steinmetz H, Pirschel J. Transcranial Doppler study of intracranial circulatory arrest. J Neurosurg. 1989;71(2):195–201.

11

Determination of neurologic death in infants and children

Thomas A. Nakagawa, Jogi V. Pattisapu

Introduction

The majority of deaths occur in intensive care units following withdrawal of life-sustaining medical therapies resulting in circulatory death.[1,2] Progress in modern medicine has limited our ability to determine death by traditional cardiopulmonary methods. Patients previously declared dead based on loss of circulation, respiration, and consciousness could now be supported with advanced technology. The advent of mechanical ventilation prevented respiratory arrest, and circulation could be restored and preserved with resuscitation procedures (i.e., external cardiac compression, electrical shock, and use of mechanical devices). Anaesthetic agents allowed patients to remain in a controlled, reversible state of unconsciousness that further complicated issues surrounding life and death. Although the general public tends to believe that death occurs when heartbeat ceases, technological advancements have required the medical community to determine a more precise and consistent definition of death.

Historical overview

In the United States of America (USA), the Harvard Ad Hoc Committee[3] defined irreversible coma as a new criterion for death in 1968. In 1981, the President's Commission for the Study of Ethical Problems in Medicine endorsed the Uniform Determination of Death Act (UDDA)[4] defining death as loss of circulatory and respiratory function or loss of function of the entire brain, including the brainstem.

The UDDA defined death but did not specifically outline how loss of circulation, respiration, or neurologic function should be determined stating, 'A determination of death must be made in accordance with accepted medical standards.' No further guidelines were offered for children less than five years of age other than the following recommendation: physicians should be particularly cautious in applying criteria to determine neurologic or brain death in children younger than five years of age. The lack of specificity to determine neurologic death (ND) in children resulted in a Special Task Force report that provided consensus-based guidelines developed by an expert panel.[5] This guideline was published in 1987 and emphasized determination of the cause of coma and the importance of the history and physical examination to ensure reversible conditions did not exist. Age-related observation periods and the need for neurodiagnostic testing were recommended specifically for children less than one year of age. ND could be based solely on a clinical basis for children older than one year of age. However little guidance was provided for infants less than seven days of age because there was a paucity of sufficient clinical experience and data in this age group.[5] In the USA, the adult guideline for the neurologic determination of death (NDD) was revised in 1995 and again in 2010.[6,7] Canadian guidelines for the NDD were published in 2006.[8] In 2011, the multi-society paediatric guidelines for the NDD in infants and children were published by the Society of Critical Care Medicine, American Academy of Pediatrics, and the Child Neurology Society.[9,10] The revised guideline provides a basis to standardize NDD in infants and children and reduce variability and diagnostic error. The consensus-based guidelines were developed with available evidence for NDD in children at the time of publication. The guideline provides the minimum criteria required to determine ND in infants and children. The guidelines did not challenge the definition of legal death as set forth by the UDDA, rather they provided guidance for clinicians to determine ND that remains a relatively rare event. The USA and Canadian guidelines recognize ND based on whole brain criteria (cortex and brainstem) while the United Kingdom recognizes ND as only the brainstem death.[8–12] Ethical issues related to ND continue to be raised and challenged by some in the medical community. However, a detailed discussion about these issues is beyond the scope of this chapter.

Determination of ND

The NDD is a clinical diagnosis.[7–9,10,13,14] An identifiable cause of irreversible coma and apnoea must co-exist to determine ND. Determination of ND requires a thorough examination of the patient. Neuroimaging studies should demonstrate evidence of an acute central nervous system (CNS) insult consistent with the loss of brain function. The aetiology of the CNS insult should be consistent with irreversible coma. Confounding variables that can interfere with the neurologic examination must be recognized and ideally corrected before performing testing for ND. Conditions that can interfere with the neurologic examination must be identified and corrected. These include adequate clearance of sedating drugs and neuromuscular blocking agents, correction of electrolyte and metabolic disturbances, consideration of end-organ dysfunction resulting in delayed drug metabolism or altered metabolic parameters, use of resuscitation medications such as anticholinergic agents that affect pupillary response, and hypothermia that can alter drug metabolism causing a comatose state imitating ND.[7–10,13,14]

Prerequisite criteria are listed in Box 11.1. Clinical criteria to determine ND may not be present on admission and may evolve over the course of several days. The neurologic examination may be unreliable immediately following resuscitation after cardiopulmonary arrest or a severe traumatic brain injury, and in those children who have sustained acute hypoxic ischemic brain injury. An observation period of 24 hours or more is recommended prior to examining the patient for ND, and serial physical examinations are routinely recommended.[7–10,13,14]

Neurologic examination

The neurologic examination of a child requires a skilled clinician to determine coma, apnoea, and loss of all brainstem reflexes.[7–10,13,14] A detailed discussion about the neurologic examination can be found in Chapter 3.

Box 11.1 Prerequisite criteria before initiating neurologic testing for death

The neurologic examination may be unreliable immediately following resuscitation after cardiopulmonary arrest or a severe traumatic brain injury. Appropriate observation of the patient should occur prior to examining the patient for ND.

Normalization of blood pressure for age
- Treatment of shock and hypotension

Normalization and maintenance of body temperature

Correction of electrolyte and metabolic disturbances
- Sodium, glucose, acidosis, hyperammonemia, uremia, inborn errors of metabolism

Adequate clearance of pharmacologic agents
- Sedatives, anesthetic agents, antiepileptic agents, alcohols, anticholinergic agents
  - Dose and duration should be determined
  - Serum drug levels should be obtained when available and be in the low to mid therapeutic range
  - Body temperature and end-organ function must be considered when determining adequate clearance of pharmacologic agents
- Neuromuscular blocking agents
  - Dose and duration should be determined
  - Adequate clearance based on body temperature and end organ function
  - A nerve stimulator can be used to determine twitch response

End-organ dysfunction or failure
- Renal failure
  - Adequate clearance of pharmacologic agents
  - Uremia
- Hepatic failure
  - Adequate clearance of pharmacologic agents
  - Hyperammonemia

Toxins should be considered and ruled out

Placement of an arterial line for hemodynamic monitoring in a critically ill patient is considered standard of care and will also assist with blood sampling during apnoea testing. The comatose patient must lack all evidence of responsiveness (absence of spontaneous or induced movements) and exhibit flaccid tone with loss of all brainstem reflexes. There should be no motor response to noxious stimulation with the exception of spinal cord mediated reflexes. Spinal reflexes including withdrawal and spinal myoclonus can be extremely pronounced. These movements can be complex and may imitate purposeful movements. Pupils should be fixed and dilated with no response to bright light. In smaller children and infants, the use of a magnifying glass may be required to determine pupillary response.[9,10] A pupilometer can be used to determine pupillary response in children older than 6 months of age. Corneal reflexes should be absent. There should be absence of bulbar musculature including facial and oropharyngeal muscle movement. Gag, cough, sucking, and rooting reflexes should be absent. Oculovestibular (cold caloric) testing should elicit no reflex. Oculocephalic (Doll's eye) testing can also be performed but caution is warranted for a patient that has suspected or confirmed cervical spine injury. The patient must also have a complete absence of documented respiratory effort following formal apnoea testing.

Apnoea testing

Apnoea testing is an essential component of the clinical examination and is considered part of the examination process to determine ND in some countries.[9, 10] Apnoea testing must be performed safely and should only occur after the patient meets prerequisite and clinical criteria for ND.[7–10,13,14] Bradycardia in the neonate, CO_2 washout and barotrauma can complicate apnoea testing in children. Testing for apnoea and allowing the partial pressure of carbon dioxide ($PaCO_2$) to rise in a patient that has not met clinical criteria for ND can result in further insult to a patient with CNS injury. The process for apnoea testing is outlined in Box 11.2. During testing, oxygenation and hemodynamics must be preserved, as respiratory acidosis will occur along with potential hypoxemia. To enhance the chances of successful completion of the apnoea test, patients should be preoxygenated with 100% oxygen. Adequate time is required

Box 11.2 Procedure for apnoea testing

- Preoxygenate the patient with 100% oxygen for 5–10 minutes
- Adjust ventilator settings to normalize the $PaCO_2$
- Obtain a baseline arterial blood gas
- Remove patient from ventilator support and attach the endotracheal tube to:
  - A self-inflating bag valve system with titration of positive end expiratory pressure
  - T-piece circuit (lung derecruitment can occur with this method)
- Monitor the patient for 5–10 minutes or longer
  - Obtain blood gases during this time interval to document targeted $PaCO_2$ threshold (typically 60 mm Hg or greater)
- The apnoea test should be aborted if:
  - Patient becomes hemodynamically unstable
  - Patient desaturates to < 85%
  - Patient takes a spontaneous breath
- Apnoea testing is consistent with ND if no respiratory effort is noted during the testing period and the $PaCO_2$ threshold is achieved
- The patient should be placed back on mechanical ventilator support with restoration of normocarbia until death is declared.

* Apnoea testing should only occur after the patient meets clinical criteria for ND. Clinicians skilled in resuscitation should only perform apnoea testing.

for the $PaCO_2$ to rise to levels that would normally stimulate the respiratory centre when removal of assisted ventilation occurs. The rise of CO_2 is approximately 3–5 mm Hg per minute.[9,10] Arterial blood gas measurements are obtained to document baseline and subsequent rise in $PaCO_2$ to the target threshold. In most countries the $PaCO_2$ threshold is 60 mm Hg or greater although a > 20 mm Hg rise above the baseline $PaCO_2$ measurement is required in some jurisdictions to account for patients with chronic respiratory disease who may only breathe in response to supranormal $PaCO_2$ levels.[7–10,14] Some countries also require the inclusion of a pH threshold.[10,15] During apnoea testing, the patient is observed for any spontaneous respiratory effort during a period of 5–10 minutes or longer while blood gases are measured to document the rise in $PaCO_2$ levels. The use of transcutaneous carbon dioxide monitoring, available in some countries, can assist with timing of blood gas analysis.[16] Apnoea testing is consistent with ND if no respiratory effort is noted during the testing period once the target $PaCO_2$ threshold has been achieved. Following completion of the apnoea test, the patient should be placed back on mechanical ventilation with restoration of normocarbia until death is confirmed.

The $PaCO_2$ threshold of 60 mm Hg is considered valid in a neonate.[9,10,14] It has been suggested that the medulla of neonates is more sensitive to hypoxemia and exposure with 100% oxygen prior to apnoea testing may inhibit the respiratory response.[9,10,17] Bradycardia during apnoea testing may be a limiting factor and precede hypercarbia in the neonate.[9,10,14] Some authors have suggested a higher apnoea $PaCO_2$ threshold for neonates during testing based on case reports.[18] Currently available evidence has not been compelling enough to suggest increasing the threshold at this time.

An arterial line should be used to ensure a normal blood pressure during apnoea testing, and to assist with blood gas sampling. Use of venous blood gas values to determine CO_2 levels have been studied; however evidence is not sufficient to validate the use of venous CO_2 measurements during apnoea testing.[19] Oxygenation can be preserved following removal from mechanical ventilation by connecting a T piece circuit to the endotracheal tube.[9,10] This method may result in de-recruitment and desaturation if lung injury is present. Patients can be connected to a self-inflating bag-valve system or anaesthesia bag with titration of positive end-expiratory pressure (PEEP) to preserve oxygenation.[9,10,14] Placement of a small-bore tube in the endotracheal tube with supplemental oxygen (tracheal insufflation) is not recommended.[9,10,14] Tracheal insufflation may cause CO_2 washout preventing adequate $PaCO_2$ rise and can potentially cause barotrauma if gas outflow is not optimal. Changing the mode of ventilation to continuous positive airway pressure (CPAP) is not recommended since modern ventilators will revert to an assist mode if apnoea is detected. Additionally, false spontaneous ventilation has been reported with patients placed on CPAP ventilation during apnoea testing.[9,10,14] The apnoea test should be aborted if the patient develops hemodynamic instability, oxygen saturations fall to 85% or less, or the patient exhibits any spontaneous breathing.[9,10,14] Only individuals skilled at resuscitation should perform apnoea testing because the patient may require medical intervention if they develop hemodynamic instability or profound oxygen desaturation.

Observation periods between examinations

Many countries require serial examinations by two different physicians to make a determination of ND in children.[8–12,15,20] The neurologic examinations may be conducted by two physicians simultaneously or separated by a period of observation depending on the jurisdiction.[8–14] A complete neurologic assessment performed by two different clinicians also avoids conflict of interest and is designed to ensure examinations are carried out independently to reduce or eliminate chances of repeated error during the clinical examination. It is recommended that apnoea testing be performed by the same clinician who is skilled at resuscitation, should the patient decompensate.[9,10,14] The neurologic examination may be unreliable immediately following resuscitation after cardiopulmonary arrest or a severe traumatic brain injury. A period of observation should occur for stabilization of the patient prior to the clinician conducting a thorough neurologic examination. Some guidelines recommend a period of at least 24 hours before initiating examination for NDD.[9,10,14] The determination of ND should only occur after prerequisite criteria have been met. Emphasis is placed on a conservative approach to determine ND especially in younger patients and patients following cardiopulmonary arrest or hypoxic ischemic brain injury.[8–14] If concerns about the neurologic examination exist, continued observation and further examinations are required to determine ND.

Ancillary studies

Ancillary studies are not mandatory to determine ND in infants and children.[8–10,13,14] Some jurisdictions or individual hospitals may have requirements mandating an ancillary study. Ancillary studies are commonly used when neurologic examination and apnoea test cannot be completed because of extenuating circumstances. Additionally, an ancillary study can be used to reduce the observation period between examinations or provide families with a better comprehension of ND.[9,10,13,14] The most commonly used ancillary studies in children are electroencephalography (EEG) and the radionuclide cerebral blood flow (CBF) study.[9,10,13,14] These studies are widely available in most countries and have been used extensively with good experience.[20] EEG and the CBF study evaluate different aspects of the CNS. EEG evaluates cortical and cellular function while the CBF study evaluates flow and uptake into the CNS. There are specific protocols for each of these ancillary studies when testing for ND.[21,22] Both of these ancillary studies require the expertise of trained and qualified individuals to interpret the test results.[9,10,13,14] Developing countries may not have readily available access to nuclear medicine studies and may rely more on the clinical examination or EEG evaluation. Four-vessel cerebral angiography to evaluate the anterior and posterior cerebral circulation remains a gold standard, but is difficult to perform in infants and smaller children.

Prerequisite criteria prior to initiating neurodiagnostic testing must be established, similar to performing the neurologic examination to determine ND.[9,10,13,14] This includes evaluation for conditions that could interfere with neurodiagnostic testing and correcting confounding variables while maintaining normothermia, and a normal blood pressure for age. Sedative agents and hypothermia can interfere with EEG testing and appropriate time should be allowed for clearance of these agents and maintenance of normal body temperature. Radionuclide CBF study to document absence of CBF is frequently used when high levels of sedating agents have been used during the cerebral resuscitation phase of patient care.[9,10,14] Reliance on EEG and CBF evaluation is discouraged because ancillary studies are not mandatory and tend to be less reliable in younger children.[9,10,13,14] Transcranial doppler study, brainstem audio-evoked potentials, computed tomography angiography have not been studied extensively or validated in children and are not recommended as ancillary studies to assist with the NDD in children.[9,10,13,14]

Determination of ND in challenging clinical situations

Technological advances continue to challenge our ability to determine circulatory death and ND. Advanced ventilator therapies, patients with congenital heart disease, and the increasing use of mechanical circulatory support have impacted the ability to determine ND by clinical criteria. The performance of apnoea testing for these patients can be complex and in some instances cannot be completed thus requiring an ancillary study to assist with the NDD. Apnoea testing for patients supported with extracorporeal membrane oxygenation therapy (ECMO) has been safely accomplished.[23,24] Rate of $PaCO_2$ rise will be affected depending on the sweep gas flow. The addition of exogenous CO_2 has been used and may reduce the duration of apnoea testing in this circumstance.[23,24] Patients with impaired oxygenation, ventilation, and hemodynamic alterations supported with advanced ventilation, such as high-frequency oscillation ventilation or airway pressure release ventilation, may not tolerate apnoea testing.[25] These patients may also require significant sedation and neuromuscular blockade that must be taken into consideration when testing for apnoea. Patients with complex congenital heart disease are typically desaturated and may not tolerate apnoea testing. Some guidelines recommend aborting apnoea testing if the patient becomes hemodynamically unstable or oxygen saturation falls to less than 85 mm Hg.[9,10] Currently, no data exists to determine the lower oxygen saturation threshold in a desaturated patient with complex congenital heart disease.

Commonly utilized pharmacologic agents can alter consciousness. The use of barbiturate therapy for refractory intracranial hypertension can pose issues with NDD. High dose infusions coupled with a prolonged half-life can result in a delayed NDD. Current paediatric guidelines recommend that sedative agents should be in the low to mid-therapeutic range if drug levels are measured.[9,10,14] Additionally, the use of targeted temperature management (TTM) and therapeutic hypothermia protocols can result in delayed drug metabolism. When high dose barbiturate therapy or hypothermia protocols are utilized, an ancillary study such as a radionuclide CBF study can be used to assist with determination of death.[9,10,14] Barbiturates and hypothermia will decrease cerebral metabolic rate but will not affect CBF. TTM and hypothermia protocols are commonly employed in neonates following neonatal birth asphyxia and occasionally used for paediatric patients following cardiac arrest and traumatic brain injury. Prognostication of neurologic outcomes following the use of TTM or hypothermia protocols should be approached with caution.[26] Patients should be adequately rewarmed and body temperature maintained at normothermia for at least 24 hours or longer prior to neurologic prognostication or initiating testing for NDD. Reasonable neurologic outcomes in adult patients following cardiopulmonary arrest have been reported 72 hours or more following TTM or therapeutic hypothermia.[27–29]

Children with non-fused cranial sutures, open craniocerebral trauma, or decompressive craniotomy can have altered intracranial pressure dynamics. In such instances, limited regional circulation can be maintained and the increased intracranial pressure commonly seen in a closed skull may not occur. Preserved regional circulation and altered intracranial pressure dynamics may affect radionuclide CBF studies.[30] Anencephalic infants have no cortex although they can have brainstem reflexes, and therefore ND based on whole brain death criteria cannot be determined in this population of patients.

Documentation of ND and other important considerations

The NDD has profound consequences and requires precision to ensure that all components of the physical examination and apnoea test have been performed properly. Utilizing a checklist or established protocol can help standardize the process to determine and document ND and reduce the chance of diagnostic error. If there is any concern that the patient does not fulfil the criteria, the observation period should be extended and additional examinations should occur. Patients should continue to be medically supported until death has been determined or a decision to withdraw life-sustaining medical therapies has been agreed upon.

Determination of ND should not be rushed or take priority over the needs of the patient or the family. However, NDD should occur in a timely fashion and appropriate emotional support should be provided to the family.[9,10] Delaying the NDD can have profound consequences for the family and care providers. This includes resource allocation, confusion of care provider duties and needs for other critically ill patients, moral distress for the staff, delayed grieving for the family, and cost implications for ongoing medical care. There may be instances where ND cannot be determined such as a critically ill patient who cannot undergo apnoea testing or complete an ancillary study to assist with NDD. In these instances, withdrawal of life-sustaining medical therapies and death following circulatory arrest can occur. The death of any child is highly emotional for families and staff. Appropriate support for all the involved parties should be available for assistance following the death of any child.

Appropriate training should occur for clinicians tasked with NDD in children. ND in children is a rare occurrence. Opportunities for clinicians in training to develop expertise in the neurologic examination and apnoea testing to determine ND are becoming less prevalent.[31] The NDD requires the expertise of the most skilled clinician who can perform a complete neurologic examination and effectively communicate the death of a child to parents and guardians. Training programmes exist to assist clinicians in developing and maintaining their skills to determine ND.[32,33]

Conclusion

Determination of ND is a clinical diagnosis with criteria that are consistent across all ages and should be uniformly applied to all patients. Guidelines outline the minimum criteria that must be met to determine ND in infants and children. However, the younger the child, the more cautious and conservative the clinician should be when making the determination of ND. Apnoea testing is required to make a determination of death and must be performed safely. Apnoea testing should only occur after the patient meets the prerequisite and clinical criteria for ND. Ancillary studies, such as EEG and radionuclide CBF studies are not required to make a determination of ND. These studies may be utilized when the clinical examination or apnoea test cannot be completed or to reduce the observation period between examinations. Regional resources, local customs, and hospital policy will dictate use of ancillary studies, specialist involvement, and additional requirements to make the NDD.

Determination of ND in children is highly reliable when performed by trained individuals, with well-accepted worldwide criteria. A standardized checklist should be used for the clinical examination and documentation of ND to improve compliance and reduce diagnostic errors. There are instances where NDD may not be confidently made, and supportive medical therapies should be continued until plans are established regarding withdrawal of life-sustaining therapies. The death of a child is highly emotional for families and staff, requiring appropriate support for all parties involved during these crucial times. The NDD requires the expertise of the most skilled clinician available, who can perform a complete neurologic evaluation, effectively communicate the death of a child to parents and guardians while guiding them through this process.

Highlights

- Diagnosis of ND in children is made by a complete and well-documented clinical examination.
- Clinical criteria to determine ND are consistent across all ages.
- ND can be determined in infants.
- Ancillary studies are not required to make a determination of ND.
- A conservative approach to determine ND is recommended for infants and younger children.
- Special circumstances such as ECMO, complex congenital heart disease, advanced modes of ventilation, and hypothermia protocols can complicate determination of ND for infants and children.
- A standardized checklist for the clinical examination and documentation of ND can improve compliance and may reduce diagnostic error.
- Regional resources, local customs, and hospital policy will dictate use of ancillary studies, specialist involvement, and additional requirements to make a determination of ND.

References

1. Burns JP, Seller DE, Meyer EC, Lewis-Newby M, et al. Epidemiology of death in the pediatric intensive care unit at five US teaching hospitals. Crit Care Med 2014;42:2101–2108.
2. Meert KL, Keele L, Morrison W, et al. Eunice Kennedy Shriver National Institute of Child Health and Human Development Collaborative Pediatric Critical Care Research Network. End-of-life practices among tertiary care PICUs in the United States: A multicenter study. Pediatr Crit Care Med. 2015;16(7):e231–238.
3. A definition of irreversible coma. Report of the Ad Hoc Committee of the Harvard Medical School to examine the definition of brain death. JAMA. 1968;205:85–88.
4. President's Commission for the Study of Ethical Problems in Medicine. Defining death: Medical, legal, and ethical issues in the determination of death. JAMA. 1981;246(19):2184–2186. Library of Congress card number- 81-600150. U.S. Government Printing Office Washington, D.C. 20402.
5. Report of Special Task Force. Guidelines for the determination of brain death in children. American Academy of Pediatrics Task Force on brain death in children. Pediatrics. 1987;80:298–300.
6. Practice parameters for determining brain death in adults (summary statement). The quality standards subcommittee of the American Academy of Neurology. Neurology. 1995;45: 1012–1014.
7. Wijdicks EF, Varelas PN, Gronseth GS, et al. Evidence-based guideline update: Determining brain death in adults: Report of the Quality Standards Subcommittee of the American Academy of Neurology. Neurology. 2010;74:1911–1918.
8. Shemie SD, Doig C, Dickens B, et al. Severe brain injury to neurological determination of death: Canadian forum recommendations. CMAJ. 2006;174(6):S1–S13.
9. Nakagawa TA, Ashwal S, Mathur M, et al. Guidelines for the determination of brain death in infants and children: An update of the 1987 Task Force recommendations. Crit Care Med 2011;39(9):2139–2155.
10. Nakagawa TA, Ashwal S, Mathur M, et al. Clinical report—Guidelines for the determination of brain death in infants and children: an update of the 1987 task force recommendations. Pediatrics 2011;128(3):e720–740.
11. Royal College of Pediatrics and Child Health. The diagnosis of death by neurological criteria in infants less than 2 month old. April 2020. https://www.rcpch.ac.uk/improving-child-health/clinical-guidelines/find-paediatric-clinical-guidelines/published-rcpch/diagn Accessed June 8, 2019.
12. Academy of Medical Royal Colleges. A Code of Practice for the Diagnosis and Confirmation of Death. 2018 Mar;30(1):71–89. doi: 10.1007/s10730-016-9307-y. https://bts.org.uk/information-resources/publications/. 2008. Accessed June 8, 2019.
13. Mathur M, Ashwal S. Pediatric brain death determination. Semin Neurol. 2015 Apr;35(2):116–124.
14. Nakagawa, TA. The determination of brain death in infants and children. A review of the updated brain death guidelines for infants and children. Clin Pulm Med. 2012;19:119–126.

15. Society AaNZIC. The ANZICS statement on death and organ donation (Edition 3.2) 2013.
16. Sochet AA, Bingham L, Sreedhar S, Teppa B, Vose LA, Nakagawa TA. Transcutaneous carbon dioxide monitoring during apnea testing for determination of neurologic death in children: A retrospective case series. Pediatr Crit Care Med. 2020;21:437–442.
17. Joffe AR, Anton NR, Duff JP. The apnea test: Rationale, confounders, and criticism. Journal of Child Neurology. 2010;25:1435–1443.
18. Sosa T, Berrens Z, Conway S, Stalets EL. Apnea threshold in pediatric brain death: A case with variable results across serial examinations. J Pediatr Intensive Care. 2019;8(2):108–112.
19. Fathi A, Lake JL Use of venous Pco_2 in determination of death by neurological criteria in children. Pediatr Neurol. 2019;93:17–20.
20. Nakagawa TA, Jacobe S. JAMA. Pediatric and Neonatal Brain Death. World Brain Death Project. Determination of Brain Death/Death by Neurologic Criteria. 2020 Sep 15;324(11):1078–1097. Supplement Doi:10.1001/jama.2020.11586.
21. Stecker M, Sabau D, Das R, et al. American Electrophysiology Society Guideline 6: Minimum technical standards for EEG recording in suspected cerebral death. J Clin Neurophysiol 2016; 33:324–327.
22. Donohoe KJ, Agrawal G, Frey KA, et al. SNM practice guideline for brain death scintigraphy 2.0. J Nucl Med Technol 2012; 40:198–203.
23. Jarrah RJ, Ajizian SJ, Agarwal S, et al. Developing a standard method for apnea testing in the determination of brain death for patients on venoarterial extracorporeal membrane oxygenation: A pediatric case series. Pediatr Crit Care Med 2014;15(2):e38–43.
24. Harrar DB, Kukreti V, Dean NP, et al. Clinical determination of brain death in children supported by extracorporeal membrane oxygenation. Neurocrit Care. 2019;31(2):304–311. [epub adhead of print] pp 1–8.
25. Gillson N, Weisleder P, Ream MA. A brain death dilemma: Apnea testing while on high-frequency oscillatory ventilation. Pediatrics 2015;135(1):e5–6.
26. Souter MJ, Blissett PA, Blosser S, et al. Recommendations for the critical care management of devastating brain injury: Prognostication, psychosocial, and ethical management: A position statement for healthcare professionals from the neurocritical care society. Neurocrit Care. 2015 Aug;23(1):4–13. doi: 10.1007/s12028-015-0137-6.
27. Mulder M, Gibbs HG, Smith SW, et al. Awakening and withdrawal of life-sustaining treatment in cardiac arrest survivors treated with therapeutic hypothermia. Crit Care Med 2014;42(12):2493–2499.
28. Gold B, Puertas L, Davis SP, et al. Awakening after cardiac arrest and post resuscitation hypothermia: Are we pulling the plug too early? Resuscitation 2014;85(2):211–214.
29. Grossestreuer AV, Abella BS, Leary M, et al. Time to awakening and neurologic outcome in therapeutic hypothermia-treated cardiac arrest patients. Resuscitation 2013;84(12):1741–1746.
30. Frisardi F, Stefanini M, Natoli S, et al. Decompressive craniectomy may cause diagnostic challenges to assess brain death by computed tomography angiography. Minerva Anestesiol. 2014;80:113–118.

31. Ausmus AM, Simpson PM, Zhang L, et al. A needs assessment of brain death education in pediatric critical care medicine fellowships. Pediatr Crit Care Med. 2018;19:643–648.
32. AAP brain death toolbox. Pediatrics September 2011;128(3):e720–e740. https://pediatrics.aappublications.org/content/128/3/e720
33. AAN toolkit. https://www.pathlms.com/ncs-ondemand/courses/1223 Accessed 20 July 2019.

12

Simulation-based training for determination of paediatric brain death

Takashi Araki

Introduction

Brain death (BD) is a physiological state described as a complete and irreversible loss of brain function. However, a social consensus has not yet been reached regarding whether or not BD can be considered human death in some countries. The mistrusted event in the first heart transplant surgery, which was held in 1968, has led to confusion in the Japanese society regarding the diagnosis of BD and organ transplants. Historically, a debate regarding BD has been strongly linked to organ transplantation in Japan, and the significance of BD in the terminal phase of neurological diseases has been recognized not only as a topic of scientific debate but also as an unresolved ethical issue. Japan's progress with organ transplantation legislation was delayed and the first organ transplantation from a brain-dead donor was performed in 1999, thirty years after the first unsuccessful experience.[1] In order to medically evaluate the limits of intensive care for patients with severe central nervous disease, it is necessary to make a strict diagnosis of BD, and education on medical knowledge and procedures concerning BD are essential.

In the past, related academic societies have independently made statements regarding the general significance of a diagnosis of BD, and the following proposal was made in 1998 by the Japan Neurosurgical Society: 'the determination of BD is an important basic part of medical practice for grasping status and determining prognosis that should be based on sufficient understanding of the family of the patient after the medical team gives them an appropriate explanation. In addition, if BD is determined with an appropriate procedure, the medical team manages the issue regarding the subsequent treatment, taking the patient's living will and wishes of their family into consideration. The Japan Neurosurgical Society considers it vital that the important medical practice of BD determination continues not to be subject to restrictions in the future.'[2]

In 2006, in a document titled 'Proposal for views on determining BD and treatment after determining BD', the Japan Association for Acute Medicine stated that 'BD is human death and is a medical phenomenon that is unrelated to social and ethical issues.'[3]

In 2015, the organ donation system maintenance committee of the Japan Council of Organ Transplantation Related Academic Societies (JCOTRAS) stated that 'knowledge and technical perspective of clinical neurology, electrophysiology, and neurocritical care are required for definite diagnosis of BD. Moreover, all healthcare providers must be carefully considerate toward patients who were diagnosed with BD and their family.'[4]

Based on very specific discussions on organ transplantation, education for BD diagnosis in Japan has been needed and built to achieve uniform and rigorous goals.

Historical background

The BD determination criteria (Takeuchi criteria) proposed by the Japanese Ministry of Health and Welfare (MHW; called the Japanese Ministry of Health, Labour and Welfare [MHLW] in 2001) originally excluded children under six years of age from being subjected to BD determination.[5]

In 2008, the Declaration of Istanbul,[6] which recommended the restriction of transplant tourism and self-supply of organs, was adopted. As a result, there was growing public concern that Japanese recipients under the age of six would have difficulty in getting a travel transplant and would not be able to receive any treatment with organ transplantation. In response to this, the revised organ transplant law[7] was established in 2009 after many discussions (Box 12.1). The MHLW's special scientific study project 'Research Regarding Determination of BD in Children and Organ Donation' was written as the basic guideline for maintaining this system and reported on the following: (1) criteria for paediatric BD determination,[8] (2) facilities for

Box 12.1 Historical background of brain death diagnosis in Japan

Historical Background

- **1985: The Ministry of Health, Labour and Welfare's Special Scientific Study Project, "Brain Death Research Group" for Standard Brain Death Determination Criteria" (Takeuchi criteria)**
- **1999: Research group for brain death determination criteria in children**
- **2000: Brain Death Determination Criteria for Children (The Journal of the Japan Medical Association: 124/11)**
    - **Based on Takeuchi criteria**
    - **Infants under adjusted age of 12 weeks excluded**
    - **Determination interval time: 24 h for children under 6 years of age**
    - **Computed tomography used to diagnose underlying diseases**
- **2003: Recommendation by Japan Pediatric Society's Ethics Review Committee**
    - **Expression of patient's own intention**
    - **Training of coordinators specializing in pediatric organ transplantation**
    - **Avoidance of organ donation from brain-dead abused children**
- **2008: The WHO Istanbul Declaration**

organ donation by brain-dead children,[9] and (3) the role of cerebral blood flow (CBF) testing in BD determination.[10] However, low competency for determination of BD and unfamiliarity with BD criteria among paediatricians were highlighted in previous nationwide studies.[7]

Considering the historical backgrounds that paediatricians who were not greatly involved in BD diagnosis were required to participate after the revision of the law, BD education for paediatricians has become very important. Therefore, the importance of off-the-job training using simulation can be described by explaining educational attempts in Japan.

Criteria for determining BD in children in Japan

BD determination is conducted on children aged twelve weeks or older and younger than six years using paediatric BD determination criteria.[8] (For children born before forty weeks' gestation, twelve weeks or older is calculated from the due date of their birth.) For children aged six years or older, the adult criteria are used. In most cases, diagnosis by CT is sufficient, but if the cause of severe brain damage is not clear, MRI may be considered for a definitive diagnosis. Cases that shall be excluded are abused children; children with hypothermia, metabolic disorders, or endocrine diseases; and those affected by drugs. In addition, criteria were established to determine blood pressure disproportionate for the child's age. Furthermore, the volume of ice-water injection (25 ml) for the vestibular reflex, judgement interval (at least 5 min), and methods for brain wave measurement and apnoea testing are changed slightly for children.

Simulation training for BD determination

Over the past years, specific information has been collected on how healthcare professionals think about organ donation from BD donors in simulation training on BD determination conducted at the annual meeting of the Japanese Society of Emergency Pediatrics.[(11)]

Simulation training course contains structured simulation stations, lectures, and case studies presented by expert faculty members. A simulation-based role play discussion was chosen to improve specific clinical decision-making for organ donation after determining BD. This structure also allowed evaluating the participants' familiarity with the BD determination and their understanding of related issues by self-scoring tests at the end of the training. The course was designed to train especially paediatric healthcare providers in determining BD in two separate modules: a multi-station round session and a group discussion session.

Baseline knowledge assessment

All participants took 20-question pre- and post-tests. The pre-test was taken before the keynote lectures to assess baseline knowledge, and the post-test was performed after the group discussion to assess improvement in knowledge. All questions were related to the entire programme content (see Figure 12.1).

Keynote lecture

Two lectures were provided for improving baseline knowledge: (1) the current situation of organ donation from BD donors in Japan; and (2) the history, definition, and pathophysiology of BD.

Q1: The revised Organ Transplant Act was enacted in 2009, allowing organ donation under brain death from all children under the age of 15.
Q2: In children younger than 18 years, even if there is suspicion of child abuse in the past, organ donation under brain death is possible.
Q3: If the person's intention is displayed if he is over 15 years old, treat it as valid.
Q4: When determining brain death under 15 years old, wait at least 24 hours after completing the first brain death determination.
Q5: If deep coma, flat EEG, and pupil dilation can be confirmed, brain death can be determined even if the underlying disease leading to brain death has not been diagnosed.
Q6: Even if the patient is under 6 years old, brain death can be determined if the core body temperature is 32 degrees or higher.
Q7: If a spinal cord reflex is observed, it cannot be said to be brain death.
Q8: Brainstem reflex confirms the seven items: light reflex, corneal reflex, ciliospinal reflex, oculocephalic reflex, vestibular reflex, pharyngeal reflex, cough reflex.
Q9: When eardrum damage is confirmed, ice water cannot be injected, so vestibular reflex testing is impossible.
Q10: For vestibular reflexes, immediately after the inspection of one ear, complete the inspection with the other ear.
Q11: Apnea test is a test to see if patient is breathing spontaneously when PaCO2 value is raised over 80mmHg.
Q12: If the continuation is judged to be dangerous during the apnea test due to desaturation or hypotension, the test will be discontinued.
Q13: The apnea test is not necessarily done at the end of the brain death determination.
Q14: Give artificial respiration with 100% oxygen for 5 minutes before the apnea test.
Q15: In children under 6 years of age, in order to prevent hypoxia during the apnea test, place a suction tube in the trachea and allow oxygen to flow at 6 L / min.
Q16: Electroencephalograms under 6 years of age take at least 5 cm between electrodes.
Q17: As for the sensitivity of EEG, it is necessary to record not only the standard sensitivity of 10μV / mm but also the high sensitivity of 2.5μV / mm (or higher sensitivity).
Q18: Brain death cannot be determined without confirming the flat EEG and disappearance of ABR (auditory brainstem-induced response) after the II wave.
Q19: There is a report that the peak of grief reaction is up to 6 months after bereavement and then gradually reduced to 27% by 24 months.
Q20: Children with disabilities who cannot effectively express their intentions must obtain the consent of their parents, grandparents and relatives living together.

Figure 12.1. Baseline knowledge assessment; sample questions

Multi-station round

This session covered six different topics of BD determination for paediatric patients: (1) clinical examination of BD following the criteria, (2) apnoea testing, (3) ancillary testing using electroencephalogram (EEG), (4) psychological care for family members, (5) the process of organ donation, (6) and how to detect abused children. The participants rotated among these stations every 35 minutes with a predetermined time schedule.

For hands-on skill development, we used the Sim Junior 3G™ simulation mannequin (Laerdal Medical, Wappingers Falls, NY, USA).[12] This model is accompanied by a monitor that can display various vital signs such as heart rate, oxygen saturation, blood pressure, temperature, respiratory rate, and end-tidal CO_2.

Preparation

The mannequin was intubated with a 6.0-mm endotracheal tube and provided a flashlight for pupillary reflex assessment, cotton swabs for corneal reflex assessment, an 18-G needle as noxious stimuli to the neck for ciliospinal reflex assessment, a 30-cc syringe with a suction catheter for oculovestibular reflex assessment, and a laryngoscope and suction catheter for gag reflex assessment. A suction catheter, an oxygen tube, and a Jackson-Rees circuit were provided for the apnoea test. An EEG machine (Nihon Kohden, Tokyo, Japan) was used for a practical presentation about the artefacts of EEG recordings. Staff members prepared the environment in each station and the timekeeper strictly managed the timetable for comfortable rotation. The experts conducted the session from orientation to debriefing.

All participants were given a booklet that included copies of all session slides for self-study, six case scenarios for group discussion, and a self-scoring sheet.

1. *Clinical examination*

After hearing a brief summary of BD criteria, the participants were told to perform a complete BD examination while verbalizing their thorough examination process. The apnoea test was performed last. The facilitator instructed the participants to track the BD criteria in the booklet and to self-evaluate their performance (see Figures 12.2 and 12.3).

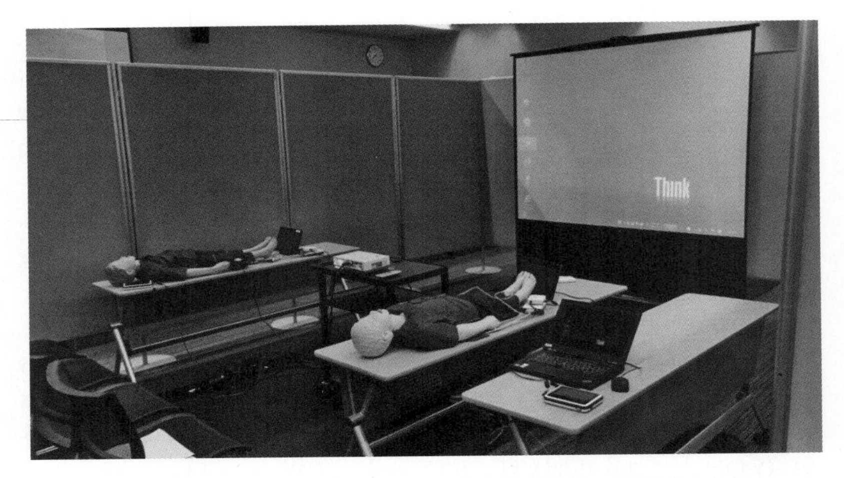

Figure 12.2. Clinical examination using the Sim Junior 3G™ simulation mannequin

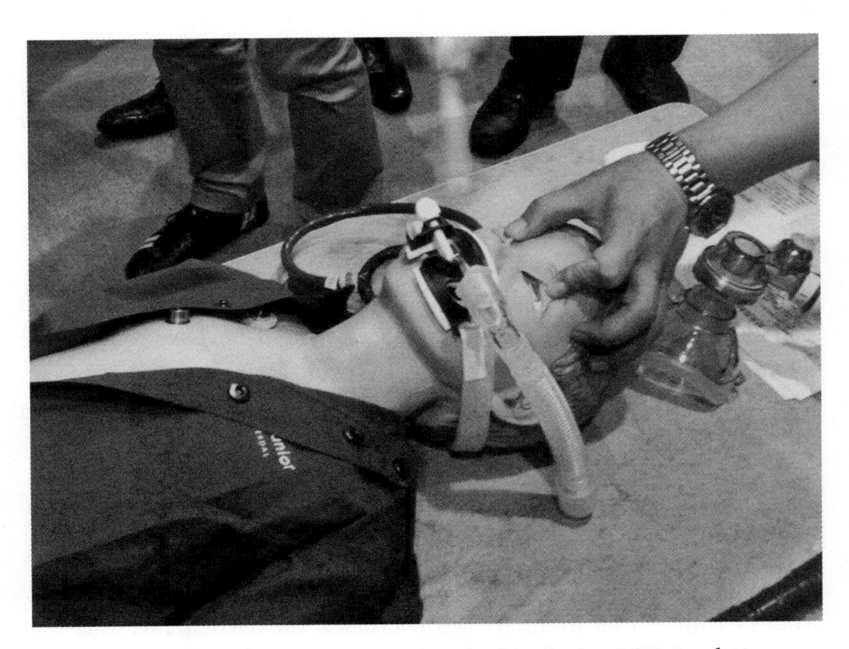

Figure 12.3. Clinical examination using the Sim Junior 3G™ simulation mannequin

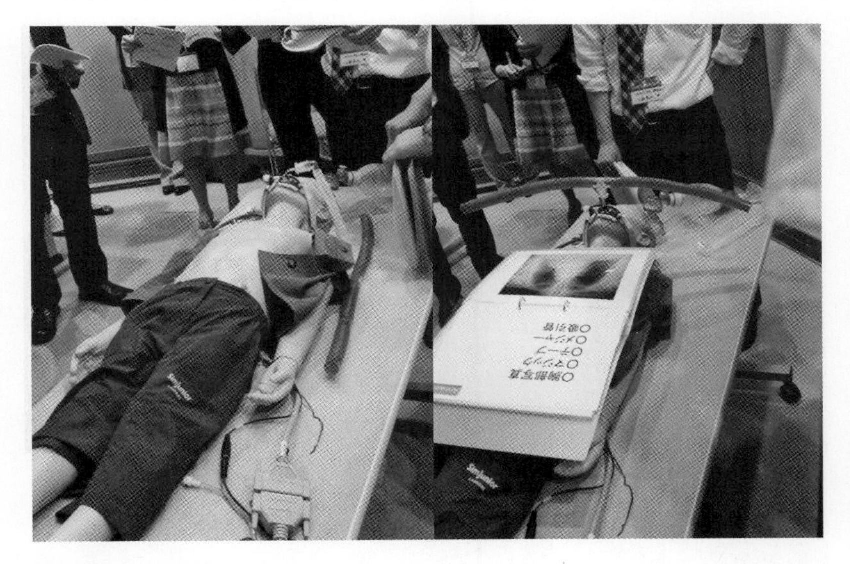

Figure 12.4. The apnoea test

2. *The apnoea test*

After a short orientation regarding the appropriate apnoea testing procedure, the facilitator demonstrated the entire procedure with a child mannequin. The participants were asked to answer brief questions about the pitfalls of apnoea testing (see Figure 12.4).

3. *EEG recording*

In a hands-on session, the participants were asked to place the electrodes on a partner's arm to learn the effect of recording artefacts on the fivefold sensitivity of the EEG. After this demonstration, the participants could recognize that the EEG recording requires a sophisticated technique to obtain a flat line on brain-dead patients (see Figure 12.5).

4. *Psychological care for the family*

Based on the results of lecturers' interviews with the family members of brain-dead patients, the participants received a short lecture about the

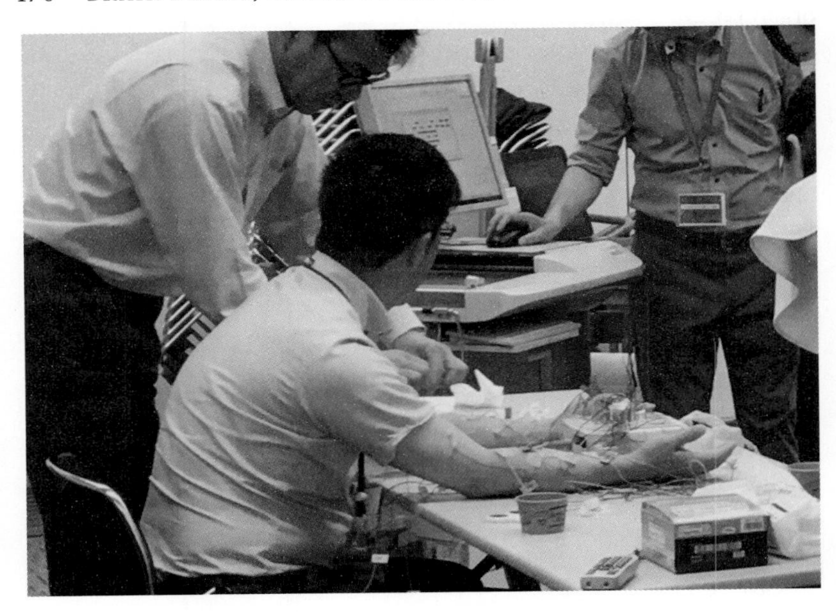

Figure 12.5. EEG recording

psychological process of the patient's family to accept the BD determination. The participants were instructed to be aware of the importance of psychological support of medical staff.

5. *Role of the Japan Organ Transplant Network (JOTNW)*

JOTNW is the only organization in Japan that acts as an intermediary and mediator between organ donors and patients waiting for transplants. The participants received detailed information about the role of the JOTNW[13] and the epidemiology of organ transplantation in Japan to understand the correct process for contacting this organization when potential donors are identified.

6. *How to determine a case of child abuse*

As per the Japanese BD criteria, parents who are suspected to have abused their children cannot act as legal representatives. Therefore, organ procurement from children with a history of child abuse will not be performed even if a clinical determination of BD is made. The clinical approach to child abuse is not always straightforward and requires multidisciplinary investigation. After this session, the participants were expected to have the comprehensive knowledge necessary for the diagnosis of child abuse.

Group discussion

A clinical vignette of a child with a history of devastating brain injury was provided to each group for discussion of whether the patient would be an appropriate candidate for BD determination. The participants were required to consider various related issues to relay their final decision.

Case presentation example:
An 11-year-old girl with a long and complex history of glioblastoma multiforme required four tumor resection operations and postoperative chemotherapies for 12 months. The patient's current prognosis is terminal and she has been prescribed full-time bed rest. She is able to open her eyes and move her limbs but is not able to communicate verbally; she does not have any evidence of systemic organ failure. She has been living in her home receiving end-of-life care. One day, a family member called 911 after she suffered a seizure at home that lasted for more than five minutes. By the time paramedics arrived, she had stopped breathing. The patient was resuscitated and transferred to the nearest emergency center, where she was intubated and taken to the intensive care unit for further care. The next day, the patient's pupils were fixed and dilated, and EEG results showed total electrocerebral silence. The patient had no advance directive, and her family was unable to decide whether to ask to stop current treatment. Two days later, the patient's family showed a memo from her desk at her home. The note read: 'I would like to donate all my organs and tissues for patients affected by organ failure when I become brain dead.' It was written a month ago by the patient.

Self-scoring and questionnaires

At the end of the course, all participants answered questionnaires (see Figure 12.6). The post-course questionnaires comprised three parts: (1) comprehension level, (2) evaluation, and (3) feedback comments. The comprehension level was scored in five aspects on a scale of 1–3: (i) significance of BD determination and related issues, (ii) skill in determining BD upon examination, (iii) recording of EEG and apnoea testing,

Post-course questionnaire

ID Number

Name

1. Comprehension Level

You understood the following topics:	Very well (1)	Moderately (2)	Not well (3)
① Significance of BD determination and issues	□	□	□
② Skill and pitfalls of BD examinations	□	□	□
③ Recording of EEG and apnea testing	□	□	□
④ Interaction with mourning family members	□	□	□
⑤ Organ donation and BD determination	□	□	□

2. Evaluation

① Value of this course

Not valuable (1) little (2) average (3) good (4) excellent (5)

② Duration of this course

Too short (1) More in details (2) Appropriate (3)

③ Difficulty of this course

Too difficult (1) Difficult (2) Appropriate (3) Easy (4) Too easy (5)

④ Please score the value of this course after it was completed.

LOW← 1 2 3 4 5 6 7 8 9 10 11 →HIGH

3. Free feedback comments about the positive aspects of this course

➢

4. Free feedback comments about the negative aspects of this course

➢

Figure 12.6. Sample of post-course questionnaire

(iv) interaction with mourning family members, and (v) knowledge of organ procurement. For course evaluation, the participants were asked to score in three aspects: value and difficulty of the course on a scale of 1–5, duration of the course on a scale of 1–3. Finally, the entire programme of this course was scored on a scale of 1–11. In the post-course feedback comments, various opinions were received from participants. The data were presented as mean score ± standard deviation (SD). In group discussions, participants were provided with simulated case scenarios and discussed family care in particular. They had to derive problems that were to be solved from the background of the case and consider how to deal with them. Similarly, the exclusion of abused children was discussed. The data used as the basis for the discussion is an analysis of test results for participants, and does not handle information that leads to individual identification. There is no involvement in medical practice beyond normal practice. This is a study with no assignment. There is no invasion of patients, and it is an exploratory clinical study by data analysis.

Statistical analysis

Test scores between groups were compared using Student's t-test for continuous variables. Statistical significance was established at $p < 0.05$.

Results

The test results of 520 students from 2010 to 2019 were collected. The questions were classified into six categories: general knowledge (GN), confounders (CF), prerequisites (PR), clinical examination (CE), apnoea test (ApT), and ancillary test (AT), and the percentage of correct answers was calculated for each of these items, and the changes before and after taking the course were compared.

The overall percentage of correct answers on the test improved from 64% before the course to 80% after the course, a statistically significant difference ($p < 0.001$). GN 65% improved to 82% ($p < 0.01$), CF 72% to 75% ($p = 0.25$), PR 64% to 69% ($p < 0.01$), CE 66% to 86% ($p < 0.01$) and both were effective. ApT was improved by 59% to

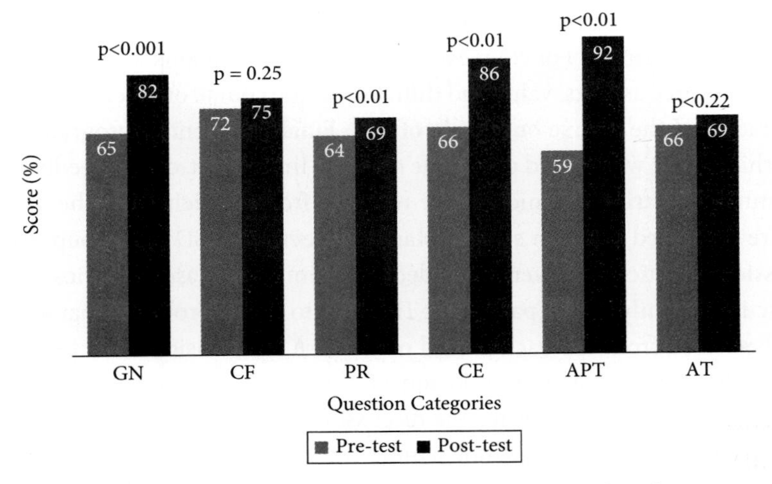

GN: general knowledge, CF: confounders, PR: prerequisites, CE: clinical examination, ApT: apnea testing, AT: ancillary test

Figure 12.7. Pre-test and Post-test scores by question categories

92% ($p < 0.01$). AT was 66% and 69% ($p = 0.22$). In the categories of confounders and prerequisites, there was no significant increase in scores, but participants improved in other categories such as general knowledge, clinical examination, apnoea testing, and ancillary test (see Figure 12.7).

Next, a simulated case was presented and interviewed about family care from a discussion. In the group discussion section, two of the six groups (33% of participants) in 2011 decided that the presented case should be considered for BD determination for organ donation. In 2012, four of the six groups (66% of participants) agreed with organ donation. All groups in 2013 (one of one; 100% of participants) and 2014 (six of six; 100% of participants) determined that the presented case should be considered for BD determination for organ donation (see Figure 12.8).

The course was also evaluated in three aspects: (1) value (4.58 ± 0.64), (2) time schedule (2.40 ± 0.61), and (3) difficulty (2.89 ± 0.43). Overall, the average score on the 11-point evaluation was very high (9.64 ± 1.69), and the course continued to receive positive evaluations over the four years (see Figure 12.9).

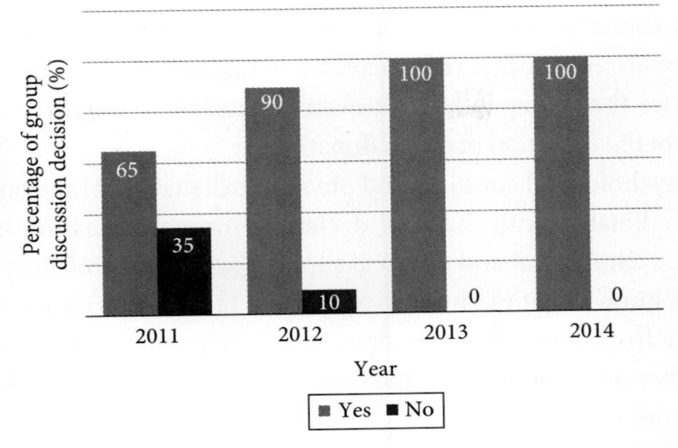

Figure 12.8. Group discussion decision: Should the presented case advance to BD determination for organ donation?

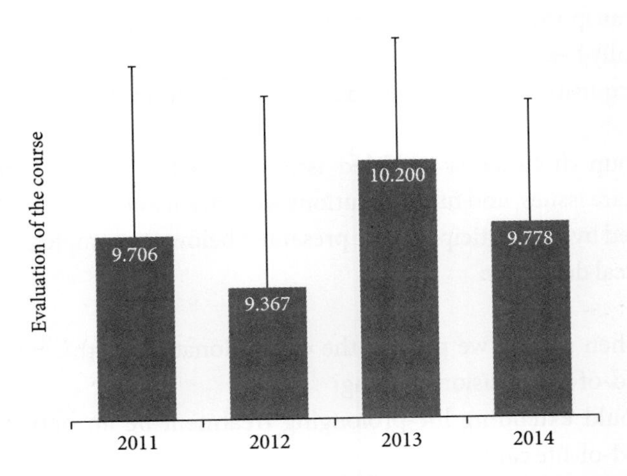

Figure 12.9. Results (average score) from the 11-point post-course evaluation from 2011 to 2014.

Discussion

After the 2010 revision of the Organ Transplant Act, organ donations from BD donors from patients under the age of eighteen have counted thirty-four cases (as of 16 October 2019), and experience has been accumulating in Japan. It has been pointed out that an increase in the number of organ transplants for children is an educational effect for healthcare professionals. Also, BD is recognized as an important medical event that determines the therapeutic limit even in paediatric intensive care, regardless of the intention of organ donation.

The psychological conflicts and physical exhaustion of the family are easily predictable until the final decision on organ donation is made, so both psychological and physical support are considered very important. It is known that the burden on patient families varies when organ donation from paediatric BD donors is implemented. The following points were raised as issues in the system of organ donation from paediatric BD donors.

① Family care
② Building trust with patient families
③ Transportation system for critically ill emergency patients (especially head trauma)
④ Acquisition of knowledge necessary for determining BD

The group discussions included issues related to medical decisions, family care issues, and future solutions were discussed. Some of the views presented by the participants are presented below as examples.

Medical decisions:

① When should we present the organ donation to the family as an end-of-life decision-making?
② Could extending life-prolonging treatment be an option for the end-of-life care?
③ It is necessary for the medical staff to discuss why the family expressed emotional reactions.
④ It is necessary to look back at how much the family understood the contents of the family explanation.
⑤ Was BD strictly diagnosed?

Family care issues:

① Parents' opinions should be respected
② The vocabulary of BD is too strong

③ The answer that cannot be decided is also a good answer
④ The time required for acceptance may be infinite
⑤ An atmosphere that promptly asks for an answer increases the mental burden of the family
⑥ It is important to talk about child's dignity

Future solutions:

① Build relationships of trust with patient families
② Trying to settle with the patient's family
③ Integration, sharing, and agreement with patient families
④ Make opportunities for multiple occupations
⑤ Bridging the distance between medical terms and common sense

To our knowledge, two previous nationwide studies of paediatric BD in Japan have been conducted and have revealed low competency for determining BD and unfamiliarity with BD criteria among paediatricians.[(14)] In addition, those studies highlighted the need for paediatricians to learn about BD determination in Japan. We assume that this course may be beneficial for paediatric healthcare providers to learn about BD. In his review, Mizuguchi[(15)] speculated that Japanese paediatricians believe the following and are unlikely to perform BD determination: (1) strict determination of BD is unnecessary when the patient is younger than fifteen years because the previous law prohibited organ transplant from paediatric BD donors, (2) apnoea testing is not required because BD determination without apnoea test is sufficient to understand the extent of brain damage and to inform the family of the child's prognosis, (3) several case reports show that apnoea testing can be invasive and can cause deterioration after implementation, and (4) obtaining informed consent for apnoea testing from the parents is very difficult because of the possibility of complications. However, since organ donation from paediatric BD donors was legally permitted, the Japanese Society of Pediatrics (JPS)[(16)] has issued a position statement on organ donation from paediatric BD donors. The JPS also agreed with the importance of educating Japanese paediatricians about BD determination. It is expected that this educational course will be recognized as a very useful opportunity for paediatric healthcare providers to learn about BD and related issues in the near future.

The Sim Junior 3G™ simulation mannequin, used for hands-on skill development in the clinical examination and apnoea testing sessions, is accompanied by a monitor that can display various vital signs such as heart rate, oxygen saturation, blood pressure, temperature, respiratory rate, and end-tidal CO_2. This mannequin model was quite useful for simulating the patient's physiological reactions during a BD examination, as evidenced by the high evaluation scores in the clinical examination section and apnoea testing. Comments were provided about the benefits of this mannequin, particularly for the clinical examination section.

The section entitled *Psychological Care in Brain Death Diagnosis* was highly rated. Many participants commented that this section was quite informative and offered information that is useful to understand the psychological stress of the patients' family members as well as staff members who had cared for the patients. The contents of this section were meticulously prepared based on the lecturer's original interview results. In the simulation, problems related to family care were extracted through discussions on simulated cases. First, opinions were divided as to whether accurate BD diagnosis was a prerequisite for end-of-life medical judgement. Depending on the facility, BD diagnosis including apnoea test may not be feasible, and there was a tendency to tell the end of life to the family at the 'state that can be considered BD' where apnoea test has not been performed yet. When reporting the fact of BD to the family, it is necessary to evaluate whether or not the psychological conflict of the person with confusion and grief, the stage/procedure for psychological recovery, and the explanation from the medical side are correctly understood. If there is a clinical psychologist intervention available, higher quality family care can be started.

Excluding child abuse, victims as candidates for organ donors are a very specific requirement in the BD criteria in Japan. The use of a checklist for detecting a suspected child abuse case is assumed as a useful tool, but no data exist regarding the accuracy and the sensitivity of determination of child abuse using this procedure, and further investigation is also needed. Given the complexity of the examination and the medicolegal ramifications of a child abuse determination, this laxity is a matter of grave significance.[17]

Participants valued this course, felt that the schedule was appropriate, and that the course contents were valuable. Although some negative feedback was received, the post-course questionnaire showed the participants' comprehension level as high overall.

Conclusion

Attending a BD diagnosis seminar was considered to be clearly useful for clarifying the uncertainties in the organ donation system from BD donors, a good opportunity to solve technical questions in BD diagnosis and to master judgement techniques. In particular, the improvement in the accuracy rate of pre- and post-test about the apnoea test is remarkable compared to other items, which seems to be the result of the non-daily demand for the apnoea test itself and the lack of general knowledge. With continuous effort, we will research and improve our intervention to ensure its effectiveness upon implementation, with the hope of firm social reliability on BD determination and subsequent organ donation from paediatric patients.

Highlights

- As for the education of BD diagnosis for healthcare providers, there is a limit to the acquisition of knowledge only by on-the-job training because of its rare opportunity.
- The simulation training course contains structured simulation stations, lectures, and case studies presented by expert faculty members to improve specific clinical decision making for organ donation after determining BD.
- The mannequin model was quite useful for simulating the patient's physiological reactions during a BD examination in the clinical examination section and apnoea testing.
- Attending simulation-based training course for BD diagnosis is considered to be useful for clarifying the uncertainties in the organ donation system, and a good opportunity to solve technical questions in BD diagnosis.
- The improvement in the accuracy rate of pre- and post-test about the apnoea test is remarkable compared to other items, which seems to

be the result of the non-daily demand for the apnoea test itself and the lack of general knowledge.

- The section entitled *Psychological Care in Brain Death Diagnosis* was highly rated and participants commented that this section was quite informative and mentioned that it is useful to understand the psychological stress of the patients' family members as well as staff members who had cared for the patients.

Acknowledgements

The author is deeply grateful to Toshio Osamura, Akira Satomi, Tomomitsu Tsuru, Minoru Umehara, Takehiro Niitsu, Tsuyoshi Yamamoto, Kazutaka Nishiyama, Hiromichi Taneichi, Tadafumi, Ishihara, Sho Kimura and Midori Yasuda, the Exploratory Committee members for Brain Death Determination and Related Issues, the Japanese Society of Emergency Pediatrics.

Reference

1. Kita Y, Aranami Y, Aranami Y, Nomura Y, Johnson K, Wakabayashi T, Fukunishi I. Japanese organ transplant law: A historical perspective: Review. Prog Transplant 2000;10(2):106–108.
2. The Basic Stance and Requests of the Japan Neurological Society regarding Organ Transplant Law: July 29, 1997, Steering Committee of the Japan Neurosurgical Society, 1997.
3. Japanese Association for Acute Medicine: Proposals for Terminal Care in Emergency Medicine (Guidelines), November 16, 2007.
4. The Japan Council of Organ Transplantation Related Academic Societies (JCOTRAS): Proposals from The Organ Donation System Maintenance Committee, January 14, 2015.
5. MHW special scientific study project, General Study Report (1999) Research regarding Standard Criteria for Pediatric Brain Death Determination (Principal Investigator: Kazuo Takeuchi).
6. The Declaration of Istanbul on Organ Trafficking and Transplant Tourism. International Summit on Transplant Tourism and Organ Trafficking. Clin J Am Soc Nephrol. Sep 2008, 3(5):1227–1231.
7. Tanizawa T. Japan Pediatric Society Ethical Committee Report, 'Results of an Internet Survey of General Members regarding Pediatric Organ Transplantation' Journal of the Japan Pediatric Society 2001;105: 1250–1252.

8. 2009 MHLW Special Research Grant (Health and Labour Sciences Research Project) Research Report regarding Determination of Brain Death in Children and Organ Donation: 'Investigation of Criteria for Determining Legal Brain Death in Children' (Co-researcher: Fujiko Yamada), 2009.
9. 2009 MHLW Special Research Grant (Health and Labour Sciences Research Project) Research Report regarding Determination of Brain Death in Children and Organ Donation: 'Research on Facilities for Organ Donation by Brain-Dead Children' (Co-researcher: Hiroyuki Yokota), 2009.
10. 2009 MHLW Special Research Grant (Health and Labour Sciences Research Project) Research Report regarding Determination of Brain Death in Children and Organ Donation: 'Cerebral Blood Flow Testing Group' (Co-researcher: Jun Hatazawa), 2009.
11. Araki T, Yokota H, Ichikawa K, Osamura T, Satomi A, Tsuru T, Umehara M, Niitsu T, Yamamoto T, Nishiyama K. Simulation-based training for determination of brain death by pediatric healthcare providers. Springerplus 2015;4:412 eCollection.
12. Sim Junior 3G [online] Available at:<https://laerdal.com/jp/products/simulation-training/obestetrics-pediatrics/simjunior/> [Accessed 2 July 2020].
13. Japan Organ Transplant Network. 2020. Japan Organ Transplant Network. [online] Available at: <https://www.jotnw.or.jp/> [Accessed 1 July 2020].
14. Takeuchi K (2000) Study on the criteria for the determination of brain death in children. Ministry of Health, Labour and Welfare Sciences Research Grant Special Research Project. Report on General Research. (in Japanese)
15. Mizuguchi M (2010) Brain death in children. Rinsho Masui 34:17–25. (in Japanese)
16. Igarashi T (2010) A position statement on organ donation from pediatric brain-dead donors. http://www.jpeds.or.jp/modules/guidelines/index.php?content_id=49 The Japanese Society of Pediatrics. (in Japanese).
17. Araki T, Yokota H, Fuse A. Brain death in pediatric patients in Japan: Diagnosis and unresolved issues; Review. Neurol Med Chir (Tokyo) 2016;56:1–8.

13

Variability of brain death determination around the world: The need for an international consensus

Francesca Fossi, Giuseppe Citerio

Brief history of brain death determination

In the past, death was defined as the cessation of cardiopulmonary function, but advances in resuscitation led to patients supported in intensive care units (ICUs) with irreversible loss of brain function.[1] In 1959, in Europe, both Mollaret and Goulon[2] and Wertheimer[3] respectively described 'le coma depassé' and 'the death of the nervous system' as states without brainstem reflexes, persistent apnoeic coma and electrically silent brains.

In 1968, after the first heart transplant a multidisciplinary panel convened at Harvard and published 'A definition of irreversible coma' where the committee concluded that with certain criteria, a patient could be defined dead and care interrupted before the cessation of cardiopulmonary function.[4] Since then, death determined by neurologic criteria was accepted all over the world and defined by law in each country, generally as 'irreversible cessation of circulatory and respiratory functions' or 'irreversible cessation of all functions of the entire brain, including the brainstem'.[4] The first European country to define brain death (BD) legally was Finland in 1971.

In the US, cardiac death and BD converged in 1981 with the Uniform Determination of Death Act,[5] which defined death as:

- Irreversible cessation of circulatory and respiratory functions, or
- Irreversible cessation of all functions of the entire brain including brainstem

Medical criteria to diagnose BD were also defined in 1981 in the 'Report of the Medical Consultants on the Diagnosis of Death to the President's Commission for the Study of Ethical Problems in Medicine and Biomedical and Behavioural Research.[5] The prerequisites were irreversible loss of all brain function (both brainstem and cortical) and in particular, the following:

- Unresponsiveness and unreactivity
- Absence of brainstem function (fixed and unreactive pupils; absence of corneal, vestibular-ocular, and gag reflexes; absence of motor movements in response to stimulation of somatic areas within the cranial nerve distribution)
- Absence of brainstem respiratory reflexes (absence of respiratory movements after the increase of arterial partial pressure of carbon dioxide over 60 mmHg)

Confounding factors should be evaluated and effects of CNS depressant or paralytics, hypothermia, severe acid-base, electrolyte, and endocrine abnormalities, and hypotension or shock necessarily excluded. The observation period is meant to be at least 6 hours (24 hours after post-anoxic brain damage in cardiac arrest). This text was designed to be the legal foundation for BD and it has been documented that the minimum clinical requisites necessary to diagnose BD are, in general, well-standardized all over the scientific community.[6]

Greer et al.,[7] in 2008, showed differences between various US centres in Brain Death Determination (BDD) dealing with prerequisites, clinical examination, and apnoea test. After the publication of this paper, the following guidelines were updated in 2010[8] (see Figure 13.1).

- There is no report of recovery after clinical, correctly performed diagnosis of BD.
- There is not enough evidence to determine the minimal duration of observation period.
- Non-brain-mediated spontaneous movements can mimic spontaneous movements similar to the mimicking of auto-triggered ventilator cycling to spontaneous breathing.

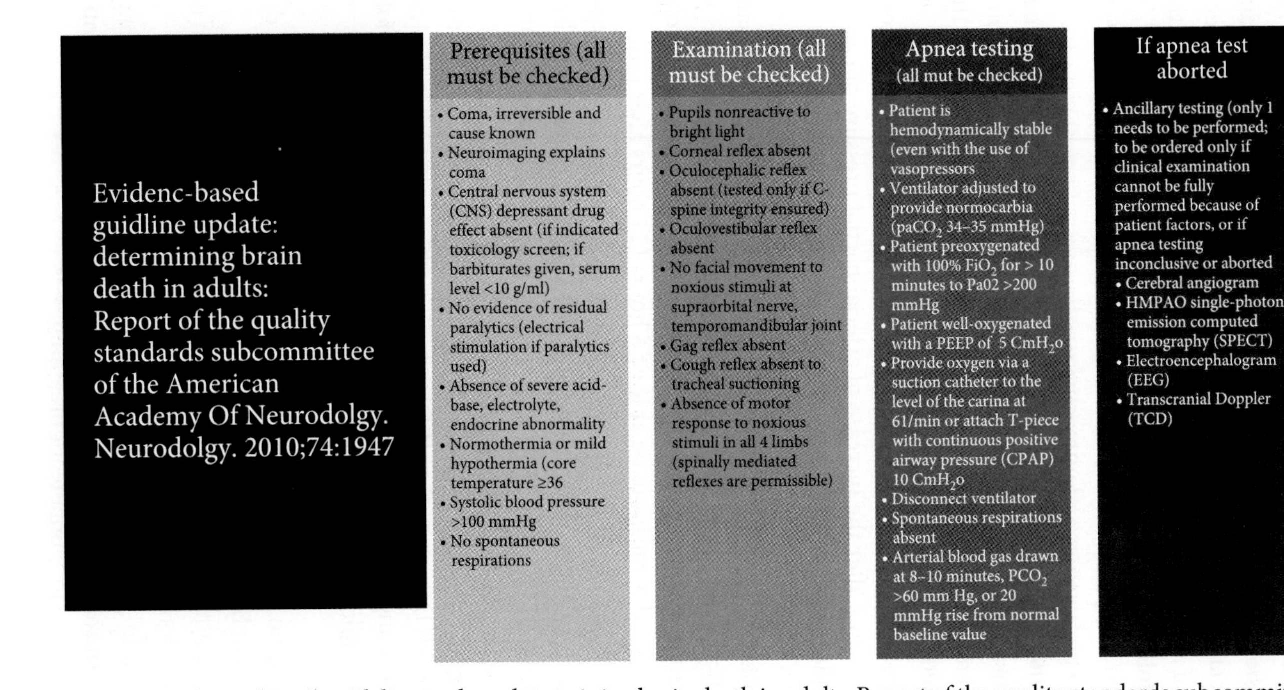

Figure 13.1. Evidence-based guideline update: determining brain death in adults: Report of the quality standards subcommittee of the American Academy of Neurology [8].

- Many techniques for apnoea testing are represented all over the world: no superiority has been demonstrated.
- There is no evidence that shows newer ancillary tests can determine the cessation of function of the brain more accurately.

BDD is essentially a clinical, bedside assessment. Beyond the basic clinical criteria, extra exams and evaluations can be added (these are the so-called ancillary tests). Some aspects of the assessment, such as the duration and timing of the observation period and professionals to be involved, were not specified in the guidelines.

In the course of the development of the BD concept, despite the updated guidelines, variability between countries arose. This variability correlates with socio-economic, cultural, and religious differences.

In 2010, Wijdicks et al[8] observed that, while BD had been accepted worldwide, diagnostic criteria were not uniform and they reported huge differences in different aspects. Guidelines were absent in many countries. Number of physicians involved and observation time were even more variable.

Consistent elements

BDD includes, in a central evaluation, the core of the diagnosis, and additional evaluations (Table 13.1). The core elements are usually consistent and not variable between different countries and centres.

In a recent research conducted by CENTER-TBI collaboration,[6] a full agreement on the clinical evaluation of BD was found between sixty-seven academic centres participating across Europe. Clinical evaluation

Table 13.1. Consistent elements vs variable elements

Common points	Differences
• unresponsiveness and unreactivity	Observation period
• absence of brainstem function	Number of operators
• absence of brainstem respiratory reflexes	Professions involved
	Ancillary testing

included: Glasgow Coma Scale (GCS) 3, absence of brainstem reflexes, no respiratory efforts in response to an apnoea test and absence of confounding factors.

Similarly a different recent review shows full agreement in Europe regarding comas with known cause, no spontaneous breathing, normothermia, and no effects of CNS depressant nor paralytics.[8]

Citerio et al[10] described that 100% of centres determined BD with coma (GCS 3), apnoea test, and cough and corneal reflexes. Pupillary, oculocephalic, and oculovestibular reflexes were tested in 98% of the centres. The number of clinical examinations was two in the large majority of countries.

Variable elements

Additional elements are often variable. Variability is usually due to national laws. Countries can be classified according to which anatomical region is required to be irreversibly dead in order to understand about BDD:

1. whole brain
2. only brainstem

The United Kingdom (UK) represents an exception in Europe because it follows the 'brainstem' concept of BD.[9] In the UK, the diagnosis of BD requires the confirmation of brainstem death, while whole-brain cessation of functions is not mandatory (no electrocerebral silence is needed, for example). The difference is more formal than practical, because the clinical determination of BD happens identically[10]; while it could be asserted that one patient might be 'brainstem dead' with cortical functions still present, this has no clinical relevance because death is a process and not an event. The death of each part of an organism cannot be independently assessed (hypothalamic–pituitary responses are never evaluated even in the 'whole brain' countries, for example). Brainstem death should be seen as an irreversible point in the process of dying.

In the US, less than 50% of practices strictly follows the '2010 American Academy of Neurology (AAN) guidelines' about BDD.[11] However, adherence to US guidelines is improving as shown by Greer et al., even regarding ancillary tests.[12]

BD was incorporated into China's legal definition of death in October 2018. Asian countries generally follow the 'whole-brain' concept of BD, with the exception of countries with past colonial links to the UK.[13] As far as it is known, protocols for BDD are not common in lower-income countries (in particular, countries without a transplant network).[14] The law of South Africa, Brazil, Malta, Slovenia, and some regions in Canada does even not define BD.

In Europe, differences exist regarding qualifications of examiners (Figure 13.2A), prerequisite for blood pressure and drug levels, number and timing of evaluations[12,14,15] (Figure 13.2B). Just 70% of the examined centres checks for acid-base balance and blood pressure in BD.[8]

Clinical evaluation is quite homogeneous. On the contrary, ancillary tests follow different indications (Figure 13.2C). In centres from Northern Europe and the UK, ancillary tests were rarely used for BDD. Some of these differences are region specific, but other aspects have variability within a single country. Variability within a region might be due to a lack of knowledge or ambiguous legislation. Among the recruiting centres of CENTER-TBI,[6] just 64% used ancillary tests in BDD.

Ancillary tests are used differently in different institutions and countries.[16] Sometimes, ancillary tests are conducted when confounding factors persist, otherwise they are strictly employed when required by law (half of the countries of European Union for example and a quarter of the states in the US).[15,17]

Ancillary tests work by evaluating either cortical functionality or blood flow:

1. Evaluating cortical functionality: Cortical functions can be assessed with EEG. Electrocerebral silence is defined as 'absence of EEG activity exceeding 2 μV in amplitude, when recording from scalp electrode pairs 10 or more centimetres apart, with interelectrode impedance below 10,000 Ohms'.[18] EEG is a part of ancillary tests, because BD is defined by the death of brainstem evaluated clinically through cranial nerves testing, while EEG is just an indirect evaluation.

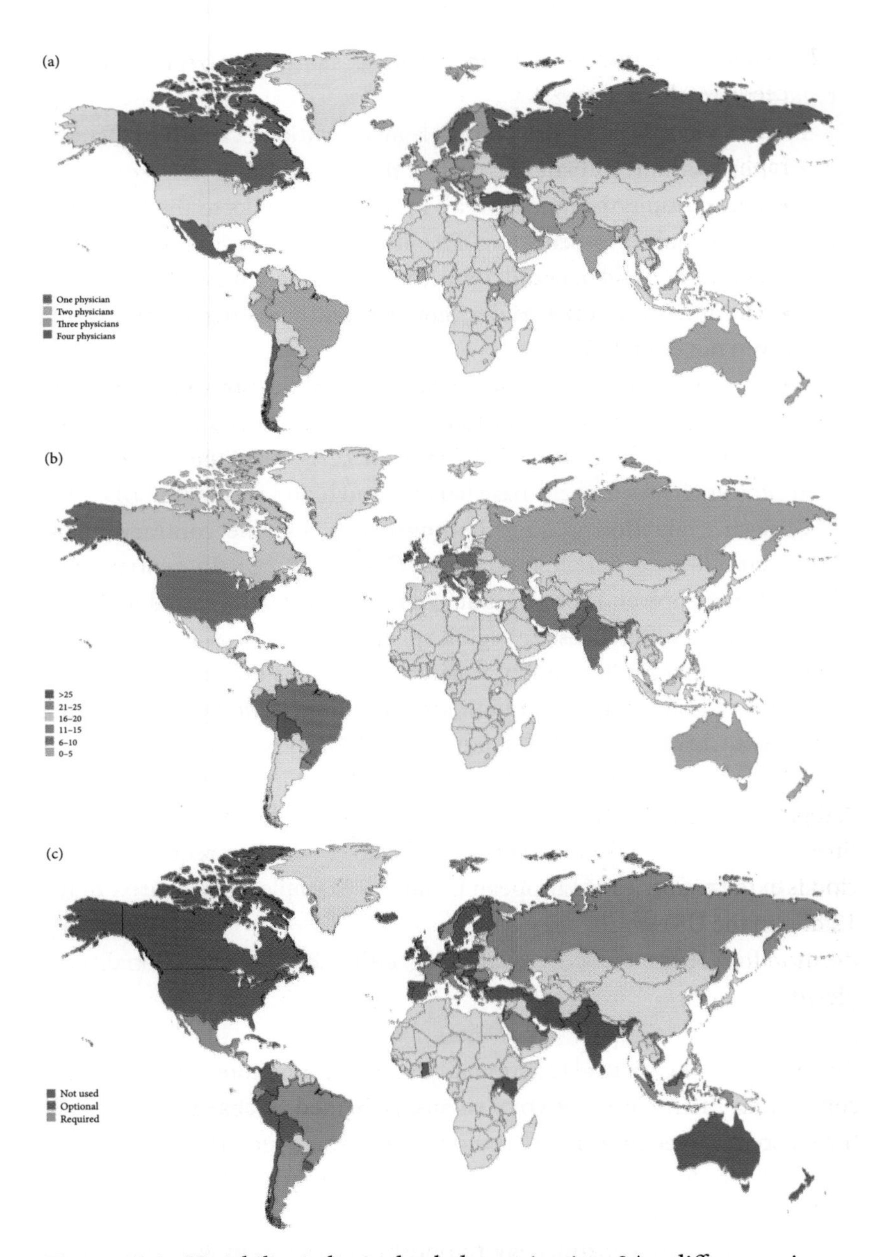

Figure 13.2. Variability in brain death determination: 2A—differences in timing and observation period; 2B—differences in the use of ancillary tests; 2C—differences in the number of physician. (data from Wahlster et al[15])

2. Evaluating blood flow: High ICP (intracranial pressure) that exceeds MAP (mean arterial pressure) stops cerebral blood flow and can be measured with different methods (angiography, CT angiography, radionuclide imaging, Transcranial Doppler)
   - Angiography is considered the gold standard, but it's invasive and not always available. It's currently used in Europe, but far less common in North America.[15,17]
   - In North America radionuclide imaging appears to be more frequently used.[17]
   - CT angiography has many advantages, being fast and frequently available, but there is no agreement about indications for this method.
   - Transcranial Doppler (TCD) examination is extremely cheap and convenient, can be conducted bedside and poses no risk to patients, but at least 10% of the population does not have a suitable bone window.[19] Analysing twenty-four studies, estimated sensitivity is 86% and specificity 98%.[20] Kramer et al reported the usefulness of TCD once the instability of the patient is too high to allow neither transport nor apnoea testing.
   - Somatosensory and auditory evoked potentials, which are not affected by sedatives and have high sensitivity, but low specificity.

A separate mention should be reserved to children, where the first guidelines were written in 1987[21] and revised in 2011.[22] The observation period is extended to 24 hours for term newborns up to 30 days of age, and 12 hours for infants and children from 31 days up to 18 years.[23] The indication for ancillary tests is the cases when apnoea test cannot be completed, if neurologic examination leaves doubt of any nature, in case of possible medication effect, or to reduce the observation period. The legal time of death in children is usually considered as the time of the second confirming examination. This is different from adults where the legal time of death is the time of the first confirming examination.

Consequences of variability in BDD

The incidence in the diagnosis of BD ranges in Europe from 3.2% in the northern countries to 7.6% in central Europe and 12.4% in southern countries.[8] On the other hand, the incidence of withdrawing life-sustaining treatments has an opposite trend,[24] possibly due to religious beliefs (well-rooted Catholicism vs protestant and agnostics). Moreover, it has been well documented that the societal acceptance of BD is related to the availability and access to advanced health care.[25]

Differences in BDD might have consequences on economic and legal aspects (practitioners could be persecuted by law for discontinuing resuscitative care). For these reasons, ethical decisions must be supported by a consensus between practices in different hospitals and countries.

Once dead, a patient is a dead body and no more a patient, so care must be discontinued, otherwise be considered as mistreatment.[26] Treatment can be prolonged in case of organ donation and in the necessity of psychological support for the family (short-term accommodation periods as a compassionate measure).[27] In current literature, cases seeking damages are described either for religious objections or denying diagnosis or emotional distress.[1] Limitations in advances are due to difficulties in performing research in this field, considering cultural and religious beliefs, emotional involvement, and a lack of awareness in the general public.[25] Religious objections to BD exist in Israel and New Jersey, where BD cannot be declared if there is an objection by a person's family member, either due to religious or moral beliefs.[28][29] In some states such as Nevada and New York, definition of death and guidelines were revised in order to underline that no consent is required for BDD.[30]

Terminology has to be uniformed. According to the difference in terminology and definitions, it would be useful to define BD functionally and not anatomically.[25] Death should be considered as a permanent loss of capacity for consciousness and loss of all brainstem functions. This may result either from permanent cessation of circulation and/or after catastrophic brain injury (CBI).[25]

Secondly, indications for ancillary tests have to be protocolled. Different tests should be compared and gold standard defined. Strict instructions for proper testing and the use of checklists could reduce variability in assessing BD.

The indication for ancillary tests might be conditions that may depress the consciousness (drugs or metabolic derangements), conditions preventing evaluation of cranial nerves (for example facial trauma), instability interfering with apnoea testing, and unclear aetiology of BD.[16]

It seems true that ancillary tests could help families to better understand BD; the level of satisfaction is higher when BD is proved also by the absence of cerebral blood flow.[19] Moreover, wrong diagnoses as far as misdiagnosis are reported in current literature.[31] Therefore, two contrasting opinions have been described: some clinicians believing that ancillary tests are often useful and others asserting that a single ancillary test may have important limitations.

New methods in order to make BDD more uniform could be simulation models; BDD is quite rare in clinical daily practice and the accuracy should be improved by simulation models of BD scenarios as recently proved by Hocker et al[32] (see Chapter 12).

Conclusion

There are descriptions in current literature about discrepancies. Goshal[33] in 2015 resumed major findings of articles describing differences in BDD; he confirmed that discrepancies were concentrated in observation time duration, number of examiners, and indication of ancillary tests.

Beyond these differences, each study shows consistency in the core elements of BDD. Everywhere the diagnosis is clinical and it requires always the same key elements: unresponsive coma with an established aetiology, absence of reversible conditions, absence of cortical or brainstem-mediated motor responses, absent brainstem reflexes, and loss of the capacity to breathe.

To let the reader understand why it is important to focus on the core of the evaluation and not on the differences, one has to start from physiology (see Chapter 5).

The neurological dying sequence starts from a well-diagnosed CBI. When preconditions exist, confounders should be excluded and the clinician has to take time to exclude them, because errors are mainly due to underestimation of confounders. After CBI occurs, the deterioration continues with progressive loss of brainstem function despite intervention. Finally, CBI brings upon the cessation of brain function and withdrawal of life-sustaining therapies is considered. In this phase, minimum clinical standards, as defined in 2010 checklist,[8] are always respected. Beyond these, additional testing might be considered by clinician due to uncertainty or law itself and each evaluation has to be repeated at the end of an observation period. The goal is to prove cessation of brain function with no possibility to resume by any means by:

- Preconditions fulfilled
- Confounding conditions excluded or addressed
- Refractory to all applied interventions
- Intervention not available or indicated

If the concept and the physiology of CBI and BD are well understood, it becomes clear that the minimum clinical standards are sufficient to prove the irreversibility of the conditions. Focusing on variability about details is confounding for the public and not useful to the scientific community according to the author's opinion.

Recently, JAMA published a consensus statement of recommendations on determination of brain death based on review of literature and expert opinions. This underlines the importance of this topic and stands out the first international consensus document in order to uniform the minimum clinical standards for determination of brain death/death by neurologic criteria in different settings.[34]

To conclude, variability is acceptable if the fundamentals are respected and if the certainty of the diagnosis comes at the end of a rigorous path of carefully conducted, repeated evaluations.

Highlights

- The core elements are usually consistent and not variable between different countries and centres.
- Variability within a region might be due to lack of knowledge or ambiguous legislation.
- Differences in BDD might have consequences on economic and legal aspects.
- Limitations in advances are due to difficulties in performing research in this field, cultural and religious beliefs, emotional involvement and lack of awareness in the general public, variability inter-countries.

- Discrepancies were concentrated in observation time duration, number of examiners, and indication of ancillary tests.
- Variability is acceptable if the fundamentals are respected.

References

1. Burkle CM, Pope TM. Brain death: Legal obligations and the courts. Semin Neurol. 2015 Apr;35(2):174–179.
2. Mollaret P, Goulon M. The depassed coma (preliminary memoir). Rev Neurol (Paris). 1959 Jul;101:3–15.
3. Wertheimer P, Jouvet M, Descotes J. Diagnosis of death of the nervous system in comas with respiratory arrest treated by artificial respiration. Presse Med. 1959 Jan 17;67(3):87–88.
4. A Definition of Irreversible Coma: Report of the Ad Hoc Committee of the Harvard Medical School to Examine the Definition of Brain Death. JAMA. 1968 Aug 5;205(6):337–340.
5. Guidelines for the determination of death. Report of the medical consultants on the diagnosis of death to the President's Commission for the Study of Ethical Problems in Medicine and Biomedical and Behavioral Research. JAMA. 1981 Nov 13;246(19):2184–2186.
6. van Veen E, van der Jagt M, Cnossen MC, Maas AIR, de Beaufort ID, Menon DK, et al. Brain death and postmortem organ donation: Report of a questionnaire from the CENTER-TBI study. Crit Care. 2018 16;22(1):306.
7. Greer DM, Wang HH, Robinson JD, Varelas PN, Henderson GV, Wijdicks EFM. Variability of brain death policies in the United States. JAMA Neurol. 2016 Feb;73(2):213–218.
8. Wijdicks EFM, Varelas PN, Gronseth GS, Greer DM, American Academy of Neurology. Evidence-based guideline update: Determining brain death in adults: Report of the Quality Standards Subcommittee of the American Academy of Neurology. Neurology. 2010 Jun 8;74(23):1911–1918.
9. Citerio G, Murphy PG. Brain death: The European perspective. Semin Neurol. 2015 Apr;35(2):139–144.
10. Citerio G, Crippa IA, Bronco A, Vargiolu A, Smith M. Variability in brain death determination in Europe: Looking for a solution. Neurocrit Care. 2014 Dec;21(3):376–382.
11. Wijdicks EFM. The transatlantic divide over brain death determination and the debate. Brain. 2012 Apr;135(Pt 4):1321–1331.
12. Smith M. Brain death: The United Kingdom perspective. Semin Neurol. 2015 Apr;35(2):145–151.
13. Nikas NT, Bordlee DC, Moreira M. Determination of death and the dead donor rule: A survey of the current law on brain death. J Med Philos. 2016 Jun;41(3):237–256.
14. Chua HC, Kwek TK, Morihara H, Gao D. Brain death: The Asian perspective. Semin Neurol. 2015 Apr;35(2):152–161.

15. Wahlster S, Wijdicks EFM, Patel PV, Greer DM, Hemphill JC, Carone M, et al. Brain death declaration: Practices and perceptions worldwide. Neurology. 2015 May 5;84(18):1870–1879.
16. Kramer AH. Ancillary testing in brain death. Semin Neurol. 2015 Apr;35(2):125–138.
17. Shappell CN, Frank JI, Husari K, Sanchez M, Goldenberg F, Ardelt A. Practice variability in brain death determination: A call to action. Neurology. 2013 Dec 3;81(23):2009–2014.
18. American Clinical Neurophysiology Society. Guideline 3: Minimum technical standards for EEG recording in suspected cerebral death. Am J Electroneurodiagnostic Technol. 2006 Sep;46(3):211–219.
19. Soldatos T, Karakitsos D, Wachtel M, Boletis J, Chatzimichail K, Papathanasiou M, et al. The value of transcranial Doppler sonography with a transorbital approach in the confirmation of cerebral circulatory arrest. Transplant Proc. 2010 Jun;42(5):1502–1506.
20. Monteiro LM, Bollen CW, van Huffelen AC, Ackerstaff RGA, Jansen NJG, van Vught AJ. Transcranial Doppler ultrasonography to confirm brain death: a meta-analysis. Intensive Care Med. 2006 Dec;32(12):1937–1944.
21. Report of special Task Force. Guidelines for the determination of brain death in children. American Academy of Pediatrics Task Force on Brain Death in Children. Pediatrics. 1987 Aug;80(2):298–300.
22. Nakagawa TA, Ashwal S, Mathur M, Mysore M, Society of Critical Care Medicine, Section on Critical Care and Section on Neurology of American Academy of Pediatrics, Child Neurology Society. Clinical report—Guidelines for the determination of brain death in infants and children: an update of the 1987 task force recommendations. Pediatrics. 2011 Sep;128(3):e720–740.
23. Mathur M, Ashwal S. Pediatric brain death determination. Semin Neurol. 2015 Apr;35(2):116–124.
24. Sprung CL, Cohen SL, Sjokvist P, Baras M, Bulow H-H, Hovilehto S, et al. End-of-life practices in European intensive care units: The Ethicus Study. JAMA. 2003 Aug 13;290(6):790–797.
25. Shemie SD, Baker A. Uniformity in brain death criteria. Semin Neurol. 2015 Apr;35(2):162–168.
26. Clarke MJ, Remtema MS, Swetz KM. Beyond transplantation: Considering brain death as a hard clinical endpoint. Am J Bioeth. 2014;14(8):43–5.
27. Verheijde JL, Rady MY, McGregor JL. The United States Revised Uniform Anatomical Gift Act (2006): New challenges to balancing patient rights and physician responsibilities. Philos Ethics Humanit Med. 2007 Sep 12;2:19.
28. Religion, organ transplantation, and the definition of death. Lancet. 2011 Jan 22;377(9762):271.
29. Setta SM, Shemie SD. An explanation and analysis of how world religions formulate their ethical decisions on withdrawing treatment and determining death. Philos Ethics Humanit Med. 2015 Mar 11;10:6.
30. Verheijde JL, Rady MY, McGregor JL. Brain death, states of impaired consciousness, and physician-assisted death for end-of-life organ donation and transplantation. Med Health Care Philos. 2009 Nov;12(4):409–21.
31. Busl KM, Greer DM. Pitfalls in the diagnosis of brain death. Neurocrit Care. 2009;11(2):276–87.

32. Hocker S, Schumacher D, Mandrekar J, Wijdicks EFM. Testing confounders in brain death determination: A new simulation model. Neurocrit Care. 2015 Dec;23(3):401–408.
33. Ghoshal S, Greer DM. Why is diagnosing brain death so confusing? Curr Opin Crit Care. 2015 Apr;21(2):107–112.
34. Greer DM, Shemie SD, Lewis A, et al. Determination of brain death/death by neurologic criteria: The World Brain Death Project. JAMA. 2020;324(11):1078–1097. doi: 10.1001/jama.2020.11586.

SECTION 2.

ORGAN DONATION ALL OVER THE WORLD: CHALLENGES AND PERSPECTIVES

14

The Spanish model of organ donation

Rafael Badenes, Valentina Della Torre, Beatriz Domínguez-Gil

Historical overview

Organ shortage is the main obstacle that precludes the full expansion of transplantation therapies. According to the Global Observatory on Organ Donation and Transplantation, almost 136,000 solid organ transplants were performed in 2016 worldwide.(1) However, this barely covers 10% of transplantation needs. Consequently, every year, thousands of patients die or deteriorate, while waiting for an organ. Shortages of organs are also the cause of organ trafficking and transplant tourism, practices that violate fundamental human rights and threaten robust transplant programs.

Through Resolution 63.22, issued in 2010,(2) the World Health Assembly (WHA) urged countries *'to strengthen national and multinational authorities and/or capacities to provide oversight, organization and coordination of donation and transplantation activities, with special attention to maximizing donation from deceased donors and to protecting the health and welfare of living donors with appropriate health-care services and long-term follow up'*. The Spanish Government anticipated the WHA's resolution by twenty years. In 1989, the Spanish National Transplant Organization (Organización Nacional de Trasplantes—ONT) was created as a technical agency, embedded within the Ministry of Health, with the responsibility of overseeing, organizing, and coordinating donation and transplant activities in Spain. It is a national network of coordinators, specifically trained, with a high degree of motivation and with a specific profile. In Spain there is a public health system, a good transplant Law (first issued in 1979), innovative and

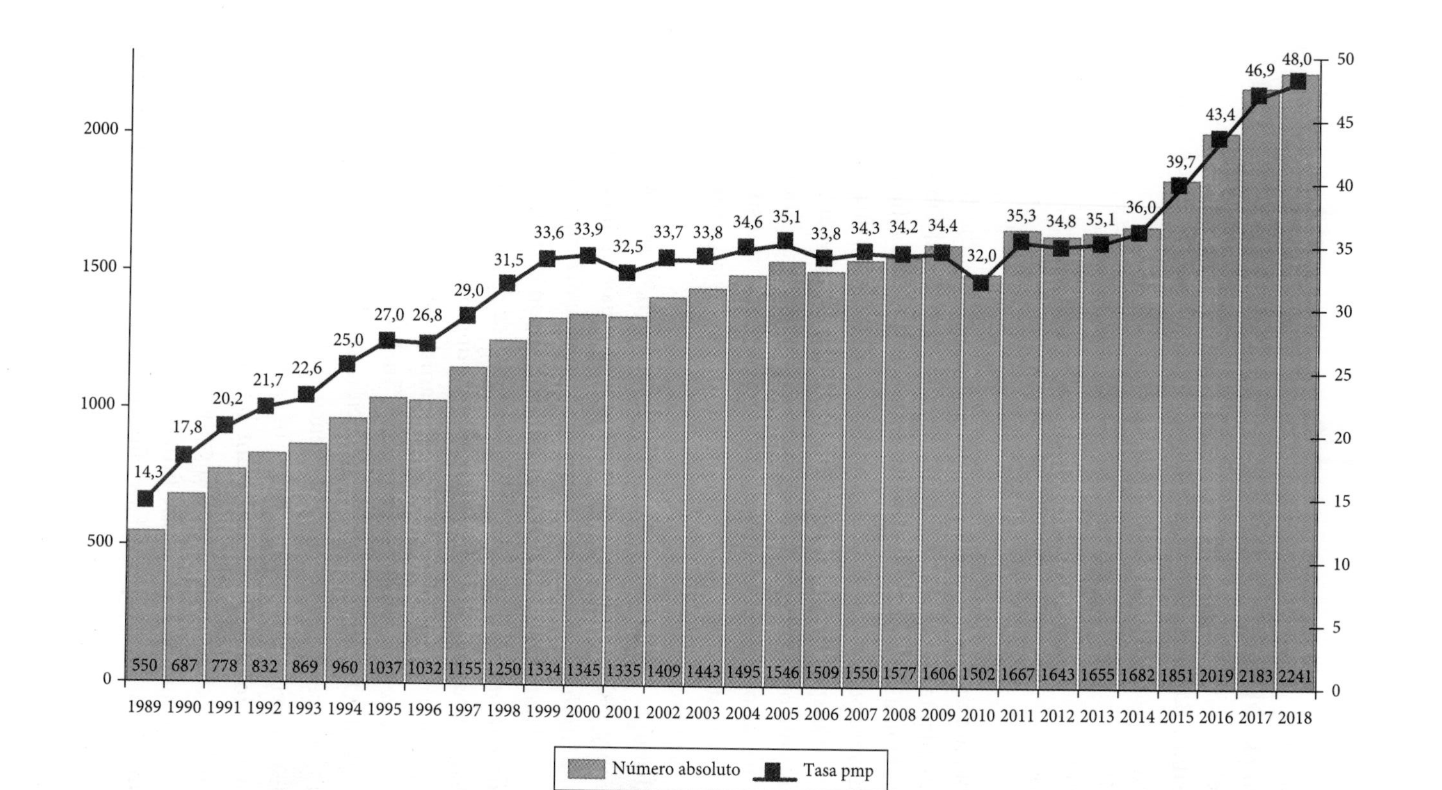

Figure 14.1. Numbers and rates of organs donations in Spain, since foundation of the ONT (1989–2017)—Número absoluto = absolute number. Tasa pmp = rate of population per million

experienced transplant teams, and a decentralized system across seventeen autonomous regions.[3]

The Spanish National Transplant Organization (ONT) conceived and implemented an organ coordination strategy, the so-called 'Spanish Model', leading the country from fourteen donors per million people to more than thirty donors, in under a decade. Since then, Spain has led deceased donation and transplantation activities worldwide. In 2018, the country achieved 48.0 donors per million—rates that by far are the most elevated in the world[4] (see Figures 14.1 and 14.2). The Spanish Model is appropriate for the legislative, technical and health framework of the country, and is recognized worldwide as a model of high effectiveness to combat the shortage of organs.

This chapter describes the main features of the Spanish model and the latest initiatives in place to further progress towards self-sufficiency in transplantation.

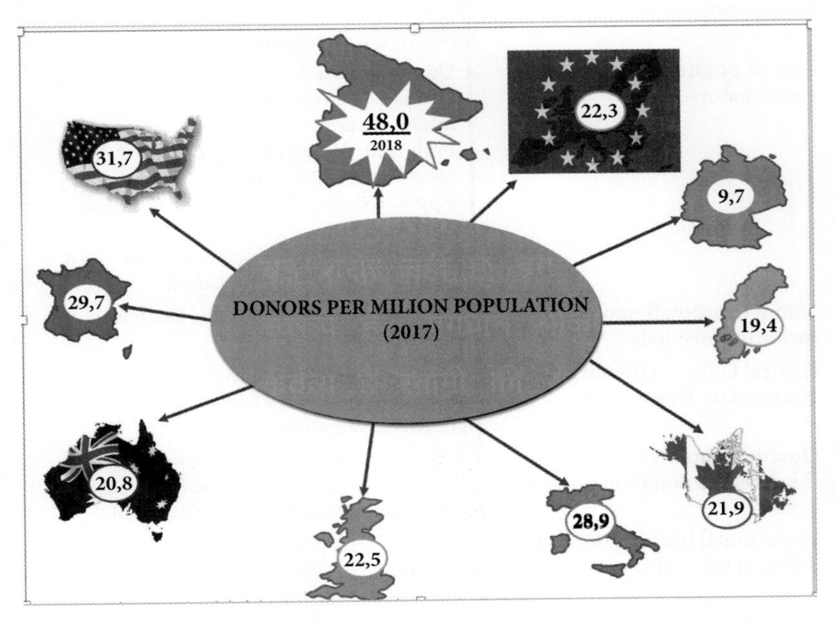

Figure 14.2. Deceased donation and transplantation 2017 rates worldwide

Current status of organ donation and transplantation in Spain

The main elements of the Spanish Model are shown in Table 14.1 and detailed as follows:

The donor coordination network

The network is structured at three inter-related levels: national (ONT), regional (17 Regional Coordination Units), and hospital-based; the first two levels are designated by and report to the national and regional authorities, respectively. They act as an interface between technical and political authorities, in support of the donation and transplantation system.[5] Any

Table 14.1 Main elements of the Spanish Model

Donor coordinator network	Organized at three inter-related levels: national, regional, hospital
Special profile of donor coordinators	• Units composed of physicians and nurses, but lead by physicians, mostly from intensive care • Part- time dedication to the donor coordination activities • Appointed by and reporting to hospital managers • Main objective: deceased donation—with pro-active donor identification
Donor coordination units inside the hospitals	DC members of the staff of the Hospital, mainly in the ICU
Central Office—Organization Nacional de Trasplantes	Not only an organ sharing office, but agency working in continuous support of the process of deceased donation
Quality Assurance Program in the deceased donation process	Continuous clinical chart review of deaths at intensive care units of procurement hospitals. Two phases: internal and external audits
Professional training through different types of courses	• Covered with governmental funds • Targeted to donor coordinators, professionals from intensive and emergency care, non-health-care professionals.
Close attention to the media	Specific communication policy
Hospital Reimbursement	For all activities related to donation and transplantation

national decision in the field is agreed upon by the National Transplant Committee, which comprises the ONT, as chair, and seventeen regional coordinators. The third level of coordination is a network of hospitals authorized for organ procurement by the regional authorities. Each hospital has a donor coordinator (DC), in charge of donation and transplantation activities at the institution.

The donor coordinator's profile

The profile of the DC is a paradigm of the Spanish model. DC teams are composed of nurses and physicians; the team leader is always a physician. The majority of these leaders are intensive care doctors, as it is in the intensive care units (ICUs) where they gain first-hand information about donation opportunities. DCs are in-house figures; they are designated by and report to hospital directors, which empower their role in the hospital. Most DCs are part-time dedicated to this activity, while they perform hospital responsibility as physicians at ICUs as well, enabling the system to also count on a DC at small hospitals, with limited donor potential. The main responsibility of every DC unit is to develop a proactive donor identification system and to facilitate the transition of deceased potential organ donors into actual ones.[6]

The Spanish National Transplant Organization

The ONT aids hospital and regional DCs in the process of organ donation, by providing support to all individual regional procedures and to national initiatives that target increment of deceased donation. ONT establishes the regulatory framework of practice, ensures continuous professional training, designs national protocols to improve practice, and conceives strategies, aimed at identifying opportunities for improvement. The central office of the ONT based in Madrid acts as a support structure for the entire system. It is responsible for the distribution of organs, the organization of transport, the management of waiting lists, statistics and databases, and in general any action that can contribute to improving the organ donation and transplant process. The support provided by the central office and some of the regions is essential, especially to small hospitals, where it is not possible to carry out the entire process without assistance. The general philosophy of the Spanish Model is an integrated approach to the donation process, which culminates with transplant, and where improvisation is avoided.

The Quality Assurance Program in Deceased Donation

The *Quality Assurance Program in Deceased Donation* has been in place since 1999,[7] and it has inspired national, regional, and local strategies for continuous improvement.[8] Focused on the process of donation after brain death (BD), the program monitors the potential donor pool, evaluates performance in donation after BD, and identifies areas for improvement. The program is based on a continuous audit of clinical charts of dead patients in ICUs, aiming for identification of potential BD donors, evaluation of their transition to actual donors and reasons if such transition would not have occurred. It includes:

- Internal audits: performed by the DC at each hospital and reported to ONT, which provides national indicators of reference to the network.
- External audits: performed at the request of regional coordinators by DC experts. These audits represent a valuable opportunity for exchanging best practices and producing recommendations to the DC team and the hospital director.

Professional training and continuous development

The Spanish government and the regional authorities promote annual courses for all professionals participating in the deceased donation process—DCs, intensive and emergency care professionals, neurologists, judges, coroners, and journalists. Since 1991, over 20,000 healthcare professionals have been trained with the government funds.[6]

The ONT and media

The ONT is devoted to providing the media with any data they need, as well as producing reports on every relevant development. In doing so, ONT increases the level of public knowledge on donation and transplantation, and the confidence in the system. The following practices have been set up: a 24-hours telephone line for consultation, and easy access to the media; relationships with journalists are built through meetings to establish mutual needs, and messages are directly reported. Therefore, the media are true allies in promoting organ donation.[6]

Reimbursement of donation and transplant activities

Hospitals are reimbursed for donation and transplantation activities. A specific budget is allocated to cover both human and material resources for the effective development of these activities at every institution.[6]

Exporting the Spanish Model worldwide

Experiences in the translation of all (e.g. Australia, Croatia, Latin American countries) or some of the elements (e.g. engagement of the intensive care community in Canada and the United Kingdom) of the Spanish Model to other countries and regions are a tangible proof that this system and its management can be reproduced, if properly adapted to the local system.[8] Some factors are necessary to export the Spanish Model: a National Public Health System, availability of doctors and nurses, availability of ICU beds and beds equipped with ventilators.[9]

Challenges for improvement of the Spanish Model

Despite the excellent activity and rate of donors and transplants, Spain is still far from properly covering the transplantation needs. Every year

5–10% of patients in need of vital organs die or get too sick to be transplanted while they are on the waiting list. Pre-emptive kidney transplantation barely represents 5% of overall activity. This exists along with a steady reduction in the potential for donation after BD due to a decrease in events that lead to catastrophic brain injury (e.g. traffic accidents and cerebrovascular events) and improvements in neurocritical care. Important changes have also implemented within the patterns of end-of-life care (e.g. withdrawal of life-sustaining therapies). Moreover, potential donors are older, due to general ageing of population, and with substantial comorbidities.[(9)]

These factors have challenged the Spanish system's capacity to innovate and modernize itself and set a framework for action plan implementation. In 2008, ONT launched the forty donors per million population (pmp) plan, aiming to reach the target by 2020, they already achieved it in 2016.[(4)] The 50x22 plan has the objective of reaching fifty donors pmp and more than 5,500 transplants by 2022. To further increase the availability of organs for transplantation, particularly from deceased organ donors, specific strategies have been implemented and are detailed below.

Intensive care to facilitate organ donation

Intensive care to facilitate organ donation (ICOD) is defined[(10)] as initiation or continuation of life-sustaining measures, such as mechanical ventilation and inotropes/vasopressor support, with the aim of enabling organ donation, in patients with a devastating brain injury (DBI), in whom active treatment has been considered futile, with the purpose of incorporating the option of donation after BD into their end-of-life care plans. In 2008, the ONT launched a benchmarking strategy, which identified a group of hospitals with outstanding results in deceased donation. Dedicated visits to these excellent hospitals identified unique practices, based on cooperation between DC units, emergency departments and hospital wards. Organ donation was systematically offered to patients with a DBI, when the decision had been made to shift from active treatment to palliative end-of-life care. The DC assessed if organ donation was consistent with the patient′s will, through Advanced Directives and dedicated interviews with families. In such cases, intensive treatment was initiated or continued, so death could be determined by neurological criteria and donation after BD developed afterwards. A so-called 'Plan, Do, Study, Act' cycle to promote ICOD at hospital level has been developed in more than 100 hospitals in Spain. As a result, 24% of actual donors were admitted to ICU to incorporate organ donation into their end-of-life plans.[11]

Donors with expanded criteria and non-standard risk donors

- Donors with expanded criteria

To guarantee continuous advances in the organ donation process, Spain has been focusing on maximizing the use of organs from donors with characteristics that fall within expanded criteria.[12]

The points considered when assessing expanded criteria are as follows:

1. Ageing: The utilization of kidneys or livers coming from aged donors is variable between Spanish teams. With regard to kidneys, the utilization of aged organs makes more sense in elderly than in young recipients, given that graft survival is expected to cover the life expectancy. However, as for livers, an existing belief contrary to the validity of organs from aged donors must be overcome. In this sense, a review seems to be required for the indications and criteria for their use.
2. Donors with positive test to certain viral serologies: There is great variability and it is difficult to explain the transplantation of organs from donors with positive serology for certain viral agents. Centres performing such practices achieve good results based on a correct assessment of the donor, an appropriate selection of the recipient, and an individualized therapeutic approach. Increasing the belief of various teams in the usefulness of these organs should probably be the first step.
3. Donors with rare diseases: Careful consideration of each potential donor is required for cases with certain conditions such as acute intoxications, cancer or related history, and rare diseases. The mentioned conditions require us to pool and review the experiences accumulated by specific registries as a basic tool to develop and update consensus documents for the decision-making process.

In addition, there is a strategy to minimize organ injuries related to the donation process, and a plan based on the selection of a receiver appropriate to the characteristics of the organ to be transplanted; and a specific surgical and clinical management of the recipient also appropriate to the type of organ and the characteristics of its donor.

- Non-standard risk donors (NSRDs)

The NSRDs' project provides information on the results of transplants from NSRDs (extreme age group, presence of infection, or history of cancer) that will allow the ONT to make an adequate risk-benefit assessment, always complying with quality and safety standards and based on evidence. The ONT makes annual reports and publishes those for the donation and transplant network.(13)

Improving use of organs from expanded criteria and NSRD

In the early '90s, the main cause of donor death was brain trauma, while in recent years more than 60% of donors die due to stroke.(9) Donor age has also increased; in 2019, 50% of donors are over the age of sixty, 30% over seventy, and 9% over eighty.(9) Therefore, a new approach is needed in terms of both DCs tackling the complex assessment of donor eligibility, and transplant teams making challenging decisions about organ utilization. A significant number of transplants have been performed with organs from old age groups with excellent results.(14) Specific allocation strategies, whereby these organs are preferentially allocated into recipients of an advanced age ('old-for-old' strategy), have been critical.(15)

External audits reveal that 22% of Spanish patients in a BD condition are not considered suitable organ donors, due to medical contraindications, which, on numerous occasions, have been inappropriately established (meaning they are suitable but established as unsuitable). This situation has led the ONT to establish a system for the DC to obtain a second opinion, available 24/7. In addition, to better define the safety limits in the utilization of organs for transplantation, a prospective follow-up of recipients of organs from NSRDs (e.g. donors with a history of malignancy or infection) was started in 2014. Information derived from this initiative has become critical for decision-making in matters of donors assessment and organs utilization.[16]

Donation after circulatory death

Donation after circulatory death (DCD) in Spain was first developed in the 1980s by pioneer teams that made donation possible in the complex scenario of death following an unsuccessfully resuscitated cardiac arrest, i.e. uncontrolled DCD (uDCD). However, donation after death following the decision to withdraw life-sustaining treatment (WLST), i.e. controlled DCD (cDCD), had not been accommodated into the Spanish regulatory framework until 2012.[17] The pressing reality of a significant number of patients dying in Spanish ICUs under these circumstances compelled the adoption of measures to make cDCD possible.[16] It was following a pilot cDCD experience in the city of Vitoria in 2012 that the regulatory framework was modified.[17] By 2019, more than 100 hospitals have functioning DCD programs. In 2017, there were 573 DCD donors, representing 26% of deceased donation activity and almost 1,000 patients received a DCD organ, with excellent post-transplant outcomes (Figure 14.3).

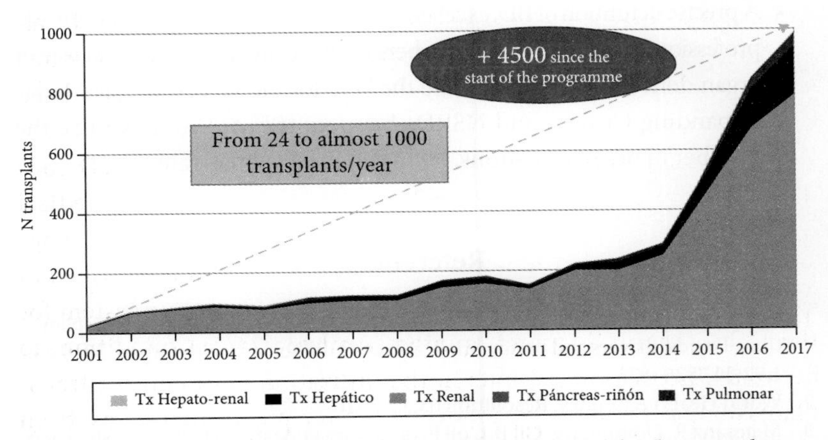

Figure 14.3. Donation and Transplantation after DCD (absolute number and rate per million population)—data updated up to 2017.

Conclusion

The Spanish Model is an example of a management system designed to facilitate the systematic identification of organ donation opportunities and their transition to actual donation. The model has been successfully replicated, either partially or totally, in other countries. Currently, the need for organs for transplantation is expected to increase, while the number of potential BD donors is expected to decrease. Novel strategies, such as ICOD, organs from expanded donors or with a non-standard risk, use of donors in asystole, NSRDs, and DCD have been implemented in Spain with good results. This might provide a model for other countries, based on measures that will increase organ availability at a time of shortage, and allow more patients to become organ donors.

Highlights

- The National Organization of Transplants (ONT), which is a national network of donor coordinators, was founded in Spain in 1989. Not only an organ sharing office, but agency working in continuous support of the process of deceased donation.
- Spain has reached forty-eight donors per million population, the highest rate worldwide.
- A precise definition of BD, excellent collaboration with media, continuous professional training for all members of the team, and the central role of organ donation coordinators are the keys for the success of this Model.
- Expanding Criteria and NSRDs have contributed to maximize the number of organ donations, increasing transplants rate.

References

1. White SL, Hirth R, Mahíllo B, et al. The global diffusion of organ transplantation: Trends, drivers and policy implications. Bull World Health Organ. 2014 Nov 1;92(11):826–835.
2. World Health Assembly. Resolution 63:22. 2010
3. Matesanz R, Domínguez-Gil B, Coll E, de la Rosa G, Marazuela R. Spanish experience as a leading country: what kind of measures were taken? Transplant Int 2011; 24(4): 333–343.

4. Matesanz R, Marazuela R, Domínguez-Gil B, Coll E, Mahillo B, de la Rosa G. The 40 donors per million-population plan: An action plan for improvement of organ donation and transplantation in Spain. Transplant Proc 2009; 41(8): 3453–3456.
5. Matesanz R, Domínguez-Gil B, Coll E, Mahíllo B, Marazuela R. How Spain reached 40 deceased organ donors per million. Am J Transplant 2017; 17(6): 1447–1454.
6. Matesanz R. 2008. El Modelo español (The Spanish Model) de Coordinación y Trasplantes. http://www.ont.es/publicaciones/Documents/modeloespanol.pdf
7. Sánchez-Vallejo A, Gómez-Salgado J, Fernández-Martínez MN, Fernández-García D. Examination of the brain-dead organ donor management process at a Spanish hospital. Int J Environ Res Public Health. 2018 Oct 4;15(10): 2173. doi: 10.3390/ijerph15102173.
8. Kramer AH, Hornby K, Doig CJ, et al. Deceased organ donation potential in Canada: A review of consecutive deaths in Alberta. Potentiel des dons d'organes après décès au Canada: un compte rendu de décès consécutifs en Alberta. Can J Anaesth. 2019;66(11):1347–1355. doi:10.1007/s12630-019-01437-1
9. Rosa G, Domínguez-Gil B, Matesanz R, et al. Continuously evaluating performance in deceased donation: The Spanish quality assurance program. American Journal of Transplantation 2012; 12: 2507–2513.
10. Martín-Delgado MC, Martínez-Soba F, Masnou N, et al. Summary of Spanish recommendations on intensive care to facilitate organ donation. Am J Transplant. 2019;19(6):1782–1791. doi:10.1111/ajt.15253
11. Martín-Delgado MC, Martínez-Soba F, Masnou N, ET AL. Summary of Spanish recommendations on intensive care to facilitate organ donation. Am J Transplant. 2019 Jun;19(6):1782–1791.
12. Matesanz R, Marazuela R, Dominguez-Gil B, Coll E, Mahillo B, de La Rosa G. The 40 donors per million population plan: An action plan for improvement of organ donation and transplantation in Spain. Tranplantation Proceedings 2009;41:3453–3456.
13. Annual Report Organ Donation and Transplantation. 2018. http://www.ont.es/infesp/Memorias/Actividad%20de%20Donación%20y%20Trasplante.pdf.
14. Pérez-Sáez MJ, Lafuente Covarrubias O, Hernández D, et al. GEODAS Group. Early outcomes of kidney transplantation from elderly donors after circulatory death (GEODAS study). BMC Nephrol. 2019 Jun 26;20(1):233.
15. Arcos E, Pérez-Sáez MJ, Comas J, Lloveras J, Tort J, Pascual J. Catalan renal registry. Assessing the limits in kidney transplantation: Use of extremely elderly donors and outcomes in elderly recipients. Transplantation 2020 Jan;104(1):176–183. 2019 Apr 8. [Epub ahead of print].
16. Domínguez-Gil B, Coll E, Elizalde J, et al. ACCORD-Spain study group. Expanding the donor pool through intensive care to facilitate organ donation: Results of a Spanish multicenter study. Transplantation. 2017 Aug;101(8):e265–e272.
17. Real Decreto 1723/2012, de 28 de diciembre, por el que se regulan las actividades de obtención, utilización clínica y coordinación territorial de los órganos humanos destinados al trasplante y se establecen requisitos de calidad y seguridad- http://www.ont.es/infesp/Legislacin/BOERD1723-2012.pdf. 2012.

15

Organ donation in Europe

Marta López-Fraga, Beatriz Domínguez-Gil

Introduction

Organ transplantation is a story of remarkable achievement. Ever since the first successful kidney transplant in 1954, organ transplantation has saved and improved the quality of life of thousands of patients. Medical procedures that were unimaginable a generation ago are a reality today due to advances in surgery, organ preservation techniques, and immunosuppressive treatment, as well as technical and organizational progress. These developments have unquestionable benefits, but the utilization of human organs, tissues, and cells also poses questions of safety, quality, and efficacy and presents new ethical dilemmas.

Today organ transplantation is the best life-saving treatment for end-stage organ failure and is performed in more than 100 countries all over the world.[1] According to the Global Observatory on Organ Donation and Transplantation, 135,860 solid-organ transplants (kidney, liver, heart, lung, pancreas, small bowel) were performed in 2016.[2] However, it is estimated that this represents less than 10% of global needs. Long periods on the waiting list for organs may result in patients deteriorating or dying before transplantation. By the end of 2016, 142,388 patients were waiting for a transplant in member states of the Council of Europe,[3] nearly six new patients were being included to the waiting list every hour and, dramatically, nineteen patients on the waiting list died every day because there was no organ available. Shortage of organs for transplantation is also the root cause of organ trafficking and transplant tourism, practices that violate fundamental human rights and pose serious risks to individual and public health.[4]

This situation is not likely to get easier in the coming years. The ageing of the general population, the increasing prevalence of diabetes mellitus and hypertension, the decrease in road deaths and improved survival rates following cerebrovascular accidents, among other factors, will affect the number of patients that will need an organ transplant, as well as the availability of organs.

This situation calls for effective measures to ensure that all possible organ donors are identified and as many as possible converted into effective donors. Furthermore, to ensure good post-transplant outcomes, donation and transplantation programmes need to comply with high quality and safety standards and rely on adequate allocation criteria. In order to support this, a number of initiatives have taken place in Europe in the recent years. This chapter describes the current situation of donation and transplantation programmes in Europe, and summarizes the strategies that have been developed by the Council of Europe and the European Union (EU) to confront the challenges of organ donation and transplantation in the European setting.

Current status of organ donation and transplantation programmes in Europe

Transplantation activities are highly variable across European countries as a result of differences in deceased and living donation rates (Figure 15.1).[1] Deceased donation has not yet been developed in some European countries, while others have reached rates beyond forty donors per million population (pmp). While it is certain that a minimum degree of development is required to build a deceased donation programme, such differences persist when comparing countries with a similar human development index (Figure 15.2). Although some scholars hypothesize about the influence of consent policies (opt-in vs opt-out)[5] or, of mortality rates relevant to organ donation,[6] variations in transplantation activities largely derive from the way countries have organized the realization of the deceased donation process within their healthcare systems. Models based on in-house donor coordinators and engaging the intensive care community represent the most

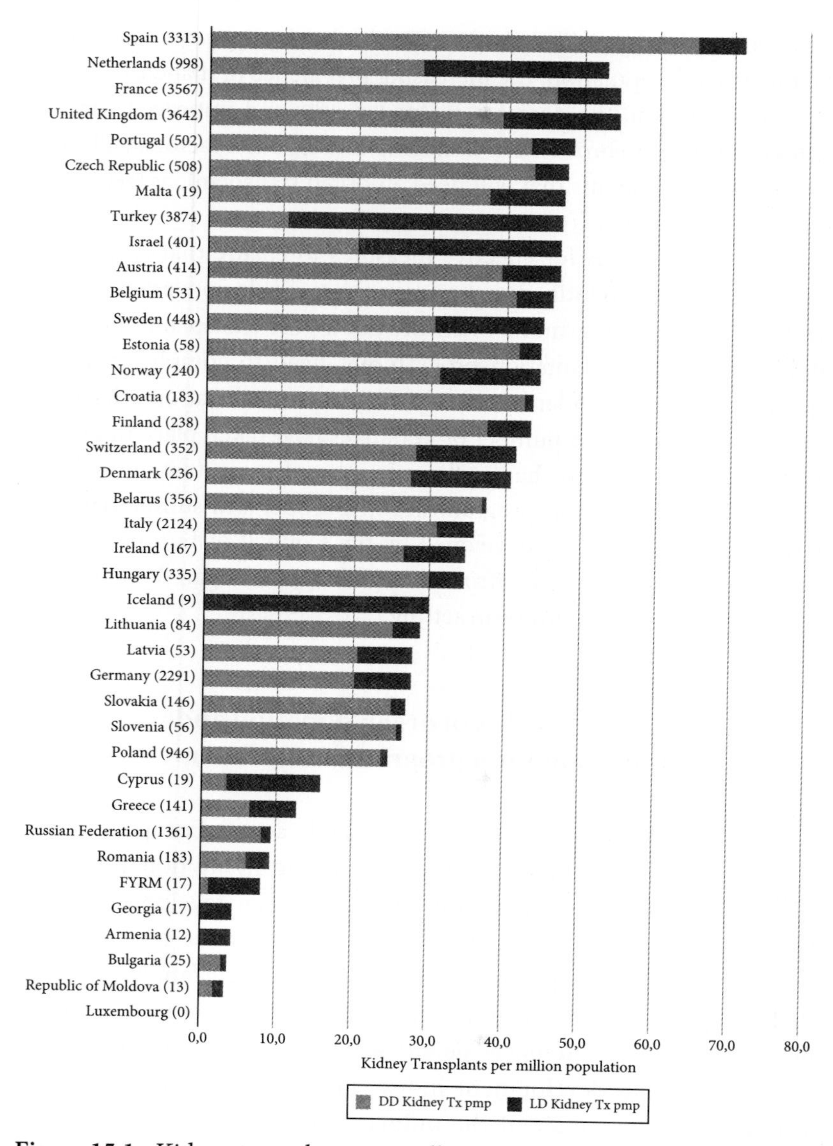

Figure 15.1. Kidney transplants per million population (pmp) in European countries in 2018. Deceased donor (DD) and Living Donor (LD) activities. (Source: International Figures on Donation and Transplantation. Newsletter Transplant 2019. (Available at: http://www.ont.es/publicaciones; https://register.edqm.eu/freepub). *Absolute number of kidney transplants is shown in brackets*

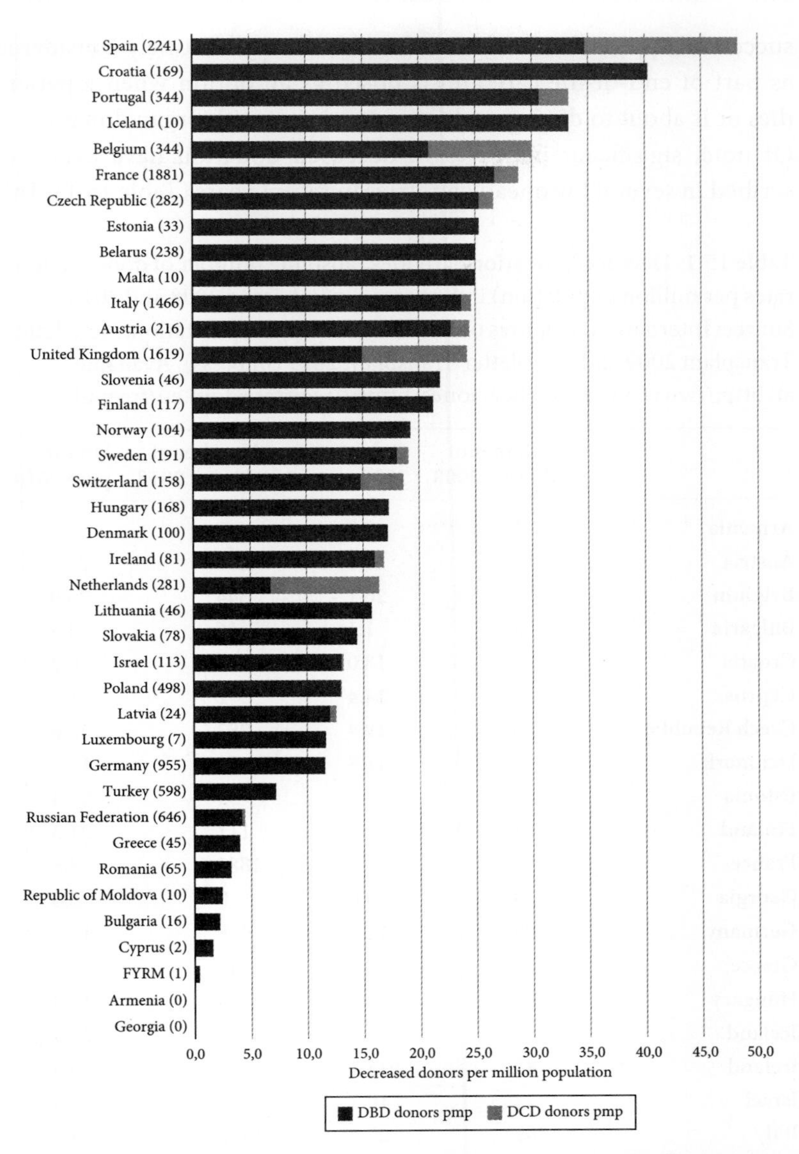

Figure 15.2. Deceased donors per million population (pmp) in European countries in 2018. Donation after Brain Death (DBD) and Donation after Circulatory Death (DCD) activities. Source: International Figures on Donation and Transplantation. Newsletter Transplant 2019. (Available at: http://www.ont.es/publicaciones; https://register.edqm.eu/freepub). *Absolute number of deceased donors is shown in brackets*

successful approaches to ensure that donation is routinely considered as part of end-of-life care and is posed as an option when a patient dies or is about to die in conditions consistent with organ donation.[7,8] Of note, significant increases in deceased donation have been described in several European countries in recent years (Table 15.1). This

Table 15.1 Deceased donation activities (absolute number of donors and rates per million population) in European countries in 2008 and 2018. Source: International Figures on Donation and Transplantation. Newsletter Transplant 2009 and Newsletter Transplant 2019 (in press). Available at: http://www.ont.es/publicaciones; https://register.edqm.eu/freepub

	Number of donors 2008	Donors pmp 2008	Number of donors 2018	Donors pmp 2018
Armenia	0	0.0	0	0.0
Austria	172	20.5	216	24.5
Belgium	274	26.1	344	29.9
Bulgaria	8	1.1	16	2.3
Croatia	83	18.0	169	40.2
Cyprus	13	14.4	2	1.7
Czech Republic	198	19.4	282	26.6
Denmark	65	11.8	100	17.2
Estonia	31	23.8	33	25.4
Finland	81	15.3	117	21.3
France	1610	26.0	1881	28.8
Georgia	0	0.0	0	0.0
Germany	1199	14.5	955	11.6
Greece	98	8.8	45	11.1
Hungary	148	14.8	168	17.3
Iceland	2	6.7	10	33.3
Ireland	81	18.4	81	16.9
Israel	72	10.3	113	13.3
Italy	1201	20.4	1466	24.7
Latvia	30	13.0	24	12.6
Lithuania	33	9.7	46	15.9
Luxembourg	9	18.0	7	11.7
Netherlands	210	12.7	281	16.4
Norway	98	20.9	104	19.3
Poland	427	11.2	498	13.1

Table 15.1 *Continued*

	Number of donors 2008	Donors pmp 2008	Number of donors 2018	Donors pmp 2018
Portugal	283	26.4	344	33.4
Republic of Moldova	0	0.0	10	2.5
Romania	60	2.8	65	3.3
Russian Federation	–		646	4.5
Slovakia	77	14.3	78	14.4
Slovenia	37	18.5	46	21.9
Spain	1577	35.4	2241	48.3
Sweden	152	16.5	191	19.1
Switzerland	90	12.0	158	18.6
North Macedonia	0	0.0	1	0.5
Turkey	262	3.5	598	7.3
United Kingdom	885	14.5	1619	24.3

increase results from the efforts of countries to progress towards self-sufficiency in transplantation and makes evident the beneficial effect of international cooperation fostered by European organizations, as described in this section.

Differences in deceased donation activities also derive from a considerable variation in the use of organs from expanded criteria donors. The transplantation of organs from donors beyond the age of sixty, seventy, or even eighty years occurs in response to the progressive ageing of potential organ donors and in the context of old-for-old allocation strategies.[9,10] However, it entails challenges such as high organ discard rates and inferior post-transplant outcomes compared with those obtained with organs from younger donors. This precludes several European countries from expanding donor-acceptance criteria. A limited number of countries have developed donation after circulatory death (DCD) programmes (Figure 15.2), and the situation is highly heterogeneous with regard to the type of programme in place (controlled or uncontrolled), the regulatory framework, and the procedures applied.[11,12] Ethical and legal barriers are the most important obstacles that prevent DCD from becoming standard practice in all European countries.

International cooperation agreements have emerged in Europe to better meet the transplantation needs of patients. To increase the chances of transplantation of patients, cross-border exchange of organs is a routine practice among countries belonging to well-established European Organ Exchange Organizations, such as Eurotransplant and Scandiatransplant.[13] Countries also exchange surplus organs (local use of organs was not possible because of the lack of suitable recipients) in the framework of bilateral or multilateral agreements (e.g. South Alliance for Transplantation, FOEDUS).[14] Patients travel for transplantation in the context of official cooperation agreements established between countries that are based on the concept of reciprocity, by which the country of origin of the patient contributes to the donor pool at the country of destination. This is particularly the case for specific types of transplants for which programmes do not exist in every country (e.g. lung transplantation).

International initiatives to promote organ donation and transplantation

In addition to an individual country's effort to develop organ donation and transplantation programmes, two large international organizations have developed ambitious international initiatives to support their member states and foster cooperation and exchange expertise.

The Council of Europe, based in Strasbourg (France) and founded in 1949, includes forty-seven member states and encompasses 820 million citizens. It is an entirely separate body from the EU. The latter, based in Brussels (Belgium), comprises twenty-eight member states that have conferred some national legislative and executive powers from the national to the EU level with the aim of achieving a higher level of integration. In contrast, Council of Europe member states maintain their sovereignty, but cooperate on the basis of common values and political decisions and commit themselves through conventions.

Following the *Third Conference of European Health Ministers on the Ethical, Organisational and Legislative Aspects of Organ Transplantation*,[15] held in Paris (France) in 1987, the Council of Europe Committee of Experts on the Organisational Aspects of Co-operation in Organ

Transplantation (SP-CTO) was created. In 2007, the Secretariat responsible for activities related to organs, tissues, and cells was transferred to the European Directorate for the Quality of Medicines and HealthCare (EDQM) of the Council of Europe, and the newly appointed European Committee on Organ Transplantation (CD-P-TO) took over as the Steering Committee.[16] This move to the EDQM facilitated closer collaboration and synergies with the EU and aimed, amongst other objectives, to avoid duplication of efforts. This was a real danger after 2004 when, following adoption of its new competencies, the EU started issuing Directives and sets of technical requirements in the fields of organs and tissues and cells.[17]

Currently, the CD-P-TO is composed of internationally recognized experts and actively promotes the non-commercialization of organ donation, the fight against organ trafficking, the development of ethical, quality, and safety standards in the field of organs, tissues, and cells, and the transfer of knowledge between member states and organizations. The work of the CD-P-TO revolves around five pillars of action: legislative initiatives, aimed at producing legal instruments to guide member states; international cooperation programmes, to foster the transfer of knowledge between countries; monitoring activities, to benchmark donation and transplantation practices in member states; projects aimed at improving professional practices through the elaboration of guidance documents; and activities targeted at the public to raise awareness and provide balanced information.

Over the years, a set of *Resolutions and Recommendations* in the field has been produced by the CD-P-TO and subsequently adopted by the Council of Europe Committee of Ministers.[18] Whereas agreements and conventions are binding on the states that ratify them, resolutions and recommendations are policy statements to governments that propose a common course of action to be followed. Although not legally binding, they have profoundly impacted national legislation, ethical frameworks, strategic plans, organizational aspects, and professional practices.

The *Convention on Human Rights and Biomedicine*[19] was opened for signature in 1997 and was the first legally binding international text designed to preserve human dignity, fundamental rights, and freedom through a series of principles against the misuse of biological and medical applications. It specifically prohibits that the body and its parts, as such, give rise to financial gain. This Convention was extended further by an *Additional Protocol to the Convention on Human Rights and Biomedicine concerning Transplantation of Organs and Tissues of Human Origin*,[20] which was opened for signature in 2002 and establishes principles for the protection of donors and recipients.

The *Council of Europe Convention on Action against Trafficking in Human Beings* and its Explanatory Report,[21] which was opened for signature in 2005, address the trafficking of persons for the purpose of organ removal. The *Council of Europe Convention against Trafficking in Human Organs*[22] and its Explanatory Report,[23] which opened for signature in 2015, identify for the first-time distinct activities that constitute 'trafficking in human organs', strengthen existing mechanisms for cooperation, and include provisions to protect and assist victims. This is of the utmost importance considering that, according to the WHO, 5–10% of all transplants performed worldwide are the result of organ trafficking.[24]

To complement the existing legal framework addressing transplant-related crimes, through the establishment of an *International Network of National Focal Points* and an *International Database on Travel for Transplantation*,[25] the Council of Europe will gain a better knowledge of these crimes and have the valuable opportunity to provide comprehensive and integrated information and recommendations on these matters at national and international level.

The CD-P-TO has also implemented some projects that support the development of effective legislative frameworks and the establishment of national transplant authorities and transplant programmes in various countries. In 2004, in cooperation with the European Commission, a Joint Programme for the Republic of Moldova resulted in a new law on transplantation, adopted by the Moldovan Parliament in 2008, and the establishment of a Transplant Agency that is now responsible for all organizational aspects in this field. Following this experience, a dedicated programme in Armenia, Azerbaijan, Bulgaria, Georgia, Moldova, Romania, the Russian Federation, Turkey, and Ukraine was launched—referred to as the *Black Sea Area Project*—which has shown great success in some of these countries.[26] The Black Sea Area Project contributed to the development of transplantation activities in the participant countries by providing expertise and guidance.

It has become evident that monitoring of practices in the member states is needed for the sake of transparency and international benchmarking. With this goal in mind, the CD-P-TO together with the Spanish Organización Nacional de Trasplantes (ONT) has, since 1996, prepared the *Newsletter Transplant,*[27] which currently provides information from almost seventy countries worldwide. The newsletter summarizes, on a yearly basis, comprehensive data on donation and transplantation activities, management of waiting lists, organ donation refusals and authorized centres for transplantation activities and has evolved into a unique official source of information that continues to inspire policies and strategic plans globally.

In addition, the EDQM/Council of Europe is responsible for the publication of the *Guide to the Quality and Safety of Organs for Transplantation* and the *Guide to the Quality and Safety of Tissues and Cells for Human Application.*[28] World-renowned experts and the most important professional associations in the field have actively participated in the preparation and dissemination of these guides, which serve as invaluable tools for regulators and health professionals throughout Europe and beyond.

As part of its public outreach activities, the CD-P-TO has also chosen topics of relevance and produced thematic booklets to provide the public with balanced and clear information so each person can make informed decisions based on strong scientific evidence tailored to their needs and values. Some of the recent titles include *Umbilical cord blood banking: A guide for parents, Exercise your way to better post-transplant health* and *Donation of oocytes, a guide for women to support informed decisions.*[29]

Finally, with the aim of drawing public attention to organ donation and transplantation, the Council of Europe celebrates the *European Day for Organ Donation and Transplantation* (EODD)[30] in a different member state every year, usually on the second Saturday of October. The main objectives are to raise public awareness and encourage public debate; to establish trust among the general public towards responsible, ethical, non-commercial, and professional organ donation and transplantation; and to engage policy-makers and the medical community. EODD is also an opportunity to honour all organ donors and their families and to thank transplantation professionals throughout Europe whose hard work helps to save lives and improve the quality of life of many people.

The EU operates through a system of European institutions (including the European Commission, the Council of the EU, and the European Parliament) and intergovernmental decisions negotiated by the member states. Not only in the field of organs, but also tissues and cells and blood, the Council of Europe/EDQM and the European Commission[31] have a standing collaboration aimed, amongst other objectives, at avoiding duplication of efforts and at increasing the dissemination and exchange of knowledge and expertise.

Acknowledging that organ transplantation is an expanding medical field that offers important opportunities for the treatment of organ failure, the EU aims for a common approach to regulation across Europe. Article 168 of the Treaty on the Functioning of the EU[32] (previously Article 152 of the Treaty of Amsterdam) gives the EU a mandate to establish high quality and safety standards for substances of human origin, such as blood, organs, tissues, and cells. *Directive 2010/53/EU*[33] lays down the quality and safety standards for organs. It covers all steps in the transplant process from donation, procurement, testing, and handling to distribution; it provides for the appointment of Competent Authorities in all member states for the authorization of procurement and transplantation centres and activities, and for the establishment of traceability systems, as well as for the reporting of serious adverse events and reactions. To help implement this basic act, the Commission proposed and adopted *Commission Directive 2012/25/EU*[33] regarding the procedures that particularly apply to the cross-border exchange of human organs intended for transplantation, between EU member states. This last Directive refers only to organs exchanged across borders and does not cover patients travelling to another country for transplantation purposes, which should only be done in the strict framework of bilateral or multilateral cooperation agreements between member states and/or organ exchange organizations.

The EU has addressed three different challenges in the field of organ donation and transplantation in the European setting[34]: increasing organ availability, enhancing quality and safety, and making transplantation systems more accessible. This has been done by the EU by supporting its member states in their efforts to implement *Directive 2010/53/EU* and the *Commission's Action Plan on Organ Donation and Transplantation (2009–2015)*.[35] To mark the mid-term period of the Action Plan, in December

2012, EU member states adopted the conclusions of the Council of the EU on organ donation and transplantation,[36] recalling the main principles and objectives. In addition, based on the ACTOR Study,[37] the Commission issued document mapping efforts at national and European levels.[38]

Moreover, to improve cooperation between EU member states in this field, several projects have been funded by the European Commission under the *Research Programme*—6th and 7th[39] Framework Programmes (FP), Horizon 2020[40]—and under the *(Public) Health Programmes*[41] run by the Consumers, Health, Agriculture, and Food Executive Agency (CHAFEA).

Finally, the *European Centre for Disease Prevention and Control* (ECDC)[42] closely supports the European Commission and the National Competent Authorities in the field to strengthen Europe's defences against communicable diseases.

Challenges and future perspectives

Despite important advancements in the field, challenges persist in the European setting. As in other regions of the world, countries shall continue to progress towards self-sufficiency in transplantation.[43] This is a shared governmental and professional responsibility to develop preventive strategies to decrease the need for organs and increase organ availability, particularly by developing deceased donation to its maximum therapeutic potential. Organizational models to ensure the systematic identification and referral of possible organ donors and optimize their transition to utilized organ donors needed implementation in every member state.[44] Overcoming ethical and legal barriers that preclude the development of DCD programmes is a must, since thousands of patients die following an unsuccessfully resuscitated cardiac arrest or the decision to withdraw life-sustaining therapies that are no longer deemed beneficial.[11] There is also the need to build evidence on the safety and quality limits when using organs for transplantation.

High quality and safety standards need to be promoted and harmonized as much as possible in the European setting. Procedures, qualification and certification initiatives, quality assurance, and training programmes must be implemented in every country. An important challenge ahead is the proper post-transplant (and post live donation) assessment in Europe. Solid pan-European registries must be designed and implemented, upholding a mandatory requirement of data reporting from authorized centres to national authorities and to international registries.

Advances in transplantation cannot be understood without active pre-clinical and clinical research in the field. Europe must play a pivotal role in elucidating how to induce tolerance, reduce the occurrence of chronic rejection, and improve post-transplant outcomes in the short, mid and long term. With DCD and expanded criteria donors becoming essential to expand the donor pool, organ preservation strategies must be supported and robust trials conducted. Bioengineering and the creation of bioartificial organs should be in the pipeline of European research projects as a future alternative for organ replacement.

Organ trafficking and transplant tourism have become a global phenomenon, and Europe must be recognized as an active region in combatting transplant-related crimes that violate individual human rights and erode ethical transplant programmes. More efforts are required to understand the realities of organ trafficking, to create frameworks for professionals to report trafficking cases to the relevant authorities, and to harmonize legal frameworks. The *Council of Europe Convention against Trafficking in Human Organs*[19] represents a great opportunity in this regard.

Highlights

- There is a very heterogeneous scene in European countries, with some countries operating very effective deceased and living donation programmes while others rely on limited numbers of living donors to meet the needs of their patients, or have no donation programmes at all.
- In spite of recent efforts, no country has been able to reach self-sufficiency in organ donation and transplantation. There is still a shortfall in the number of suitable organs for transplantation.
- In all European countries, there is potential to obtain and use more organs for transplantation, through the development of

new programmes and the optimization of existing resources, and learning to cooperate with neighbouring countries.

- In order to support individual country efforts, the Council of Europe and the EU have launched ambitious work programmes to strengthen donation and transplantation programmes throughout Europe and foster cross-border and multi-sectorial cooperation. They have implemented an effective approach by providing detailed technical guidance to ensure safety and quality in organ, tissue, and cell donation and transplantation. In addition, they add value by defining ethical principles and practical programmes to support the development of transplantation programmes in areas where they are in their early stages.

References

1. International figures on donation and transplantation 2018. Newsletter Transplant 2018; 23 (1), available at https://register.edqm.eu/freepub
2. Global observatory on donation and transplantation, available at www.transplant-observatory.org
3. Newsletter Transplant 2017. Available at: https://www.edqm.eu/en/reports-and-publications
4. Martin DE, Van Assche K, Domínguez-Gil B, et al. A new edition of the Declaration of Istanbul: Updated guidance to combat organ trafficking and transplant tourism worldwide. Kidney Int. 2019; 95(4): pp. 757–759.
5. Arshad A, Anderson B, Sharif A. Comparison of organ donation and transplantation rates between opt-out and opt-in systems. Kidney Int 2019; 95(6): pp. 1453–1460. doi: 10.1016/j.kint.2019.01.036.
6. Weiss J, Elmer A, Mahíllo B, et al. Evolution of deceased organ donation activity versus efficiency over a 15-year period: An international comparison. Transplantation. 2018; 102(10): pp. 1768–1778. doi: 10.1097/TP.0000000000002226.
7. Matesanz R, Domínguez-Gil B, Coll E, de la Rosa G, Marazuela R. Spanish experience as a leading country: What kind of measures were taken? Transpl Int. 2011; 24(4): pp. 333–343. doi: 10.1111/j.1432-2277.2010.01204.x.
8. Manara A, Procaccio F, Domínguez-Gil B. Expanding the pool of deceased organ donors: The ICU and beyond. Intensive Care Med. 2019; 45(3): pp. 357–360. doi: 10.1007/s00134-019-05546-9.
9. Matesanz R, Domínguez-Gil B, Coll E, Mahíllo B, Marazuela R. How Spain reached 40 deceased organ donors per million population. Am J Transplant. 2017; 17(6): pp. 1447–1454. doi: 10.1111/ajt.14104.
10. Boesmueller C, Biebl M, Scheidl S, et al. Long-term outcome in kidney transplant recipients over 70 years in the Eurotransplant Senior Kidney Transplant Program: A single center experience. Transplantation. 2011; 92(2): pp. 210–216. doi: 10.1097/TP.0b013e318222ca2f.

11. Domínguez-Gil B, Haase-Kromwijk B, Van Leiden H, et al. Current situation of donation after circulatory death in European countries. Transpl Int. 2011; 24(7): pp. 676–686. doi: 10.1111/j.1432-2277.2011.01257.x.
12. Smith M, Dominguez-Gil B, Greer DM, et al. Organ donation after circulatory death: Current status and future potential. Intensive Care Med. 2019; 45(3): pp. 310–321. doi: 10.1007/s00134-019-05533-0.
13. www.eurotransplant.org www.scandiatransplant.org
14. Study on the set-up of organ donation and transplantation in the EU Member States, uptake and impact of the EU Action Plan on Organ Donation and Transplantation (2009-2015). Available at: https://ec.europa.eu/health/sites/health/files/blood_tissues_organs/docs/organs_actor_study_2013_en.pdf
15. Conclusions of the Third Conference of European Health Ministers (1987) 16–17 November 1987, available at https://rm.coe.int/CoERMPublicCommonSearchServices/DisplayDCTMContent?documentId=09000016804c6d07
16. European Committee on Organ Transplantation (CD-P-TO), available at http://www.edqm.eu/en/organ-transplantation-work-programme-72.html
17. EU policy in the field of organs, tissues and cells, available at http://ec.europa.eu/health/blood_tissues_organs/policy/index_en.htm
18. Organs, Tissues and Cells of Human origin. Council of Europe resolutions, recommendations and reports—3rd Edition (2017). Available at https://register.edqm.eu/freepub
19. Council of Europe (1997) Convention for the Protection of Human Rights and Dignity of the Human Being with regard to the Application of Biology and Medicine: Convention on Human Rights and Biomedicine, available at http://conventions.coe.int/Treaty/en/Treaties/Html/164.htm
20. Council of Europe (2002) Additional Protocol to the Convention on human rights and biomedicine, on transplantation of organs and tissues of human origin, available at http://conventions.coe.int/Treaty/en/Treaties/Html/186.htm
21. Council of Europe Convention on action against trafficking in human beings and its Explanatory Report, available at http://conventions.coe.int/treaty/en/Treaties/Html/197.htm
22. Council of Europe Convention against Trafficking in Human Organs, available at http://www.coe.int/en/web/conventions/search-on-treaties/-/conventions/treaty/216
23. Explanatory Report to the Council of Europe Convention against Trafficking in Human Organs, available at https://rm.coe.int/CoERMPublicCommonSearchServices/DisplayDCTMContent?documentId=09000016800d3840
24. Shimazono, Y. The state of the international organ trade: A provisional picture based on integration of available information. Bull World Health Organ. 2007; 85(12): pp. 955–962.
25. Proceedings of the II Workshop for National Focal Points on Transplant-Related Crimes, available at www.edqm.eu/freepub
26. Arredondo E, López-Fraga M, Chatzixiros E, et al. Council of Europe Black Sea Area Project: International cooperation for the development of activities related to donation and transplantation of organs in the region. Transplant Proc. 2018 Mar; 50(2): pp. 374–381.

27. *Newsletter Transplant* and past editions (Archives) available at https://register.edqm.eu/freepub
28. More information available at: https://www.edqm.eu/en/organs-tissues-and-cells-technical-guides
29. CD-P-TO thematic booklets for the general public available at https://www.edqm.eu/en/reports-and-publications
30. European Day for Organ Donation and Transplantation (EODD). More information available at https://www.edqm.eu/en/events/european-day-organ-donation-and-transplantation
31. European Union: European Commission General Directorate on Public Health, Organ Transplantation Section, available at http://ec.europa.eu/health/blood_tissues_organs/organs/index_en.htm
32. Treaty on the Functioning of the European Union, available at https://eur-lex.europa.eu/legal-content/EN/TXT/PDF/?uri=CELEX:12012E/TXT
33. Commission Implementing Directive 2012/25/EU of 9 October 2012 laying down information procedures for the exchange, between Member States, of human organs intended for transplantation Text with EEA relevance Available at: https://eur-lex.europa.eu/legal-content/EN/TXT/?uri=celex%3A32012L0025
34. European Commission Campaign 'Europe for Patients' on organ donation and transplantation: Commission Action plan on Organ Donation and Transplantation (2009-2015), available at http://ec.europa.eu/health-eu/europe_for_patients/organ_donation_transplantation/index_en.htm
35. Communication from the Commission: Action plan on Organ Donation and Transplantation (2009–2015): Strengthened Cooperation between Member States, available at http://ec.europa.eu/health/archive/ph_threats/human_substance/oc_organs/docs/organs_action_en.pdf
36. Council conclusions on organ donation and transplantation (2012/C 396/03) of EU Member States, available at http://ec.europa.eu/health/blood_tissues_organs/docs/organs_council_ccl_2012_en.pdf
37. ACTOR study: Study on the set-up of organ donation and transplantation in the EU Member States, uptake and impact of the EU Action Plan on Organ Donation and Transplantation (2009-2015), available at http://ec.europa.eu/health/blood_tissues_organs/docs/organs_actor_study_2013_en.pdf
38. Commission Staff Working Document on the mid-term review of the EU Action Plan on Organ Donation and Transplantation, available at http://ec.europa.eu/health/blood_tissues_organs/docs/midtermreview_actionplan_organ_en.pdf
39. EU Research and Innovation, 7th Framework Programme, available at https://ec.europa.eu/research/fp7/index_en.cfm
40. Horizon 2020, available at https://ec.europa.eu/programmes/horizon2020/en
41. EU Health Programmes, available at https://ec.europa.eu/health/funding/programme_en
42. European Centre for Disease Prevention and Control, available at https://ecdc.europa.eu/en/home

43. Delmonico FL, Domínguez-Gil B, Matesanz R, et al. A call for government accountability to achieve national self-sufficiency in organ donation and transplantation. Lancet. 2011; 378(9800): pp. 1414–1418. doi: 10.1016/S0140-6736(11)61486-4.
44. Domínguez-Gil B, Delmonico FL, Shaheen FA, et al. The critical pathway for deceased donation: Reportable uniformity in the approach to deceased donation. Transpl Int. 2011; 24(4): pp. 373–378. doi: 10.1111/j.1432-2277.2011.01243.x.

16

Organ donation in UK

Ajay Kumar Sharma, Ahmed Halawa

Historical perspective

Since its inception in July 1948, the National Health Scheme (NHS) in UK has been the torch-bearer of innovations and application of key advancements of medical sciences. Transplantation has evolved through NHS with epoch-making contributions from a number of scientists and medical professionals. Irradiation and high doses of steroids were used as immunosuppressant in late fifties and early sixties, but it was associated with high mortality among those transplanted with kidneys. In 1960, UK's first successful kidney transplant, between identical twins, was carried out by Sir Michael Woodruff in Edinburgh.[(1)] The donor returned to work after three weeks while the recipient took fifteen weeks to recover. Five years later, the first kidney transplant from a 'non-heart beating' donor was carried out in Edinburgh. In the period 1960–1974, 127 patients were transplanted in Nuffield Transplant Centre at Edinburgh referred as 'Fort Woodruff'.[(1)]

Roy Calne reported that azathioprine was more effective and less toxic than 6-mercaptopurine in preventing acute rejection.[(2)] The combination of azathioprine and prednisolone, known as conventional immunosuppression in 1960s, remained the backbone of immunosuppression for the next two decades until cyclosporine arrived in 1980s. Clinical application of cyclosporine was possible by contributions from Roy Calne once again. It made an impact by significantly reducing early graft loss due to acute rejection, a major hurdle for a successful liver, heart, and lung transplantation.[(2)] In 1990s, a number of key innovations from UK included trials of immunosuppressive drugs, inventions in immunology, progress in virology and ever-improving technology that transformed the outcomes in transplantation.

From the point of view of ethics of organ donation, it is worth mentioning about the 'Exeter Protocol' (elective ventilation), a distinctive British experience.(3) Driven by a well-meaning utilitarian ethos to benefit as many people in society, in Exeter Protocol, those patients who were in deep coma as a result of extensive cerebrovascular accident (CVA) but without all the features of brainstem death, were ventilated electively (range: 3 and 41 hours) in intensive therapy unit (ITU) to offer whatever minuscule chance they would have to survive.(3) Those who would not recover and evolve into full-blown brainstem death would become candidate for organ donation. The limitations of Exeter Protocol were two-fold: the lack of ethical correctness and unpragmatic use of ITU beds, a precious resource indeed, for patients who had low likelihood of poor outcomes. Such patients, having developed a life-threatening CVA, would not have been in a position to decide about utility (or futility), such an intervention that prolonged their life by only a few hours. Since Exeter Protocol did not satisfy the ethical standards it was proclaimed to be unlawful in 1994.(3)

Human Organ Transplants Act was promulgated in 1989 to encourage living organ donation to related needy family members and to regulate organ donation (living and cadaveric) to the highest ethical standards.(4) Unrelated Live Transplant Regulatory Authority (ULTRA) was constituted to assess requests by unrelated donors, such as spouses and living partners, in order to ensure that there is no coercion.(4) ULTRA was disbanded in 2006 and its responsibilities were transferred to Human Tissue Authority (HTA).(4)

Current scenario of organ donation in UK

Until 2009, there has been a consistent rise in the gap between demand and supply of organs for transplant in UK. Eight dedicated regional multi-organ retrieval teams cover the whole of UK and proactive identification of potential donors and placement of specialist nurses for organ donation (SNODs) has turned around this situation. In UK, 5,699 patients were on the waiting list for solid organ transplant as on

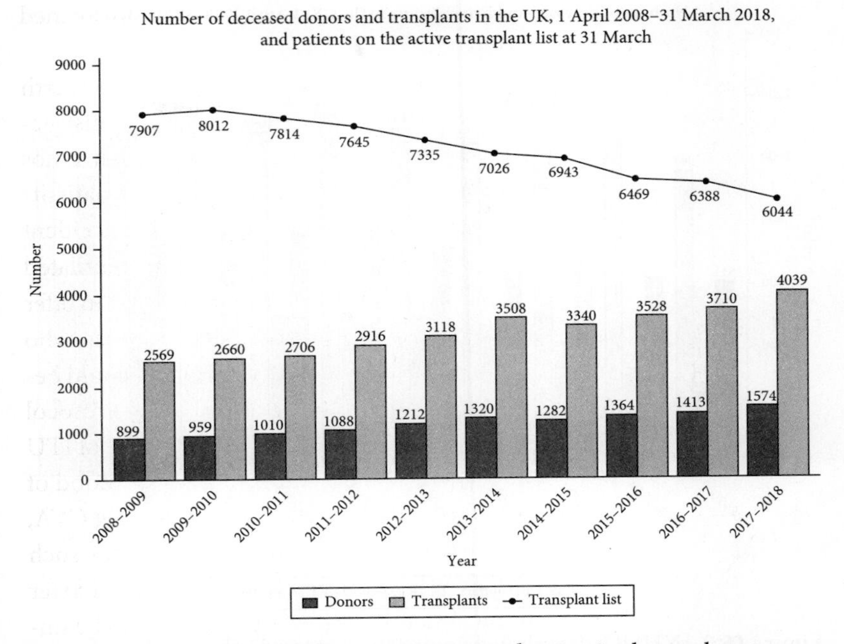

Figure 16.1. NHSBT data shows consistent reduction in the gap between the demand and supply as a result of initiatives implemented in 2008.[5]

31st March 2020, Figure 16.1 taken from National Health Scheme Blood and Transplant (NHSBT) data shows consistent reduction in the gap between the demand and supply as a result of initiatives implemented in 2008.[5] Each year, about 1100 living donors undergo a major operation to donate a kidney or part of liver to help their loved one survive.[5] Figure 16.2 from NHSBT data shows significant increase in the number of living donors since the laparoscopic donor nephrectomy became a routine procedure.[5] More than 600 altruistic kidney donors have donated their kidney to someone totally unknown to them. Currently, there are more than 52,000 patients with functioning allograft in UK. In spite of all the efforts, on an average, three patients die every day as they do not receive solid organ transplant. One major hurdle is that only 57% of families agree to consent for donation of organs of their loved ones if they are not aware of their wishes expressed before death even though 82% people support organ donation. However, only 37% have registered their choice on NHS Organ Donor Register.[6] In Wales, the

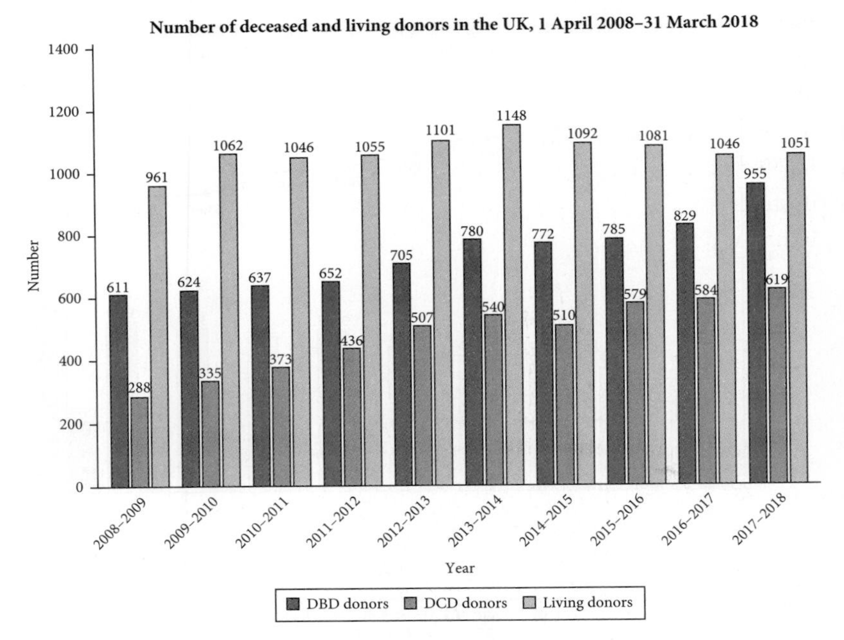

Figure 16.2. NHSBT data shows significant increase in the number of living donors since the laparoscopic donor nephrectomy because a routine procedure.[5]

opt-out system (also known as deemed consent) was implemented in 2015. Similar efforts are being made in Northern Ireland. The Scottish Parliament passed the opt-out system of organ donation in June 2019, an amendment to Human Tissue (Scotland) Act 2006, which was an opt-in system.[7] The Scottish Bill (Human Tissue Authorization Scotland Bill) allows the parents and guardians to register their children under the age of twelve (under eighteen in England, Wales, and Northern Ireland), and allows children over twelve years to make a declaration (or withdraw that declaration) to participate in the opt-out scheme. The Scottish Bill has been given Royal Assent in July 2019 and will be implemented in March 2021. There is a marker in relation to their registration that will be removed once that person attains the age of twelve in Scotland (or at eighteen in the rest of UK). In England, the opt-out system has been implemented in May 2020 and it is called Max and Keira's Law.[7] Opt-out system means that one is deemed to be an organ donor after death if one has not expressed desire not to donate on NHS Organ Donor Register (a computerized national register). Figure 16.3 shows a picture of 165th altruistic donor whose most inspiring campaign led to registration of more than 10,000 people in organ donor registry. The current legislation in Northern Ireland is for opt-in system, that allows one to nominate up to two representatives to make the decision oneself. These could be family members, friends, or one's faith leader.

GIVE A KIDNEY
Did you know
that 687 people
(so far) have
donated one of
their kidneys to a
complete stranger?
Could you be № 688 ?
in common?
Find out more about living kid
donation, visit
call 0300 123 23 23 or
Yes

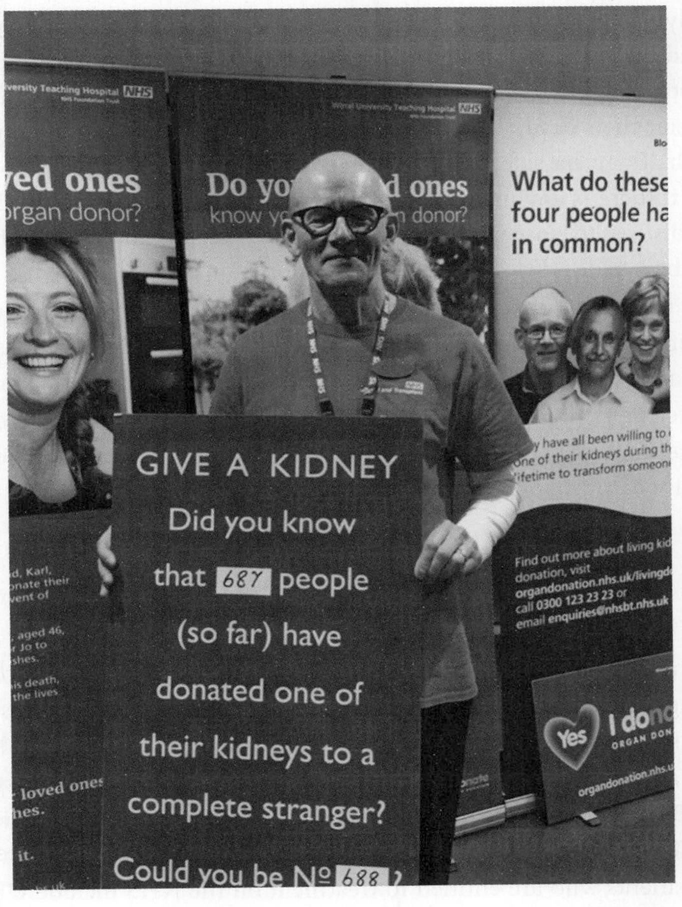

Figure 16.3. This picture of Paul Dixon, 165th altruistic donor in UK, whose most inspiring campaign led to registration of more than 10,000 people in organ donor registry

Soft opt-out versus hard opt-out system

Many countries in Europe, such as Austria and Belgium, follow the system of presumed consent for organ donation. That means everyone after death is deemed as an organ donor unless there an evidence to the contrary. In UK, the opt-out system would be 'soft opt-out' system that allows the next-of-kin to override if they had reason to believes that the donor may have had views against donation.[7] In Wales, one can nominate up to two representatives (either the religious leader, friend, or family members) who can decide on one's behalf after death. In England, any adult who does not wish to donate can register to express his/her wish to opt-out of organ donation. Any adult can record on UK Organ Donor Register their desire to donate or nominate someone to decide on one's behalf. There are safeguards to ensure that organ retrieval does not proceed if there is any inkling that the organ retrieval would cause significant distress to close family members. Therefore, it is far easier for family members to decide for or against organ donation if a discussion has taken place in a family. The families are twice as likely to agree to organ donation if there have been discussions on this issue. NHSBT provides support and guidance through website and telephonic advice for anyone registering as organ donor.[6] SNODs do always phone UK organ donor register to look for any objection or expression of interest to donate irrespective of opt-in or opt-out system.

Usage of donor organs in UK

For the best recipient of a donated organ, a matching run is performed through the computerized database at NHSBT in order to correspond to blood group, age, body weight, clinical urgency (in case of heart, lung, and liver), and tissue typing of the patients waiting for transplant. NHSBT has nationwide information of all the prospective recipients.[5–7] The donors are notified to NHSBT on a 24/7 basis and 365 days a year. The patients who are entitled to treatment on the NHS include UK citizens, armed forces personnel and those foreign nationals who have reciprocal arrangement with the Department of Health. Those patients being managed in private sector and not entitled to NHS treatment can be offered an organ if there were no suitable patients in NHS. Moreover, when there is a specific permission from donor or donor family, the organs can be used for research purposes.

Confidentiality of donor information

It is the responsibility of all the members of transplant team to ensure confidentiality of cadaveric and non-directed altruistic donors. If the donor family has expressed a wish to know some details of recipient, then the age (rounded off to a decade) and sex is made known to them. Likewise, the recipients can be given similar information about their donor. The donor and recipient families may exchange anonymous letters of expressing gratitude or greetings through SNODs.

Views of different faiths and religions in relation to organ donation

The ethnic minorities such as Asians and Blacks are twice as likely to be on waiting list for a renal transplant than the Caucasians. In UK all the major faiths (Christians, Muslims, Hindus, Jews, Jains, Buddhists, and Sikhs) support or are neutral to organ donation and transplantation. Only exceptions are Shintoists, Rastafarians, and Romany Gypsies, whose are rather minuscule in numbers among UK inhabitants. It is very important to appreciate that the outcomes of transplant are much better if the ethnic origin of donor and that of the recipient is same.[(8)]

Commonly arising doubts in organ donation

The major doubts in the minds of those contemplating to join the organ donor registry are as follows:[(9–11)]

1. *Will the process of organ donation cause disfigurement?*

No. After corneal donation from a cadaveric donor, the eye balls are replaced by an artificial one. The abdomen and thorax are operated as for any other operation in theatres with paramount important given to asepsis and dignity.

2. *Is it possible to declare someone dead before death just to facilitate organ donation?*

There are strict procedures, checks, and balances in place in the NHS to ensure that such a scenario would never happen. Two sets of brainstem death tests are performed to certify brain death (DBD, i.e. donation after brain death) by two experts (anaesthetists, intensivists, or neurologists). The decision about the futility of treatment and the irreversibility of recovery in a situation of potential donation after circulatory death (DCD), is taken by the experts who are independent of the transplant team. The doctors must wait until 5 minutes after potential DCD donor's heart has stopped before the death is confirmed, and another 5 minutes before the operation for retrieval of organs is commenced.

3. *Organs might be sold?*

In UK, this cannot happen. The laws in UK absolutely prohibit the sale of human organs or tissue. It is not unlawful to seek a donor online or through an advertisement in a newspaper, only if there is no offer of a reward, payment, or material advantage to the potential donor or a supplier. A transplant department, because of resource constraints, is not obliged to test all those who may come forward in response to an advertisement.

Paired or pooled organ donation to share living donor kidneys

About 30% of living donors are not able to go ahead with directed donation (i.e. to their relative or friend) because of blood group incompatibility or due to incompatibility as a result of anti-donor antibodies against recipient's human leucocyte antigens (HLA). Paired or pooled exchange of kidneys allows the transplantation between such donor-recipient combinations who otherwise could not proceed. Furthermore, this organ share of kidneys is being used for providing a better matched kidney. Usually the operation of two or more donors involved in this organ sharing scheme commences at the same time, followed by transportation of organs between hospitals.

Altruistic organ donation

If a suitable donor (after detailed psychological and physical assessment) is considered fit to donate then an organ can be offered to the best possible match on national waiting list. This is called non-directed altruistic organ donation. There are situations when one of the potential recipients in a chain of pooled donor-recipients pairs does have incompatibility to any available donor and; as a result, the chain is stuck at that point. Often an altruistic donor is used to trigger a chain of pooled organ donation that would benefit more than one recipient. Less often, an altruistic donation can be directed to a specific potential recipient who has come up in response to the donor's wish to donate or in response to the recipient's advertisement.

Reimbursement for the expenses incurred by the donor

Payment of fee, material exchange, or a reward to anyone for an organ transplant is an offence in UK.[11,12] All the donors must sign to confirm that there is no financial or material reward before or after donor operation. However, UK law allows for direct payment to the donor for the loss of salary (living), for travel, and for expenses incurred (if any) in post-operative period. Although there is no obligation on NHS for the recipient or the recipient's family to pay for these expenses, it is seen as a good practice for NHS to pay. The process for this reimbursement needs to be initiated well in advance so that non-payment of expenses does not become an impediment to donation of organ. If there is such a situation, it is acceptable for the recipient's family to reimburse to the donor directly. If requested by HTA, the donor and recipient must be able to furnish the proofs that the donor has not materially benefitted from any point of view. This issue is of particular importance when the donor is coming from overseas. Such a claim for reimbursement should be made to the NHS Commissioning Board through the living donor co-ordinator. British Transplant Society forbids the transplant departments to accept any living donor that has been found (matched) from a website advertisement that registers recipients for a fee.

Challenges in organ retrieval and organ usage

Studies demonstrate that there is a drop in numbers at each and every step in the process of organ retrieval and organ usage and, therefore, there is a significant scope of improvement.[5] Only 37% people in England are aware of a change in organ donation law. We need to appreciate that only around 1% of people in UK die in a setting (such as in intensive care unit, possibly in high dependency unit, and rarely in emergency department) where organ donation is feasible.[13] Therefore, increasing the intensive care beds might have one more benefit, i.e. the possibility of increased number of potential organ donors from those who are brain-dead or have an irreversible loss of cardiac or pulmonary function after cardiac arrest. Figure 16.4 taken from NHSBT website shows the flow diagram that depicts the numbers of potential donors reaching fruition.[5] It has been observed that a number of donors could have been DBD, but their brainstem tests could not be organized or were inconclusive, resulting in those donors been offered as DCD. It is worth highlighting that the number of organs per donor are lesser from DCD in comparison to DBD, and 30–50% of potential DCD donors do not reach fruition.[7] An organ donor card that is carried by a potential donor makes it much easier for SNODs to discuss with their respective family (Figure 16.5).

Guidance for transplant teams and Independent Assessors in regards to living organ donation

After the medical team has assessed a prospective donor and the fitness to donate the organ is confirmed, an independent assessment by a suitably

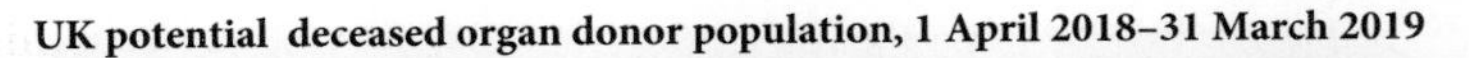

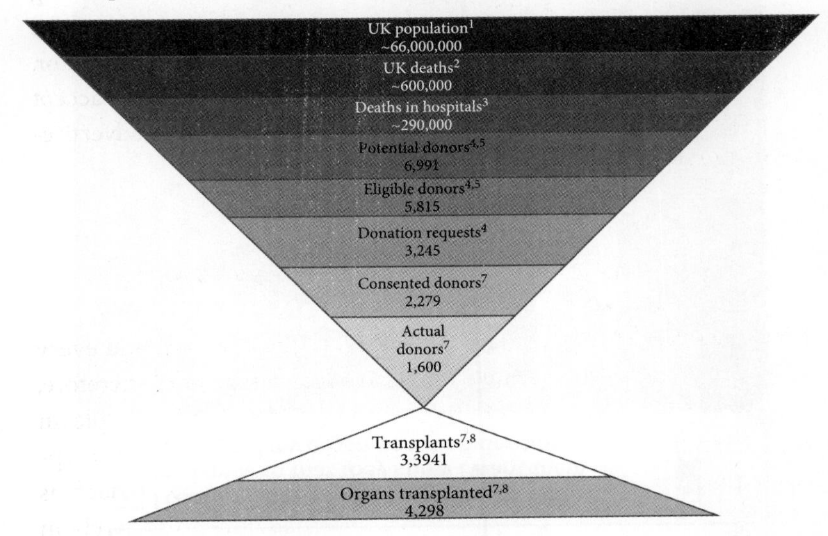

[1] Mid 2017 estimates: www.ons.gov.uk
[2] 2017 data: England & Wales www.ons.gov.uk; Scotland www.gro-scotland.gov.uk; Northen Ireland www.nisra.gov.uk
[3] 2017 data: England & Wales www.ons.gov.uk; Scotland www.isdscotland.org; Northern Ireland www.nisra.gov.uk
[4] 2018/2019 data, NHSBT, Potential Donor Audit
[5] Potential donor-patients for whom death was confirmed following neurological tests or patients who had treatment withdrawn and death was anticipated within four hours
[6] Eligible donor-Potential donor with no absolute medical contraindications to solid organ donation
[7] 2018/2019 deceased donor data: NHSBT, UK Transplant Registry
[8] Using organs from actual donors in the UK

Figure 16.4. NHSBT figure shows the flow diagram that depicts the numbers of potential donors reaching fruition.[5]

trained and accredited Independent Assessor (IA) is required.[14,15] The IA would interview the prospective donor and recipient separately on behalf of HTA to ensure that there is no coercion or payment. The IA must be able to establish that the decision to donate is a well-informed one. Evidence in the form of documents, old letters, and photographs to prove the relationship should be provided to the IA. If there is a need for translator, the living donor co-ordinator would arrange that in advance. This interview often lasts for 30 minutes to an hour. The IA would submit a report to HTA within ten working days. In some cases, HTA staff may need to do further assessment themselves or might refer to a panel of three investigators, who have to reply, respectively in five and ten working days. The HTA would communicate their decision to the transplant unit. The living donor co-ordinator has the duty to convey HTA's decision to the donor and recipient.

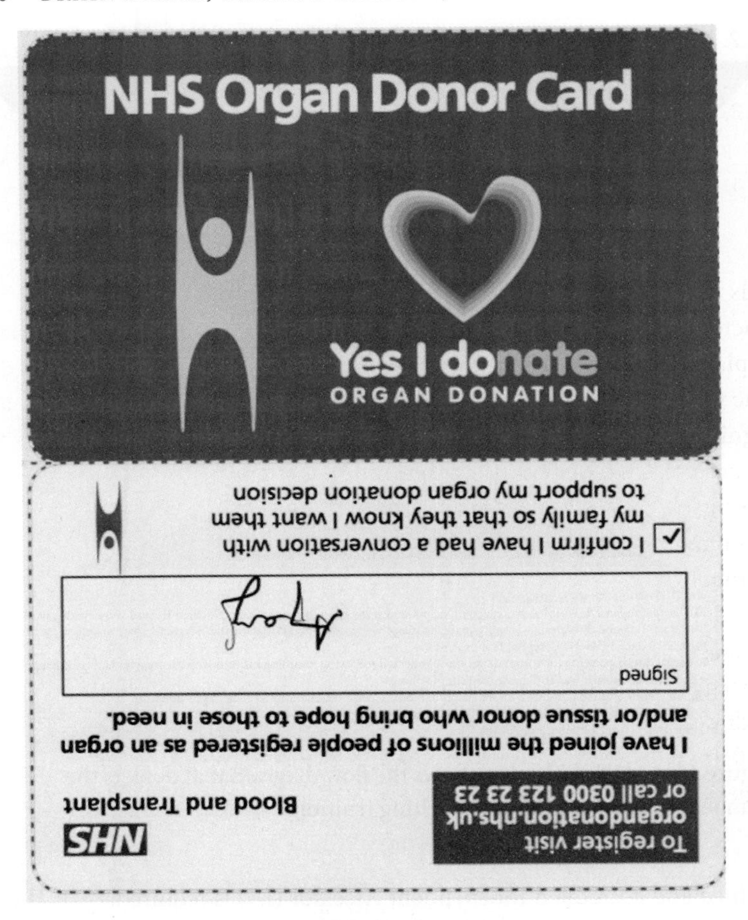

Figure 16.5. A donor card showing registration of keenness to donate after death

Future perspectives

The NHSBT and Department of Health document aims to achieve the following by 2020:[(16)]

1. To define strategies to increase consent rate to 80% from a current figure of 57% that includes increasing awareness among Blacks, Asians, and other minority ethnic communities.

2. To increase cadaveric donors to 26 per million population (pmp); which is currently at 19.1 pmp.
3. To increase the number of organs transplanted by 5% more from those donors whose families have consented.
4. To raise the number of cadaveric transplant to 74 pmp from a current figure of 49 pmp.

It is debated whether a sustained awareness campaign and training the doctors and nurses to engage in conversation about opt-out scheme is the explanation for a possible increase in organ donation rather than directly due to implementation of opt-out system.[(17)] It is too early to notice any significant influence of opt-out system, but there is no doubt it has increased the awareness among public.[(7)]

Organ donation from cadaveric donors in paediatric age group in UK has remained static at 50–57 between the years 2014 and 2019, while the number of children waiting for transplantation is consistently about 138–183 during the same period. Therefore, a strategy ought to be evolved to increase the availability of paediatric organs.[(18)] Public education is the key strategy to increase organ donation, and it will be possible if efforts are made to discuss the philosophy, science and ethics of organ donation system with all faiths and religious groups. The lessons need to be learnt from Australian experience, where organ donation is part of curriculum at schools.[19]

Highlights

- In UK, only 57% of families agree to give consent for donation of organs of their loved ones.
- 82% of public support the organ donation.
- In UK, the opt-out system would be 'soft opt-out' system that allows the next-of-kin to override.
- A strategy ought to be evolved to increase the availability of paediatric organs.
- Public education is the key to discuss the philosophy, science and ethics of organ education system with all faiths and religious groups.
- Payment of fee, material exchange, or a reward to anyone for an organ transplant is an offence in UK

References

1. The history of dialysis and kidney transplantation in Edinburgh. 2001. http://edren.org/ren/unit/history/the-history-of-dialysis-and-kidney-transplantation-in-edinburgh/ Modified April 3, 2019.
2. Hurst J. A modern Cosmas and Damian: Sir Roy Calne and Thomas Starzl receive the 2012 Lasker~Debakey Clinical Medical Research Award. J Clin Invest. 2012;122(10):3378–3382.
3. Riad Hany, Nicholls Anthony. An ethical debate: Elective ventilation of potential organ donors BMJ 1995; 310 :714
4. Choudhry S, Daar AS, Radcliffe Richards J, et al. Unrelated living organ donation: ULTRA needs to go. Journal of Medical Ethics 2003;29:169–170.
5. ODT Clinical: Annual Activity report. 2019–20. https://www.odt.nhs.uk/statistics-and-reports/annual-activity-report/
6. ODT Clinical: Register to be an organ donor. 2019–20. https://www.odt.nhs.uk/information-for-patients/register-to-be-an-organ-donor/
7. Organ donation law in England is changing. 2019. https://www.organdonation.nhs.uk/uk-laws/organ-donation-law-in-england/
8. Medcalf JF, Andrews PA, Bankart J, et al. Poorer graft survival in ethnic minorities: results from a multi-centre UK study of kidney transplant outcomes. Clin Nephrol. 2011;75(4):294–301. doi:10.5414/cn106675
9. Michielson P. Presumed consent to organ donation: ten years' experience in Belgium. Journal of the Royal Society of Medicine 1996;89: 663–666.
10. David Price (2000) Legal and Ethical Aspects of Organ Transplantation Cambridge University Press. Cambridge.
11. Bell M D D. Non-heart beating organ donation—clinical process and fundamental issues. Br J Anaesth 2005; 94: 474–478.
12. Bell M D D. The UK Human Tissue Act and consent: Surrendering a fundamental principle to transplantation needs? J Med Ethics. 2006; 32 (5); 283–286.
13. 2019. https://www.nhsbt.nhs.uk/news/pass-it-on-campaign/#:~:text=Only%2037%25%20of%20over%2016s%20in%20England%20currently,have%20told%20their%20family%20they%20want%20to%20donate
14. Living donor kidney transplantation. 2019. https://bts.org.uk/wp-content/uploads/2016/09/19_BTS_RA_Living_Donor_Kidney-1.pdf
15. Human Tissue Authority. https://www.hta.gov.uk/policies/guidance-transplant-teams-and-independent-assessors. Updated on 24 August 2021.
16. Taking organ transplantation to 2020- UK Strategy, 2020. https:// nhsbtdbe.blob.core. windows.net/umbraco-assets-corp/4241/nhsbt_organ_donor_strategy_summary.pdf.
17. Veronica English and Brian L Sadler. Head to head: Is an opt-out system likely to increase organ donation? BMJ 2019; 364: 392–393.
18. Campaign for more child organ donors launched. News: Seven Days in Medicine. BMJ 2019; 364: 381.
19. For teachers: donate life school resources. 2021. https://donatelife.gov.au/resources/school-resources/teachers.

17

Organ donation in USA

Amit Sharma, Brianna Ruch, Iolanda Russo-Menna

Introduction

Organ transplantation has become the optimal treatment for many end-stage organ-specific diseases and the total number of transplanted organs has gradually increased over the last few decades. Despite this, more than 120,000 people in the United States are waiting to receive a life-saving organ transplant. It is estimated that more than 7,000 candidates die annually while on the waitlist, or within thirty days of leaving the list, without receiving an organ transplant.(1) An understanding of these processes allows us to recognize the unique challenges and opportunities facing organ transplantation in the United States.

Transplantation is one of the most regulated aspects of healthcare in the United States. In 1984 the National Organ Transplant Act (NOTA) was passed by Congress to establish a centralized registry, the Organ Procurement and Transplantation Network (OPTN) for matching and placing organs for transplantation.(2) The Omnibus Budget Reconciliation Act of 1986 requires that all medical centres performing organ transplantation participate in the OPTN or forfeit their eligibility for federal Medicare and Medicaid payments. The United Network for Organ Sharing (UNOS), based in Richmond, Virginia, has held and administered the OPTN contract continuously since 1986.(3)

The Uniform Anatomical Gift Act (UAGA) was promulgated in 1968 by the National Conference of Commissioners with the intent of simplifying the process of obtaining organs from deceased persons and promoting uniformity among states.(4) It should be noted that the UAGA and subsequent revisions are not federal laws, but rather templates that various states can use in developing their own laws governing anatomical gifts. The act allows individuals to give authorization to make an anatomical gift in several forms, including through a statement or symbol on a driver's license or a donor card or via a donor registry.[5]

All hospitals engaged in transplantation must meet the federal Medicare Conditions of Participation and also the accreditation requirements of the Joint Commission, both of which contain provisions related to organ donation. Following transplantation, organ recipients receive extensive follow-up care and transplant programmes are mandated to submit their perioperative and follow-up data to OPTN/UNOS. This data is then analysed by the Scientific Registry of Transplant Recipients (SRTR).[6] The data (without any individual identifiers) is then made available to the general public, clinicians, researchers, policymakers, and regulatory agencies. Overall, this protocol creates a multi-tiered, federally regulated and nationwide system for the procurement and allocation of organs within the United States.

Old organ allocation system

The OPTN membership in the U.S was historically divided into eleven geographic regions (Figure 17.1) referred to as donation services areas

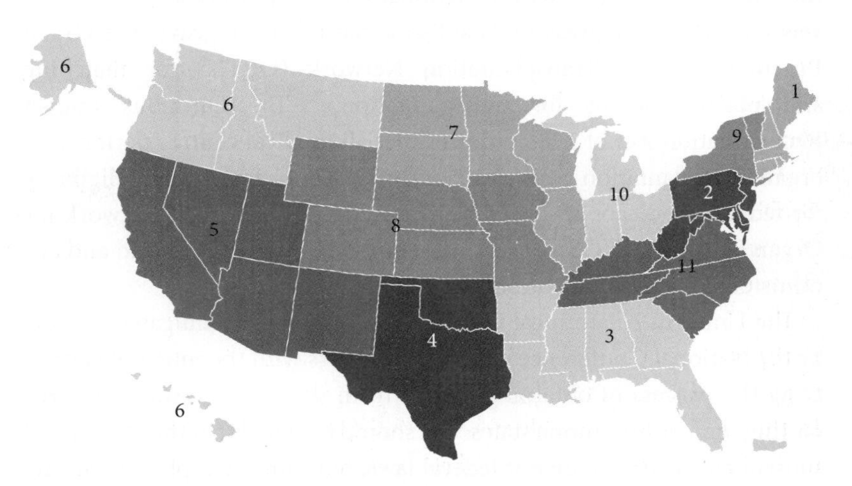

Figure 17.1. Donation service areas (now defunct) in the United States. (Adapted with permission from Scientific American Surgery, Decker.)[10]

(DSA). Each DSA encompassed Organ Procurement Organizations (OPO), the donor hospitals contracted to work with the OPO, and the assigned transplant hospitals, transplant programmes, and histocompatibility laboratories that serve the area. Members belonged to the region in which they were located. The OPTN still oversees the OPOs, which are local, non-profit organizations responsible for the evaluation and procurement of organs for transplantation. Currently there are fifty-eight such organizations in the United States.(7) The OPOs serve as the first line of contact with hospitals and donor families and their outcomes are monitored by donation rates (eligible donors per eligible deaths) and donor yield measure (organs per donor).(2) Until recently, the DSAs functioned to procure and transplant organs within their area. However, in attempts to reduce geographic disparities, a new organ allocation system has been approved so that it increasingly works on a national scale.(8, 9) This has been discussed later in this chapter.

A national computerized network, UNet^{SM}, is used to match donated organs with potential recipients and links all 58 OPOs, 254 transplant hospitals, and 150 histocompatibility laboratories. All patients awaiting an organ from a deceased donor are placed in the UNet^{SM} waiting list database. Each time an organ is donated within an OPO service area, the allocation system matches the donor with the database of waiting transplant candidates. The UNOS policy permits patients to be considered for organs that become available in other areas if the patient has been evaluated and listed at more than one centre. This may help reduce the waiting time in some cases.

After an eligible donor has been identified in a hospital, the local OPO representative is informed by the intensive care team and takes over management of the donor. The donor family is contacted and informed consent for organ or tissue donation is obtained. Organ donation in the United States operates by an 'opt-in' model in contrast to several European (e.g., Spain, Austria, Belgium, France) and South American (e.g., Argentina, Colombia) countries that utilize an 'opt-out' system. In the former, the individual, while alive, or their next of kin after the individual's death, choose to donate organs, while the latter system presumes donor authorization and participation in the absence of any clear objection.(11, 12)

The UNOS generates a list of potential recipients and notifies the appropriate transplant centre of the available organ. The centre will then consider the offer (with a one hour time limit) and either accept or decline. Should they decline, the organ is then offered to the next centre until it is placed. Once all intended organs from the deceased donor have been matched, the OPO, in collaboration with the donor hospital, arranges for the organ recovery surgery. Typically, multiple teams in various combinations including heart, lungs, intestine, liver, pancreas, and kidneys will procure multiple organs. Seamless collaboration between the procuring teams and the OPO is essential during procurement. The perioperative management and the surgical techniques for procurement may vary across states and transplant centres and are beyond the scope of this chapter.(13–16)

Current status and challenges

In 2017, 82% of organs transplanted in the United States were from deceased donors (28,582 organs from 10,286 deceased individuals) while only 6,182 organs were transplanted from living donors.(17) Therefore, in this section we discuss the current status of organ donation in the United States with focus on deceased donors.

Organ shortage

A majority of deceased donor organs are procured following declaration of brain death, determined after irreversible cessation of brainstem activity that is documented by bedside neurologic tests (donation after brain death). Over the past decade there has been an increase in donation after cardiac death (DCD) donors from 7% in 2005 to 18% in 2017 of all deceased donors.(17) The total number of transplantations performed in the United States have continued to slowly increase, with 19,613 kidneys, 8,082 livers, 213 pancreases, 3,244 hearts, 2,449 lungs, and 109 small bowel transplants performed in 2017.(18,19) Despite this gradual increase, more than 1,15,00 patients remain on the waitlist and over 6,400 patients died while on the waitlist never having received a transplant (Figure 17.2).(18, 20)

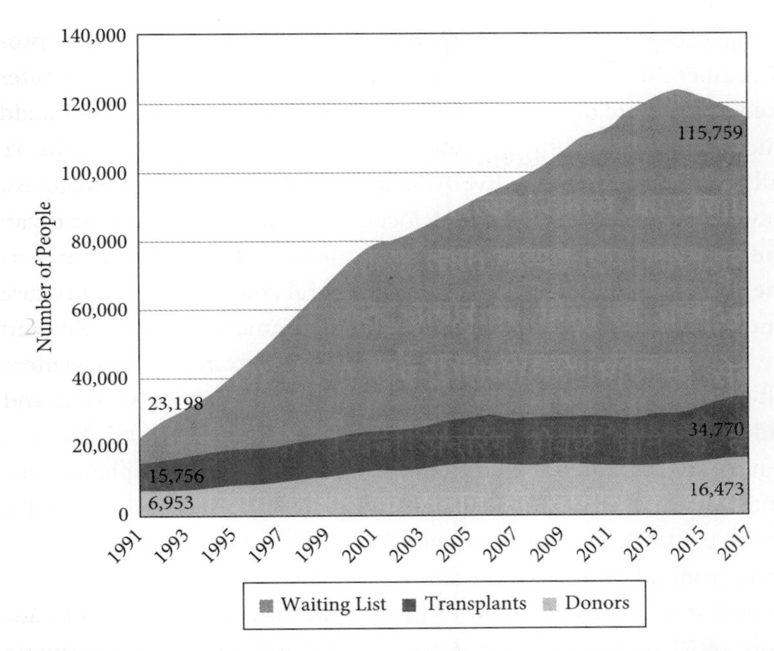

Figure 17.2. Widening gap between available organ donors, transplanted organs and wait-listed candidates. (Source: Freely available at Organdonor.gov, U.S. Government Information on Organ Donation and Transplantation.)[20]

Geographic disparities and the new organ allocation system

Until recently, the organ allocation system in United States had focused primarily on local or regional allocation along the respective DSAs. However, some regions have longer waiting lists than others, and there is now the possibility of moving towards allocation algorithms that prioritize candidates across the country rather than those who are local. The OPTN Final Rule sets the requirements for allocation policies developed by the OPTN/UNOS, including sound medical judgement, best use of organs, ability for transplant hospitals to decide whether to accept an organ offer, avoiding wasting organs, promoting patient access to transplant, avoiding futile transplants, and promoting efficiency. The Final Rule also includes a requirement that allocation policies 'shall not be based on the candidate's place of residence or place of listing, except to the extent required'. The OPTN Board of Directors, in December 2018, approved a continuous distribution model to replace fixed geographic boundaries with statistical models incorporating distances along with clinical parameters. However, this proposal was legally challenged by some liver transplant centres that felt the proposal may deprive their recipients of locally procured organs and provide undue advantage to larger centres in densely populated areas.[21–24] The controversy was resolved when a federal court ruling issued on 16 January 2020 removed the potential for an injunction that would delay the implementation of the new policy.[25] The new system replaced the old geographic boundaries of fifty-eight donation service areas (DSAs) and eleven transplant regions. For example, livers from all deceased donors are currently offered to the most urgent liver transplant candidates (Status 1A and 1B) listed at transplant hospitals within a radius of 500 nautical miles of the donor hospital.[26] After these candidates, livers from adult donors are offered to patients with a MELD (model for end-stage liver disease) or PELD (paediatric end-stage liver disease) score of 37 or higher listed at transplant hospitals within a radius of 150, 250, and 500 nautical miles from the donor hospital respectively. If the organ is still not placed, progressive offers are made to candidates at transplant hospitals within 150, 250, and 500 nautical miles of the donor hospital with ranges of MELD or PELD scores from 33 to 36, from 29 to 32, and from 15 to 28. In order to reduce the preservation time, livers from deceased donors older than age seventy, and/or those who die as a result of cardiorespiratory failure (DCD), are offered differently. After considering Status 1A and 1B candidates within a 500 nautical mile radius of the donor hospital, they are offered to candidates with a MELD or PELD score of 15 or higher at transplant hospitals within 150 miles of the donor location. In addition, livers from deceased donors younger than age eighteen are first offered to paediatric candidates (younger than age eighteen) listed at any transplant hospital within a 500 nautical-mile radius of the donor hospital. It is expected that this new policy based on these 'acuity circles' will save more lives annually by providing increased transplant access for the most urgent candidates as well as increase the number of paediatric liver transplants. Policy details and other updates can be freely accessed from the OPTN website (https://optn.transplant.hrsa.gov/).[27]

Organ discards

Many organs recovered from deceased donors are not transplanted.[28] These organs may either be used for research or discarded. In 2015, 4,370 organs were discarded, including 3,157 kidneys, 311 pancreases, 703 livers, 30 hearts, and 214 lungs. In many cases the organs are deemed unsuitable for transplantation while being assessed by the procuring surgeon at the time of recovery. The reasons for discard may include intrinsic disease in the organ concerned, longer than expected cold ischemia time, poor flush, surgical damage or incidentally discovered cancer.[29] Organ donor intervention research presents an opportunity to discover methods to improve organ quality and viability leading to increased utilization.[30–33]

State policies and registration for organ donation

While 95% of Americans endorse positive opinions regarding organ donation, only 58% are officially registered as organ donors.[34] In addition, family consent rates for donation when approached by an OPO professional vary widely.[35] If a family member is registered as an organ donor prior to being a donor candidate, the family is significantly more likely to proceed with donation.[36,37] Overall, the revised UAGA (1987 and 2006) has been pivotal in allowing the development of state organ donor registries with many of these registries linked to drivers' licenses. The application of the revised UAGA (2006) is determined at the state level and remains inconsistent. As a result various states may still differ on what qualifies as authorization for donation. Hence, there is a need for a unified, secure national donor registry that is easily accessible to organ procurement organizations.[28,38]

Organ donation in minority populations

In order to increase organ donation rates, adequate education must be provided to potential donors, family members, providers, and organ procurement organizations. Initiatives like the National Minority Organ

Tissues Transplant Education Program, which was established in 1991 to target African-American, Hispanic, Asian, and other ethnic groups, have yielded positive results. A review of the UNOS database (1990 to 2010) showed that Black organ donors per million had gradually increased and totalled 35.4 versus 27 for white, 25.6 for Hispanic and 14.7 for Asian donors.[39] At the same time, it has been shown that in the United States racial minorities encounter barriers throughout the entire process from initial education, referral, and in-person evaluation. This disparity is particularly apparent in terms of living donation[40] and decreases with increased individual education level, with those having received a college level or greater education more likely to undergo transplantation with post-operative outcomes similar to the Caucasian population.[41,42]

Obesity epidemic

The American population struggles with widespread obesity, with 39.8% of adults being considered obese and 7.6% being morbidly obese.[43] The increasing prevalence of obesity and metabolic syndrome will likely contribute to an increase in chronic conditions that lead to end-stage organ diseases and widen the demand-supply gap for organ transplantation.[44–46] Therefore, long-term measures are needed to address the epidemic of obesity in the general population.[47] In the short-term, transplant centres and OPOs will need to devise innovative strategies to use these marginal organs. From an organ recipient perspective, several studies have shown that although obese patients are at a higher risk of complications, they still benefit from transplantation.[48, 49]

Opportunities and future directions

Organ donation is a complex process especially in a large, heterogeneous nation like the United States. Each step in this process of organ donation presents opportunities to devise strategies that could increase donation rates.

Increasing registrations for organ donation

Attempts to increase the number of registered potential donors are an ongoing endeavour. A 2017 poll for why people did not register as organ donors showed that up to 30% indicated uncertainty or perceived disqualification.[50] This subset of the population may be receptive to further education and reconsideration. Education-based initiatives aimed at the Department of Motor Vehicles (DMV) have had modest success at increasing the registration rates.[51] The most significant effects occurred when interventions were aimed at those applying for their first license and while educating the employees at the DMV.[52,53] Other initiatives to increase the donor registration may include education at primary care physician offices, schools, and use of social media.[54,55]

Increasing the number of actual donors

Organ procurement organizations pursue many more cases, including eligible deaths and potential (imminent) donors, than the approximately 8,000 actual donors per year in the United States. It is postulated that these additional cases could increase the number of actual and potential donor cases to over 18,300. However, donation may not be realized because the 'imminent' category includes patients who may still exhibit brainstem reflexes, and therefore cannot be declared brain dead and also may not be viable DCD candidates. The integration of organ donation with end-of-life care has been recommended to allow the donation process to start before the occurrence of the donor's death.[56] Delayed referral from the medical teams taking care of potential donors in the hospital may also negatively impact organ donation. It is therefore recommended that the potential donor be referred early and the determination of the suitability for donation should be deferred to the OPO rather than to the intensive care team. This provides the OPO adequate time to medically evaluate the potential donors, manage unstable donors, and subsequently approach the family for consent.[14]

Donor families and consent rates

Unlike in other nations, organ donation in the United States is based on explicit rather than presumed consent. The family (or nearest kin) of any registered donor is always contacted before organ procurement. The current consent rate ranges between 62% and 93% across all OPOs.[57] Factors that are associated with low consent rates include extreme age of the donor; time elapsed between certification of brain death and approach to the family; the amount of time spent by the OPO coordinator with the family; and ethnicity of the donor.[58,59] Some barriers to donation in ethnic minorities include lack of awareness of transplantation, distrust of the medical community due to religious or cultural reasons along with fear of racism and consequently medical abandonment. Therefore, culturally sensitive communication and education are imperative to overcome these barriers.[60,61]

Increased use of infectious risk donors

The perceived risk of contracting donor-derived infections from 'high risk donors' may prompt patients and physicians to decline organs that may otherwise be suitable for transplantation. It has been shown that the risk of transmission of infectious diseases from such donors is low.[62] In the past, the use of Hepatitis C organs was limited to recipients with a previous diagnosis of Hepatitis C.[63,64] Currently due to the availability of highly efficacious antiviral therapies,[65] transplantation of organs from Hepatitis C positive donors to Hepatitis C negative recipients is being accepted as a means to increase organ utilization and significantly reduce the wait-list times for liver, kidney, heart, and lung recipients.[63,66] The long-term effects of this strategy are still under investigation.

Salvaging marginal organs

While expanded-criteria organs may carry an increased risk of graft failure or dysfunction, they still provide better long-term health outcomes for a recipient than would be expected from not receiving an organ transplant at all.[67,68] Existing and emerging technologies like hypothermic[69,70), (32] and normothermic[30] pulsatile pump perfusion of organs may allow optimization and evaluation of function prior to transplantation, thus potentially reducing discard rates. Donor intervention research offers the use of medications, procedures, or other interventions to improve the quality of donated organs for transplantation. Such research is unique because: (a) the outcomes of interventions in the deceased donor may directly affect the transplant recipient, (b) the timeframe for interventions is limited to maintain organ viability, and (c) organs from one donor may go to multiple recipients in different transplant centres and this adds to the complexities and scope of this research. These factors also stress the need for an ethical framework with oversight mechanisms.[28]

Transportation of organs is one of the most crucial aspects of the transplantation process. The amount of time an organ can remain viable while in transit is critical and reduction of the cold ischemia times could result in utilization of many organs that may otherwise be discarded. Drones could provide organ deliveries that are faster, safer and more widely available than the currently used methods (road transportation, use of commercial aircrafts) of transporting organs. In 2019, a kidney was transported using a drone and subsequently transplanted successfully.[71] Widespread application of unmanned aircraft systems to deliver organs appear exciting but will require collaboration among engineers, pilots, the Federal Aviation Administration, surgeons, organ procurement specialists, and patients.

Legal and policy framework

The existence of heterogeneity and inconsistencies across DMVs, OPOs, and individual coordinators continue to handicap organ donation from deceased donors in the United States. It is recommended that template language should be used by all organ donor registries to obtain authorization for organ donation. The talking points should be standardized when interacting with donor families while taking into account the wide variations in health literacy. State legislations should be enacted to ensure a single, secure national donor registry that is easily accessible to organ procurement organizations.[28]

Promoting live organ donation

Despite the modest increase seen with deceased donor transplants, living organ donation (kidneys and liver) in the United States has largely remained stagnant. A majority of transplant centres now have websites or Facebook pages to help endorse the programme and educate patients. While such efforts may help encourage living donations, they may also serve as conduits of excessive pressure and coercion on donors.[72] In addition to inadequate education, part of the limitation to living donation is attributed to the financial burden incurred during the process. In 2006, the Department of Health and Human Services established the National Living Donor Assistance Center (NLDAC) which allocated up to $6,000 reimbursement for travel and lodging expenses incurred from donation.[73] Despite this assistance, living kidney donors may have more than one out-of-pocket expense in addition to lost work hours, the majority of which remain unpaid. As a result, 89% of kidney donors have an overall net financial loss in the year of the donation.[74,75] To help rectify the current problems faced by living donors, the Living Donor Protection Act of 2019 is currently under review by Congress with aims to (a) prohibit life, disability insurance companies from denying or limiting coverage based on organ donor status and (b) amend the Family and Medical Leave Act of 1993 to specify living organ donation as a serious health condition.[76]

Conclusion

Organ donation from living and deceased donors is a multi-step process that, despite some challenges, works efficiently in the United States. There is a renewed interest to bridge the gap between organ demand and supply. New strategies focus on reducing organ discards and organ rejuvenation. Discussions to allocate deceased donor organs at a national level have resulted in a new organ allocation system. This system is based on 'acuity circles' rather than the historical donation service areas. The goal is to make organ transplantation accessible to candidates based on their medical condition rather than their geographical location. The long-term impacts of this policy change remain awaited.

Highlights

- Organ transplantation in the United States is a multi-tiered, federally regulated system.
- Organ donation operates by an 'opt-in' model, in which the individual while alive or their next of kin after the individual's death choose to donate organs.
- Organ allocation has been remodelled to reduce geographic disparities by eliminating allocation based regional donor service areas and switching to a continuous national distribution model based 'acuity circles'.
- Organ donation rates from living donors have remained largely stagnant. There are several new political initiatives that are being introduced to promote live organ donation.
- Future directions include the reduction of organ discards through marginal organ salvage, increasing use of organs from high infection-risk donors including transplantation of Hepatitis C positive organs to Hepatitis C negative recipients and the possible use of drones for efficient long-distance organ transportation to curtail cold ischemia times.

References

1. OPTN. Organ Procurement and Transplantation Network. 2019 Annual Report of the U.S. Organ Procurement and Transplantation Network and the Scientific Registry of Transplant Recipients: Transplant Data 2008–2019. Department of Health and Human Services, Health Resources and Services Administration, Healthcare Systems Bureau, Division of Transplantation, Rockville, MD; United Network for Organ Sharing, Richmond, VA; University Renal Research and Education Association, Ann Arbor, MI.
2. 42 USC 274: Organ procurement and transplantation network, (1984).
3. United Network for Organ Sharing [Available from: https://unos.org. Accessed on 2019].
4. Goodwin M. Black Markets: The Supply and Demand of Body Parts. 1st ed. United States of America: Cambridge University Press; 2006.
5. Anatomical Gift Act, (1968, revised in 1987 and 2006, and amended in 2007).
6. Scientific Registry of Transplant Recipients [Available from: https://www.srtr.org/about-the-data/the-srtr-database/ Accessed on 2021.
7. Association of Organ Procurement Organizations [cited 2019 07/12/2019]. Available from: http://www.aopo.org/ Accessed on 2021.

8. Davies RR, Farr M, Silvestry S, Callahan LR, Edwards L, Meyer DM, et al. The new United States heart allocation policy: Progress through collaborative revision. J Heart Lung Transplant. 2017;36(6):595–596.
9. Davis AE, Mehrotra S, McElroy LM, Friedewald JJ, Skaro AI. The extent and predictors of waiting time geographic disparity in kidney transplantation in the United States. Transplantation. 2014;97(10):1049–1057.
10. Nazarian SH, J; Gupta, M; Goldshore, M. Transplantation for the general surgeon: History of transplantation, end-organ disease, organ donation and allocation, and transplantation regulation and ethics 2018 08/11/2019. 2018. Available from: https://www.deckerip.com/decker/surgery/chapter/4017/pdf/.
11. Shepherd L, O'Carroll RE, Ferguson E. An international comparison of deceased and living organ donation/transplant rates in opt-in and opt-out systems: A panel study. BMC Med. 2014;12:131.
12. Samuel L. To solve organ shortage, states consider 'opt-out' organ donation laws.2017 08/09/2019. 2017. Available from: https://www.statnews.com/2017/07/06/opt-solution-organ-shortage
13. Copeland H, Copeland J, Hayanga JWA. Cardiac and pulmonary donor procurement. Curr Opin Organ Transplant. 2018;23(3):281–285.
14. Kotloff RM, Blosser S, Fulda GJ, Malinoski D, Ahya VN, Angel L, et al. Management of the potential organ donor in the ICU: Society of Critical Care Medicine/American College of Chest Physicians/Association of Organ Procurement Organizations Consensus Statement. Crit Care Med. 2015;43(6):1291–1325.
15. Rosenthal JT, Shaw BW, Jr., Hardesty RL, Griffith BP, Starzl TE, Hakala TR. Principles of multiple organ procurement from cadaver donors. Ann Surg. 1983;198(5):617–621.
16. Starzl TE, Hakala TR, Shaw BW, Jr., Hardesty RL, Rosenthal TJ, Griffith BP, et al. A flexible procedure for multiple cadaveric organ procurement. Surg Gynecol Obstet. 1984;158(3):223–230.
17. Israni AK, Zaun D, Rosendale JD, Schaffhausen C, Snyder JJ, Kasiske BL. OPTN/SRTR 2017 Annual data report: Deceased organ donation. Am J Transplant. 2019;19 Suppl 2:485–516.
18. Hart A, Smith JM, Skeans MA, Gustafson SK, Wilk AR, Castro S, et al. OPTN/SRTR 2017 Annual data report: Kidney. Am J Transplant. 2019;19 Suppl 2:19–123.
19. Kim WR, Lake JR, Smith JM, Schladt DP, Skeans MA, Noreen SM, et al. OPTN/SRTR 2017 Annual data report: Liver. Am J Transplant. 2019;19 Suppl 2:184–283.
20. U.S. Government Information on Organ Donation and Transplantation: Health Resources & Services Administration; 2019. [Available from: https://www.organdonor.gov.
21. Kowalczyk L. A nation divided, even on organ transplants. The Boston Globe [Internet]. December 2016 07/12/2019. Available from: https://www.bostonglobe.com/metro/2016/12/24/you-want-increase-your-chances-getting-liver-transplant-move-georgia/TbfleFMkaYqUzW11TSpl7I/story.html.
22. Naugler WE. California has long wait lists for liver transplants, but not for the reasons you think. Los Angeles Times [Internet]. 2016 12/2016. Available from: http://www.latimes.com/opinion/op-ed/la-oe-naugler-liver-transplant-rules-20161213-story.html

23. Network OPaT. Liver Policy Organ Procurement and Transplantation Network. Updated 2020. [Available from: https://optn.transplant.hrsa.gov/governance/policy-initiatives/liver/.
24. Network OPaT. Eliminate the use of DSAs and regions from kidney and pancreas distribution 2019. [Available from: https://optn.transplant.hrsa.gov/governance/public-comment/eliminate-the-use-of-dsas-and-regions-from-kidney-and-pancreas-distribution/.
25. Updated liver and intestinal organ allocation policy to be implemented Feb. 4, 2020 UNOS News2020. 2020. [Available from: https://unos.org/news/updated-liver-and-intestinal-organ-allocation-policy-to-be-implemented-feb-4-2020/).
26. https://optn.transplant.hrsa.gov/news/optnunos-board-approves-updated-liver-distribution-system/ Board approves updated liver distribution system [press release]. Organ Procurement and Transplantation Network, 12/04/2018 2020. 2018.
27. Organ Procurement and Transplantation Network Policies: Organ Procurement and Transplantation Network; 2021. [updated 07/14/2020. Available from: https://optn.transplant.hrsa.gov/media/1200/optn_policies.pdf.
28. In: Liverman CT, Domnitz S, Childress JF, editors. Opportunities for Organ Donor Intervention Research: Saving Lives by Improving the Quality and Quantity of Organs for Transplantation. Washington (DC)2017.
29. Israni AK, Zaun D, Bolch C, Rosendale JD, Schaffhausen C, Snyder JJ, et al. OPTN/SRTR 2015 Annual Data Report: Deceased Organ Donation. Am J Transplant. 2017;17 Suppl 1:503–542.
30. Ravikumar R, Jassem W, Mergental H, Heaton N, Mirza D, Perera MT, et al. Liver transplantation after ex vivo normothermic machine preservation: A phase 1 (First-in-Man) clinical trial. Am J Transplant. 2016;16(6):1779–1787.
31. Quillin RC, 3rd, Guarrera JV. Hypothermic machine perfusion in liver transplantation. Liver Transpl. 2018;24(2):276–281.
32. Guarrera JV, Henry SD, Samstein B, Reznik E, Musat C, Lukose TI, et al. Hypothermic machine preservation facilitates successful transplantation of 'orphan' extended criteria donor livers. Am J Transplant. 2015;15(1):161–169.
33. Burra P, Zanetto A, Russo FP, Germani G. Organ preservation in liver transplantation. Semin Liver Dis. 2018;38(3):260–269.
34. Schulz PJ, van Ackere A, Hartung U, Dunkel A. Prior family communication and consent to organ donation: Using intensive care physicians' perception to model decision processes. J Public Health Res. 2012;1(2):130–136.
35. Rodrigue JR, Cornell DL, Howard RJ. Organ donation decision: Comparison of donor and nondonor families. Am J Transplant. 2006;6(1):190–198.
36. Rodrigue JR, Cornell DL, Howard RJ. Organ donation decision: Comparison of donor and nondonor families. Am J Transplant. 2006;6(1):190–198.
37. Shah MB, Vilchez V, Goble A, Daily MF, Berger JC, Gedaly R, et al. Socioeconomic factors as predictors of organ donation. J Surg Res. 2018;221:88–94.
38. Verheijde JL, Rady MY, McGregor JL. The United States revised uniform Anatomical Gift Act (2006): New challenges to balancing patient rights and physician responsibilities. Philos Ethics Humanit Med. 2007;2:19.
39. Callender CO, Koizumi N, Miles PV, Melancon JK. Organ donation in the United States: The tale of the African-American journey of moving from the bottom to the top. Transplant Proc. 2016;48(7):2392–2395.

40. Reed RD, Sawinski D, Shelton BA, MacLennan PA, Hanaway M, Kumar V, et al. Population health, ethnicity, and rate of living donor kidney transplantation. Transplantation. 2018;102(12):2080–2087.
41. Goldfarb-Rumyantzev AS, Sandhu GS, Baird B, Barenbaum A, Yoon JH, Dimitri N, et al. Effect of education on racial disparities in access to kidney transplantation. Clin Transplant. 2012;26(1):74–81.
42. Goldfarb-Rumyantzev AS, Sandhu GS, Barenbaum A, Baird BC, Patibandla BK, Narra A, et al. Education is associated with reduction in racial disparities in kidney transplant outcome. Clin Transplant. 2012;26(6):891–899.
43. Hales CM, Fryar CD, Carroll MD, Freedman DS, Ogden CL. Trends in obesity and severe obesity prevalence in US youth and adults by sex and age, 2007–2008 to 2015–2016. Jama. 2018;319(16):1723–1725.
44. Engin A. The definition and prevalence of obesity and metabolic syndrome. Adv Exp Med Biol. 2017;960:1–17.
45. Mathews SE, Kumar RB, Shukla AP. Nonalcoholic steatohepatitis, obesity, and cardiac dysfunction. Curr Opin Endocrinol Diabetes Obes. 2018;25(5):315–320.
46. Riaz H, Khan MS, Siddiqi TJ, Usman MS, Shah N, Goyal A, et al. Association between obesity and cardiovascular outcomes: A systematic review and meta-analysis of mendelian randomization studies. JAMA Netw Open. 2018;1(7):e183788.
47. LeBlanc ES, Patnode CD, Webber EM, Redmond N, Rushkin M, O'Connor EA. Behavioral and pharmacotherapy weight loss interventions to prevent obesity-related morbidity and mortality in adults: Updated evidence report and systematic review for the US preventive services task force. JAMA. 2018;320(11):1172–1191.
48. Nicoletto BB, Fonseca NK, Manfro RC, Goncalves LF, Leitao CB, Souza GC. Effects of obesity on kidney transplantation outcomes: A systematic review and meta-analysis. Transplantation. 2014;98(2):167–176.
49. Spengler EK, O'Leary JG, Te HS, Rogal S, Pillai AA, Al-Osaimi A, et al. Liver transplantation in the obese cirrhotic patient. Transplantation. 2017;101(10):2288–2296.
50. Reynolds-Tylus T, Quick BL, King AJ, Moore M. Illinois department of motor vehicle customers' reasons for (not) registering as an organ donor. Prog Transplant. 2019;29(2):157–163.
51. Rodrigue JR, Fleishman A, Fitzpatrick S, Boger M. Organ donation video messaging in motor vehicle offices: results of a randomized trial. Prog Transplant. 2015;25(4):332–338.
52. Harrison TR, Morgan SE, Di Corcia MJ. Effects of information, education, and communication training about organ donation for gatekeepers: Clerks at the Department of Motor Vehicles and organ donor registries. Prog Transplant. 2008;18(4):301–309.
53. Thornton JD, Alejandro-Rodriguez M, Leon JB, Albert JM, Baldeon EL, De Jesus LM, et al. Effect of an iPod video intervention on consent to donate organs: A randomized trial. Ann Intern Med. 2012;156(7):483–490.
54. Cameron AM, Massie AB, Alexander CE, Stewart B, Montgomery RA, Benavides NR, et al. Social media and organ donor registration: The Facebook effect. Am J Transplant. 2013;13(8):2059–2065.

55. Thornton JD, Sullivan C, Albert JM, Cedeno M, Patrick B, Pencak J, et al. Effects of a video on organ donation consent among primary care patients: A randomized controlled trial. J Gen Intern Med. 2016;31(8):832–839.
56. Institute of M. Organ Donation: Opportunities for Action. James FC, Catharyn TL, editors. Washington, DC: The National Academies Press; 2006.
57. Girlanda R. Deceased organ donation for transplantation: Challenges and opportunities. World J Transplant. 2016;6(3):451–459.
58. Brown CV, Foulkrod KH, Dworaczyk S, Thompson K, Elliot E, Cooper H, et al. Barriers to obtaining family consent for potential organ donors. J Trauma. 2010;68(2):447–451.
59. Ebadat A, Brown CV, Ali S, Guitierrez T, Elliot E, Dworaczyk S, et al. Improving organ donation rates by modifying the family approach process. J Trauma Acute Care Surg. 2014;76(6):1473–1475.
60. Bratton C, Chavin K, Baliga P. Racial disparities in organ donation and why. Curr Opin Organ Transplant. 2011;16(2):243–249.
61. Davis BD, Norton HJ, Jacobs DG. The organ donation breakthrough collaborative: Has it made a difference? Am J Surg. 2013;205(4):381–386.
62. Gupta G, Kang L, Yu JW, Limkemann AJ, Garcia V, Bandyopadhyay D, et al. Long-term outcomes and transmission rates in hepatitis C virus-positive donor to hepatitis C virus-negative kidney transplant recipients: Analysis of United States national data. Clin Transplant. 2017;31(10): e13055–e13057.
63. Levitsky J, Formica RN, Bloom RD, Charlton M, Curry M, Friedewald J, et al. The American society of transplantation consensus conference on the use of Hepatitis C Viremic donors in solid organ transplantation. American Journal of Transplantation. 2017;17(11):2790–2802.
64. Vargas HE, Laskus T, Wang LF, Lee R, Radkowski M, Dodson F, et al. Outcome of liver transplantation in hepatitis C virus-infected patients who received hepatitis C virus-infected grafts. Gastroenterology. 1999;117(1):149–153.
65. Lagging M, Wejstal R, Duberg AS, Aleman S, Weiland O, Westin J, et al. Treatment of hepatitis C virus infection for adults and children: Updated Swedish consensus guidelines 2017. Infect Dis (Lond). 2018;50(8):569–583.
66. Woolley AE, Singh SK, Goldberg HJ, Mallidi HR, Givertz MM, Mehra MR, et al. Heart and lung transplants from HCV-infected donors to uninfected recipients. N Engl J Med. 2019;380(17):1606–1617.
67. Rao PS, Ojo A. The alphabet soup of kidney transplantation: SCD, DCD, ECD--fundamentals for the practicing nephrologist. Clin J Am Soc Nephrol. 2009;4(11):1827–1831.
68. Doshi MD, Hunsicker LG. Short- and long-term outcomes with the use of kidneys and livers donated after cardiac death. Am J Transplant. 2007;7(1):122–129.
69. Jochmans I, Moers C, Smits JM, Leuvenink HG, Treckmann J, Paul A, et al. Machine perfusion versus cold storage for the preservation of kidneys donated after cardiac death: A multicenter, randomized, controlled trial. Ann Surg. 2010;252(5):756–764.
70. Moers C, Smits JM, Maathuis MH, Treckmann J, van Gelder F, Napieralski BP, et al. Machine perfusion or cold storage in deceased-donor kidney transplantation. N Engl J Med. 2009;360(1):7–19.

71. Preidt R. World First: Drone Delivers Kidney for Transplant 2019. 2019. Available from: https://www.webmd.com/a-to-z-guides/news/20190429/world-first-drone-delivers-kidney-for-transplant#1.
72. Henderson ML, Clayville KA, Fisher JS, Kuntz KK, Mysel H, Purnell TS, et al. Social media and organ donation: Ethically navigating the next frontier. Am J Transplant. 2017;17(11):2803–2809.
73. Warren PH, Gifford KA, Hong BA, Merion RM, Ojo AO. Development of the national living donor assistance center: Reducing financial disincentives to living organ donation. Prog Transplant. 2014;24(1):76–81.
74. Rodrigue JR, Kazley AS, Mandelbrot DA, Hays R, LaPointe Rudow D, Baliga P, et al. Living donor kidney transplantation: Overcoming disparities in live kidney donation in the US—Recommendations from a consensus conference. Clin J Am Soc Nephrol. 2015;10(9):1687–1695.
75. Rodrigue JR, Schold JD, Morrissey P, Whiting J, Vella J, Kayler LK, et al. Direct and indirect costs following living kidney donation: Findings from the KDOC study. Am J Transplant. 2016;16(3):869–876.
76. Living Donor Protection Act of 2019, 116th Congress, 1st Session Sess. (2019).

18

Organ donation in India: Life after death exists

Deepak Gupta, Abhay Singh, Sanjeev Lalwani, Chhavi Sawhney, SS Kale, AK Banerji

Introduction

Organ transplantation is often the only option to save the lives of patients with end-stage organ failure. One donor can possibly give 'gift of life' to many terminally ill patients and can save the lives of eight people on average and enhance the lives of many more through tissue donations. Globally a new patient is added to the organ transplant list every 10 minutes.(1) Counselling the family plays an important role in the organ donation process and transplant coordinator needs to look at various psychosocial aspects of the family during the counselling process.

The Transplantation of Human Organs and Tissues Act (THOA), 1994, has undergone major and minor changes in the past three decades in the form of addition of rules and amendments.(2,3) However, most public hospitals with busy neurological and trauma services have had no donations in the twenty-five years since the Transplant Act was passed.(4)

The national organ donation rate in India is 0.08% (0.34 donors per million population (pmp)) which is one of the lowest in the world.(5) It is estimated that organ requirements could be met if 5–10% of potential deceased organ donors become actual organ donors.(6) Attempts to increase organ donation have focused on public education and starting organ donor registries.(7,8) Public education through media is expensive and has not impacted the organ donation drive in India so far.(4)

One needs to analyse and intervene both in the practices of the professionals involved in the process of organ generation and address attitudes of general population to increase organ donation rates in India.

Historical perspectives

The Hindu mythology and its relation to organ transplantation have been described in Box 18.1.

As previously stated, the first Indian legislation on organ transplantation came in the year 1994 (THOA) to provide regulation, removal,

Box 18.1 Hindu Mythology

It is believed that 'Rishi Dadhichi' donated his own bones for making weapons in order to help the Gods in the war between the gods and demons to defeat the demons and reclaim heaven. It is also noted that King Shibi donated his own flesh to a hawk in order to save the life of a dove.[9] King Daksha organized a huge yagna (religious ceremony) and intentionally omitted inviting Shiva and Sati, the divine couple. Shiva discouraged Sati, daughter of Daksha to attend the ceremony as they were not invited. However, the parental bond made Sati ignore her husband's wishes and she went to the ceremony alone. She was snubbed and insulted by Daksha in front of the guests. Sati, unable to bear the insult, ran into the sacrificial fire and immolated herself. Shiva, upon learning about the terrible incident, in his wrath, sent his followers to the site of the ceremony and Daksha was decapitated. However, he was later forgiven by Shiva and given life by fixing a male goat's head. In another Hindu mythological story, Ganesha (the son of Parvati [Sati] and Shiva) was beheaded by Shiva. Shiva was going to enter the room where Parvati (Sati) was bathing and was stopped by their son Ganesha whom Parvati had asked to guard the door and not allow anyone to enter. Shiva in a rage decapitated the head of Ganesha. However, on Parvati's pleading, he took an elephant's head and transplanted it on the neck of the headless Ganesha.[10] (Figure 18.1).

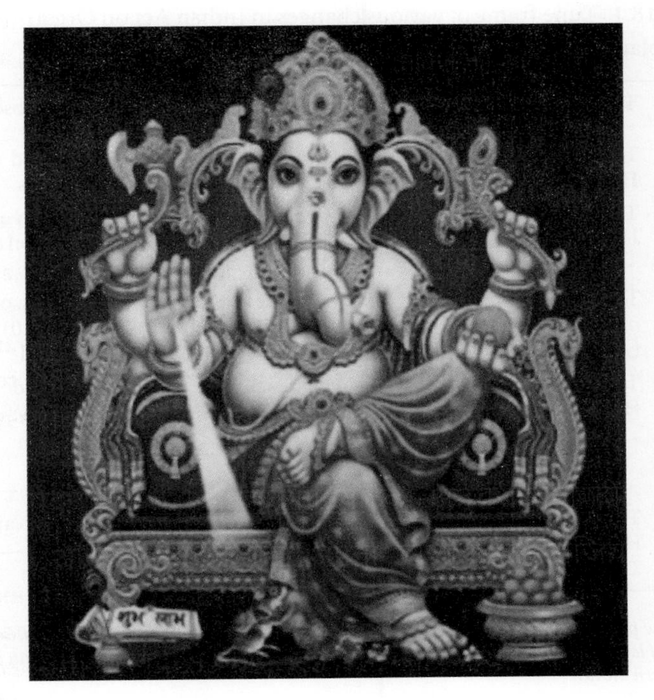

Figure 18.1. Lord Ganesha

storage, and transplantation of human organs for therapeutic purposes and for prevention of commercial dealings in human organs. Series of changes via amendments/rules were made in this act over the next few years (Tables 18.1 and 18.2). It redefined a donor as a person who voluntarily authorizes the removal of his/her human organs and tissues or both for therapeutic purposes. A hospital was identified as Human Organ Retrieval Centre (provided it had adequate facilities for treating seriously ill patients who could then be potential donors of organs in the event of death; such a hospital should be registered under the act with the appropriate authority).

Table 18.1 Time frame of various changes in Indian Act on Organ Transplantation between 1994 and 2014

Year	Title	Issuing authority	Sections/Subsections
1994	The Transplantation of Human Organs Act	President assent Approved by Parliament	Sections and Subsections
1995	Transplantation of Human Organ Rules	Ministry of Health and Family Welfare	Notification of rules Introduction of Forms
2008	Transplantation of Human Organs (Amendment) Rules	Ministry of Health and Family Welfare	Notification of rules Forms (1–10) were Modified
2011	The Transplantation of Human Organs Act	President assent Approved by Parliament Ministry of Law, Justice and Company Affairs	Sections and Subsections
2014	Transplantation of Human Organs and Tissues Rules	Ministry of Health and Family Welfare	Notification and rules

**Act: Law passed by legislature. # Amendments: Minor change or addition to improve some subsection of legislation. $ Rules: Certain provisions are left by legislature wherein rules can be laid to help govern the law.*

Table 18.2 Key differences between Indian THOA 1994 Act and THOTA 2011 Act

	THOA (Act:1994,Rules:1995, Amendment: 2008)	**THOTA (Act: 2011, Rules: 2014)**
Introduction of Advisory committee for guiding authorization committee	No	Yes
Proof of genetic relationship to authorization committee	No	Yes, Defined further in 2014.
Appropriate authority	Mentioned	Defined: Who and What
Scope of work and limits of Authorization committee and its composition	Centre and State	Centre, State and Included hospitals of >25 transplants/ year (in 2014)
National Registry	No	Yes, Defined further the scope and work at national/ regional level
Video recording of interview	Not required	Video recording added in 2014

Table 18.2 *Continued*

	THOA (Act:1994,Rules:1995, Amendment: 2008)	THOTA (Act: 2011, Rules: 2014)
Definition of brain death	Yes	Yes
Expansion of Brain death declaration team	Neurology/ Neurosurgeon	Added, anaesthetist, intensivist, and intensivist/ doctor on duty (added in 2014)
Hospitals	Transplantation centres	Added non transplant retrieval centres
Which hospital: Prerequisites of infrastructure in hospitals which can declare potential brain deaths	–	Any hospital with RMP and ICU facility
Registration of hospital	For Organ retrieval registration required	Yes for organ retrieval but not needed for tissues
Expansion of Near relative category	'Near relative' means spouse, son, daughter, father, mother, brother or sister	'Near Relatives' included grandparents, grandchildren
Swap donations	No	Yes, should also be approved by authorization committee
Pledge	No	Yes form 7
Counselling for donation	Mentioned	Mandatory
Medicolegal cases	Not Defined	Simplified
Number of forms	13	21
Role of doctor	Needed for organ retrieval	Yes for organ retrieval, not for tissue
Defining the scope of work and role of Transplant coordinators	Mentioned	Mandatory
Organ retrieval charges	Not mentioned	Recipient/Govt/NGO
Organ allocation priority	No	Mentioned (2014)
Foreign national transplant	No	Yes, Defined further in 2014.
Inclusion of Tissues (Yes or No)	Organs Only (Tissues No)	Organs and Tissues (Yes) Concept of Tissue bank, prerequisites of the same added. Registration of tissue bank.
Penalties	Less	More

(*continued*)

Table 18.2 *Continued*

	THOA (Act:1994,Rules:1995, Amendment: 2008)	THOTA (Act: 2011, Rules: 2014)
Offences and Punishments	–	Redefining the offences and punishments, 21 forms were added in 2014.
Concept of maintenance of national Registries	No	Yes
	Changes in the Act 1995 (Rules) Defined duties of medical practitioner Form 8 for brain death declaration added Test for HLA, DNA probe and donor authorization forms added Joint application by donor and recipient in live renal transplantation in Form 10. Payment details of registration and renewal of hospitals. Conditions for grant of permission: General requirement, infrastructure, personnel. Details of appeal in case of authorization committee rejection. Changes added in the act 2008 (Amendments) Definition of NABL accredited labs. Replacement of Form 1 with Form 1A, Form 1B, Form 1C. Composition of authorization committee.	Amendments and Rules made in the act 2011 Inclusion of tissues along with organs in the act Expansion of near relative category: Inclusion of grandchildren, grandparents Concept of tissue bank, prerequisites of the same Defining the scope of work and role of transplant coordinator Prerequisites of infrastructure in hospitals which can declare potential brain deaths. Expansion of team of brain death declaration: Inclusion of physician, anaesthetist and surgeon, intensives in brain death declaration team. Scope of work and limits of authorization committee. Composition of authorization committee. Introduction of advisory committee for guidance to authorization committee Concept of maintenance national registry Registration of tissue bank Forms in THOTA 2011: 11

Table 18.2 *Continued*

	THOA (Act:1994,Rules:1995, Amendment: 2008)	THOTA (Act: 2011, Rules: 2014)
	Addition of hospital-based authorization committee. The documents for evaluation by the authorization committee in case of other than near relative transplant. Checklist document evaluation by competent authority in case of near relative transplant. Introduction of process of senior embassy official certification of relationship in case of foreigners. Video graphing the procedure of interviewing. Mandatory transplant coordinator in hospitals performing organ transplant. 24-h availability of infrastructure and personnel in the hospitals applying for registration. Qualifications of the skilled expertise of doctors involved in organ transplantation. No mention of forms in THOA 1994.	Forms in THOTA 2014 (1-21) 1 For organ or tissue donation from identified living near related donor 2 For organ or tissue donation by living spousal donor 3 For organ or tissue donation by other than near relative living donor 4 For certification of medical fitness of living donor 5 For certification of genetic relationship of living donor with recipient 6 For spousal living donor 7 For organ or tissue pledging 8 For declaration cum consent 9 For unclaimed body in a hospital or prison 10 For certification of brain stem death 11 Application for approval of transplantation from living donor 12 Application for registration of hospital to carry out organ or tissue transplantation other than cornea 13 Application for registration of hospital to carry out organ/tissue retrieval other than eye/cornea retrieval

(*continued*)

Table 18.2 *Continued*

	THOA (Act:1994,Rules:1995, Amendment: 2008)	THOTA (Act: 2011, Rules: 2014)
		14 Application for registration of tissue banks other than eye banks 15 Application for registration of eye bank, corneal transplantation center, eye retrieval center under Transplantation of Human Organs Act 16 Certificate of registration for performing organ/ tissue transplantation/ retrieval and/or tissue banking 17 Certificate of renewal of registration 18 Certificate by the authorization committee of hospital (If hospital authorization committee is not available then the authorization committee of the district/state) where the transplantation has to take place 19 Certificate by competent authority (as defined at rule 2©) for Indian near relative, other than spouse, cases (In case of spousal donor, Form 6 will be applicable) 20 Verification certificates in respect of domicile status of recipient or donor 21 Certificate of relationship between donor and recipient in case of foreigners

Organ donation process in India

The actual organ donation rates of India are low as compared to USA, 26% and Spain, 40%.[11] Legislation made deceased organ donation a possibility in India since 1994. Deceased organ donation and transplantation was almost non-existent in India before 1994.

Irreversible cessation of circulatory and respiratory functions is universally acceptable for cremation/burial or for insurance claims. One doctor is needed to certify cardiopulmonary death while four doctors are needed for certification of brain death. UK criteria of brainstem death are followed in India. If the person of a family declared brain dead, agrees for organ donation, organs are retrieved, after which the ventilator is turned off. If for any reason they say 'No' to donation after brain death is certified the patient continues on the ventilator till the heart stops. Declaration of brain death was made mandatory in Government Medical College Hospitals in Chennai in 2008. It was noted that several patients who were brain dead were kept on life support systems that could have been utilized by other patients who have a better chance of recovery. Tamilnadu government order gave permission to remove ventilators in brain dead patients in three of the largest teaching public hospitals of Chennai. This is a heartening initiative and needs to be expanded to other states of India.[12] Many such patients continue to be ventilated despite being brain dead as there are no universal guidelines about disconnecting ventilators in such situations. False and misleading stories in the media of a person making a 'miraculous recovery' from a coma or a 'dead person coming alive' exist.[13] Continuing the ventilation of a brain-dead patient also prevents care of another critical patient when ICU beds are full, and leads to ethical dilemmas among clinicians.[14] In this context, there is an urgent need to delink brain death from organ donation in India.[15,16]

National or state authority checks the waiting list of potential recipients after being informed of the brain-dead donor availability. They decide, according to objective criterion, i.e. blood group, size of the organ, medical urgency of the organ, time on waiting list, tissue type, and more. The recipient is not selected based on status/religion/gender. After finding the compatible recipient, the state authority contacts the hospitals and potential recipients receive call from the hospitals. The major donor organs and tissues are heart, lungs, liver, pancreas, kidneys, eyes, heart valves, skin, bones, bone marrow, connective tissues, middle ear, and blood vessels.

Treating doctors inform relatives of the patient without ambiguity and equivocation, the fact of the patient's brain death which is synonymous to death. Brain death is confirmed by performing an apnoea test twice by a panel of four doctors. All the phases of brain death determination are clearly documented. After the second apnoea test, the team starts counselling the family members regarding organ donation. The harvesting team is not involved in counselling the relatives. The process of counselling the relatives and obtaining consent for organ donation progresses while the intensivist tries to keep the donors' organ systems viable for donation.

Preparation in the recipient operation room starts before the harvesting team begins its task in a timely fashion. The transplant team is informed about the timing of arrival of organs, the organs to be retrieved and specific plans for each organ, along with the harvesting team. Harvesting team then notifies the transplant centre (of available organs) and gives an estimate of cross-clamp time (for heart) and travel time to allow planning so as to minimize ischemic time, particularly if prolonged preparation is necessary. Green corridors (special road route that facilitates the transportation of harvested organs meant for transplantation to the desired hospitals; street signals are manually operated to avoid stoppage at red lights and to divert the traffic) are set up to ensure a rapid transportation of the desired organs to transplant centres.

Organ donation in Indian states

The first successful cardiac transplant in India was carried out in All India Institute of Medical Sciences, New Delhi on a 42-year-old patient with a history of dilated cardiomyopathy by P. Venugopal et al on 2 August 1994 from a 35-year-old brain-dead donor.(17) The first successful multiorgan transplant was facilitated by K. Ganpathy in December 1995 in Chennai after certifying brain death in a head injury patient.(18) Various programmes are running in different parts of India to increase organ donor rate (ODR); Andhra Pradesh has the Jeevandan programme (www.jeevandan.gov.in), Karnataka has the Zonal Coordination Committee of Karnataka for Transplantation (www.zcck.in), and Maharashtra has the Zonal Transplant Coordination Center in Mumbai (www.ztccmumbai.

org), Kerala government has 'Mritha-sanjeevani' and the Kerala Network for Organ Sharing (www.knos.org.in), and Rajasthan has Rajasthan Network for Organ Sharing (www.rnos.org). In a recent study from Northeast part of India, a low organ donation rate was attributed to lack of awareness and attitudes amongst doctors.[19] According to 2014 data, Puducherry had the highest ODRs with 10.4 organ donations pmp, followed by Chandigarh with ODRs of 5.7 pmp[5,16]

Public–private partnership models

The public-private partnership (PPP), with help of transplant coordinators, have significantly contributed to improving organ-procuring rates in India recently, especially in southern states of India (Tamil Nadu, Kerala, Andhra Pradesh, and Puducherry). MOHAN (Multi-Organ Harvesting and Networking) foundation was started in 1997 as a philanthropic, not for profit, non-governmental organization (www.mohanfoundation.org) by a group of like-minded and concerned medical and non-medical professionals committed to increasing the reach of the THOA with a mission to ensure that every Indian who is suffering from end-stage organ failure be provided with the 'gift of life' through a life-saving organ. Major objectives of MOHAN foundation are to create public awareness, to train health care professionals in transplant coordination, to counsel families of 'brain dead' victims to donate their loved ones' organs, to create a computerized network for logistic support for organ donation in hospitals and the utilization of organs, to liaise with Government (State and Central) to pass favourable legislation that will help increase organ donations in India, networking with other organ procuring organizations in the country and raising resources to promote organ donation efficiently. It also promulgates system of organ sharing system in India by establishing the Indian Network for Organ Sharing (INOS) in the year 2000.[20] Table 18.3 shows the deceased organ donations in India over five-year period.

Organ donation at All India Institute of Medical Sciences (AIIMS, Delhi)

The Organ Retrieval Banking Organization (ORBO) coordinates the entire process of deceased organ donation and transplantation at AIIMS,

Table 18.3 Deceased organ donation in India (2012-17)

State	No. of deceased organ donors	Kidney	Liver	Heart	Lung	Pancreas	Intestine	Hand	Larynx	Total Organs
Tamil Nadu	839	1525	789	300	208	18	2	0	0	2842
Maharashtra	477	819	387	107	2	3	0	0	0	1318
Telangana	345	553	329	64	9	5	0	0	0	960
Andhra Pradesh	196	354	177	42	31	4	0	0	0	608
Kerala	269	460	211	49	3	6	2	8	1	740
Karnataka	272	439	248	53	4	8	1	0	0	753
Gujarat	269	512	235	20	0	1	0	0	0	768
Delhi- NCR	153	264	449	46	2	0	1	0	0	442
Chandigarh	116	208	55	16	4	11	0	0	0	294
Uttar Pradesh	37	70	22	2	0	0	0	0	0	94
Madhya Pradesh	52	96	36	18	0	0	0	0	0	150
Puducherry	47	92	11	9	0	0	0	0	0	112
Rajasthan	24	43	23	13	1	1	0	0	0	81

(Source: www.mohanfoundation.org)

New Delhi. The transplant coordination team carries out the entire process till the relatives receive the body of the deceased. The ORBO networks with all the hospitals of Delhi, including private and government hospitals. Currently, ORBO has 101,715 brain death donor registries available in India (www.orbo.org.in). At the JPN apex trauma centre in New Delhi, a total of fifty-three patient families, after clinical diagnosis of brainstem death of patient were counselled for organ donation between 2017 and 2019. However, organ donation could be done only in twelve of these fifty-three cases while in forty-one cases, the family members refused for various reasons.

Medico-legal issues

Important medico-legal issues of concern in Indian legislations are related to consent process, brainstem death certification, and hospital/ tissue bank registration process (Table 18.4).

Table 18.4 Important aspects of medicolegal issues of concern in Indian Laws related to Organ Donation

Consent
Who can be a donor in India: Anyone regardless of age, race or gender can become an organ and tissue donor. Voluntary authorization during life (Form-7—this can be done by any person >18 years of age by filling up the form prescribed under the Act.
If he/she is under the age of 18 years, then the consent of parent or legal guardian is essential.
Near relatives, as defined in law, includes spouse, son/ daughter, mother/father, brother, sister, grandparents and grandchildren.
Consent is 'explicit' involving a system of 'opting in'. Expressed consent of the deceased person, during his or her lifetime, is required in the form of a written document. The form is also to be signed by two witnesses, of which one should be near relative. However, in case of death, near relatives may not agree for organ or tissue donation in spite of voluntary authorization. The relatives can be counselled and in case of refusal, their decision against donation needs to be respected.
Medical suitability for donation is determined at the time of death. During lifetime, a person can pledge for organ donation by filling up a donor form.
After demise, the relatives give a written consent and the organs are harvested within a few hours. No Authorization by the person during life (Form-8)—in the absence of voluntary authorization during life, near relatives can give consent for organ or tissue donation by filling up the form prescribed under the Act in case of deceased donor.

(continued)

Table 18.4 *Continued*

Brain Stem Death Certification (Form-10) Brainstem death is certified by a board of medical experts comprising of four doctors by conducting a series of tests in a prescribed format. The names of such doctors must be from the panel approved by the appropriate authority under the Act. The team of doctors includes: – Registered Medical Practitioner in charge of Hospital where brain stem death has occurred – Registered Medical Practitioner treating the person whose brainstem death has occurred. – Any independent Registered Medical Practitioner – a Neurologist/ Neurosurgeon/ Physician/ Anesthetist/ Intensivist/ Surgeon can be nominated only if they are not members of transplantation team for the recipient. The certification is legally valid after conducting series of tests twice within a gap of 6 hours in case of adults and 12–24 hours in case of children.
Registration of Hospital/Tissue Bank All the activities in regard to tissue/organ retrieval (except Cornea), storage in bank and transplantation must be carried out at a place registered for this purpose under this act. However, the blood bank is not in the purview of this act.
Special Situations The body of a person can be sent for post-mortem examination due to medico-legal purposes by reason of the death which include accident or any other unnatural cause. In such cases, the removal of any human organ and tissue or both from such dead body has to be permitted by a competent authority/police after consent of family and proper certification of death/brainstem death, in belief that such human organ and tissue or both will not be required for the medico-legal post-mortem examination. The assistance of autopsy surgeon in such cases can also be sought as and when felt. Unknown unclaimed deceased person (Form-9)—The authority for the removal of any human organ and tissue or both from the dead body can be given only after 48 hours from the time of the death of the concerned person. However, the period of 48 hours can be extended in belief that some relative may come or in view of other criteria like police rules etc.

THOA1994: Transplantation of human organs act. THOTA 2011: Transplantation of Human Organs and Tissues Act

National programmes on organ donations in India

A National Programme of Organ and Tissue Transplantation (NOTP) has been approved under which a national networking system and a tissue bank is being developed under NOTTO (National level Organ and Tissue Transplant Organization). NOTTO plans to develop five such mini-centres in different regions of the country under Regional

Organ and Tissue Transplant Organization (ROTTO) and State level networking system in other states using six AIIMS like medical institutions under State level Organ and Tissue transplant Organization (SOTTO). The results of organ transplantation continue to improve in India as a consequence of the improvements in methods of donor optimizations. Transplant Coordinators have an important role in the development of a successful transplantation programme and are involved in the fulfilment of both on-call responsibilities and work related to identification, evaluation, management, and coordination of donor activity related documentations. Most centres conducting organ transplant programmes have Transplant Coordinators earmarked for this work in India now.

NOTTO is a National level organization set up under Directorate General of Health Services, Ministry of Health and Family Welfare, Government of India (www.notto.gov.in) with two divisions: 'National Human Organ and Tissue Removal and Storage Network' and 'National Biomaterial Centre'. Presently, twenty-four centres in Delhi are authorized by NOTTO for organ retrieval and transplantation. It is estimated if each of these centres facilitates do one cadaveric donation in one year, it will increase the ODR to 9–10 times than its present rate. With the existing infrastructure, the donation rates can be increased substantially by increasing awareness and by motivating healthcare workers in the care of the brain-dead patients.

'National human organ and tissue removal and storage network'

This has been mandated as per the Transplantation of Human Organs (Amendment) Act 2011 and is the nodal networking agency for Delhi. The network performs procurement, allocation, and distribution of organs and tissues in Delhi (Capital of India). National Network division of NOTTO functions as the apex centre for All India activities of coordination and networking for procurement and distribution of Organs and Tissues and registry of Organs and Tissues Donation and Transplantation in the country. It lays down policy guidelines and protocols for various functions, compiles all registry data from states and regions, coordinates procurement of organs and tissues, monitors transplantation activities in the regions and states, maintains data-bank and assists in data management for organ transplant surveillance and organ transplant and organ donor registry. NOTTO website (www.notto.gov.in) enlists all the hospitals (registered under THOA 2011 act of India) where retrievals/transplants are done in India. Individual donors can also pledge online at the website.

National biomaterial centre (National Tissue Bank)

The Transplantation of Human Organs (Amendment) Act 2011 has included the component of tissue donation and registration of tissue banks. It becomes imperative under the changed circumstances to establish National level Tissue Bank to fulfil the demands of tissue transplantation including activities for procurement, storage, and distribution of biomaterials. The main thrust and objective of establishing the centre is to fill up the gap between 'Demand' and 'Supply' as well as 'Quality Assurance' in the availability of various tissues including bone and bone products, skin graft, cornea, heart valves, and blood vessels.

Current scenario of organ donation in India

Despite advances in medicine and technology and increased awareness of organ donation and transplantation, the number of people waiting for organ transplants is increasing. Each year over 100,000 die in India from road traffic accidents and over half of these die from Traumatic Brain Injury (TBI).[21] Though India is a thickly populated country (1.32 billion population), organ scarcity is prevalent in every hospital. The national average organ donation rate is 0.08% (0.34 per million) compared to 70–80% (36 per million population) in countries like Spain and Belgium.[22] In India, Tamil Nadu state has 1.9 pmp while Kerala state has 1.03 pmp deceased organ donation rates.[23,24] Lack of or negligible brain death declaration in many hospitals across the states is considered as one of the major reasons for poor organ donation rates in India. Much of the problem surrounds the lack of registered donors.

The real reason behind a living person's interest in donating organ is important to determine but it is often difficult to recognize. As per the current Indian legislation, though a strong personal will of an individual pledging to donate his organs after death might be considered, the family decision after the person's death is only taken into consideration (opt-in consent system). Opt-out system wherein one is automatically assumed to give consent for the donation of his/her organs in the event of death unless he/she removes him/herself from the organ donor register is currently in practice in few countries across the world and has been shown to have increased ODRs to 10–30 pmp.[27,26] The maximal rate of organ donation is estimated to be 50 donors pmp, in Western Europe, it is 12–20 pmp.[1,28]

In India, less than 2–5% of population are registered as organ donors. A study from AIIMS, New Delhi, on the attitudes of 352 subjects from the general public in Northern India by Panwar et al revealed that only 1.4% of subjects willing to donate organs actually registered their names for organ donation.[29] Gender of a person affects his or her decision to donate organs. Men being the main source of income may be reluctant to donate whereas women's decision to donate is heavily influenced by their parents and spouse. Darlington et al in their study on 480 medical students noted that females fared worse than males in knowledge and attitude but they fared better than males in practice scores.[30] A huge gap noted in knowledge about organ donation and transplantation among medical community can be bridged by introducing radical changes in the medical curriculum and the intelligent use of social media.[31,30]

Patient's families often have reservation of accepting brain death due to fear of harvesting organs for pecuniary benefits or sheer carelessness. In a recent survey conducted over reasons of low organ donations in India, lack of faith in health care system (42.9%) was one of the major reasons.[32] The main reason for organ shortage in India is ignorance about the benefits of organ donation. People with co-morbidities, who wish to donate, do not even sign up for organ donation pledge thinking they are not eligible. This is compounded by existing myths and superstitions in various societies. In a country where religion influences public as well as personal decisions, many believe that their faith does not allow for organ donation. Hinduism and Islam (the major religions in India) do not oppose the practice of organ donation as Hinduism leaves the decision to the individual, while Islam, by the principle of valuing and saving human life, implies support. In Hinduism, the body belongs to the heirs and successors to dispose of as they want. Even if a person wishes to donate his body or wishes his organs to be donated, often the family doesn't consent. However, religious belief has not been found to impact an individual's decision to donate organs in several studies from India. Emphasis on public awareness is the key.

The absence of cultural, regional, or religious bias against eye donation in India is a good surrogate marker for social acceptability of deceased organ donation.(7,33,8) Even when everything is done perfectly, conversion from recognition of brain death to actual organ donation is distressingly low at most centres.(34) A recent study (2007–2012) showed a conversion rate of 10 out of 205 brain dead patients only (< 2%).(34) The reasons for non-organ donation in the remaining 195 cases were lack of consent, procedural problems, patients not counselled, too unstable for donation, age, and co-morbidities. The CENTRE TBI (Collaborative effectiveness in Neurotrauma Research and Education in Traumatic brain injury) group noted agreement on the clinical evaluation for brain death determination and post mortem organ donations in 100% of the centres (CENTER-TBI, www.center-tbi.eu). Brain death diagnosis for non-donor patients was deemed mandatory in 18% of the centres before withdrawing life-sustaining measures (LSM). In 45% of the centres organ donation after circulatory arrest was forbidden.(35) A cross-sectional study among professional drivers in coastal south India on 300 participants to assess knowledge, attitude, and practices regarding organ donation revealed nearly half of the participants having unsatisfactory knowledge and attitude scores.(36) The authors conducted this study as professional taxi drivers are at an increased risk of road traffic accidents and therefore a large proportion of organ deficit could be addressed by drivers who are educated and aware of the need for organ donation.(36) Previous studies on awareness on organ donation were mainly done on medical students, healthcare workers, and patient families.

Factors contributing to limited organ donation in India

1. Lack of awareness, religious, and other issues
   - Brain death is synonymous to death is not widely understood or recognized by the public. Also, there is hesitation on the part

of the medical fraternity to certify brain death as it is often presumed to be a complex procedure.
- Religious beliefs and superstitions also may be a reason for families not to agree to deceased organ donation. The idea of charity and perceptions about donation varies from one community to another.
- Lack of family support and fear of donated organs going into medical research were the key barriers to organ donation.

2. Infrastructural and skilled personnel problems
   - ICU beds or ventilators for maintaining brain dead persons are not available as there is high influx of trauma patients and always the first priority goes to the salvageable patients.
   - Lack of training for intensive-care unit personnel to maintain brain dead person. A large percentage of medical professionals are unaware of the process as a whole and about the idea of brain death since it is not part of their formal education.
   - In the case of deceased organ donations, only a few intensive care specialists declare brain deaths and are not in place to counsel families, both of which lead to a poor conversion rate.

Organ donations are more likely to result from structured hospital programmes based on good ICU care and counselling of families of patients with fatal traumatic brain injuries, than from additional public education to promote deceased organ donations. Management of deceased organ donations should not be left to neurosurgeons and neurologists, they must gradually shift care from 'patient-centred care' to 'donation-centred care'. Structured hospital programmes in large hospitals (involving recruitment of transplant surgeons, ICU counsellors, transplant coordinators, and transplant administrators) could change the approach to counselling process by recognizing/conveying to family about the acceptance of death using verbal and non-verbal cues and identification of a power person in the family set up. Nursing education, ICU counselling, and Organ Donation team group meetings taking place after every five failed attempts at eliciting organ donation in a centre in South India increased the organ donations from zero to eighty-five and positive family consents in thirty-two out of thirty-eight cases (84%) in a two-year period.[(4)] A collective approach with political

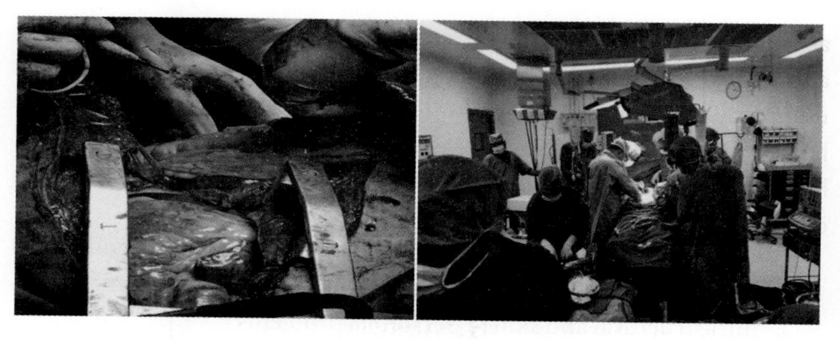

Figure 18.2. Intraoperative picture of Organ harvesting process at JPN apex trauma Centre, in Delhi

and administrative will, with sensitization campaigns in print/electronic/social media and active involvement of stakeholders from health sector including doctors might help increase the number of people signing for these organ donation programmes. Lack of sensitization, family refusal, and fear of mutilation of the body after death are a few possible factors responsible for not getting enough organ donors from the southern part of the country. Cumbersome official paper work or insufficient knowledge about the procedure might be some of the other pertinent factors.

Conclusions

A good relationship with health care workers and patients' family's faith in treatment have played a great role in increasing donation rates. The shortage of available organs can be reduced if people choose to donate their organs after they die. If all the people pledge while living to donate their organs under circumstances like brain death and also convince their families, then probably the issue regarding organ shortage can be minimized. Medical and nursing curriculum should have a symposium on brain death with intensivists, neurologists/neurosurgeons, psychologists, and forensic specialists focusing on when to declare brain death, break the news to family, and counselling regarding organ donation. There is an urgent need for a widespread campaign to spread awareness about organ donation in India and to bridge the gap between the supply and demand. The numbers that are mentioned are estimates and real numbers could be far more than this. As organ donations take place in hospitals, a hospital-based approach is the key to success and aim must be to set up multispecialty consensus-based protocols towards the organ donation process along with public education.

Highlights

- All major religions support organ and tissue donation. Organ donations do not happen unless an effort is made to make them happen.
- Change term 'Brain dead' to 'Cadaver with heartbeat' in regard to counselling family. No consent is required from families before brainstem diagnosis.
- Preliminary test for brain death should be done early (as soon as brainstem clinical reflexes are noted to be absent and there is no spontaneous respiration) as delays result in body decomposition.
- If apnoea test done early is positive, one should proceed with formal testing for confirmation of brain death diagnosis. There is a wide-spread perception that this can be done only with family consent if they are willing for organ donation. However, the same is not true as family consent is required for willingness of family to donate organs and not for confirmation of diagnosis of brain death.
- Anyone can and every one should donate organs. One organ donor can save up to eight lives and enhance the lives of many others through tissue donation.
- We burn or bury. Why not donate? Sale and purchase of organs are illegal and one can be jailed for this.
- Is there life after death? Yes.

Acknowledgements

The authors are thankful to the entire team at ORBO and JPN apex trauma centre (AIIMS) for their dedication towards organ donation. We are also thankful to Ms Ayushi Taneja (Research Scholar, AIIMS), Ms Kaveri Sharma (Research Scholar, AIIMS), and trauma nurse coordinator Ms Rachna Trehan from JPN apex trauma centre, for their support in compiling this manuscript.

References

1. Organ Donor | Organ Donor [Internet]. [cited 2019 Dec 29]. 2019. Available from: https://www.organdonor.gov/
2. Yadla M. Legal policies of organ transplantation in India: Basics and beyond. Saudi J Kidney Dis Transplant Off Publ Saudi Cent Organ Transplant Saudi Arab. 2019 Aug;30(4):943–952.
3. Lobo Gajiwala A. Regulatory aspects of tissue donation, banking and transplantation in India. Cell Tissue Bank. 2018 Jun;19(2):241–248.
4. Thomas PG, Aswathy C, Joshy G, Mathew J. Elements of a successful hospital-based deceased donation programme in India: Zero to eighty-five in two years. Natl Med J India. 2018 Aug;31(4):201–205.
5. Srivastava A, Mani A. Deceased organ donation and transplantation in India: Promises and challenges. Neurol India. 2018 Mar 1;66(2):316.
6. Shroff S. Legal and ethical aspects of organ donation and transplantation. Indian J Urol IJU J Urol Soc India. 2009 Jul;25(3):348–355.
7. Vania DK, Randall GE. Can evidence-based health policy from high-income countries be applied to lower-income countries: Considering barriers and facilitators to an organ donor registry in Mumbai, India. Health Res Policy Syst. 2016 Jan 13;14:3.
8. Balwani MR, Gumber MR, Shah PR, Kute VB, Patel HV, Engineer DP, et al. Attitude and awareness towards organ donation in western India. Ren Fail. 2015 May;37(4):582–588.
9. Dasgupta S. Hindu Mysticus : Six lectures. New York F Ungar Pub Co; 1959.
10. Kansupada KB, Sassani JW. Sushruta: The father of Indian surgery and ophthalmology. Doc Ophthalmol Adv Ophthalmol. 1997;93(1–2):159–167.
11. India's rate of organ donation compares poorly with other countries—Times of India [Internet]. [cited 2019 Dec 28]. 2019. Available from: https://timesofindia.indiatimes.com/edit page/Indias-rate-of-organ-donation-compares-poorly-with-other-countries/articleshow/21559260.cms
12. Health and Family Welfare (Z1) Department. Brain death—Declaration of brain death made mandatory in Government Medical College Hospitals in Chennai—Orders Issued. 2008 Aug. Report No.: G.O. (Ms) No. 6.
13. LifeSiteNews.com. NY woman declared 'brain dead' woke up moments before organs harvested [Internet]. LifeSiteNews. [cited 2020 Jan 8]. 2020. Available from: https://www.lifesitenews.com/news/ny-woman-declared-brain-dead-woke-up-moments-before-organs-harvested
14. Swinburn JM, Ali SM, Banerjee DJ, Khan ZP. Ethical dilemma: Discontinuation of ventilation after brain stem death. BMJ. 1999 Jun 26;318(7200):1753–1754.

15. Defining death legally: indialegalonline.com [Internet]. [cited 2020 Jan 8]. 2020. Available from: https://www.indialegallive.com/cover-story-articles/il-feature-news/defining-death-legally-14973
16. Sumana Navin, Sunil Shroff, Sujatha Niranjan. Deceased organ donation in India [Internet]. 2020. Available from: https://www.mohanfoundation.org/organ-donation-transplant-resources/organ-donation-in-india.asp
17. Venugopal P. The first successful heart transplant in India. Natl Med J India. 1994 Oct;7(5):213–215.
18. Ganapathy K. Brain death revisited. Neurol India. 2018 Apr;66(2):308–315.
19. Tamuli RP, Sarmah S, Saikia B. Organ donation—'attitude and awareness among undergraduates and postgraduates of North-East India'. J Fam Med Prim Care. 2019 Jan;8(1):130–136.
20. Ganapathy K. Brain death revisited. Neurol India. 2018 Mar 1;66(2):308.
21. Kamalakannan SK, Gudlavalleti ASV, Murthy Gudlavalleti VS, Goenka S, Kuper H. Challenges in understanding the epidemiology of acquired brain injury in India. Ann Indian Acad Neurol. 2015;18(1):66–70.
22. Life after death: On Organ Donation Day, let's resolve to donate as well as set up an effective policy mechanism [Internet]. Times of India Blog. 2015 [cited 2019 Dec 25]. Available from: https://timesofindia.indiatimes.com/blogs/toi-editorials/life-after-death-on-organ-donation-day-lets-resolve-to-donate-as-well-as-set-up-an-effective-policy-mechanism/
23. Kerala Network for Organ Sharing (KNOS). Annual Report 2013 for Kerala, Deceased Donor Organ Transplantation. [online] [Internet]. 2013. Available from: http://knos.org.in/pdf/Knos Report 2013.pdf
24. Mekkodathil A, Asim M, Sathian B, Rajesh E, Kumar RN, Simkhada P, et al. Current scenario of organ donation and transplantation in Kerala, India. Nepal J Epidemiol. 2019 Jun 30;9(2):759–760.
25. glorep2017.pdf [Internet]. [cited 2019 Dec 25]. 2019. Available from: http://www.transplant-observatory.org/wp-content/uploads/2019/11/glorep2017.pdf
26. Arshad A, Anderson B, Sharif A. Comparison of organ donation and transplantation rates between opt-out and opt-in systems. Kidney Int. 2019 Jun;95(6):1453–1460.
27. Matesanz R, Domínguez-Gil B, Coll E, Mahíllo B, Marazuela R. How Spain reached 40 deceased organ donors per million population. Am J Transplant Off J Am Soc Transplant Am Soc Transpl Surg. 2017 Jun;17(6):1447–1454.
28. Bugge JF. Brain death and its implications for management of the potential organ donor. Acta Anaesthesiol Scand. 2009 Nov;53(10):1239–1250.
29. Panwar R, Pal S, Dash NR, Sahni P, Vij A, Misra MC. Why are we poor organ donors: A survey focusing on attitudes of the lay public from Northern India. J Clin Exp Hepatol. 2016 Jun;6(2):81–86.
30. Darlington D, Anitha FS, Joseph C. Study of knowledge, attitude, and practice of organ donation among medical students in a tertiary care centre in South India. Cureus. 2019 Jun 13;11(6):e4896.
31. Basavaraj Patthi, Swati Jain, Ashish Singla, Shilpi Singh, Hansa Kundu, Khushboo Singh. Beliefs and barriers for organ donation and influence of educational intervention on dental students: A questionnaire study. J Indian Assoc Public Health Dent. 2015;13(1):58–62.

32. Srivastava A, Mani A. Deceased organ donation and transplantation in India: Promises and challenges. Neurol India. 2018 Apr;66(2):316–322.
33. Patil R, E RP, Boratne A, Gupta SK, Datta SS. Status of eye donation awareness and its associated factors among adults in rural pondicherry. J Clin Diagn Res JCDR. 2015 Feb;9(2):LC01–04.
34. Sawhney C, Kaur M, Lalwani S, Gupta B, Balakrishnan I, Vij A. Organ retrieval and banking in brain dead trauma patients: Our experience at level-1 trauma centre and current views. Indian J Anaesth. 2013;57(3):241–247.
35. van Veen E, van der Jagt M, Cnossen MC, Maas AIR, de Beaufort ID, Menon DK, et al. Brain death and postmortem organ donation: Report of a questionnaire from the CENTER-TBI study. Crit Care Lond Engl. 2018 16;22(1):306.
36. Jagadeesh AT, Puttur A, Mondal S, Ibrahim S, Udupi A, Prasanna LC, et al. Devising focused strategies to improve organ donor registrations: A cross-sectional study among professional drivers in coastal South India. PloS One. 2018;13(12):e0209686.

19

Organ donation in South Africa

David Thomson, Elmi Muller, Tinus Du Toit

Historical overview

The place of South Africa (SA) is cemented in transplantation history by the pioneering work of Christian Barnard who performed the first heart transplant on 3 December 1967.(1) As with all leaps forward in transplantation, it was built on the work of many others.(2) The first patient, Louis Washkansky, only lived eighteen days after the procedure, succumbing to pneumonia and septicaemia related to immunosuppression(3) (Figures 19.1 a and b). A significant factor in the race to perform the first heart transplant was that death determination on neurological grounds was accepted to the prevailing medical standards of the time in SA.(4)

More than the first case, it was the second patient, Philip Blaaiberg, a dentist, transplanted two weeks later who generated more medical interest. He lived for nineteen months post-transplant. Outcomes from many heart transplant centres were poor in an era when the expected outcomes of cardiac transplantation were unknown.(3) With the fifth and sixth South African transplant recipients who lived thirteen and twenty-three years respectively, the true potential of cardiac transplantation was demonstrated.

An important step taken by Dr Barnard was that the treating clinical team had to certify neurological/brain death of the potential donor, independent of the transplant team. In Japan, there was a widespread outcry following the first Japanese heart transplant in 1968 with the speculation around the independence of the death certification and the surgeon charged with murder for performing the donor operation.(6) Japan permitted brain death legally only in 1997.(7)

(a)

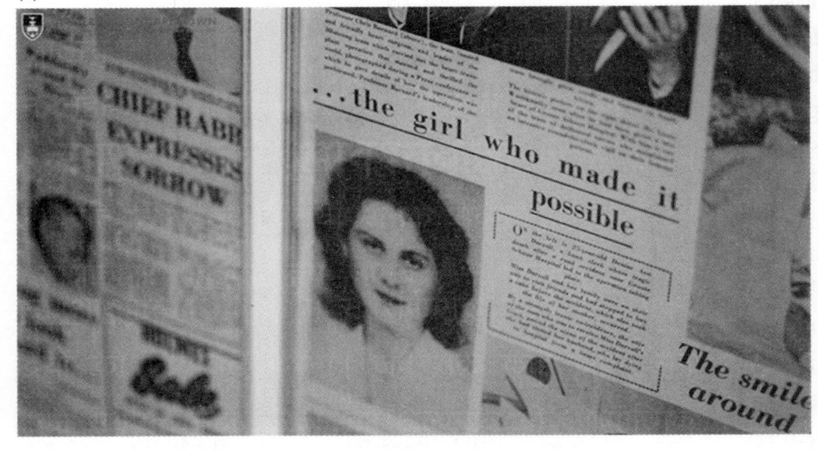

(b)

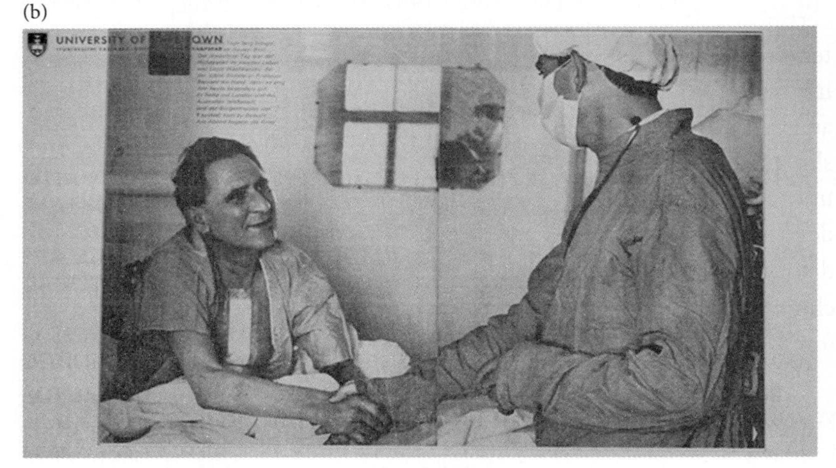

Figure 19.1A. The girl who made it possible

Figure 19.1B. Louis Washkansky and Chris Barnard after the first heart transplant

Screenshots from online course Organ Donation: From Death to Life by the University of Cape Town[5]

One of the last medical acts in SA by Sir Raymond Hoffenberg, future President of the Royal College of Physicians in the United Kingdom, was to certify the neurological/brain death of a patient.[8] On the day before a banning order from the apartheid government, prevented him from seeing patients or entering a teaching facility, he was asked to certify a donor. He described the inherent pressures of making such a determination at that time.[8] That patient was the donor of the heart transplanted to Phillip Blaaiberg.

The clinical situation of brain death or 'coma dépassé' had been recognized since 1959 following the development of mechanical ventilation. A subset of patients supported on ventilators never recovered any signs of life. The creation of guidelines to assist clinicians was spearheaded by the publication of the Harvard Ad Hoc Committee[9] to examine the definition of brain death in 1968. The Committee outlined a rationale containing the core standards that make up the principles of brain death certification.[9] Other bodies around the world followed suit with the core tenets of death determined by neurological criteria—the permanent and irreversible ability of the person to interact with their environment and an inability to breathe.[10] While different countries and jurisdictions use slightly different criteria, the core tenets are the same and have remained unchanged over fifty years since.[11] Although not the sole reason for the development of these guidelines, organ transplantation requires a clear definition of death. The 'dead donor rule' states all deceased donors are clinically certified dead to agreed-upon medical and legal standards before any organ or tissue recovery operation.

The first renal transplant in SA preceded the first heart transplant by a year and was performed by Professors Thomas Starzl and Bert Myburgh in Johannesburg in 1966.[12] Dr Chris Barnard performed the first renal transplant in Cape Town in the same year as the first heart transplant. In the politically charged atmosphere of the time, one kidney from the first heart donor, Denis Darval, went to a young, non-white boy and the donor for Phillip Blaaiberg was a non-white male.

Further pioneering transplants

Other pioneering research carried on in the field of cardiac transplantation in the 1970s included several donor hearts used in heterotopic positions (an extra heart added) in the hope that the patient's existing ailing heart would recover function after a temporary period of assistance from the heterotrophic transplant.[3] As with all other transplanted organs expressing HLA antigens, it was only with the advent of cyclosporin in 1984 that substantial long-term outcomes could be achieved as the norm from deceased donors.

South African surgeons have continued to innovate in transplantation, especially in research with HIV positive donors. The first HIV positive deceased donor to HIV positive recipient kidney transplant programme in the world showed good results.[13,14] In SA, 7.52 million people (13.2% of the population) are infected with HIV. This research has led to other countries taking steps to ensure that the HIV positive deceased donors are not lost (Figure 19.2).

A case of living related liver donation from an HIV positive mother to her HIV negative child with decompensated end-stage liver disease has also been reported after the child had been unable to secure a deceased donor liver.[15] It is important to note that such programmes in SA and in other countries form part of ongoing research within ethically approved protocols contributing to peer-reviewed academic research.

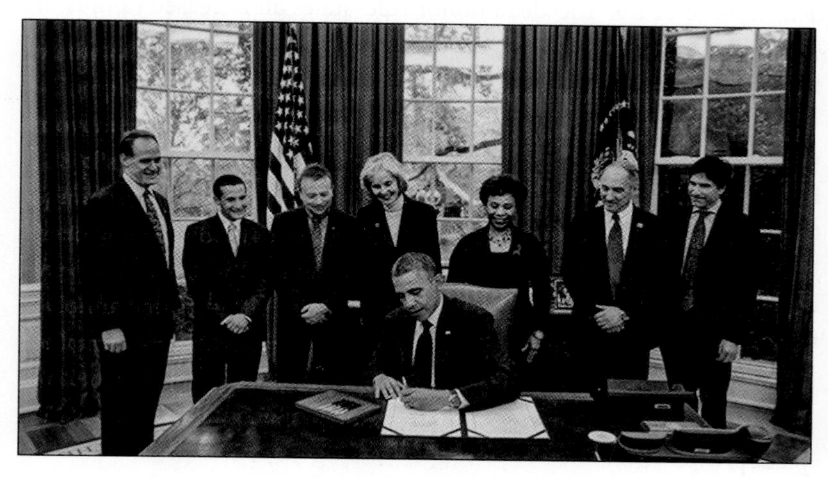

Figure 19.2. President Barack Obama signing the HIV Organ Policy Equity (HOPE) Act on 21st November 2013. (Official White House Photo by Lawrence Jackson)

In another initiative of using deceased donor organs to treat a local disease, a 21-year-old man who had lost his penis to sepsis following a traditional circumcision received a penile allotransplant from a brain-dead multi-organ donor. Ritual circumcisions of African men are considered a rite of passage and are often conducted in rural settings away from healthcare facilities which unfortunately results in penile amputation for an estimated 250 young men per year with a mortality rate of 9% in those admitted to hospital. A successful penis transplant was performed in 2015 with restoration of sexual function, penile sensation, and normal urination. As per the donor family's wishes, a reconstruction of the penis was fashioned in the deceased donor using the rectus muscle in order to recreate a phallus. Unfortunately, this penile transplantation programme was essentially shut down due to withdrawal of local government support over funding concerns.(16)The cold ischaemic time of 16 hours in this case driven by a lack of available theatre time are some challenges faced by centres conducting novel research in the developing world.

All these innovations in transplantation were driven by a pioneering spirit and disease burden in SA that is markedly different from the rest of the world. None of these advances would have been possible without donation of the organs.

Current status of organ donation in SA

Legally organ donation is governed by Chapter 8 of the National Health Act of 2003.(17) Brain death is accepted as death; and in cases of organ donation, brain death is required to be determined by two doctors, one with more than five years' experience, and both not involved in the transplant team. The definition of death is set to accepted medical standards and not legally defined beyond the clinicians who certifies death and their independence from the transplant team. This is different from the rest of Africa where there is often no legislation to support deceased donation, which is a major stumbling block to developing deceased donor transplant programmes.

SA has deceased donor heart, liver, lung, kidney, and pancreas transplant programmes and living donor kidney and liver transplant programmes. These programs co-exist across two disparate healthcare systems. South African hospitals are either funded by the South African government (state hospitals) or by private companies. The former provides healthcare to all citizens which is free for those who earn less than a specified minimum amount, whereas the latter are available to patients who have private medical insurance or the finances to pay for treatment.

The state sector provides healthcare services to 84% of the population with 30% of the doctors while the remaining 16% population are serviced by 70% of the doctors.(18) Access to transplantation is limited with expertise and resources concentrated in a few major metropolitan centres. Renal transplants are the most widely performed, occurring in seven state-funded and eight privately funded centres located in four of the nine provinces in SA.(19) Living donor renal transplants in SA comprise between 35% and 100% of transplant activity, depending on the geographic region. The total volume of renal transplants was 254 in 2015 with 95 in the state sector (from 38 deceased donors and 19 living donors) and 159 in the private sector (from 41 deceased donors and 77 living donors).(21) The ability of the private sector to expand their capacity by relying more on living donors show that this area is a relatively low hanging fruit in terms of expanding access to transplantation, while improving deceased donation is a more challenging undertaking. Only one state hospital has been able to expand deceased donation to include donors after circulatory death in SA and in the whole of Africa.(22)

In the state sector, dialysis spots are limited and one of the criteria used for acceptance to the dialysis programme is an assessment of the patient's ability to safely tolerate a transplant operation and their willingness to undergo such an operation. This is because renal transplantation is the most cost-effective method of treating renal failure. In a setting where only 25% of patients are able to be accepted for dialysis, a single deceased donor, through kidneys alone, allow two patients to be taken off dialysis and two new patients to access dialysis.(23)

In the private sector, access to dialysis is less restricted and increases in the waiting list have been driven exclusively by this sector. The development of a National Health Insurance plan is designed to address the disparity in health care access in SA. It is essential that a national resource such as deceased organ donation be treated equitably, especially in a society with a history of apartheid and ongoing socio-economic inequality.

Allocation of organs from a deceased donor follows the practices endorsed by the South African Transplantation Society.

Organ allocation across a multi-cultural society, with considerable genetic diversity and historically (and ongoing) disadvantaged ethnic groups, is done with a greater focus on justice than utility. The HLA matching of deceased donor kidneys is done but not heavily weighted in renal allocation to prevent potential racial discrepancies in allocation. Deceased donor kidneys are allocated within blood groups to patients with a negative crossmatch. Time on the waiting list is the major determinant in allocation with immunosuppression tailored to the degree of HLA mismatches.

Organs are shared between state and private healthcare systems with allocation of heart, liver, and lungs based on national medical urgency. Kidneys are allocated within provinces. In the Western Cape Province, one kidney is allocated to the healthcare system that cares for the donor while the other is allocated to a combined (state and private) provincial waiting list. In the rest of the country, one kidney is allocated to state and one to private from each deceased donor.

Liver transplantation is offered in two programmes, one in Cape Town (since 1988) and one in Johannesburg (since 2005).[24] The Johannesburg programme, initially operated on a small scale similar to Cape Town, has improved access to liver transplantation with a targeted strategy to aggressively split deceased donor livers and expand into a living donor program in order to accommodate for the shortage of deceased donor organs.[25] Living donor liver transplantation is only offered in Johannesburg, initially only in the private sector but now offered to patients in state sector as well. Around seventy liver transplants are performed annually in SA.

Cardiac transplants are still performed in the state sector at Groote Schuur Hospital in Cape Town and in private centres in Cape Town and Johannesburg with a smaller programme in Durban. Approximately ten to fifteen cardiac transplants are performed annually in the country. Lung transplantation is offered in two centres, one in private (Milpark Hospital in Johannesburg) and the other in state (Groote Schuur Hospital in Cape Town) with small volumes of less than ten transplants per year.

There is no national coordinating body for organ donation and transplantation in SA. Special transplant coordinators are hospital based, as are the surgical teams. A potential deceased donor is referred to a local transplant coordinator. Unfortunately, transplant coordinators cover many, different hospitals across vast distances. The transplant coordinator facilitates the discussion with the family about organ donation, medically manages the deceased donor, and arranges all logistics of the procurement. Deceased donation relies heavily on these transplant coordinators, with only 22 (8 in state and 14 in private) in a country of 52 million in 2015.[19] Many provinces do not have transplant coordinators, and a local untrained doctor or nurse will cover the responsibilities of a coordinator when a potential donor is identified. The lack of education and standardization of procedures related to organ donation is a major problem in SA.

Public awareness is conducted by the Organ Donor Foundation, a non-governmental organization (NGO). Transplant statistics are collected by this group and reported to the Global Observatory for Transplantation Activity. Other NGOs and patient support groups also help to inform the public about the benefits of organ donation and transplantation.

Challenges of organ donation

Organ donation faces many challenges in SA. Low numbers of donor referrals (in the private sector) and a low consent rate (in the state sector) are postulated reasons.[20] In SA, there is currently no national strategy in place for advancing organ donation. As there is currently no central database of donor referrals, transplant volumes and outcomes mean that quality assessment and improvements are difficult to implement. High performing systems, such as Spain, use ongoing quality assurance mechanisms to ensure that all potential donors are identified, referred, and managed appropriately with specifically trained professionals making an appropriately timed and sensitive approach to the family for consent.[26] Other countries have been able to improve their deceased donation rates through a number of initiatives while the South African deceased donation figures have unfortunately remained stagnant (Table 19.1).

To improve donor referrals to transplant teams, better donor identification and education are needed. In countries such as the United Kingdom where there are 'minimum notification criteria' and the United States of America where there are 'clinical triggers for referral', hospitals and their clinicians are required to refer all potential donors. End of life

Table 19.1 Global Observatory on Donation and Transplantation—Deceased Donor Rates per million population (pmp)[27]

Country	Population	Number of deceased donors in 2017	Deceased donation rate 2017	Deceased donation rate 2007	Change in donor rate over 10 years
Australia	24.5 million	510	20.82	9.61	11.21
Brazil	209.3 million	3 420	16.34	5.48	10.86
South Africa	56.7 million	91	1.6	1.3	0.3
Spain	47.05 million	2 183	47.05	35.55	12.5
United Kingdom	66.2 million	1 492	22.54	13.22	9.32
United States	324.5 million	10 286	31.7	26.6	5.1

care practices are audited to allow quality improvements to be made to ensure due consideration of organ and tissue donation is always done.[28]

Education is of paramount importance for meeting the challenges and removing misperceptions that exist about organ donation in the developing world. A major step forward in improving access to educational materials for medical students, professionals and the lay public is the ability of internet-based teaching to reach a broad audience with quality teaching materials.

A massive, open, four week, online course entitled 'Organ Donation: From Death to Life' hosted freely on Coursera.org (Table 19.2) has been running worldwide since July 2017 and providing knowledge to lay public and medical students about the fundamentals of deceased donation[29] (Figure 19.3).

Consent for deceased donation in SA is by the deceased donor's next of kin, with a very small organ donor registry. Informed consent is always required from a grieving family. Consent rates vary depending on socio-economic status, education, religious beliefs, and cultural traditions. Religious and cultural engagement in SA is required to increase the acceptance of organ donation across all communities. In African culture, organ donation is often not viewed favourably. The Muslim Judicial Council of SA only supports donation after circulatory death. The use of donor organs after circulatory arrest is often proposed as a

Table 19.2 Curriculum of the massive open online course 'Organ Donation: From Death to Life'[5]

Week and title	Lessons (video content)	Number of videos	Assessments
Week 1: Brain Death and Consent	The Prerequisites for Deceased Organ Donation Brain Death: The History, The Mechanism, The First Heart Donor Informed Consent and Communicating Effectively with a Grieving Family	17	4 Practice quizzes 1 Graded MCQ (20 questions with 75% pass mark)
Week 2: Donation after Circulatory Death	End of Life Care: Principles in Medical Ethics, Withdrawal of Treatment, A Good Death, An Approach to Withdrawal of Non-beneficial Treatment Donation after Circulatory Death: Circulatory death certification, Types of donation after circulatory death, consent for donation after circulatory death Donation of tissues and bones, What happens to the body?	12	4 Practice quizzes 1 Graded MCQ (20 questions with 75% pass mark) 1 peer reviewed assignment (optional)
Week 3: The Organ Donation Process	The Organ Donation Process: Who can donate what? Work-up and Management, Organ Procurement, Preservation and Transport The Waiting List and Organ Allocation The Recipient Operations, Interviews with Recipients	14	4 Practice quizzes 1 Graded MCQ (20 questions with 75% pass mark)
Week 4: Ethical Issues in Transplantation	Money and Transplantation, Travel and Organ Trafficking Religion and Culture Improving Deceased Donation, Assessing the Potential, Deceased Donation Models, Public Awareness Campaigns	9	4 Practice quizzes 1 Graded MCQ (20 questions with 75% pass mark) 1 peer reviewed assignment (optional)

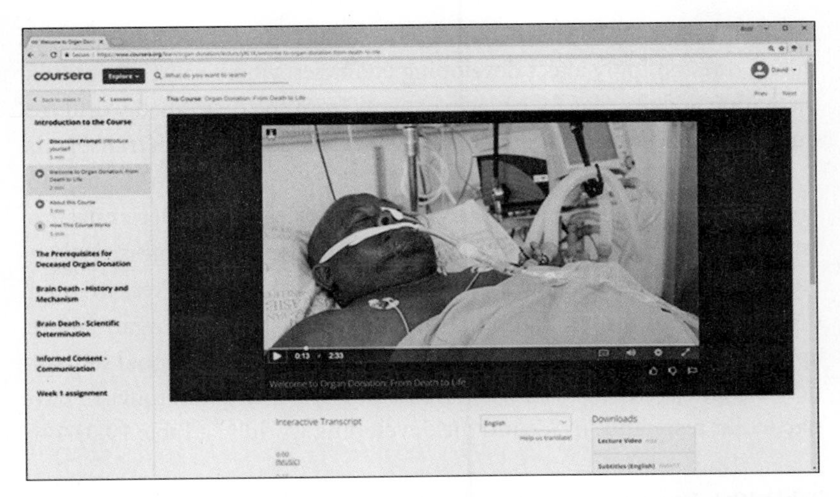

Figure 19.3. Screenshot of brain death testing re-enactment video from the massive open online course 'Organ Donation: From Death to Life'[5] (www.coursera.org/learn/organ-donation)

more culturally acceptable way to support organ donation in communities where brain death is not widely accepted. This has not been the experience in SA where the DCD program had only thirteen donors after circulatory death in ten years (from 2007 to 2016) with only kidneys transplanted from these donors.[22]

Organ trafficking

Following an organ trafficking scandal in Durban, SA, where Israeli patients were transplanted kidneys from living, unrelated Romanian and Brazilian persons, the transplantation service in the second-most populous province in the country collapsed. In 2010, a private hospital group pleaded guilty to receiving R3.8 million (US $342,000) from illegal organ transplants between June 2001 and November 2003.[30] The limited success of the prosecutorial team in punishing the perpetrators further highlights the problem across the world where inadequate legislation leads to a lack of appropriate punishment.

Organ trafficking takes many forms and all countries must be aware of this. It does not only affect developing countries, where most illicit transplantation activity may take place; patients from the developed world frequently seek to leverage their better financial position to obtain transplants.

The National Department of Health, the South African Transplant Society, and the SA Renal Society are signatories of the Declaration of Istanbul, a guiding document that gives countries and professional societies a set of principles and definitions to guide policymakers in organ donation and transplantation.[31] Focus on prevention of organ failure, appropriate legislative framework, equitable allocation, national self-sufficiency and prohibition of organ trafficking and transplant tourism have particular resonance in SA and the developing world[32] (Table 19.3).

Table 19.3 Principles of the Declaration of Istanbul on Organ Trafficking and Transplant Tourism[31]

1.	Governments should develop and implement ethically and clinically sound programs for the prevention and treatment of organ failure, consistent with meeting the overall healthcare needs of their populations.
2.	The optimal care of organ donors and transplant recipients should be a primary goal of transplant policies and programs.
3.	Trafficking in human organs and trafficking in persons for the purpose of organ removal should be prohibited and criminalized.
4.	Organ donation should be a financially neutral act.
5.	Each country or jurisdiction should develop and implement legislation and regulations to govern the recovery of organs from deceased and living donors and the practice of transplantation, consistent with international standards.
6.	Designated authorities in each jurisdiction should oversee and be accountable for organ donation, allocation and transplantation practices to ensure standardization, traceability, transparency, quality, safety, fairness and public trust.
7.	All residents of a country should have equitable access to donation and transplant services and to organs procured from deceased donors.
8.	Organs for transplantation should be equitably allocated within countries or jurisdictions, in conformity with objective, non-discriminatory, externally justified and transparent rules, guided by clinical criteria and ethical norms.
9.	Health professionals and healthcare institutions should assist in preventing and addressing organ trafficking, trafficking in persons for the purpose of organ removal, and transplant tourism.
10.	Governments and health professionals should implement strategies to discourage and prevent the residents of their country from engaging in transplant tourism.
11.	Countries should strive to achieve self-sufficiency in organ donation and transplantation.

In SA, the approval of the Minister of Health is required for all living unrelated transplants from anyone further than a first cousin (including from a spouse to spouse). This entails sending the workup of donor and recipient to a Ministerial Advisory Committee of clinicians and ethicists who review the work-up and advise the minister on the appropriateness of the transplant. For foreign nationals needing transplants, an application needs to be made to Minister of Health for written approval prior to the transplant operation. It is hoped that, with ongoing vigilance and these safeguards in place, SA will never have a recurrence of such organ trafficking.

Challenges with infectious diseases

Infectious diseases are a challenge in SA. In donors the infectious work-up needs to take heed of endemic transmissible diseases such as tuberculosis (TB), HIV, and hepatitis. Tuberculosis is the most common cause of death in SA. Deceased donors are screened with X-rays and rapid diagnostic tests. Transplant recipients are routinely given prophylaxis.

HIV is screened with the most sensitive nucleic acid tests available to minimize the window period and risk for recipients. In the time sensitive context of deceased donor transplants, false-positive results may not have time to be retested and donor allocation will proceed to HIV + recipients.

Immunosuppression in a developing country with a high burden of infectious diseases is a challenge. The home circumstances of transplant recipients are taken into consideration when they are assessed for transplantation. Adequate social support, access to healthcare, and sanitation are requirements to be listed. The dysregulated immune system of HIV + recipients predisposes them to more instances of rejection and these patients need intensive monitoring as they require heavy immunosuppression at the time of transplant.

Future perspectives

Organ donation is a reflection of a well-functioning healthcare system. A deceased donor can only be a patient who has access to the healthcare system and can be supported with mechanical ventilation while a family is taken through an informed consent process about organ donation.

The donor pool for deceased donation is the entire population and the lifesaving benefits of transplantation need to be available to the whole population. SA needs a central coordinating body endorsed by the national government. Adequate data collection systems are required to help inform policy and to ensure transparency for a population that has lived through the destruction wrought by colonial and apartheid rule.

Organ donation and transplantation expertise exist in isolated pockets and the challenge is to scale up services, while ensuring equitable access to transplantation for the entire population. An official organ procurement organization supported by all stakeholders, including the government and legislative backing has the potential to provide a giant step forward in organ donation, with improved education, quality assurance, and outcome monitoring by one body.

International collaboration with professional bodies such the International Society for Organ Donation and Procurement (ISODP), the Transplantation Society (TTS) and the International Society of Nephrology (ISN) can facilitate change. As with any collaboration with the developing world, self-sustaining systems need to be set up within the country.

The financial challenge of reforming and growing resource intensive organ donation and transplant services in SA is substantial. Many changes can, however, be made in terms of organization, regulation, and legislation with minimal capital investment. Deceased donation could be improved by employing more transplant coordinators throughout the different regions of SA. This measure would help to streamline donor referrals and markedly improve consent rates for organ donation.

World-leading innovation is possible in resource-constrained environments in the developing world, and takes into account relevant local factors in disease burden and pragmatic limitations in service delivery. Better organizational structures and funding is, however, required to move organ donation in this region of the world forward and ensure equitable access for all citizens.

While the challenges to improvement may seem huge, they have been successfully achieved by other countries around the world. SA, with its unique position as a world leader in transplant innovation and African perspectives on health care challenges, must grow from its current position to a centre of excellence and training in Africa.

Highlights

- SA has a proud history in transplantation with numerous firsts, the most recognized of which was the first heart transplant in 1967.
- Ongoing innovation and research in organ donation are taking place in SA with HIV + donation changing practices around the world and helping expansion of the donor pool.
- The realities of lower- and middle-income countries with limited financial resources and competing primary healthcare priorities impact directly on organ donation and transplantation services.
- Organ trafficking is a real concern across the world and is limited through ethical safeguards, ongoing vigilance and adherence to the Declaration of Istanbul.
- Online education initiatives provide a cost-effective way to educate about deceased organ donation on a large scale to a diverse audience.
- Donation and allocation practices across a multi-ethnic society and two healthcare systems must ensure equitable access to transplantation with improvement measures needed at various points.

References

1. Barnard CN. Human cardiac transplant: an interim report of a successful operation performed at Groote Schuur Hospital, Cape Town. South African Medical Journal. 1967;41(48):1271–1274.
2. Hassoulas J. Heart transplantation: Research that led to the first human transplant in 1967. SAMJ: South African Medical Journal. 2011;101(2):97–101.
3. Brink JG, Cooper DK. Heart transplantation: The contributions of Christiaan Barnard and the University of Cape Town/Groote Schuur Hospital. World journal of surgery. 2005;29(8):953–961.
4. Kantrowitz A. America's first human heart transplantation. ASAIO journal. 1998;1(2):244–252.
5. University of Cape Town. Online course: Organ donation: From death to life available at https://www.coursera.org/learn/organ-donation July 2017.

6. Morioka M. Bioethics and Japanese culture: Brain death, patients' rights and cultural factors. Eubios Journal of Asian and International Bioethics. 1995;5:87–90.
7. Kita Y, Aranami Y, Aranami Y, Nomura Y, Johnson K, Wakabayashi T, et al. Japanese organ transplant law: A historical perspective. Progress in Transplantation. 2000;10(2):106–108.
8. Watts G. Sir Raymond Hoffenberg. The Lancet. 2007;369(9576):1854.
9. A definition of irreversible coma. Report of the Ad Hoc Committee of the Harvard Medical School to examine the definition of brain death. Jama. 1968;205(6):337–340.
10. Michael A. History of brain death as death: 1968 to the present. Journal of Critical Care. 2014;29(4):673–678.
11. Wahlster S, Wijdicks EF, Patel PV, Greer DM, Hemphill JC, 3rd, Carone M, et al. Brain death declaration: Practices and perceptions worldwide. Neurology. 2015;84(18):1870–1879.
12. Schreiber L, Gillwald J. Johannesburg Hospital/Hospitaal 1890–1990: history of the hospital: Johannesburg Hospital Board; 1990.
13. Muller E, Barday Z, Mendelson M, Kahn D. HIV-positive–to–HIV-positive kidney transplantation—results at 3 to 5 years. New England Journal of Medicine. 2015;372(7):613–620.
14. Muller E, Kahn D, Mendelson M. Renal transplantation between HIV-positive donors and recipients. New England Journal of Medicine. 2010;362(24):2336–2337.
15. Botha J, Conradie F, Etheredge H, Fabian J, Duncan M, Mazanderani AH, et al. Living donor liver transplant from an HIV-positive mother to her HIV-negative child: Opening up new therapeutic options. AIDS (London, England). 2018;32(16):F13.
16. Van der Merwe A. In response to an argument against penile transplantation. Journal of Medical Ethics. 2020 Jan;46(1):63–64. doi: 10.1136/medethics-2018-104795. Epub 2019 Feb 8. PMID: 30737254. medethics-2018-104795.
17. McQuoid-Mason D. Medicine and the law Human tissue and organ transplant provisions: Chapter 8 of the National Health Act and its Regulations, in effect from March 2012—What doctors must know. SAMJ: South African Medical Journal. 2012;102(9):730–732.
18. Mayosi BM, Benatar SR. Health and health care in South Africa—20 years after Mandela. New England Journal of Medicine. 2014;371(14):1344–1353.
19. Muller E, Thomson D, McCurdie F. Transplantation in South Africa. Transplantation. 2015;99(4):643–645.
20. Bookholane, H et al. Factors influencing consent rates of deceased organ donation in Western Cape Province, South Africa. South African Medical Journal, [S.l.], Feb 2020;110(3):204–209.
21. Davids MR, Marais N, Jacobs JC. South African renal registry annual report 2015. African Journal of Nephrology. 2017;20(1):201–213.
22. Du Toit T, Manning K, Thomson D, Muller E. Kidney transplantation utilising donors after circulatory death–The first report from the African continent. Transplantation. 2018;102:S493–S4.
23. Moosa MR, Maree JD, Chirehwa MT, Benatar SR. Use of the 'accountability for reasonableness' approach to improve fairness in accessing dialysis in a middle-income country. PLoS One. 2016;11(10):e0164201.

24. Botha J, Spearman C, Millar A, Michell L, Gordon P, Lopez T, et al. Ten years of liver transplantation at Groote Schuur Hospital. South African medical journal = Suid-Afrikaanse tydskrif vir geneeskunde. 2000;90(9):880–883.
25. Song E, Fabian J, Boshoff P, Maher H, Gaylard P, Bentley A, et al. Adult liver transplantation in Johannesburg, South Africa (2004–2016): Balancing good outcomes, constrained resources and limited donors. South African Medical Journal. 2018;108(11):929–936.
26. Rodriguez-Arias D, Wright L, Paredes D. Success factors and ethical challenges of the Spanish Model of organ donation. Lancet (London, England). 2010;376(9746):1109–1112.
27. WHO-ONT. Data of the WHO-ONT Global Observatory on Donation and Transplantation. http://www.transplant-observatory.org/: World Health Organization and Organizacion Nacional de Trasplantes, Nov 2019.
28. Bleakley G. Implementing minimum notification criteria for organ donation in an acute hospital's critical care units. Nursing in critical care. 2010;15(4):185–191.
29. Thomson D, Muller E, Jaffer T, Nkgudi B, Du Toit T, Edwardes K, et al. Teaching principles of deceased organ donation through a massive open online course—It's place in the world. Transplantation. 2018;102:S192–S3.
30. https://mg.co.za/article/2011-04-29-kidneygate-what-the-netcare-bosses-really-knew/ 29 April 2011.
31. The declaration of Istanbul on organ trafficking and transplant tourism (2018 Edition). Transplantation. 2019;103(2):218–219.
32. Martin DE, Van Assche K, Domínguez-Gil B, López-Fraga M, Gallont RG, Muller E, et al. Strengthening global efforts to combat organ trafficking and transplant tourism: Implications of the 2018 edition of the Declaration of Istanbul. Transplantation direct. 2019;5(3):e433. Published 2019 Feb 22. doi:10.1097/TXD.0000000000000872

20

Organ donation in Pernambuco and Brazil

Artur Henrique Galvão Bruno Da Cunha,
Tereza Eickmann Bruno Da Cunha

Introduction

Organ transplants have become more frequent and safer in the last forty years in Brazil. Consequently, the indications for transplants and the number of potential receivers have been increasing. However, in the opposite direction of technological evolution, the number of potential donors does not keep up with the growth in demand. The failure to identify possible donors, often due to the lack of diagnosis or notification of brain death, has led to the emergence of long waiting lists for the scarcity of organs available for donation.(1) The procurement of organs for transplants in Brazil is still far from the needs. Brazilian transplantation rates are 5–10 times lower when compared to developed countries.(2,3)

The diagnosis of brain death and its acceptance still creates many doubts and concerns in the general public. When the relatives are immediately approached about a possible organ donation, it arouses their insecurity and fear. Many factors contribute or hinder family understanding and acceptance regarding organ donation. Though a good relationship of trust exists between doctors and family members, acceptance rates vary from 22% to 62%.(1)

The phenomenon of death is not a static condition, but a cascade of physiological and pathophysiological occurrences that can often be reversed at an early stage. However, the demarcating line between the possibility of reversibility and the irreversible is not always evident. It should be remembered that the protocols for brain death diagnosis are not just aimed at including the patient in an organ donation programme. Throughout the world, efforts have been made to establish more reliable diagnostic protocols for the central nervous system's death. They are important in the real evaluation of the patient's health conditions, avoiding unnecessary therapies and allowing rational management of the intensive care beds.

After much discussion about the ethical aspects and the variety of diagnostic criteria that existed, a protocol was created. Apart from medical and technological challenges, there was also a great deal of legal insecurity. In Brazil, the Federal Council of Medicine (CFM) established the criteria for brain death diagnosis, through Resolution 1480 (dated 21 August 1997), and made it mandatory. The Central de Notificação, Captação e Distribuição de Órgãos (Central Notification, Procurement and Distribution of Organs) (CNCDO) is a national organization that is responsible for registering patients who need transplants, drawing up a waiting list, taking into account the date of notification and priorities. This organization is linked to the Ministry of Health of the Federal Government and has representation in all states in the form of State transplant centres. The CFM established that notification of brain death is compulsory with the CNCDO. The CNCDO is also responsible for drafting guidelines for identifying possible donors and fast and efficient transport of organs to the transplant site.[4]

Brazilian protocol

To include a patient in the protocol of brain death diagnosis, the following criteria must be obeyed. The patient has to be classified as scoring a cumulative of three on the Glasgow Coma Scale assessment, should be in apnoea and have potentially irreversible brain damage, documented through complementary examinations. Conditions such as hypothermia, use of drugs that depress the central nervous system, and endocrine, metabolic and hydro-electrolyte disturbances should be excluded.

Once included in the protocol, the patient should undergo two clinical evaluations at age-appropriate intervals. These assessments could not be made by physicians involved in the treatment of the patient or members of the transplant teams. Recently, a new regulation has been created that requires clinical evaluations to be performed only by credited physicians, specially trained through courses to diagnose brain death.

In addition to clinical evaluation, the brain death diagnostic protocol requires some additional tests and examinations. Apnoea evaluation is one of the tests to be performed. The patient is ventilated to 100% oxygen saturation and then disconnected from the ventilator to observe the presence or absence of breathing movements while PCO_2 is elevated.

The Brazilian protocol requires two electroencephalographic (EEG) examinations at intervals of 12 to 48 hours, using at least twenty-one channels.[2] The requirement to perform the EEG brings some difficulties. The examination has to be done in the intensive care unit (ICU) bed, and many hospitals do not have portable devices. Besides, there is a possibility of cerebral electrical tracing being influenced by the presence of numerous electronic devices connected to the patient in the ICU.[4,5]

Transcranial Doppler ultrasonography can assess blood flow in the large cerebral vessels. Although it is a non-invasive exam and easy to perform on the patient's bedside, it requires a lot of experience on the part of the examiner. This diagnostic tool requires proof of results by other means.[4–6]

Cerebral scintigraphy using the technetium 99m radioisotope is also part of the brain death diagnostic protocol. However, it is not a widely used tool due to the cost and the need for patients shifting to access specialized services.

In Brazil, more value is given to the results of cerebral arteriography in the diagnosis of brain death. Arteriography is very effective in observing the presence or absence of cerebral blood flow, after contrast injection to study the carotid and vertebrobasilar system. However, due to its high cost and the need for a hemodynamic service, cerebral arteriography is not always a viable test; especially for the public health system in Brazil.

The Brazilian protocol requires only positive and unquestionable complimentary examination, with a final examination being repeated after 24 hours. The diagnosis is confirmed only after the second clinical examination, a positive apnoea test, and a complementary brain death-compatible exam, and the process of evaluating the patient for a possible organ donation is initiated.[4,5]

Challenges in organ donation

Upon completion of the brain death diagnostic protocol, detailed clinical and laboratory evaluation is still required to determine whether the patient may be a possible organ donor or not. Knowledge of the determinants of death and potential comorbidities is indispensable. Organ donors cannot be seropositive patients with AIDS (HIV, HTLV-1 and -2), septic patients (bacteria, viruses or fungi) or patients with some neoplasms. Patients with malignant tumours in the nervous system are also excluded from the group of possible donors.

After undergoing all screening, a potential organ donor is submitted to a new series of laboratory tests for further clinical and compatibility evaluation. Parallel to this process, a team of social workers and psychologists approach the family members in order to obtain consent to include the patient in the organ donation programme. In Brazil, obtaining family consent is still a major challenge.

Despite the numerous institutional campaigns through the various media, according to data from the Brazilian Ministry of Health, about 50% of all families approached deny the donation.[1,4,5] In Brazil, even if patients, while alive, have stated their wish to be donors, or in cases where this wish was made explicit in the identification document, the consent and authorization of the family members are still necessary. If potential donors are under the age of eighteen, the family authorization must be signed by parents or guardians. The signature of witnesses is also recommended to avoid any legal problems. Patients not correctly identified or whose family members do not have complete documentation will not be included in the donor programme.[1,4,5]

Beyond the sceptical stance regarding the diagnosis of brain death, Brazil is a country with a vast cultural, ideological, and religious variety. One cannot ignore the low educational level of about 30% of the population, which makes it difficult for them to understand the state of brain death and that organ donation can save or improve the quality of another patient's life.[1,2] Another significant difficulty for the organ donation and transplantation programme is the size of the country. Brazil has a continental dimension, and medical care is still poorly distributed in both quantitative and qualitative terms. Capturing organs and reaching recipients on time often requires complex and costly operations, as is the case for the heart and lungs.[1,2,4]

According to the Ministry of Health, nearly 45,000 people expect transplants, with half of them expecting a kidney transplant and around 500 expect a heart transplant. Despite all the difficulties, in 2016, 24,000 transplants were performed in Brazil (14,641 corneas, 5,492 kidneys, 2,362 bone marrow, 1,880 livers, and 357 hearts).[4,5] The National Transplant System of the Brazilian Ministry of Health, together with the State Transplant Centers, has a registry of all services and professionals involved with organ and tissue transplants, maintains and updates data for all patients waiting for organs, and arranges organ distribution according to internationally accepted scientific and ethical protocols.[4,5]

Located in the northeast of Brazil, Recife, the capital city of Pernambuco state, is recognized as one of the leading medical centres in the country. Despite economic difficulties and negative family acceptance of up to 46%, the number of transplants performed has been growing year by year. According to the Secretariat of Health of Pernambuco, between 2017 and 2018, the number of transplants grew from 6% to 15%, depending on the required organ. The highest growth was registered in kidney and liver transplants. For corneal transplants, there is virtually no waiting list. Despite the encouraging numbers, there are still about 1,150 people waiting for organ donation in Pernambuco alone.[7]

Conclusion

Organ transplants are procedures of high complexity and cost, and the development of an efficient programme depends on political and social changes. Public awareness campaigns should be developed effectively and continuously. Public policies for the improvement and maintenance of the system must be continually developed. Through investments in the training of specialized personnel and infrastructure, Brazil promises important advances in the organ donation programme in the coming years.

Highlights

- Encephalic/brain death diagnosis may create a feeling of concern and fear in family members, followed by insecurity when an organ donation team approaches them about organ donation.

- Brazil has established protocols for brain death diagnosis, with a variety of criteria.
- The protocol includes two clinical trials and a series of exams and tests.
- The protocol will only have a positive result in the case of unquestionable results.
- Detailed clinical and laboratory evaluations are necessary to determine if a patient is a possible organ donor.
- Difficulties faced regarding organ donation in Brazil include cultural aspects, low education levels, and weak infrastructure.

References

1. Schelemberg AM, Andrade J, Boing AF. Notificações de mortes encefálicas ocorridas na Unidade de Terapia Intensiva do Hospital Governador Celso Ramos à Central de Notificação, Captação e Distribuição de Órgãos e Tecidos: análise do período 2003–2005. Arquivos Catarinenses de Medicina. 2007;36(1):30–36.
2. Santiago-Delpin EA. Organ donation and transplantation in Latin America. Transpl Proc. 1991 Oct;23(5):2516–2518.
3. Annual report of the U.S. Scientific Registry for transplant Recipients and the organ Procurement and Transplantation Network: transplant, U.S. Department of Health and Human Services, Public Health Resources and Services Administration, Rockville M D, United Network for Organ Sharing (UNOS), Richmond, VA, 1999. 2018. Available at www.unos.org.
4. Tannous LA, Yazbek VMC, Giugni JR, Garbossa MCP, da Camara BMD. Secretaria de Estado da Saúde do Paraná. Sistema Estadual de Transplantes. Manual para Notificação, Diagnóstico de Morte Encefálica e Manutenção do Potencial Doador de Órgãos e Tecidos—Curitiba: SESA/SGS/CET, 2018. P. 1–68.
5. Conselho Federal de Medicina, Portal Médico (portal.cfm.org.br), 15/01/2018.
6. Lange M C, Zétola V H F, Miranda-Alves M, Moro C H C, Silvado C E, Rodrigues D L G, di Gregorio E G, Silva G S, Oliveira-Filho J, Perdatella M T A, Pontes-Neto O M, Fabio S R C, Avelar W M, Freitas G R. Brazilian guidelines for the application of transcranial ultrsound as a diagnostic test for the confirmation of brain death. Arquivos de Neuropsiquiatria. 2012;70(5):373–380.
7. Transplantes: PE bate recorde de rim e fígado. Secretaria Estadual de Saúde de Pernambuco, portal.saude.pe.gov, 30/01/2019.

21

Organ donation in Colombia

Laura Pastor, Juan S. Montealegre, Nicolle Simmonds, Killiam D. Mora, David S. Vera, José A. González-Soto, María N. Suarez, Andrés M. Rubiano

Historical overview

The practice of transplants in Colombia dates from the 1960s of the 20th century.[1] The first kidney transplant in Colombia was carried out in 1963, at the San Juan de Dios Hospital which was unsuccessful. However, it wasn't until 1973 when the first successful kidney transplant was performed; it was a resounding success for the patient, who lived twenty-nine more years until he died in a traffic accident.[2,3]

In 1976, the first liver transplant was successfully performed.[1] From then on, transplants of different anatomical components increased in number, becoming a routine practice in the country. All these surgical and scientific advances were accompanied by Colombian legislation, with a variety of bills submitted to the Congress of the Republic seeking to regulate these procedures.[1]

On the other hand, in 1988, the first simultaneous kidney and pancreas transplant was achieved, as well as the first heart transplant.[4] Later in 2003, the first trachea transplant was carried out, but the patient died a few days later due to a cerebral ischemia.[1]

In 2004, the first small bowel transplant was performed and in 2005, the oesophagus transplant. Additionally, in 2008 the first face transplant was realized in the central military hospital,[1] the patient was a soldier who was hit by a rocket in combat. More historical facts are summarized in Table 21.1.

Table 21.1 Chronology of transplants in Colombia

Year	Transplant	Place
1963	Kidney transplant without success	San Juan de Dios Hospital
1973	First successful renal transplant with living donor	San Vicente de Paul University Hospital
1974	First successful renal transplant with cadaveric donor	San Vicente de Paul University Hospital
1976	First bone marrow transplant in Latin America	San Vicente de Paul University Hospital
1976	First liver transplant	San Vicente de Paul University Hospital
1988	First simultaneous kidney and pancreas transplant	San Vicente de Paul University Hospital
1988	First heart transplant	San Vicente de Paul University Hospital and Santamaria Cardiovascular Clinic
1993	First bone marrow transplant	San Vicente de Paul University Hospital
2001	First umbilical cord cell transplant	San Vicente de Paul University Hospital
2002	Second larynx transplant in the world	San Vicente de Paul University Hospital
2003	First trachea transplant in the world	San Vicente de Paul University Hospital
2004	First small bowel transplant in Colombia	San Vicente de Paul University Hospital
2005	First oesophageal transplant in Colombia	San Vicente de Paul University Hospital
2008	First total face transplant in Colombia	Central Military hospital

Source: Homemade. Data from Niño-Murcia, A., Pinto Ramirez, J.L., & Nino-Torres, L. 2018. Organ Transplantation in Colombia. Transplantation, 102, 1779–1782.

Legislation

The legal framework that regulates transplant processes in Colombia had its beginning in the late 1970s with the Law 9 of 1979 of the Colombian Congress, which regulated 'the donation or transfer and receipt of organs, tissues and organic fluids usable for therapeutic purposes'.[(5)]

The definition of brain death was seen for the first time in the Decree of 'brain death' on 6 June 1989. This was later amended by the Decree 1546 of 1998, which also required legal medical guidelines, as the necessary signs to perform the diagnosis.[6]

Subsequently, due to the problem of donor shortages, the Decree 2493 of 2004 emerged, with the aim of boosting organ donation.[7] However, this purpose was never achieved successfully because family denial persisted. Therefore, the Law 1805 of 2016 was created, which currently governs the country in relation to obtaining organs and tissues for transplants.[8]

From then to now, the concept of legal presumption of donation was modified. It is presumed that a person is a donor after death if during life they have refrained from exercising the right to oppose the removal of organs, tissues, or anatomical components from their body. This eliminates the requirement of consent authorizing the donation by the determinations[8]:

— Everyone has the right to oppose the legal presumption of donation. It must be expressed in writing, authenticated before a Notary Public and filed with the National Institute of Health.
— Minors become donors of organs and tissues, if within the next 8 hours of brain death, their parents give informed consent for the donation.
— The severity of the patient's disease and the anatomical compatibility is defined as the only national criteria for distribution and allocation of organs and tissues, according to the List of Persons Waiting for Donation.
— Transplantation of organs and tissues is prohibited to foreigners, who are not residents of the country, unless the donor is the spouse, relative up to fourth degree of consanguinity, second of affinity, or first civilian, in which case the service will be provided.

Currently, the most intense aspect of debate has been to expand the legal presumption of donation through the abolition of family rejection.[9]

Transplant network in Colombia

The 'Organ and Tissue Donation and Transplant Network' was created by the Social Protection Ministry (now Ministry of Health) in 2004, through the Decree 2493.[10] It is an integrated system of Tissue and Bone Marrow Banks, IPSs (*Institución Prestadora de Salud*—Health Provider Institution) enabled with transplant programmes or implants, the National Institute of Health, the Departmental and District Health Directorates, and other entities of the system.

It seeks the coordination of activities related to the promotion, donation, extraction, transplantation, and implantation of organs and tissues, in order to make them accessible in quality conditions, in a timely and sufficient manner to the population, following the principles of cooperation, effectiveness, efficiency, equity, and solidarity.

The National Institute of Health, coordinator of the Network, performs its national coordination functions. For its operation, the country was divided into six regionals as shown in Figure 21.1[11]:

- **Regional 1**: based in Bogotá, D.C., it is integrated by the states of Cundinamarca, Tolima, Boyacá, Casanare, Meta, Caquetá, Vichada, Vaupés, Guaviare, Guainía, Putumayo, and Amazonas.
- **Regional 2**: based in Medellín, it is integrated by the states of Antioquia, San Andrés and Providencia, Chocó, Córdoba, and Caldas.
- **Regional 3**: based in Santiago de Cali, it is integrated by the states of Valle del Cauca, Cauca, Nariño, Risaralda, and Quindío.
- **Regional 4**: based in Bucaramanga, it is integrated by the states of Santander, Norte de Santander, Cesar, and Arauca.
- **Regional 5**: based in Barranquilla, it is integrated by the states of Atlántico, Bolívar, Magdalena, La Guajira, and Sucre.
- **Regional 6**: based in Neiva, integrated by the state of Huila alone.

Each regional has its own coordination and, in a joint work with operational transplant coordinators of the main cities and the national ones, monitor the proper functioning of the network.[11]

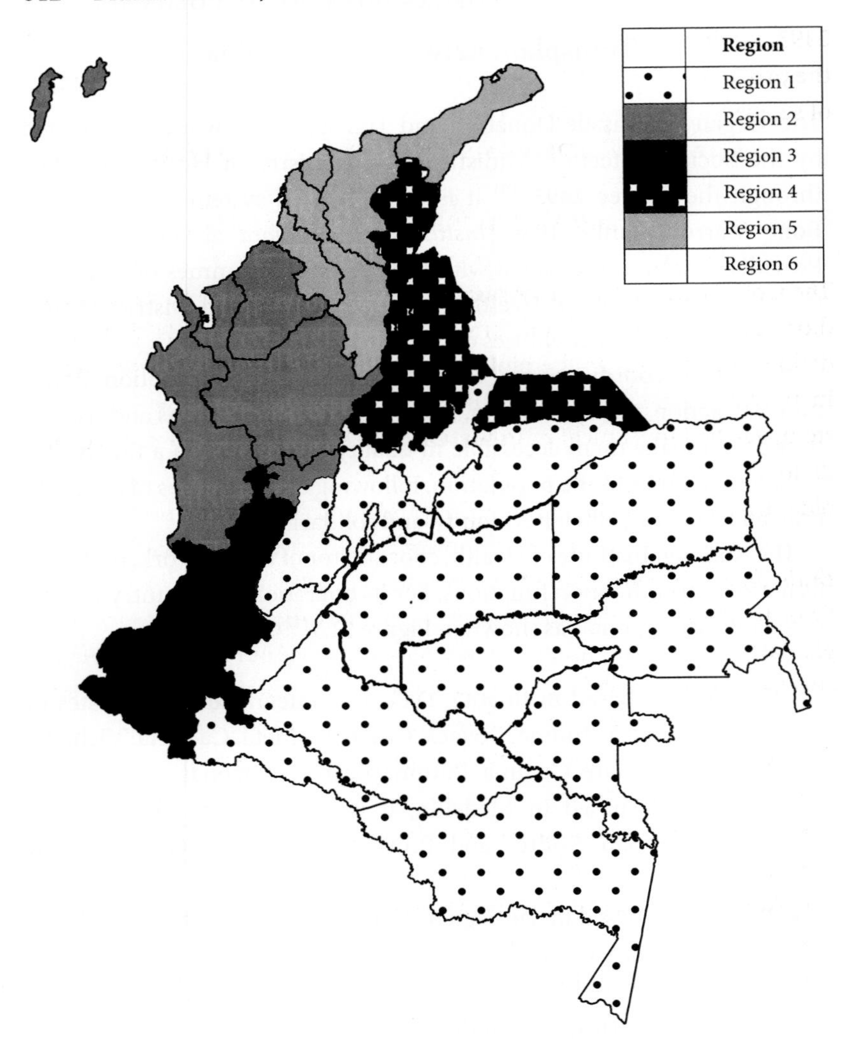

Figure 21.1. Transplant Network in Colombia. (Source: https://images.app.goo.gl/Y7J5gyCGXXx98JfV7)

The IPSs is a potential organ donor and must notify the regional transplant network through the medical staff responsible for the patient. Likewise, they must allow the procedures required by the operating medical coordinators and by the medical and paramedical personnel, who perform the rescue of said organs and tissues (Decree

2493, Article 23).[10] This regulation strengthens the development of the procedure throughout the Colombian territory, generating a scope of security and clarity in the IPS.[12–14]

Brain death determination in Colombia

The Colombian way of determination of death in a patient includes cardiorespiratory criterion and brain criterion. The Decree 2493 of 2004 defines brain death as the biological fact that occurs in a person when in an irreversible way there is an absence of the functions of the brainstem, verified by clinical examination.[10] Criteria for determination are divided into two categories according to age—two years and under, and older than two years.

Brain death in people older than two years

Prior to any procedure for the use of anatomical components for transplantation purposes in patients older than two years, it is necessary to check the presence of the following signs:

- Absence of spontaneous breathing (Apnoea Test)
- Permanent dilated pupils
- Absence of the pupillary reflexes to light
- Absence of corneal reflex
- Absence of oculovestibular reflexes
- Absence of pharyngeal or gag reflex
- Absence of cough reflex

The signs of encephalic death in the adult must be positive in at least two different examinations without specific time frames. Commonly, it is separated by a period of 6 to 12 hours. If the patients were sedated with long action medications or if there is renal or liver failure, this period can be prolonged.

The diagnosis of brain death is not appropriate when any of the following causes or conditions simulating it exists, but reversible:

- Toxic (exogenous) alterations.
- Reversible metabolic alterations.

- Alteration by drugs or depressants of the central nervous system and muscle relaxants.
- Hypothermia.

The diagnosis of brain death and the verification of the presence or absence of brainstem signs must be done by two or more non-interdependent doctors who are not part of the transplant programme, one of whom must have the status of specialist in neurological sciences. Said actions must be recorded in writing in the corresponding clinical record, indicating the date and time of the same, their result and final diagnosis, which will include the verification of the seven signs that determine the said rating.

When it is not possible to corroborate any of the established signs, a test of certainty must be applied. These tests include imaging, perfusion, or electric function tests.

Brain death in children of two years of age or below

The data that allows the determination of brain death in children of two years and under are similar as adult population but include additional requirements: Clinical history, physical examination, observation period, and complementary examinations should be recorded in a detailed and clear manner, including all members of the healthcare team that had acted simultaneously in obtaining the data. This data includes[10]:

1. Clinical history:
   a. Coma of known aetiology and irreversible characteristics.
   b. Clinical or neuroimaging evidence of a destructive lesion in the central nervous system compatible with the situation of encephalic death.
2. Clinical physical examination:
   a. Immediately before starting the clinical neurological examination, it is necessary to check whether the patient has the following prerequisites:
      - Hemodynamic stability
      - Oxygenation and adequate ventilation
      - Central body temperature greater than 32°
      - Absence of metabolic alterations

- Absence of substances or drug depressants of the central nervous system, which may be causing coma
- Absence of neuromuscular blockers
- Alterations of electrolytes

b. The unreactive coma state should be established in which no type of motor or vegetative responses are found to the painful stimulus produced in the territory of the cranial nerves; there must not be decerebrate or decortication postures.

c. Absence of reflexes of the brainstem:
   - Pupils in medium or dilated position
   - Absence of the photo-motor reflex
   - Absence of eye movements: neither spontaneous nor provoked
   - Absence of spontaneous flicker
   - Absence of corneal reflex
   - Absence of facial movements
   - Absence of spontaneous muscle movements
   - Absence of oculovestibular reflexes
   - Absence of oculocephalic reflexes
   - Absence of gag reflex
   - Absence of cough reflex
   - Absence of spontaneous breathing

d. The presence of spontaneous or induced motor activity of spinal origin does not invalidate the diagnosis of encephalic death.

e. The exam must be compatible with brain death during the entire observation period and the practice of complementary tests.

3. Observation period: It is recommended and depends on the age of the patient and the complementary tests used.
   a. Seven days to two months of age:
      - Two clinical examinations and electroencephalograms separated by at least 48 hours
   b. Two months to two years of age:
      - Two clinical examinations and electroencephalograms separated by at least 24 hours;
      - In hypoxic ischemic encephalopathy, the observation period should be 24 hours
   c. In children over two years of age, it is assimilated to the adult.
4. Confirmatory paraclinical tests:

If the medical team have the possibility to perform certain tests that evaluate cerebral blood flow, these can be used to shorten the observation time.[15] The following are some of them in order of relevance:

- Gammagraphy with Technetium 99 HMPAO (SPECT) provides information about neural metabolism.
- Radionuclide angiography and 4-vessel angiography, which are capable of demonstrating the absence of circulation in the brain. There are reports of false positives due to unobservable normal blood flow in the brainstem; false negatives could happen because the presence of intracranial circulation doesn't exclude the diagnosis of brain death.
- Transcranial Doppler for evaluating presence or absence of cerebral blood flow. It will depend on the operator expertise.
- Electroencephalogram has a lot of false negative and false positive reported.
- Magnetic Resonance Spectroscopy is expensive, impractical and with many false positive and false-negative results.
- Tomography by Emission of Positrons might be great to visualize the metabolism in the brain, but it is excessively expensive and not practical.
- Auditory Evoked Potentials is unhelpful due to low specificity and sensitivity.

None of these paraclinical tests are diagnostic themselves and neither are necessary to diagnose encephalic death. However, they can be useful in situations of doubt.

Maintenance of the deceased donor

When brain death has been diagnosed, maintenance and support procedures for the deceased donor may be carried out by artificial means in order to maintain the optimum viability of the anatomical components that are destined for transplants.

The death certificate will be issued by any of the treating doctors, or the forensic doctor in case of brain death caused by violent aetiologies. This certificate cannot be issued by any of the doctors who belong to the transplant programme.

Transplants data from Colombia

According to figures from the National Institute of Health of Colombia, in 2015 there were a total of 405 real organ donors, a national rate of 8.4 donors per million population, mostly at the expense of cadaveric donors.(16)

The waiting list of the National Institute of Health in 31 December 2015 reported 2,029 patients who needed solid organs for transplantation. There were practised only 1,204 transplants in the country in that year, putting in evidence the lack of organ donation to meet the needs. Figures 21.2 and 21.3 show the variation of the donor and transplant rate and increasing the active waiting list for transplants in the last years in Colombia.(17)

As shown in the Table 21.2, the evolution of the transplant rate in Colombia has meant a discreet increase in organ donation.

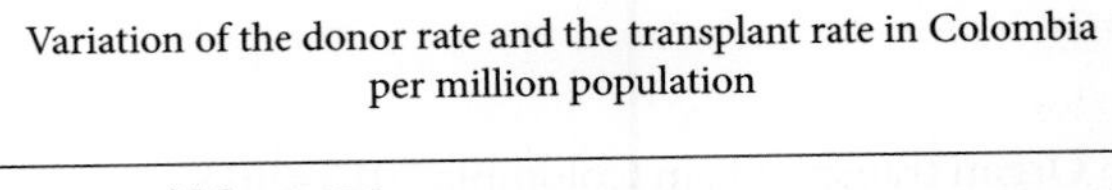

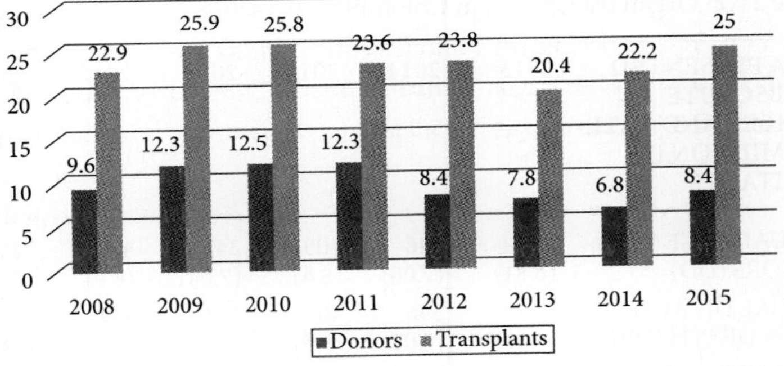

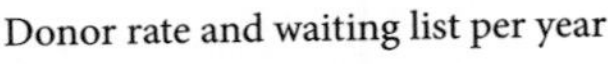

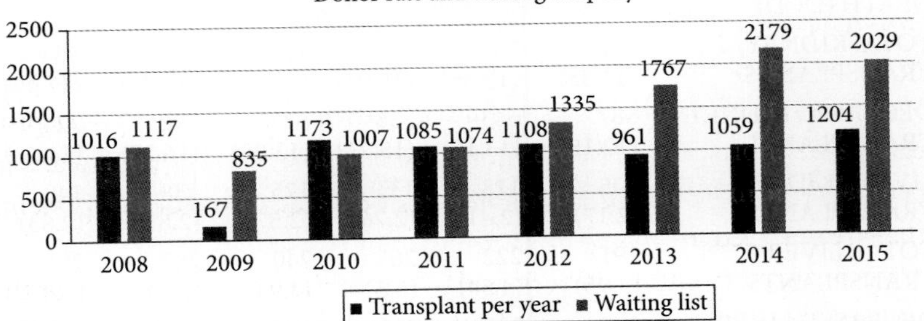

Figure 21.2. Variation of donor rate and transplant rate in Colombia per million population. (Source: National Institute of Health Colombia)

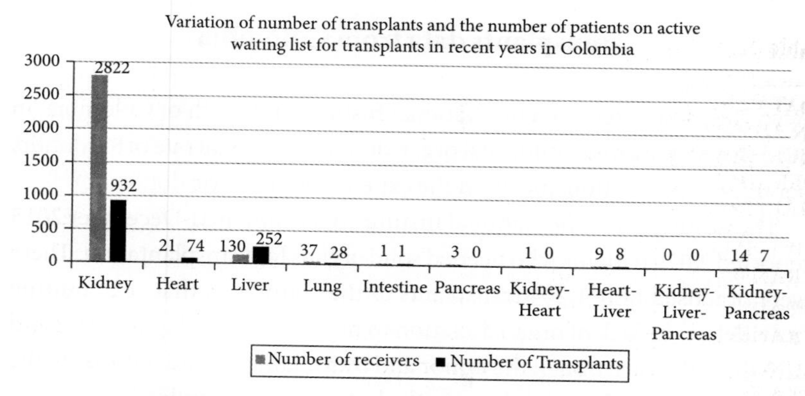

Figure 21.3. Variation of the number of transplants and the number of patients on active waiting list for transplants in recent years in Colombia. (Source: National Institute of Health Colombia)

Table 21.2 Organ transplants in Colombia 2015–2018

DATA PRESENTED IN ABSOLUTE NUMBER AND RATE PER MILLION IN HABITANTS	2013	2014	2015	2016	2017	2018
ACTUAL DECEASED DONORS (DD)	329 (6.81)	346 (7.08)	405 (8.4)	343 (7.04)	437 (8.9)	398 (8.04)
ACTUAL DD AFTER BRAIN DEATH (DBD)	329 (6.81)	346 (7.08)	405 (8.4)	343 (7.04)	437 (8.9)	398 (8.04)
ACTUAL DD AFTER CIRCULATORY DEATH (DCD)	(-)	(-)	(-)	(-)	(-)	(-)
TOTAl KIDNEY TRANSPLANTS	692 (14.33)	761 (15.56)	869 (18.03)	762 (15.65)	936 (19.06)	864 (17.45)
DECEASED KIDNEY TRANSPLANTS	587 (12.15)	643 (13.15)	736 (15.27)	637 (13.08)	798 (16.25)	724 (14.63)
LIVING KIDNEY TRANSPLANTS	105 (2.17)	118 (2.41)	133 (2.76)	125 (2.57)	138 (2.81)	140 (2.83)
TOTAL LIVER TRANSPLANTS	191 (3.95)	222 (4.54)	265 (5.5)	240 (4.93)	282 (5.74)	251 (5.07)
DECEASED LIVER TRANSPLANTS	178 (3.69)	201 (4.11)	232 (4.81)	199 (4.09)	243 (4.95)	201 (4.06)

Table 21.2 *Continued*

DATA PRESENTED IN ABSOLUTE NUMBER AND RATE PER MILLION IN HABITANTS	2013	2014	2015	2016	2017	2018
LIVING LIVER TRANSPLANTS	13 (0.27)	21 (0.43)	33 (0.68)	41 (0.84)	39 (0.79)	50 (1.01)
HEART TRANSPLANTS	82 (1.7)	82 (1.68)	65 (1.35)	58 (1.19)	75 (1.53)	57 (1.15)
LUNG TRANSPLANTS	8 (0.17)	10 (0.2)	17 (0.35)	16 (0.33)	24 (0.49)	17 (0.34)
PANCREAS TRANSPLANTS	4 (0.08)	3 (0.06)	11 (0.23)	5 (0.1)	13 (0.26)	10 (0.2)
SMALL BOWEL TRANSPLANTS	2 (0.04)	5 (0.1)	3 (0.06)	3 (0.06)	(-)	(-)
TOTAL ORGAN TRANSPLANTS	979 (20.27)	1,083 (22.15)	1,230 (25.52)	1,084 (22.26)	1,330 (27.09)	1,199 (24.22)

(-): Data Not Available or Not Applicable

Source: http://www.transplant-observatory.org/summary/

Future perspectives

In general, Colombia is suffering a shortage of cadaveric donors, the same trend as seen in other regions of the world. Advances in neurocritical care in well-resourced areas and limitations in neurocritical care in lower resourced areas generate shortage of donors because of opposite causes: improving survival with high quality treating therapies, or losing potential donors due to lack of supportive therapies in the brain death patients. Additionally, decrease in social violence related injuries has been a trend in the last couple of years, associated to the peace process. As a general response, the increasing community awareness for early donation in diagnosed brain death patients is an actual trend. Additionally, early supportive therapy for catastrophic central nervous system injuries (mostly related to motorcycle accidents) and expansion of inclusion criteria for potential donors (specially related to CNS or systemic oncological diseases) have been discussed recently by actors of the transplant network connected with international networks of transplant experts. In this perspective, it seems like new strategies for increasing organ donation culture will be required in order to decrease the list of transplant requirements in the country.

Highlights

- The establishment of a transplant network and changes in legislation has been the main strategy to increase the donation of anatomical organs and components in Colombia.
- In the Law 1805 of 2016, it is presumed that a person is a donor unless he/she has officially rejected it during your life.
- Despite the most recent regulations, organ donation rates continue to be low, mainly due to family refusal.
- Additional strategies from social, economic, and political approaches are required to boost organ donation in Colombia.

References

1. Bermeo S, Ostos H, Cubillos J. Transplantes de órganos perspectiva histórica y alternativas futuras. Rev Fac Salud—RFS. 2015;1(2):63–71.
2. Nino-Murcia A, Pinto Ramirez JL, Nino-Torres L. Organ transplantation in Colombia. Transplantation. 2018;102(11):1779–1783.
3. Fundación, H. (2019). 40 años del primer trasplante de órgano en Colombia. [online] Hospitaluniversitario.sanvicentefundacion.com. Available at: http://hospitaluniversitario.sanvicentefundacion.com/index.php/comunidad-online/noticias/107-noticias-del-hospital-universitario/648-40-anos-primer-trasplante-de-organo [Accessed 31 August 2019].
3. López-Casas JG. La donación y el trasplante de componentes anatómicos en Colombia: siete décadas de logros. Biomedica. 2017;37(2):145–146.
4. Chaparro GR. La presunción de la donación de órganos en Colombia: reflexiones para el debate. Rev Latinoam Bioética [Internet]. 2017 [cited 2019 August 31];17(33-2):92–106. Available from: http://dx.doi.org/10.18359/rlbi.2178.
5. Ley 9 de 1979 [Internet]. 2019 [cited 5 September 2019]. Available from: https://www.minsalud.gov.co/Normatividad_Nuevo/LEY%200009%20DE%201979.pdf
6. Ley 73 de 1988 Nivel Nacional [Internet]. Compilación de la Legislación Aplicable al Distrito Capital: Régimen Legal de Bogotá. 2016. Available from: https://www.alcaldiabogota.gov.co/sisjur/normas/Norma1.jsp?i=14524
7. Ley 919 de 2004 Nivel Nacional [Internet]. Compilación de la Legislación Aplicable al Distrito Capital: Régimen Legal de Bogotá. 2004. Available from: https://www.alcaldiabogota.gov.co/sisjur/normas/Norma1.jsp?i=15507

8. Ley 1805 de 2016 [Internet]. 2016. Available from: http://es.presidencia.gov.co/normativa/normativa/LEY 1805 DEL 04 DE AGOSTO DE 2016.pdf
9. Pinto B. Boris Pinto [Internet]. Razón Publica. 2017. Available from: https://razonpublica.com/index.php/economia-y-sociedad/10028-la-nueva-ley-de-trasplantes-en-el-país-un-paso-importante-pero-insuficiente.html
10. Decreto 2493 de 2004 [Internet]. Minsalud.gov.co. 2019 [cited 5 September 2019]. 2004. Available from: https://www.minsalud.gov.co/Normatividad_Nuevo/DECRETO%202493%20DE%202004.pdf
11. Coordinaciones Regionales de Donación y Trasplantes de Colombia. 2020. https://www.dssa.gov.co/index.php/organigrama/item/939-coordinaciones-regionales-de-donacion-y-trasplantes-de-colombia
12. Aristizábal AM, Castrillón Y, Gil T, Restrepo D, Solano K, Guevara M, et al. Manejo actual del donante potencial de órganos y tejidos en muerte cerebral: guía de manejo y revisión de la literatura. Rev Colomb Cirugía. 2017;32(2):128–145.
13. Secretaria de Salud [Internet]. Saludcapital. 2019 [cited 31 August 2019]. 2020. Available from: http://www.saludcapital.gov.co/DDS/Paginas/QuienesSomos_DonacionyTrasplantes.aspx
14. Salinas Nova MA, Rojas Meneses Á, Restrepo Gutierrez JC. Liver Transplant in Colombia. Liver Transplant. 2019;25(4):658–663.
15. Centanaro G. 'Guía para el diagnóstico de muerte encefálica'. En: Uribe Granja M., ed., Guía Neurológica. Neurología en las unidades de cuidado intensivo (UCI), Bogotá: Asociación Colombiana de Neurología, 2004, 251–258.
16. Instituto Nacional de Salud—Coordinacion Nacional red donación y trasplantes 2015. https://www.ins.gov.co/Direcciones/RedesSaludPublica/DonacionOrganosYTejidos/Estadisticas/Informe%20Red%20de%20Donaci%C3%B3n%20y%20Trasplante%202015.pdf
17. GODT. 2020. Available from: http://www.transplant-observatory.org/summary

22

Organ donation in Australia

Lucinda Barry, Helen Opdam

Historical overview

Australia has an excellent healthcare system and is a world leader in clinical outcomes for transplantation. Despite this, it has historically ranked poorly when compared to other developed countries in terms of donation and transplantation rates.

Pre-national reform programme (2000–2008)

Deceased donation rates were relatively static during the period 2000–2008, averaging 10 donors per million population (dpmp). Demand for transplantation continued to outstrip the supply of deceased donor organs, with more than 1,800 Australians waitlisted for an organ transplant.(1)

Australia's Health Ministers recognized the importance of transplantation and agreed that a new approach was needed if the country should narrow the widening gap between the demand for, and availability of, organs for transplantation. In 2006, a National Clinical Taskforce on Organ and Tissue Donation(1) was established to consider expert advice and to widely consult with clinicians and other stakeholders with a view of recommending practical initiatives for reform. The final report was delivered in 2008.(1)

Concurrently, the National Organ Donation Collaborative was established. During 2006–2009, staff from twenty-eight hospitals across Australia, including executive, medical, and nursing representation from intensive care and emergency medicine, came together four times a year to share best donation practices.

These initiatives informed the elements of the national reform programme, with the National Clinical Taskforce recommendations forming the blueprint, and the learning from the Collaborative informing its subsequent implementation.

National reform programme (from 2009)

In 2008, the Australian Government announced a national reform programme which was agreed by the Council of Australian Governments (COAG). *A World's Best Practice Approach to Organ and Tissue Donation for Australia*[2] aimed to improve practices related to deceased donation to achieve a significant and lasting increase in the number of life-saving transplants.

The foundations of this programme were drawn from countries leading the world with successful practices in donation and transplantation as adapted to the Australian environment. This evidence demonstrated that a coordinated national approach and system, focused on clinical practice reform in hospitals, improves organ donation and transplantation rates.

The two objectives of the national programme are to:

- increase the capability and capacity within the health system to maximize donation and transplantation rates.
- raise community awareness and stakeholder engagement across Australia to promote organ and tissue donation.

There was a clear division of government responsibilities under the national programme. The Australian Government provided resources to enhance organ and tissue donation, while the state and territory governments managed downstream services, including tissue typing, retrieval surgery, and transplant services.[3]

The national programme was framed by nine measures which are outlined in Figure 22.1.

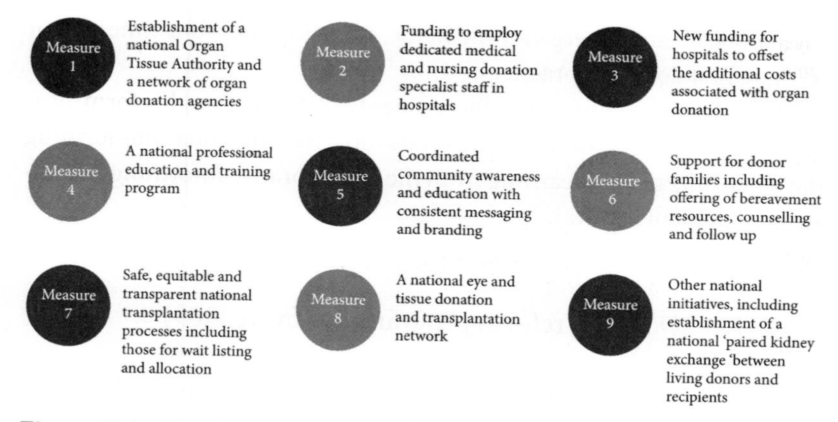

Figure 22.1. Nine measures of the nation reform program

The national programme commenced in 2009 with the establishment of the Australian Organ and Tissue Donation and Transplantation Authority, referred to as the Organ and Tissue Authority (OTA).

This chapter provides an overview of the changes that have occurred in deceased organ donation in Australia since the national reform, highlighting the elements that have been crucial to its success as well as the challenges.

Current status of organ donation in Australia

In 2018, Australia reached 22.2 dpmp[4]—the highest rate achieved to date, as shown in Figure 22.2.

This translated into 1,544 Australians receiving an organ transplant from 554 deceased organ donors.[5]

The improvement in Australia's donation and transplantation outcomes follows a decade of reform under the national programme. Since 2009, the number of deceased organ donors has more than doubled (124% increase) resulting in a 93% increase in the number of transplant recipients, with the trajectory suggesting potential for further increase as outlined in Figure 22.3. Over the past ten years, 11,000 Australians have been given a second chance at life due to the generosity of 4,018 organ donors and their families.[4]

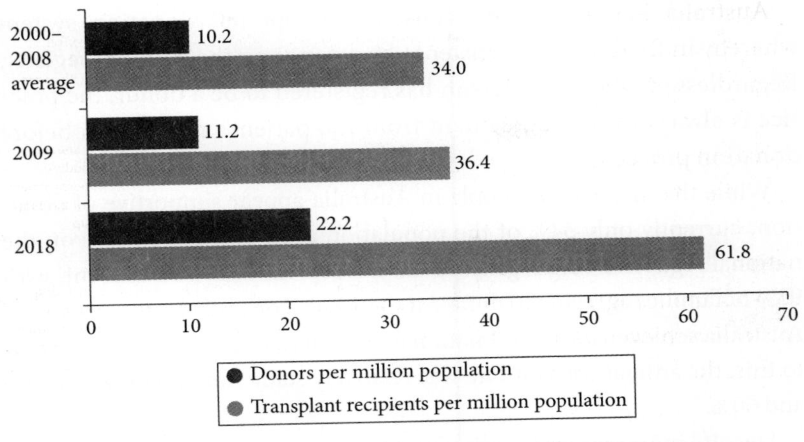

Figure 22.2. Australian organ donation and transplantation rates 2000–2008, 2009, and 2018. (Source: Australian and New Zealand Organ Donation (ANZOD) Registry)

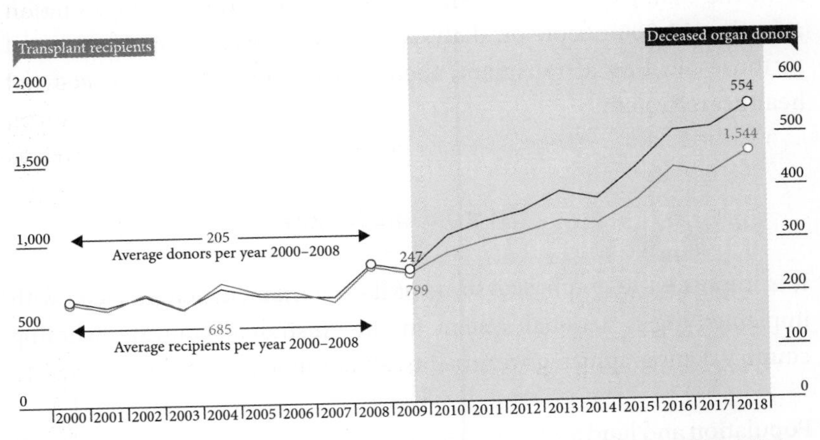

Figure 22.3. Deceased organ donors and transplant recipients 2000-2018. (Source: Australian and New Zealand Organ Donation (ANZOD) Registry)

The OTA leads the national programme in partnership with the state and territory governments; the Donate Life Network consisting of a donation agency in each state and territory, and hospital donation specialist staff; the donation and transplantation clinical sectors; eye and tissue banks; and the community. This collaboration has been integral to the success of the programme.

Australia has an explicit consent (or 'opt in') donation system whereby individuals can register to be a donor on the national register. Regardless of whether a person has registered to be a donor, the practice is always to seek agreement from the patient's next of kin before donation proceeds.

While the majority of people in Australia appear supportive of donation, currently only 34% of the population aged over sixteen are on the national register. Being registered has a direct influence on consent, with 93% of families agreeing to donate if their loved one was on the register.[(4)] Australia achieved its highest national consent rate of 64% in 2018.[(6)] Prior to this, the annual consent rate was relatively static ranging between 55% and 60%.

Despite increases in donation and transplantation rates, the demand for organ transplantation exceeds the supply of donor organs. There are currently around 1,400 Australians waitlisted for a transplant, with the majority being patients with chronic kidney failure[(7)]; with a further 11,000 people on dialysis.[(8)] This comes at a significant cost to those needing a transplant, their family, the community, and the healthcare system.

External challenges

It is important to emphasize some of the external challenges faced with implementing a national system in the Australian context including country demographics, governments, and healthcare system.

Population and land size

Australia is sparsely populated with 25.1 million people.[(9)] It is the sixth largest country in land area and the only nation to govern an entire continent (7.69 million square kilometres). It is thirty-two times larger than the United Kingdom and 80% the size of the United States.

Distance poses challenges when providing health services. Not all states and territories have their own retrieval or transplant units; so clinical staff and organs travel, sometimes, long distances by air.

Three per cent of the population (760,000) comprises Indigenous Australians—Aboriginal and Torres Strait Islander people—many of whom live in remote areas. Indigenous Australians experience much poorer health and well-being than the general population across many key measures, including the incidence of chronic disease. The rate of end-stage kidney disease for Indigenous Australians is especially high.

Australia is a country with a rich history of migration with 44% of all Australians born in another country and more than 300 languages spoken and a vast number of religious faiths practised.[(10)] Public education about the importance of donation needs to be tailored to this highly multicultural society as does the communication in hospitals with families who are faced with making a decision about donation.

Federated system of government

Australia is a federation with powers divided between a central government (the Australian Government) and regional governments (six state and two territory governments). Under this system, the states and territories have legislative power over all matters that occur within their borders, including public hospitals as well as organ and tissue donation and transplantation.[(11)] In the federated system, while the OTA, as a federal Agency, has national leadership over the programme, states, and territories have the responsibility of delivering donation and transplantation services in hospitals and changes to be made in policy, funding or data requires collaboration, and often agreement, between the federal, state, and territory governments.

Healthcare in Australia

In Australia, healthcare is provided by both the public and private health sectors. Medicare is Australia's public health system. Under this system, free public hospital care and subsidies are provided for primary care, meaning Australians have access to a broad range of quality health services at little or no cost to the individual patient. The Australian Government provides substantial funding for the health system, including significant contributions to state and territory governments who have the responsibility of delivery of hospital services. A private health sector complements the public system.[(12)] The majority of donation and transplantation services are provided in the public system.

Increasing organ donation over the past decade

A number of key initiatives have been crucial to the success of the national programme.

Establishment of the OTA and the DonateLife network

The establishment of the OTA enabled, for the first time, the provision of national leadership to drive, implement, and monitor initiatives and system improvements for organ donation.

The OTA established the DonateLife Network through funding agreements with each of the state and territory governments to deliver donation services consistent with the national programme. Each state and territory have a donation agency; a clinical leadership team and hospital-based medical and nursing donation specialist staff. Agency staff includes educators, communication officers, donor family support officers, and data and audit personnel.

The OTA leads the national programme working in partnership with the DonateLife Network to develop strategies and implement processes that enhance donation practice including national guidelines; community engagement and awareness; data analysis, monitoring and reporting; and professional education programmes.

To inform the national program, the OTA established a number of key national advisory committees with representation from across governments, the donation, transplantation, and community sectors. These committees provide the necessary expertise and jurisdictional input to inform the development and implementation of key initiatives.

National community messaging

Prior to the national programme, numerous community groups promoted a variety of messages about donation, so it was important at the outset to engage with community advocates to agree on a national brand and consistent public messaging. The DonateLife name and logo was launched in September 2009.[13]

Community engagement aims to build public support for donation with a focus on encouraging all Australians to register as a donor and discuss their wishes with their family.

Noting Australia's population demographics, a key priority of the community programme is engagement with faith and multicultural communities, Aboriginal and Torres Strait Islander people; and development of appropriate resources. There are Statements of Support for organ and tissue donation from the majority of religious groups in Australia; and culturally appropriate resources in eighteen languages, including resources for Aboriginal and Torres Strait Islander communities.[14]

In addition to the use of media, social media and website channels to raise awareness of donation in Australia, a national community awareness campaign—DonateLife Week[13]—is held annually. A national Thank You Day is also held each year to publicly acknowledge all deceased and living organ and tissue donors and their families who agreed to donate.

Driving clinical practice change within hospitals

A number of successful initiatives have been introduced to embed optimal donation practices within hospitals.

Donation specialists in hospitals

Key to the success of the national program has been the employment of donation specialist medical and nursing staff in all major public hospitals.

Historically, donation staff in Australia were largely based outside of the hospitals. Donor identification and family request were usually undertaken by intensive care medical staff who contacted the external donation agency when a family expressed willingness to donate. Donor Coordinators then attended the hospital to undertake the donation process. Now DonateLife staff are embedded in all major hospitals. Medical Donation Specialists are usually intensive care specialists who dedicate a part of their employed time to donation activities. They work as a team with Nurse Donation Specialists who may be employed full or part-time in this role with varied staffing models in smaller and regional hospitals. Donation specialists have the role of implementing best practices within their hospital, particularly in donor identification and referral;

monitoring processes and providing quality assurance; and family communication to offer a donation. Their role has been particularly crucial in the implementation of donation after circulatory death and donor assessment is given expanded medical suitability criteria.

Medical Donation Specialists have a greater focus on peer influence and overcoming barriers to implement new initiatives, whereas Nurse Donation Specialists are increasingly holding the donation conversation with the family; and undertaking donor coordination, audit and data collection, and professional education.

Clinical Governance Framework and Clinical Practice Improvement Program

Essential to guiding change in hospitals has been the development of a Clinical Governance Framework and Clinical Practice Improvement Program (CPIP).[15] These were a key recommendation of the Mid-point Implementation Review of the National Reform Agenda conducted in 2011. The review recommended greater emphasis on roles and accountabilities for DonateLife hospital-based teams.[16]

The CPIP is used as a vehicle for driving clinical practice change and ensuring accountability in the donation sector. It has evolved over time with three phases.

The initial CPIP (Phase 1) focused on guiding hospital teams in developing a hospital plan around twelve components of best clinical practice in donation. CPIP Phase 2 included group learning forums and paired donation team visits between hospitals from different states and territories to exchange ideas and learn from each other. The most recent CPIP (Phase 3), implemented in 2018, is focused on achieving routine referral of all intensive care unit and emergency department patients with planned end-of-life care to DonateLife staff, as well as embedding best practice for family approach to offer a donation.[17]

Improved family communication

The OTA collaborated with the Gift of Life Institute (Philadelphia) between 2011 and 2014 to develop a family donation conversation (FDC) workshop tailored to the Australian environment. The workshop was designed to provide professionals with communication skills to support families in making an informed decision about donation. Acceptance and uptake of the workshop were assured by close consultation in its development with the DonateLife Network, key clinical stakeholders and donor family and community representatives. The Australian two-day core FDC workshop was finalised in March 2012 and is regularly revised. It is complemented with post e-learning and a one-day practical skill-based workshop; and is deemed mandatory by the College of Intensive Care Medicine as part of intensive care specialist training.

A key performance indicator under CPIP phase 3 is having an FDC trained person conduct the donation conversation with families.

Collaborative requesting model

The OTA and the DonateLife clinical leadership met in 2012 to review international family approach models and experience. It was considered that a collaborative approach involving both the treating clinician and a separate requester who had undertaken FDC training—ideally a donation specialist—was the ideal approach for raising donation with families in Australia.

Given the historical practice in Australia of donation being raised by intensive care medical staff, the change required an evidence-based and inclusive approach.

A pilot of a collaborative model of request was undertaken through the engagement of external researchers to evaluate the pilot and fifteen hospitals collecting data over a twelve month period between March 2013 and March 2015.[18] The study found an association between higher consent rates and the involvement of an FDC trained requester; with a consent rate of 68% compared with 45% if there was no FDC trained person involved.

More recent data further supports the collaborative model of involvement of donation specialist requesters with 75% of families in 2018 agreeing to donation when they were supported by a donation specialist compared with 45% if there was no trained donation specialist involved.[19]

Best practice guideline for offering organ and tissue donation

The *Best Practice Guideline for Offering Organ and Tissue Donation in Australia*[20] outlines the preferred process for family approach about donation. This includes early referral to DonateLife staff for provision of donation specialist support; checking the Australian Organ Donor Register before approaching the family; and involving staff who have undertaken the FDC training to plan and undertake the family communication, and the subsequent team review.

National performance and reporting framework

The collection, analysis and reporting of data to monitor, assess, and inform the national programme is a key focus for the OTA. Across the sector, data analysis informs donation processes including medical suitability assessments; organ allocation and transplant practice; and development of FDC training for hospital-based staff.

There has been a significant enhancement of the national performance and reporting framework since the programme started.

Today, key performance indicators for each element of clinical focus are monitored and reported at the national, jurisdictional and hospital levels through dashboards produced by the OTA. These reports are provided to the DonateLife Network and state and territory health departments to inform the identification of processes that can improve clinical practice.

A range of epidemiological analyses and predictive modelling has also been developed to identify factors that impact donation and to assist in directing focus where change may further increase organ donation.

Vigilance and Surveillance Framework

The initial work to develop a national vigilance and surveillance system for organ donation and transplantation commenced in Australia in 2011. A national system was launched in October 2017.[21] The national system involves notification of serious adverse events and/or reactions (SAERs) to the OTA for retrospective review and rating and monitoring by the Vigilance and Surveillance Expert Advisory Committee (VSEAC). This committee comprises high-level technical specialists with relevant expertise from key clinical, government, and professional organizations. De-identified outcomes from the VSEAC's review are shared in the form of reports and communiques that aim to raise awareness and educate clinicians regarding best practices and also inform protocols and guidelines with the aim of improving practice and patient outcomes. Annual reports that quantify the small proportion of transplant recipients adversely affected by donor-derived disease transmission relative to the volume of donation and transplantation are important for the transparency and maintaining community trust in the system. Communiques are used to highlight specific risks, for example, the risk of severe donor allergy transmission through organ transplantation and in such circumstances the importance of instructing recipients to avoid certain allergens.

Collaboration with the transplantation sector

Collaboration with the transplantation sector is essential to ensure that appropriate systems and policies are in place to optimize the use of all available organs for transplantation. Engagement with the Transplantation Society of Australia and New Zealand (TSANZ) and the National Health and Medical Research Council (NHMRC) has resulted in the development of clinical and ethical guidelines that provide guidance on the eligibility and assessment criteria for organ transplantation, and the allocation of deceased donor organs to waitlisted patients.[22,23]

In April 2019, a new state-of-the-art organ allocation software platform, known as OrganMatch,[24] was launched. It has the capacity to facilitate complex allocation algorithms supporting optimal donor organ and recipient matching as well as providing a range of reporting and modelling capabilities.

Donor family support service

The DonateLife Network, supported by the OTA, provides a nationally consistent service to support donor families after donation. This service is coordinated by a dedicated position in each DonateLife Agency and involves the offer of donor family follow-up; bereavement resources and access to counselling; facilitation of the exchange of anonymous correspondence between donor family and transplant recipients; and hosting annual services of remembrance.

Donor families are invited to participate in the biennial Donor Family Study[25] to provide feedback on their experiences of organ and tissue donation, with results used to inform the national programme.

Future direction for Australia

Much has been achieved in the past ten years as a result of the national programme in Australia. Further increases in donation and transplantation are possible and contingent on close collaboration between the donation and transplantation sectors. Areas of focus include further embedding best practices in our hospital system, particularly routine referral and the family approach to offer donation; as well as the development of processes to further expand the donor pool and support optimal use of organs for transplantation.

In 2018, the government commissioned a review of the Australian organ donation, retrieval, and transplantation system. The Final Report[26] found that increased donation activity has created significant pressure on downstream retrieval and transplant services and on the capacity of the health system. A key finding was that enhancements to the current system are required to sustain and continue deriving optimal transplantation outcomes. This includes adequate resourcing, workforce planning, and systems improvements. A future national strategy is currently being developed to address key priorities identified by the review.

Highlights

- A nationally coordinated system has increased deceased organ donation and almost doubled access to transplantation for Australians over the past ten years.

- A clinical practice improvement programme in hospitals driven by dedicated donation specialist roles has been crucial to improving donation practices and outcomes.
- Key elements of clinical focus have included: introducing routine referral of all patients with planned end of life care in intensive care units and emergency departments; and embedding best practice for offering organ donation that involves trained, skilled staff.
- National data collection, monitoring and analysis, with regular feedback and reporting, have been essential to driving clinical practice change.

References

1. National Library of Australia [Internet]. Canberra ACT: Department of Health and Ageing; 2008. National Clinical Taskforce on Organ and Tissue Donation final report: think nationally, act locally; [cited July 2019]. Available from: http://pandora.nla.gov.au/tep/82729
2. Parliament of Australia [Internet]. Canberra ACT: Parliament of Australia; 2008. $136.4 million national plan to boost organ donation and save lives; [cited July 2019]. Available from: https://parlinfo.aph.gov.au/parlInfo/search/display/display.w3p;query=Id:%22media/pressrel/6NYQ6%22
3. Council of Australian Governments [Internet]. Sydney NSW: Council of Australian Governments; 3 July 2008. COAG Meeting Communique, 3 July 2008; [cited July 2019]. Available from: https://www.coag.gov.au/sites/default/files/communique/2008-03-07.pdf
4. Organ and Tissue Authority [Internet]. Canberra ACT: Organ and Tissue Authority; 2019. National performance data 2018 Donation and Transplantation Activity Report; [cited July 2019]. Available from: https://donatelife.gov.au/about-us/strategy-and-performance/national-performance-data
5. Organ and Tissue Authority [Internet]. Canberra ACT: Organ and Tissue Authority; 2019. National performance data 2018 Donation and Transplantation Activity Report; [cited July 2019]. Available from: https://donatelife.gov.au/about-us/strategy-and-performance/national-performance-data
6. Organ and Tissue Authority [Internet]. Canberra ACT: Organ and Tissue Authority; 2019. National performance data 2018 Donation and Transplantation Activity Report; [cited July 2019]. Available from: https://donatelife.gov.au/about-us/strategy-and-performance/national-performance-data
7. Organ and Tissue Authority [Internet]. Canberra ACT: Organ and Tissue Authority; 2019. National performance data 2018 Donation and Transplantation Activity Report; [cited July 2019]. Available from: https://donatelife.gov.au/about-us/strategy-and-performance/national-performance-data

8. Organ and Tissue Authority [Internet]. Canberra ACT: Organ and Tissue Authority; 2019. National performance data 2018 Donation and Transplantation Activity Report; [cited July 2019]. Available from: https://donatelife.gov.au/about-us/strategy-and-performance/national-performance-data
9. Australian Bureau of Statistics [Internet]. Canberra ACT: Australian Bureau of Statistics; 2019. Australian Demographic Statistics, Dec 2018; [cited July 2019]. Available from: https://www.abs.gov.au/AUSSTATS/abs@.nsf/mf/3101.0
10. Australian Bureau of Statistics [Internet]. Canberra ACT: Australian Bureau of Statistics; 2017. Census reveals a fast changing, culturally diverse nation; 27 June 2017 [cited July 2019]. Available from: https://www.abs.gov.au/ausstats/abs@.nsf/lookup/Media%20Release3
11. Australia.gov.au [Internet]. Canberra ACT: Australian Government; [date unknown]. Federation; [cited July 2019]. Available from: https://www.australia.gov.au/about-government/how-government-works/federation
12. Department of Foreign Affairs and Trade [Internet]. Canberra ACT: Department of Foreign Affairs and Trade; [date unknown]. Society and culture [cited July 2019]. Available from: https://dfat.gov.au/about-australia/society-culture/Pages/health-care.aspx
13. Organ and Tissue Authority [Internet]. Canberra ACT: Organ and Tissue Authority; October 2010. Organ and Tissue Authority 2009-10 Annual Report Available from https://donatelife.gov.au/sites/default/files/annualreports/2009-10/OTA_annual_report_2009-10.pdf
14. Organ and Tissue Authority [Internet]. Canberra ACT: Organ and Tissue Authority; [date unknown]. Multicultural and faith communities [cited July 2019]. Available from: https://donatelife.gov.au/resources/multicultural-and-faith-communities
15. Organ and Tissue Authority [Internet]. Canberra ACT: Organ and Tissue Authority; October 2018. Organ and Tissue Authority 2017-18 Annual Report [cited July 2019]; 62-72. Available from: https://donatelife.gov.au/about-us/strategy-and-performance/annual-report-0
16. Organ and Tissue Authority [Internet]. Canberra ACT: Organ and Tissue Authority; July 2011. Final Report: Mid-point Implementation Review of the national reform package - A World's Best Practice Approach to Organ and Tissue Donation [cited July 2019]. Available from: https://donatelife.gov.au/file/1425/download?token=mqDBStmc
17. Organ and Tissue Authority [Internet]. Canberra ACT: Organ and Tissue Authority; October 2018. Organ and Tissue Authority 2017-18 Annual Report [cited July 2019]; 1-16. Available from: https://donatelife.gov.au/sites/default/files/ota_ar2018-19_13.pdf
18. Lewis VJ, White VM, Bell A, Mehakovic E. Towards a national model for organ donation requests in Australia: evaluation of a pilot model. Critical Care and Resuscitation. 2005 [cited July 2019]; 17(4): 233–238.
19. Organ and Tissue Authority [Internet]. Canberra ACT: Organ and Tissue Authority; 2019. National performance data 2018 Donation and Transplantation Activity Report; [cited July 2019]. Available from: https://donatelife.gov.au/about-us/strategy-and-performance/national-performance-data

20. Organ and Tissue Authority [Internet]. Canberra ACT: Organ and Tissue Authority; 2017. Best Practice Guideline for Offering Organ and Tissue Donation in Australia; [cited July 2019]. Available from: https://donatelife.gov.au/resources/clinical-guidelines-and-protocols/best-practice-guideline-offering-organ-and-tissue
21. Organ and Tissue Authority [Internet]. Canberra ACT: Organ and Tissue Authority; [date unknown]. Available from https://donatelife.gov.au/resources/clinical-guidelines-and-protocols/australian-vigilance-and-surveillance-system-organ
22. Organ and Tissue Authority [Internet]. Canberra ACT: Organ and Tissue Authority; [date unknown]. National Donor Family Study; [cited July 2019]. Available from: https://donatelife.gov.au/resources/donor-families/national-donor-family-study
23. The Transplant Society of Australia and New Zealand [Internet]. Sydney NSW: The Transplant Society of Australia and New Zealand; May 2019. Clinical Guidelines for Organ Transplantation from Deceased Donors, Version 1.3; [cited July 2019]. Available from: https://www.tsanz.com.au/organallocationguidelines/index.asp
24. Organ and Tissue Authority [Internet]. Canberra ACT: Organ and Tissue Authority; 2019. Available from https://donatelife.gov.au/organmatch
25. National Health and Medical Research Council [Internet]. Canberra ACT: National Health and Medical Research Council; April 2016. Ethical Guidelines for organ transportation from deceased donors [cited July 2019]. Available from: https://www.nhmrc.gov.au/about-us/publications/ethical-guidelines-organ-transplantation-deceased-donors
26. Department of Health. Australian government. Review of the Australian organ donation, retrieval and transplantation system. Final Report [December 2018] Available from https://www.health.gov.au/resources/publications/review-of-the-organ-donation-retrieval-and-transplantation-system-final-report

23

Organ donation in Saudi Arabia

Faissal AM Shaheen, Mohamed F Shaheen, Abdulla A Al Sayyari

Introduction

The first kidney transplant in Saudi Araba took place in 1979 AD. It was a living-related kidney transplantation.[1] Back then, the Saudi Arabian organ transplantation regulations adhered strictly to using only living donor transplants including donation between blood relatives, spousal donation, and transplantation between persons who were nurtured by the same mother, i.e. breast milk-based kinship. The latter is a recognized and permissible concept in Islam by which children breastfed by the same women are deemed to have strong kinship.[2] It wasn't until many years later, after extensive discussion by relevant stakeholders in light of organ shortage, that the authorities in the Kingdom of Saudi Arabia (KSA) passed a formal law, in 2004, allowing non-related living donation under stringent conditions. The process included interviewing the potential donors to ensure their altruistic motives, examining their psychiatric and psychological make-up and scrutinizing any potential financial or social circumstances that could ethically confound donation. Donors would go through at least two interviews in a gap of at least two weeks by carefully selected standing committee members whose primary function is to be the donors advocate, ensuring the absence of any potential ethical conflicts beyond any reasonable doubt. In order to prevent any abuse of expatriate workers by their Saudi employers, an important precondition for living non-related donation programme dictated that the donor should be of the same nationality as his/her recipient. Further elaboration has been provided through a paper titled 'A proposed Saudi approach to the ethical utilization of living unrelated kidney donation'.[3]

The current magnitude of the contribution to the total living kidney transplant pool performed in Saudi Arabia can be judged by the figures of kidney transplantation done in 2017, which revealed that out of a total 776 kidney transplantations performed from living donors in that year, 671 (86%) were from living related donors and 105 (14%) from living unrelated donors.[4]

History of organ transplantation

The organ transplantation history in Saudi Arabia went through several phases. During the 1970s, Saudi patients were sent to the USA to undergo kidney transplantation using deceased donor kidneys. At the time, deceased donor organs were still accessible for non-US citizens. This phase allowed transplant physicians in Saudi Arabia to have early exposure to the then new immunosuppressive agents (cyclosporine, and later tacrolimus) and to actively participate in providing post-transplant patient care.[5]

The second phase involved the performance of living-related transplantation within Saudi Arabia by a visiting team from St-Thomas's Hospital, London, UK who would perform a few transplants every few weeks. This phase spanned from 1979 to 1981, during which time, Saudi transplant physicians and surgeons were being trained.[1]

The third phase started in 1981 which consisted of obtaining deceased donor kidneys from Eurotransplant, besides continuing the local living-related transplantation programme. This phase was made possible via an agreement with Eurotransplant Organization that lasted for three years, thereby providing Saudi Arabia with deceased kidneys that, for some reason, were not utilized in their country of origin in Europe. This experience was of enormous benefit to the Saudi programme as it introduced the important challenges of logistics and coordination in organ procurement and started the Saudi deceased donor kidney transplantation experience. Although the kidneys offered were often suboptimal, by virtue of the agreement, a total of sixty-four kidneys were utilized during this period.[6] This experience also led to several publications describing the acceptable results of utilizing many, of the then often discarded, 'marginal' kidneys. A lot of those kidneys were what would presently be labelled as 'expanded pool' kidneys, and thus were rejected by European centres as per their clinical practice at the time. Such expanded pool kidneys are now routinely used in European and USA centres. Among the kidneys utilized, half were 'horseshoe' kidney, a 'third-hand' kidney,[7] and kidneys with cold ischemic time as long as 72 hours.[8]

The fourth phase involved the use of kidneys from deceased donors procured locally. The very first deceased donor kidney transplant took place in December 1984.[9]

The fifth phase witnessed the establishment of the Saudi Center for Organ Transplantation (SCOT) as the multi-organ donation organization and the spread of renal transplantation with the founding of ten transplantation centres serving all the regions of the country. SCOT has also been spearing a wide range of national efforts that included: boosting of donations from living and deceased donors, meticulous gathering of data on patients with end-stage organ failure, and the development of the ethical standards that are used to guide organ allocation. SCOT also carries out the important task of enabling the coordination between donor hospitals and transplant centres by providing coordinators, procuring teams, and overseeing the consenting process. SCOT has published a directory that regulates the practice of organ donation and transplantation in the KSA.[10]

Since its inception, SCOT has been pivotal in developing and implementing strategies to increase awareness in both the medical community and the public with frequent school visits and participation in public awareness campaigns. SCOT also focused on providing education for medical staff in intensive care units (ICUs) and emergency departments. The SCOT has developed strong collaborative links and communication with international bodies involved in organ donation and transplantation and contributed to international guidelines in these fields as well. Hence, SCOT has become a model and prototype for an organ procurement organization (OPO) in the Muslim world.

Socio-religious factors affecting organ donation

For deceased organ donation and transplantation to be a reality in Saudi Arabia, the organ transplant medical community needed fatwas (theological opinion) from the highest religious authorities in the country. The goal was to establish the correct understanding of brain death as a concept and equating the diagnosis of brain death—from a religious perspective—to death and end of life. This Islamic theological opinion would ease the permissibility of performing transplantation using organs from brain dead donors and be vital to push forward the national deceased donor programme. Indeed, a decisive fatwa came about in 1982 (Decision No. 99, dated 25-8-1982). The fatwa stated that according to Islamic Jurisprudence, it is permissible to perform deceased donor transplantation. This important advance paved the way to start the national deceased donor renal transplant programme. Another landmark fatwa issued during the Islamic Jurisprudence Conference in 1986 in Amman opined that the diagnosis of brain death is permissible and can be used to diagnose an irreversible process. Another landmark fatwa issued in Saudi Arabia in 1988 allowed cessation of therapy, including ventilation, in hopeless cases with irreversible brain damage.(11)

Islamic teachings and jurisprudence are important to Saudis. They are an integral component permeating and guiding their daily living. Consideration of these socio-religious factors is vital to the success of obtaining consent for organ donation and providing care for the transplant recipients in Saudi Arabia. In fact, several specific socio-religious features that should be considered during the processes involved in organ donation and transplantation in the Saudi community have been previously documented.(12)

Among these are:

1. **Donor's suicide as cause of death:** Islamic teaching prohibits committing suicide, and views it as a sinful act that is punished after death by going to hell. There has been a case of a cardiac transplant recipient who, on learning that his donor's cause of death was suicide, became immensely depressed and despondent and stopped the immunosuppressive medication leading to the rejection of the heart and his subsequent demise.
2. **Local Imam influence:** In Sunni Islam, there is no pastoral hierarchy and Muslims can ask any scholar they trust for a fatwa. It follows that even in the presence of positive fatwas from 'official fatwa councils',

many people, nevertheless, may still resort to their local Imam opinion, which further stresses the importance of spreading public understanding of concepts of organ donation and brain death.

3. **Departure of the Soul**: Muslims believe that death occurs when the soul of a person departs from her/his body. Some believe that there is a metaphysical linkage between the 'soul' and 'breathing' (the Arabic language uses a similar word for 'soul' and 'breathing'). In this context, a person asking the relatives for organ donation needs to emphasize to the family that the patient has ceased to breathe on his own and is merely assisted by a machine.
4. **Timing of death:** The timing of death is crucial in Islamic Sharia and it has implications on inheritance and dictates the widow's time-frame of abstinence from engaging in subsequent relationship with another partner. It is crucial that those caring for the brain dead specify the exact time of their issuance of the death certificate and inform the person's relatives.
5. **Disfigurement of body**: Islamic teaching abhors the disfiguring of bodies after death. The same rules apply to disfiguring animals as well. When asking for consent for organ donation from the relatives, the requester needs to explain what exactly is being done when recovering the organs and that no disfigurement of the body occurs.
6. **Extended family:** In Western countries, typically, the immediate next of kin such as the spouse or a parent makes the decision to donate or not. In Saudi Arabia, the decision often is a joint familial decision involving all the close relatives including the siblings and parents. Any of the adult relatives may have the 'veto power' against donation even if other family members are in favour, or do not oppose donation. This important extended family dynamics should be taken into account when approaching a family for donation.
7. **Quick Burial:** Islamic teachings view quick burial after death as a sign of respect to the deceased. Hence, relatives are commonly uncomfortable with the unnecessary delays. This aspect should be considered with care and understating while addressing the consent for donation.

Awareness and willingness of organ donation and transplantation

In one study that explored why some Saudi families consented to organ donation on behalf of their deceased loved ones, it was found that the consenting families were more educated, had positive feelings about donation, possessed knowledge on the topic of organ donation, were familiar with the formal Islamic viewpoint about donation and they also had higher awareness of the need and the results of organ transplantation.(13) On the other hand, no differences in economic status, relationship to the deceased person or age between consenters and non-consenters were noted. Interestingly the consent was less likely when death was caused by a motor vehicle accident when compared to other causes leading to death.(13)

A recent study on awareness and altruism in organ transplantation among Saudi health college students revealed a high degree of awareness, particularly about the concept of brain death (86.4%). Female respondents had a higher degree of awareness and altruism score than the male students (59.90% vs 45.60%). Awareness was higher among students in their final academic year.(14) Another recent study among Saudi medical students showed that while the majority understood that the Islamic teachings do not oppose donation after death, 27.1% believed that Saudi Society is unlikely to accept it.(15)

Overview of organ donation and transplantation in the KSA

There are 142 ICUs in the KSA, of which 74% participate in the brain death diagnosis and organ donation programme. The active involvement and close collaboration of these ICUs with SCOT have become a central component in the organization of organ recoveries in the KSA during the past thirty years. By the end of 2015, a total of 11,220 potential deceased were reported to SCOT.

Kidney transplantation

Organ transplantation programme in the KSA started in 1979 when the first kidney from a living donor was transplanted in Riyadh Military Hospital. By the end of 2017, a total of 11,509 kidneys were transplanted; 7,838 from living related donors, 3,108 from deceased donors, and 563 from living unrelated donors.[11] In 2017 alone, a total of 921 kidneys were transplanted; 776 from living donors and 145 from deceased donors. Among the 145 deceased kidneys, 26 were used for paediatric recipients and 119 for adults.[15] In 2017, consents from 123 deceased donor cases were obtained for kidney donation, which resulted in 177 kidney transplantations (145 were transplanted inside the Kingdom, 26 in Kuwait, and 6 in the United Arab Emirates). Out of the 145 deceased kidneys transplanted in the Kingdom in 2017, (83%) were from standard criteria donors (SCD) and (17%) were from expanded criteria donors (ECD). Kidney Donor Risk Index (KDRI) for deceased donors ranged between 0.73 and 2.58 with an average of 1.23. It is worth mentioning that 23 (31%) of the cases has a KDRI less than one, 38 (51%) were between (1.0 and 1.5), and 14 (18%) had a KDRI above 1.5. The mean cold ischemia time (CIT) was 10 hours with 75% of the cases below 12 hours.[11]

In 2017, a total of 776 living donor kidney transplantations were performed (86%) from living related and 14% from living unrelated donors.[11]

Kidneys were not recovered from donors after obtaining donation consent in twenty-seven cases. This was due to medical reasons, such as presence of sepsis or acute renal failure, (52%), donor's sudden cardiac arrest (41%), and technical reasons (7%). A total of 194 kidneys were discarded after recovery due to a variety of reasons, the commonest being; congenital and vascular anomalies (18%), evidence of chronic kidney disease (13%), and presence of renal trauma (13%).[4]

Liver transplantation

Liver transplantation programme in the Kingdom was started in 1990 and by the end of 2017, four centres transplanted 2,233 livers (1,133 from living related donors, 95 from living unrelated donors and 1,005 from deceased donors). In 2017, 147 livers were transplanted from living donors and 79 from deceased donors.[4]

In a survey on liver transplantation in the Arab world published on 2014,[16] it was noted that Saudi comes only after Egypt in terms of the volume of liver transplants done in the Arab World (35% in Saudi Arabia, 56% in Egypt, and 9% in the rest of the Arab World combined). However, almost all the liver transplants performed in Egypt were from living liver donors and hardly any from deceased donors, the donors in Saudi Arabia were equally divided between living and deceased donors.[16]

In 2017, 142 deceased cases were consented for liver donation; of which 74 were utilized (79 livers, including 5 split livers). An 87% of the deceased livers were transplanted in adults and 13% in paediatric recipients. The mean CIT was 7 hours 48 minutes with CIT of <6 hours in 58% of the cases. Livers were not retrieved from thirty-five cases while in thirteen cases livers were discarded after the organ recovery. The main reason for livers not recovered in thirty-five cases was donor's sudden cardiac arrest (31%), deeming the organ unsuitable for transplant (20%), donor's active infection (14%), and donor's hemodynamic instability (9%).[4]

Heart transplantation

The first heart transplant in the Kingdom was performed in 1986 at Riyadh Military Hospital. During the period between 1986 and 2017, a total of 376 whole heart transplantations were done inside the Kingdom, in addition to 650 hearts used as a source for valves.[11]

A total of 117 consents were obtained for heart donation in 2017 (94% of total consents), 37 whole hearts were recovered and transplanted inside the Kingdom. In addition, twenty-one hearts were also harvested to be used as a source for valves.[4] Some hearts were discarded due to the absence of suitable recipients.[11]

Lung transplantation

Lung transplantation in the Kingdom was started in 1991 at King Fahd Hospital, Jeddah. And by the end of 2017, a total of 285 lungs were transplanted to 160 recipients as single or double.[11]

During 2017, a total of 117 consents were obtained for lung donation (94% of total consents) and 37 donors were utilized to transplant 72 lungs; 70 as double lungs for 35 recipients and two as single for another two recipients. Lungs were not recovered from seventy-six deceased donors while in other four cases, lungs were discarded after retrieval.[4]

Pancreas transplantation

A total of sixty-four pancreata were transplanted since the inception of the programme in 1990. During 2017, a total of 118 consented for pancreas donation; 97 were from inside the Kingdom, and 21 were from Gulf Cooperation Council (GCC) countries. Eighteen pancreata were recovered and transplanted; eleven as simultaneous kidney-pancreas transplantation (SKP), and seven as pancreas alone transplantation (PTA).[4]

Tissue transplantation

Tissue donation programme (cornea, bones, and other connective tissue) was started in 1983 for cornea and in 2009 for bones and musculoskeletal connective tissue. A total of 700 corneas, 410 bones, and 144 musculoskeletal connective tissues were recovered. In 2017, seventy-nine bones, twenty-seven musculoskeletal connective tissues, and two corneas were recovered.

GCC collaborative organ procurement programme

As a result of the organ sharing programme between the Kingdom and GCC countries, a total of 67 kidneys, 156 livers, 24 whole hearts, 60 hearts for valves, 56 lungs, and 3 pancreata were shared and were transplanted inside the Kingdom since the start of the programme in 1996.[11]

In 2017, thirty-seven organs were transplanted inside the Kingdom through the organ sharing programme including two kidneys, fourteen livers, three whole hearts, two heart valves, sixteen lungs, and two pancreata.

Challenges and obstacles

Like other countries, Saudi Arabia faces the pertinent problem of organ shortage with ever-increasing gap between supply and demand (Figure 23.1), an ever-lengthening waiting time for patients with end-stage organ disease and an increasing death rate among those on the waiting list. Furthermore, the implementation of strict policies preventing Saudis with organ failure from seeking commercial organ transplanting abroad increased the local demand for organs in the face of ongoing shortage. The number of Saudis travelling abroad for commercial transplantation dropped 69.0% between 2003–2005 and 2013–2016.(17)

Trends in deceased donor kidney availability and utilization

In a recent study, the authors looked into the trends in deceased donor kidney availability and utilization in Saudi Arabia, waitlist changes, and

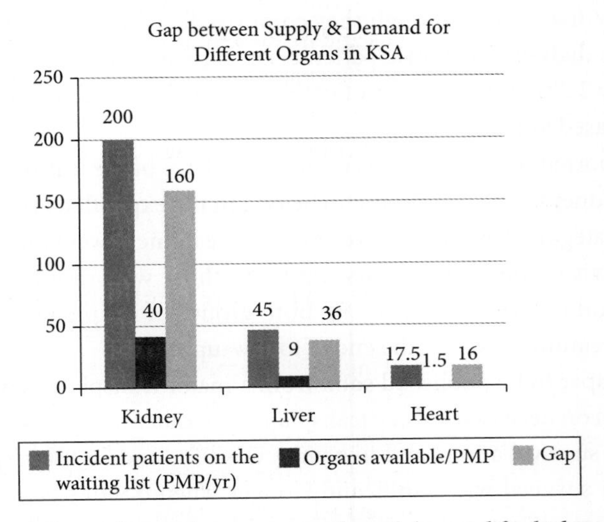

Figure 23.1. shows the gap between supply and demand for kidney, liver and heart transplants in Saudi Arabia

* PMP = per million population

recipient characteristics over the previous ten years registry data from the SCOT.[17] This study revealed that the annual number of deceased donor transplants performed remained almost constant (mean of 129 cases). It also revealed that the use of kidneys from expanded criteria donors increased from 16% to 28%. This was associated with an increased frequency of delayed graft function from 16% to 36.2% and acute rejection from 5.4% to 19.6%.

Donor consent rate remained fairly constant throughout the ten year period (34%) as did the cold ischemic time (12.3 hours). While the absolute number of patients on the waiting list for kidney transplantation remained constant (mean of 2825 patients), the percentage of dialysis patients dropped from 24% to 17%. Between 2008 and 2016, the prevalence of patients aged > 65 and >75 years rose by 4.2% and 2.4%, respectively. The prevalence of diabetes mellitus in dialysis patients had also increased by 59.2%.

Of kidneys available for organ recovery after obtaining donation consent by the next of kin, 14.7% were not recovered in 2016, mainly because of sudden cardiac arrest (60%). Of the total transplanted kidneys, the proportion of organs utilized from deceased donors decreased from 51% (2008–2010) to 22.1% (2014–2016). Only 13% of recipients were older than fifty-five years, although they comprised 25% of the number of patients on dialysis. Paediatric patients, i.e. patients < 18 years, compromised only 2.2% of the number of patients on dialysis and received 15% of the deceased kidneys.[17]

As reported by others, it was found that 21.8% of the utilized deceased donor kidneys were considered to belong in the expanded criteria donor kidney category. Patients who received those kidneys were found to have graft survival rates at two years similar to those who received standard criteria kidneys (93.3% vs 94.6%). Both groups of recipients had similar serum creatinine levels at the end of follow-up.[18]

In a paper to be published soon from a major transplant centre in the Kingdom on deceased kidney transplantation outcome, it was found that the graft survival at one and five years was 95% and 73.8% respectively. The graft survival was significantly longer when donor's death resulted from trauma compared to a cerebrovascular event (5.9 and 5.3 years respectively ($p = 0.029$). The median graft survival was significantly reduced when the donors developed terminal acute kidney injury before kidney operative recovery (6.97 and 8.16 years respectively, $p = 0.0062$). There was also a negative correlation between graft survival and donor age ($r = 0.17$, $p = 0.01$) and one-year serum creatinine level ($r = 0.17$, $p = 0.01$).[19]

Over a five-year period ending in 2015, SCOT's registry showed that for all deceased kidney organ transplantation, CIT > 24 hours occurred in 27.1%, delayed graft function in 33.4% and biopsy proven acute rejection 16.5% of cases. The overall one- and five-year graft survival rates were 88% and 79.8% respectively. Inferior graft function was found to be associated with DGF (OR 7.74 (95% [CI] 6–13.4; $P = .0001$), CIT > 20 hours, non-traumatic donor death, and donor ICUs bed capacity <20 beds ($P = 0.03$).[20]

Observations on Saudi living-related donors

It is of note that there are some differences in the nature of the Saudi living donor pool when compared to what is reported from the Western countries.[21] One paper shows that there are more male than female kidney donors in Saudi Arabia.[22] The authors of that paper speculate that this may be related to the traditional Saudi Arabian Bedouin tribal culture, which is overprotective of women. It is thought to be less related to the religious teachings of Islam as this trend is also different when compared to other countries with Muslim majority. Particularly, Saudi Arabia has a better economic safety net which reduces any possible financial loss, as opposed to the financial situation in other Islamic countries where such financial loss would be severe.[22] Another difference found was that Saudi kidney donors tend to be younger. While only one-tenth of the Saudi male donors were between fifty and seventy years, almost half of the Swedish male donors were in that age range. On the other hand, the Saudi recipients were older than those in some Western countries.

These discrepancies in donor and recipient ages are due to the fact that Saudi kidney donations are primarily from offspring to parents or between siblings, whereas, in the Western countries it's primarily parent to child. This difference could be explained by socio-religious and cultural differences between the Saudi and the Western societies.[22] Additionally, due to familial and societal pressures present in the Saudi community, covert coercion on a vulnerable relative could compel him/her to become a potential living donor. Al Khader et al describes some fascinating examples of such coercive forces.[23]

In one paper, the author, who has a long experience with living donors, suggests that Saudi relatives who are unwilling to donate an organ, would—very often—not admit to it, as this might be viewed as a shameful behaviour by the society. The authors propose that the assessment of unwillingness to donate an organ should be pursued with care and a great understanding of the surrounding circumstances. The physician should never show signs of hostility towards the potential donor especially if he/she reveals his unwillingness to donate late in the process, albeit the disappointment due to wasted time and resources. The authors developed a scoring system that grades willingness to donate early on, and is based on objective measures and inculcates the impact of being a vulnerable donor in the scoring system.[23]

Actions for the future

We believe that there are many factors that affect organ donations worldwide including religious, legislative, and economic factors, OPO, culture issues, and the presence of commercial transplantation. Some other factors may be hidden, yet can also affect the outcome of transplantation.

As for the religious factors, we find a wide difference in donation rates between countries with the same religious backgrounds, which may indicate that the impact is not big or that is not due to the religious background per se. The same implies to the legislative factor as we see countries carrying similar legislations but difference in organ donation rates. The economic factor seems to play a more obvious role. Organ donation rates tend to increase in countries with higher average incomes to its citizens. However, that is not as consistent and there are countries with similar average income but a wider difference in donations rates. The cultural factors seem to be an important factor to consider. It is difficult for the organ donation rate to improve in rigid cultures that do not readily accept brain deaths as an equivalent to end of life. An attempt to change these cultural views should be sought via fostering education and awareness of adopting brain death to reflect the end of a person's life. The factor that seems to be of utmost important is the presence of a well-recognized OPO. All the countries that tend to have high donations rate possess an OPO that works to facilitate and improve the process. The availability of commercial transplantation or transplant tourism is considered a major obstacle to the improvement of a national transplantation programme and in turn, can impose a problem to organ donation on a global scale.

In order to improve organ donation rates, a strategic approach needs to be undertaken to tackle its root causes. This will in turn improve the donation rates and contribute to the development of a successful organ transplantation programme. Judging from the global experiences, we believe that the first element to enhance organ donation is the establishment of the OPO to perform and orchestrate organ transplantations efforts. Additionally, teaching the medical community about the process and need is vital, as well as tackling the cultural dogmas through education and collaboration with authoritative national institutions. Negotiating legislations aimed at increasing donation rates can be helpful. The other factors mentioned are difficult to modify and seem to be less impactful.

The ideal model is to have national organizing OPO for transplantation efforts, approved legislations, sufficient government funding, the support of authorities of religion or cultures, and to directly approach and train the medical community for organ donation.

In 2018, Saudi Arabia instituted five initiatives to increase organ donation in the Kingdom as per the author's personal communication with the Director General of the SCOT.

1. Establish advanced training and simulation centre for deceased donation programme.
2. Maximize cooperation between ICUs and SCOT.
3. Advance national web-based registry system for end-stage organ failure and donor-recipient transplant patients.
4. Advance national public campaign to promote organ donation and transplantation.
5. Establish a national auditing system for donor and transplant hospitals.

Highlights

- Saudi Arabia is the leading Islamic Country in Organ Donation and Transplantation.
- The Supervisory Organization for Organ Donation and Transplantation is the Saudi Centre for Organ Transplantation (SCOT).
- Saudi Arabia has multiple multi-organ donation and transplantation centres (including kidney, liver, heart, lung, and pancreas).
- Saudi Arabian Organ Donation and Transplantation is sensitive to the socio-religious and cultural background of the Saudi population.
- Saudi Arabian Organ Donation and Transplantation abides by strict ethical standards as outlined by international transplantation bodies and WHO.
- The Saudi Arabian Government remains fully supportive of Organ Donation and Transplantation.

References

1. Al Sayyari AA. The history of renal transplantation in the Arab world: A view from Saudi Arabia. Am J Kidney Dis. 2008;51(6):1033–1046.
2. El-Khuffash A, Unger S. The concept of milk kinship in Islam: Issues raised when offering preterm infants of Muslim families donor human milk. Journal of human lactation: official journal of International Lactation Consultant Association. 2012;28(2):125–127.
3. Shaheen FA, Kurpad R, Al-Attar BA, Al-Khader AA. A proposed Saudi approach to the ethical utilization of living unrelated kidney donation. Transplant Proc. 2005;37(5):2004–2006.
4. Organ transplantation in Saudi Arabia; 2017. Saudi Journal of kidney diseases and transplantation. 2018;29(6):1523–1536.
5. Al-Khader A, Chang R, Jawdat M, Abomelha M, Etaibi K, Al-Hasani MK, et al. Cyclosporine in living related renal transplantation—single unit experience. Transplant Proc. 1987;19(5):3669.
6. Al-Khudair WK, Huraib SO. Kidney transplantation in Saudi Arabia: A unique experience. World J Urol. 1996;14(4):268–271.
7. Al-Hasani MK, Saltissi D, Chang R, Van Goor H, Tegzess AM. Successful regrafting of an explanted transplant kidney. Transplantation. 1987;43(6):916–917.
8. Chang RW, Saltissi D, Al-Khader A, Abomelha M, Jawdat M. Survival of suboptimal cadaver renal grafts with prolonged cold ischaemic times using cyclosporin. Nephrology, dialysis, transplantation: Official publication of the European Dialysis and Transplant Association—European Renal Association. 1987;1(4):246–250.

9. Al-Sayyari AA. The story of the first deceased donor kidney donation in Saudi Arabia—by a firsthand witness. Saudi journal of kidney diseases and transplantation: An official publication of the Saudi Center for Organ Transplantation, Saudi Arabia. 2017;28(5):983–991.
10. Shaheen FA, Souqiyyeh MZ, Al-Swailem AR. Saudi center for organ transplantation: Activities and achievements. Saudi journal of kidney diseases and transplantation: An official publication of the Saudi Center for Organ Transplantation, Saudi Arabia. 1995;6(1):41–52.
11. SCOT. Annual Report for Organ Transplantation in Kingdom of Saudi Arabia 2017 [updated 12/04/2019. Available from: https://www.scot.gov.sa/en/Home/Home
12. Al-Khader AA, Shaheen FA, Al-Jondeby MS. Important social factors that affect organ transplantation in Islamic countries. Experimental and clinical transplantation: Official journal of the Middle East Society for Organ Transplantation. 2003;1(2):96–101.
13. Al Shehri S, Shaheen FA, Al-Khader AA. Organ donations from deceased persons in the Saudi Arabian population. Experimental and clinical transplantation: Official journal of the Middle East Society for Organ Transplantation. 2005;3(1):301–305.
14. AlHejaili W, Almalik F, Albrahim L, Alkhaldi F, AlHejaili A, Al Sayyari A. Scores of awareness and altruism in organ transplantation among Saudi health colleges students—impact of gender, year of study, and field of specialization. Saudi journal of kidney diseases and transplantation: An official publication of the Saudi Center for Organ Transplantation, Saudi Arabia. 2018;29(5):1028–1034.
15. AlShareef SM, Smith RM. Saudi medical students knowledge, attitudes, and beliefs with regard to organ donation and transplantation. Saudi journal of kidney diseases and transplantation: An official publication of the Saudi Center for Organ Transplantation, Saudi Arabia. 2018;29(5):1115–1127.
16. Khalaf H, Marwan I, Al-Sebayel M, El-Meteini M, Hosny A, Abdel-Wahab M, et al. Status of liver transplantation in the Arab world. Transplantation. 2014;97(7):722–724.
17. Hejaili F, Attar B, Shaheen FAM. Trends in Deceased Donor Kidney Availability and Utilization in the Kingdom of Saudi Arabia. Experimental and clinical transplantation: official journal of the Middle East Society for Organ Transplantation. 2017;15(4):381–386.
18. Shaheen FA, Attar B, Hejaili F, Binsalih S, Al Sayyari A. Comparison of expanded criteria kidneys with 2-tier standard criteria kidneys: Role of delayed graft function in short-term graft outcome. Experimental and clinical transplantation: Official journal of the Middle East Society for Organ Transplantation. 2012;10(1):18–23.
19. Alenazi SF, Almutairi GM, Sheikho MA, Al Alshehri MA, Alaskar BM, Al Sayyari AA. Nonimmunologic factors affecting long-term outcomes of deceased—donor kidney transplant. Experimental and clinical transplantation: official journal of the Middle East Society for Organ Transplantation. 2019 Dec 1;17(6):714–9.
20. Shaheen MF, Shaheen FA, Attar B, Elamin K, Al Hayyan H, Al Sayyari A. Impact of recipient and donor nonimmunologic factors on the outcome of deceased donor kidney transplantation. Transplant Proc. 2010;42(1):273–276.

21. Guella A, Mohamed E. Donor and recipient gender distribution in a Saudi kidney transplant center. Transplant Proc. 2011;43(2):415–417.
22. Hejaili F, Juhani A, Flaiw A, Ghamdi G, Jondeby M, Eid A, et al. Is there a bias against women in kidney transplantation practices in Saudi Arabia? Experimental and Clinical Transplantation 2006;4(2):571–573.
23. Al-Khader A, Jondeby M, Ghamdi G, Flaiw A, Hejaili F, Querishi J. Assessment of the willingness of potential live related kidney donors. Annals of transplantation. 2005;10(1):35–37.

24

Organ donation in United Arab Emirates

Fayez Alshamsi, Walid Zaher, Bashi Sankari, Shiva Kumar, Ayman Ibrahim, Zain Ali Al Yafei, Asma Al Mannaei, Gehad ElGhazali, Ali Al Obaidli

Introduction

Historically, the UAE was established by unification of seven emirates on 2 December 1971. In 2018, the total population of UAE was estimated to be 9.6 million.[1] Of which, 1.4 million are Emirati citizens and 8.2 million are expatriates. A total of 42.8% population resides in Dubai, 29.0% in Abu Dhabi, 24.7% in Sharjah (Table 24.1). The UAE culture is one that empowers women, embraces diversity, encourages innovation, and welcomes global engagement.[1] The UAE is committed to encouraging values of inclusion and coexistence with a designated 'Ministry of Tolerance' to implement programmes that foster respect, peaceful coexistence, and mutual understanding among people in the UAE.[2]

The UAE has made substantial investments in healthcare infrastructure and saw an incremental increase in healthcare spending since established especially in recent years with the introduction of mandatory health insurance and universal access to care since 2007. This introduction of mandatory health insurance allowed further investment into the healthcare infrastructure for both public and private sectors which enhanced their healthcare delivery operations. There are ongoing plans aimed at ranking healthcare providers according to their outcomes with tailor-made reimbursements for each rank to further augment the quality of provided healthcare services.

Table 24.1 UAE demographics and population statistics(1)

Area[1]	83,600 Km
Capital	Abu Dhabi
Population[1]	9,682,088
Three most populated cities:	1.Dubai (4,177,095) 42.8% of the poulation 2.Abu Dhabi (2,784,490)29.0% of the population 3.Sharjah (2,374,132)24.7% of the population
Official language	Arabic
Official currency	UAE dirham (AED)

Cardiovascular disease is the principal cause of death in the UAE, constituting 28% of total deaths(3); other major causes are road traffic accidents and its related injuries, malignancies, and congenital anomalies.(4) According to World Health Organization data from 2014, 37.2% of adults in the UAE are clinically obese, with Body Mass Index (BMI) score of 30 or more.(5,6) The overall improvement in healthcare services and public health of UAE has been impressive. The average life expectancy rose from 60.5 years in 1978 to 73 years in 2004 and currently is estimated at 78.5 years. The average crude birth rate is 18.4% and crude death rate is 2.9%. The persons below fifteen years old form 19.7% of the total population, while those older than sixty-five years of age comprise only 1.6% of the population.(1)

A brief look at the organ transplantation in the UAE

The organ transplantation in UAE can be described in three phases. The initial or first phase extended from 1985, when kidney transplantation began, till 2006. The second phase began with the declaration of Istanbul and continued till 2015 with the expansion of living transplant services. The third phase was marked by the deceased organ donation and continues till present.

First phase (1985–2006)

Donation and transplantation in UAE started in 1985 with the first live-related kidney transplant at Mafraq hospital in Abu Dhabi. Subsequently there were two cadaveric transplants in 1989 where the kidneys were donated to UAE from the European Union. A total of sixty-two kidney transplants were performed intermittently over the next few years.[7] The increasing demands of kidney failure patients were met by getting support for transplantation in USA and Europe as was the practice in most of the Gulf Cooperation Council (GCC) countries.

A UAE Presidential decree on transplantation was issued in 1993 and a federal National Transplant committee was established soon after to work on needed bylaws and policies. Nevertheless, and like many other countries, commercial transplantation was a major ethical challenge as many patients living in UAE (UAE nationals and Expats) were travelling outside for unethical form of transplantation.[8] Desperate patients with kidney failure were often having post-transplant poor outcomes with high mortality and life-threatening infections and primary graft non-function.[8,9] In these situations, both poor individuals and patients with organ failure were victims of middlemen involved in orchestrating organ trafficking.

Second phase (2007–2015)

The declaration of Istanbul on organ trafficking and transplant tourism (2008) was truly transformational for UAE organ donation and transplantation programme as it was for many other countries.[10] The preparatory work for the declaration summit by worldwide organ donation and transplantation community representatives of the Transplantation Society (TTS) and International Society of Nephrology (ISN) forming the steering committee of the declaration took place in UAE in December 2007. Plans of action were discussed to try to put an end to commercial transplantation, support ethical forms of transplantation, and call for countries and regions to work towards organ donation and transplantation self-sufficiency. This was a timely support in the UAE to align the resources and vision and in addition to getting governmental support for meeting the demand for patients with organ failure. That great momentum was used in three ways.

1. The new Cleveland Clinic Abu Dhabi hospital (CCAD) which was in the design phase during that time (2008) was tasked to plan for

and develop an adult multiorgan transplant capacity and complement the capacity for kidney transplantation for the UAE and the broader region as will be highlighted in the next section.[7]

2. UAE Federal decree law No. 5 (13) was formulated in accordance with best international standards and ethical principles addressing needed support for deceased donation, criminalizing organ trafficking and transplant commercialism. The new transplantation law regulating transfer and transplant of human organs and tissues was signed by His Highness Shaikh Khalifa Bin Zayd, the President of the country. This was in parallel with investments into the healthcare capacity and infrastructure in general and organ donation and transplantation specifically.[7]
3. In 2008, Shaikh Khalifa Medical City (SKMC) (part of Abu Dhabi Health Services company—SEHA) supported by Department of Health of Abu Dhabi re-established a kidney transplantation programme.[7] The programme included living-related paediatric and adult kidney transplantation for all residents in UAE which was sponsored by the government of Abu Dhabi with either mandatory health insurance coverage or coverage through governmental mandated funds. Since 2008, SKMC was the only hospital in the country providing living and deceased donor kidney transplants (for both adults and paediatrics) with clinical outcomes that are equivalent to international standards with one- and three-years graft survival of 98% and 96% respectively. To ensure the quality of transplant services, SKMC was a part of the Transplants-Specific Quality Improvement program (Trans QIP) of the American Society of Transplants Surgeons (ASTS), and American College of Surgeons (ACS) from Alpha phase. The reported quality outcomes provided needed assurance to build the required trust of patients and families in the living-related transplantation services.[11]

Third phase (2017 onwards):

The passing of the new organ donation and transplantation law[7] in 2016 and the Ministry of Health and Prevention (MOHAP) approved guidelines to define the declaration of brain death[7] on 5 May 2017 were crucial milestones that led to the initiation of UAE deceased donation programme. Since the activation of deceased donation in UAE in 2017, a total of twenty-one deceased donations took place, permitting seventy-nine organ transplantations, sixty transplanted in the UAE, and nineteen in Kingdom of Saudi Arabia, in collaboration with the Saudi Center of Organ Transplant. This was achieved through activation of organ sharing schemes that exist between GCC countries in order to maximize utilization of organs (Table 24.2).

With the introduction of new transplantation law in 2016, two hospitals in Dubai under the academic umbrella of Mohammed Bin Rashid University of Medicine and Health Sciences (MBRU) started offering kidney transplantation services, including Al-Jalilah hospital offering paediatric transplants and Mediclinic City Hospital offering adult kidney transplantation.(7) Both programmes attracted expert and highly qualified staff and formed a multidisciplinary team, which further augmented patient access to kidney transplantation across UAE. As of 2018, there are four licensed facilities for organ transplantation in the UAE, Sheikh

Table 24.2 UAE total number of deceased cases from 2017 to May 2019 demographics in UAE

UAE TOTAL number of Deceased Cases from 2017 to May 2019

2017	2018	May 2019	Total
3	8	3	14

UAE number of Donated Deceased Organs from 2017 to May 2019

	Heart	Lungs	Liver	Pancreas	Kidneys	Total
2017	3	3	3	1	3	13
2018	3	4	6	0	7	20
2019	1	1	1	0	3	6
Total	7	8	10	1	13	39

UAE total number of Transplanted Successful cases from 2017 to May 2019

	2017	2018	2019	Total	Percentage
Total	12	66	30	108	100%
Successful	9	58	27	94	87.0%
Unsuccessful	3	8	3	14	13.0%
Percentage of success cases	25.0%	12.1%	10.0%	13.0%	

Khalifa Medical City (SKMC), Cleveland Clinic Hospital (CCAD), Mediclinic (Dubai Healthcare City), and Al Jalila Specialist Hospital for Children. So far, over thirty nationalities have benefitted from the programme (e.g. Emirati, American, Saudi Arabian, Indian, Bangladeshi, Syrian, Jordanian).

In 2014, the Department of Health in Abu Dhabi introduced a comprehensive quality index (Jawda) that measures the quality of healthcare services, patient safety, and patient experience. It is in compliance with the international regulations and according to consistent objectives and quality standards ensuring that the health sector in Abu Dhabi complies with international standards concerning organ donation and organ failure prevention. Organ donation programme specific key performance indicators (KPIs) was introduced in Jawda with plans to expand it to all other emirates that enable the monitoring of performance on donation and transplantation. All hospitals and related healthcare services such as 'future' organ procurement organizations (OPO) are mandated to report their KPIs to ensure adherence to the international best practice. The reporting of Jawda is validated through audit visits and third-party inspections.

Establishment of multi-organ transplant programme

The establishment of CCAD hospital was a key milestone towards building the capacity for the organ transplantation. This was the result of a partnership between Mubadala Healthcare, a government company in Abu Dhabi and the Cleveland Clinic Foundation in Cleveland, Ohio. It began clinical operation in early 2015 with one of the main mandates being the establishment of a comprehensive adult multi-organ transplant centre and an additional capacity for kidney transplant programme. A meticulous and thoughtful collaborative approach identifying key operational needs resulted in the establishment of transplant services within only two and half years of the hospital's opening. Perhaps this was the fastest initiation of a liver, heart, and lung transplant programme within two and a half years in a young hospital.[7]

The first heart transplant was done in UAE at CCAD on 5 December 2017. Since then, a total of eleven heart transplants were done so far with 100% patient and graft survival. Liver transplant programme for both deceased and living donors was initiated at CCAD with the first successful deceased donor liver transplant done in UAE in February 2018 and living related transplant on July 2018. By the end of 2019, a total of seventeen deceased and nine living-related (three right lobe and six left lobe grafts) donor liver transplants were done with 100% graft and patient survival.[7] The first single and double lung transplants were performed at CCAD on 11 February 2018 and 10 June 2018, respectively. A total of ten lung transplants were performed till 2019 (one single and three double) with patient and graft survival of 100%.[7] Establishing the liver, heart, and lung transplant programmes began in the early phase of the hospital activation with early plans which lead to a number of aligning steps being taken such as building an institute model for involved services, and ensuring a high referral base for complex diseases in related fields to care for patients with end-stage organ disease.

Tissue transplantations such as corneas, bones, and valves are already practised in many specialized centres in UAE although these are from external donation sources. Considerations to build capacity for tissue donations and expansion of solid organ transplantations to include pancreas and small bowel are anticipated in the future with the formal establishment of UAE Organ Donation Program (OPO) and needed infrastructure.

Organ donation and transplantation are supported by the Histocompatibility and Immunogenetics laboratory at SEHA which was first established in 1998 to support live-donor renal transplants and to screen Bone Marrow Transplant (BMT) donors and recipients. The laboratory was further expanded in 2008 to provide high-quality services for the newly reestablished kidney transplant programme in Abu Dhabi. In addition, the human leucocyte antigen (HLA) lab does typing by the Luminex-based technology and calculates the panel reactive antibody (PRA) screen and specific HLA class I and Class II single antigen identification in addition to the flow cytometry cross-match for immunological risk- assessment.[12] Currently, the HLA laboratory continues to serve all living and deceased programs in UAE and developed tests based on the HLA phenotypes of the unique multinational UAE population.[13] This is done to assess the sensitization levels in potential transplant recipients and to avoid the possibility of encountering an incompatible donor for transplant recipients. The Histocompatibility and Immunogenicity laboratory is internationally accredited by both the College of American Pathologists (CAP) (since 2010) and the ISO 15189 (since 2017).

GCC collaborative organ procurement programme

The GCC countries share a unified organ donation and transplantation guidebook and have an existing organ sharing scheme. Since the activation of the deceased donation in UAE in 2017, a total of twenty-one deceased donations took place, permitting seventy-nine organ transplantations. Nineteen organs were transplanted in the Kingdom of Saudi Arabia and sixty in UAE. The number of transplanted organs per deceased donation for UAE till 2019 is 3.8.

In UAE, the first deceased donor became a five-organ donor (Figure 24.1). This is a great aspirational goal and key performance indicator target for all programmes as the best international data from International Registry on Organ Donation and Transplantation (IRODaT) (2014) that indicates Norway having the highest ratio of 3.5 transplanted organs per deceased

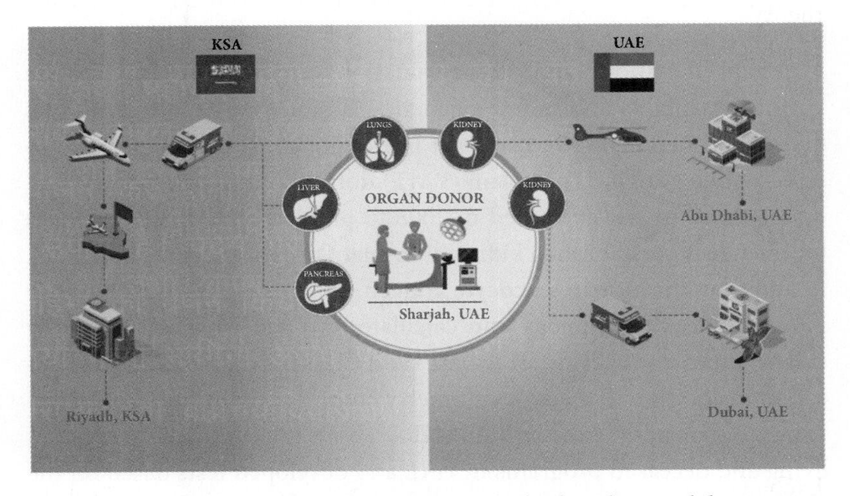

Figure 24.1. Schematic diagram representing the first deceased donation

donor followed by Austria (3.4).[14] Achieving a maximum transplanted organ per deceased donor requires adopting the best organ maintenance practices, addressing logistics of regional collaboration and organ sharing as well as better use of Expanded Criteria Donors (ECD) to increase the donor pool. Most importantly, there is a special value to the family of the deceased to know that their personal loss and tragedy saved the maximum possible number of lives through the great heroic act of their loved one's donation.

Organ donation capacity building

UAE has a positive environment for academic activities hosting a large number of regional and international medical conferences including those related to organ donation and transplantation. Such activities are very important for building human capacity and raising awareness of organ donation and transplantation among the medical community. Key examples include hosting the 'Middle East Society for Organ Transplantation' (MESOT) in 2012 (https://www.mesot-tx.org/history/held.php), 'The Transplantation Society (TTS) workshop on deceased organ donation' in 2018 (https://tts.org/news/tribune-pulse-weekly-newsletter/557-tribune-pulse-march-22-2019-volume-iii-issue-13), and the 'International Society of Organ donation and Procurement' (ISODP) meeting in 2019. In addition, Abu Dhabi was planning to host the 'World Congress of Nephrology' in 2020, canceled due to pandemic. Furthermore, there have been significant training programmes using state of art simulation centres to train physicians, nurses, and allied medical staff on organ donation protocols. Moreover, there have been many capacity building initiatives in collaboration with international centres such as the Donation and Transplantation Institute (DTI) in Spain and others with plans underway to establish an OPO dedicated to organ donation in the country.

With the UAE 2020 vision and transformation plans, the UAE has taken huge leaps in its digital transformation journey and healthcare is no exception. The UAE healthcare has already adopted a digital healthcare and electronic medical records system in most public sector hospitals since the last decade. An advanced and unique Health Information Exchange (HIE) introduced in 2019 will further enable healthcare providers to build efficient care systems by linking all public and private hospitals in a unified database that allows information exchange and democratization of data sharing which could be used for many great initiatives including enhancing organ donation efforts.

In relation to organ donation, a pilot project is initiated to use the digital healthcare database and electronic medical records as a Deceased Alert System (DAS). This is a prospective registry for potential donors with enabled electronic medical records (EMR) decision support and artificial intelligence, and ensures maximum organ donation support is aligned once a referral is triggered. In addition, four major hospitals are supported to reach an accreditation level based on compliance following best international potential organ donation referral and practices in accordance with UAE standardized pathway at each step with the hope of presenting the right to donate to maximum eligible donors' families and increase organ donation rates.

Future perspectives

A UAE unified standardized critical care notification pathway has been created that incorporates support for brain death diagnosis to ensure uniformity of practice and the building of complimentary support services between critical care units and hospitals (Figure 24.2). The applied protocol lays a huge emphasis on the needed support for families to help them understand the prognosis and implication of brain death and provision of second opinion from other ICUs if needed. In cases where families are not living in UAE, if needed relatives are invited, sponsored, and supported to travel to the UAE regardless of their decision to consent for organ donation or not to ensure that they are given all information needed to consider the act of donation and to maintain public trust.

Additionally, our approach emphasizes the importance of early notification with Glasgow Coma Scale (GCS) score of less than 8 to ensure maximum referral and support as needed (Figure 24.3). The total population size in a country and percentage of people dying in hospitals defines the ideal donation after brain death (DBD) potential. Furthermore, it is estimated that 2–4% of hospital deaths, 8–16% of ICU deaths, and 50–60% of deaths with acute cerebral damage could be in the potential DBD

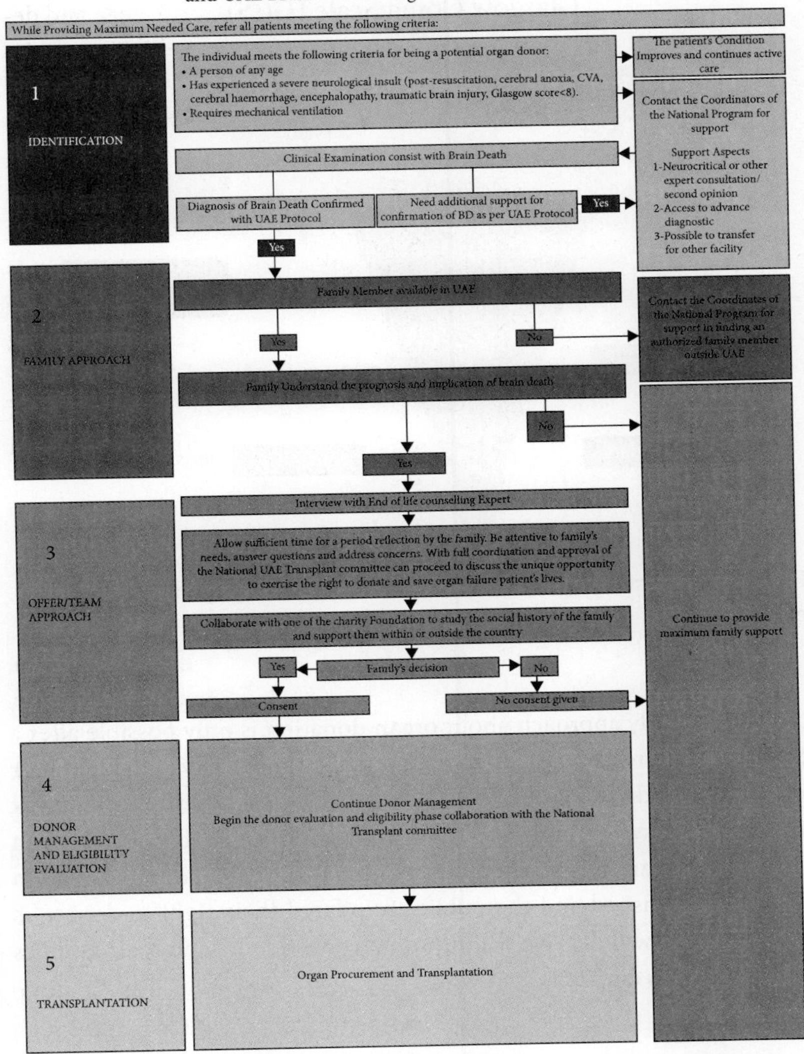

Figure 24.2. Standardized critical care case notification and UAE brain death diagnosis protocol

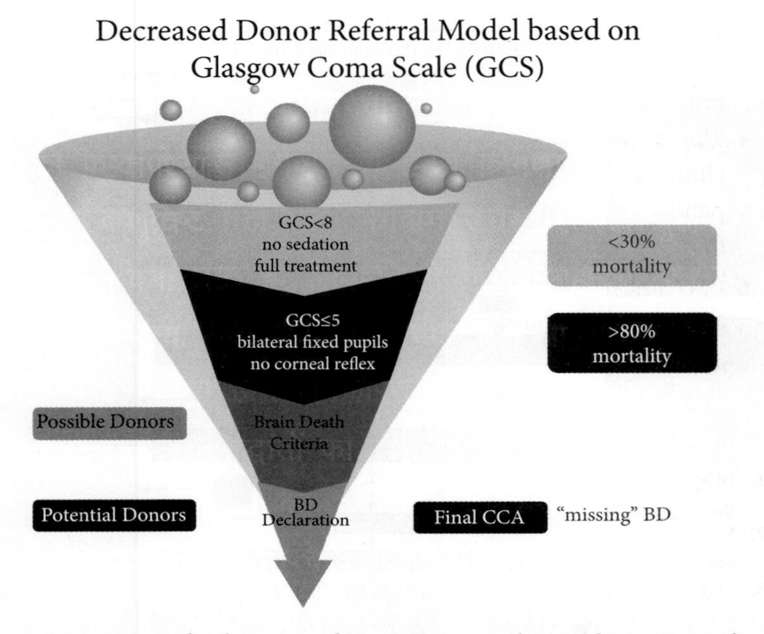

Figure 24.3. Brain death versus Glasgow Coma Scale population/mortality pyramid

category. Family approach about organ donation is only possible after a potential donor becomes an eligible donor (a medically suitable donor who has been declared dead based on neurological criteria). Alignment of the health system and oversight of hospital leadership jointly with OPO support are important factors to ensure that maximum donation potential is grasped and the public are offered their right to donate as misalignment will deprive willing and eligible donors and their families of their right to donate.

Highlights

- A highly developed country such as the UAE has taken substantial strides in healthcare system and delivery including addressing end of life matters and is on the path to achieve self-sufficiency in organ donation soon.

- UAE DBD programme started in 2017 after Federal Law enactment on organ donation in 2016. The first multi-organ transplant from brain deceased donor in the UAE was achieved in 2017.
- The challenges ahead include the expansion of donor pool to include deceased cardiac donation, paired exchange donation, and expanded critical donation which requires the stakeholders alignment for its initiation and proper implementation.
- Another key challenge facing organ donation in UAE is the need for a broader community awareness and engagement.

References

1. https://www.worldometers.info/world-population/united-arab-emirates-population/, accessed November 2020
2. https://uaecabinet.ae/en/details/cabinet-members/his-excellency-sheikh-nahayan-mabarak-al-nahayan, accessed November 2020
3. Hajat C, Harrison O, Al Siksek Z. Weqaya: A population-wide cardiovascular screening program in Abu Dhabi, United Arab Emirates. Am J Public Health. 2012;102: 909–914. doi: 10.2105/AJPH.2011.300290
4. Hajat C, Harrison O, Shather Z. A profile and approach to chronic disease in Abu Dhabi. Glob Health. 2012;8: 18 doi: 10.1186/1744-8603-8-18
5. Alhyas L, McKay A, Balasanthiran A, Majeed A. Prevalences of overweight, obesity, hyperglycaemia, hypertension and dyslipidaemia in the Gulf: Systematic review. JRSM Short Rep. 2011;2: 55 doi: 10.1258/shorts.
6. Saadi H, Carruthers SG, Nagelkerke N, Al-Maskari F, Afandi B, Reed R, et al. Prevalence of diabetes mellitus and its complications in a population-based sample in Al Ain, United Arab Emirates. Diabetes Res Clin Pract. 2007;78: 369–377. doi: 10.1016/j.diabres.
7. Kumar, S, Sankari, BR, Miller, CM, Obaidli, AAKAl, Suri, RM. Establishment of solid organ transplantation in the United Arab Emirates, Transplantation April 2020;104 (4): 659–663.
8. Martin, DE, Van Assche, K, Domínguez-Gil, B, López-Fraga, M, García Gallont, R, Muller, E, Capron, AM. Strengthening global efforts to combat organ trafficking and transplant tourism: Implications of the 2018 edition of the declaration of Istanbul. Transplantation direct, 2019;5(3), e433. doi:10.1097/TXD.0000000000000872
9. Delmonico, Francis L. The implications of Istanbul Declaration on organ trafficking and transplant tourism. Current Opinion in Organ Transplantation: April 2009;14(2): 116–119 doi: 10.1097/MOT.0b013e32832917c9
10. Steering Committee of the Istanbul Summit. Organ trafficking and transplant tourism and commercialism: the Declaration of Istanbul. Lancet. 2008;372(9632):5–6.

11. Parekh J, Ko C, Lappin J, Greenstein S, Hirose R. A Transplant-Specific Quality Initiative-Introducing TransQIP: A Joint Effort of the ASTS and ACS. Am J Transplant. 2017;17(7):1719–1722.
12. Lachmann N, Terasaki PI, Budde K, Liefeldt L, Kahl A, Reinke P, Pratschke J, Rudolph B, Schmidt D, Salama A, Schönemann C. Anti-human leukocyte antigen and donor-specific antibodies detected by luminex posttransplant serve as biomarkers for chronic rejection of renal allografts. Transplantation. 2009;87(10):1505–1513.
13. Valluri V1, Mustafa M, Santhosh A, Middleton D, Alvares M, El Haj E, Gumama O, Abdel-Wareth L. Frequencies of HLA-A, HLA-B, HLA-DR, and HLA-DQ phenotypes in the United Arab Emirates population. Tissue Antigens. 2005;66(2):107–113.
14. IRODaT Preliminary Numbers 2014 (August 2015) https://docplayer.net/49772585-Organ-donation-performance-improvement-measurement-and-kpis.html

25
Organ donation in Turkey

Mehmet Haberal

Historical overview

Solid-organ transplantation in Turkey was first attempted with two heart transplants in 1969. By the early 1970s, experimental studies on liver transplantation in pigs and dogs had already been initiated by our team.[(1)] The first successful living-related renal transplant from a mother to her 12-year-old child was performed by our team at Hacettepe University Hospital on 3 November 1975.[(2)]

In those days, there was no legislation in Turkey governing organ transplantation or organ donation. Throughout the 1980s, the only alternative for transplant candidates on waiting lists in Turkey was grafting from first-degree living-related donors. It was, therefore, necessary to show the public that deceased-donor kidneys could also be used successfully for the treatment of patients, but this could only be possible with organs brought from abroad. In an attempt to make deceased-donor organs available to Turkish patients, the author contacted and worked in cooperation with the Eurotransplant Foundation (Leiden, The Netherlands). The first deceased-donor kidney transplantation was carried out at our centre on 10 October 1978, using an organ supplied by Eurotransplant.[(3)] It is important to note that in those years kidneys were not preserved for more than 12 hours and anything beyond that was considered unusable. However, the kidney received for the first deceased-donor transplant had already undergone more than 24 hours cold ischemia time. Despite the long ischemia time and the organ transported in a simple storage vessel, the surgery was successful and the kidney functioned. This was a breakthrough for the team. Subsequently, a telex was sent to Bernard Cohen and Guido Persijn at Eurotransplant and Gene Pierce at the South-Eastern

Organ Procurement Foundation (Richmond, VA, USA) requesting them to send any kidneys with longer than 12 hours cold-ischemia time.

The organs received from these organ procurement foundations reached us often after having undergone more than 48 hours, and sometimes even more than 100 hours of cold ischemia time and were also anatomically defective. However, we found that deceased-donor kidneys that are well preserved at 4°C, imported with a simple storage system and a warm ischemia time of lower than 5 minutes were still viable and these kidneys could be with a high success rate. We performed more than 100 transplants with these kidneys, and one of our patients survived twenty-five years with the organ that had a cold ischemia time of 110 hours 44 minutes (Figure 25.1).[3,4,5]

Laws on organ transplantation

During the early periods, the absence of laws on organ procurement was a significant barrier to further progress in transplantation activities in Turkey. To overcome this problem, we made attempts to convince members of Parliament, the Presidency of Religious Affairs, and the Ministry of Health that transplantation was a life-saving procedure worth developing. Our efforts became successful and law on organ and tissue transplantation was drafted and passed on 3 June 1979.[6,7,8,9] This law was deemed to be used as a model by many countries. Immediately afterwards, on 27 June, our team performed the first local deceased-donor kidney transplantation.[10]

We also worked with the Turkish public to provide education about the benefits, and social responsibilities involved in organ donation. In addition, we founded the Turkish Organ Transplantation and Burn Treatment Foundation on 4 September 1980, to advance these interests. Organ Donation Cards were printed as well, with the aim to promote organ donation and bring this concept to life in people's minds (Figure 25.2).

On 21 January 1982, an addendum was made to Law 2238 with the passing of Law 2594, which allowed for deceased donation without consent in cases where next-of-kin does not exist or cannot be located, and the termination of life has taken place as a result of an accident or natural death.[6]

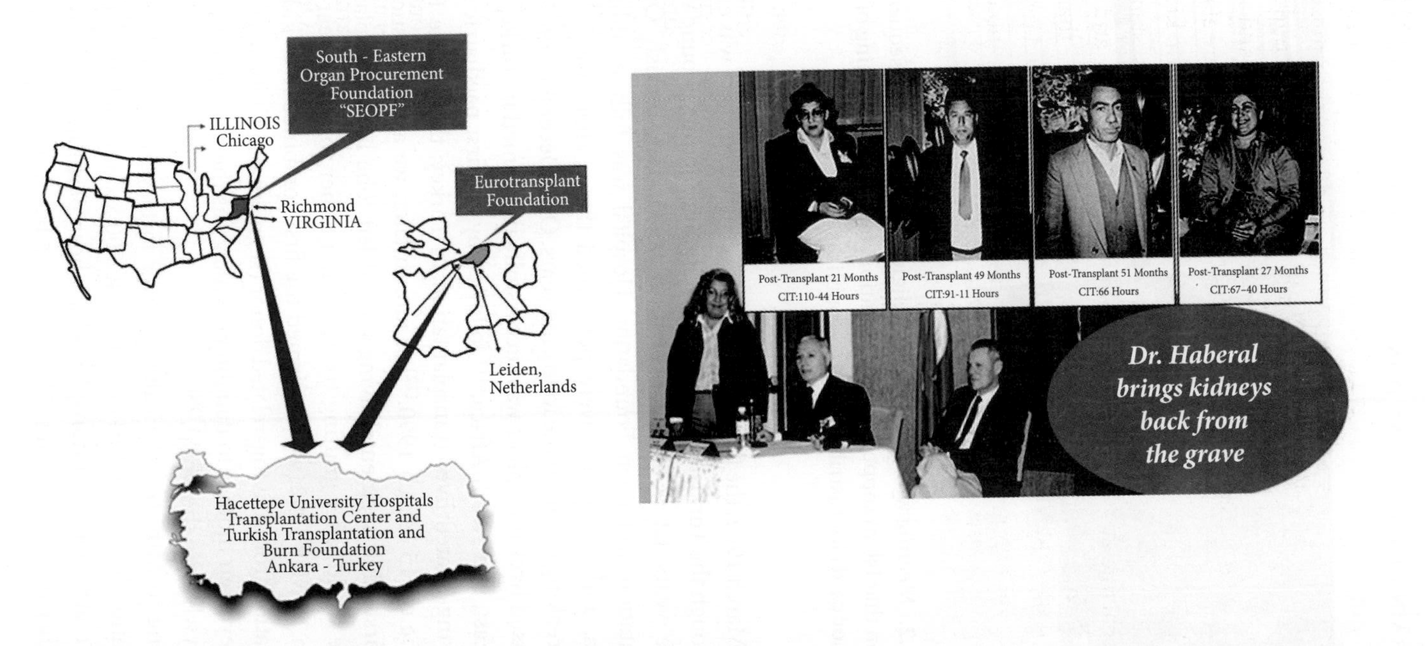

Figure 25.1. Patients who received organs from Eurotransplant

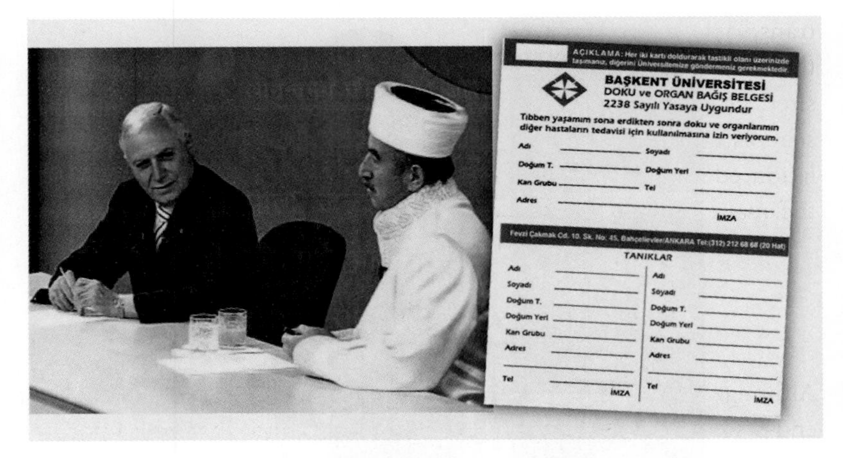

Figure 25.2. Meeting with President of Religious Affairs and subsequent declaration that Islam supports organ donation, followed by printing of organ donor cards for distribution to the public

On 12 March 1982, the first haemodialysis centre in Ankara was established through the Turkish Organ Transplantation and Burn Foundation. Just three years later, on 16 September 1985, the Turkish Organ Transplantation and Burn Foundation Hospital was fully established in Ankara, and transplants were performed there. There were many ground-breaking events in the following years. On 8 December 1988, the first deceased liver transplant was successfully performed in Turkey, the Middles East, and North Africa,[(11)] followed by the first paediatric segmental living-related liver transplantation in Turkey, the Middle East, and Europe on 15 March 1990.[(12)] A month later, we achieved success with the first adult segmental living-related left-lobe liver transplantation in the world, after grafting tissue from a father to his 22-year-old son.[(13)] On 16 May 1992, we performed the first combined liver-kidney transplantation from a living-related donor (segmental left-lobe liver and right kidney from mother to daughter), which was the first operation of its kind anywhere in the world.[(14)]

According to Ministry of Health, in over forty years of solid organ transplantation history in Turkey, almost 40,000 kidney, and more than 14,000 liver and 1000 heart transplants have been performed nationwide in over eighty different centres (77 kidneys, 46 livers, 16 hearts, 4 lungs transplant centres). Transplantation activities are accelerating day by day throughout the country, but deceased donors are still far below the desired rates. Efforts to increase awareness continue through the media, schools, and many public and private institutions. Improvements in legislation, education, and coordination are the primary factors for improving the quality and the number of transplantation activities in Turkey.

Current status of organ donation in Turkey

Although organ transplantation has become the treatment of choice for end-stage organ disease, it is essential to recognize that with improved outcomes, the number of transplant candidates has also increased. Unfortunately, there is insufficient supply to meet the demand, and organ shortage has become the most significant challenge facing the field of organ transplantation today. This shortage of organs is particularly true for countries in the Middle East, Africa, and Mid Asia, where deceased donation rates are very low or, as in some regions, non-existent.

Organ transplantation is possible through two sources: (1) transplantation from deceased donors after determination of either brain death or circulatory death; (2) living donors. Living donor organ transplantation is generally a safe practice that is acceptable as long as it is performed within ethical and legal boundaries. However, the widespread acceptance of living donation means live donors carry much of the burden of organ transplantation.

The vast majority of organ transplants in Turkey are from living donors, with most of these organs typically coming from first- and second-degree family members (although the law allows living transplantation from family members up to and including the fourth degree and spouses). In recent years, paired organ exchange has also been initiated with excellent results.

Transplantation activity in Turkey is among the highest in the world. The 2016 Global Observatory on Donation and Transplantation (GODT) data reveals that Turkey is within the top twenty most active countries in transplantation in the world with a total organ transplantation rate of 62 per million population (pmp).[(15)] In addition, the 2017 figures collected by the International Registry in Organ Donation and

Transplantation and published in December 2018 shows that Turkey has the highest rate of worldwide living donor transplants with a rate of 47.49 pmp.[16] In 2018 alone, 5597 organ transplants (3871 kidneys, 1588 livers and 91 hearts transplants) were performed in Turkey.[17] Based on these numbers, it is clear that Turkey is very active in organ transplantation.

However, it is insufficient to meet the demand for organs. As of April 2019, more than 26,000 patients are on the waiting list for organs, with 22,670 patients need a kidney, 2184 a liver, and 1114 a heart.[17] Despite the high number of living donor organ transplants that are taking place each year in Turkey, it is in no way sufficient to meet the demand for organs. Besides, those waiting for a heart have no option other than deceased donation.

Further data by the International Registry on Organ Donation and Transplantation (IRODaT) reveal that deceased donation rates are suffering in comparison to living donation. Figure 25.3 shows the actual living and deceased donor kidney and liver transplants performed in Turkey in 2018.[18] The picture clearly demonstrates that living donor transplantation constitutes about three-quarters of all kidney and liver transplants in Turkey today.

2018	Kidney (n = 3870)	Liver (n = 1588)
Deceased	859	438
Living	3011	1150

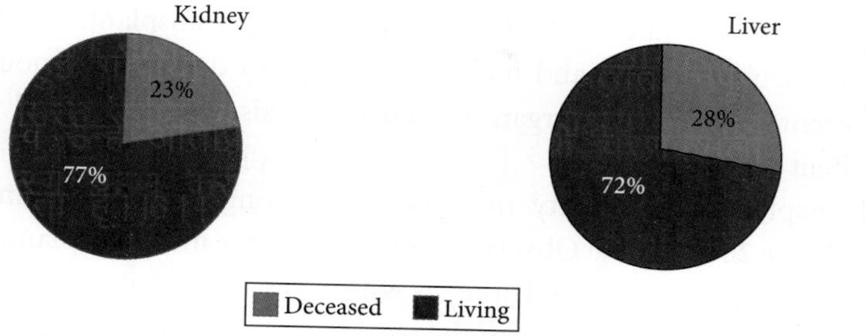

Figure 25.3. Comparison of living and deceased organ transplant rates in Turkey in 2018

The council of Europe published a similar report with the data collected in 2017, which showed the transplantation rates (pmp) in Turkey for kidney transplants from all sources (41.4), living donors (32.8), and deceased donors (1.5).[(19)] These rates are unfortunately significantly lower than many other countries in Europe and the USA.

Increasing deceased donation rates has been a priority in our country for many decades. Our team initiated a national organ sharing programme in 1989, which facilitated the distribution of organs nationwide and improved communication among the transplantation centres, thereby increasing the number of deceased-donor organ transplants. Later, in 2001, the 'National Organ and Tissue Transplantation Coordination System' was set up under the control and coordination of the Ministry of Health. The objective of this system is to ensure that, with fair allocation and in conformity with scientific rules and medical ethics, organs and tissues from deceased donors are matched to the most suitable patients and delivered to the transplantation centres in the shortest time possible.

These efforts have made some impact on donation rates. Official Ministry of Health figures show that deceased donation rates have increased 5-fold from 111 donations in 2011 to 598 in 2018 (Figure 25.4).[20]

Nevertheless, deceased donation rates are far lower than where they potentially could be. In 2018, 2178 deceased donors were reported, and of these only 598 received approval from the next-of-kin for transplantation. This report indicated that just over a third of viable deceased donor organs are being transplanted into patients on the waiting lists. It is clear that apart from the identification of potential deceased donors, the real issue lies with receiving consent for the organs from next-of-kin.

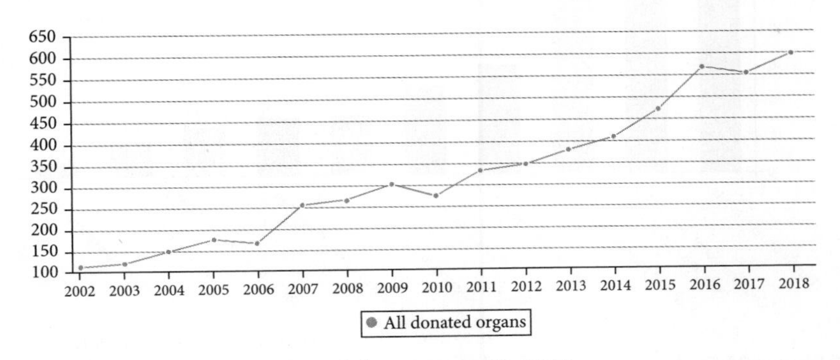

Figure 25.4. Rates of deceased donation 2002–2018.

These numbers show the sad reality of deceased donation rates in our country, which are in stark contrast to the transplant activity and the rates of living donation that support it. It is, therefore, crucial to identify barriers to consent and analyse the attitudes of the families towards donation.

Challenges

In recent years, limited organ availability has become one of the major problems in organ transplantation. Lack of donors is a significant problem for organ transplantation on a global scale, not only faced by Turkey.

Multiple steps in the process of deceased organ donation can be targeted to increase the number of organs suitable for transplant, from the ICU specialist to the transplant coordinator to the next of kin. There is a recognized need for both health professionals and members of the community to become better educated about donation and transplantation. In particular, public attitudes about organ donation and volunteerism are essential factors in the lack of donors. A study performed by the Ministry of Health identified that the biggest obstacle standing in the way of deceased donations in Turkey is family disagreements (Figure 25.5).

Although socio-cultural reasons continue to play a role in donation decisions all around the world, since the Presidency of Religious Affairs in

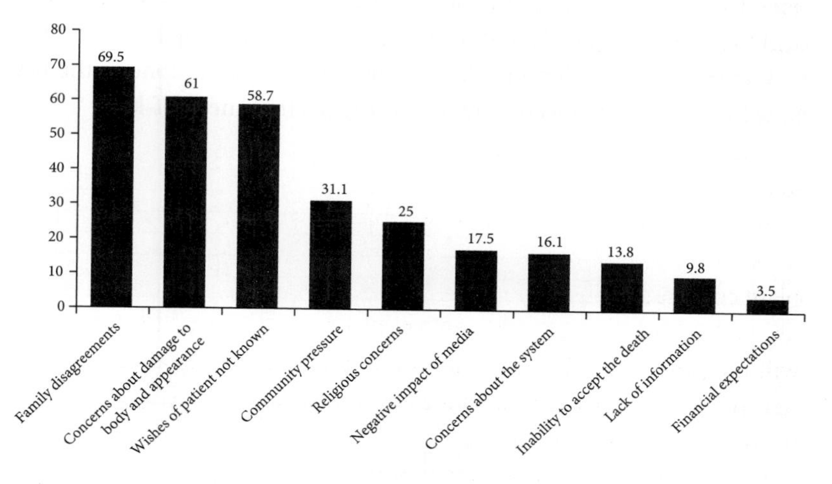

Figure 25.5. Reasons for refusal to donate

Turkey voiced its support for organ donation in the late 1970s, this is no longer an issue of vast proportion. The problem lies in the lack of knowledge about the procedure and what it means for the donor and the recipient. With social awareness projects (through use of the media, classes in schools, etc.), as well as more vigorous efforts to promote the use of donor cards, the low rates of deceased donation can be increased considerably.

Future perspectives

The successful melding of legal, ethical, medical, social, psychological, technological, economical, and religious aspects is mandatory for any transplantation organization. It is nearly impossible to create or run an effective system without regard for all these components.

In recent years, limited organ availability has become one of the major problems in organ transplantation. Each country has a responsibility to assess the transplantation needs of its people and, as such, the goal that we must strive for is the establishment of self-sufficiency regarding organ donation and procurement. This lack of deceased donors is a particularly significant problem for organ transplantation in Turkey and the region as a whole. But there is considerable effort to turn this around as can be seen in Shiraz, Iran, where they have succeeded in establishing deceased donation programmes that rival those in Europe and the rest of the world.

We must realize that thousands of our citizens die each year with healthy organs that are not donated and are therefore unable to provide the opportunity for transplant to many patients with end-stage organ failure.

Although living donation can be a safe and acceptable source of organs if performed within ethical and legal guidelines, our aim as the transplant community should now be to work towards a system of meeting the organ demand as much as possible with a deceased donation. This action will not only result in the reduction of unethical transplantation activities. It will also make an enormous difference to those patients awaiting transplants in which living organ donors are not an option.

It is essential to support ongoing educational, legal, regulatory, ethical, and public health challenges in collaboration with the Ministries of

Health and Education, as well as national medical societies related to and involved in transplantation to achieve these goals.

Among our primary concerns must be the means of meeting the growing demand for organs through ethical organ donation and procurement, and promoting scientific understanding and equality in standards of clinical practice and patient care. Transparency must be ensured in transplantation activities, and educational programmes are required to meet the needs of transplant programmes in our country.

Highlights

- Organ transplantation started in Turkey in 1975, and since 1979 these activities are being carried out within a medical, legal, and ethical framework established by laws 2238 and 2594, as well as various directives set out by the Ministry of Health.
- Today, there are over eighty transplant centres in Turkey authorized for kidney, liver, heart, and lung transplants. Thousands of organ transplants that are performed each year in these centres making Turkey one of the most active countries in transplantation as well as the country with the highest rate of living-donor organ transplants in the world.
- Organ Transplantation legislation in Turkey permits living donation from relatives up to the fourth degree, spouses, paired kidney exchange, and deceased donation.
- Unfortunately, deceased donation has suffered dramatically with >70% of kidney and liver transplants being performed from living-related donors.
- National Organ and Tissue Transplantation Coordination System has been set up under the control and coordination of the Ministry of Health in order to increase deceased donation. Despite a fivefold increase in deceased donation rates since 2001, the numbers are still below the desired rates.
- Support for organ donation by religious leaders, social awareness projects (through use of the media, classes in schools, etc.), as well as more vigorous efforts to promote the use of donor cards can be effective in significantly increasing the rates of deceased donation.

References

1. Haberal M, Bilgin N, Sanac Y, et al. Köpekte baypas kullanilmadan yapilan ortotopik karaciger homotransplantasyonu. Hacettepe Tip Cerrahi Bülteni. 1972;5:462.
2. Haberal M, Sert S, Aybasti N, et al. Living donor kidney transplantation. Transplant Proc. 1988;20(1 Suppl 1):353.
3. Haberal M, Oner Z, Karamehmetoglu M, et al. Cadaver kidney transplantation with cold ischemia time from 48 to 95 hours. Transplant Proc. 1984;16(5):1330–1332.
4. Haberal M, Aybasti N, Arslan G, Bilgin N. Cadaver kidney transplantation cases with a cold ischemia time of more than 100 hours. Clin Transpl. 1986:126–127.
5. Haberal M, Moray G, Bilgin N, Karakayali H, Arslan G, Büyükpamukçu N. Ten-year survival after a cold-ischemia time of 111 hours in the transplanted kidney. Transplant Proc. 1996;28(4):2333.
6. http://www.lawsturkey.com/law/2238-organ-transplantation-law. Accessed 19 April 2019.
7. Haberal M, Kaynaroğlu V, Bilgin N. Ethics in organ procurement in Turkey. Int J Artif Organs. 1992;15(5):261–263.
8. Haberal M, Moray G, Karakayali H, Bilgin N. Ethical and legal aspects, and the history of organ transplantation in Turkey. Transplant Proc. 1996;28(1):382–383.
9. Haberal M, Moray G, Karakayali H, Bilgin N. Transplantation legislation and practice in Turkey: A brief history. Transplant Proc. 1998;30(7):3644–3646.
10. Haberal M, Demirağ A, Cohen B, et al. Cadaver kidney transplantation in Turkey. Transplant Proc. 1995 Oct;27(5):2768–2769.
11. Haberal M, Tokyay R, Telatar H, et al. Living related and cadaver donor liver transplantation. Transplant Proc. 1992;24(5):1967–1969.
12. Haberal M, Büyükpamukçu N, Bilgin N, et al. Segmental living related liver transplantation in pediatric patients. Transplant Proc. 1994;26(1):183–184.
13. Haberal M, Buyukpamukcu N, Telatar H, et al. Segmental living liver transplantation in children and adults. Transplant Proc. 1992;24(6):2687–2689.
14. Haberal M, Abbasoğlu O, Büyükpamukçu N, et al. Combined liver-kidney transplantation from a living-related donor. Transplant Proc. 1993;25(3):2211–2213.
15. GODT organ donation and transplantation activities 2016 report. File:///c:/users/rektorluk/downloads/datos%202016fw.pdf. Accessed 22 April 2019.
16. International Registry in Organ Donation and Transplantation 2017 Newsletter. http://www.irodat.org/img/database/pdf/IRODaT%20Newsletter%202017.pdf. Accessed 22 April 2019.
17. Ministry of Health Blood, Organ and Tissue Transplantation Services website organ transplant data. https://organ.saglik.gov.tr/0TR/70Istatistik/OrganNakilIstatistikKamusal.aspx. Accessed 19 April, 2019.
18. International Registry in Organ Donation and Transplantation Turkey data. http://www.irodat.org/?p=database&c=TR#data. Accessed 22 April 2019.

19. *EDQM Newsletter Transplant: International figures on donation and transplantation 2017*. Volume 23, 2018.
20. Ministry of Health Blood, Organ and Tissue Transplantation Services website organ donation data. https://organ.saglik.gov.tr/0TR/70Istatistik/OrganBagisIstatistikKamusal.aspx. Accessed 19 April 2019.

26

Organ donation in Iran

Seyed Ali Malek-Hosseini, Farrokh Habibzadeh

Brief historical overview

The first organ transplantation performed in Iran in 1967 was a live donor kidney transplant at Namazi Hospital in Shiraz, Southern Iran.[1] Later on, transplantation progressed slowly. Some of the wealthy patients, who could afford the expenses incurred, went abroad to receive living-related transplants; though the outcomes were commonly poor. A total of 114 renal transplantations was performed before the 1979 Iranian Revolution.[2] The Revolution and the Iran-Iraq war retarded the already slow pace; only a few attempts were made to move transplantation forward.

The Iranian government established the 'paid living-unrelated donation' model in 1988 and started the programme first in Tehran.[2] The model soon gained acceptance by almost all kidney transplant centres in the country. The Shiraz transplant centre, nonetheless, adopted another policy and emphasized on 'deceased donation'.[3] The transplant community (and the transplant centres) divided into two parties—those mostly in favour of paid living-unrelated donation and those practising in Shiraz emphasizing deceased donation.

Current status of organ donation in Iran

Transplantation depends crucially on the availability of transplant organs. Because of organ donor shortage, 10–30% of patients with end-stage organ disease on organ transplantation waitlist die.[4] The only countries in the world where paid donation is allowed are Iran, Singapore, and Saudi Arabia.[5] Although the paid-donation model, first established by Iran government in 1988, is the only known system that could eliminate the kidney waitlist, the financial incentives for organ donation including the direct monetary relations between the donor and recipient have raised specific ethical concerns.[6]

The US economic sanctions and organ donation

Although the US economic sanctions imposed on Iran were not supposed to affect the health of Iranian people, it has caused serious health problems.[7] The altruistic motives are not the only reason for organ donation in Iran.[8] The chronic economic crisis and inflation in Iran, mainly caused by long-lasting sanctions imposed on the country, and the relatively high unemployment rate have led some poor people to donate their organs.[6] More than four-fifth of the paid organ donors, but only half of the recipients, belong to low socio-economic groups.[2,9] In a recent study on donors in Iran, almost 70% of paid living-unrelated kidney donors interviewed mentioned that poverty was an important reason to donate their organs.[10] However, no evidence of coercion or imposed pressure on women to be potential donors was reported; there were no prisoners or mentally impaired donors. Despite false accusations suggesting that Iran retrieves organs from executed prisoners, herein, we affirm that there have not been and will not be organs procured from executed prisoners in Iran. This is strictly illegal in Iran.[11]

Pros and *cons* of the paid-donation model

The system works well anyway, and both recipients and donors look happy. Almost all recipients are glad they were given the opportunity to pay for the organ instead of waiting in a long waitlist; and many donors are happy to legally earn enough money to solve part of their problems, though they regret not asking for more.[6] Some authors believe that if there were no financial incentives, many transplantation centres would collapse.[8,12]

The inconvenient truth, however, is that most of the paid donors are, indeed, afflicted in this process. Almost all of them prefer not to be identified as organ donors for the fear of experiencing social stigma of selling their organs.[6, 8, 10] Most of them do not have satisfactory education to realize the complications associated with nephrectomy.[2] According to the law, the paid donors are provided health insurance only for one year. Most of them are not even aware that they would need a longer follow-up, perhaps life-long. Paid living-unrelated donors have usually a significantly lower-than-normal quality of life; microalbuminuria develops in more than a third of paid living-unrelated but none of the living-related donors.[5]

The programme, although, supposed to be strictly monitored by the government, has only been partly regulated and found to be open to abuse. The paid-donor model was supposed to help only those patients with no living-related donor. However, it came out that more than 80% of the recipients had a potentially living-related donor at the time of transplantation and that they received paid-donation merely because they could afford it.[13] Another problem is the possible direct monetary relationship between the donor and recipient without any safeguard against mediation of organ brokers, even transplant tourism. There are many reports of non-Iranian patients from Iraq, Saudi Arabia, Azerbaijan, and other countries who tried to pay to receive organs from Iranian donors using forged documents.[2]

Deceased donation programme at Shiraz

While other transplant centres in Iran mainly focused on a paid living-unrelated donation, the transplant team at Shiraz was exploring every avenue towards the establishment of a deceased-donor programme.[3] Paying too much attention to paid living-unrelated donation and the incentives offered to donors further hampered the development of deceased donation in other centres.

After overcoming numerous daunting challenges, deceased donation has become fully operational in Shiraz since 2000 after the necessary religious edicts and legislations had been issued. The rate of liver transplant from deceased donors in Shiraz has increased exponentially from 0.2 donations per million people (pmp) in 2000 to more than 11 donations pmp in 2017, representing an average annual growth rate of 21% (Figure 26.1). A parallel, exponential increasing trend can also be seen in the number of liver transplantations performed at Shiraz centre. With the acceptable religious decrees obtained and the necessary legal legislations into effect on one hand, and the problems of paid living-unrelated donations mentioned, on the other hand, the deceased donation has become more prevalent in other centres too (Figure 26.2). Nearly, all transplantations performed in Shiraz have had deceased donors (Figure 26.3). Contribution of living liver transplant donors has declined from 25% in

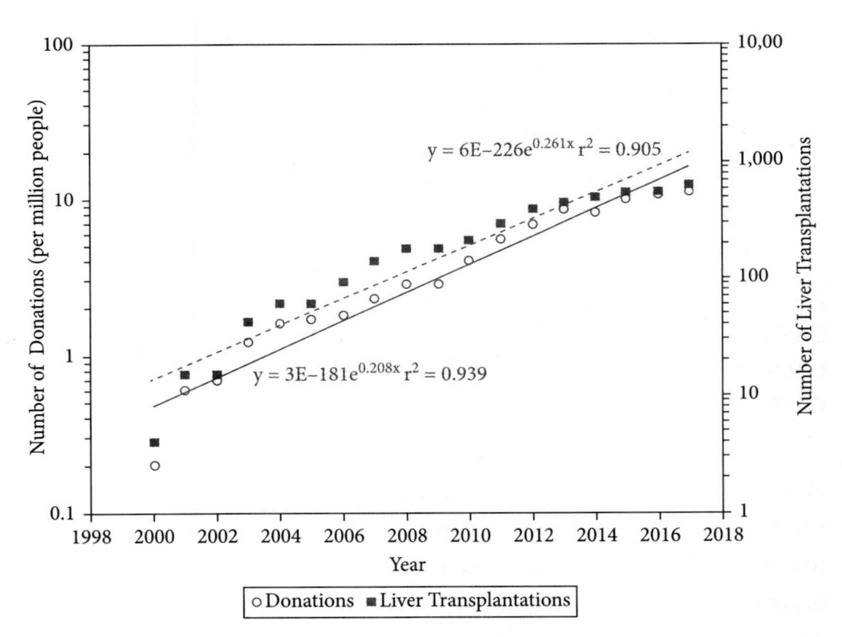

Figure 26.1. Trends of organ donation (open circles), mostly deceased donations, and liver transplantations performed in Shiraz Transplant Center (solid squares) between 2000 and 2017. Both vertical axes have logarithmic scale, meaning that the trends for the number of organ donations (solid line) and liver transplantations (dashed lines) are indeed exponential with average annual growth rates of 21% and 26%, respectively. The two lines are parallel reflecting the obvious dependency of transplantations on donor availability

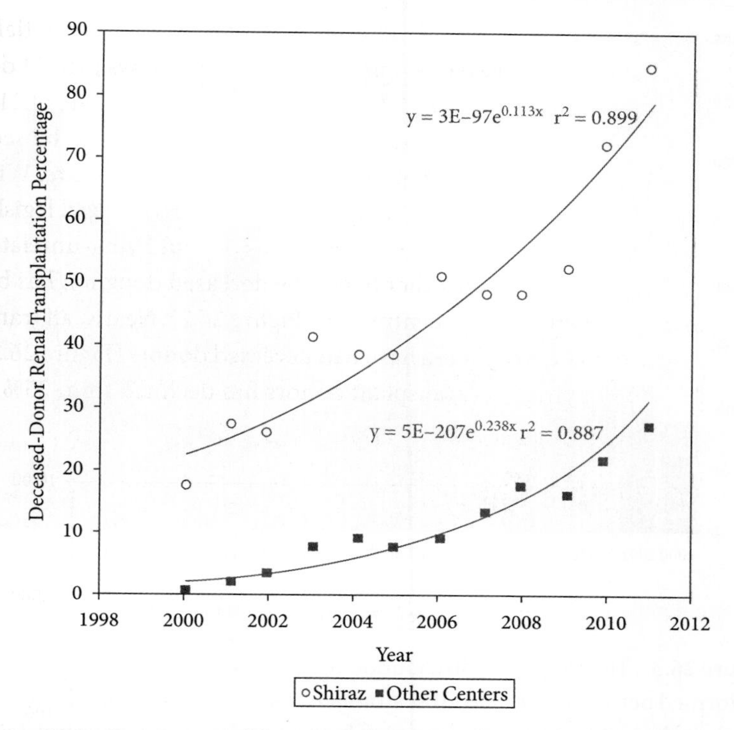

Figure 26.2. Percentage of deceased-donor renal transplantation from 2000 to 2011 in Shiraz Transplant Center and other centres in Iran. Note the exponentially increasing trend in the percentage of deceased donation in all centres over the time

2000 to almost 8% in 2017.[3] This decrease would not have been possible, however, without tireless work of not-for-profit organizations that manage to raise public awareness about deceased donation. One of these organizations, very active in Iran since 2015, is *Nafas*, literally meaning 'breath'.

Organ donation rate in Iran

The mean organ donation rate in Iran is 11.7 donations pmp. The rate has increased over the past two decades throughout the country.[14] However, it varies significantly from place to place from a maximum

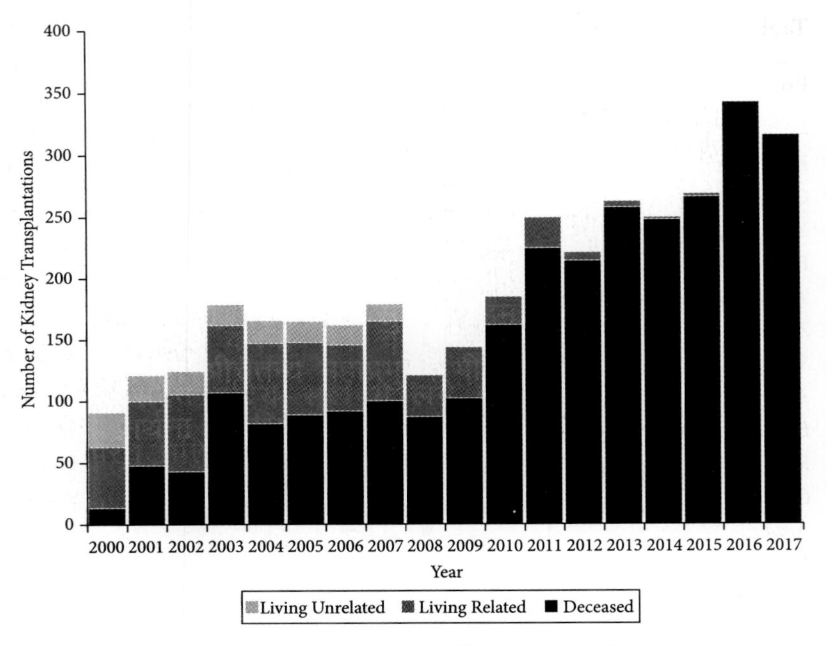

Figure 26.3. The frequency distribution of kidney transplantations performed between 2000 and 2017 stratified by type of donation. The trend is although increasing, the frequency of living-unrelated and living-related donors had substantially decreased—no living-unrelated donation since 2008; living-related donations have become a rarity since 2016. In clear contrast to what is practiced in many other centres in the region, Shiraz Transplant Center only relies on deceased donation

of 35 donations pmp in *Kohgiluyeh va Boyer-Ahmad* province, Western Iran, to none in *Hormozgan*, Southern Iran, based on 2018 statistics (Table 26.1). *Hormozgan*, nonetheless, has become active since early 2019.

With an increasing rate of deceased donor procurements, a reliable transport system had to be established to quickly transfer the procured organs from any hospital in Iran to another. Iran is divided into seven zones. *Fars* province (the capital of which is Shiraz) and its five neighbouring provinces have the highest average deceased organ donation rate of 20 pmp; Tehran zone (11 provinces) with 15 pmp ranks second in the country.[3] Undoubtedly, the success of Shiraz could not have been

Table 26.1 Population and donation rates in 31 provinces of Iran in 2018

Province	Population ($\times 10^6$)	Donors per million people
Kohgiluyeh va Boyer-Ahmad	0.7	34.93
Chaharmahal va Bakhtiari	0.9	28.75
Yazd	1.1	26.00
Fars	4.9	23.40
Tehran	13.3	21.63
Zanjan	1.1	19.05
Semnan	0.7	17.14
Alborz	2.7	16.61
Bushehr	1.2	15.52
Razavi Khorasan	6.4	15.40
Qom	1.3	13.95
Ardabil	1.3	13.39
Isfahan	5.1	10.74
Mazandaran	3.3	9.45
Guilan	2.5	8.30
Hamedan	1.7	8.09
Kerman	3.2	7.59
South Khorasan	0.8	6.49
North Khorasan	0.9	5.81
Kermanshah	2.0	5.13
Ghazvin	1.3	4.72
Ilam	0.6	3.45
West Azerbaijan	3.3	3.37
Golestan	1.9	3.23
Khuzestan	4.7	3.18
East Azerbaijan	3.9	2.56
Markazi	1.4	2.10
Lorestan	1.8	1.70
Kurdistan	1.6	0.63
Sistan va Baluchestan	2.8	0.36
Hormozgan	1.8	0.00

Source: Iranian Society for Organ Transplantation

possible without its enthusiastic transplant coordinators and their painstaking efforts in identifying brain-dead donors and convincing their relatives to grant permission for organ donation.[3] Shiraz Transplant Center is now one of the most active centres and the largest liver transplant facility (in terms of volume) in the world.[3]

Types of solid transplants performed in Iran

Although in the early days, more emphasis was placed on kidney and liver transplantations, various types of solid organ transplantations (heart, lung, pancreas, intestine, etc.) are nowadays routinely performed in many transplant centres of Iran.[15] For instance, Shiraz Transplant Center performs a wide variety of transplantations (Figure 26.4).

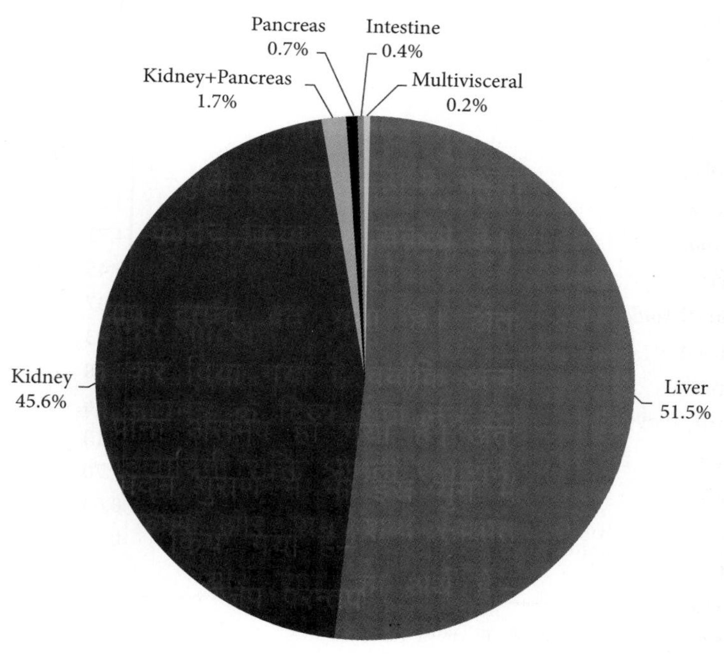

Figure 26.4. Relative frequency distribution of various types of transplantations performed between 1993 and late 2018 at Shiraz Transplant Center

Challenges

Among the important barriers, we had to overcome at the beginning, were lack of financial support due to severe economic depression after a prolonged devastating war; severe shortage of dialysis facilities across the country; shortage of available space including hospital beds, well-equipped operation rooms; lack of qualified supporting units (e.g. gastro-enterology, radiology, and immunopathology); lack of trained transplant staff including surgeons, physicians, coordinators, and nurses; lack of transportation facilities such as private plane and even a well-equipped ambulance; and finally lack of awareness of the 'brain death' entity, even among the well-educated people.

All these problems have been solved satisfactorily through entering into negotiations with charity foundations. These organizations raise money for establishing well-equipped dialysis centres and healthcare facilities; training enthusiastic transplant surgeons, anaesthesiologists, nephrologists, gastroenterologists, pathologists, and nurses to organise an efficient transplant team; and establishing a national procurement network consisting of seven zones to arrange for smooth transfer of the procured organs among centres. In addition, the organizations are also involved in promoting awareness among people through holding meetings at universities, hospitals, high schools, and contacting eminent scholars and celebrities for support.

For deceased donation, the situation was much more complicated. One of the main challenges deceased donation faced with then was significant religious and legal issues about providing an operational definition for death, not required for living donation for obvious reasons.(16) Islam, the prevailing religion in Iran, does not give any verdict on the exact time the soul separates from the body, hence, on the exact time of death. Islam respects a dead body. Saving a life is also highly respected in Islam. Therefore, it was expected that the religious authorities could be convinced to give the necessary decrees for deceased donation if the importance of organ donation and transplantation was communicated convincingly.(3) After delicate multilateral negotiations, the decrees on brain death were finally issued by the clergy in 1989, and the legislation on brain death and organ transplantation was ultimately passed by the Iranian parliament in 2000.(3, 16) Thereafter, deceased donation has progressed at a high pace and the number of deceased donations and transplantations has had an exponential increasing trend.

Another serious problem faced is the transplant tourism. Although against the law, there were many private healthcare centres that performed this illegal act. The recent law passed prohibiting transplantation in private healthcare centres was meant to control this illegal, unethical practice.

Future perspectives

Considering the extensive experience we have in Shiraz Transplant Center, particularly in deceased-donation model and liver transplantation, we have been sharing our knowledge with other centres in Iran and abroad. Every year, we train many fellow surgeons and nurses from local, national, and regional transplant centres.[3] So far, we have witnessed unparalleled success. Nowadays, we have good active dialysis centres in many remote cities. Transplantation teams are also active in most centres of Iran.

Currently, the transplant team approaches only one-third of brain-dead patients' families to obtain their consent to grant permission for transplantation.[3] It has been shown that adopting a more active practice of identification of brain-dead patients would not only increase the number of organs donated, but also improve the chance of obtaining consent from the patient's family.[4] Further efforts should therefore be made in effective training of transplant coordinators in communication skills. More research should also be done into identifying the motivation of Iranian families with brain-dead patients to agree to donate their organs for transplantation. Finally, we will try our best to totally eliminate the paid living-unrelated donation, which is unethical in our view, and replace it completely with deceased-donation, paired-donation, and domino-donation models. In paired-donation living donors are not compatible with their recipients; however, the donor in each pair is compatible with the recipient of another pair. Under such a circumstance, if both living donors and recipients agree, a paired-donation can be considered. Domino-donation is more complicated and involves more than two pairs of donors and recipients. It may happen in various ways and get very complicated and involve many pairs of living donors and recipients across a country or even continent; it may involve a volunteer living donor who begins the domino and donates organ based on altruistic motives. Just imagine a world where nobody becomes that desperate to sell a part of his or her body.

Highlights

- The Iranian government established the 'paid living-unrelated donation' model, the only known system that could eliminate the kidney waitlist.
- Parallel to the paid living-unrelated donation model, Shiraz adopted deceased-donation model, which has become fully operational after the necessary religious edicts and legislations have been issued.
- Having an exponentially increasing trend in the number of deceased donations, the model has gained acceptance in other centres too.
- The mean organ donation rate in Iran is 11.7 donations per million people.
- Efforts should be made to eliminate the paid living-unrelated donation and replace it with deceased-donation, pair-donation, and domino-donation models.

References

1. Saidi RF, Broumand B. Current challenges of kidney transplantation in Iran: Moving beyond the 'Iranian Model'. Transplantation. 2018 Aug;102(8):1195–1197. DOI: 10.1097/TP.0000000000002212.
2. Ghahramani N. Paid living donation and growth of deceased donor programs. Transplantation. 2016 Jun;100(6):1165–1169. DOI: 10.1097/TP.0000000000001164.
3. Malek-Hosseini SA, Habibzadeh F, Nikeghbalian S. Shiraz organ transplant center: The largest liver transplant center in the world. Transplantation. 2019 Aug;103(8):1523–1525. DOI: 10.1097/TP.0000000000002581.
4. Sadegh Beigee F, Mohsenzadeh M, Shahryari S, Mojtabaee M. Role of more active identification of brain-dead cases in increasing organ donation. Exp Clin Transplant. 2017 Feb;15(Suppl 1):60–62. DOI: 10.6002/ect.mesot2016.O42.
5. Bruzzone P. Paid organ donation: An Italian perspective. Transplant Proc. 2015 Sep;47(7):2109–2112. DOI: 10.1016/j.transproceed.2015.01.032.

6. Hamidian Jahromi A, Fry-Revere S, Bastani B. A revised Iranian model of organ donation as an answer to the current organ shortage crisis. Iran J Kidney Dis. 2015 Sep;9(5):354–360.
7. Habibzadeh F. Economic sanction: A weapon of mass destruction. Lancet. 2018 Sep 8;392(10150):816–817. DOI: 10.1016/S0140-6736(18)31944-5.
8. Ghods AJ. Governed financial incentives as an alternative to altruistic organ donation. Exp Clin Transplant. 2004 Dec;2(2):221–228.
9. Ghods AJ, Savaj S. Iranian model of paid and regulated living-unrelated kidney donation. Clin J Am Soc Nephrol. 2006 Nov;1(6):1136–1145. DOI: 10.2215/CJN.00700206.
10. Fry-Revere S, Chen D, Bastani B, Golestani S, Agarwal R, Kugathasan H, et al. Coercion, dissatisfaction, and social stigma: An ethnographic study of compensated living kidney donation in Iran. Int Urol Nephrol. 2020 Dec;52(12):2403–2414. DOI: 10.1007/s11255-018-1824-y.
11. Habibzadeh F, Malek-Hosseini SA. Retrieving organs of executed prisoners in Iran? Transplantation. 2020 Jun;104(6):e185. DOI: 10.1097/TP.0000000000003116.
12. Mahoney JD. Should we adopt a market strategy to organ donation? In: Shelton W, Balint J (ed.) The Ethics of Organ Transplantation. Amsterdam: Elsevier Science Ltd; 2001. p. 65.
13. Ghahramani N, Rizvi SA, Padilla B. Paid donation: A global view. Adv Chronic Kidney Dis. 2012 Jul;19(4):262–268. DOI: 10.1053/j.ackd.2012.05.002.
14. Donation & Transplantation Institute. International Registry in Organ Donation and Transplantation (IRODaT) Preliminary Numbers 2019 [Internet]. 2020 Jun. Available from *https://www.irodat.org/img/database/pdf/Newsletter%20June%202020%20.pdf.*
15. Broumand B. Transplantation activities in Iran. Exp Clin Transplant. 2005 Jun;3(1):333–337.
16. Habibzadeh F. Transplantation in the Middle East. Lancet [Internet]. 2012 November 9, 2018; 379. Available from: *https://els-jbs-prod-cdn.literatumonline.com/pb/assets/raw/Lancet/global-health/middle-east/Mar12_MiddleEastEd_Transplantation-1507541850093.pdf?elsca1=050312&elsca2=MIDDLEEADTED&elsca3=segment.*

27

Organ donation in Russia

Sergey V. Gautier, Artem Monakhov, Olga M. Tsiroulnikova, Sergey Khomyakov, Marina G. Minina, Deniz Dzhiner

Historical perspective

The founder of the World's experimental transplantology was a talented Soviet scientist Vladimir Demikhov (Figure 27.1). His experiments inspired many other gifted physicians and scientists worldwide to study his approaches, master them, create new approaches, and finally apply them on people.

Demikhov conducted numerous experiments on laboratory animals. In 1946, he performed the first heterotopic heart transplant into a dog's thoracic cavity and the first heart-lung complex transplant and the first lung transplant in the following year. In 1948, he started experiments in liver transplant and in 1951 he transplanted a donor heart to a dog proving that surgeries of such kind are possible. In 1960, Demikhov published a monograph 'Experimental Transplantation of Vital Organs' which was subsequently translated into several foreign languages and for a long time, remained the only transplant manual in the world.(1,2)

In 1933, Yurii Voronoy made his first attempt to perform deceased donor kidney transplantation in clinical settings. He managed to perform the first human allograft kidney transplantation from a deceased donor to a woman with acute kidney failure after a suicide attempt. The graft remained functional for one day. Unfortunately, on the second postoperative day, the recipient died. Voronoy made three more attempts of human allograft kidney transplantation, all of which failed.(3)

On 15 April 1965, a famous Soviet surgeon, Boris V. Petrovsky performed the first successful kidney transplantation from a living donor. In 1969, based on his initiative, Institution of Organ and Tissue

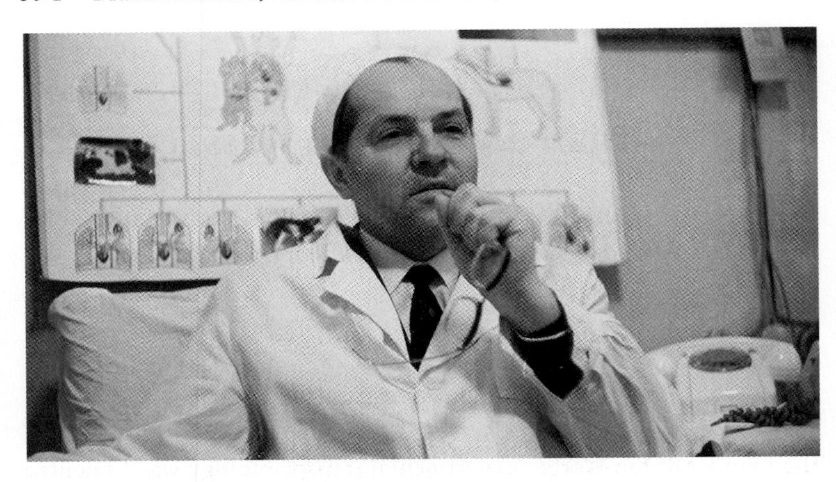

Figure 27.1. Vladimir Demikhov

Transplantation, USSR Academy of Medical Science, was formed. This hospital is still functioning under the name of National Medical Research Center of Transplantology and Artificial Organs named after V.I. Shumakov and remains the leading transplant centre in Russia.

For a long time, definition of brain death and a law regulating organ explantation from a brain-dead individual were absent in the USSR. Only in 1987, the lawful criteria for brain death diagnosis were formed. In the same year, on 12 March, Valery Shumakov performed the first successful heart transplantation in the USSR (Figure 27.2). This pushed forward the development of Soviet heart surgery.

Another important transplant centre in Russia is the Russian Research Center of Surgery where on 14 January 1990, a group of specialists under the leadership of Alexander Eramishantsev performed the first deceased donor liver transplantation.

Despite the economic and social crisis faced by Russia in the early 1990s, transplant medicine continued to develop and grow. In 1997, Sergey Gautier performed the first successful right lobe liver transplant from a living donor. From the year 2000, the number of transplant centres in Russia began to increase. Over twenty years, different types of solid organ transplantations have become a routine practice; cell technologies started to develop as well. In 2008, the Russian Transplant Society was founded to aim the consolidation of Russian transplant professionals,

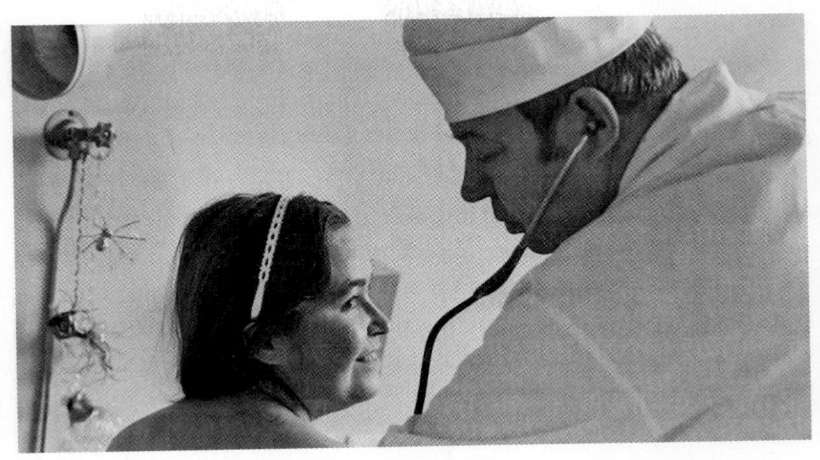

Figure 27.2. Valery Shumakov during a physical exam of first soviet heart recipient

development of transplant medicine as a science, implication of research results in Russian environment and also to strengthen international relationships.[4]

General structure of organ procurement

One of the main goals of Russian Healthcare is the provision of the population with affordable high-quality transplant assistance. For that reason, a new, more effective network of capable transplant clinics is being created. Organ donation and transplantation is financed by the State and by the system of Compulsory Health Insurance.

Russia employs a two-step system of organ donation coordination. The first step is carried out by the main transplant coordinator of a region who arranges and controls the activities of regional transplant departments of accredited hospitals. The second step is the work of National Transplant Register. The Register offers its data to a number of international registers such as International Registry of Organ Donation and Transplantation (IRODaT), Registry of the European Renal Association—European Dialysis and Transplant Association, (ERA EDTA Registry), and Registries of the International Society for Heart and Lung Transplantation

(ISHLT Registries). Since 2016, the Russian National Register is used as a tool for quality and transplant data collection control.[5] Data collection is performed via responsible executives of all Russian transplant centres and department surveillance.

Considerable progress in National transplant medicine has been achieved in the past decades; however, many serious issues still persist. Among the issues are uneven distribution of donor resources between the regions, insufficient promotion of the deceased organ donation ideas, and virtual lack of public awareness of organ deficit problem. It is worth mentioning the absence of under-aged deceased donor organ donation programme as an independent issue.[6]

Legislative aspects

The first version of Russian organ transplant law was issued in 1992 with subsequent editions in the years 2000, 2006, 2007, and finally, 2016.[7]

Russia uses the opt-out system, but if a potential donor had not made a request prohibiting organ extraction before death, their relatives can decline the procedure. The law does not prohibit organ extraction from deceased under-aged donors if their caregivers permit; however, all the deceased donors in Russia have always been at least eighteen years of age.

A living donor cannot be less than eighteen years of age or lack the medical decision-making capacity. In the latter case, even a legal caregiver cannot consent if a donor is not competent. Also a living donor of a solid organ must be a genetic relative to the recipient. The law does not mention the strength of kinship, though only specifies that a relation must exist.

Both a living donor and a recipient give an informed consent before the surgery. All living donors must consent themselves. In case of a recipient lacking medical decision-making capacity temporarily, transplantation still can be performed without a signed consent form. If a recipient is a minor or incompetent their legal guardian can consent for them.

Currently, a sustained effort is being made on a new, improved law edition. In foreseeable future, this new version will be released and hopefully successfully implemented by transplant centres nationwide.

Transplant programmes and the waiting lists

Currently, there are sixty operating transplant centres in Russia located across thirty-two federative subjects (there is a total of eighty-five subjects in Russia) with a population of 99.4 million people (a total of 144.5 million). Out of these centres, fifteen centres function in Moscow and Moscow Oblast and seven centres in Saint Petersburg and Leningrad Oblast. In 2018, transplant programmes were launched for the first time in Ryazan Oblast (1.1 mln people), Tula Oblast (1.5 mln people), and Stavropol Krai (2.8 mln people).[8]

With the widening of the geography of transplant programmes in Russia, the vector of administrative solutions for enhancing the availability and quality of transplant medical assistance will shift from extensive multiplying of transplant programmes in remote federative subjects to improving the efficiency of already existing centres.

During 2018, there were 6,219 potential recipients in the kidney transplant waiting list, which is 13.8% of the total pool of dialysis patients in Russia (according to the data of Russian Dialysis Society, there were approximately 45,000 of these patients). Out of these potential recipients, 1,728 people were included in the waiting list for the first time in 2018. There were 2,229 potential kidney recipients (35.8% of national waiting list) in Moscow and Moscow Oblast. Mortality rate among kidney transplant waiting list patients list was 0.9% (57 patients).

In 2018, liver transplant waiting list had 1,830 patients, 579 of which have been included in 2018. In Moscow and Moscow Oblast, there were 610 potential liver recipients (35.8% of national waiting list) and about 8.5% (154 patients) of waiting list patients died.

Heart transplant waiting list had 823 potential recipients in 2018; 397 of them were included in the list in 2018. In Moscow, there were 403 patients (49.0% of national waiting list). Mortality rate among potential heart recipients in 2018 was 5.8% (48 patients).[8]

Organ donation

In 2018, solid organ transplant surgery was available in twenty-nine (out of eighty-five) federative subjects with a total population of 94.2 million

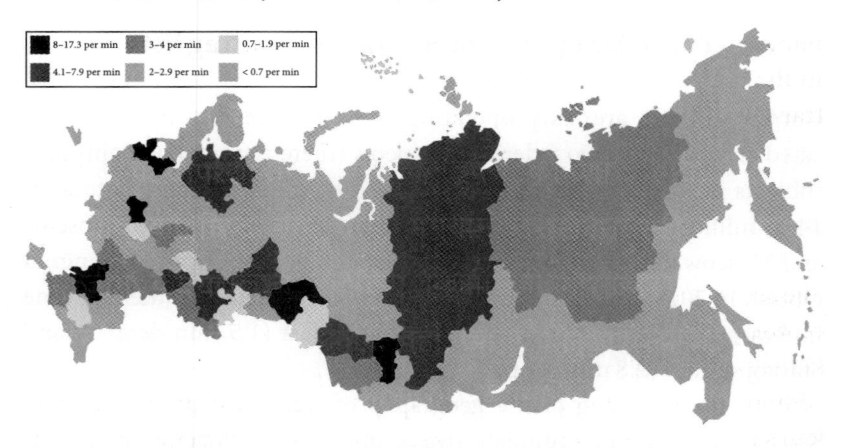

Figure 27.3. Organ donations per million in Russian regions (2018)

people (Figure 27.3). In addition, in three subjects (Tula Oblast, Perm Krai, Ulyanovsk Oblast) only living donor kidney transplantation programs were in progress.

Moscow and Moscow Oblast accounted for 44.7% (286) of effective donors (comparing to 47.9% (270) in 2017). There were 6.8 effective donors per million people in regions with functioning transplant centres. The best results have been shown in Moscow (17.3 per 1 mln people), Kemerovo Oblast (11.1), Moscow Oblast (9.1), Tyumen Oblast (8.7), Leningrad Oblast (8.3), Samara Oblast (7.2), Saint Petersburg (6.3), Novosibirsk Oblast (6.1), Sverdlovsk Oblast (5.6), and Krasnoyarsk Krai (5.5), respectively.[(8)]

The mean number of solid organs obtained from one deceased donor was 2.9 (2.8 in 2017). The best results have been observed in the regions with advanced extra-renal transplant programs and/or developed interregional organ coordination such as in Ryazan Oblast (3.5), Moscow (3.3), Novosibirsk Oblast (3.2), Moscow Oblast, Leningrad Oblast, and Altai Krai (3.1). A low index of 1.9 was recorded only in Volgograd Oblast.

There were 364 living donor explantations in 2018 which account for 36.3% of total explantations (1003). In 2017, living donor explantation rate was 332 or 37.0% of 896 in total (Figure 27.3).[(9)]

Since 2006, the number of effective donors in Russia has increased 1.5 folds; number of donors with the diagnosis of brain death increased 2.9 folds, and their fraction in the total donor pool increased by 49.3%. The number of multi-organ donors increased seven folds and their fraction in the total donor pool increased by 45.6%. The number of extra-renal transplantations increased 6.8 folds.[8,10,11]

Kidney transplantation

The activity of Russian kidney transplant centres varies significantly. Five centres perform approximately fifty surgeries a year, about thirty to fifty kidney transplants are accomplished in another ten centres every year, additional fifteen to twenty-nine transplants are performed in another fourteen centres in a year, whereas the rest twenty centres account only for fifteen surgeries annually.

Moscow and Moscow Oblast house fourteen kidney transplant centres which account for 50.3% (685) of all the kidney transplantations occurring in the country (in 2017—53.5% or 629 surgeries).

In 2018, twenty-eight of forty-nine centres performed living donor kidney transplantations, a total of 200 living donor surgeries were conducted (in 2017—201 surgeries). Moscow and Moscow Oblast have nine centres which performed 117 living donor kidney transplants in 2018 (58.5% of all living donor kidney transplants in Russia). Paediatric kidney transplant was practised in nine centres in 2018 with cumulative result of 89 kidney transplant surgeries (in 2017—105 surgeries); 85 (95.5%) of them were performed in Moscow. In general we can observe a steady increase in kidney transplant surgeries.[8,9]

Extra-renal transplantation

Since 2006, the amount of extra-renal transplant surgeries increased 7.8 folds, (Figure 27.4). The fraction of extra-renal transplantations, however, increased only by 22.0%.

In 2018, 282 heart transplants were performed (1.9 per 1 million people), out of them only 9 recipients were underaged. Heart transplant programme is ongoing in eighteen centres. National Medical Research Center of Transplantology and Artificial Organs named after V.I. Shumakov (Moscow) performed 68.8% (194) of all heart transplant

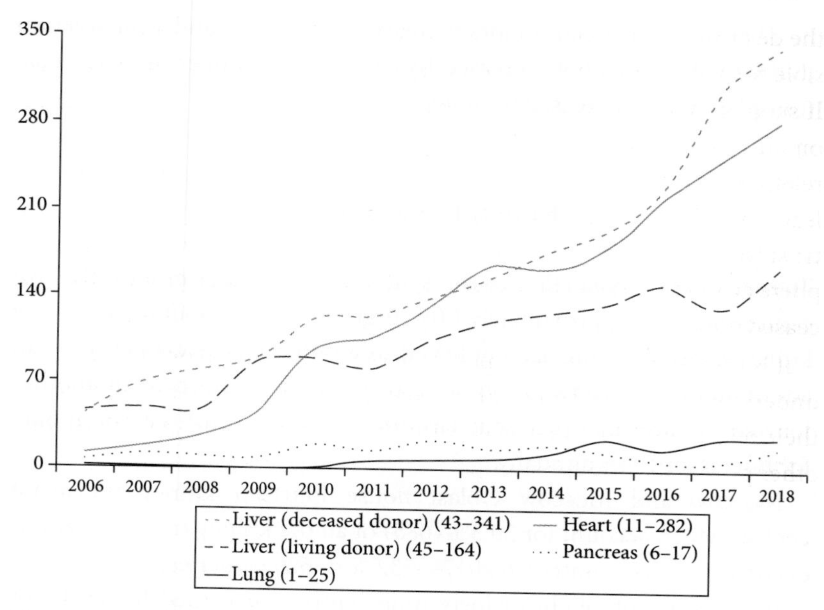

Figure 27.4. Transplantation of extrarenal organs

surgeries in the country. Successful heart transplant programmes in this centre along with new programmes in other clinics continue to show general positive tendency of increase in the number of heart transplantations in Russia from 2009 to 2018.

Liver transplantation is practised in twenty-eight centres. Moscow accounts for almost 70% of the surgeries. Living donor liver donation programmes are ongoing in only nine centres and these programmes account for approximately 30% of the total liver transplants. Paediatric liver transplantations are performed only in three centres with cumulative result of 100–130 surgeries per year.

According to the official data, pancreas transplantation is practised in six clinics. In 2018, a total of seventeen transplantations of pancreas have been performed, sixteen of them in combination with a kidney.

Current issues in promotion of organ donation

The solution of current problems in modern transplant assistance depends on social attitude and perception of transplant medicine, and on the desire of people to become donors. There is no organization responsible for promotion of positive image of transplant medicine in Russia. If such an organization was created, it would make a possible influence on information current, and provide decent communication with media, relatives of a donor and all the people in general. This, in turn, would lead to normalization of informational background, straightening of trust to transplant medicine in Russia and creation of a peaceful atmosphere around the concept of brain death and organ transplant from a deceased donor.

It is important to talk with people about controversial or incompletely understood topics in transplant medicine, to educate them and answer their questions. This is possible with the cooperation of physicians and other professionals such as religion workers, sociologists and teachers.(12)

Conclusion

Uneven development of transplantation and organ donation in Russia continues to be a serious issue. Organ demand in Russia keeps exceeding the abilities of transplant assistance. The number of patients in the waiting lists in 2018 was more than 9000 and continues to rise. This tendency demands particular attention to the arrangement of decent medical help for the patients in the expanding waiting lists, in particular, the need for special rates in the compulsory health insurance for this category of patients.

Donor organ deficit is exaggerated by the lack or insufficiency of regional transplant activity. This raises a question of responsibility of the regional executives, regional healthcare, and medical facilities for the organization of transplant assistance.

The crucial factor determining the national transplant help volume is the state financing as well as its source and methods of funds delivery to medical organizations participating in organ donation and transplantation. One of the opportunities to improve access to kidney grafts, as an example, would be an integration of kidney transplant into a basic programme of compulsory health insurance with preservation of financial normative. Therefore, the state would create uniform financing of different kidney replacement therapy types and the patients would be able to pick a preferable option according to their own needs and requirements.

Highlights

- Organ transplant is one of the top priorities of Russian Healthcare.
- Despite the rich history of organ procurement, originating in the beginning of 1930s, a number of socio-economic issues interfered with the development of transplant medicine in USSR and Russia.
- Currently, one of the most important problems is uneven distribution of organ donation programs among Russian regions.
- Present-day Russia is in the process of achieving an ambitious goal of providing the most remote regions of the country with up-to-date transplant technologies.
- In order to develop organ donation programmes nationwide, complex measures from transplantology promotion among lay people to conducting audits in regional healthcare facilities are implemented.

Reference

1. Werner, A, Glyantsev, SP, Demikhov, VP. 'Transplantation of vital organs in experiment' (1960) in foreign scientific press [to the 50th anniversary of the first heart transplantation in human]. Transplantologiya. 2017;9(4):360–370. (in Russ.) DOI:10.23873/2074-0506-2017-9-4-360-370.
2. Chzhao, Alexey V. From history to up-to-date realities of organ transplantation in Russia. Transplantologiya. The Russian Journal of Transplantation. 2013;(3):34–38. (In Russ.)
3. Voronoi, Uriy U. Peresadka konservirovannoy trupnoy pochki kak method biostimulyacii pri tyajelykh nephritah. Vracheb. delo. 1950; (9): 813–816. (In Russ.)
4. Transplantologiya i iskusstvennye organy: uchebnik / Edited by. S.V. Gautier. M.: Laboratoriya znaniy, 2018, pp. 16–25 (In Russ.)
5. Gautier SV, Khomyakov SM. Organ donation and transplantation in the Russian Federation in 2016 9th report of the National Registry. Russian Journal of Transplantology and Artificial Organs. 2017;19(2):6–26. (In Russ.) https://doi.org/10.15825/1995-1191-2017-2-6-26
6. Minina, M. To some organizational aspects of organ donation. Russian Journal of Transplantology and Artificial Organs 12.3 (2014): 81–88.
7. Law of the Russian Federation of December 22, 1992 No. 4180-I About organ transplantation and (or) tissues of the person (as amended on 08-12-2020)
8. Gautier SV, Khomyakov SM. Organ donation and transplantation in Russian Federation in 2018 11th report of the national registry. Russian Journal of Transplantology and Artificial Organs. 2019;21(3):7–32. (In Russ.) https://doi.org/10.15825/1995-1191-2019-3-7-32

9. Gautier SV, Khomyakov SM. Organ donation and transplantation in Russian Federation in 2017 10th report of the national registry. Russian Journal of Transplantology and Artificial Organs. 2018;20(2):6–28. (In Russ.) https://doi.org/10.15825/1995-1191-2018-2-6-28
10. Gautier SV, Moysyuk YG, Khomyakov SM, Ibragimova OS. Progress in organ donation and transplantation in Russian Federation in 2006–2010. Report of national registry. Russian Journal of Transplantology and Artificial Organs. 2011;13(2):6–20. (In Russ.) https://doi.org/10.15825/1995-1191-2011-2-6-20
11. Gautier SV, Moysyuk YG, Khomyakov SM, Ibragimova OS. Organ donation and transplantation in Russian Federation in 2011. Russian Journal of Transplantology and Artificial Organs. 2012;14(3):6–18. (In Russ.) https://doi.org/10.15825/1995-1191-2012-3-6-18
12. Reznik ON, Reznik AO. Promotion of organ donation: Current practices, issues, perspectives. Russian Journal of Transplantology and Artificial Organs. 2018;20(4):112–120. (In Russ.) doi.org/10.15825/1995-1191-2018-4-112-120

28

Organ donation in China

Wenshi Jiang, Li Li, Chao Li, Xiangxiang He

The 'Chinese Model' of organ donation and transplantation

Organ transplantation was found to be the most effective treatment for organ failure in the 20th century, saving the life of more than 130 thousand patients annually worldwide.[1] With the rapid development of surgery, immunosuppressive drugs, organ preservation and cell separation techniques and immunological basis of transplantation, considerable progress has been made in organ transplantation technology.[2]

In 2007, the State Council promulgated *the Regulations on Human Organ Transplantation*, the first organ transplant law in China, to govern the clinical practices under the legal framework for organ transplant in China. With over a decade of strenuous efforts, China has made remarkable achievements in organ donation and transplantation. Based on the guiding principles of the World Health Organization (WHO) on organ transplantation[3] and conforming to the cultural traditions and current socio-economic conditions of the country, China has established a scientific, ethical system to foster the sound development of organ donation and transplantation practices. This system, referred to as the 'Chinese model' by the WHO,[4] is well received by the public and widely praised at home and abroad. Promising outcome was demonstrated by a trend of rapid increase in the annual number of organ donations after citizens' death in China, starting from 34 cases (donation per million population: 0.03) in 2010 to 5222 cases (donation per million population: 3.7) in 2020.[5] As shown in Figure 28.1, China has become the second largest country in terms of the absolute number of organ donations worldwide since 2015.

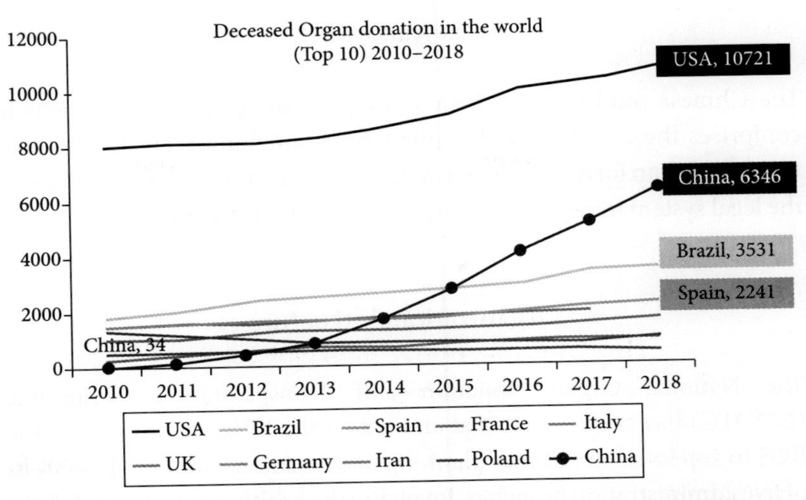

Figure 28.1. Deceased Organ donation in the world 2010–2018 (TOP 10). (Data source: International Registry on Organ Donation and Transplantation and China Organ Donation Administrative Center)

The Chinese model is unique, which takes into consideration the regional characteristics of Chinese society, politics, economy, and culture and is gradually formed and constantly improved on the basis of practices. As being well summarized by Prof. Jiefu Huang, Chairman of China Organ Donation and Transplantation Committee, the Chinese model has the following characteristics.(6)

Governmental support

The reform of organ transplantation in China was carried out under the strong leadership of the central committee of the communist party and the State Council, with the participation of National Health Commission (NHC) of the People's Republic of China, the Red Cross Society of China (RCS), and the Department of Transportation and other departments. The mechanism ensures smooth progress of the organ donation and transplantation process.

Legal framework

The Chinese model is based on a comprehensive legal system, which comprises the core laws and regulations on human organ transplantation, more than forty supporting system documents and the provisions of the legal system in regard to organ donation and transplantation.

Organizational structure

The National Organ Donation and Transplantation Committee (NODTC) has been established and led by the NHC and joined by the RCS to supervise the overall planning of the national system. It consists of five administration branches, involving the health commission authorities and Red Cross societies at all levels—China Organ Transplantation Development Foundation, Chinese Hospital Association, Chinese Medical Association, Chinese Medical Doctor Association, and medical institutions engaged in organ transplantation.

Donation classification and process

There are two main types of deceased organ donation in the world, namely Donation after Brain Death (DBD) and Donation after Circulatory Death (DCD). The DCD accounted for about 22.8% of organ donation globally in 2019.[(1)]

Due to the absence of legislation and the lack of clinical practice in place for brain death diagnosis, the clinical application of DCD in China is more common than other countries in the world (Figure 28.2). The Chinese model defines the standards and procedures of deceased organ donation in three categories, and follows the traditional culture and socialist core values, which is conducive to promoting the development of organ donation in China. The three categories for organ donation are described as follows:[(7)]

China category I (C-I) is DBD, which meets the existing international brain-death standard and the latest national brain-death standard in all indices upon strict medical examination, is determined by relevant

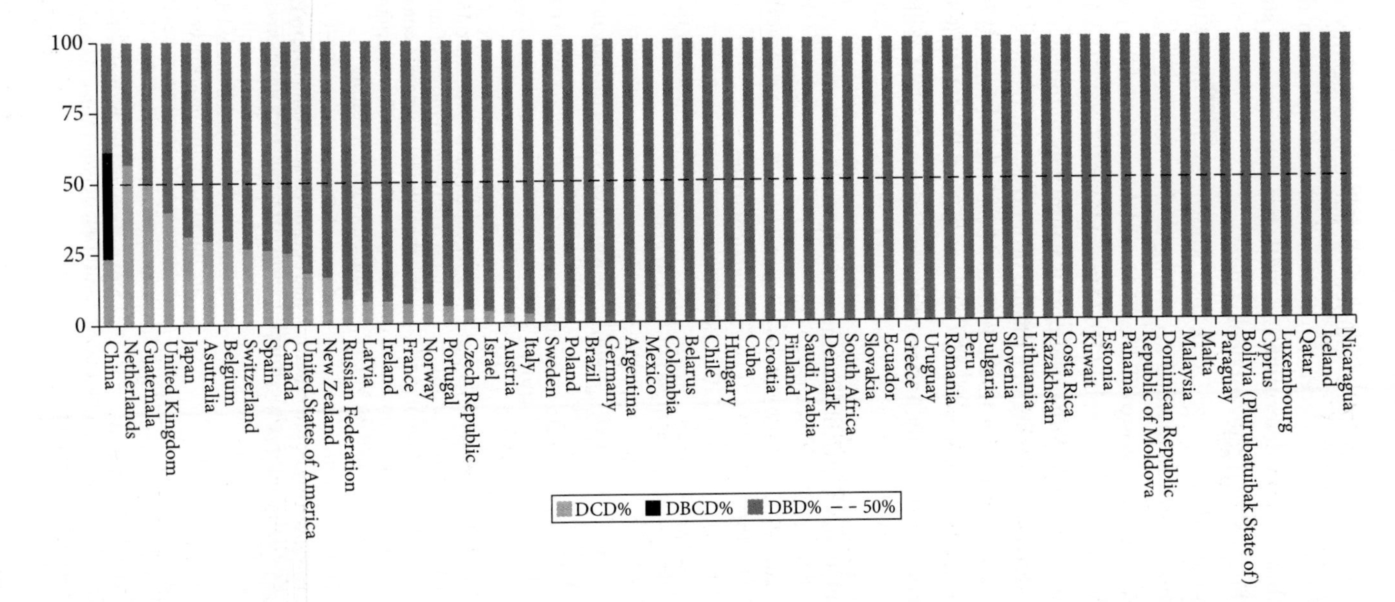

Figure 28.2. Proportion of DCD and DBD in countries. (Data source: Global Observatory on Donation & Transplantation).

*: Chinese data are shown by Chinese categories

experts with training certificate granted by authorized agency of the NHC.[8] The family of the deceased understood and agreed to donate organs after brain death determination, with the approval and support given by the hospital and relevant department.

China category II (C-II) is DCD, also known as non-heart-beating donors (NHBD), they are divided according to the modified Maastricht classification into five categories (Table 28.1), which can further be reduced to two main groups: (1) Controlled DCD (categories III and IV), wherein circulatory and respiratory organ support is voluntarily withdrawn by the medical provider, in the setting of a dismal prognosis that renders cardio-respiratory support no longer in the patient's best interest and survival is deemed futile; and (2) Uncontrolled DCD (categories I, II, and V), in which cardiac death occurs suddenly, and resuscitation is unsuccessful or absent.

Table 28.1 Updated Maastricht Classification of non-heart-beating donors[9,10]

Classification	Description	Particularities
I	Dead on arrival. Resuscitation attempts not possible	Uncommonly used (mainly in Spain and France)
II	Unsuccessful resuscitation (a) Out-of-hospital refractory circulatory arrest (b) In-hospital refractory circulatory arrest	Uncommonly used (mainly in Spain and France)
III	Awaiting death by cardiorespiratory arrest Hospitalized patients with life-threatening conditions or who are planned for WLST	Most commonly used. The time elapsed between removal of support and mechanical asystole is one of the main determinants of organ suitability for harvesting
IV	Death by cardiorespiratory arrest during or after brain death diagnostic procedures	Unusual. Resuscitation efforts may be permitted according to family's wishes. If circulatory function is restored and brain death confirmed, donation protocols following DBD are pursued, or the protocol is switched to DCD in case resuscitation attempts are unsuccessful
V	Medically assisted cardiorespiratory arrest in a terminally ill patient	Not recognized in the majority of countries as constitutes euthanasia

China category III (C-III) is Donation after Brain Death followed by Cardiac Death (DBCD), which means that the patient meets the brain death criteria, but objectively it is implemented according to the DCD procedure. In China, there is no brain death legislation and the brain death concept and practice have not been the norm of Chinese society. To develop a national system of deceased-organ donation that respects Chinese culture, DBCD was introduced by the NHC with the initiation of the pilot organ donation programme.

Humanitarianism and humanism

Based on the Chinese model, a humanitarian assistance policy was put forward to guarantee people's rights and interests, to ensure voluntary donation, and to embody the socialist core values and the traditional virtues of the Chinese nation.

Construction of China Organ Procurement Organization

To further regulate the clinical practice of organ donation, as of February 2019, China established more than 110 organ procurement organizations (OPOs) across the country at the hospital level. The OPOs have been playing a key role in the whole success. An OPO team is founded by different groups of professionals from various fields such as transplant surgeons, neurosurgeons, intensive medical practitioners, emergency physicians and nurses, and social workers. The OPOs are similar to the 'Transplant Procurement Management (TPM) unit' adopted in many European counties, originally created in Spain. In 2018, China's first provincial OPO was established in Shanxi Province. Independent from the transplant hospital, the centre is a public institution approved by the provincial health commission. As the pilot province, Shanxi explored a feasible and up-to-date organ procurement structure coordinating organ donation, recovery, and allocation within the province. The 'Shanxi experience' has shown how organ donation can advance in parallel to establishing professionalism, thus serving as reference procurement model for other regions in China in support of the country's effort of self-sufficiency.

If we consider OPOs as a bridge connecting donation hospital and transplant centres, the organ donation coordinator should be considered as a messenger connecting 'Death' and 'Life'. Their work reflects the 'humanitarian, fraternity and dedication' spirit of the RCS, bearing great social significance. To ensure the quality of donation service, the OPOs are required to organize a team of donation coordinators with expertise and qualification. By the end of 2020, the China organ donation administrative centre has trained and certified more than 2800 coordinators. Among them, 34% were from the Red Cross system with multidisciplinary background and 66% were staffs from the medical institutes.(1)

The Article 22 of *the Regulations on Human Organ Transplantation* stipulates: 'The ranking of the patients receiving human organ transplantation shall be in conformity with medical needs and in adherence to the principles of fairness, impartiality and transparence.' Currently, China has issued the national allocation rules for deceased livers, kidneys, hearts, and lungs.

Challenges and opportunities

The success of the reform of organ donation in China was only the first step in a long-term journey. We are still facing many difficulties ahead.

1. The shortage of organs in China is particularly prominent:

The data released by China's National Renal Data System showed that by the end of 2019, the number of dialysis patients nationwide had increased from 331,000 in 2013 to 735,000 in 2019.(11) However, only 11,037 kidney transplants were performed in 2020. That is to say, only one of the sixty-six dialysis patients can receive a kidney transplant within one year.

2. Brain death has not yet been legislated:

China has established the Brain Injury Evaluation Quality Control Centre and issued the criteria and practical guidance for determination of brain death in adults and children. With the development and deepening of human understanding of life science, advocating brain death as the criterion of death has become an important symbol of civilization development and international social progress. The legislation of brain death can also promote the development of medicine and law, as well as make full use of the limited medical resources and reduce the risk for health care staff performing the brain death diagnosis.

3. The awareness and professional skills of medical staffs on organ donation shall be increased:

The professionalization of medical staff can ensure that the wishes of donors are fully respected and effectively implemented, and ensure the safety of transplant patients and the long-term effectiveness of transplantation. In reality, donor loss will occur due to several factors. From the international experience, the conversation rate of organ donors is around 50%. The deceased organ donation critical pathway published by WHO points out that the common causes for donor loss are the failure to identify potential donors, medical contraindication to donation, failure to implement the brain death diagnosis, family refusal, and improper donor maintenance.(12) Except the medical contraindication to donation, other causes can be addressed by enhancing the awareness and professional skills of medical staff. In China, around 0.76 million hospital deaths occurred in 2016 but only 0.062% of these hospital deaths were converted to actual organ donors.(13) A few studies have indicated a lack of awareness among Chinese medical staff regarding brain death and organ donation. These studies implied the causes of low donor identification rate.(14) Much is left to be improved. Therefore, we need to increase the awareness of medical staff, especially those working in the OPO and in the donor generating units.

4. The surveillance and quality management system for organ donation and transplant shall be implemented:

The annual number of organ donations in China has leapt to the second highest level in the world. More attention should be paid to establish a solid quality management system for the process management and quality improvement of organ donation.

5. The publicity and popularization of organ donation shall be increased:

The Confucian concept supports organ donation. By using the Application Programming Interface (API) to randomly crawl 16 million users' registration information and all their messages posted in weibo (a social media similar to Twitter) in 2017, after cleaning and analysing the data of 1,755 representative messages, we found that although public attention towards organ donation needs to be enhanced, the majority of people mentioning organ donation have a positive attitude (88%). Public attention to topics of organ donation usually needs to be aroused by specific events. People with negative attitudes towards organ donation mainly fear that the patient may not be saved. The second reason why people say no to organ donation is their distrust in the medical system. Distrust of the medical system result in conspiracy theories against organ donation as well as misunderstanding about the organ transplantation process. In addition to promoting donor registration, actions should be taken to popularize the relevant scientific knowledge of organ donation and transplantation so as to eliminate those misunderstandings. More explanation should be given to demonstrate to the voluntaries based on the system and eliminate their fears of being thought as selling the organ of their loved ones or the fears of selling their own organs by their family.

Conclusion

The WHO recognized the efforts made by the Chinese society to promote self-sufficiency for organ transplantation. China has established a scientific, ethical system to foster the sound development of organ donation and transplantation practices.[(4)] Under 'The Belt and Road' Initiative, the prospect for cultural cooperation and exchanges between China and other countries is much more promising. China will keep on working. The next step is to further improve the legal system and the working mechanism, strengthen supervision, and promote the exchanges among professionals. China will work hand in hand with other countries to create a better future in this regard.

Highlights

- As Chinese model has been introduced to the world, China participated in drafting the summit's statement that provided guidance to organ transplantation development across the world.
- It is a model that combines the regional characteristics of society, politics, economy, and culture in China, and gradually forms and constantly improves based on practices.
- The OPO system has been created to increase efficiency and quality of the procurement service, with different models being explored in different regions.
- In the future, we should not only continue to increase the publicity and popularization of organ donation to let more people understand and play their part in organ donation, but also to strengthen the education of organ donation among medical staff, especially those working in the donor generating units.

References

1. GODT. Global Observatory on Donation and Transplantation 2017 [Available from: http://www.transplant-observatory.org/. Published 2021. Accessed August 30 2021.
2. Haiying Shi. Study On Organ Transplantation in China: Shandong University; 2009.
3. Sixty-Third World Health Assembly WHO. WHO guiding principles on human cell, tissue and organ transplantation. Transplantation. 2010;90(3):229.
4. Guo Y. The 'Chinese Mode' of organ donation and transplantation: Moving towards the center stage of the world. Hepatobiliary Surgery and Nutrition. 2018;7(1):61–62.
5. CODAC. China Organ Donation Administrative Center [Available from: http://www.rcsccod.cn/. Published 2021. Accessed April 10 2021.
6. Huang J. The 'China Model' of Organ Donation and Transplantation. China Medical News. 2017;32(9):6.
7. Huang J, Wang H, Fan ST, Zhao B, Zhang Z, Hao L, et al. The national program for deceased organ donation in China. Transplantation. 2013;96(1):5–9.
8. Brain Injury Evaluation Quality Control Center of National Health Commission. Criteria and practical guidance for determination of brain death in adults (BQCC version). Chinese medical journal. 2013;126(24):4786–4790.
9. Kootstra G, Daemen JH, Oomen AP. Categories of non-heart-beating donors. Transplant Proc. 1995;27(5):2893–4.
10. KeTLOD. China-EU Organ Donation Management (Bilingual Edition). Beijing: Science Press; 2018.

11. National Health Commission of the People's Republic of China. National Report on the Services, Quality and Safety in Medical Care System 2017. Beijing: Scientific and Technical Documentation Press; 2018.
12. Dominguez-Gil B, Delmonico FL, Shaheen FA, Matesanz R, O'Connor K, Minina M, et al. The critical pathway for deceased donation: Reportable uniformity in the approach to deceased donation. Transplant international: official journal of the European Society for Organ Transplantation. 2011;24(4):373–378.
13. National Bureau of Statistics. Statistical Bulletin on National Economic and Social Development 2016 of China 2017 [Available from: http://www.stats.gov.cn/tjsj/zxfb/201702/t20170228_1467424.html. Published 2018.
14. Yilin Jiao, Li Gao, Yanhong Jin. Investigation of the status of the experience of persuading to donate and the willingness toward organ donation for ICU nurses. Chinese Journal of Modern Nursing. 2013;19(15):1745–1748.

29

Organ donation in Japan

Kaori Kuramitsu, Hiroto Egawa

History of organ donation in Japan

In Japan, transplantation from cardiac arrest donors started around 1970s.[1] In 1979, 'Cornea and Kidney Transplantation Law' was established. However, brain death was not accepted as legal death by Japanese general citizens. In 1997, Japanese Organ Transplantation Law was established. However, because prior living and written consent for organ donation after brain death were mandatory, the number of organ donation from brain death donors remained around ten per year.

After clinical introduction of the immunosuppression regimen consisting of cyclosporin in 1978, the outcomes of kidney, liver, and heart transplantation improved by up to 80% and demand of transplantations dramatically increased all over the world.[2–5] However, donor scarcities produced transplant tourism and organ trafficking. In 2004, the World Health Organization,[6] called on member states 'to take measures to protect the poorest and vulnerable groups from transplant tourism and the sale of tissues and organs, including attention to the wider problem of international trafficking in human tissues and organs'. To address the urgent and growing problems of organ sales, transplant tourism and trafficking in organ donors in the context of the global shortage of organs, a Summit Meeting of more than 150 representatives of scientific and medical bodies from around the world, government officials, social scientists, and ethicists, was held in Istanbul in 2008.[7] This Istanbul Declaration reflects the importance of international collaboration and global consensus to improve donation and transplantation practices.

At the time many Japanese patients went abroad for organ transplantation. Until 2013, a total of thirty-one patients underwent successful liver

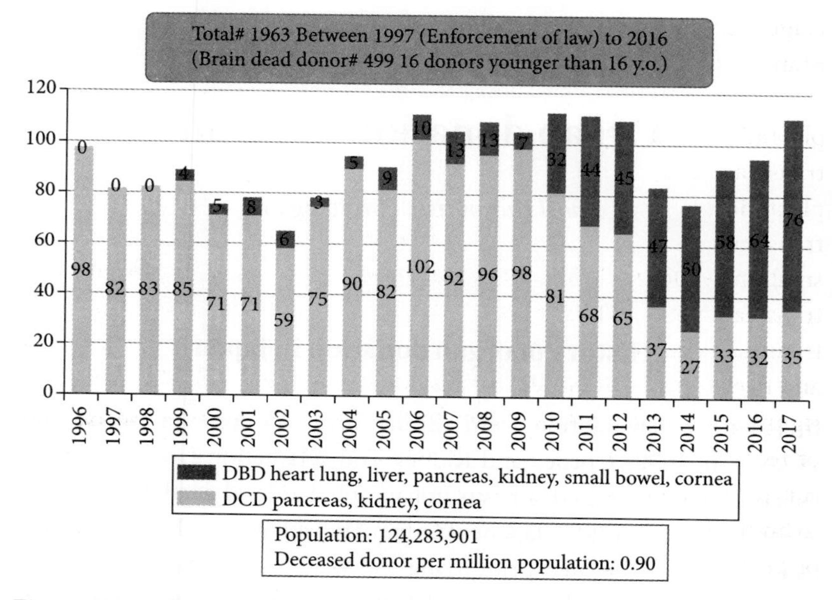

Figure 29.1. Changes of number of deceased donor

transplantation in other countries. The total number for kidney transplantation is not available, and Japan was accused of international organ trafficking by international medical societies.

The Istanbul Declaration pushed Japanese Government and medical professionals to revise the Japanese Organ Transplantation Law in 2010. Since the prior living and written consent for organ donation after brain death became non-mandatory, the number of deceased organ donors increased gradually thereafter, up to sixty-eight cases in 2018 (Figure 29.1). On the other hand, the number of Donation after Cardiac Death (DCD) for kidney transplantation decreased. The total number of deceased and DCD donors remains around 100.

Present status of deceased donor transplantation in Japan

Based on the International Registry in Organ and Transplantation data, deceased donor per million population in 2017 was 0.88 in Japan

(Figure 29.1), while it was 9.7 in Germany, 23.05 in England, 26.9 in France, and 31.96 in United States of America.[(8)]

On 31 March 2019, there were 732 patients registered for heart transplantation, 348 for lung transplantation, 3 for both heart and lung transplantation, 308 for liver transplantation, 12,055 for kidney transplantation, 22 for both liver and kidney transplantation, 41 for pancreatic transplantation, 172 for both pancreas and kidney transplantation, 1 for small intestine transplantation, and 1 for both liver and small intestine transplantation.[(9)] On 31 March 2019, there were ten institutions for heart transplantation, ten for lung, twenty-five for liver, nineteen for pancreatic, and twelve for small intestine transplantations respectively.[(10)] The most significant characteristics of Japanese transplantation are high number of recovered organs from one donor and superior recipient, and graft survivals. Japanese distinguished medical consultant system contributed to both of the characteristics. Since 2002, one or two transplant surgeons or physicians were sent to the recovery hospital as a medical consultant or consultants to assess organ condition and to stabilize donor hemodynamics to improve cardiac and lung function as much as possible.[(10)] As a result, the availability of organs became higher in Japan compared to other countries. In 2018, 5.5 organs from one donor were transplanted in Japan while 3.5 organs were being transplanted in United States based on the Organ Procurement and Transplantation Network (OPTN) national data.[(11)] By 31 March 2019, five-year survival (patient/graft) was 92.5/92.5% for heart transplantation, 73.4/72.2% for lung transplantation, 82.0/81.3% for liver transplantation, 91.1/78.1% for kidney transplantation, 94.9/76.0% for pancreas transplantation, and 73.2/65.1% for small intestine transplantation in Japan.[(9)] In comparison to Japanese national data, the OPTN national data revealed five-year survival (patient/graft) was 79.1/78.3% for heart transplantation, 55.0/52.5% for lung transplantation, 75.0/71.9% for liver transplantation, 83.2/74.4% for kidney transplantation, 81.3/59.2% for pancreas transplantation, and 56.1/47.7% for small intestine transplantation.[(11)] Average waiting time of patients who underwent heart transplantation in 2017 was 1,173 days, that of patients who had lung transplantation until 2017 was 1,284 days, patients who had liver transplantation until 31 May 2014 was 377 days, patients who had kidney transplantation in 2017 was 4,850 days, and that of patients who had pancreas transplantation in 2017 was 1,287 days in Japan.[(9)] In contrast, based on OPTN national data, median waiting time of patients listed from 2011–2014 and had heart transplantation in Status 1A (the candidate who has a life expectancy without a liver transplant of less than 7 days) was 87 days, that of patients who had lung transplantation was 125 days, that of patients who had liver transplantation in Status 1 was 6 days, that of patients who had kidney transplantation was 1,460 days, that of patients who had pancreas transplantation was 306 days, and that of patients who had small intestine transplantation was 109 days.[10]

Current strategies to facilitate donor hospitals

To increase deceased donors, there are two approaches: to facilitate donor hospitals, and to motivate general citizens including medical staff. Based on the guidelines authorized by Japanese Ministry of Health, Labour and Welfare, organ recovery from brain death donors is allowed in the hospitals belonging to following five facility types: (1) university hospitals, (2) leading hospitals certificated by the Japanese Association of Acute Medicine, (3) leading hospitals certificated by the Japanese Society of Neurosurgery, (4) certificated acute medicine centres, and (5) certificated children's hospitals. On 31 March 2017, there were 896 certificated hospitals. Of these, 269 (30.0%) hospitals were ready for all ages of deceased donors, 166 (18.5%) were ready for only adult deceased donors, and 461 (51.5%) were not ready for deceased donors. In-house system maintenance project was started in 2013 to educate hospitals not ready for donations. Expert donor coordinators were sent to such hospitals, for example, to establish ethical committees, to prepare manuals, and to hold simulation of brain death diagnosis. However, only sixteen to seventeen hospitals participated in these projects for the first three years and the number of brain death donors did not increase, because hospitals required recommendation of prefectural and city governments to participate in the project as per the initial plan. Government changed the recruit system to expand the project, in which all willing hospitals could participate without nomination by local governors and finally, eighty-nine hospitals participated in 2018.

Current strategies to motivate general citizen and medical staffs

In August 2017, an opinion poll was performed by the cabinet office. A national survey was performed on 3,000 general citizen aged more than eighteen years, and the collection rate was 63.7%. To the question 'Do you want to donate your organs when you become brain dead?' 41.8% of all ages answered yes. Of note, the percentage was the highest, 69.6% among the youngest generations, aged eighteen to twenty-nine years, compared to the lowest percentage, 29.7% among the oldest generations, aged more than seventy years. The higher percentage among younger generations partly resulted in the increased number of paediatric donors. Importantly, more than 60% of Japanese adult citizens younger than fifty years wanted to donate their organs when they became brain dead. To motivate general citizen further, the Japanese Ministry of Health, Labour and Welfare produces pamphlets for public awareness of organ donation and distributes to junior high students every year. In addition, October is set as a promotion month for spreading awareness on transplantation. Several events such as green light up of locally famous monuments like Tokyo tower, holding a popular mass meeting, and sport games by transplant recipients are organized widely. From April 2018, live-action to indicate self-intention for donation was included in the video which all the drivers watch at the timing of driver's license renewal. As another novel approach to create public awareness, education of organ donation and transplantation for school children has been just started. In Japan, moral education was set as a must subject for elementary school children in 2018 and for junior high school students in 2019 and education of organ donation and transplantation is included as one of the sections in moral education textbooks. Since school teachers do not have enough experience to teach this subject, in 2019, the government began sessions for teachers every month as a pilot in which eight to ten teachers were selected from several schools to discuss how to educate children on gift of life. Development of nationwide education tools for school teachers is planned.

In the past, brain death was considered as a loss by medical staff in the field of critical care and neurosurgery and the concept of brain death was unfamiliar in public, and they hesitated to let family know about organ donation. Moreover, determination of brain death gave them a heavy burden of both human and financial resources. Big efforts were made to increase incentives and to decrease burden on donor hospitals. Currently about 30,000 USD is paid to a donor hospital per donor. Under the revised law, two brain specialists making brain death diagnosis had to be regular employees. To avoid decline due to this regulation, one doctor was allowed from another hospital for help since 2017. Setting of a new kind of medical professionals began to reduce mental and physical stress of attending doctors and nurses of critical patients and to increase the quality of hospital stay of patient and family. They take care of the family of a patient with unexpected critical conditions immediately after admission and communicate with family and may introduce donor coordinators if they desire. To improve skills and to reduce fatigue through the process, hands-on seminars are held on a regular basis during annual congress of acute medicine, clinical acute medicine, and intensive care medicine. As a research project funded by Japanese Ministry of Health, Labour and Welfare from 2017 to 2019, entitled 'Improvement of satisfaction of donor family and construction of efficient system for organ donation', simplification and standardization of organ procurement process was also studied. The study group consists of eight specialists who were recommended from Japanese Association for Acute Medicine, Japanese Society for Emergency Medicine, Japanese Society of Intensive Care Medicine, and Japan Neurosurgical Society. As a product, they made a practical manual (handbook) for organ procurement for the beginners which cover the entire process from the treatment of acute injuries to organ recovery surgery.

Future strategies to increase deceased donors

Transplant surgeons are the only doctors who could possibly deliver the greatness of transplant medicine. From 2016, Japanese Society for Transplantation started to struggle with two agendas; stay close to professionals of acute medicine field and the government which is in charge of transplant medicine. Free from historical conflict, the first symposium with expert presenters from all the four acute medicine-related societies was held at the annual meeting of Japanese Society for Transplantation in 2018. Furthermore, Japanese Society for Transplantation selected three doctors and one coordinator among more than fifty Japanese who graduated the international course of DTI (Donation & Transplantation Institute) and sent them to DTI again to understand human resources, strategies, structures, and finance of the Spanish model in 2018. Based on their experiences, a novel strategy to increase donor hospitals was launched in 2019. Hospitals with no experience of brain death donor can build up the scheme beforehand by participating in-house system maintenance business. However, it is more convincing if they could have some specialists for the treatment, examination, and control of the entire process. As a result, it was decided to develop organ and tissue donation support system at one prefecture in Japan with a national budget of $500,000. The system consists of mother hospitals and daughter hospitals. The mother hospital had doctors and technicians who have experience in performing several organ donations procedures. Daughter hospitals had a few or no medical staff with experience in performing organ donations procedures. A mother hospital and daughter hospitals perform regular meetings to share their experiences and to constitute a better support system (Figure 29.2). Additionally, an education programme for both donor management and donor coordinators are also developed. A mother hospital sends doctors and technicians to a daughter hospital to help, if necessary, in case of organ donation.

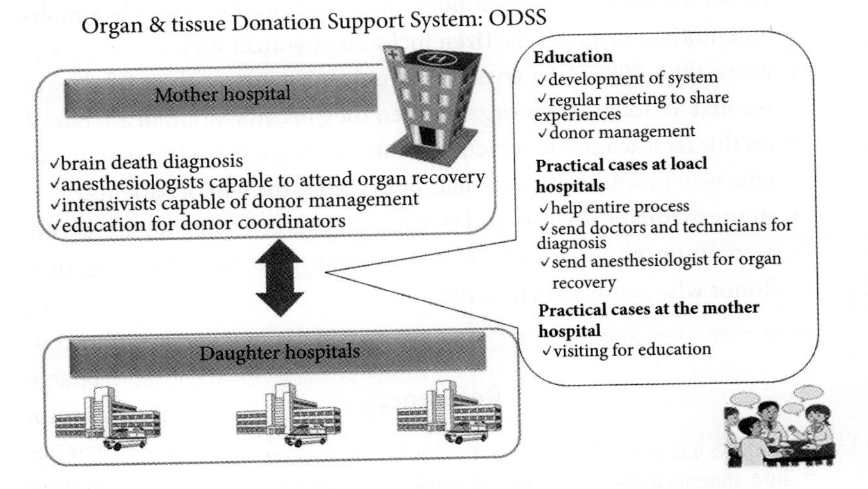

Figure 29.2. Organ and tissue Donation Support System: ODSS

Organ transplantation is performed to fulfil the hope of a donor who wants to help somebody. To fulfil the wish of donors, all doctors should do their best. Acute medicine doctors handle organs to transplant surgeons safely, and, the transplant surgeons let the organs survive as long as possible. As a result, the recipients can enjoy their newly given lives. Historically, organ donation in Japan did not work well. The cooperation structure with academic societies of acute medicine and transplantation and government will definitely change organ donation in Japan.

Highlights

- Japanese Organ Transplantation Law was established in 1997 and the number of DBD remains under ten per year. Japanese Organ Transplantation Law was revised in 2010.
- Since the prior living and written consent for organ donation after brain death became not mandatory, the number of deceased organ donors was increased gradually thereafter, up to sixty-eight cases in 2018.
- Although the number of decreased donors is less, more organs are recovered from one donor compared to other countries and outcomes of organ transplant is excellent in Japan.
- Japanese Ministry of Health, Labour and Welfare is making a big effort of increase deceased donors such as facilitating donor hospitals, and motivating general citizen including medical staffs.
- More than 60% of Japanese adult citizens younger than fifty years wanted to donate their organs when they became brain dead. Based on this fact, academic societies of intensive care fields began to make efforts to promote organ donation to realize the will of patients.
- Acute medicine doctors and transplant surgeons can cooperate with a common philosophy that their mission is to fulfil the hope of a donor who wants to help somebody.

References

1. Tsuji K, Takahashi T, Shiwaku Y, Akiyama N, Inou T. The first report of the human renal transplant registry in Japan. Transplant Proc 1979; 11(1): 107–114.

2. Flechner SM, Payne WD, Van Buren C, Kerman R, Kahan BD. The effect of cyclosporine on early graft function in human renal transplantation. Transplantation 1983; 36(3): 268–272.
3. Merion RM, White DJ, Thiru S, Wvans DB, Calne RY. Cyclosporine: Five year's experiences in cadaveric renal transplantation. N Engl J Med 1984; 19: 310(3): 148–154.
4. Iwatsuki S, Starzl TE, Shaw BW et al. Long-term use of cyclosporine in liver recipients. Reduction of dosages in the first year to avoid nephrotoxicity. Transplantation 1983; 36(6): 614–613.
5. Bolman RM 3rd, Elick B, Olivari MT, Ring WS, Arentzen CE. Improved immunosuppression for heart transplantation. J Jeart Transplant 1985; 4(3): 315–318.
6. Resolution on human organ and tissue transplantation. Geneva: WHO; 2004 (WHA 57.18)
7. Steering Committee of the Istanbul Summit. Organ trafficking and transplant tourism and commercialism: the Declaration of Istanbul. Lancet 2008; 372(9632):5–6.
8. accessed from IRODaT homepage in 2019 July. http://www.irodat.org
9. accessed from Japan Organ Transplant Network Homepage in March 2019. https://www.jotnw.or.jp/english/data.html
10. Fukushima N, Ono M, Nakatani T, Minami M, Konaka S, Ashikari J. Strategies for maximizing heart and lung transplantation opportunities in Japan. Transplantation Proceedings 2009; 41: 273–276.
11. Accessed from Organ Procurement and Transplantation Network in July 2019. https://optn.transplant.hrsa.gov/data/view-data-reports/national-data

SECTION 3.
THE ORGAN DONOR

30

Pathophysiological changes at the moment of brain death

Anna Teresa Mazzeo, Deepak Gupta

Introduction

Central nervous system (CNS) is recognized as the central regulator of systemic homeostasis and its interconnections with the heart, the lungs, the kidneys, the gut have been widely investigated in literature during the last decades.[1–5]

A well-settled cross-talk between the brain and each of the other organs and systems is critical for the functionality of the whole human being. Hemodynamic, respiratory, metabolic, and endocrine systems are all maintained in equilibrium through finely regulated interconnections which are essential for a proper functioning of each of these systems.

When organs in such a finely tuned system don't talk any more, the extraordinary artwork of human being will disintegrate and each small piece of this mosaic will not be able to connect anymore in the brilliant music of life. Brain death will therefore result in a disintegrated collection of organs.[6]

In the critical phases of transition from a catastrophic brain injury to the loss of all functions of the brain including the brainstem, a cascade of events will occur and will be responsible for an irreversible derangement of functions that were earlier maintained in equilibrium, be it delicate, or robust. At bedside, the intensivist will recognize in advance that brain death is occurring, as clinical events such as sudden hemodynamic changes, hypothermia, polyuria, and failure to increase heart rate in response to intravenous injection of atropine, among others, will occur.

Once brain death has occurred, the objective of intensive care management should move from the care of the critically ill patient to the care of a potential organ donor, maximizing the number and quality of transplantable organs. Therefore, only by understanding, anticipating and correcting the pathophysiological changes which will occur at the moment of brain death, the intensivist will be able to allow the gift of new lives for the patients in waiting list to happen. It is, in fact, recognized that organs from deceased potential donors are frequently refused because they are considered not suitable for transplantation.(7) This may occur if inevitable progressive changes will not be timely detected and corrected. Conversely, the number of transplantable organs is more if donor management goals are met.(8–10) Achieving optimal organ perfusion and cellular oxygenation should be, therefore, the crucial aim of management of the deceased potential organ donor.

Hemodynamic changes

Hemodynamic dysfunction is the most frequent alteration occurring at the moment of brain death and, compromising systemic perfusion, is frequently responsible for the deterioration of organ function. Therefore, the occurrence of such alterations should be adequately monitored, anticipated, and promptly corrected.

Hemodynamic changes typically mirror the rostrocaudal evolution of cerebral ischemia and blood flow arrest.(11) As pontine ischemia develops, vagal and sympathetic stimulation with short period of bradycardia and hypertension will occur. With the progression of ischemic damage to medulla oblongata and involvement of vagal nucleus, unopposed sympathetic stimulation will occur. This sympathetic storm with release of high levels of catecholamines will be responsible for severe hypertension and tachycardia. At this time, the occurrence of hypertension is the expression of the attempt to preserve cerebral perfusion pressure in the face of severe intractable intracranial hypertension. During autonomic storm, only short-acting drugs should be considered, as this phase will be rapidly followed by severe persistent hypotension. With further caudal evolution of ischemia to spinal cord, subsequent loss of sympathetic tone and decrease of peripheral vascular resistance will occur. Relative intravascular hypovolemia, decreased pre-load, reduced coronary perfusion, and severe hypotension will follow. Distributive, hypovolemic, and cardiogenic shock may all be present when brain death occurs. The correct identification of the main cause of hemodynamic impairment, whether secondary to hypovolemia, stress cardiomyopathy or vasoparalysis, will allow the proper treatment to be administered. To this extent, close hemodynamic monitoring is important to guide treatment.

Neurogenic stress cardiomyopathy

Neurogenic cardiac injury plays a crucial role among all the hemodynamic pathophysiological changes occurring in the patients with catastrophic injury evolving to brain death, because it can affect not only the treatment, but also the decision whether heart is suitable or not for transplantation.[12]

The autonomic storm occurring at the moment of brain death resembles the one observed in patients with acute neurological damage, most often after subarachnoid haemorrhage, and known as neurogenic stress cardiomyopathy (NSC). Variably reported with an incidence of 20–75%, NSC can manifest either with elevation in serum markers of cardiac injury and of the B-type natriuretic peptide or as ECG alterations (QT interval prolongation, T wave and ST segment anomalies, cardiac arrhythmias), or in terms of regional or global wall motion abnormalities at echocardiography. The pathogenesis of NSC seems to be multifactorial, though catecholamine-mediated direct myocardial injury due to massive discharge of catecholamines following a sudden increase in intracranial pressure is the most accepted theory.[3,13–17]

It is also possible that a spectrum of pathogenetic factors, not mutually exclusive, ranging from coronary artery spasm or cardiac microvascular dysfunction or a particular genetic basis with polymorphisms of β1, β2, and α2 receptors, Gs or Gi proteins, adenyl-cyclase to other downstream components of the biochemical adrenergic pathways, may play a role in stress-related cardiomyopathy syndrome, along with the excess of catecholamines.[3] In a study to evaluate the catecholamine surge and the histologic lesions in hearts procured from brain death donors, in whom hearts had been rejected for transplant because of donor age, weight, or recipient blood group incompatibility, the authors demonstrated the presence of contraction bands in 54% of these donors. Furthermore, 62% were positive for apoptotic cells. Affected areas never exceeded 5% of the total area examined and, therefore, were unlikely to have had any major detrimental effect on post-transplant cardiac function.(18) Contraction band necrosis is a typical feature of NSC, as cell dies in a hypercontracted state with early myofibrillar damage and anomalous irregular cross-band formations. The authors demonstrated that while epinephrine peaked at only 2.36 fold at the moment of brain death, norepinephrine peaked 8.56 times the standard value 1 hour after brain death and dopamine, 54.76 times. After this marked rise at the time of brain death, circulating catecholamine levels fell.(18) It has been suggested that local release of norepinephrine from myocardial sympathetic nerve terminals is also a key in the pathogenesis of contraction band necrosis.(19)

Further research in this field is ongoing, trying to identify the subjects at risk for developing these cardiac complications, as genetically more susceptible to stress, or more susceptible to the administration of pharmacologic agents active on the adrenergic receptors. Specifically, several significant associations between beta adrenergic receptor polymorphisms and the presence of left ventricular dysfunction after brain death have been reported.(20)

Clinical experience and research data have demonstrated that NSC is functional in nature and reversible over days/weeks. Whether or not stress cardiomyopathy is the underlying cause of ventricular dysfunction associated with brain death has been recently a matter of intense debate.(21)

Therefore, occurrence of NSC at the moment of brain death should not preclude consideration of possible suitability of a heart for transplantation. Successful transplantation of hearts with regional wall motion abnormalities related to brain death associated with catecholamine storm has been reported in literature, showing that cardiac dysfunction in NSC is reversible even after the heart has been transplanted to another patient.(22) Recently, an amendment to current recommendations on donor cardiac function has been proposed by Redfors et al, suggesting that a donor heart with regional wall motion abnormalities and/or ejection fraction below 40% should be considered for transplantation if coronary angiography shows no obstructive coronary artery disease and criteria for NSC are met.[22]

Therefore, better research to evaluate the extent of possible reversible cardiac dysfunction should be prompted and means to buy more time for the improvement of dysfunctional heart offered for transplantation should be considered,[21] only after ruling out other causes of cardiac dysfunction such as ischemia or myocarditis. As stunned myocardium is potentially a reversible cause of cardiac dysfunction, the possibility to prolong maintenance period should be considered, allowing to identifying the contractile reserve of dysfunctional myocardium.[23,24]

Respiratory dysfunction

The occurrence of lung injury after an acute brain injury is well described in literature and represents one of the most frequent extracranial complications in these patients,[25–35] with many proposed pathogenetic mechanisms.[31,36,37]

The eventuality of brain-lung interplay has been increasingly addressed in experimental models and in humans and has been related to an increased morbidity and mortality.[2,38–43]

Aspiration, pneumonia, neurogenic pulmonary oedema, massive increase in sympathetic activity and increased production of proinflammatory cytokines then released into the systemic circulation are among the several mechanisms that have been proposed to play a role in the occurrence of lung injury in a neurological critically ill patient.[31,36,37]

A sympathetic storm caused by an acute increase in intracranial pressure is the crucial mechanism of the 'blast injury theory', proposed by Theodore in 1976, and recognized as the pathogenetic mechanism of neurogenic pulmonary oedema.[36] At respiratory level, high levels of catecholamine determine an increase in vascular hydrostatic pressure and lung capillary permeability. This will eventually cause endothelium damage allowing protein-rich plasma to escape into the interstitial and alveolar spaces causing the clinical picture of acute lung injury.[2]

Furthermore, neuroinflammation has been involved in the pathogenesis of this pathologic process.[32,43] Several inflammatory mediators (IL-1, IL-6, and TNF-alfa, among others) are involved in this mechanism and, if neuroinflammatory response represents initially a coordinated effort to protect the brain after injury, it may then become dysregulated and cause activation of the secondary injury cascade leading to single or multiple organ dysfunctions.[44,45] Additionally, it has been hypothesized that increased sympathetic activity and increased production of proinflammatory cytokines create a systemic inflammatory environment responsible for the increased lung susceptibility to subsequently occurring injurious events, such as mechanical ventilation, or others.[43] Therefore, careful, protective mechanical ventilation and strategies to reduce ventilation associated mortality after acute brain injury[46] have been proposed to prevent further injury. Mechanical ventilation strategies in the potential organ donor are specifically discussed in Chapter 32 of this book.

Diabetes insipidus and electrolyte imbalance

Diabetes insipidus occurs in up to 75% of patients evolving to brain death[47] and sudden polyuria, the main clinical sign, is a frequent bedside indicator of impending brain death. If not promptly treated with fluid infusion and hormone replacement therapy, loss of vasopressin will determine inappropriate diuresis, severe hypovolemia, and hypernatremia. The posterior pituitary lobe receives blood from the hypophyseal arteries which have extradural origin from internal carotid artery and, therefore, its damage is usually secondary to direct damage rather than from hypoperfusion.

As diabetes insipidus will contribute to severe hemodynamic derangements, timely detection of its occurrence is crucial. Measurements of plasma and urine sodium concentration and osmolality, and tight fluid balance determination, together with clinical signs remain the most important diagnostic parameters. Hypotonic polyuria (>50ml/kg/day), serum sodium > 145mmol/L, serum osmolality >295 mmol/Kg H2O, and urine osmolality <200 mmol/Kg H2O are the diagnostic criteria.[48]

Renal changes

Although less investigated, brain-kidney cross-talk has been hypothesized and is potentially responsible for acute kidney injury (AKI) in brain death patients.[5] The inflammatory response associated to acute brain injury and determining damage to several organs can affect the kidneys also. An increase in renal sympathetic nervous system activity, affecting renal blood flow and glomerular filtration, and altered vasopressin release can lead to changes in sodium and water balance and should be promptly anticipated and treated.

Kidney function may be compromised not only by inflammatory response, but also by haemodynamic impairment and neurohormonal changes occurring after acute brain damage.[5]

Possible negative impact of acute brain damage on allograft outcome should be considered and prevented.

Hypothermia

At bedside, rapidly evolving hypothermia is among the early signs which will indicate the clinician that something has changed and brain death may be impending. Hypothermia is multifactorial: loss of central thermoregulation after brain death, heat loss due to vasoplegia, and decreased metabolic rate are the main contributors. Temperature loss will progress to deep values if not promptly corrected and, therefore, should be anticipated and actively treated.

Hypothermia is a great mimic of brain death and can suppress neurologic function. As hypothermia will physiologically develop after brain death and will hinder neurologic examination, maintenance of normothermia is a mandatory prerequisite for brain death examination. Furthermore, apart from interfering with clinical examination, hypothermia can also worsen concomitant coagulopathy and increase the risk of cardiac arrhythmias.

Endocrine changes

Endocrine changes are well recognized among the pathophysiological changes occurring at the time of brain death.[49] Nevertheless, results from clinical data are mainly observational in design, and are not so robust to clearly dictate a secure strategy of treatment.

Although critical illness itself has profound effects on the pituitary function, neuroendocrine dysfunction may represent a distinct secondary damage after acute brain injury and it can jeopardize systemic homeostasis. Endocrine dysfunction occurring after acute brain damage and at the moment of brain death will contribute to hemodynamic instability and organ deterioration.

Pituitary function is at particular risk after an acute brain injury because of the vulnerable anatomic location of the gland within the sella turcica, as well as its delicate infundibular hypothalamic structure and its fragile vascular supply. In several neuropathological studies, haemorrhage, necrosis, and fibrosis of the pituitary gland and hypothalamus have been recorded after acute brain injury.[50]

Thyroid axis suppression may alter vascular reactivity and reduce response to vasopressor. The hypothesis that endocrine dysfunction can alter vascular tone further increasing the burden of secondary insults responsible for brain damage, and that hormonal replacement can reverse it, led to the proposal of hormonal therapy to achieve hemodynamic stability, even if with controversial results. However, alterations in pituitary hormone levels have been demonstrated after brain death, especially affecting the hypothalamic-hypopituitary-adrenal axis and the hypothalamic-hypopituitary-thyroid axis, thus, whether or not hormonal replacement therapy could be beneficial remains an unsolved question.[51–57] Actual consensus statements recommend to consider thyroid hormone replacement either alone or as part of a combination hormone therapy for hemodynamically unstable donors.[58]

In 2019, the author's research group in Torino, Italy, investigated, over the first five days of admission, the neuroendocrine alterations in a population of 113 critically ill patients including patients with acute respiratory distress syndrome (ARDS), severe TBI, subarachnoid haemorrhage (SAH), and a group of neurocritically ill patients at the moment of brain death.[59] In the brain death group, the pituitary axes were severely depressed with low level of copeptin (the C-terminal part of the AVP precursor pro-AVP), thyroid deficiency (30%) and the absence of HPA activation (90%). The ACTH and cortisol levels were lower than in the other critically ill patients with ARDS, SAH, and TBI.

Large randomized controlled trials are urgently needed to further explore this complex arena.

Inflammatory and complement response

An intense inflammatory response, linked to immunologic and endocrine cascades, has been described in severe neurologic damage evolving to brain death.[60,61] Increased release of Interleukins (IL-1, IL-6, IL-8) and tumour necrosis factor alpha has been described at the moment of brain death.[62]

In an observational study on severe TBI patients, our group hypothesized that a specific pattern of cytokines and chemokines was related to secondary insults and might identify patients who die early because of brain herniation. The study demonstrated that median plasma cytokine levels were significantly higher in patients evolving to brain death when compared to both favourable and unfavourable outcome groups, and that IL-6 was the most important cytokine associated with raised ICP and low CPP insult.[63]

Furthermore, the complement system is also triggered. It has been suggested that complement is not only activated later during transplantation, but it is already activated in the potential organ donor.[64] Systemic complement activation may also trigger local inflammation, and production of damage-associated molecular pattern molecules (DAMPs) has been documented as a consequence of hypoxia in deceased organs.[64]

There is literature investigating the role of complement response not only in donors after brain death but also in Donation after Circulatory Death (DCD) donors. While inflammatory cascade is prevalent after brain death, apoptosis seems to be the most important pathway of injury in DCD donors.

Therefore, the possibility to target the complement system has been proposed as a new mode of treatment in the deceased organ donor[65,66] even if peculiarities of organ dysfunction would require a well-tailored treatment. The role of complement activation as a cause of deteriorating organ function and the possibility to target it by the use of novel therapies has been recently revised in a comprehensive review.[64]

The inflammatory reaction occurring after brain injury may contribute to distal organ injury although underlying mechanisms have not been completely elucidated.

Coagulation impairment

Along with intense inflammatory response, activation of coagulation and a prothrombotic state is associated with brain death. Occurrence of disseminated intravascular coagulation due to plasminogen activator release after acute brain injury may negatively affect organ function. Low platelet levels and alteration in coagulation factors have been described and need close monitoring and correction to avoid bleeding disorders in the potential organ donor.

Conclusion

The occurrence of brain death following a catastrophic brain injury is mainly induced by rapidly spreading ischemic events,[67] despite intensive brain monitoring in the neuro-intensive care unit.[68–72] The transition phase to brain death determines, over a short period of time, several changes which can potentially affect all organ functions. During this phase and during the period of brain death determination by neurological criteria,[73,74] the number and intensity of organ dysfunction may be variable, but they should be anticipated and promptly corrected in order to avoid irreversible alterations in organ function which could compromise the eventuality of subsequent organ donation.

Highlights

- The evolution from a severe acute brain injury to brain death is characterized by several sudden pathophysiological changes which may compromise organ perfusion and function.
- Identification of the potential organ donor is the first crucial step in organ donor management.

- A continuum of care from the treatment of acute brain injury to the management of the potential organ donor is essential to expand donation pool.
- Adequate management of brain death organ donors is crucial to maximize number and function of the donated organs.
- Understanding the changes in hemodynamic, respiratory, endocrine, and metabolic function, among others, is important for a proper management of the potential organ donor in the intensive care unit.

References

1. Samuels MA. The brain-heart connection. Circulation 2007;116:77–84.
2. Mazzeo AT, Fanelli V, Mascia L. Brain-lung crosstalk in critical care: How protective mechanical ventilation can affect the brain homeostasis. Minerva Anestesiol. 2013;79:299–309.
3. Mazzeo AT, Micalizzi A, Mascia L, Scicolone A, Siracusano L. Brain-heart crosstalk: The many faces of stress-related cardiomyopathy syndromes in anaesthesia and intensive care. Br J Anaesth. 2014;112:803–815.
4. Civiletti F, Assenzio B, Mazzeo AT, et al. Acute tubular injury is associated with severe traumatic brain injury: In vitro study on human tubular epithelial cells. Sci Rep. 2019;9:6090.
5. Nongnuch A, Panorchan K, Davenport A. Brain–kidney crosstalk. Critical Care 2014, 18:225 doi: 10.1186/cc13907.
6. De Georgia MA. History of brain death as death: 1968 to the present. J Crit Care. 2014;29:673–678.
7. Meyfroidt G, Gunst J, Martin-Loeches I, et al. Management of the brain-dead donor in the ICU: General and specific therapy to improve transplantable organ quality. Intensive Care Med. 2019;45:343–353.
8. Patel MS, Zatarain J, De La Cruz S, et al. The impact of meeting donor management goals on the number of organs transplanted per expanded criteria donor: A prospective study from the UNOS Region 5 Donor Management Goals Workgroup. JAMA Surg. 2014;149:969–975.
9. Malinoski DJ, Patel MS, Daly MC, Oley-Graybill C, Salim A; UNOS Region 5 DMG workgroup. The impact of meeting donor management goals on the number of organs transplanted per donor: Results from the United Network for Organ Sharing Region 5 prospective donor management goals study. Crit Care Med. 2012;40:2773–2780.
10. Floerchinger B, Oberhuber R, Tullius SG. Effects of brain death on organ quality and transplant outcome. Transplant Rev (Orlando). 2012;26:54–59.
11. Drake M, Bernard A, Hessel E. Brain Death. Surg Clin North Am. 2017;97:1255–1273. doi: 10.1016/j.suc.2017.07.001.
12. Madias JE. Donor hearts, hearts of resuscitated cardiac arrest victims, hearts of patients with neurogenic stress cardiomyopathy, and hearts of patients

with Takotsubo syndrome: Any commonalities? Int J Cardiol. 2015;199:33. doi: 10.1016/j.ijcard.2015.06.184

13. Nguyen, H, Zaroff, JG. Neurogenic stunned myocardium. Curr. Neurol. Neurosci. Rep. 2009;9:486–491.
14. Ripoll JG, Blackshear JL, Díaz-Gómez JL. Acute cardiac complications in critical brain disease. Neurosurg. Clin. N. Am. 2018;29:281–297.
15. Bybee KA, Prasad A. Stress-related cardiomyopathy syndromes. Circulation 2008;118;397–409.
16. Gopinath R, Ayya SS. Neurogenic stress cardiomyopathy: What do we need to know. Ann. Card. Anaesth. 2018;21:228–234.
17. Tahsili-Fahadan P, Geocadin RG. Heart-brain axis: Effects of neurologic injury on cardiovascular function. Circ Res. 2017;120:559–572.
18. Pérez López S, Otero Hernández J, Vázquez Moreno N, et al. Brain death effects on catecholamine levels and subsequent cardiac damage assessed in organ donors. J Heart Lung Transplant. 2009;28:815–820.
19. Novitzky D, Wicomb WN, Cooper DK, Rose AG, Reichart B. Prevention of myocardial injury during brain death by total cardiac sympathectomy in the Chacma baboon. Ann Thorac Surg. 1986;41:520–524.
20. Khush KK, Pawlikowska L, Menza RL, et al. Beta-adrenergic receptor polymorphisms and cardiac graft function in potential organ donors. Am J Transplant. 2012;12:3377–3386.
21. Berman M, Ali A, Ashley E, Freed D, Clarke K, Tsui S, Parameshwar J, Large S. Is stress cardiomyopathy the underlying cause of ventricular dysfunction associated with brain death? J Heart Lung Transplant. 2010;29:957–965.
22. Redfors B, Råmunddal T, Oras J, et al. Successful heart transplantation from a donor with takotsubo syndrome. Int J Cardiol. 2015;195:82–84. doi: 10.1016/j.ijcard.2015.05.137
23. Zaroff JG, Babcock WD, Shiboski SC, Solinger LL, Reosengard BR. Temporal changes in left ventricular systolic function in heart donors: Results of serial echocardiography. J Heart Lung Transpl 2003;22:383–388.
24. Maciel CB, Greer DM. ICU management of the potential organ donor: State of the art. Curr Neurol Neurosci Rep. 2016;16:86. doi: 10.1007/s11910-016-0682-1.
25. Aisiku IP, Yamal JM, Doshi P, Benoit JS, Gopinath S, Goodman JC, Robertson CS. Plasma cytokines IL-6, IL-8, and IL-10 are associated with the development of acute respiratory distress syndrome in patients with severe traumatic brain injury. Crit Care. 2016;20:288. doi: 10.1186/s13054-016-1470-7
26. Chen GS, Liao KH, Bien MY, Peng GS, Wang JY. Increased risk of post-trauma stroke after traumatic brain injury-induced acute respiratory distress syndrome. J Neurotrauma. 2016;33:1263–1269.
27. Holland MC, Mackersie RC, Morabito D, et al. The development of acute lung injury is associated with worse neurologic outcome in patients with severe traumatic brain injury. J Trauma 2003;55:106–111.
28. Bratton SL, Davis RL. Acute lung injury in isolated traumatic brain injury. Neurosurgery 1997;40:707–712.
29. Piek J, Chesnut RM, Marshall LF, et al. Extracranial complications of severe head injury. J Neurosurg 1992;77:901–907.

30. Zygun DA, Kortbeek JB, Fick GH, Laupland KB, Doig CJ. Non-neurologic organ dysfunction in severe traumatic brain injury. Crit Care Med 2005;33:654–660.
31. Lopez-Aguilar J, Villagra' A, Bernabe' F, et al. Massive brain injury enhances lung damage in an isolated lung model of ventilator-induced lung injury. Crit Care Med 2005;33:1077–1083.
32. Mascia L. Ventilatory setting in severe brain injured patients: Does it really matter? Intensive Care Med 2006;32:1925–1927.
33. Mascia L, Sakr Y, Pasero D, Payen D, Reinhart K, Vincent JL; Sepsis Occurrence in Acutely Ill Patients (SOAP) Investigators. Extracranial complications in patients with acute brain injury: A post-hoc analysis of the SOAP study. Intensive Care Med 2008;34:720–727.
34. Caricato A, Conti G, Della Corte F, et al. Effects of PEEP on the intracranial system of patients with head injury and subarachnoid hemorrhage: The role of respiratory system compliance. J Trauma 2005;58:571–576.
35. Pelosi P, Severgnini P, Chiaranda M. An integrated approach to prevent and treat respiratory failure in brain-injured patients. Curr Opinion Crit Care 2005;11:37–42.
36. Theodore J, Ronin E. Speculation on neurogenic pulmonary edema (NPE). Am Rev Resp Dis 1976;113:405–411.
37. Smith WS, Matthay MA. Evidence for a hydrostatic mechanism in human neurogenic pulmonary edema. Chest 1997;111:1326–1333.
38. Koutsoukou A, Perraki H, Raftopoulou A, et al. Respiratory mechanics in brain-damaged patients. Intensive Care Med 2006;32:1947–1954.
39. Mascia L, Grasso S, Fiore T, Bruno F, Berardino M, Ducati A. Cerebro-pulmonary interactions during the application of low levels of positive end-expiratory pressure. Intensive Care Med 2005;31:373–379.
40. Mascia L, Zavala E, Bosma K, et al. Brain IT group. High tidal volume is associated with the development of acute lung injury after severe brain injury: An international observational study. Crit Care Med 2007;35:1815–1820.
41. Quilez ME, Lopez-Aguilar J, Blanch L. Organ crosstalk during acute lung injury, acute respiratory distress syndrome, and mechanical ventilation. Curr Opin Crit Care 2012;18:23–28.
42. Zygun DA, Zuege DJ, Boiteau PJ, Laupland KB, Henderson EA, Kortbeek JB, Doig CJ. Ventilator-associated pneumonia in severe traumatic brain injury. Neurocritical Care 2006;5:108–114.
43. Mascia L. Acute lung injury in patients with severe brain injury: A double hit model. Neurocrit Care 2009;11:417–426.
44. Kelley BJ, Lifshitz J, Povlishock JT. Neuroinflammatory responses after experimental diffuse traumatic brain injury. J Neuropathol Exp Neurol 2007;66:989–1001.
45. Hutchinson PJ, O'Connell MT, Rothwell NJ, et al. Inflammation in human brain injury: Intracerebral concentration of IL-1α, IL-1β, and their endogenous inhibitor IL-1ra. J Neurotrauma 2007;24:1545–1557.
46. Asehnoune K, Mrozek S, Perrigault PF, et al. BI-VILI study group. A multi-faceted strategy to reduce ventilation-associated mortality in brain-injured patients. The BI-VILI project: A nationwide quality improvement project. Intensive Care Med. 2017;43:957–970.

47. Smith M. Physiologic changes during brain stem death–lessons for management of the organ donor. Journal of Heart and Lung Transplantation 2004;23(9 Suppl): S217–S222.
48. Winzeler B, Zweifel C, Nigro N, et al. Postoperative copeptin concentration predicts diabetes insipidus after pituitary surgery. J Clin Endocrinol Metab 2015;100:2275–2282.
49. Ranasinghe AM, Bonser RS. Endocrine changes in brain death and transplantation. Best Pract Res Clin Endocrinol Metab. 2011;25:799–812.
50. Harper CG, Doyle D, Adams JH, Graham DI. Analysis of abnormalities in pituitary gland in non-missile head injury: Study of 100 consecutive cases. J Clin Pathol 1986;39:769–773.
51. Novitzky D, Mi Z, Sun Q, Collins JF, Cooper DK. Thyroid hormone therapy in the management of 63,593 brain-dead organ donors: A retrospective analysis. Transplantation. 2014;98:1119–1127.
52. Macdonald PS, Aneman A, Bhonagiri D, et al. A systematic review and meta-analysis of clinical trials of thyroid hormone administration to brain dead potential organ donors. Crit Care Med. 2012;40:1635–1644.
53. Rosendale JD, Kauffman HM, McBride MA et al. Aggressive pharmacologic donor management results in more transplanted organs. Transplantation 2003;75:482–487.
54. Rosendale JD, Chabalewski FL, McBride MA, Garrity ER, Rosengard BR, Delmonico FL, Kauffman HM. Increased transplanted organs from the use of a standardized donor management protocol. Am J Transplant. 2002;2:761–768.
55. Rosendale JD, Kauffman HM, McBride MA et al. Hormonal resuscitation yields more transplanted hearts, with improved early function. Transplantation 2003;75:1336–1341.
56. Venkateswaran RV, Steeds RP, Quinn DW et al. The haemodynamic effects of adjunctive hormone therapy in potential heart donors: A prospective randomized double-blind factorially designed controlled trial. European Heart Journal 2009;30:1771–1780.
57. Salim A, Martin M, Brown C et al. Using thyroid hormone in brain-dead donors to maximize the number of organs available for transplantation. Clinical Transplantation 2007;21:405–409.
58. Kotloff RM, Blosser S, Fulda GJ et al. Management of the potential organ donor in the ICU: Society of critical care medicine/American College of Chest Physicians/Association of Organ Procurement Organizations Consensus Statement. Crit Care Med 2015;43:1291–1325.
59. Mazzeo AT, Guaraldi F, Filippini C, et al. Activation of pituitary axis according to underlying critical illness and its effect on outcome. J Crit Care. 2019;54:22–29.
60. Watts RP1, Thom O, Fraser JF. Inflammatory signalling associated with brain dead organ donation: From brain injury to brain stem death and posttransplant ischaemia reperfusion injury. J Transplant. 2013;2013:521369.
61. Barklin A. Systemic inflammation in the brain-dead organ donor. Acta Anaesthesiol Scand. 2009;53:425–435.
62. Birks EJ, Yacoub MH, Burton PS et al. Activation of apoptotic and inflammatory pathways in dysfunctional donor hearts. Transplantation 2000;70:1498–1506.

63. Mazzeo AT, Filippini C, Rosato R, et al. Multivariate projection method to investigate inflammation associated with secondary insults and outcome after human traumatic brain injury: A pilot study. J Neuroinflammation. 2016;13:157.
64. van Zanden JE, Jager NM, Daha MR, Erasmus ME, Leuvenink HGD, Seelen MA. Complement therapeutics in the multi-organ donor: Do or don't? Front Immunol. 2019;10:329. doi: 10.3389/fimmu.2019.00329
65. Damman J, Bloks VW, Daha MR, et al. Hypoxia and complement-and-coagulation pathways in the deceased organ donor as the major target for intervention to improve renal allograft outcome. Transplantation. 2015;99:1293–300.
66. Damman J, Seelen MA, Moers C, et al. Systemic complement activation in deceased donors is associated with acute rejection after renal transplantation in the recipient. Transplantation. 2011;92:163–169.
67. Mazzeo AT, Kunene NK, Choi S, Gilman C, Bullock RM. Quantitation of ischemic events after severe traumatic brain injury in humans: A simple scoring system. J Neurosurg Anesthesiol. 2006;18:170–178.
68. Mazzeo AT, Gupta D. Monitoring the injured brain. J Neurosurg Sci. 2018;62:549–562.
69. Kitagawa R, Yokobori S, Mazzeo AT, Bullock R. Microdialysis in the neurocritical care unit. Neurosurg Clin N Am. 2013;24:417–426.
70. Mazzeo AT, Bullock R. Monitoring brain tissue oxymetry: Will it change management of critically ill neurologic patients? J Neurol Sci. 2007;15;261:1–9.
71. Naldi A, Provero P, Vercelli A, et al. Optic nerve sheath diameter asymmetry in healthy subjects and patients with intracranial hypertension. Neurol Sci. 2020;41:329–333.
72. Mazzeo AT, Bullock R. Effect of bacterial meningitis complicating severe head trauma upon brain microdialysis and cerebral perfusion. Neurocrit Care. 2005;2:282–287.
73. Lewis A, Bakkar A, Kreiger-Benson E, et al. Determination of death by neurologic criteria around the world. Neurology 2020, Jul 21;95(3):e299–e309.
74. Greer DM, Shemie SD, Lewis A, et al. Determination of brain death/death by neurologic criteria. The World Brain Death Project. JAMA. 2020;324:1078–1097. doi: 10.1001/jama.2020.11586.

31

Management of the potential organ donor in the intensive care unit

Anna Teresa Mazzeo, Rosario Urbino, Raffaele Potenza,
Francesco Puliatti, Deepak Gupta

Introduction

Organ transplantation represents one of the most important successful accomplishments of modern medicine and is the result of a well-integrated system involving hospital managers, procurement coordinators, intensivists, and transplant surgeons. Hard clinical work, together with efforts dedicated to education,[1] training and research in this area allowed the most experienced centres to achieve the actual results, in terms of increased activity and improved outcomes.

In a well-organized system, it is essential to recognize organ procurement as an integral component of clinical pathways inside the hospital, so that the opportunity to donate is offered to any patient dying in the hospital. To allow this, the procurement process needs to be involved in all clinical time sensitive pathways inside the hospital (such as head injury, cerebrovascular accidents, and cardiac arrest). Therefore, organ donation is to be considered not as a success of a single person but as the result of the entire hospital.

Analysis of data reported in literature and, especially, the big gap existing between the number of transplanted organs and the number of patients in the waiting lists is the evidence that procurement system does not operate to its full potential and efficiency, with rare exceptions all over the world.[2]

Though donation rates may vary between structures, an increased awareness on organ donation among healthcare personnel and citizens should be recognized as a main target of any hospital in the modern era. Failure to timely identify the potential organ donor, failure to certificate brain deaths, and failure to maintain a potential organ donor are all recognized as the main obstacles to a successful transplantation.

As 'brain-oriented' intensive care describes the complex of care dedicated to a patient with acute brain injury inside the intensive care unit (ICU), 'organ-oriented' intensive care describes the complex of care dedicated to a potential organ donor. When brain death has occurred, the mission of the intensivist is to move from the care of a salvageable, critically ill patient to the care of a potential organ donor. Maintenance of adequate organ perfusion and evaluation of organ suitability for transplantation are critical steps for a successful transplant programme.

Only by understanding the pathophysiological changes occurring in the transition from acute brain damage to brain death, the intensivist will be able to timely detect and correct derangements in organ homeostasis, which will unavoidably deteriorate their function. The pathophysiological changes occurring when brain death is impending have been extensively described in Chapter 30 of this book to which we refer the readers; the basis of this chapter will directly address the management of a potential organ donor in the ICU.

The importance of targeting donor management goals

Literature demonstrates that a rigorous systematic application of organ donor management strategies can reduce progressive derangement of organ function occurring after brain death and increase the rate of organs suitable for transplantation. The main objective of treatment at this stage is the maintenance of systemic homeostasis, preservation and improvement of organ function, and eventually organ procurement. In order to achieve these objectives, it is important to rely on bedside checklists which include, among others, specific targets of hemodynamic, ventilatory, metabolic, and temperature management. The use of checklist may help in improving adherence to management goals. Training of ICU team involved in the care of the potential organ donor on the proper application of protocols is critical. Each intervention, such as fluid selection, vasopressor or inotropes selection, hormonal replacement therapy, ventilation strategy, and monitoring selection, should be based on the identification of relevant pathophysiological determinants, as illustrated in Chapter 30, 'Pathophysiological changes at the moment of brain death' of this book, to which we refer.

Literature demonstrates that targeting donor management goals (DMG), which are normal cardiovascular, pulmonary, renal, and endocrine end points, is crucial to increase the number and quality of transplanted organs.[3–5] In a prospective study hypothesizing that meeting DMGs during the organ donation process would be associated with more organs transplanted per donor, it was demonstrated that meeting donor DMGs (defined as having met seven of nine critical care end points) was independent predictors of ≥4 organs transplanted per donor.[4] When expanded criteria donors (ECD) (who are typically older donors with more significant comorbidities) were later investigated in 2014, Patel et al demonstrated that meeting DMGs prior to organ recovery was associated with a 90% higher chance of obtaining three or more organs transplanted per ECD.[5] Investigated DMGs were: Mean arterial pressure 60–110 mmHg; Central venous pressure 4–12 mmHg; Ejection fraction ≥50 %; Low-dose vasopressors (dopamine at 10 µg/kg/min or less, neosynephrine at 60 µg/min or less, and norepinephrine at 10 µg/min or less) with number of agents ≤1; Arterial blood gas, pH 7.3–7.5; PaO2:FIO2 ratio ≥300; Serum sodium ≤155 mEq/L; Urine output ≥0.5 mL/kg/h over 4 h; Glucose ≤150 mg/dL.[5]

The application of institutional checklists with specific DMGs should, therefore, be considered as the standard of care in the management of potential organ donor.

Indeed, the implementation of an intensive lung donor-treatment protocol succeeded in increasing the lung procurement rate in centres with and without lung transplant programmes.[6] The proposed protocol in the study by Minambres et al comprehended: Apnoea test performed with ventilator (continuous positive pressure mode); Mechanical ventilation with PEEP 8–10 cm H2O and tidal volume 6–8 ml/kg; Recruitment manoeuvres once per hour and after any disconnection from the ventilator; Bronchoscopy with bilateral bronchoalveolar lavage immediately after brain death; Close hemodynamics monitoring; goal extravascular lung water of <10 ml/kg (with administration of diuretics if necessary) and CVP (objective) of <8 mmHg; Methylprednisolone (15 mg/kg) after brain-death declaration; Alveolar recruitment manoeuvres; in those lung donors with PaO2/FIO2 <300 mmHg, semilateral decubitus position plus recruitment manoeuvres.[6]

A consensus statement of the process for donor heart and lung procurement has been published in 2020 to standardize the procurement process and to prevent graft failure.[7]

Competing targets for organ perfusion could theoretically call for antagonistic strategies such as fluid replacement or high positive end-expiratory pressure. Nevertheless, recent studies demonstrated that judicious application of lung management protocols has no negative impact on the recovery rates of other grafts or on early survival of heart, liver, pancreas, or kidney recipients.[8] On the other hand, the multicentre randomized MOnIToR trial, to determine whether protocolized fluid therapy increases the number of organs transplanted, demonstrated that protocolized fluid therapy was not superior to usual care in increasing the number of organs transplanted.[9]

A modified version of the VIP approach (Ventilation, Infusion, and Pumping strategy) and the inclusion of the additional initials, 'P' and 'S', referred to Pharmacological treatment of shock and Specific management of the etiologic cause of shock, has been favourably proposed.[10]

Recently, the ongoing Donation Network to Optimise Organ Recovery (DONOR) Study, a planned, cluster, randomized controlled trial that aims to evaluate the effectiveness of the implementation of an evidence-based, goal-directed checklist for brain-dead potential organ donor management in ICUs, in reducing the loss of potential donors due to cardiac arrest has been proposed and will give, in the near future, results of such an implementation of care.[11]

Introducing a pathway to stop the early withdrawal of life-sustaining treatments in patients with devastating brain injury admitted to emergency department and to transfer all such patients to ICU, allows time for more accurate prognostication and improves end of life care. Recent evidences demonstrate that the devastating brain injury pathway increased the potential for organ donation and the proportion of donors after brain death to donors after circulatory death, with only a small negligible impact on ICU resources.[12]

Better communication among professionals involved in different stages of the process at the hospital level (ICU personnel, donor

Box 31.1 Cardiovascular Management

Challenge: Hemodynamic dysfunction is very frequent in the potential organ donor. Potential causes are reduction of preload due to hypovolemia, reduction of afterload due to distributive shock, and reduced myocardial contractility either related to primary cardiac injury, or congestive heart failure, neurogenic stress cardiomyopathy, or hypothermia.

Endpoints of treatment:

- To achieve optimal organ perfusion and cellular oxygenation.
- To maintain hemodynamic stability.

Consider:

- Specific management of the relevant underlying cause/s of shock.
- Detection and prompt correction of hypovolemia
- Fluid replacement using hemodynamic parameters and guided by monitoring; isotonic crystalloids being the preferred choice.
- Target mean arterial pressure ≥60 mmHg, urine output ≥1 mL/kg/h, left ventricle ejection fraction ≥45%.
- Target lower number and dose of vasopressors (Dopamine, dobutamine, or epinephrine may be preferred in primary cardiac pump dysfunction; Norepinephrine or phenylephrine may be preferred to treat distributive shock due to low systemic vascular resistance; vasopressin in the case of refractory shock).
- In the case of unmet hemodynamic goals, or if left ventricular ejection fraction <45%, consider the use of hormonal replacement therapy to improve vascular responsiveness to vasopressors.

Monitoring: Invasiveness of hemodynamic parameters is guided by clinical status, vasopressor doses, and responsiveness to treatment.

Serial measurements of lactate, venous oxygen saturation, acid-base balance, and central venous pressure are recommended. ECG monitoring and biologic markers are measured for myocardial necrosis.

Echocardiography is required for determination of the suitability of the heart for transplantation, to guide hemodynamic management, to exclude functional, reversible, stress-related cardiomyopathy.

Pulmonary artery catheter monitoring or minimally invasive hemodynamic monitoring techniques for cardiac output measurement should be considered, in selected cases, if cardiovascular restoration guided by basic monitoring fails, to allow for assessment of volume, pump or resistance goals.

Box 31.2 Pulmonary Care

Challenge: Acute lung injury secondary to inflammatory response, neurogenic oedema, ventilator-associated pneumonia, or prolonged injurious ventilation is very frequent and can jeopardize lung procurement.

Endpoints of treatment:

Avoid lung injury and maintain optimal oxygenation. Maintain negative or neutral fluid balance.

Lung protective ventilation strategy:

Tidal volumes 6–8 ml/Kg predicted body weight

PEEP 8–10 cmH_2O

Closed circuit for suctioning

Consider CPAP (equal to previous PEEP) for apnea tests

Recruitment manoeuvres after disconnections from ventilator

Monitoring: Oxygen saturation, capnography, arterial and venous blood gas analysis, lung compliance, bronchoscopy, chest XR.

Box 31.3 Diabetes Insipidus Treatment

Challenge: Loss of antidiuretic hormone incretion (arginine vasopressin, AVP) is very frequent and can induce severe hypovolemia, electrolytic imbalance and hemodynamic instability.

Diagnostic criteria for diabetes insipidus are hypotonic polyuria (>50ml/kg/day), serum sodium >145 mmol/L, serum osmolality >295 mmol/Kg H_2O, urine osmolality <200 mmol/Kg H_2O or urine specific gravity < 1.005.

Endpoints of treatment: Intravenous dose of 1–4 μg of desmopressin titrated to response (expected reduction in serum sodium, osmolarity, and urine output) and repeated as required. Correct hypovolemia in order to maintain normovolemia and preserve organ perfusion. When diabetes insipidus is associated with hypotension that persists despite adequate fluid resuscitation, intravenous AVP at 0.01–0.04 IU/min may be used.

Monitoring: Strictly monitor hourly diuresis. Closely monitor natremia. Check plasma and urine osmolality. Closely monitor and replace as required serum electrolytes to avoid hypokalemia, hypophosphatemia, hypomagnesemia.

Box 31.4 Hormonal Replacement Therapy

Challenge: Dysfunction of the anterior pituitary gland after acute brain injury and at the moment of brain death has been variably reported in literature. Neuroendocrine dysfunction may alter peripheral vascular tone and contribute to hemodynamic instability and organ deterioration.

Endpoints of treatment:

- *Thyroid hormones* should be considered for hemodynamically unstable donors or for potential cardiac donors with abnormal (< 45%) left ventricular ejection fraction.

Administration of intravenous (IV) T4: 20-μg bolus, followed by an infusion at 10 μg/hr, or IV T3: 4.0-μg bolus, followed by an infusion at 3 μg/hr.

- *Steroids* have been proposed to reduce the inflammatory cascade following brain death.

High-dose corticosteroid administration (methylprednisolone 1000 mg IV, 15 mg/kg IV, or 250 mg IV bolus followed by infusion at 100 mg/hr; or Hydrocortisone 50 mg IV bolus and 10 mg/h IV maintenance or 300 mg/d IV).

When indicated, hormonal replacement therapy should only be administered after blood sampling for tissue typing, as it can reduce human leukocyte antigen expression.

Monitoring: Hemodynamic monitoring

Box 31.5 Renal Care

Challenge: Immunological and non-immunological damage to the kidneys and impaired autoregulation of renal blood flow and glomerular filtration may jeopardize the maintenance of adequate organ perfusion and diuresis. Potential additional effect of nephrotoxic drugs is possible.

Endpoints of treatment:

- Hemodynamic stabilization
- Judicious fluid resuscitation to maintain end-organ perfusion
- Maintain normovolemia
- Maintain urine output 0.5–2.5 ml/Kg/h
- Maintain acid-base equilibrium
- Monitor and replace serum electrolytes as required

Monitoring: Hemodynamic monitoring, serial measurements of lactate, serial monitoring of electrolytes, blood gas analysis, renal function monitoring, hourly urine output measurement.

Box 31.6 Liver Care

Challenge: Elevated serum sodium concentration determine the accumulation of idiogenic osmoles within the liver cells, which, after the transplantation into recipients with relatively normal serum sodium concentration cause intracellular water accumulation, cell lysis, and cell death. This can cause hepatic dysfunction and graft loss.

Endpoint of treatment:

Liver protecting strategy:

- Correct serum sodium level with a target below 155 mmol/L
- Maintain CVP between 8 and 10 mmHg
- Maintain adequate nutrition to restore liver glycogen stores

Monitoring: Hemodynamic monitoring, serial measurements of lactate, serial monitoring of electrolytes and glycemia, liver function laboratory tests

Box 31.7 TEMPERATURE MANAGEMENT

Challenge: Loss of thermoregulation, peripheral vasodilatation, and reduction in metabolic activity are the main causes of hypothermia which can obstacle neurological examination and determine cardiac and coagulation alterations.

Endpoints of treatment:

- Reduce heat loss
- Use humidified ventilatory circuit
- Actively correct hypothermia to maintain normothermia.

Monitoring: Continuous monitoring of temperature

Box 31.8 General management measures

Challenge: Systemic homeostasis is rapidly threatened after brain death and can compromise organ function.

Endpoint of treatment:

Simple ICU care measures are indicated to maintain systemic homeostasis and avoid organ dysfunction. Early involvement of transplant coordinator and team can share experience and increase organ procurement rate.

- Proper communication and support of family should also be considered part of the treatment.
- Treatment of infections
- Maintenance of normoglycemia according to local institutional protocols
- Monitoring and correction of coagulation alterations
- Monitoring and correction of anaemia
- Elevation of head of the bed

coordinators, clinicians involved in time-depending pathways, radiologists, cardiologists, neurologists, neurosurgeons, among others) can help in improving final results. Outcome will be measured inside each hospital as a decreased number of brain death donors lost by cardiac arrest, an increased number and quality of organ recovered, and better long-term outcome in the recipients, measured as improved graft function, survival and quality of life. The implementation of a goal-directed checklist for the care of the potential organ donor is a critical step to achieve at the hospital level.

Specific targets of treatments, coming from the best available evidence in literature, are proposed in Boxes 31.1–31.8 to guide daily practice in the care of potential organ donors.[6,13–23]

Conclusion

Understanding the pathophysiological changes occurring at the moment of brain death is critical to better anticipate, detect, and treat organ dysfunctions commonly accompanying this phase. Specific targets of treatments, known as DMGs, may help to preserve organ function and can increase the number of organs transplanted per donor. The use of bedside management algorithms and checklists can assist the intensivists to achieve better results in organ donor management.

Highlights

- In order to understand organ donor management, it is essential to understand pathophysiological changes occurring at the moment of brain death.
- Donor management has to be considered as a continuum of care, from the critical care management of the acute brain injured patient to the care of a potential organ donor.
- 'Organ-oriented' intensive care describes the complex of care dedicated to the potential organ donor.
- Meeting DMG is an independent predictor of organ transplanted per donor.

- The application of institutional checklists with specific DMG should be considered as standard of care in the management of potential organ donor.

References

1. Hakeem AR, Dave R, Prasad KR, Menon KV, Lewington A, Fernando B, Sanfey H, Ahmad N. An imperative need to change organ donation and transplant curriculum results of a nationwide United kingdom junior doctor survey. Transplantation. 2015;99:771–785.
2. Tullius SG, Rabb H. Improving the supply and quality of deceased-donor organs for transplantation. N Engl J Med 2018; 378:1920–1929.
3. Malinoski DJ, Daly MC, Patel MS, Oley-Graybill C, Foster CE 3rd, Salim A. Achieving donor management goals before deceased donor procurement is associated with more organs transplanted per donor. J Trauma. 2011;71:990–995.
4. Malinoski DJ, Patel MS, Daly MC, et al. The impact of meeting donor management goals on the number of organs transplanted per donor: Results from the United Network for Organ Sharing Region 5 prospective donor management goals study. Crit Care Med 2012;40:2773–2780.
5. Patel MS, Zatarain J, De La Cruz S, et al. The impact of meeting donor management goals on the number of organs transplanted per expanded criteria donor: A prospective study from the UNOS Region 5 Donor Management Goals Workgroup. JAMA Surg. 2014;149:969–975.
6. Miñambres E, Pérez-Villares JM, Chico-Fernández M, et al. Lung donor treatment protocol in brain dead-donors: A multicenter study. J Heart Lung Transplant. 2015;*34*:773–780.
7. Copeland H, Hayanga JWA, Neyrinck A, et al. Donor heart and lung procurement: A consensus statement. J Heart Lung Transplant. 2020 Jun; 39(6):501–517.
8. Miñambres E, Pérez-Villares JM, Terceros-Almanza L, et al. An intensive lung donor treatment protocol does not have negative influence on other grafts: A multicentre study. Eur J Cardiothorac Surg. 2016;49:1719–1724.
9. Al-Khafaji A, Elder M, Lebovitz DJ, et al. Protocolized fluid therapy in brain-dead donors: The multicenter randomized MOnIToR trial. Intensive Care Med. 2015;41:418–426.
10. Westphal GA. A simple bedside approach to therapeutic goals achievement during the management of deceased organ donors—An adapted version of the 'VIP' approach. Clin Transplant. 2016;30:138–144.
11. Westphal GA, Robinson CC, Biasi A, Machado FR, et al. DONORS (Donation Network to Optimise Organ Recovery Study) Investigators and the BRICNet. Study protocol to evaluate the implementation of an evidence-based checklist for brain-dead potential organ donor management in intensive care units, a cluster randomised trial. BMJ Open. 2019;9:e028570. doi: 10.1136/bmjopen-2018-028570

12. Rivers J, Manara AR, Thomas I, Derrick E. Impact of a devastating brain injury pathway on outcomes, resources, and organ donation: 3 years' experience in a regional neurosciences ICU. Neurocrit Care. 2020;33:165–172. doi: 10.1007/s12028-019-00879-1.
13. Kotloff RM, Blosser S, Fulda GJ, et al. Society of Critical Care Medicine/American College of Chest Physicians/Association of Organ Procurement Organizations Donor Management Task Force. Management of the Potential Organ Donor in the ICU: Society of Critical Care Medicine/American College of Chest Physicians/Association of Organ Procurement Organizations Consensus Statement. Crit Care Med. 2015;43:1291–1325.
14. Rosengard BR, Feng S, Alfrey EJ, et al. Report of the Crystal City meeting to maximize the use of organs recovered from the cadaver donor. Am J Transplant. 2002;2:701–711.
15. Dictus C, Vienenkoetter B, Esmaeilzadeh M, Unterberg A, Ahmadi R. Critical care management of potential organ donors: our current standard. Clin Transplant. 2009;23 Suppl 21:2–9.
16. Citerio G, Cypel M, Dobb GJ, et al. Organ donation in adults: A critical care perspective. Intensive Care Med. 2016;42:305–315.
17. Meyfroidt G, Gunst J, Martin-Loeches I, Smith M, Robba C, Taccone FS, Citerio G. Management of the brain-dead donor in the ICU: General and specific therapy to improve transplantable organ quality. Intensive Care Med. 2019;45:343–353.
18. Dupuis S, Amiel JA, Desgroseilliers M, et al. Corticosteroids in the management of brain-dead potential organ donors: A systematic review. Br J Anaesth. 2014;113:346–359.
19. Macdonald PS, Aneman A, Bhonagiri D, et al. A systematic review and meta-analysis of clinical trials of thyroid hormone administration to brain dead potential organ donors. Crit Care Med. 2012;40:1635–1644.
20. Mascia L, Pasero D, Slutsky AS, et al. Effect of a lung protective strategy for organ donors on eligibility and availability of lungs for transplantation: A randomized controlled trial. JAMA. 2010;304:2620–2627.
21. McKeown DW, Bonser RS, Kellum JA. Management of the heartbeating brain-dead organ donor. Br J Anaesth. 2012;108 Suppl 1:i96–i107. doi: 10.1093/bja/aer351.
22. Novitzky D, Mi Z, Sun Q, Collins JF, Cooper DK. Thyroid hormone therapy in the management of 63,593 brain-dead organ donors: A retrospective analysis. Transplantation. 2014;98:1119–1127.
23. Rosendale JD, Chabalewski FL, McBride MA, Garrity ER, Rosengard BR, Delmonico FL, Kauffman HM. Increased transplanted organs from the use of a standardized donor management protocol. *Am J Transplant.* 2002;2:761–8.

32

Protective mechanical ventilation in the potential organ donor

Andrea Costamagna, Vito Fanelli, Luciana Mascia

Introduction

Lung transplantation is a lifesaving treatment for end-stage respiratory failure. Statistics from the Organ Procurement and Transplantation Network and the Scientific Registry of Transplant Recipients confirm that donor shortage remains a concern, despite continuous improvement in donor management.(1,2) Brain dead donors (BDD) experience impairment in gas exchange, mainly due to neurogenic pulmonary oedema (NPE) and atelectasis.(3,4) Nevertheless, organ donor after cardiac death (DCD) experience peculiar pathological changes mainly due to warm ischemic time period.(1,5) Ex vivo lung perfusion (EVLP) has emerged, in the last ten years, as an effective strategy to expand lung donor pool allowing to further evaluate suboptimal lungs, either from BDD or DCD donors.(1,6,7)

BDD's pathophysiology carries a complex and predictable multi-organ derangement, which is mainly driven by increments in intracranial pressure (ICP). Cushing reflex, characterized by tachycardia and compensatory arterial hypertension to sustain cerebral perfusion pressure (CPP), is accompanied by massive endogenous catecholamine release, followed by loss of autonomic vascular tone and hypotension. Consequence is that brain death can be followed by cardiovascular collapse due to myocardial injury and multiorgan ischaemia, due to both vasoconstriction and hypoperfusion, together with NPE. Pathophysiology of NPE has not been fully elucidated; catecholamine release with raised pulmonary arterial pressure, capillary leak due to increased pulmonary capillary permeability, and cytokines release can lead to the emergence of NPE. Essentially, NPE shares radiological and clinical features with acute respiratory distress syndrome (ARDS), such as arterial hypoxia and non-cardiogenic pulmonary oedema with bilateral chest X-ray infiltrates. Multiorgan dysfunction is complicated by loss of posterior pituitary function with the onset of diabetes insipidus, together with significative electrolyte abnormalities and fluid (free water) loss, hypothyroidism, hypothalamic temperature control derangement with hypothermia, inflammation, and coagulopathy.[3,4]

During the time period required for diagnosis of brain death, lungs have to be managed with the aim to preserve the organ itself to be evaluated for lung donation and to avoid ventilator-induced lung injury (VILI). The VILI may theoretically be detrimental also for distal organs, through cytokine-meditated systemic inflammation.[8–11]

Protective mechanical ventilation is one of the most effective sustaining therapies for lung preservation during donor management in ICU.[1,7] It is based on low tidal volume protective mechanical ventilation strategies with positive end-expiratory pressure (PEEP) application and recruitment manoeuvres. In BDD patients, particular attention has to be paid to hemodynamic and homeostatic interactions between the need to use relatively high PEEP with potentially frequent recruitment manoeuvres and the theoretical rise in carbon dioxide (CO_2) and the need to manage ICP and to preserve cardiac function.[3,4]

The objective of this chapter is to summarize the current evidence and provide clinical guidance about BDD lung ventilatory management. Furthermore, special concerns about DCD patients and during EVLP strategies will be discussed (Figure 32.1).

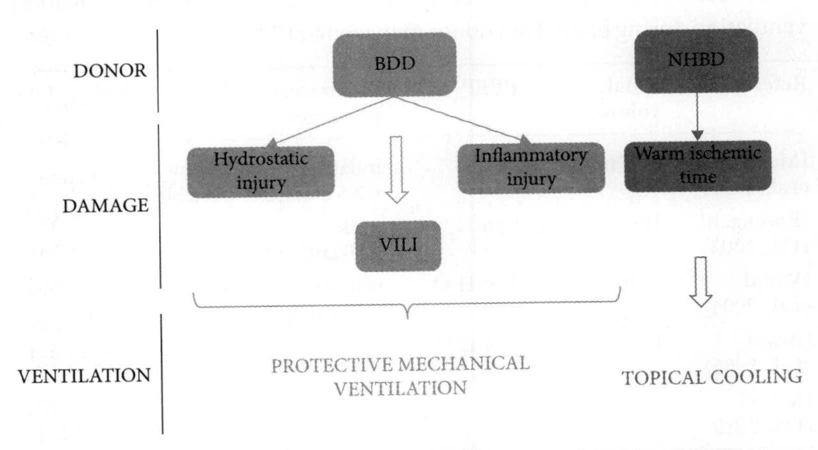

Figure 32.1. Physiopathology of lung injury and ventilatory strategies during BDD and non-heart beating donors (NHBD) management

Historical overview

Recommendation about ventilatory management of the potential BDD has extensively changed over the last twenty years, focusing both on avoiding VILI to preserve lung function and on minimizing multiorgan dysfunction (Table 32.1).[4]

In a review from 1997, the authors suggested to ventilate lungs with low rates, low inspiratory pressures but highest tidal volumes as possible, up to 15 ml/Kg, and with the lowest inspired fraction of oxygen (FiO_2). However, the author did not make difference between close chest ventilation in ICU during BDD observation period and donor surgery during organ harvesting.[12] In 2002, a consensus meeting held by the American Society of Transplant Surgeons and the American Society of Transplantation to maximize organ retrieval from cadaver donors recommended to ventilate lungs with 10–12 ml/Kg with a fixed PEEP of 5 cm H_2O and avoiding peak inspiratory pressures (PIP) of more than 30 cmH_2O.[13] All other parameters being equal, Wood et al suggested, in 2004, to set a tidal volume of 8 to 10 ml/Kg, focusing mainly on the concept of standardizing organ management protocols.[14] As part of an active donor lung management protocol, Angel et al proposed to introduce active recruitment manoeuvres for patients with impaired oxygenation parameters and pulmonary oedema or atelectasis to expand

Table 32.1 Historical overview of recommended changes about mechanical ventilation during brain dead donor management[12–16]

Reference	Tidal volume	PEEP	Inspiratory pressures	FiO_2	RM	FBS
(Maclean et al., 1997)	≤ 15 ml/Kg	-	inflation < 7.5 cmH_2O	lowest possible	-	-
(Rosengard et al., 2002)	10–12 ml/Kg	5 cmH_2O	peak < 30 cmH_2O	0.40	-	Yes
(Wood et al., 2004)	8–10 ml/Kg	5 cmH_2O	plateau < 30 cmH_2O	0.40	-	Yes
(Angel et al., 2006)	10 ml/Kg	5 cmH_2O	-	-	Yes	Yes
(Kotloff et al., 2015)	6–8 ml/Kg	8–10 cmH_2O	-	-	Yes	Yes

RM=recruitment manoeuvres; FBS= fiberoptic bronchoscopy; FiO2= inspiratory oxygen fraction donor pool, without changing conventional ventilation parameters. This strategy allowed to, significantly, target lung donor pool increment.[15] More recently, a document developed through the efforts of the Society of Critical Care Medicine, the American College of Chest Physicians, and the Association of Organ Procurement Organizations suggested to strongly consider using ventilatory strategies based on low stretch protocols and recruitment manoeuvres.[16] The authors report, in support of this affirmation, the results of a European multicentre randomized controlled trial (RCT) which compared a traditional, conventional mechanical ventilation strategy with a protective protocol using 6–8 mL/kg of tidal volumes together with 8 to 10 cmH_2O PEEP and recruitment manoeuvres whenever appropriate, limiting disconnection from ventilator.[8] This protocol, based on the ARDS network protective ventilatory strategy,[17] allowed to significantly increase lung donor pool and to limit the amount of circulating pro-inflammatory cytokines in the protective ventilation group.[8]

Lung damage in the brain-dead donor

To explain the development of lung failure associated with brain injury evolving to brain death, a 'double hit' model has been proposed integrating experimental and clinical evidence.[3,18,19] The first or primary hit is represented by the systemic consequences of the sympathetic storm and the pro-inflammatory environment caused by brain injury eventually evolving to brain death.[3] Once 'primed' the respiratory system is then vulnerable to further inflammatory insults caused by mechanical stress induced by mechanical ventilation.[11] A vicious circle may, therefore, be activated where the deterioration of the respiratory function may worsen the damage of the central nervous system that will result in distal organs failure. In this prospective, the lungs represent an organ particularly susceptible to receive further insults if mechanical ventilation is not applied with a protective modality.[19] This model has been validated by experimental and clinical data.

In a model of traumatic brain injury, membrane lipid peroxidation, nuclear chromatin degeneration, vacuolar degeneration of sub-cellular organelles, and down-regulation of anti-apoptotic genes have been demonstrated in type II alveolar cells.[20,21] In a rat model of intra-cerebral haemorrhage, Wu and coworkers showed increased expression of inflammatory mediators and neutrophil infiltration in both brain and lung.[22] In an experimental model of ischemic stroke, lung water content was significantly increased compared to control.[23] Kalsotra et al, in an experimental model of cortical impact injury, found altered lung permeability, marked migration of neutrophils and activated macrophages in the alveolar space.[24] More recently, Quilez and coworkers revealed that injurious mechanical ventilation may induce neuronal activation in amygdala, thalamus, and paraventricular hypothalamic nuclei in intact animals.[25] Heuer and colleagues showed neuronal shrinkage in hippocampus region of previously healthy animals with acid aspiration-induced lung injury.[26]

In patients with cerebral haemorrhage, evidence of acute lung oedema has been demonstrated by extra vascular lung water (EVLW) accumulation,[27] while in patients dying soon after and within 96 hours of acute brain injury, evidence of elevations in lung weights have been shown.[28] In a small series of twelve patients with acute cerebrovascular accident who developed acute pulmonary oedema, Smith and coworkers showed that hydrostatic mechanisms accounted for NPE formation.[29] More recently, Mascia and associates demonstrated that patients with acute brain injury are more susceptible to develop respiratory failure than a general population of critically ill patients.[30]

Brain death, as the final evolution of many causes of acute brain injury, may induce lung injury, as demonstrated by several experimental settings. In a rat model, Tang et al. illustrated that brain death can induce lung injury through apoptosis enhancement, mediated by endoplasmic reticulum stress.[31] Hemodynamic derangement immediately following brain death, with increase in capillary wedge pressure and pulmonary venous resistance, was associated to lung injury and cytokine storm in a porcine model by Belhaj and associates.[32] Vascular permeability plays also a pivotal role in brain death-induced lung injury. Animal experimental data show that the administration of a molecule able to activate the sphingosine 1–phosphate receptor resulted in a significant reduction of vascular permeability and consequent lung protection following brain death.[33] Lung histology and oxygenation improvement, and reduction of inflammatory molecules were achieved by Zhou et al. with the administration of carbon monoxide to brain dead rats.[34] On the contrary, Methylprednisolone,[35] aprotinin and inhaled nitric oxide[36] did not result in donor lung protection in experimental animal models of brain death. Naloxone, although promising for oxygenation improvement in BDD based on experimental[37] and human retrospective studies,[38] did not result, when tested in a RCT, in oxygenation nor donation rate improvement.[39]

Ventilator-induced lung injury

The main indication for ventilatory support in patients with severe brain injury is to treat the respiratory dysfunction consequent to cerebral damage. Under these circumstances, an adequate ventilatory setting to guarantee tight control of blood gas exchange helps in preventing secondary brain insults. However, there has been increasing evidence that the mechanical forces necessary to inflate the lungs during ventilatory support can cause damage—called as Ventilator-Induced Lung Injury, VILI and this damage may worsen outcomes by multiple mechanisms (Figure 32.2).[11] This phenomenon is more evident in pulmonary conditions characterized by a non-homogeneous distribution of lung damage such as

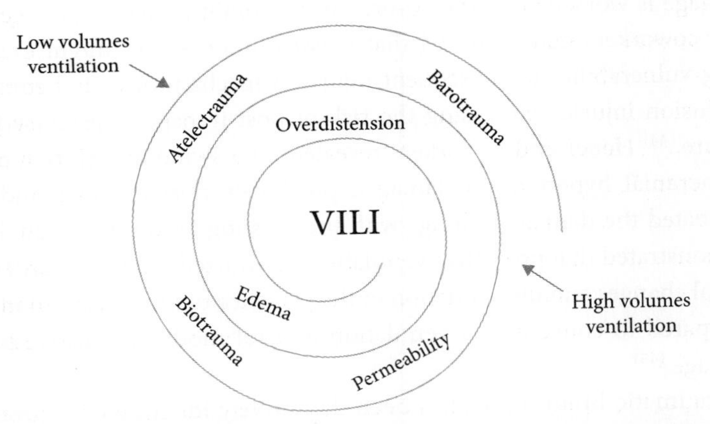

Figure 32.2. Ventilator-induced lung injury pathophysiology, represented as a spiral in which both high and low volumes ventilation, without applying appropriate positive end-expiratory pressure and recruitment manoeuvres, can trigger mechanical and biological damage, leading to increased alveolar capillary permeability and inflammatory pulmonary oedema

ARDS.[11] In these patients, it is well established that a ventilatory strategy designed to minimize VILI applying a tidal volume of 6 ml/kg of predicted body weight (PBW) and plateau pressure < 30 cmH2O improves the outcome.[17] Later, the hypothesis that VILI may occur in 'normal' lungs as well has been made. A new meta-analysis, involving 2822 patients who underwent mechanical ventilation for elective surgery, demonstrated that protective ventilation strategy with low tidal volume significantly reduced mortality, pulmonary infection and atelectasis.[40] In a recent control trial, surgical patients randomized to receive protective ventilation developed less pulmonary (atelectasis, pneumonia) and extra-pulmonary (sepsis) complications in the postoperative period and lower hospital length of stay compared to conventional ventilation.[41] Not long ago, a Cochrane systematic review aiming to assess the benefits of perioperative low tidal volume ventilation on post-operative pulmonary complications showed that pneumonia and post-operative need for ventilatory support were reduced in patients ventilated with protective settings.[42]

Recent experimental studies showed that VILI may also impact brain structure and function. Lung stretch-induced hippocampal apoptosis has been denoted in mechanically ventilated animals with high pressure.[43] Models of coexisting lung and brain acute injuries show that lung damage is worsened by the co-presence of brain injury. Lopez-Aguilar and coworkers demonstrated that massive brain injury might escalate lung vulnerability to subsequent injurious mechanical or ischemia-reperfusion injuries increasing the risk of post-transplant primary graft failure.[44] Heuer and coworkers revealed, in a swine model, that acute intracranial hypertension damaged previously normal lungs and exacerbated the damage in lungs with pre-existing lesions.[26] Krebs et al demonstrated that protective ventilation minimized lung morpho-functional changes and inflammation in the presence of massive brain injury compared to conventional ventilation in a rat model of massive brain damage.[45]

Traumatic brain injury has been definitively identified as a predisposing factor for ARDS.[46] In 2012, Rincon et al reported that the occurrence of this complication carried a higher risk of in-hospital death after brain injury.[47] Pelosi et al described that acute neurologically ill patients received a mean VT equal to 9 ml/PBW with a PEEP equal to

4 cmH2O and that ventilator settings applied to neurological patients were undistinguishable from that used for non-neurological critically ill.[48] In a prospective observational study in patients with severe brain injury, Mascia and coworkers demonstrated that injurious mechanical ventilation was a contributing factor to the development of ARDS and that, patients with this complication were more dependent on ventilatory support and spent more days in ICU.[49] Most recently, ARDS incidence was estimated to be 3% in a prospective cohort of 986 mechanically ventilated patients, due to brain injury.[50] Pro-inflammatory (IL6 and IL8) and anti-inflammatory (IL10) cytokines were found to be significantly higher in a prospective cohort of patients with traumatic brain injury who developed ARDS, compared to patients without associated lung damage.[51]

Similar results were also demonstrated in potential organ donors. In an observational study conducted in fifteen Italian ICUs, after diagnosis of brain death, cardiovascular management was modified to preserve peripheral organ perfusion while ventilatory management was not modified from a 'cerebral protective' to a 'lung protective' strategy, and no manoeuvres for recruiting the lung and preventing mechanical stretch were performed. Consequently, during the six hours period required by the Italian law for brain death confirmation, 50% of potential lung donors became ineligible for lung donation due to deterioration in oxygenation.[52]

These data strongly support the notion that activation of the innate immune system after brain injury causes distal organ injury through the release of inflammatory mediators, even without macroscopic evidence of organ damage. The data suggests that mechanical ventilation may affect the lung function of potential organ donors predisposing to post-transplant primary graft failure. Therefore, the lungs primed by an inflammatory response elicited by brain injury could be further injured by sequential noxious stimuli leading to lung failure. Since the 'primary hit' is constituted by the severity of brain injury, clinical interventions are limited and unlikely to be successful. On the other hand, appropriate supportive therapies are likely to influence the occurrence and intensity of 'secondary hits' that may impair distal organ function.

Mechanical ventilation: Protective strategy

Lungs from BDD may suffer a decline in their function because of the progression of the primary neurological injury and up to 60% of these lungs will be not considered suitable for transplantation.[1,52,53] Although lung failure may result from the detrimental consequences of brain death,[30,54] recent evidences suggest that injurious mechanical ventilation may further contribute to deterioration of susceptible lungs.[9,49]

Mechanical ventilation for patients with severe brain injury is oriented to a 'cerebral protective' strategy in order to avoid hypoxemia and hypercapnia, thus limiting secondary insults to the brain. According to previously available guidelines[55] a $PaCO_2$ between 35 and 40 mmHg is usually obtained with high tidal volumes and low respiratory rates, while a PaO_2 > 90 mmHg should be obtained with high FiO_2 and low level of PEEP to avoid interference with cerebral venous drainage. More recently, the consensus statement of the Society of Critical Care Medicine, the American College of Chest Physicians, and the Association of Organ Procurement Organizations suggests the use of ventilatory strategies based on low stretch protocols and recruitment manoeuvres.[16]

If patients with severe brain injury evolve to brain death, critical care management of the potential organ donors suggests that the priority should be shifted from a 'cerebral protective' strategy to an 'organ protective' strategy, able to optimize organs donation. The lungs are responsible for maintaining systemic homeostasis, optimal oxygenation and optimal acid-base balance (pH), while the heart is responsible for optimal perfusion of peripheral organs. However, the lungs also act as potential organs to be donated and, as such, should be protected by further 'hits' that can impair their function. Traditionally, clinical management of potential organ donors is oriented to guarantee optimal oxygenation and perfusion rather than to primarily protect the cardiothoracic organs.

Following this approach, in the past, international guidelines for potential organ donors management recommended the following ventilatory strategy: tidal volume between 8 and 15 mL/Kg to maintain $PaCO_2$ between 35 and 40 mmHg and peak pressure lower than 30 cmH_2O; PEEP levels equal to 5 cmH_2O and elevated fraction of inspired oxygen (FiO_2) in order to guarantee O_2 saturation higher than 95%. Bronchoscopy, frequent suctioning, and aspiration precautions were also recommended.[1,16] These guidelines are not substantially different from the Brain Trauma Foundation guidelines for management of traumatic brain injury patients.[55] The adherence to previous international guidelines for organ donor management has been verified in a multicentre observational study which confirmed that the ventilatory and hemodynamic management of potential organ donors was coherent with published recommendations and might have been suboptimal in preserving lung function.[52] Therefore, a potential conflict of interest may exist between the priority to maintain systemic homeostasis (optimal gas exchange and acid-base balance) and the priority to protect the lungs based on the robust evidence that VILI may also occur in 'normal' lungs at risk to develop ARDS, predisposing to post-transplant primary graft failure.

In 2010, a multi-centre RCT compared the use of a protective ventilatory strategy to the conventional strategy previously proposed by the international guidelines in potential organ donors. The protective strategy included low VT (6–8 mL/kg of PBW), PEEP equal to 8–10 cm H2O, use of closed circuit for tracheal suction, alveolar recruitment manoeuvres after any disconnection and the use of continuous positive airways pressure during apnoea test. The application of this strategy increased the number of eligible and transplanted lungs while the number of transplanted hearts, livers, and kidneys were similar in both groups.[8]

In the same prospective, several studies have proposed to extend lung donor criteria and to apply protocols to fully recruit the lungs. Angel and coworkers proposed the San Antonio Lung Transplant (SALT) protocol applying levels of PEEP up to 15 cmH_2O, limiting inspiratory pressure to 25 cmH_2O with neutral fluid balance, head elevation at 30° and inflation of the endotracheal cuff at pressure of 25 cmH_2O. This approach, compared to the standard of care in the four years period before the implementation of the protocol, increased the rate of lung procurement from 12% to 26%.[15] Noiseux and coworkers demonstrated that lung recruitment manoeuvres with two deep inflations at pressure of 30 cmH_2O for 30 seconds followed by 1 hour of mechanical ventilation with peak pressure < 30 cmH_2O and PEEP of 10 cmH_2O resulted in a significant increase in rate of transplanted lungs from 20% to 33%, without affecting the homeostasis of other organs.[56] Paries and associates, in a case-control study, showed that the application of one lung recruiting manoeuvre performed just after apnoea test (35 cmH_2O x 40 seconds) improved oxygenation with transient side effects on systemic hemodynamics. Compared to the historical control, this manoeuvre improved the rate of lungs that met eligibility criteria for transplantation.[57] Minambres and coworkers, in a cohort study with historical control, demonstrated that a protocol with VT of 8 ml/kg, PEEP of 8–10 cmH_2O, apnoea test performed with continuous positive airways pressure, recruitment manoeuvres performed every 2 hours and after disconnection from the ventilator, negative fluid balance and hormonal replacement therapy, increased the rate of lungs eligible for transplant without adverse effect on kidney graft survival.[58] Moretti et al confirmed that the use of VT equal to 6 ml/Kg, PEEP higher than 7 cmH_2O, recruiting manoeuvres and negative fluid balance increased the number of eligible lungs compared to historical control.[59] Routine application of PEEP to avoid de-recruitment and hypoxia also proved to be feasible and safe in a retrospective analysis of 169 BDD subjects, including patients on ECMO.[60] Recently, a meta-analysis on management of brain-dead organ donors underlined the concept that aggressive donor management should rely on strong pathophysiologic evidence. In their analysis of the available literature, Rech et al concluded that the best evidence in the management of organ donor refers to protective mechanical ventilation,[8,61] while other strategies such as hormonal replacement are weak. Similar conclusions were recently reached by Slutsky and Ranieri that recommended the use of protective lung strategy in heart-beating organ donors.[11]

In conclusion, a strong line of evidence suggests that: (a) brain injury evolving to brain death is a predisposing factor for ARDS; (b) an injurious mechanical ventilation enhances the risk of VILI in vulnerable lungs of potential organ donors; and (c) the application of protective ventilation significantly increases the number of transplanted lungs without affecting other grafts survival. Nevertheless, it is important to note that the available guidelines of organ procurement organizations do not suggest anymore the use of high tidal volume and low level of PEEP, accepting the strong line of evidence that support the application of a protective mechanical ventilation in potential organ donors.[16]

Further studies are required to elucidate if a multi-faceted protective ventilatory strategy may be helpful also in marginal potential organ donors to increase the number of transplanted lungs without affecting the homeostasis of other organs.

Mechanical ventilation and donation after cardiac death

Donation after cardiac death (DCD) represents a relatively brand-new pathway to overcome the problem of organ donor shortage. Although limited by a variable 'no touch' period after declaration of death and subsequent assessment, donor organs are not subjected to the intense hormonal and hemodynamic derangements following brain death.[4,5,62,63] However, warm ischemic time still limits organ suitability. Non-heart beating donors (NHBD) can be classified according to Maastricht classification and subsequently proposed modifications[64] into 'uncontrolled' and 'controlled' donors, depending on the timing and circumstances of death and on warm ischemic time duration, which are quantifiable and foreseeable for controlled donors only.[5,62]

Lung management during NHBD evaluation and organ retrieval focuses mainly on topical intra-thoracic cooling techniques. Worldwide programmes to manage controlled NHBD involve the perfusion of abdominal organs with a veno-arterial ECMO circuit and descending thoracic aorta clamping, after completing the assessment of death process. During this phase, lungs are cooled by in-vivo flush with cold preservation solutions, often accompanied by topical cooling with cold crystalloids and lungs re-inflation by recruitment manoeuvres or mechanically ventilated with protective protocols.[65–71]

Lungs from uncontrolled NHDB have been managed with topical in vivo cooling through chest tubes. After consent is obtained, the patient is transferred to the operative room, fluid is drained and protective mechanical ventilation with low tidal volumes is resumed for organ evaluation.[66,72–74] Conversely, Valenza et al. reported a case report of an uncontrolled NHBD successfully managed with a protocol involving the application of recruitment manoeuvres, protective MV and CPAP after the 20 minutes of asystole on electrocardiogram required in Italy for death assessment.[75]

Normothermic EVLP represents an innovative technique also in the field of NHDB to determine lung suitability, both controlled and uncontrolled, after organ retrieval.[1,66]

Mechanical ventilation during EVLP

Normothermic EVLP represents a platform to evaluate and theoretically optimize suboptimal donor lungs that have been defined 'marginal' during donor assessment.[6] In fact, EVLP allowed clinicians to expand donor pool preventing the potential harm to the recipient in using lungs with sub-optimal criteria for tansplantability.[1]

During EVLP, donor lungs are perfused and ventilated according to a standardized protocol and periodically evaluated. Although different in terms of re-perfusion settings, the three existing described EVLP procedures used worldwide (the Toronto,[6] Lund,[76] and OCS[77] protocols respectively) are concordant about the use of protective mechanical ventilation, with tidal volumes (VT) which ranges from 5 to 7 ml/Kg of donor's PBW and low PEEP from 5 to 7 cmH_2O. They differ mostly in terms of respiratory rate (from 7 bpm to 20 bpm in Toronto and Lund protocols, respectively) and FiO_2 (from 12% to 50% in OCS and Lund protocols, respectively). In the Toronto protocol, during lung function assessment, VT and FiO_2 are increased to 10 ml/Kg and 100%, respectively, without changes in PEEP levels.[6] In Lund experience, increments of PEEP for short periods with the aim to recruit atelectatic alveolar units are described.[76]

The common feature regarding mechanical ventilation during EVLP is the use of low tidal volumes to prevent and avoid VILI, translating current recommendations for ARDS patients.[11,17] However, for some patients, the use of protective ventilatory settings may not be enough to prevent ventilator-induced damage.[11,78] For this reason, Terragni et al. in a preliminary study quantified the risk of VILI during EVLP by using the 'stress index' parameter.[79] The authors showed that about two-thirds of lungs were non-protected, and that the stress index during EVLP directly correlates with increase in circulating cytokines and clinical outcomes.[80] However, due to the lack of high quality evidence-based literature on this specific matter, it is not possible to draw conclusions and suggest clinicians to modify current ventilatory settings during EVLP.

Conclusions

Brain injury evolving to brain death is a predisposing factor for ARDS; furthermore, injurious mechanical ventilation enhances the risk of VILI. Protective mechanical ventilation is a cornerstone of respiratory management for BDD and during EVLP.

DCD and EVLP represent valuable strategies to overcome organ donor shortage. Recent evidences suggest that: (a) lungs are the most susceptible organs to the deleterious effect of warm ischemia, (b) variable time needed to declare cardiac death (ranging from 5 to 60 min) that differs among several countries extensively affects organs homeostasis, (c) Protective mechanical ventilation associated to the application of lung recruitment manoeuvres and continuous positive airway pressure may limit graft deterioration, (d) EVLP technique is a valuable strategy to objectively evaluate graft function in order to expand the organ donor pool, (e) Protective mechanical ventilation tailored on lung mechanics may potentially improve graft function after transplantation.

Further studies are needed to elucidate if more protective settings should be used in specific sub-populations and to clarify optimal settings during apnoea test in BDD evaluation.

Highlights

- To explain the development of lung failure associated with brain death, a 'double hit' model has been proposed integrating experimental and clinical evidence.
- Mechanical forces necessary to inflate the lungs during ventilatory support can cause damage (Ventilator-Induced Lung Injury), which may also impact brain structure and function.
- The application of a protective ventilation significantly increases the number of transplanted lungs without affecting other grafts' survival.

- DCD represents a relatively brand-new pathway to overcome the problem of organ donor shortage.
- Normothermic EVLP represents an innovative technique to evaluate suboptimal donor lungs, and also in the field of DCD.

References

1. Sales G, Costamagna A, Fanelli V, Boffini M, Pugliese F, Mascia L, et al. How to optimize the lung donor. Minerva Anestesiologica [Internet]. 2018 Feb [cited 2019 May 12];(2). Available from: https://www.minervamedica.it/index2.php?show=R02Y2018N02A0204
2. Valapour M, Lehr CJ, Skeans MA, Smith JM, Uccellini K, Lehman R, et al. OPTN/SRTR 2017 Annual Data Report: Lung. American Journal of Transplantation. 2019;19(S2):404–484.
3. Busl KM, Bleck TP. Neurogenic Pulmonary Edema: Critical Care Medicine. 2015 Aug;43(8):1710–1715.
4. McKeown DW, Bonser RS, Kellum JA. Management of the heartbeating brain-dead organ donor. British Journal of Anaesthesia. 2012 Jan;108:i96–i107.
5. Fanelli V, Geraci PM, Mascia L. Donation after cardiac death: Is a 'paradigm shift' feasible in Italy? Minerva Anestesiol. 2013 May;79(5):534–540.
6. Cypel M, Anraku M, Sato M, Madonik M, Hutcheon M, Yasufuku K, et al. Normothermic ex vivo lung perfusion in clinical lung transplantation. The New England Journal of Medicine. 2011;10(364):1431–1440.
7. Meyfroidt G, Gunst J, Martin-Loeches I, Smith M, Robba C, Taccone FS, et al. Management of the brain-dead donor in the ICU: General and specific therapy to improve transplantable organ quality. Intensive Care Med. 2019 Mar;45(3):343–353.
8. Mascia L, Pasero D, Slutsky AS, Arguis MJ, Berardino M, Grasso S, et al. Effect of a lung protective strategy for organ donors on eligibility and availability of lungs for transplantation: A randomized controlled trial. Jama. 2010;304(23):2620–2627.
9. Ranieri VM, Suter PM, Tortorella C, Tullio RD, Dayer JM, Brienza A, et al. Effect of mechanical ventilation on inflammatory mediators in patients with acute respiratory distress syndrome: A randomized controlled trial. JAMA. 1999 Jul 7;282(1):54–61.
10. Ranieri VM, Giunta F, Suter PM, Slutsky AS. Mechanical ventilation as a mediator of multisystem organ failure in acute respiratory distress syndrome. JAMA. 2000 Jul 5;284(1):43–44.
11. Slutsky AS, Ranieri VM. Ventilator-induced lung injury. N Engl J Med. 2013 Nov 28;369(22):2126–2136.
12. Maclean A, Dunning J. The retrieval of thoracic organs: Donor assessment and management. Br Med Bull. 1997 Jan 1;53(4):829–843.
13. Rosengard BR, Feng S, Alfrey EJ, Zaroff JG, Emond JC, Henry ML, et al. Report of the crystal city meeting to maximize the use of organs recovered from the cadaver donor. American Journal of Transplantation. 2002;2(8):701–711.

14. Wood KE, D'Alessandro AM. Care of the potential organ donor. The New England Journal of Medicine. 2004;10(351):2730–2739.
15. Angel LF, Levine DJ, Restrepo MI, Johnson S, Sako E, Carpenter A, et al. Impact of a lung transplantation donor—management protocol on lung donation and recipient outcomes. Am J Respir Crit Care Med. 2006 Sep 15;174(6):710–716.
16. Kotloff RM, Blosser S, Fulda GJ, Malinoski D, Ahya VN, Angel L, et al. Management of the potential organ donor in the ICU: Society of Critical Care Medicine/American College of Chest Physicians/Association of Organ Procurement Organizations Consensus Statement. Critical Care Medicine. 2015 Jun;43(6):1291–1325.
17. The ARDS Network. Ventilation with lower tidal volumes as compared with traditional tidal volumes for acute lung injury and the acute respiratory distress syndrome. The Acute Respiratory Distress Syndrome Network. N Engl J Med. 2000 May 4;342(18):1301–1308.
18. Mascia L, Mastromauro I, Viberti S, Vincenzi M, Zanello M. Management to optimize organ procurement in brain dead donors. MINERVA ANESTESIOLOGICA. 2009;75(3):9.
19. Pelosi P, Rocco PR. The lung and the brain: A dangerous cross-talk. Crit Care. 2011;15(3):168.
20. Yildirim E, Kaptanoglu E, Ozisik K, Beskonakli E, Okutan O, Sargon MF, et al. Ultrastructural changes in pneumocyte type II cells following traumatic brain injury in rats. Eur J Cardiothorac Surg. 2004 Apr 1;25(4):523–529.
21. Yildirim E, Ozisik K, Ozisik P, Emir M, Yildirim E, Misirlioglu M, et al. Apoptosis-related Gene Bcl-2 in lung tissue after experimental traumatic brain injury in rats. Heart, Lung and Circulation. 2006 Apr;15(2):124–129.
22. Wu S, Fang CX, Kim J, Ren J. Enhanced pulmonary inflammation following experimental intracerebral hemorrhage. Experimental Neurology. 2006 Jul;200(1):245–249.
23. Toung T, Chang Y, Lin J, Bhardwaj A. Increases in lung and brain water following experimental stroke: Effect of mannitol and hypertonic saline*. Critical Care Medicine. 2005 Jan 1;33(1):203–208.
24. Kalsotra A, Zhao J, Anakk S, Dash PK, Strobel HW. Brain trauma leads to enhanced lung inflammation and injury: Evidence for role of P4504Fs in resolution. J Cereb Blood Flow Metab. 2007 May;27(5):963–974.
25. Quilez ME, Fuster G, Villar J, Flores C, Martí-Sistac O, Blanch L, et al. Injurious mechanical ventilation affects neuronal activation in ventilated rats. Crit Care. 2011;15(3):R124.
26. Heuer JF, Pelosi P, Hermann P, Perske C, Crozier TA, Brück W, et al. Acute effects of intracranial hypertension and ARDS on pulmonary and neuronal damage: a randomized experimental study in pigs. Intensive Care Med. 2011 Jul;37(7):1182–1191.
27. Touho H, Karasawa J, Shishido H, Yamada K, Yamazaki Y. Neurogenic pulmonary edema in the acute stage of hemorrhagic cerebrovascular disease. Neurosurgery. 1989 Nov;25(5):762–768.
28. Rogers FB, Shackford SR, Trevisani GT, Davis JW, Mackersie RC, Hoyt DB. Neurogenic Pulmonary Edema in Fatal and Nonfatal Head Injuries. The Journal of Trauma: Injury, Infection, and Critical Care. 1995 Nov 1;39(5):860–868.

29. Smith WS, Matthay MA. Evidence for a hydrostatic mechanism in human neurogenic pulmonary edema. Chest. 1997 May;111(5):1326–1333.
30. Mascia L, Sakr Y, Pasero D, Payen D, Reinhart K, Vincent J-L, et al. Extracranial complications in patients with acute brain injury: A post-hoc analysis of the SOAP study. Intensive Care Med. 2008 Apr 1;34(4):720–727.
31. Tang H, Zhang J, Cao S, Yan B, Fang H, Zhang H, et al. Inhibition of endoplasmic reticulum stress alleviates lung injury induced by brain death. Inflammation. 2017 Oct 1;40(5):1664–1671.
32. Belhaj A, Dewachter L, Rorive S, Remmelink M, Weynand B, Melot C, et al. Mechanical versus humoral determinants of brain death-induced lung injury. PLoS One [Internet]. 2017 Jul 28 [cited 2019 May 1];12(7): e0181899. Available from: https://www.ncbi.nlm.nih.gov/pmc/articles/PMC5533440/
33. Sammani S, Park K-S, Zaidi SR, Mathew B, Wang T, Huang Y, et al. A Sphingosine 1–Phosphate 1 Receptor Agonist Modulates Brain Death—Induced Neurogenic Pulmonary Injury. Am J Respir Cell Mol Biol. 2011 Nov;45(5):1022–1027.
34. Zhou H, Liu J, Pan P, Jin D, Ding W, Li W. Carbon monoxide inhalation decreased lung injury via anti-inflammatory and anti-apoptotic effects in brain death rats. Exp Biol Med (Maywood). 2010 Oct 1;235(10):1236–1243.
35. Pilla ES, Pereira RB, Junior LAF, Forgiarini LF, Paludo A de O, Kulczynski JMU, et al. Effects of methylprednisolone on inflammatory activity and oxidative stress in the lungs of brain-dead rats,. J Bras Pneumol. 2013;39(2):173–180.
36. Avlonitis VS, Wigfield CH, Kirby JA, Dark JH. Treatment of the brain-dead lung donor with aprotinin and nitric oxide. The Journal of Heart and Lung Transplantation. 2010 Oct;29(10):1177–1184.
37. Peterson BT, Ross JC, Brigham KL. Effect of naloxone on the pulmonary vascular responses to graded levels of intracranial hypertension in anesthetized sheep. Am Rev Respir Dis 1983 Dec;128(6):1024–1029. doi: 10.1164/arrd.1983.128.6.1024.PMID: 6650974 DOI: 10.1164/arrd.1983.128.6.1024
38. Eagan C, Keller CA, Baz MA, Thibault M. Effects of administration of intravenous naloxone on gas exchange in brain-dead lung donors. Prog Transplant. 2009 Sep;19(3):267–271.
39. Dhar R, Stahlschmidt EB, Paramesh A, Marklin G. A randomized controlled trial of naloxone for optimization of hypoxemia in lung donors after brain death. Transplantation. 2019 Jul;103(7):1433–1438. doi: 10.1097/TP.0000000000002511.
40. Neto AS, Cardoso SO, Manetta JA, Pereira VGM, Espósito DC, Pasqualucci M de OP, et al. Association between use of lung-protective ventilation with lower tidal volumes and clinical outcomes among patients without acute respiratory distress syndrome: A meta-analysis. JAMA. 2012 Oct 24;308(16):1651–1659.
41. Futier E, Constantin J-M, Paugam-Burtz C, Pascal J, Eurin M, Neuschwander A, et al. A trial of intraoperative low-tidal-volume ventilation in abdominal surgery. New England Journal of Medicine. 2013 Aug;369(5):428–437.
42. Guay J, Ochroch EA, Kopp S. Intraoperative use of low volume ventilation to decrease postoperative mortality, mechanical ventilation, lengths of stay and lung injury in adults without acute lung injury. Cochrane Database of Systematic Reviews [Internet]. 2018 [cited 2019 May 19];(7). Available from: http://www.cochranelibrary.com/cdsr/doi/10.1002/14651858.CD011151.pub3/full

43. González-López A, López-Alonso I, Aguirre A, Amado-Rodríguez L, Batalla-Solís E, Astudillo A, et al. Mechanical ventilation triggers hippocampal apoptosis by vagal and dopaminergic pathways. Am J Respir Crit Care Med. 2013 Aug 20;188(6):693–702.
44. López-Aguilar J, Villagrá A, Bernabé F, Murias G, Piacentini E, Real J, et al. Massive brain injury enhances lung damage in an isolated lung model of ventilator-induced lung injury*. Critical Care Medicine. 2005 May;33(5):1077.
45. Krebs J, Tsagogiorgas C, Pelosi P, Rocco PR, Hottenrott M, Sticht C, et al. Open lung approach with low tidal volume mechanical ventilation attenuates lung injury in rats with massive brain damage. Crit Care. 2014;18(2):R59.
46. Gajic O, Dabbagh O, Park PK, Adesanya A, Chang SY, Hou P, et al. Early identification of patients at risk of acute lung injury. Am J Respir Crit Care Med. 2011 Feb 15;183(4):462–470.
47. Rincon F, Ghosh S, Dey S, Maltenfort M, Vibbert M, Urtecho J, et al. Impact of acute lung injury and acute respiratory distress syndrome after traumatic brain injury in the United States. Neurosurgery. 2012 Oct 1;71(4):795–803.
48. Pelosi P, Ferguson ND, Frutos-Vivar F, Anzueto A, Putensen C, Raymondos K, et al. Management and outcome of mechanically ventilated neurologic patients*: Critical Care Medicine. 2011 Jun;39(6):1482–1492.
49. Mascia L, Zavala E, Bosma K, Pasero D, Decaroli D, Andrews P, et al. High tidal volume is associated with the development of acute lung injury after severe brain injury: An international observational study*: Critical Care Medicine. 2007 Aug;35(8):1815–1820.
50. Tejerina E, Pelosi P, Muriel A, Peñuelas O, Sutherasan Y, Frutos-Vivar F, et al. Association between ventilatory settings and development of acute respiratory distress syndrome in mechanically ventilated patients due to brain injury. Journal of Critical Care. 2017 Apr;38:341–345.
51. Aisiku IP, Yamal J-M, Doshi P, Benoit JS, Gopinath S, Goodman JC, et al. Plasma cytokines IL-6, IL-8, and IL-10 are associated with the development of acute respiratory distress syndrome in patients with severe traumatic brain injury. Crit Care [Internet]. 2016 Sep 15 [cited 2019 May 26];20. Available from: https://www.ncbi.nlm.nih.gov/pmc/articles/PMC5024454/
52. Mascia L, Bosma K, Pasero D, Galli T, Cortese G, Donadio P, et al. Ventilatory and hemodynamic management of potential organ donors: An observational survey*: Critical Care Medicine. 2006 Feb;34(2):321–327.
53. Ware LB, Wang Y, Fang X, Wamock M, Sakuma T, Hall TS, et al. Assessment of lungs rejected for transplantation and implications for donor selection. The Lancet. 2002;360(9333):619–620.
54. Treggiari MM, Hudson LD, Martin DP, Weiss NS, Caldwell E, Rubenfeld G. Effect of acute lung injury and acute respiratory distress syndrome on outcome in critically ill trauma patients. Crit Care Med. 2004 Feb;32(2):327–331.
55. Brain Trauma Foundation, American Association of Neurological Surgeons, Congress of Neurological Surgeons, Joint Section on Neurotrauma and Critical Care, AANS/CNS, Bratton SL, Chestnut RM, et al. Guidelines for the management of severe traumatic brain injury. XIV. Hyperventilation. J Neurotrauma. 2007;24 Suppl 1:S87–S90.

56. Noiseux N, Nguyen BK, Marsolais P, Dupont J, Simard L, Houde I, et al. Pulmonary recruitment protocol for organ donors: A new strategy to improve the rate of lung utilization. Transplant Proc. 2009 Oct;41(8):3284–3289.
57. Paries M, Boccheciampe N, Raux M, Riou B, Langeron O, Nicolas-Robin A. Benefit of a single recruitment maneuver after an apnea test for the diagnosis of brain death. Crit Care. 2012 Jul 3;16(4):R116.
58. Miñambres E, Coll E, Duerto J, Suberviola B, Mons R, Cifrian JM, et al. Effect of an intensive lung donor-management protocol on lung transplantation outcomes. The Journal of Heart and Lung Transplantation. 2014 Feb;33(2):178–184.
59. Moretti MP, Betto C, Gambacorta M, Vesconi S, Scalamogna M, Benazzi E, et al. Lung procurement for transplantation: New criteria for lung donor selection. Transplant Proc. 2010 May;42(4):1053–1055.
60. Giani M, Scaravilli V, Colombo SM, Confalonieri A, Leo R, Maggioni E, et al. Apnea test during brain death assessment in mechanically ventilated and ECMO patients. Intensive Care Med. 2016 Jan 1;42(1):72–81.
61. Rech TH, Moraes RB, Crispim D, Czepielewski MA, Leitão CB. Management of the brain-dead organ donor: A systematic review and meta-analysis. Transplantation Journal. 2013 Apr;95(7):966–974.
62. Ceulemans LJ, Inci I, Van Raemdonck D. Lung donation after circulatory death. Current Opinion in Organ Transplantation. 2019 Jun;24(3):288–296.
63. Snell G, Levvey B, Levin K, Paraskeva M, Westall G. Donation after brain death versus donation after circulatory death: Lung donor management issues. Semin Respir Crit Care Med. 2018 Apr;39(02):138–147.
64. Thuong M, Ruiz A, Evrard P, Kuiper M, Boffa C, Akhtar MZ, et al. New classification of donation after circulatory death donors definitions and terminology. Transplant International. 2016;29(7):749–759.
65. Barbero C, Messer S, Ali A, Jenkins DP, Dunning J, Tsui S, et al. Lung donation after circulatory determined death: A single-centre experience. Eur J Cardiothorac Surg. 2019 Feb 1;55(2):309–315.
66. Erasmus ME, Raemdonck D van, Akhtar MZ, Neyrinck A, Antonio DG de, Varela A, et al. DCD lung donation: Donor criteria, procedural criteria, pulmonary graft function validation, and preservation. Transplant International. 2016;29(7):790–797.
67. Inci I, Hillinger S, Schneiter D, Opitz I, Schuurmans M, Benden C, et al. Lung transplantation with controlled donation after circulatory death donors. Annals of Thoracic and Cardiovascular Surgery. 2018;24(6):296.
68. Machuca TN, Mercier O, Collaud S, Tikkanen J, Krueger T, Yeung JC, et al. Lung transplantation with donation after circulatory determination of death donors and the impact of ex vivo lung perfusion. American Journal of Transplantation. 2015;15(4):993–1002.
69. Oniscu GC, Randle LV, Muiesan P, Butler AJ, Currie IS, Perera MTPR, et al. In situ normothermic regional perfusion for controlled donation after circulatory death—The United Kingdom experience. American Journal of Transplantation. 2014;14(12):2846–2854.
70. Stéphanie I. De Vleeschauwer, Shana Wauters, Lieven J. Dupont, Stijn E. Verleden, Anna Willems-Widyastuti, Bart M. Vanaudenaerde, Geert M. Verleden, Dirk E.M. Van Raemdonck. Medium-term outcome after lung

transplantation is comparable between brain-dead and cardiac-dead donors. The Journal of Heart and Lung Transplantation. 2011 Sep 1;30(9):975–981.

71. Zych B, Popov A-F, Amrani M, Bahrami T, Redmond KC, Krueger H, et al. Lungs from donation after circulatory death donors: An alternative source to brain-dead donors? Midterm results at a single institution. Eur J Cardiothorac Surg. 2012 Sep 1;42(3):542–549.
72. Domínguez-Gil B, Duranteau J, Mateos A, Núñez JR, Cheisson G, Corral E, et al. Uncontrolled donation after circulatory death: European practices and recommendations for the development and optimization of an effective programme. Transplant International. 2016;29(8):842–859.
73. Gomez-de-Antonio D, Campo-Cañaveral JL, Crowley S, Valdivia D, Cordoba M, Moradiellos J, et al. Clinical lung transplantation from uncontrolled non-heart-beating donors revisited. The Journal of Heart and Lung Transplantation. 2012 Apr;31(4):349–353.
74. Suberviola B, Mons R, Ballesteros MA, Mora V, Delgado M, Naranjo S, et al. Excellent long-term outcome with lungs obtained from uncontrolled donation after circulatory death. American Journal of Transplantation. 2019;19(4):1195–1201.
75. Valenza F, Citerio G, Palleschi A, Vargiolu A, Fakhr BS, Confalonieri A, et al. Successful transplantation of lungs from an uncontrolled donor after circulatory death preserved *in situ* by Alveolar recruitment maneuvers and assessed by *ex vivo* lung perfusion. Am J Transplant. 2016 Apr;16(4):1312–1318.
76. Ingemansson R, Eyjolfsson A, Mared L, Pierre L, Algotsson L, Ekmehag B, et al. Clinical transplantation of initially rejected donor lungs after reconditioning ex vivo. The Annals of Thoracic Surgery. 2009 Jan;87(1):255–260.
77. Warnecke G, Moradiellos J, Tudorache I, Kühn C, Avsar M, Wiegmann B, et al. Normothermic perfusion of donor lungs for preservation and assessment with the Organ Care System Lung before bilateral transplantation: A pilot study of 12 patients. The Lancet. 2012;380(9856):1851–1858.
78. Terragni PP, Rosboch G, Tealdi A, Corno E, Menaldo E, Davini O, et al. Tidal hyperinflation during low tidal volume ventilation in acute respiratory distress syndrome. Am J Respir Crit Care Med. 2007 Jan 15;175(2):160–166.
79. Terragni PP, Filippini C, Slutsky AS, Birocco A, Tenaglia T, Grasso S, et al. Accuracy of plateau pressure and stress index to identify injurious ventilation in patients with acute respiratory distress syndrome: Anesthesiology. 2013 Oct;119(4):880–889.
80. Terragni PP, Fanelli V, Boffini M, Filippini C, Cappello P, Ricci D, et al. Ventilatory management during normothermic ex vivo lung perfusion: Effects on clinical outcomes. Transplantation. 2016 May;100(5):1128–1135.

33

Pharmacological considerations in the potential organ donor

Russell Dixon, Brittny Medenwald, Gretchen M. Brophy

Introduction

It is essential that the diagnosis of brain death be made with accuracy and urgency to ensure the highest level of success for organ retrieval and transplantation. Practitioners must consider the impact of pharmacotherapy during brain death diagnosis and leading up to organ retrieval. When brain death is being considered, the effects of medication must be excluded. For example, sedatives are commonly used in the critically ill population and can interfere with apnoea testing by causing respiratory depression. It is imperative that the pharmacokinetic and pharmacodynamic properties of all centrally active medications are accounted to accurately interpret brain death testing results. After the declaration of brain death, hospital practitioners should work closely with organ procurement organizations to ensure ideal pharmacologic management of patients to augment the chance for successful organ transplantation.[1] This chapter focuses on the pharmacologic management of patients with non-survivable, devastating brain injury and highlights the medication considerations necessary prior to determination of brain death in adults.

Pathophysiologic changes influencing medical management in brain injured patients

The Centers for Medicare and Medicaid Services and the Neurocritical Care Society support resuscitation of the potential organ donor after devastating brain injury to allow for the opportunity of organ donation.[2,3] The Association of Organ Procurement Organizations has developed management goals for donor optimization, which has shown to increase the number of organs recovered per donor.[4–6] The support and efforts of these organizations combined with the 'Management of the Potential Organ Donor in the Intensive Care Unit Consensus Statement' set a strong foundation to levy institutions into action to help provide healthy organs to those in need of this potentially lifesaving gift.[7] In addition, utilization of the best available evidence is essential to developing a good pharmacologic management strategy for the most commonly used medications surrounding brain death.

Management of patients after devastating brain injury prior to and after declaration of brain death can be challenging for many reasons. Paucity of well-designed research, variations in brain injuries, lack of a systematic care plan, ethical dilemmas, and poor communication between providers are some of the barriers to successful management of this population. Therefore, the provider must be fluent in understanding the potential complications surrounding brain death and have a good comprehension of the mechanism of brain injury and extent of injury in order to make good therapeutic decisions about care for these patients, regardless of whether the patient becomes an organ donor or not. This foundation of knowledge facilitates the stabilization of patients which will allow for prognostication as well as the exploration of the opportunity for organ donation.

Understanding the mechanism of brain injury is the key to developing a resuscitation plan and anticipating complications. The array of brain injuries, including but not limited to traumatic, cerebrovascular, and anoxic injury, provides unique challenges for the provider. One of the unique challenges with penetrating injury into the cranial vault is the specific loss of brain function during the initial phases of injury depending on the trajectory of the missile. Patients with severe brain injury progress through two distinct pathophysiologic phases during advancement towards brain death and are worthy of differentiation as the expected complications and management of each is distinctly different. These two phases include the brain ischemia phase and the brain death phase.[7] The practitioner may find themselves managing either phase at any point of time including the emergency room, operating room, and intensive care unit (ICU).

Hormone resuscitation therapy

Hormone resuscitation therapy (HRT), which typically includes thyroid medication, insulin, vasopressin, and corticosteroids, is commonly used to help stabilize patients who are declared brain dead and are potential organ donors, in an effort to increase the success of organ recovery.[8–10] Thyroid replacement therapy is typically needed as euthyroid sick syndrome commonly occurs, which contributes to hemodynamic instability. The options for thyroid replacement consist of free thyroxine (T4) or triiodothyronine (T3). T4 is typically converted in the body to the more potent form T3, which has a faster onset of action. There are exogenous factors that can impair the conversion of T4 to T3, but this can be overcome by administering large doses of T4. Either of these formulations of thyroid hormone are acceptable.[8,11] In countries where intravenous formulations of T4 are not available, oral therapies are being administered. A crossover study of thirty-four organ transplant patients compared oral T4 formation at doses of 2 mcg/kg to the intravenous formulation administered over 15 minutes. The oral formulation had a bioavailability of 91–93% of the intravenous group at 6 hours after the dose and similar hemodynamic effects up to 13 hours after the dose.[12] Therefore, an oral dosage form may be considered when intravenous formulations are not available. It is noted that oral T4 (levothyroxine) concentrations can be decreased if given with food or enteral nutrition.[13]

In an effort to build a case that corticosteroid treatment may improve transplant outcomes, Watts et al. describe three main time frames leading to inflammatory cascade activation from brain injury resulting in organ damage.[14] The first is the initial damage to organs due to traumatic injury, cerebrovascular accidents, or anoxic brain injury. The second occurs at the time of brain death and the third is ischemia reperfusion injury and occurs when organs are harvested and subsequently transplanted. Another consideration for corticosteroid treatment was described by Dimopoulou et al. who found decreased cortisol production in brain dead potential organ donors when patients were administered adrenocorticotropic hormone.[15] Thirteen of the seventeen brain dead patients (76%) did not respond to the stimulation test dose.

Corticosteroid use to facilitate hemodynamic stabilization, reduce organ damage as a result of inflammatory cascade activation due to interleukins or cytokines, or reduce harmful effects of ischemia reperfusion injury has not been studied well enough to definitively understand if steroid administration improves outcomes related to organ donation. Corticosteroids effects on each organ transplanted including the heart, lungs, kidneys, liver, pancreas, and small intestine as well as the host response to inflammatory inciting injuries must be considered when reviewing this data. The potential beneficial effect of corticosteroid treatment appears to outweigh any observed detrimental effects. The current consensus statement recommends administration of corticosteroids at doses listed in Table 33.1.[7] Research from three groups did not show improvement in outcomes for liver transplant, minimization of the incidence or duration of acute renal failure for kidney transplant patients, or improvement in hemodynamics after corticosteroid administration.[16–18] However, two authors were able to show decreased accumulation of water in lung tissue and improved yields for transplanted lungs as well as suppression of the immune system decreasing the rate of acute rejection during liver transplant.[18,19]

Immediately prior to brain death there is often a significant increase in endogenous catecholamines in an effort of the brain to maintain perfusion as intracranial pressure (ICP) increases. This catecholamine storm induced by endogenous dopamine, norepinephrine, and epinephrine significantly affect cardiac tissue.[20] Profound tachycardia > 140 beats per minute and hypertension with systolic blood pressure > 200 mmHg ensue pushing the cardiac tissue to exhaustion similar to Tokotsubo like cardiomyopathy. One group studied the potential of using pharmacologic agents to ameliorate the effect of the catecholamine storm on cardiac tissue by using esmolol and urapidil. They were able to show improvement in left ventricular ejection fraction and increase the probability of cardiac transplantation in the treatment group.[21] However, many experts do not recommend initiating organ donor management strategies until brain death has been diagnosed. It is important to note that not all potential organ donors progressing to brain death experience high levels of catecholamines and therefore would not likely benefit from treatment with cardiac protective medications. Those potential organ donors that experience a catecholamine storm will often have profound hypotension and bradycardia immediately after brain death has occurred. This is the time that many potential organ donor opportunities are lost due to cardiovascular collapse. Table 33.1 summarizes the physiologic changes that often occur following devastating brain injury and the medical management strategies that should be considered.

Table 33.1 Potential Physiologic Derangements that may occur in patients during Devastating Brain Injury and Potential Management Strategies(7,13,22)

Brain injury	Physiologic changes	Prevalence	Brain Injury Phase	Potential Therapeutic Strategy	Dosing	Pearls
Activation of inflammatory cascade	Capillary vasodilation and damage; vasoplegia; pulmonary oedema; acute blood volume diversion	13–18%	Ischemia and Death	Methylprednisolone sodium succinate	15mg/kg IV bolus, or 1000mg IV bolus, or 2000mg IV bolus, or 250 mg IV bolus followed by 100mg/hr continuous infusion	Methylprednisolone may be given independently or as part of hormonal resuscitation therapy following brain death If not using continuous infusion, repeat bolus dose daily.
Catecholamine storm	Hypertension, tachycardia, arrhythmias, myocardial damage; reduced coronary blood flow	25–32%	Ischemia	Careful use of β1 selective β blockers (esmolol) for cardiac protection	Esmolol 50–200 mcg/kg/min continuous infusion	Use of short acting β blockers may be considered; however, many experts do not recommend these agents due to the potential for initiation of organ donor management prior to diagnosis of brain death

Table 33.1 *Continued*

Brain injury	Physiologic changes	Prevalence	Brain Injury Phase	Potential Therapeutic Strategy	Dosing	Pearls
Hypothalamic damage	Poikilothermia; reduced metabolic rate; vasodilatation and heat loss	Inevitable if not prevented	Ischemia and death	Temperature regulation with heating or cooling blankets/devices; or IV heating and cooling catheters		Hyperthermia increases metabolic rate which increases the rate of elimination for many medications; hypothermia decreases metabolic rate which prolongs the rate of elimination for many medications and brain death testing should not be conducted until 24–48 hours after rewarming the patient to ensure drug clearance.
Myocardial dysfunction; Takotsubo like cardiomyopathy	Hypotension; hypovolemia; reduced coronary blood flow; reduced cardiac output (left ejection fraction < 45%)	81–97%	Death	Ensure euvolemia; vasopressors; hormone resuscitation therapy (HRT)	HRT; See table 33.3 for regimen; see table 33.2 for vasopressor dosing	HRT should be considered if vasopressor resistant shock or left ventricular ejection fraction < 45 %.

(continued)

Table 33.1 *Continued*

Brain injury	Physiologic changes	Prevalence	Brain Injury Phase	Potential Therapeutic Strategy	Dosing	Pearls
Diabetes Insipidus (DI) due to damage to the posterior pituitary structures; the hypothalamic supraoptic nuclei, or the paraventricular nuclei	Vasopressin deficiency leading to hypotension, hypovolemia, hyperosmolality and hypernatremia	46–78%	Ischemia and death	Volume replacement; Vasopressin infusion if hypotension and DI; DDAVP injection if DI only	Vasopressin 0.01–0.04 U/min; DDAVP 1–4 mcg bolus, then 1–2 mcg every 6 hours,	Titrate dose to predetermined goal urine output, serum sodium, and urine osmolality. Monitor serum sodium closely and avoid large concentration fluctuations. Monitor potassium, phosphorus, and magnesium due to high urinary loss associated with DI Consider DI if one or more of the following: 1) Urine output > 3–4 L/d or 2.5-3 ml/kg/hr 2) Dilute urine: specific gravity < 1.005, urine osmolality < 200 mOsm/kg H20 3) Hypernatremia: Na+ > 145 mmol/L

Table 33.1 *Continued*

Brain injury	Physiologic changes	Prevalence	Brain Injury Phase	Potential Therapeutic Strategy	Dosing	Pearls
Tissue factor release from brain and other tissue injury	Disseminated intravascular coagulation; clotting factor consumptive coagulopathy	29–55%	Ischemia and death	Frozen plasma 24 (FP24), fresh frozen plasma (FFP), prothrombin complex concentrates (PCC)	Transfuse FP 24 or FFP if bleeding per institutional policies.	Monitor for clotting and bleeding. May consider FFP, FP 24, or PCC if: INR > 1.5 or aPTT > 1.5 times control

Hemodynamic therapies

Patients with devastating brain injury may experience hemodynamic instability as a result of hypovolemia, catecholamine store depletion, catecholamine release dysregulation, adrenal insufficiency, or vasopressin deficiency. Once brain death occurs, these patients are also at risk for cardiogenic shock due to cardiac tissue damage from extremely high levels of catecholamines experienced during the last efforts of the brain to maintain perfusion. Providers must ensure euvolemia by assessing a combination of urine output, mean arterial pressure (MAP), central venous pressure, pulmonary arterial occlusion pressure, and/or dynamic measures (stroke volume variation or pulse pressure variation) as per institution-specific protocols. Maintaining hematologic parameters including haemoglobin > 7 gm/dL to ensure oxygen-carrying capacity and consideration for administration of fresh frozen plasma if INR > 1.5 or aPTT ≥ 1.5 times control, should be considered. If MAP remains < 60 mmHg, vasopressor support is indicated. Norepinephrine is considered first line but providers should not wait long to consider vasopressin as an additional agent due to the potential for pituitary damage resulting in decreased vasopressin secretion or lack of baroreflex-mediated release of vasopressin. After brain death diagnosis, dopamine and vasopressin become the preferred agents and patients experiencing vasopressor resistant shock or left ventricular ejection fraction < 45% should be given HRT to stimulate cardiac tissue in an effort to achieve hemodynamic goals.[7,23–26] Tables 33.1 and 33.2 provide detailed information about vasopressor agents and Table 33.3 provides suggested HRT regimen.

Fluid and electrolyte management

Volume resuscitation is extremely important in all patients as hypovolemia can lead to neurological deficits; therefore, management and monitoring of fluid balance and blood pressure is the key. In patients with devastating brain injury who are potential organ donors, hemodynamic goals to achieve adequate fluid resuscitation include a MAP greater than 60 mmHg, urine output 1–3ml/kg/hr, decrease in dose of vasoactive agents (dopamine ≤ 10 μg/kg/min), and left ventricular

Table 33.2 Common Characteristics of Vasopressor Agents[7,13,27,28]

Medication	Site of action							Dosing	Pearls
	α_1	α_2	β_1	β_2	DA	V_1	V_2		
Norepinephrine	++++	++	++	0	0	0	0	0.01–3 mcg/kg/min	Increases SVR and MAP; increases CO at high doses Most effective for low SVR shock Decreased renal perfusion Reduced 1-year survival in patients receiving heart transplant Increased pulmonary capillary permeability due to α receptor stimulation
Epinephrine	++	++	++++	+++	0	0	0	0.01–0.05 mcg/kg/min	Increases CO, SVR and MAP Most effective for low SVR and low cardiac index shock Increased risk of arrhythmias
	++++	++++	+++	+	0	0	0	>0.05–1 mcg/kg/min	
Vasopressin	0		0	0	0	+++	+	0.01–0.04 units/min	Increases SVR and MAP, as a response HR and CO may decrease Most effective for low SVR shock Effective during acidosis and hypoxia due to site of action on V_1 and V_2 receptors May be considered prior to brain death if persistent hypotension combined with suspected or confirmed damage to posterior pituitary gland; or clinical signs of decreased pituitary gland function (i.e. DI) May be considered after brain death if persistent hypotension, LVEF <45%, low SVR, or if DI present. Often used in combination with HRT

(continued)

Table 33.2 *Continued*

Medication	Site of action							Dosing	Pearls
	α_1	α_2	β_1	β_2	DA	V_1	V_2		
Phenylephrine	++++	+	0	0	0	0	0	0.5–9 mcg/kg/min	Increases SVR and MAP; may induce reflex bradycardia and reduced CO Most effective for low SVR shock Decreased renal perfusion Increased pulmonary capillary permeability due to α receptor stimulation
Dopamine	0	0	+	0	++++	0	0	1–3 mcg/kg/min	May be considered first line after brain death diagnosis due to: 1. Decrease in the detrimental effects of the cytokine cascade 2. Reduces effects of ischemia reperfusion injury 3. Faster alveolar fluid clearance 4. Decreased need for dialysis after kidney transplant Increased incidence of arrhythmias compared to norepinephrine Most effective for low cardiac index shock
	+/-	0	++++	++	++++	0	0	> 3–10 mcg/kg/min	
	+++	0	++++	+	0	0	0	> 10–20 mcg/kg/min	
Dobutamine	+	0	+++	++	0	0	0	2–10 mcg/kg/min	Increased CO May be effective as add on therapy for low cardiac index shock
	++	0	++++	+++	0	0	0	>10–20 mcg/kg/min	

V_1 = Arginine vasopressin receptor 1a, V_2 = Arginine vasopressin receptor 2, DI = Diabetes insipidus, SVR = Systemic vascular resistance, HR = Heart rate, CO = Cardiac output, LVEF = Left Ventricular Ejection Fraction, HRT = Hormone replacement therapy 0 = no action, +/– = minimal to no action, + = minimal action, ++ = mild action, +++ = moderate action, ++++ = significant action

Table 33.3 Hormone Replacement Therapy for Organ Donors[27–31]

Hormone Replacement Therapy Regimen (All medications administered within 30 minutes)

Indications:

1) High suspicion for brain death, massive catecholamine cardiogenic shock
2) Left ventricular ejection fraction < 45%

Dosing:

1) Levothyroxine (T4) 20 mcg IV bolus followed by infusion of 10 mcg/h (100mcg levothyroxine in normal saline 250ml protected from light is stable 24 hours(32))
2) Alternative if shortage: Tri-iodothyronine (T3) given as a 4mcg IV bolus followed by infusion of 3 mcg/h
3) Methylprednisolone 15mg/kg IV piggy back (Maximum 2000mg)
4) Vasopressin infusion of 0.01–0.04 U/min
5) Dextrose 50% 50mL given prior to regular insulin 10 units IV push

ejection fraction of at least 45%.[7] With fluid management and physiologic changes in these patients, managing electrolytes also pose unique challenges for practitioners. Having a good working understanding of the available electrolyte solutions is essential. Part of the management for elevated ICP is facilitated by increasing the serum sodium concentration above 150 mmol/L. Unfortunately, once brain death has been diagnosed, a high sodium level may cause transplant centres to reject livers, which is a lost opportunity.[33,34] Changes in potassium concentration can also occur if acid/base disorders develop or the patient's body temperature rapidly drops below 37°C. Therefore, administering the most appropriate medication and fluid therapy is extremely important in these patients. Electrolytes should be monitored at least every 12 hours, if not more, when treating these patients to avoid rapid fluctuations that could potentiate further complications. Currently, available resuscitation fluid properties can be found in Table 33.4. Hydroxyethyl starch solutions are commonly available in the ICU and should be avoided due to the risk of significant complications including acute kidney injury, accumulation in the hepatic reticuloendothelial system, coagulopathy, and acute hypervolemia.[35,36]

Table 33.4 Characteristics of Commonly Used Intravenous Resuscitation Fluids[13,23–25]

Solution	Tonicity	Osmolarity/L	Uses	Complications
0.9% Sodium Chloride (NS)	Isotonic pH 5.7 (4.5–7.0)	308 mOsmol	Hydration/ resuscitation; replacement of sodium and chloride; alkalosis; may be used as carrier solution for blood transfusions	Hyperchloremic metabolic acidosis
0.45% Sodium Chloride (½ NS)	Hypotonic pH 5.6 (4.5–7.0)	154 mOsmol	Hydration/ resuscitation; replace sodium and chloride; hyperosmolar diabetes	May decrease blood osmolality; may cause haemolysis; elevated ICP
3% Sodium Chloride	Hypertonic pH 5.0 (4.5–7.0)	1027 mOsmol	Symptomatic hyponatremia; hyperosmolar therapy in traumatic brain injury patients	Rapid hypernatremia (osmotic demyelination syndrome); hyperchloremic metabolic acidosis; central line required for prolonged infusions
5% Dextrose (D5W)	Isotonic pH 4.3 (3.2–6.5)	278 mOsmol	Hydration/ resuscitation; provides some calories	Not recommended for these patients. Water intoxication; dilution of body's electrolytes with long infusions; hyperglycaemia; elevated ICP.
Lactated Ringer's	Isotonic pH 6.6 (6.0-7.5)	273 mOsmol	Hydration/ resuscitation; replace mild electrolyte losses; mild to moderate acidosis (lactate metabolizes to become bicarbonate)	Do not administer with blood products due to calcium content. Does not contain enough electrolytes for maintenance; patients with hepatic disease have trouble metabolizing the lactate; do not use if lactic acidosis is present; closely monitor electrolytes in patients with renal impairment

Table 33.4 *Continued*

Solution	Tonicity	Osmolarity/L	Uses	Complications
Normosol-R®	Isotonic pH 7.4 (6.5–7.6)	295 mOsmol	Hydration/ resuscitation; replace mild electrolyte losses; may be used as carrier solution for blood transfusions	Not enough electrolytes for maintenance; closely monitor electrolytes in patients with renal impairment
Plasma-Lyte A®	Isotonic pH 7.4 (6.5–8.0)	294 mOsmol	Hydration/ resuscitation; replace mild electrolyte losses; may be used as carrier solution for blood transfusions	Not enough electrolytes for maintenance; closely monitor electrolytes in patients with renal impairment

Pharmacologic characteristics of commonly used medications in brain injury patients

The pharmacokinetic and pharmacodynamic characteristics of medications administered in potential organ donors must be considered. Pharmacokinetics is described as the drug absorption, distribution, metabolism, and elimination, commonly thought of as what the body does to the medication. Pharmacodynamics is the biochemical and physiological effects of drugs in the body, commonly thought of as what the medication does to the body. In a patient with a devastating brain injury, the pharmacokinetics may vary widely due to alterations in pathophysiology, changes in volumes of distribution, and changes in the blood brain barrier.(37) Similarly the pharmacodynamics may vary widely based on if the patient is cooled due to a decrease in hepatic metabolism and drug-drug interactions, including enzyme induction and inhibition. The rate of elimination of a medication will impact the pharmacologic effect and hepatic enzyme activity determines the rate of elimination for many medications. The most common hepatic enzyme inducing medications used in neurocritical care patients are barbiturates, rifampicin, and phenytoin. By inducing the hepatic enzymes, concentrations of medication metabolized by these enzymes can be reduced faster than anticipated. The opposite is also true, if a patient is receiving an enzyme inhibitor (e.g. simvastatin, diltiazem, amiodarone, fluoxetine, fluconazole, erythromycin), the rate of medication metabolism can be decreased and the effect of the medication will be prolonged.[37]

When considering brain death testing, providers should take into consideration all medications that the patient has received at the scene of the injury, in route to the hospital, and while at the hospital. Most medications that cross the blood-brain barrier and act centrally cause some degree of respiratory depression and can impact apnoea testing. Additionally many antiepileptic medications can cause central nervous system (CNS) depression, further complicating the testing results. It is generally recommended to avoid life support termination in the presence of any CNS depressing medication.[9] Therefore, the pharmacologic properties of each medication must also be accounted to ensure the pharmacologic action of the medication will no longer impact brain death testing. A drug's elimination half-life from the plasma is the time necessary for the concentration of the drug to be reduced by half. After five half-lives the concentration of the drug is reduced by approximately 97%. Thus, experts recommend waiting for five elimination half-lives prior to brain death testing.[38]

Neuromuscular blocking agents (NMBA) should be avoided when establishing irreversible cause of coma.[38] If a patient has received an NMBA, providers should monitor using the train-of-4 device with maximal stimulation on the ulnar nerve to ensure that paralysis is no longer present.[37] It is important to recall that if the patient has been recently cooled (below 37° C), the duration of the NMBA may be clinically longer than anticipated as enzyme metabolism is slowed during cooling. It is also recommended that prior to brain death testing there should be an absence of CNS depressant medications. One common example is that of barbiturates, the recommended serum level should be < 10 mcg/mL.[38] While serum barbiturate concentrations can be determined with laboratory testing, logistically it can be troublesome. Typically, barbiturate concentrations can take days to be reported (must be sent to an outside laboratory) and clinically, these concentrations are not reflective of the actual CNS impact of the medications at the time they are received, and prolong the ICU time to brain death declaration. It is important for practitioners to realize that, specifically with continuous infusion barbiturates, the CNS half-life and clinical duration of action are shorter than the stated serum half-life, and patients may recover sooner than waiting for five serum half-lives. Generally, waiting 24–48 hours after a barbiturate has been stopped is acceptable for brain death testing. Table 33.5 depicts some

Table 33.5 Pharmacologic and Pharmacokinetic Considerations for Medications Commonly Used in Adult Traumatic Brain Injury Patients[39]

Medication	Half-life	Duration of Effect	Renal dysfunction	Liver impairment
Analgesia				
Fentanyl	3–12 hr; prolongs with infusion duration	0.5–96 hours	---	---
Remifentanil	10–20 min	3–10 min	Dialyzable	---
Sufentanil	164 min	5 min	---	---
Hydromorphone	IV: 2–3 hr ER PO: 8–15 hr	IV: 3–4 hours ER PO: ~13 hr	CrCl< 30 mL/min: terminal half-life increases to 40 hours	---
Morphine	IV: 2–4 hr Avinza®: ~24 hr Kadian® ~ 10 hr	IV: 2–5 hr ER: 8–24 hr	Active metabolites are renally eliminated and can accumulate; CNS metabolite peak concentration may be delayed up to 24 hours in ESRD	Half-life is increased in cirrhosis
Oxycodone	3.7 hr	IR: 3–6 hr ER:< 12 hr	CrC< 60 ml/min: increase by 1 hour	Mild to moderate impairment: half-life increase by 2.3 hr
Hydrocodone	ER: 7–12 hr	---	----	---
Alfentanil	90–111 min	30–60 min	---	Half-life is increased in compromised liver function

(continued)

Table 33.5 *Continued*

Medication	Half-life	Duration of Effect	Renal dysfunction	Liver impairment
Methadone	8–59 hours	4–48 hours 4–8 with single dose 22–48 with repeated	---	---
Sedation				
Propofol	Initial 40 min Terminal 4–7 hours After 10 days: 1–3 days	3–10 min	---	---
Dexmedetomidine	Up to 3 hours	60–120 min	Renal impairment, 113.4 minutes	Hypoalbuminemia, 140 minutes
Antiepileptic				
Diazepam	PO: Up to 48 hours IV: 33–45 hr Desmethyldiazepam: 100 hr Accumulation occurs with multiple doses	15–30 min	---	Prolonged 2–5 fold
Lorazepam	PO: 12 hr IV: 14 hr IM: 13–18 hr	6–8 hours	ESRD half-life 18 hr	---
Midazolam	1.8–6.8 hr	Single IV dose:< 2 hr	Accumulation and prolonged effect	Prolonged in cirrhosis
Phenytoin/ Fosphenytoin	7–42 hours	---	Displacement from albumin binding sites with high BUN, increasing free concentrations	Clearance may be decreased

Table 33.5 *Continued*

Medication	Half-life	Duration of Effect	Renal dysfunction	Liver impairment
Phenobarbital	53–118 hr	PO: 10–12 hours IV: >6 hr	Moderately dialyzable	---
Valproate sodium	9–19 hr	---	Mildly dialyzable	Extensively metabolized by the liver and clearance decreases with impairment; CYP enzyme inhibitor
Levetiracetam	6–8 hours	---	Clearance is decreased Dialyzable	---
Brivaracetam	9 hours	---	---	Potential drug interactions with CYP 2C19, inducer or inhibitors
Lacosamide	13 hours	---	Dialyzable	---
Topiramate	IR: 21hr Trokendi XR®: 31 hr Qudexy XR®: 56 hr	---	Increases half-life up to 59hr Dialyzable	Clearance may be reduced
Thiopental	3–26.1 hours	Single dose: 10–30 min Accumulates with multiple doses	---	---
Pentobarbital	15–50 hr dose dependent	IV: 15–45 min	---	---

(*Continued*)

Table 33.5 *Continued*

Medication	Half-life	Duration of Effect	Renal dysfunction	Liver impairment
Ketamine	Alpha 10–15 min Beta 2.5 hr	IV: Anaesthetic: 5–10 min Recovery: 1–2 hr IM: Anaesthetic: 12–25 min Analgesia: 15–30 Recovery: 3–4 hr	---	---
Esketamine	7–12 hr	---	---	---
Neuromuscular Blocking Agents				
Succinylcholine	< 1 min	IV: 4–6 min IM: 30 min	---	---
Rocuronium	Alpha: 1–2 min Beta: 1.4–2.4 hr	30 min	2.4 hours	4.3 hours
Pancuronium	89–161 min	22 min	Elimination half-life is doubled and plasma clearance is reduced	Elimination half-life is doubled and plasma clearance is doubled.
Vecuronium	65–75 min	~45–65 min	---	---
Cisatracurium	22–29 min	35–45 min	Half-life is increased	Half-life is increased
Atracurium	Initial: 2 min Terminal 20 min	60–70 min	---	---
Mivacurium	2 min	15–20 min	Duration is 1.5 time longer in ESRD	Duration is 3 times longer in ESRD

pharmacologic considerations for typical medications used in neurocritical care patients.[39]

Substances of abuse considerations

In addition to the medications administered during hospitalization, patients may present with recent ingestion of substances of abuse. It is not recommended to conduct brain death testing until the substance of abuse is no longer detectable. The detection time of substances of abuse and toxins is difficult to determine since there is a lack of studies that investigate illicit drugs, and the available studies are in healthy volunteers at doses much smaller than anticipated street dosing. Table 33.6 depicts pharmacologic considerations for typical substances of abuse based on the available literature.[40]

Practitioners should become familiar with the drugs of abuse screening tests at their institution as results are very important to consider prior to the diagnosis of brain death. Drug screening tests can differ from institution to institution on the drugs detected, the concentrations necessary for detection, and the medications that can cause false-positive results. These also do not detect all drugs that could depress mental status, meaning that

Table 33.6 Urine Detection Times for Substances of Abuse[40]

Medication	Typical Dose	Typical Route	Cutoff for Detection in the Urine (ng/mL)	Typical Urine Detection Time (hours)	Maximal Urine Detection Time (days)
Amphetamine	6 mg	Oral	4	46	9
Methamphetamine	10 mg	Oral	2.5	87 ± 51	6
MDMA	100 mg	Oral	20	48	–
Cannabis	1.75% 3.5%	Smoked	15 15	34 87	95
Cocaine	100 mg	Intranasal	1000	48–72	22
LSD	0.28	Oral	0.2	36–96	4
Heroin	10–15	Smoked		11–54	11.3
GHB	100 mg/kg	Oral	10000	12	–

a negative drug screen cannot fully exclude intoxication.[41] The hospital laboratory director should have information for the specific drug screen tests at the institution. In cases where very large drug over-dose of CNS depressant drugs or medications are suspected, it is recommended to wait longer than the traditional five half-lives for drug clearance prior to declaration of brain death. This is due to the fact that patients can experience delayed gastric emptying, gut hypomotility, prolonged absorption time due to hypoperfusion of the gastrointestinal tract or splanchnic vasoconstriction, or even saturable elimination kinetics. These can lead to prolonged drug effects and a clinical pharmacist and/or toxicologist should be consulted.[42]

Conclusion

Prior to brain death determination, providers must consider not only the current medication regimen of a patient but all medications that the patient has received prior to admission. It is imperative to account for the pharmacokinetic and pharmacodynamic properties of all centrally active medications as these drug characteristics will change with the pathophysiological changes occurring during the various stages of brain death. Drug-drug interactions are also likely; therefore, determination of drug concentrations and/or monitoring for prolonged clinical effects is essential prior to declaration of brain death. Substances of abuse must also be evaluated and taken into account. The detection time of substances of abuse and toxins is difficult to determine due to lack of robust data; however, practitioners should utilize the available drug screening tests at their institution. Developing a management strategy for treatment of devastating brain injury prior to brain death determination should be considered to ensure appropriate medications are given to successfully increase the opportunity for organ donation.

Highlights

- Good medication management practices increase the number of organs recovered per donor and improve the quality of organs recovered.

- Predicting, understanding, and appropriately managing complications associated with devastating brain injury patient care are essential for facilitating the best outcomes.
- Devastating brain injury may cause hemodynamic instability at any point during care and the practitioner should consider vasopressin as an addition to other vasopressor agents, or after brain death, combined with hormone replacement therapy to restore organ perfusion.
- It is imperative that the pharmacokinetic and pharmacodynamic properties of all centrally active medications are accounted to accurately interpret brain death testing results.
- Waiting five half-lives prior to brain death testing for centrally acting medications is recommended to ensure the drug elimination.
- Substances of abuse should be accounted by utilizing the available drug screen tests, which will help guide medical management.

References

1. Kennedy M, Kiloh N. Drugs and brain death. Drug Saf 1996; 14: 171–180.
2. Souter MJ, Blissitt PA, Blosser S, Bonomo J, Greer D, Jichici D et al. Recommendations for the critical care management of devastating brain injury: Prognostication, psychosocial, and ethical management : A position statement for Healthcare Professionals from the Neurocritical Care Society. Neurocrit Care 2015; 23: 4–13.
3. CMS Organ Procurement Regulations Condition of Participation: Organ, Tissue and Eye Procurement. https://www.cms.gov/Regulations-and-Guidance/Guidance/Transmittals/downloads/R37SOMA.pdf. 2019.
4. Patel MS, De La Cruz S, Sally MB, Groat T, Malinoski DJ. Active donor management during the hospital phase of care is associated with more organs transplanted per donor. Journal of the American College of Surgeons 2017; 225: 525–531.
5. Patel MS, Zatarain J, De La Cruz S, Sally MB, Ewing T, Crutchfield M et al. The impact of meeting donor management goals on the number of organs transplanted per expanded criteria donor: A prospective study from the UNOS region 5 donor management goals workgroup. JAMA Surgery 2014; 149: 969.
6. UNOS. Critical Pathway for the Organ Donor. https://www.unos.org/wp-content/uploads/unos/Critical_Pathway.pdf. 2019.
7. Kotloff RM, Blosser S, Fulda GJ, Malinoski D, Ahya VN, Angel L et al. Management of the potential organ donor in the ICU: Society of critical care medicine/American College of Chest Physicians/Association of Organ Procurement Organizations Consensus Statement. Critical Care Medicine 2015; 43: 1291–1325.

8. Mi Z, Novitzky D, Collins JF, Cooper DK. The optimal hormonal replacement modality selection for multiple organ procurement from brain-dead organ donors. Clin Epidemiol 2015; 7: 17–27.
9. Salim A, Vassiliu P, Velmahos GC, Sava J, Murray JA, Belzberg H et al. The role of thyroid hormone administration in potential organ donors. Arch Surg 2001; 136: 1377–1380.
10. Joseph B, Aziz H, Pandit V, Kulvatunyou N, Sadoun M, Tang A et al. Levothyroxine therapy before brain death declaration increases the number of solid organ donations. J Trauma Acute Care Surg 2014; 76: 1301–1305.
11. Dhar R, Stahlschmidt E, Yan Y, Marklin G. A randomized trial comparing triiodothyronine (T3) with thyroxine (T4) for hemodynamically unstable brain-dead organ donors. Clinical Transplantation 2019; 33: e13486.
12. Sharpe MD, van Rassel B, Haddara W. Oral and intravenous thyroxine (T4) achieve comparable serum levels for hormonal resuscitation protocol in organ donors: a randomized double-blinded study. Can J Anaesth 2013; 60: 998–1002.
13. Lexicomp Clinical Drug Information Version 4.6.0. 2019.
14. Watts RP, Thom O, Fraser JF. Inflammatory signalling associated with brain dead organ donation: From brain injury to brain stem death and posttransplant ischaemia reperfusion injury. J Transplant 2013. Doi:10.1155/2013/521369.
15. Dimopoulou I, Tsagarakis S, Anthi A, Milou E, Ilias I, Stavrakaki K et al. High prevalence of decreased cortisol reserve in brain-dead potential organ donors. Critical Care Medicine 2003; 31: 1113–1117.
16. Amatschek S, Wilflingseder J, Pones M, Kainz A, Bodingbauer M, Mühlbacher F et al. The effect of steroid pretreatment of deceased organ donors on liver allograft function: A blinded randomized placebo-controlled trial. Journal of Hepatology 2012; 56: 1305–1309.
17. Kainz A. Steroid pretreatment of organ donors to prevent postischemic renal allograft failure: A randomized, controlled trial. Annals of Internal Medicine 2010; 153: 222.
18. Venkateswaran RV, Steeds RP, Quinn DW, Nightingale P, Wilson IC, Mascaro JG et al. The haemodynamic effects of adjunctive hormone therapy in potential heart donors: A prospective randomized double-blind factorially designed controlled trial. European Heart Journal 2009; 30: 1771–1780.
19. Kotsch K, Ulrich F, Reutzel-Selke A, Pascher A, Faber W, Warnick P et al. Methylprednisolone therapy in deceased donors reduces inflammation in the donor liver and improves outcome after liver transplantation: A prospective randomized controlled trial. Annals of Surgery 2008; 248: 1042–1050.
20. Brain death provokes very acute alteration in myocardial morphology detected by echocardiography: preventive effect of beta-blockers – Ferrera – 2011 – Transplant International – Wiley Online Library. https://onlinelibrary-wiley-com.webproxy2.ouhsc.edu/doi/epdf/10.1111/j.1432-2277.2010.01184.x (accessed 2 August 2019).
21. Audibert G, Charpentier C, Seguin-Devaux C, Charretier P-A, Grégoire H, Devaux Y et al. Improvement of donor myocardial function after treatment of autonomic storm during brain death. Transplantation 2006; 82: 1031–1036.
22. McKeown DW, Bonser RS, Kellum JA. Management of the heartbeating brain-dead organ donor. British Journal of Anaesthesia 2012; 108: i96–i107.

23. Chen JM, Cullinane S, Spanier TB, Artrip JH, John R, Edwards NM et al. Vasopressin deficiency and pressor hypersensitivity in hemodynamically unstable organ donors. [Miscellaneous Article]. Circulation 1999; 100.
24. Pennefather SH, Bullock RE, Mantle D, Dark JH. Use of low dose arginine vasopressin to support brain-dead organ donors. Transplantation 1995; 59: 58–62.
25. Callahan DS, Neville A, Bricker S, Kim D, Putnam B, Bongard F et al. The effect of arginine vasopressin on organ donor procurement and lung function. Journal of Surgical Research 2014; 186: 452–457.
26. Plurad DS, Bricker S, Neville A, Bongard F, Putnam B. Arginine vasopressin significantly increases the rate of successful organ procurement in potential donors. The American Journal of Surgery 2012; 204: 856–861.
27. Kumar L. Brain death and care of the organ donor. J Anaesthesiol Clin Pharmacol 2016; 32: 146–152.
28. Wood KE, Becker BN, McCartney JG, D'Alessandro AM, Coursin DB. Care of the potential organ donor. N Engl J Med 2004; 351: 2730–2739.
29. Rosendale JD, Kauffman HM, McBride MA, Chabalewski FL, Zaroff JG, Garrity ER et al. Hormonal resuscitation yields more transplanted hearts, with improved early function. Transplantation 2003; 75: 1336–1341.
30. Rosendale JD, Myron Kauffman H, McBride MA, Chabalewski FL, Zaroff JG, Garrity ER et al. Aggressive pharmacologic donor management results in more transplanted organs1: Transplantation 2003; 75: 482–487.
31. Zaroff JG, Rosengard BR, Armstrong WF, Babcock WD, D'Alessandro A, Dec GW et al. Consensus conference report: Maximizing use of organs recovered from the cadaver donor: Cardiac recommendations: March 28–29, 2001, Crystal City, Va. Circulation 2002; 106: 836–841.
32. Stadalman KA, Kelner MJ, Box K, Dominguez A, Rigby JF. Stability of levothyroxine sodium 0.4 microg/mL in 0.9% sodium chloride injection. Prog Transplant 2009; 19: 354–356; quiz 357.
33. Totsuka E, Dodson F, Urakami A, Moras N, Ishii T, Lee M-C et al. Influence of high donor serum sodium levels on early postoperative graft function in human liver transplantation: Effect of correction of donor hypernatremia. Liver Transplantation and Surgery 1999; 5: 421–428.
34. Figueras J, Busquets J, Grande L, Jaurrieta E, Perez-Ferreiroa J, Mir J et al. The deleterious effect of donor high plasma sodium and extended preservation in liver transplantation. A multivariate analysis. Transplantation 1996; 61: 410–413.
35. Cittanova ML, Leblanc I, Legendre C, Mouquet C, Riou B, Coriat P. Effect of hydroxyethylstarch in brain-dead kidney donors on renal function in kidney-transplant recipients. Lancet 1996; 348: 1620–1622.
36. Perel P, Roberts I, Ker K. Colloids versus crystalloids for fluid resuscitation in critically ill patients. The Cochrane database of systematic reviews 2013; 2: CD000567.
37. Varghese JM, Roberts JA, Lipman J. Pharmacokinetics and pharmacodynamics in critically ill patients. Curr Opin Anaesthesiol 2010; 23: 472–478.
38. Wijdicks EFM, Varelas PN, Gronseth GS, Greer DM, American Academy of Neurology. Evidence-based guideline update: Determining brain death in adults: Report of the Quality Standards Subcommittee of the American Academy of Neurology. Neurology 2010; 74: 1911–1918.

39. Wijdicks EF, Varelas PN, Gronseth GS, Greer DM. Evidence-based guideline update: Determining brain death in adults Report of the Quality Standards Subcommittee of the American Academy of Neurology Neurology Jun 2010, 74 (23) 1911–1918; DOI: 10.1212/WNL.0b013e3181e242a8
40. Verstraete AG. Detection times of drugs of abuse in blood, urine, and oral fluid. Ther Drug Monit 2004; 26: 200–205.
41. Drake M, Bernard A, Hessel E. Brain death. Surgical Clinics of North America 2017; 97: 1255–1273.
42. Neavyn MJ, Stolbach A, Greer DM, Nelson LS, Smith SW, Brent J et al. ACMT position statement: Determining brain death in adults after drug overdose. J Med Toxicol 2017; 13: 271–273.

34

Challenges with organ donation in children

Thomas A. Nakagawa, Jogi V. Pattisapu

Introduction

Organs recovered from deceased donors annually impact thousands of children and adults who benefit from a life-changing or life-saving organ transplant.[1,2] On the other hand, unfortunately, many adults and children continue to die waiting for an organ that never becomes available. A persisting need to recover more organs for transplantation exists despite efforts to improve donation awareness and increase organ transplantation. This need also exists in children with end-stage organ failure where the highest death rate waiting for an organ occurs in children less than one year of age.[1,2] Additionally, more children die before an organ becomes available for transplantation because their condition deteriorates and they are removed from the waiting list.[1] The majority of children needing an organ transplant have end-stage renal failure and are waiting for a kidney transplant followed by children with liver disease who are waiting for a liver transplant.[1] The importance of organ donation is supported by the American Academy of Pediatrics and other global organizations.[2,3]

Recovery of organs for paediatric transplantation can occur following neurologic death (donation after brain death, DBD), circulatory death (donation after circulatory death, DCD), or from living donation. Most deaths in an intensive care unit occur following withdrawal of life-sustaining medical therapies (WLST).[4,5] Neurologic death is more common in paediatric intensive care units (PICU) compared with neonatal intensive care units (NICU). Mechanism of injury resulting in neurologic

Table 34.1 Organs recovered following brain death and circulatory death

Neurologic death (DBD)	Circulatory death (DCD)
Heart	Heart*
Lungs	Lungs
Liver	Liver
Kidney	Kidney
Pancreas	Pancreas
Intestines	
Tissues: bone, skin, cartilage, heart valves, cornea	

* Boucek MM, Mashburn C, Dunn SM, et al. Pediatric heart transplantation after declaration of cardiocirculatory death. N Engl J Med 2008;359(7):709–714.

*White CW, Messer SJ, Large SR, et al. Transplantation of hearts donated after circulatory death. Font Cardiovas Med. 2018;5–8.

death in children tends to be hypoxic ischemic injury or traumatic brain injury.[6] A considerable number of donor organs are recovered following neurologic death although the number of paediatric DCD donors has increased significantly.[1] Organs recovered for transplantation are dependent on the type of donation (Table 34.1).

Process of organ donation

Organ donation is a process. Like many other processes in medicine such as patient admission, discharge, and surgical procedures, organ donation requires collaboration and coordination with appropriate specialists to ensure a successful outcome. The critical care team and organ procurement organization (OPO) must engage and interact in a professional manner respecting the expertise that each group contributes to the process of organ donation. This process begins when a critically ill patient is identified as a potential donor. Development of clinical triggers alerts the medical team to contact the OPO. Early referral is considered a best practice for successful donation, allowing the critical care team and the OPO to determine patient trajectory to recovery or neurologic death, assess donation potential, and involve the family about organ donation discussions if appropriate.[7] This process evolves over time and includes: (1) identification of a potential donor, (2) determination of neurologic or circulatory death in a timely manner, (3) authorization for organ donation, (4) perioperative management of the donor, and (5) recovery of organs for transplantation.[8] Ensuring engagement of the OPO and the intensive care team's understanding of the entire donation process eliminates confusion that can disrupt successful organ recovery. This best practice improves authorization rates and assists families with understanding and dealing with end-of-life care issues for their child.[7] Challenges exist at every level related to the donation process. This chapter provides discussion and recommendations to overcome many of these challenges. The determination of neurologic death in infants and children is discussed in Chapter 11.

There are several unique challenges associated with paediatric organ donation. These challenges can result in missed or lost opportunities for donation. Some challenges include: fewer paediatric donors with less provider experience, authorization for donation, medical examiner denials, inadequate perimortem and donor management, allocation of organs, and surgical recovery of organs for transplantation. Additionally, regionalization of specialized care for critically ill children including those who become transplant recipients can present problems for families who are displaced from their home and community. Ethical issues specifically related to donation following circulatory death exist.[9,10] A discussion on ethical issues and challenges related to paediatric transplantation is beyond the scope of this chapter.

Authorization for organ donation

Organ recovery for transplantation requires a formal authorization for the process to be initiated. Unlike adults, where first person consent designates the individual's desire to become a donor, children typically are not asked about donation until they begin driving, and in most countries, they are not allowed to make this decision independently. Authorization from a parent or guardian is common in paediatrics where consent for treatments and procedures is necessary. Authorization for donation requires a coordinated approach with the OPO and the critical care team when talking to parents and families.[7] These discussions with parents or guardians may differ from spouses and relatives of adult donors. The traditional approach by an OPO coordinator decoupling the death and authorization process for adult donation may not be the best approach for parents facing end-of-life issues and donation of their child's organs. One study found that timing of organ donation discussions prior to or following determination of death did not appear to influence parents' decisions to donate their child's organs.(11) Parents may require sufficient time to discuss end-of-life care issues including donation and may prefer discussions with the paediatric intensivist or a member of the health-care team they trust before neurologic death occurs.(11) The decision to donate is made after thoughtful discussions between the medical team and the parents/guardians. It is most important to ensure this decision is made by the parents or guardians and not by the medical team. Preconceptions about donor eligibility by medical teams cause a protective stance by the medical team and may have unintended consequences such as denying families the opportunity to help or save other lives.(12) Additionally, few families of adults and children appear to suffer psychological harm after having the donation option presented to them.(12) Collaboration with the OPO and the medical team is essential to assist families with an understanding of end-of-life issues and organ donation. Engagement of palliative care specialists may provide additional family support and be a resource to assist the ICU team during end-of-life care discussions.(13,14)

Preserving the option of organ donation

Coordination of care for a critically ill or injured child with the involvement of a paediatric intensivist and the critical care team is the foundation for successful specialized centres with good outcomes. Involvement of critical care specialists throughout the donation process impacts the quality and number of organs recovered.(7,8) Care of the critically ill child and their family through all phases of illness including end-of-life issues should be a seamless transition. The continuum of care for the patient that progresses to death and becomes a donor requires the expertise of the paediatric intensivist and critical care team to preserve the option of donation.(7) Continued patient management is essential to: (1)

prevent organ systems deterioration and subsequent loss of transplantable organs, (2) help the family deal with the death of their child, and (3) facilitate the donation process and successful recovery of organs for transplantation. Best practices for deceased organ donation emphasize patient management that preserves the option of donation for potential donors prior to and after declaration of death.[2,3,7,8,15] Preserving the option of donation by providing appropriate perimortem and donor management care is essential to successful recovery of organs when the family authorizes donation. The physician is obligated to provide continued medical care to the critically ill patient until a determination of ongoing medical therapies and resuscitation status, or death has occurred. Continuing to treat the patient for purposes of preserving the potential for organ donation is consistent with attempting to save the life of the patient and benefits the patient and society.[16] If the critical care team is unable to save the life of the child, the option of donation can be presented to the parents or guardians. In the case of the dying child, ensuring palliative or end-of-life care and supporting a family's request for donation must be balanced.

Management of the paediatric organ donor

The wide age range of children from birth through adolescence can prove challenging when caring for a paediatric patient apart from the complexities of managing a paediatric donor. Specialized care for paediatric patients is best accomplished in medical centres with paediatric expertise.[8] This expertise may not be available in every community, resulting in transfer to a regional paediatric centre skilled in the unique needs of caring for critically ill infants and children. The skill of specially trained paediatric critical care specialists includes important aspects related to care of the child and the family. This expertise includes: access to age-appropriate medical equipment including selection of the appropriately sized endotracheal tube to provide airway support, securing vascular access in infants and children, weight-based drug dosing, and skilled nursing and respiratory therapist support.[17] The paediatric donor requires appropriate medical management to support organ system function following determination of death. Subsequent care differs from management prior to death. Following determination of death and once the decision to proceed with organ donation has been established, cerebroprotective efforts are abandoned and care shifts towards providing adequate circulation and oxygen delivery to preserve vital organ function for transplantation.[7,17] Intensive care staff and families must be prepared for the transition in goals of therapy from lifesaving to organ preserving. The critical care team should remain actively involved to manage the potential donor and correct existing physiologic derangements that follow neurologic death to preserve the option of organ donation for the family.[7] The existing physiologic derangements such as decreased intravascular volume to reduce cerebral blood flow, metabolic disturbances such as hypernatremia and hyperglycaemia associated with hyperosmolar therapy and catecholamine release, volume loss from hyperglycaemia and diabetes insipidus, respiratory alkalosis from over ventilation, and temperature regulation following neurologic death should be promptly evaluated and corrected.[7,8,17] Cardiovascular management goals are targeted towards maintaining normal perfusion pressure and blood pressure for age to ensure adequate end-organ perfusion. Targeting donor management goals increases organ recovery and can result in a better graft for the transplant recipient.[18] Table 34.2 lists paediatric donor management goals. As a general rule, good donor management equates to good patient management to maintain organ system function. Inadequate donor management can result in significant loss of valuable organs for transplantation.[19]

Many OPO's routinely use hormonal replacement therapy (HRT) during donor management treatment. HRT for the brain dead donor restores aerobic metabolism, replaces hormones derived from the hypothalamus and pituitary, augments blood volume, and minimizes the use of inotropic support while optimizing cardiac output.[17] Commonly used agents include thyroid hormone, steroids, and vasopressin. Studies in children are extremely limited; however, HRT is a reasonable consideration when hemodynamic instability does not improve with fluid and inotropic support.[7,8,17] There is supporting evidence that earlier institution of HRT improves outcomes resulting in greater organ procurement rates.[20]

Table 34.2 Pediatric Donor Management Goals

Pediatric Donor Management Goals

Hemodynamic Support	Blood Pressure		
• Normalization of blood pressure ○ Systolic blood pressure appropriate for age ○ Note: Lower systolic blood pressures may be acceptable if biomarkers such as lactate are normal. • CVP < 12 *(if measured)* • Dopamine< 10 mcg/kg/min • Normal serum lactate		Systolic	Diastolic
	Neonate	60–90	35–90
	Infants (6 months)	80–95	50–65
	Toddler (2 years)	85–100	50–65
	School age (7 years)	90–115	60–70
	Adolescent (15 years)	110–130	65–80
	Normal systolic blood pressure = 80 + 2 x age in years		

Oxygenation and Ventilation	Fluids and Electrolytes	
• Maintain PaO_2 > 100 mmHg • FiO_2 0.40 • Normalize $PaCO_2$ 35–45 mmHg • Arterial pH 7.30–7.45 • Tidal volumes 8–10 cc/kg • PEEP 5 cm H_2O	• Serum Na^+	130–150 meq/L
	• Serum K^+	3–5.0 meq/L
	• Serum glucose	60–150 mg/dl
	• Ionized Ca^{++} *(if measured)*	0.8–1.2 mmol/L

Thermal Regulation
• Core body temperature 36–38°C

From: North American Transplant Coordinators Organization (NATCO) Pediatric Donor Management and Dosing Guidelines. Nakagawa, TA. 2007

Management of DCD donors

Management of the DCD donor differs from DBD donors. A decision to WLST must be made before discussion and authorization for organ donation. Prior to WLST, comfort measures and palliative goals are established for the child. Specific donor management begins with WLST includes the provision of palliative treatments, and ends with death determination based on cessation of circulation or determination that the donor is ineligible.[7] Discussions with the critical care team and the OPO are essential and should include operating room personnel. Discussions should include where WLST will occur, appropriate provisions for family presence prior to death and following organ recovery, and accommodations for ongoing comfort care should the child not progress to circulatory arrest within the specified time period to determine death.[7] The location of WLST should minimize warm ischemic time that can affect graft function. Consideration of operating room schedules to minimize daily workflow requires coordination with the operating room staff. Parents and family should be prepared for rapid separation from their child once death has been pronounced. Appropriate ongoing support for the family should be immediately available. Importantly, all members of the healthcare team should be aware of these challenges and be willing to care for the child and the family. Members of the healthcare team may 'opt out' of participating in this type of donation based on their comfort level. If patients cannot be cared for, or the option of donation is impeded by hospital policies or procedures, transfer to another centre that can provide resources and accommodate the family's wishes can be considered. These challenges must be addressed for DCD to be successfully completed.

Determining suitability of donor organs

Medical teams may presume that organs are not suitable for recovery because the child is too ill or critically injured. Suitability of donor organs for transplantation is best assessed by the OPO.[7] The threshold for acceptable organ function can vary depending on the time of evaluation, comfort levels of the transplant surgeon, and the recipients' need for an organ. Disease processes may differ in children and require collaboration between the OPO, the ICU team, and paediatric specialists to determine donor suitability. Inborn errors of metabolism, complex congenital heart disease, infections, and oncologic disease are several examples where differences may exist compared with adults. Serial echocardiograms may demonstrate improved donor organ function following effective medical therapy allowing cardiac recovery for transplantation.[7] Bacterial meningitis or a positive blood culture may not preclude organ donation if antibiotic therapy has been administered.[7] Renal and hepatic function may improve following donor management strategies to correct and maintain end-organ function. Organs from HIV positive donors are being transplanted into recipients with and without HIV.[21] Additionally, donor organs with hepatitis C have been transplanted into patients with and without hepatitis C.[22,23] Continued evolution of medical advancements, treatments, and medications has allowed organs that were once unsuitable for transplantation to become organs that can be recovered and transplanted with good outcomes.

Despite the best possible donor management, many organs from paediatric donors are never transplanted and paediatric wait list recipients continue to die because an organ is not available in a timely manner. Finding a suitable recipient can be challenging because of specific issues related to children. Allocation of paediatric organs to a transplant recipient must be size and weight matched. Additionally, time constraints from organ recovery to transplantation, specifically for heart, may limit the distance an organ can be transported. Recovery of organs for transplantation requires surgical expertise, especially in younger donors with smaller vessels, etc. Injury to the organ or vasculature during recovery may preclude an organ from being transplanted. Appropriate surgical resources with paediatric expertise should be considered when dealing with a paediatric donor. The importance of utilizing paediatric medical and surgical specialists cannot be overemphasized.

Many children that die from head injuries are victims of non-accidental trauma. Medical examiner or coroner denials can impact organ recovery for transplantation.[24] Collaboration with investigative teams, medical examiners and coroners in cases of accidental or non-accidental death is imperative to determine the cause of death and allow the donation process to proceed.[7,24] These emotionally charged cases require balance to preserve the integrity of the ongoing criminal investigation while respecting the family's desire for organ donation to occur. Successful recovery of organs and the prosecution of the perpetrator can occur in most cases with close cooperation between forensic investigators, treating physicians, the transplant team, and OPO.[7,8,25] Preservation of evidence and early consultation and discussions with the coroner, medical examiner, and forensic or child abuse team may result in requests for additional testing and noninvasive imaging that can assist with the death investigation without precluding donation.

Neonatal donation

Infants waiting for an organ transplant continue to have the highest death rate on the waiting list.[1,2] Opportunities for neonatal donation are rare but can increase organ availability for transplantation. Neurologic death is a rare event in many NICU. Although brain death can occur in this population of patients, most neonates die following WLST,.[7,14,26] Organ donation following neurologic and circulatory death can occur in neonates. Specific criteria to determine neurologic death in a neonate are discussed in Chapter 11. DCD requires extensive collaboration with the medical, surgical team, and the OPO to ensure a successful outcome.[7] Organs have been recovered from anencephalic infants in rare instances.[27,28]

Liver cell transfusion therapy from neonatal donors is occurring as a bridge to transplantation for infants and children with liver disease.[29,30] Liver cells from neonatal donors are recovered and require special processing. These donor hepatocytes are infused into infants with urea cycle defects and Crigler-Najjar syndrome until the child is big enough to receive a transplant.[29,30] En-bloc kidney recovery from neonatal donors has occurred and organs are being transplanted with good success.[31,32] Infant hearts have been recovered from neonatal DCD donors and transplanted successfully.[33] The use of ex-vivo perfusion for heart recovery has been reported and may provide additional means to recover infant and paediatric DCD hearts.[34] Allocation of smaller organs is more difficult because of size and weight matching for organ transplantation and fewer waiting list recipients in this age group. More information about neonatal donation and transplantation can be found in Chapter 35, Neonatal organ donation.

Education and awareness

The increasing global education and awareness about organ donation is an important area to sustain the continued efforts to recover more organs for transplantation.[2] The rarity of neurologic death and organ donation with frequent physician, nursing, and other healthcare provider turnover requires progressing efforts to ensure the medical team is constantly aware of donation opportunities. Continued discussions between the OPO and the critical care team with ongoing provider education can enhance relationships and help create a culture where donation is integrated into end-of-life care for any patient and family cared for in the PICU.[7] This includes ongoing education with colleagues in neonatology to increase awareness and recovery of neonatal organs as an important initiative to help increase the overall pool of organ donors. Public education and awareness are another important factors, so that families of potential paediatric donors have exposure to donation prior to hospitalization. In one study, organ donation was more likely when the parent was a registered organ donor and had favourable organ donation beliefs.[11]

Conclusion

The successful recovery of organs for transplantations requires a collaborative approach that identifies and cares for the paediatric organ donor by a skilled team of specialists who must not only deal with the deceased child, but also with the family. The process of donation begins when a critically ill or injured child is identified as a potential donor with a timely referral to the OPO. Early involvement of the OPO with a timely referral allows coordination with the critical care team and other medical services to support the family and enhance the chance for the family to understand, accept the death of their child, and authorize organ donation. There are clearly challenges with organ donation that can be overcome with a shared responsibility that relies on respecting the expertise of those involved with the process of donation. Collaboration between paediatric critical care specialists, the critical care team, the OPO, and other dedicated professionals providing specialized donor management helps families heal following the death of their child. The lives of the donor family and the many potential recipients and their families are impacted by a life-saving and life-changing organ or tissue transplant. The opportunity to allow organ donation to occur is a family decision that should be honoured by the medical team that preserves this option. Organ donation provides positive meaning to the death of a child and allows the child's legacy to continue and live on through this most generous gift of saving a life.

More information and additional resources about paediatric organ donation can be found in the Organ Donation Toolbox at: https://organdonationalliance.org/resources/toolbox/

Highlights

- Challenges with paediatric donation include: fewer paediatric donors with less provider experience, authorization for donation, medical examiner denials, inadequate perimortem and donor management, allocation of organs, and surgical recovery of organs for transplantation.
- Organ donation is a process.
- Successful donation requires collaboration between the critical care team, OPO, and other medical specialists.
- Authorization for donation requires a coordinated approach with the OPO and the critical care team when talking to parents and families.
- Specialized care for children including paediatric donors is best accomplished in medical centres with paediatric staff that have expertise in the unique issues related to medical management and care for the family.
- Organ recovery for paediatric transplantation can occur following neurologic death (donation after brain death DBD), circulatory death (donation after circulatory death DCD), or from living donation.

References

1. Data. OPTN: Organ Procurement and Transplantation Network. Available at: https://optn.transplant.hrsa.gov/data/view-data-reports/national-data/. Accessed May 20, 2019.
2. Martin DE, Nakagawa TA, Siebelink MJ, et al. Pediatric deceased donation—A report of the Transplantation Society Meeting in Geneva. *Transplantation* 2015;99:1403–1409.
3. Committee on Hospital Care, Section on Surgery, and Section on Critical Care. Policy statement—pediatric organ donation and transplantation. Pediatrics 2010;125(4):822–828.
4. Burns JP, Seller DE, Meyer EC, et al. Epidemiology of death in the pediatric intensive care unit at five US teaching hospitals. Crit Care Med 2014;42:2101–2108.
5. Meert KL, Keele L, Morrison W, et al. Eunice Kennedy Shriver National Institute of Child Health and Human Development Collaborative Pediatric Critical Care Research Network. End-of-life practices among Tertiary Care PICUs in the United States: A multicenter study. Pediatr Crit Care Med. 2015 Sep;16(7):e231–e238. doi: 10.1097/PCC.0000000000000520.

6. Kirschen MP, Francoeur C, Murphy M, et al. Epidemiology of brain death in pediatric intensive care units in the United States. JAMA Pediatr. 2019; 173(5):469–476.
7. Nakagawa TA, Shemie SD, Dreyden-Palmer K, et al. Organ donation following neurologic death. Pediatric Critical Care. Death and Dying Supplement. 2018:19:S26–S32. DOI:10.1097/PCC.0000000000001518.
8. Kotloff RM, Blosser S, Fulda GJ, et al. Management of the potential organ donor in the ICU: Society of Critical Care Medicine/American College of Chest Physicians/ Association of Organ Procurement Organizations Consensus Statement. Crit Care Med 2015;43(6):1291–1325.
9. Joffe AR, Carcillo J, Anton N, et al. Donation after cardiocirculatory death: A call for a moratorium pending full public disclosure and fully informed consent. Philos Ethics Humanit Med. 2011 Dec 29;6:17. doi: 10.1186/1747-5341-6-17.
10. Nakagawa TA, Rigby MR, Bratton S, et al. A call for full public disclosure for donation after circulatory determination of death in children. Pediatr Crit Care Med. 2011 May;12(3):375–377; author reply 377-8. doi: 10.1097/PCC.0b013e31820ac30c.
11. Rodrigue JR, Cornell DL, Howard RJ. Pediatric organ donation: what factors most influence parents' donation decisions? Pediatr Crit Care Med 2008;9(2):180–185.
12. Siminoff LA, Molisani AJ, Traino. A comparison of the request process and outcomes in adult and pediatric organ donation. Pediatrics. 2015;136(1):e108–e114.
13. Owens DA. The role of palliative care in organ donation. J Hosp Palliat Nurs 2006;8(2):75–76.
14. Boss R, Nelson J, Weissman D, et al. Integrating palliative care into the PICU: a report from the Improving Palliative Care in the ICU Advisory Board. Pediatr Crit Care Med 2014;15(8):762–767.
15. Domínguez-Gil B, Murphy P, Procaccio F. Ten changes that could improve organ donation in the intensive care unit. Intensive Care Med. 2016; 42:264–267.
16. Sochet AA, Glazier AK, Nakagawa TA. Diagnosis of brain death and organ donation after circulatory death. In Mastropietro CW, Valentine KM. Pediatric Critical Care. Current Controversies. Switzerland; Springer Nature:2019: p 309–321.
17. Nakagawa TA, Mou SS. Management of the pediatric organ donor. In: LaPointe D, Ohler L, Rudow T, et al., (eds.). The clinician's guide to donation and transplantation. Lenexa, KS: North American Transplant Coordinators Organization (NATCO), 2006. p.839–845.
18. Patel MS, De La Cruz S, Sally MB, et al. Active donor management during the hospital phase of care is associated with more organs transplanted per donor. J Am Coll Surg. 2017 Oct;225(4):525–531. doi: 10.1016/j.jamcollsurg.2017.06.014. Epub 2017 Jul 21.
19. Salim A, Velmahos GC, Brown C, et al. Aggressive organ donor management significantly increases the number of organs available for transplantation. J Trauma 2005;58(5):991–994.
20. Rosendale JD, Kauffman HM, McBride MA, et al. Hormonal resuscitation yields more transplanted hearts, with improved early function. Transplantation 2003;75(8):1336–1341.

21. Botha J, Conradie F, Etheredge H, et al. Living donor liver transplant from an HIV-positive mother to her HIV-negative child: opening up new therapeutic options. AIDS. 2018;32(16):F13–F19.
22. Sise ME, Chute DF, Gustafson JL et al. Transplantation of hepatitis C virus infected kidneys into hepatitis C virus uninfected recipients. Hemodial Int. 2018;22 Suppl1:S71–S80.
23. Woolley AE, Singh SK, Goldberg JH et al. Heart and lung transplants from HCV-infected donors to uninfected recipients. N Engl J Med. 2019;380:1606–1617.
24. Webster PA, Markham L. Pediatric organ donation: A national survey examining consent rates and characteristics of donor hospitals. Pediatr Crit Care Med 2009;10(4):500–504.
25. Shafer TJ, Schkade LL, Evans RW, et al. Vital role of medical examiners and coroners in organ transplantation. Am J Transplant 2004;4(2):160–168.
26. Nakagawa TA, Ashwal S, Mathur M, et al. Guidelines for the determination of brain death in infants and children: An update of the 1987 Task Force recommendations. Crit Care Med 2011;39(9):2139–2155.
27. Nakagawa TA, Zollinger C, Chao J, Hill R, Angle S, Pilot M. Anencephalic infants as organ donors. Transplantation 2017:101;8(S-2) Supplement:S60.
28. Brierley J, Hasan A: Aspects of deceased organ donation in paediatrics. Br J Anaesth 2012; 108(Suppl 1):i92–i95
29. Meyburg J, Opladen T, Spiekerkötter U, et al. Human heterologous liver cells transiently improve hyperammonemia and ureagenesis in individuals with severe urea cycle disorders. J Inherit Metab Dis 2018;41(1):81–89.
30. Smets F, Dobbelaere D, McKiernan P, et al. Phase I/II trial of liver derived mesenchymal stem cells in pediatric liver based metabolic disorders: A prospective, open label, multicenter, partially randomized, safety study of one cycle of heterologous human adult liver-derived Progenitor Cells (HepaStem®) in urea cycle disorders and Crigler-Najjar Syndrome patients. Transplantation 2019; 103(9):1903–1915.
31. Perez R, Santhanakrishnan C, Demattos A, et al. The neonatal intensive care unit (NICU) as a source of deceased donor kidneys for transplantation: Initial experience with 20 cases (abstract #2289). Am J Transplant 2014;14(Suppl 3):134.
32. Lau KK, Berg GM, Schjoneman YG, Perez RV, Butani L. Pediatric en bloc kidney transplantation into pediatric recipients. Pediatr Transplant 2010;14(1):100–104.
33. Boucek MM, Mashburn C, Dunn SM, et al. Pediatric heart transplantation after declaration of cardiocirculatory death. N Engl J Med 2008;359(7):709–714.
34. White CW, Messer SJ, Large SR, et al. Transplantation of hearts donated after circulatory death. Font Cardiovas Med. 2018;5–8. Published online 2018 Feb 13. doi:10.33889/fcvm.2018.00008.

35

Neonatal organ donation

Colin Coulter, Joe Brierley

Introduction

While the neonatal period accounts for more child deaths than any other period, most of these deaths occur in infants who are not eligible for organ donation. Partly, this is due to many deaths occurring in premature neonates. Secondly, transplant teams are reluctant to use very small organs—so near-term/term infants are the only solid organ donors in the neonatal period. Neonatal organ donation like paediatric donation provides life-saving and transforming transplants for those on waiting lists expecting small size matched organs. Neonates and infants can donate mostly the same organs as older children.[1] For some awaiting a life-saving organ transplant, such small-sized organs are their only option, which is most clearly the case in heart transplantation due to the limitation of the thoracic cavity size and necessary vascular anastomoses. Sadly, this means many infants die on waiting lists, or are not listed, as the chance of a suitable organ is so remote. Despite this, it is surprising to many, that some organs donated by neonates are not transplanted into other infants or even children but into adults as en bloc kidneys.

Donation after both neurological determination of death (or the less preferred older term, brain death (DND/DBD) and circulatory determination of death (DCD) in neonates and small infants are feasible, but subject to national law and medical standards which vary considerably. For example, DCD in children occurs in the UK, but not in Germany and France. However, until recently in the UK, DND/DBD from infants under two-months of age was prevented due to national guidance stating the diagnosis of brain death was unsafe in infants. In contrast, it could occur in France and Germany.

Demographics of neonatal and infant death

The neonatal period is essentially the first four weeks of life; infants are children under one year outside the neonatal period. It is generally sensible to consider donation from infants who die following an acute life-threatening illness in the same context as that from older children, both being usually admitted to hospital from home via the emergency department (ED) before transfer to Intensive Care for organ support. The critical illness preceding death has similar diagnoses and pathophysiology, with identical verification of death and donation processes.

In contrast, the *neonatal* group are in NICU (Neonatal Intensive Care Unit) or another ICU having been admitted following the complications of delivery, transition from foetal to postnatal life or severe congenital abnormalities. There are specific policies and often a different clinical team involved in their care.

All organ donations in younger children, including those in the first year of life, occur in the presence of life-sustaining therapies, (LST) almost always including invasive mechanical ventilation. The LST either maintains the infant who will be diagnosed dead using neurological criteria or is withdrawn (WLST) before death is verified using circulatory criteria.

There is a crucial, ethical standard underpinning DCD. LST is never withdrawn for donation purposes. Rather, the clinical team and parents, consider doing so in the best interests of the child, with organ donation only as a secondary consideration following the decision to withdraw LST.[2]

A large group of children who die in infancy cannot become organ donors as they die without the presence of LST. For donation to be considered, a baby needs to be resuscitated to a physiologically stable condition and maintained on LST. It is possible that in the future, donation of (stem) cells as already exists for tissues such as heart valves may be viable many hours after the baby dies.

Screening of critically ill neonates for donation potential is challenging as there are many neonatal intensive care units compared to Paediatric Intensive Care Units (PICU), though very few—if any—donors within any individual unit. A considerable proportion of neonates and older infants will be receiving critical care in a PICU as they have been admitted from home, or are receiving highly specialist treatment, e.g. neurovascular embolization. Essentially, it is reasonable to refer any term neonate or infant to donation/procurement services with (i) fixed dilated pupils or (ii) for whom there is a plan to withdraw LST, with an expectation of death within a DCD-compatible time frame (often 3 hours). Even if DCD is not available in that country, this enables donor potential to be assessed and changes to law/standards to be considered.

Neurologic determination of death

The UK medical hierarchy's reluctance to accept 'brain death' in infants less than two months of age originated from concerns in the 1980s and 1990s about the reliability of the diagnosis. The Neurologic determination of death (NDD) is partly based on the loss of cranial nerve function, but at the time cranial nerve development in infancy was not fully delineated. Such a precautionary principle-type stance was less important at a time when infant DND/DBD was not feasible. However, when it became technically possible to transplant neonatal-sized organs, many other jurisdictions decided that the absence of evidence of any issue meant 'infant brain death' was safe. As a consequence, the UK recently undertook a rigorous assessment of the evidence before lately changing its position.[3]

There are legitimate issues novel to neonatal NDD: (i) the use of therapeutic hypothermia in severe birth asphyxia and (ii) the potential of the infant brain to recover from perinatal hypoxia. While it is outside the remit of this chapter to list the various policies and protocols that exist in neonatal DND/DBD, it is fair to state that many countries have specific safeguards in place that are not required in older children. These often include a prolonged period of observation to ensure the elimination of the effects of therapeutic hypothermia used in neonatal brain injury which include direct inhibitory effects on cerebral metabolism or the effects on the pharmacokinetics of sedative agents, both potentially confounding causes of the child's coma. In fact, the cause of coma in infants is usually clear: hypoxic-ischaemic encephalopathy secondary to birth asphyxia; cardiac arrest of other aetiology; infections such as GBS meningitis, or abusive/other head injuries.

The length of the prolonged periods between the two sets of bedside NDD tests, if required, and the specific time after the onset of coma when the first test can be done show significant international variability.

In older infants and older children, there is little practical difference from NDD in adults, with the same verification criteria used in most jurisdictions with the same pre-conditions, diagnostic imaging, and tests necessary. Confounding factors which may contribute to a coma such as the effects of sedative drugs, electrolyte imbalance, and hypothermia must be excluded. Once this is assured, the clinical bedside test is composed of confirmation of coma, absence of relevant cranial nerve reflexes, and the apnoea test. These vary, perhaps unhelpfully, between different jurisdictions, though with little suggestion of real variability in the outcome.

Once the baby is dead, organ donor management processes that may improve the chance of successful transplant can happen; these include changing inotropes to more cardio-protective agents and the use of hormone therapies. The circulation, and therefore, the perfusion to vital organs, remains intact until the point of retrieval.

Circulatory determination of death

Almost all neonates and infants who die have their death verified using circulatory criteria, though in only very few can DCD be considered. All neonatal DCD follows elective cessation of LST in the child's best interests; there is no uncontrolled neonatal DCD.

The most likely situation to lead to neonatal DCD is a significant neurological condition, such as birth asphyxia or neonatal meningitis, with a prognosis so poor that the withdrawal of LST is considered to be in the child's best interest.

In older infants, brain injury secondary to prolonged cardiac arrest or trauma becomes more common, and in some countries organ donation after abusive head trauma in infancy is permitted. However, any situation in which an acute withdrawal of LST is considered likely to lead to death in a compatible time frame can be suitable not just brain injury.

The most frequent LST to be withdrawn are mechanical ventilation and inotropes, though ECMO (extracorporeal membrane oxygenation) or VADs (ventricular assist devices) can also be removed. The issue is that death must occur in a suitable time frame to prevent donated organs from receiving irreversible damage due to warm ischaemia.

Another unusual LST removal concept is placental perfusion cessation at delivery in the rarely occurring perinatal cases of anencephalic DCD.

Unlike in DND/DBD, there is little material difference in the procedures and practice of neonatal and infant DCD compared with that in older children or even adults. The main ethical concern is the ability to safely verify human death in a time-frame compatible with the retrieval and effective transplantation of organs. The crucial limit is the warm ischaemia that occurs to the organs during the child's dying process, death verification process, and the surgical retrieval of organs.

The process of controlled DCD is almost identical at any age. A decision to withdraw LST in the best interest of the patient, in agreement with the relatives or, in this case, parents, must be made first with no consideration about organ donation.

Initial overall concerns about the safety of DCD, specifically the occurrence of the Lazarus phenomenon in which spontaneous circulatory return follows initial asystole, have not been borne out in studies of death, following elective cessation of LST at any age. Those opposed to DCD per se will equally oppose neonatal DCD, yet there seems no scientific reason to consider it different, despite how refractory the neonatal myocardium is to hypoxia. Once a patient of any age is verified as dead, donation is ethically acceptable, with appropriate consent.

Once LST is withdrawn, usual end-of-life medical care—such as analgesia—must be continued. The only difference in death verification during DCD compared to the usual CDD is the more intense monitoring required to ensure that the process is performed correctly. A senior clinician is present at withdrawal and throughout the dying process and verifies death after 5 minutes of continuous asystole. Despite some attempts to reduce this 5 minute time to decrease ongoing warm ischaemic damage to donate organs, it does appear to be an internationally acceptable standard at all ages. Interestingly, it was in neonatal cardiac DCD that considerably shorter stand-off times were used in Denver to minimize the critical warm ischaemic damage to the heart that occurs during the dying process.[4]

International variability in the permissibility of DCD seems to involve cultural and subsequent legal variability, rather than any legitimate medical difference in how humans die.

In countries where withdrawal of LST is generally less prevalent, DCD is rarer. Europe, perhaps due to historical events in the last century, proves a good example of profound international variability, with no scientific or physiological justification. The DCD is unlawful in Germany, paediatric DCD is lawful but not practised in Switzerland and France,[5] whereas it occurs in the Netherlands, Spain, and the UK. In most countries, DCD has only been considered in neonates after becoming well established in older children.

Size matching and limitations of neonatal organs

Neonatal DND/DBD provides similar organs to any other aged donors, though there is the specific explicit limitation of size-matching recipients for such small organs. Due to the overall scarcity of neonatal sized organs, there are limitations on the provision of LST for neonates with severe organ failure in organ systems that require transplant of size-matched vital organs, especially the heart.

Therefore, the use of ECMO followed by Berlin heart support in infants with severe cardiomyopathy given the scarcity of neonatal sized donated hearts is questionable.

Apart from the Denver experience mentioned above,[4] most of all neonatal hearts are from the very few infants who fulfil neurological criteria for death. The recent ground-breaking success in adult cardiac transplants from DCD donors[6] may be realized in neonates and infants if the significant hurdle of developing small extracorporeal resuscitation devices can be overcome.

Neonatal liver donation is increasingly feasible,[7] and for infants awaiting transplant, the possibility of a neonatal donated hepatocyte bridge to eventual liver transplant from either a deceased infant donor or reduced/partial graft from a deceased or living-related donor are viable options.[8]

Renal centres are reluctant to transplant infants with renal failure who can be successfully managed on dialysis until they are over a year/10kg.

At this stage, live-related transplant becomes a viable option due to non-anatomical extra-peritoneal organ transplant positioning. As a corollary, most donated neonatal kidneys, whether DND/DBD or DCD, are transplanted en-bloc into adults.[9]

A multi-visceral transplant from an infant-sized donor is feasible but extremely rare, possibly due to the lack of potential recipients, and surgical expertise in the required time frame, in any area.[10]

Parents' consent

The parents of any deceased child suffer unimaginable tragedy, but if they choose to donate their dying child's organs to save/transform the lives of other people, there can be long-term psychological benefits. This is equally the case for the mothers and partners of infants who donate. Whether an offer of donation leads to transplantation depends on many factors, yet surely parents have to be provided with accurate information and have donation considered, where it is possible.[11]

Antenatal considerations

Recently, the paradigm of pregnant women considering organ donation following the diagnosis of foetal anomalies likely to be associated with infant death, such as anencephaly, have appeared. While donation from infants with anencephaly was first considered in the 1980s, only DND/DBD existed, and foetal medicine with the possibility of accurate antenatal diagnosis was in its infancy. Trying to determine that these babies fulfilled the criteria for ND, followed by facilitating heart donation was neither ethically sustainable nor practical, and attempts ceased worldwide.[12] However, with the onset of high quality early prenatal imaging and DCD, an opportunity for a more prolonged consideration of donor preparation and death verification process equivalent to all other human beings for the terminally-ill newborn donor has become possible. Several successful donations have now been reported, but questions about the resources required compared to the benefits for recipients are essential considerations.[13]

Donor optimization

In DND/DBD, despite the lack of data on efficacy, donor optimization occurs in a deceased infant. However, in DCD, interventions occur in living, albeit expected to die, babies.[14] These interventions are not strictly in the baby's best interests, yet can be considered appropriate if any potential harm to the baby can be mitigated and the parents give explicit consent. Deferring extubation, use of heparin to prevent theoretical ischaemic damage due to thrombosis or instituting mechanical ventilation to postpone death until an organ retrieval team can attend represents a hierarchy of acceptable interventions.[15] Potential harms may correspondingly be survival in a severely compromised state, bleeding and the pain of non-medically beneficial intubation and ventilation. All can be readily planned for and avoided.

Resources for neonatal donation

The need for significant resources to realize neonatal donation is a serious issue. Providing the NICU with the type of screening facilities required by donation services as for older children and adults, keeping potential recipients alive waiting for an organ which may never come—as in the case of a Berlin heart or ECMO—or training surgical teams in small organ techniques requires serious healthcare economic consideration.

While recent successes in adult cardiac DCD offers a new paradigm in transplantation, sadly the specialist organ preservation devices that maintain DCD hearts for transplantation have not yet been developed in the smaller child and infants sizes required, despite infant cardiac DCD having been the bridgehead of DCD heart transplant.

Conclusion

Data has been previously published about the potential for donation in a specialist children's hospital, and perhaps the approach suggested is reasonable with support from collocated PICU colleagues to specialist children's hospital NICUs and a regional PICU approach to stand-alone NICUs.[16]

Even with this approach, there remain missed opportunities for parents to consider organ donation, and this should be addressed with education and training for neonatal teams.[17] The critical steps required for NICU and PICU teams are to ensure timely referral to organ donation/procurement services. They should also join organ donation discussion with those specialist teams to ensure accurate information about end-of-life options is provided by those with suitable expertise, with compassion for the family as this happens at a time of great sadness.

Discussions about donation as part of a child's end-of-life care are often welcomed by families even though donation may not be possible.[18] So, we recommend that as part of holistic end-of-life care in stable neonates and infants in a suitable situation a discussion about organ donation, even if it cannot happen, is appropriate and may save lives.

Highlights

- Neonatal organ donation is possible and saves lives.
- For some small-sized children, only a size-matched organ can save their life.
- Neonatal donation after neurological determination of death is possible in most countries with contemporary ICU provision.
- Neonatal donation after circulatory determination of death is also possible but practised in fewer countries based on ethical and legal standards surrounding the withdrawal of LST.
- Neonatal organ donation can provide great comfort to bereaved families but does require significant investment and support from government and from the regional Paediatric ICUs.

References

1. Nakagawa TA, Shemie SD, Dryden-Palmer K, Parshuram CS, Brierley J. Organ donation following neurologic and circulatory determination of death. Pediatr Crit Care Med. 2018 Aug;19(8S Suppl 2):S26–S32.
2. Larcher V, Craig F, Bhogal K, Wilkinson D, Brierley J; Royal College of Paediatrics and Child Health. Making decisions to limit treatment in life-limiting and life-threatening conditions in children: a framework for practice. Arch Dis Child. 2015 May;100 Suppl 2:s3–s23.

3. The diagnosis of death by neurological criteria in infants less than two months old. Royal College of Paediatrics and Child Health. Available at *https://www.rcpch.ac.uk/sites/default/files/2019-03/2015_dnc_-_full_clinical_guideline.pdf*. Accessed 08/19.
4. Boucek MM, Mashburn C, Dunn SM, Frizell R, Edwards L, Pietra B, Campbell D. Denver children's pediatric heart transplant team. Pediatric heart transplantation after declaration of cardiocirculatory death. N Engl J Med. 2008 Aug 14;359(7):709–714.
5. Leblanc C, Genuini M, Deho A, Lodé N, Philippe-Chomette P, Hervieux E, Amblard A, Pracros N, Léger PL, Jean S. Successful extracorporeal membrane oxygenation transport of a 4-month-old brain-dead infant for organ donation: A case report. Pediatr Transplant. 2019 Aug 22:e13515.
6. Page A, Messer S, Large SR. Heart transplantation from donation after circulatory determined death. Ann Cardiothorac Surg. 2018 Jan;7(1):75–81
7. Gao W, Song Z, Ma N, Dong C, Sun C, Meng X, Zhang W, Wang K, Wu B, Li S, Qin H, Han C, Li H, Shen Z. Utility of neonatal donors in pediatric liver transplantation: A single-center experience. Pediatr Transplant. 2019 Aug;23(5):e13396.
8. Iansante V, M1itry R, Filippi C, Fitzpatrick E, Dhawan A. Human hepatocyte transplantation for liver disease: Current status and future perspectives. Pediatr Res. 2018 Jan;83(1-2):232–240.
9. Wijetunga I, Ecuyer C, Martinez-Lopez S, Jameel M, Baker RJ, Welberry Smith M, Patel C, Weston M, Ahmad N. Renal transplant from infant and neonatal donors is a feasible option for the treatment of end-stage renal disease but is associated with increased early graft loss. Am J Transplant. 2018 Nov;18(11):2679–2688.
10. Cauley RP, Suh MY, Kamin DS, Lillehei CW, Jenkins RL, Jonas MM, Vakili K, Kim HB. Multivisceral transplantation using a 2.9 kg neonatal donor. Pediatr Transplant. 2012 Dec;16(8):E379–E382
11. Lechner, B. E. (2018). Of tragedies and miracles—Neonatal organ donation. New England Journal of Medicine, 379(22), 2089–2091.
12. Brierley J. Neonatal organ donation: Has the time come? Arch Dis Child Fetal Neonatal Ed. 2011 Mar;96(2):F80–F83.
13. Powers RJ, Schultz D, Jackson S. Anencephalic organ donation after cardiac death: A case report on practicalities and ethics. J Perinatol. 2015 Oct;35(10):785–787.
14. Jivraj A, Scales A, Brierley J. Elective ventilation to facilitate organ donation in infants with anencephaly: Perinatal professionals' views and an ethical analysis. Acta Paediatr. 2016 May;105(5):494–498.
15. Brierley J, Shaw D. Premortem interventions in dying children to optimise organ donation: An ethical analysis. J Med Ethics. 2016 Jul;42(7):424–428.
16. Charles E, Scales A, Brierley J. The potential for neonatal organ donation in a children's hospital. Arch Dis Child Fetal Neonatal Ed. 2014 May;99(3):F225–F229.
17. Hawkins KC, Scales A, Murphy P, Madden S, Brierley J. Current status of paediatric and neonatal organ donation in the UK, Arch Dis Child. 2018 Mar;103(3):210–215.
18. Darlington AS, Long-Sutehall T, Randall D, Wakefield C, Robinson V, Brierley J. Parents' experiences of requests for organ and tissue donation: The value of asking. Arch Dis Child. 2019 Sep;104(9):837–843

36

Infections—A contraindication to organ donation

Ahmed Halawa, Ajay Kumar Sharma

Introduction

Organ transplantation has been evolving since Joseph Murray performed the first successful kidney transplantation in 1954. Donor transmitted infection (DTI) is one of the risks an organ recipient faces, particularly if the cause of death was missed or misdiagnosed. Fortunately, the incidence of DTI is quite low; it is estimated at 1%.[1] In the setting of post-transplant immunosuppression, DTI manifests with variable severity ranging from being asymptomatic to a fatal outcome. The spectrum of the pathophysiology of DTI includes viral, bacterial, fungal, parasitic, and helminthic infections. However, the clinicians must appreciate that there would be a significant publications bias because not all cases are reported; hence all the risk factors may not be identified and hence, their impact on a transplant recipient cannot be quantified.

Undoubtedly, the understanding of the potential risk of transmitting some infections such as cytomegalovirus (CMV), Epstein-Barr virus (EBV), has helped in counselling a prospective recipient before transplantation. Some of these infections are not considered a contraindication to transplantation but require long-term surveillance, prophylactic treatment, or pre-emptive therapy.[2] Furthermore, the acceptability of the risk of transplanting a potentially infected organ varies according to the organ to be transplanted. The presence of some types of infections in a potential donor is an absolute contraindication to transplantation in non-life saving transplants such as the kidney allograft, because the maintenance dialysis is like a 'lifeboat' for such patients. On the other hand, similar infection in a potential donor is considered to be a relative contraindication in life-saving transplants such as heart transplants. Transplant clinicians must bear in mind that an infection transmitted with allograft does not necessarily originate from the donor. It could be a result of contamination during retrieval, preservation, transport, or during the transplantation operation itself, which may not be evident to the transplant team at the time of transplantation. Sharma and colleagues (2005)[3] reported that the contamination of renal allografts, as evident by positive culture of perfusion fluid, with lactose fermenting coliforms or yeasts requires pre-emptive treatment by antibiotics therapy for 5–7 days. In comparison, the contamination with a microbe of skin origin (Staphylococcus aureus, coagulase-negative Staphylococcus, and diphtheroid) does not need any treatment. This approach is possible by close co-operation between proactive microbiology teams and transplant clinicians since these patients are at the peak of immunosuppression within the first week of operation.

Donor Transmitted Infections

Every attempt is made to identify the potential organ donors who pose a risk of transmitting the infection to a prospective allograft recipient. The pre-transplant screening measures include a careful review of the patient's records, interviewing the family, and analysing the circumstances of death. Even with a negative screening test, a few cases slip through the net. It is incumbent on the lead transplant surgeon to determine the risk/benefit ratio and take informed consent from a prospective transplant recipient after discussing the possibility of undiagnosed DTIs.

The host immunity, the vaccination status, the naivety of host, the type of the organ transplanted, the type of the organism, and the magnitude and type of post-transplant immunosuppression play a vital role in the severity of the clinical presentation of DTI.[4] Non-specific signs such as altered mental status, increasing blood sugars, and worsening anion gap may be the only clue to trigger further investigations.[5] It is easy to miss infection in transplant recipients because the symptoms, signs, and laboratory features may be either subtle or even be absent in the light of immunosuppression. Therefore, clinicians must predict and pre-empt by

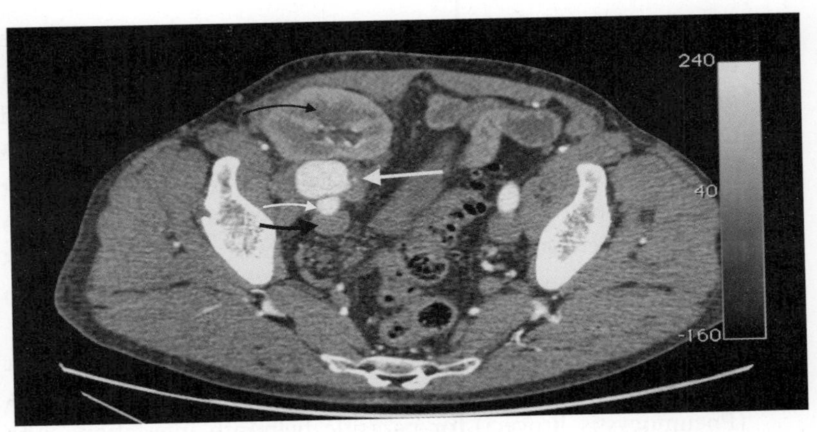

Figure 36.1. CT scan demonstrating infected pseudoaneurysm of right kidney transplant (upper black arrow). The renal vein (lower black arrow), the external iliac artery (smaller white arrow), renal transplant artery compressed and pushed by renal artery pseudoaneurysm and is located at 3 o'clock position of aneurysm (bigger white arrow). (Courtesy Dr Peter Brow, Sheffield Teaching Hospitals, UK)

being suspicious to the extent of being 'almost paranoid' in the early phase of post-transplant period. Pre-donation diagnosis of infection is possible by sensitive microbiological tests that would provide crucial clues. These infections are likely to be of nosocomial origin. There is an exhaustive list of organisms to be tested for including Salmonella, Pseudomonas, Escherichia coli, Meningococcus, Pneumococcus and Haemophilus Influenzae, Candida species and Aspergillus species. These organisms might colonize the suture line (vascular and ureteric anastomosis), colonize hematomas, or brew in fluid collections. The DTI can cause allograft failure and life-threatening complications, including anastomotic bleeding, infected pseudoaneurysms (Figure 36.1), and abscesses.[(4)]

Clinical presentations of DTI

1. Actively infected but asymptomatic donors (carriers or in the incubation phase): Diseases like the HIV, West Nile virus, rabies, herpes simplex virus, respiratory viruses, lymphocytic choriomeningitis

virus (LCMV), and hepatitis viruses (A, B, and C, possibly E) may be transmitted this way.[(4)] These infections are associated with high mortality, particularly in the setting of immunosuppression.

2. Donors with latent infections that become active after transplantation in an immunosuppressed host that include CMV, EBV, and Human Herpes viruses (HHV 6, 7, and 8). This form of transmission results in well-recognized syndromes, particularly, in those who are seronegative and receive a seropositive organ (Figure 36.2).[(5)] This type of transmission addresses the importance of screening and prevention, e.g. CMV.
3. Delayed presentation of latent infection which could present in a disseminated form such as tuberculosis, protozoal infections (Pneumocystis Jiroveci), or parasitic helminth infestations. The treatment of such infections is often complicated by drug interactions with immunosuppressive drugs.[(6)]

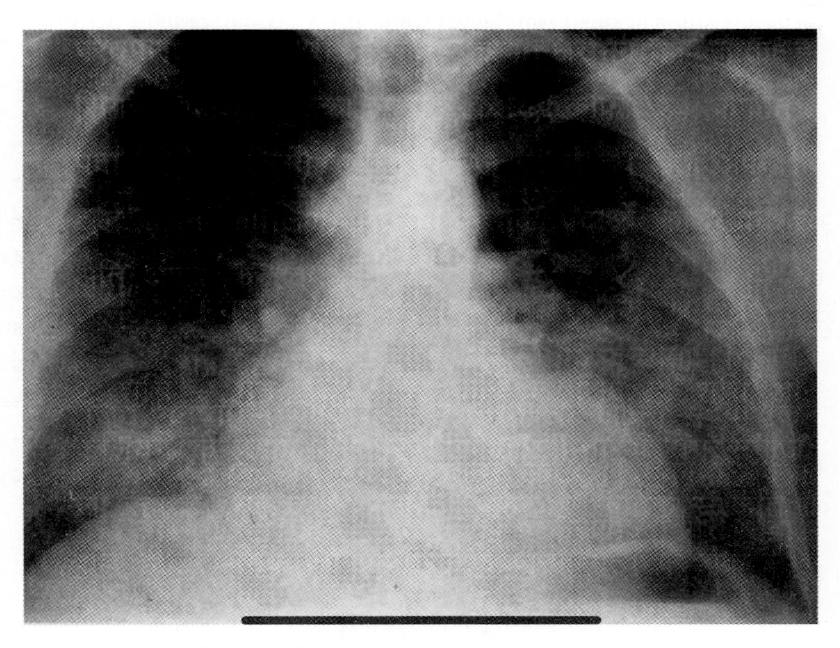

Figure 36.2. Diffuse peri-hilar infiltrate secondary to cytomegalovirus infection in an 18-year-old man with a rapidly deteriorating febrile condition 5 weeks post-transplant, after a course of anti-lymphocyte globulin for acute allograft rejection

Risk stratification

The majority of the DTIs can be predicted by careful review of the documentation (hospital notes or primary care records) and laboratory screening. Post-transplant risk-mitigation measures involve protocol-driven regular screening (BK virus infection, CMV, EBV), prophylaxis (CMV or Pneumocystis Jiroveci) or pre-emptive treatment (CMV). On occasions, the disease transmission is quite unexpected as a result of either poor sensitivity of a test, or the lack of suspicion of a pathogen that is rare, and thereby, is missed prior to organ donation. The risk stratification of potential organ donors is demonstrated in Table 36.1.[6]

Table 36.1 Risk levels for potential organ donors, as defined by the Italian National Transplant Centre[6]

Category	Definition
Unacceptable risk	This includes HIV positive donors for HIV negative recipients. Untreated sepsis, certain viral infection, e.g. encephalitis, prion disease, e.g. Creutzfeldr-Jacob disease (CJD) and its variant (vCJD).
Increased but acceptable risk	When there is a limited chance of survival without transplant, there is still a high risk of infection and transplantation is the last chance for survival. This includes patients with fulminate hepatitis, liver primary non-function. Appropriate prophylaxis and patient counselling are mandatory.
Calculated risk	This group includes donor (HBsAg+, anti-HCV+, or HBcAb+) to similarly positive recipients. There is a theoretical risk of an increase in the viral load or infection with a diffident strain of the same virus. Donors with bacterial meningitis, e.g. meningococcal meningitis, are included in this group after eradication treatment (at least 24 hours of the appropriate antibiotic therapy).
Not assessable risk	When the assessment of the donor is incomplete (absent medical records, inappropriate (using insensitive test) or completely lacking). This group include those donors with strong clinical suspicion and absent microbiology results. Every attempt has to be made to complete the missing data. In this scenario, the organ can be transplanted for those whose chance of survival is poor without the transplant after appropriate informed consent and prophylaxis (considered as increased, but acceptable risk).
Standard risk	When there is no evidence of infection based on the donor history, including patient's records, clinical assessment and laboratory results. Since there is still a risk of DTI, though small, the patient should be counselled against the potential infection risk. HIV HBV and HCV can infect during the incubation period before the seroconversion.

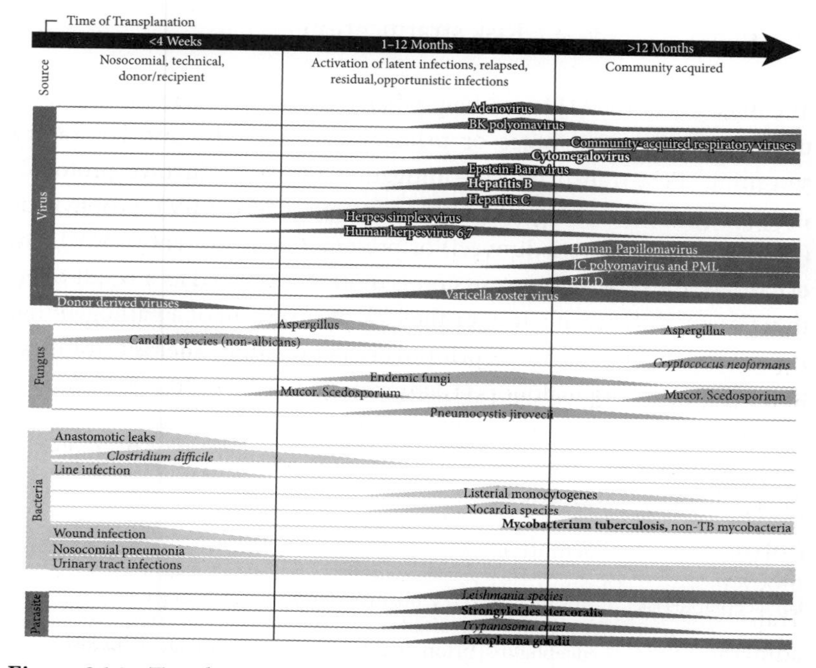

Figure 36.3. Timeline of post-transplant infection,[7] reproduced with permission

Timeline for DTI

Figure 36.3 demonstrates the timeline of different post-transplant infections,[7] irrespective of the situation where the donor or the recipient was the source of DTI.

Special considerations of infected organs

Transplantation is the victim of its own success; as a result, the gap between the supply of donor organs and the patients on the waiting list has been increasing. Some transplant units have made a careful use of organs from HIV positive donors for stable HIV-positive recipients after proper counselling. Blumberg and colleagues suggested the following criteria to use kidneys from HIV positive donors[8]:

- Viral load <50 copies/mL and CD4 count >200/μL for at least six months prior to donation.
- Exclude HIVAN by biopsy and absence of proteinuria.

Muller and colleagues (2015)[9] presented their experience with twenty-seven HIV positive Chronic Kidney Disease patients who received kidneys from HIV positive deceased donors with a median follow up for 2.4 years (Figure 36.4–36.5). They reported a modest initial decline in CD4 count in the first year, followed by an increase above the baseline at three years. They reported patient survival (Figure 36.3) of 84% at one year, 84% at three years, and 74% at five years and graft survival (Figure 36.4) of 93%, 84%, and 84% respectively.[9]

Cotrimoxazole (480 mg per day for six months) is a standard prophylaxis across all the transplant department to prevent Pneumocystis Jiroveci (a protozoa) pneumonia. Until 2008, there was no case of pneumocystis pneumonia (PCP) over thirty-five years at the regional Liverpool Transplant Unit (unpublished experience), but eighteen patients needed admission in intensive therapy unit for managing PCP over six months from the date of their transplant that triggered initiating cotrimoxazole as standard prophylaxis in all transplant patients. Cotrimoxazole would be effective against possible toxoplasmosis as well, though authors have not seen toxoplasmosis in Sheffield or in Liverpool.

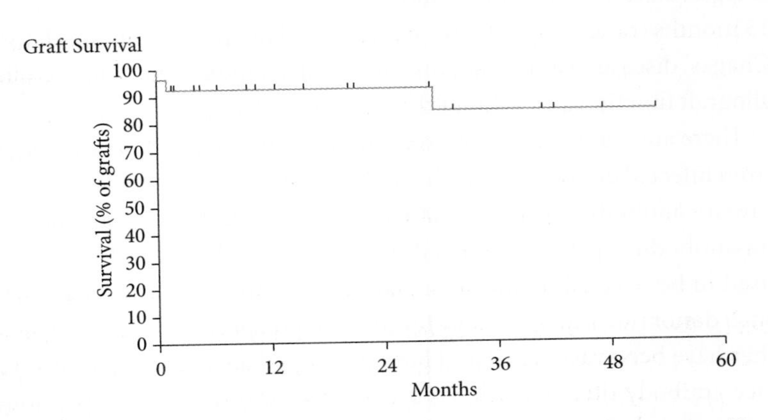

Figure 36.4. Patient survival of HIV-positive donor kidney transplant,[9] reproduced with permission

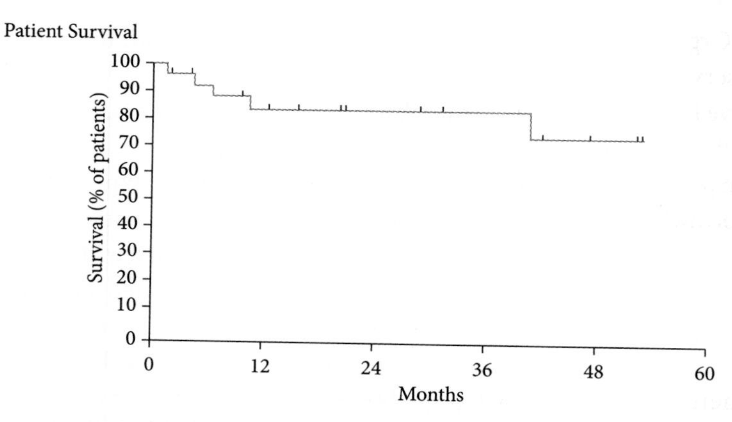

Figure 36.5. Graft survival of HIV-positive donor kidney transplant,[9] reproduced with permission

In the UK, all the transplant recipients of South Asian origin are given six months of isoniazid prophylaxis to prevent tuberculosis. However, there is no need to offer such a prophylaxis to an organ recipient if the prospective donor is of South Asian origin, nevertheless, only after careful assessment of pre-donation clinical assessment.

McCormack and colleagues (2012)[10] transplanted nine uninfected patients from donors who were seropositive Chagas' disease without prophylaxis. These patients were carefully monitored for the development of Chagas' disease. The median follow-up time of the seven live patients was 15 months (range: 13–20). Two patients died of other causes unrelated to Chagas' disease. All the patients remained symptom-free with excellent allograft function and without the evidence of Chagas' disease.

There are many reports of excellent outcomes of transplanting organs from infected donors with the hepatitis B virus (HBV) and who were positive for antibodies against hepatitis B core antigen (HBcAb) and negative for antibodies against hepatitis B surface antigen (HBsAg). These donors used to be rejected by transplant surgeons in the past. The organs from such donors are transplantable for selected prospective recipients who either have been vaccinated and have developed adequate hepatitis B surface antibody titre (HBsAb >100 U/mL), or those who were previously infected and given with specific hyperimmunoglobulin and anti-HBV antiviral agents.[11–13]

Organs from hepatitis C virus (HCV) infected donors are generally reserved for HCV positive recipients.[14,15] HCV-positive donor organs have been used in uninfected recipients on direct-acting antiviral agents with 95% success. Henceforth, judicious use of organs from donors who are positive for either hepatitis B or C to carefully selected recipients is a worthwhile approach.[11–17]

Conclusion

There are instances when it is difficult to exclude infection in a deceased donor, merely based on clinical grounds. Pre-donation screening helps to identify those donors who pose a significant risk of DTI. For the prospective recipients whose need for transplantation is relatively less urgent, a transplant surgeon should decline organs from the donors with unexplained fever, rash, clinical pictures suggestive of encephalitis, or overwhelming sepsis. Judicious use of high-risk cadaveric organ donors requires careful study of medical records of the potential organ donor that is supported by relevant laboratory tests for risk stratification. Protocol-based monitoring of post-transplant infections and standard chemoprophylaxis are key steps. All transplant recipients should be consented against DTI regardless of the degree of urgency of the operation. The clinicians need to appreciate that the risk of infection can never be zero, though we should never cease to endeavour to minimize this risk to achieve an optimal outcome in every transplant recipient.

Highlights

- Transplant clinicians have managed to provide acceptable outcomes despite pushing boundaries by accepting high-risk organ donors.
- The severity of DTIs is evaluated by a plethora of determinants: the recipient's immunity, the naivety of host, the vaccination status, the type of the organ transplanted, the type of the organism, and the magnitude and type of post-transplant immunosuppression.

- Many of these risks are preventable by careful assessment of the donors, by initiating prophylactic or even pre-emptive treatment.
- Protocol-based monitoring of post-transplant infections and standard chemoprophylaxis are the key steps.
- The clinicians need to appreciate that infective risk cannot be zero.
- Transplant clinicians should endeavour to keep the risk of the post-transplant infections to as low level as possible.

References

1. Ison MG, Hager J, Blumberg E, Burdick J, Carney K, Cutler J, et al. Donor-derived disease transmission events in the United States: Data reviewed by the OPTN/UNOS Disease Transmission Advisory Committee. Am J Transplant 2009;9:1929–1935.
2. S Pradeep, Buttigieg J, Zayan T, Sharma A, Halawa A. Infections after solid organ transplantation. J Renal Transplant Sci 2018; 1(1): 29–42.
3. Sharma AK, Smith D, Sinha S, Smith G, Rustom R, Sells RA, Hammad A, A Bakran. Outcome of cadaveric renal allografts contaminated before transplantation. Transplant International 2005;18(7):824–827.
4. Gunawansa N, Rathore R, Sharma A, Halawa A. Vaccination and renal transplantation; review of the current guidelines and recommendations world. J Transplant 2018; 8(3): 68–74.
5. Abbas F, El Kossi M, Kim JJ, Sharma A, R Pararajasingam, Halawa A. Parasitic infestation in organ transplant recipients. JESNT 2019;19(2);31–61.
6. Nanni Costa A, Grossi P, Gianelli Castiglione A et al. Quality and safety in the Italian donor evaluation process. Transplantation 2008;85: S52–S56.
7. Fishman JA. Infection in solid-organ transplant recipients. N Engl J Med 2007;357:2601–2614.
8. Blumberg EA, Rogers CC; American Society of Transplantation Infectious Diseases Community of Practice. Solid organ transplantation in the HIV-infected patient: Guidelines from the American Society of Transplantation Infectious Diseases Community of Practice. Clin Transplant 2019;33(9):e13499.
9. Muller E, Barday Z, Mendelson M, Kahn D. HIV-positive-to-HIV-positive kidney transplantation—results at 3 to 5 years. N Engl J Med 2015;372(7):613–620.
10. McCormack L, Quiñónez E, Goldaracena N, Anders M, Rodríguez V, Orozco Ganem F, Mastai RC. Liver transplantation using Chagas-infected donors in uninfected recipients: A single-center experience without prophylactic therapy. Am J Transplant. 2012;12(10):2832–2837.
11. Veroux M, Corona D, Veroux P. Kidney transplantation from donors with hepatitis. In: Veroux M, Veroux P, editors. Kidney Transplantation: Challenging the future UAE. Bentham Science Publisher 2012: 71–84.

12. Veroux M, Corona D, Ekser B, et al. Kidney transplantation from hepatitis B virus core antibody-positive donors: Prophylaxis with hepatitis B immunoglobulin. Transplant Proc 2011;43:967–970.
13. Veroux P, Veroux M, Sparacino V, et al. Kidney transplantation from donors with viral B and C hepatitis. Transplant Proc 2006; 38: 996–998.
14. Veroux P, Veroux M, Puliatti C, et al. Kidney transplantation from hepatitis C virus-positive donors into hepatitis C virus-positive recipients: A safe way to expand the donor pool. Transplant Proc 2005;37:2571–2573.
15. Morales JM, Fabrizi F. Hepatitis C and its impact on renal transplantation. Nat Rev Nephrol 2015;11:172–182.
16. Guidelines for Hepatitis B & Solid Organ Transplantation. British Transplantation Society (2018). https://bts.org.uk/wp-content/uploads/2018/03/BTS_HepB_Guidelines_FINAL_09.03.18.pdf
17. UK Position Statement on the use of Organs from Hepatitis C Viraemic Donors and Increased Infectious Risk Donors in Hepatitis C Negative Recipients. British Transplantation Society (2018). https://www.basl.org.uk/uploads/UK%20Position%20Statement%20on%20the%20use%20of%20Organs%20from%20Hepatitis%20C%20Viraemic%20Donors%20in%20Hepatitis%20C%20Negative%20Recipients%20Final%20Version%20BASL%20Website%202.pdf

37

Malignancy—A contraindication to organ donation

Antonia D'Errico, Albino Eccher, Deborah Malvi, Claudia Mescoli, Luca Novelli

Introduction

Over the years, the guidelines for donor selection have changed to expand the donor pool. People with multiorgan failure and end-stage organ failure have increased in number due to the ageing of the population and the increase in comorbidities[1,2] enlarging the gap between the patients on the waiting list and the organ pool availability. The shortage of donor organs is actually the main focus. To face this problematic issue, the use of elderly donors, resulting in a potential higher risk of cancer's transmission, and the use of donors with past history or affected by malignancies at the procurement time has been adopted as a strategy to expand the organ pool availability.[3–5] The Solid Organ Transplant community has focused its attention firstly to minimize the risk associated with unexpected neoplastic transmission to the recipients and secondarily to maximize the number of suitable organs performing a risk-benefit assessment in every single case. The risk of disease transmission has to be balanced carefully with the mortality risk keeping a recipient on the waiting list, which has huge costs and a dramatic impact on the quality of life and survival of patients.[4,6,7]

The transmission of a neoplastic disease from a donor to a recipient is an undesirable consequence of organ transplantation. Past medical history, and radiological and laboratory investigations minimize the risk but do not always uncover malignant diseases in the frequently urgent circumstances associated with the donation. On the other hand, the practice to classify donors into definite risk category has been applied in order to better stratify and manage donor's risk, also offering a clinical perspective.

Risk of malignancy transmission

By definition, a donor-transmitted malignancy is the transmission of a malignant neoplasm present in the donor prior to transplant and a donor-derived malignancy is defined as a neoplasm derived from the donor cells but not present as a clinical neoplasm at the moment or before the time of transplant.[8] Even in the absence of systematic reviewing of literature, the overall risk of transmission derived from large series appears low, ranging from 0% to 0.06%.[8–16] A relatively higher rate of transmission is reported in the series from Israel Penn International Transplant Tumor Registry (IPITTR). But this finding must take into account that this registry is based on voluntary reporting to IPITTR, which means that only a selected cohort and a small number of patients are included and they are more likely to be reported if they suffered a transmission event.[17–19] Therefore, literature data are considered to overestimate the transmission risk.[3] National and international efforts have been made to better estimate the risk of transmission, leading to various position statements and recommendations.[3,20–22]

Donor risk assessment

In order to better stratify and define the donors' risk category, the Italian Transplant Network and the National Transplant Centre (Centro Nazionale Trapianti, CNT) have applied their guidelines.[22] A donor is defined as 'suitable' or 'non-suitable' depending upon the risk factors associated. 'Suitable donors' are considered 'standard risk' when no risk factors are found in the donor's past medical history and during the organ procurement. The donors that fall in the 'non-standard risk' category are further subdivided into 'negligible risk' and 'acceptable risk', when risk factors are present but the risk of neoplastic transmission is lower than the potential benefit of transplantation. In these circumstances, the donor organs can be used with informed consent and recommendations regarding recipient follow-up. A 'non-suitable donor' is the one affected by any condition resulting in an unacceptable risk. Neoplasms making a donor 'non-suitable' are malignancies present at the time of donation for which there is a documented high risk of metastasis in their natural history, with actual metastases or past history of malignancy shorter than ten years (with exception of malignancies which fall into 'non-standard, negligible/acceptable risk'). When the malignant potential of neoplasm cannot be assessed, the risk class is 'not assessable' and decision on whether to use the organs has to be done by the single-centre according to the transplant benefit/risk ratio (Table 37.1).

Overall, the final judgement of donor organ suitability is based on past medical history, physical examination, laboratory analyses and radiological, and any other instrumental investigation. Furthermore, when the donor is in the operating theatre room, the surgeon examines thoracic and abdominal organs, looking for unidentified potentially malignant lesions. In some cases, the finding of lesions unidentified at the previous levels of investigation prompts the need for a histopathological rapid frozen section examination to assess the nature of the newly discovered lesion. Specimens sent for histopathological examination may include whole organs, biopsies or fine-needle aspiration samples based on the judgement of the surgeon. In these cases, the diagnosis is made by the on-call pathologist and could be further managed by the Second Opinion consultation service.

The involvement of on-call general pathologists in transplantation activity is required for donor risk assessment but the necessity to answer specific questions within the forcedly limited time represents the main problem. To face this difficulty, in Italy a Second Opinion consultation service was created in 2004 by the National Italian Transplant Centre, to manage all questions related to neoplasm in donors, concerning both past medical history and currently or *de novo* neoplastic diseases. The 24/7 duty system ensures a permanent and fast consultation service, charged by the Ministry of Health, based on the expertise of endorsed pathologists in the field of oncology and risk transmission. Second Opinion Pathologist helps centres to evaluate the medical history of donors and to plan the clinical-radiological-pathological investigations, representing a pivotal figure in the donation process leading to a refinement of the risk profile. Undeniably, the impact of a correct risk assessment is of great

Table 37.1 Risk definition criteria for the most common donor's neoplasia according to the Italian's Guideline of CNT, 2017.

STANDARD	NEGLIGIBLE RISK	ACCETABLE	INACCETABLE*
- all dysplastic and pre-cancerous lesions with the exception of intraductal papillary mucinous neoplasm (IPMN) of the pancreas.	- in-situ carcinomas of all sites (with exception of high grade in-situ carcinoma of the breast), - ***low-grade IPMN*** of the pancreas according WHO; - basal cell and squamous cell carcinoma of skin; - ***low grade*** urothelial intraepithelial or chorion infiltrating papillary carcinoma (pTa or pT1); - ***high grade*** intraepithelial urothelial papillary carcinoma (pTa); -prostatic adenocarcinoma with Gleason score ≤ 6; - encapsulated papillary microcarcinoma of the thyroid; - low grade renal cell carcinoma (pT1a); - benign central nervous system neoplasia and WHO grade 1, 2 and 3 malignant tumours.	- ***high grade IPMN*** of the pancreas according WHO; - central nervous system malignancies grade 4 according to WHO without clinical risk factors (such as long course of the disease, previous surgical interventions, radiotherapy).	- ***high grade*** in-situ carcinoma of the breast; -invasive carcinomas of all sites (with the exception of prostate gland acinar carcinomas, urothelial papillary carcinomas, renal cell carcinomas); -central nervous system malignancies grade 4 according to WHO with clinical risk factors; - glioblastoma; - gliosarcoma; -embrional tumours; - melanoma; -lymphomas and leukaemia; - melanoma; -metastases.

* These are the most recent guidelines. In the presence of the malignant WHO grade 4 central nervous system neoplasia with clinical risk factors, together with glioblastoma, gliosarcoma, embrional tumours, melanoma, lymphomas, leukaemia, melanoma, and metastases, the definition of inacceptable donor has to be given by the Second Opinion.

importance, considering the potential recovery of organs which would have been discarded on the basis of only malignancy history and conversely, correct discard of organs with an unacceptable risk profile.

Donors with neoplastic history

As far as the Italian experience is concerned, a total of 595 donors with a past or current history of neoplasia, malignant or benign, have been evaluated from a total number of 11271 donors (5%), recorded in CNT databases from 2006 to 2015.[(7)] The average percentage of donors per year with neoplasm was 5% (ranging from 4% to 7%). The 595 donors had a total number of 618 neoplasia, as 23 donors had more than one. Cases with past history of neoplastic processes were 313 (50.65%) while current neoplastic processes were discovered in 305 donors (49.35%). The risk profile of the 595 donors was considered 'standard' in 173 cases (29.08%), 'non-standard, negligible' in 364 cases (61.18%), 'non-standard, acceptable' in 51 cases (8.57%), and 'not assessable/not recorded' in 8 (1.34%) cases. Among all donors with neoplasm, 464 (77.98%) were recognized before organ procurement, 118 (19.84%) before transplantation procedure and 13 (2.18%) after transplantation, during donor's autoptic examination. Donors presented a benign neoplasm in 173 (29.08%) cases, a malignant one (with a variable risk of transmission) in 415 cases (69.75%) and in the remaining 8 cases (1.34%), a definite indication of a diagnosis of the neoplastic process was not available. The donor's neoplasia arose from the urinary system (40%) followed by central nervous system (CNS, 17%), gastrointestinal tract (11%), gynaecological (9.2%), endocrine (6.96%), thoracic and head and neck regions (5.50%), with a minor percentage of neoplastic processes arising from the skin (4.37%), hematopoietic system (1.13%), soft tissue (0.85%), testis (0.65%), and others locations (3.24%).

Prostate tumours

Prostate gland was the most affected organ, representing more than 20% of all the neoplasia evaluated (n=129, 20.87%) and more than 50% of all the urinary tract lesions. Prostate tumours comprised acinar adenocarcinoma in 112 cases and not otherwise specified benign lesions in 17 cases. This data is in line with the literature that reports the incidence of prostate adenocarcinoma ranging from 3 to 18, 5%, according to the different series.[23] Despite the high probability to find prostatic adenocarcinoma in older donors, the transmission of the neoplastic disease is extremely rare. Doerfler et al. analysed more than 120 transplantations from neoplastic donors affected by prostate adenocarcinoma without no neoplastic transmission to the recipients (with a follow-up ranging from 16 to 53 months).[23] Literature reported just one case of donor-derived prostate cancer in a heart recipient, albeit the donor was suspected to have metastatic disease at the time of explant.[24] In Italy, guidelines for the evaluation of donors with prostate cancers have been applied since 2001 and the CNT has been a pioneer in the International scenario to have a protocol for donors with prostate cancer, allowing to expand the donor pool and to recover about 30% of the evaluated donors, affected by prostatic adenocarcinoma.[25]

Kidney tumours

The second most commonly affected organ, overall, was the kidney (a total of 77 lesions, 12.46%). In particular, kidney tumours were mostly represented by clear cell renal cell carcinoma (ccRCC) in 46 cases (7.44% of all the neoplasia and 59.44% of renal tumours) and papillary renal cell carcinoma (pRCC) in 17 cases (2.75% of all the neoplasia and 22.08% of renal tumours). Oxyphilic-cell lesions, such as chromophobe carcinomas and oncocytomas accounted for 8 lesions (1.29% of all the neoplasia and 10.39% of renal tumours) while other 5 lesions (0.81% of all the neoplasia and 6.49% of renal tumours) comprised angiomyolipoma and papillary adenomas. Even though renal tumours are very frequently found in donors, data of the literature suggest that there is a very low risk of cancer transmission to recipients (generally in low-grade and low-stage cases).[19] Moreover, Xiao et al. noted that RCC may have the best prognosis among the donor-transmitted neoplasia probably due to the fact that it is generally organ-confined and small size lesion.[26]

Transmission of kidney carcinoma has been described in many studies. Sack et al., in 1997, described a case of renal cancer transmission in a heart transplanted recipient,[27] while Barrou et al. described the transmission of a very small renal papillary carcinoma to a kidney and heart recipient (the recipient had an undifferentiated renal cell carcinoma without any evidence that the tumour transmitted was really a papillary renal cell carcinoma).[28] More recently in 2009, Llamas et al[29] reported the case of a sarcomatoid carcinoma in two kidney recipients after transplantation, but without any evidence of a tumour at the time of the organ removal. The RCC is the most frequent donor-derived tumour according to the report of Organ Procurement and Transplantation Network.[8] However, there is uniform consent in the international transplant setting to the favourable use of donors with small cancers, stratifying the donor risk according to the cancer dimension and nucleolar grade.[3,20]

CNS tumours

Meningioma was the most common CNS lesion with a total of 52 cases (49.52%), followed by glial-cell tumours further subdivided in 11 cases (10.46%) of astrocytomas, 8 cases (7.62%) of oligodendrogliomas; in other 8 cases (7.62%) the diagnosis was of not otherwise specified benign lesions. According to the literature, CNS tumours are associated with a low risk of extraneural spreading[30] even though cases of tumour transmissions have been reported.[4,9,10,31,32] In these series, there were, however, many high-grade tumours including grade IV gliomas (glioblastoma multiforme) and medulloblastomas. Better refinement of risk of transmission for different CNS neoplasms is of particular importance, given that an important quota of donors with CNS tumours is young adults or paediatric patients whose organs are almost always suitable for transplant and of high quality from a functional point of view.

Other tumours

Gastrointestinal and gynaecological districts accounted for about 10% each of the overall neoplastic pathology, with large bowel and stomach and uterine corpus respectively representing the majority in these regions.

Thyroid gland neoplasm accounted for 65.12% of all endocrine gland pathology and about 5% of the total cases with 28 cases. Very rare cases of thyroid cancer transmission are reported in the literature[33,34] and the need for reassessment of risk, particularly for papillary thyroid cancer, has emerged recently.[35] Though not present in the Italian registry, melanoma is a known malignancy with a high risk of transmission according to other series[36–38]; together with breast cancer.[39] The recognized hematologic diseases were monoclonal gammopathy of uncertain significance (MGUS) in all cases.

The Italian experience

During a study period (2006–2015), a total of 29858 transplants had been performed, 1198 patients (4,01%) received an organ from a neoplastic donor. In the considered period, five cases of neoplastic transmission from a donor had been recorded, involving a total of ten recipients: this data represents 0.03% of all transplantation procedures. Noteworthy, none of these cases derived the disease from the 595 donors with a known neoplastic process, but all the 5 cases of neoplastic transmissions derived from donors with no recorded history of neoplasm and any elements of the suspicion on the surgeon table; so they were considered donors with no need for further investigation. Nine out of the ten recipients involved died, while one recipient is still alive and underwent medical treatments for the neoplastic disease.

The Italian experience shows that the use of neoplastic donors can be safe, as no cases of transmission were recorded from this donor pool and let to expand the pool of donor organs, with great effort by the Italian National Health Institute to collect and review data. Overall, the low rate of neoplastic transmission (0.03%) is in line with the data in the literature,[4,8,9,11,13,16] demonstrating the efficacy and accuracy of established protocols of donor assessment.

Conclusion

Most of the cases of neoplastic transmission in Italy involved an unrecognized hematologic disease and this data push towards the improving of laboratory tests to exclude hematologic diseases. Limitations in the data collection are mainly due to the non-homogenous reporting of the different Italian Transplant Centers about medical history, and imaging investigation or histological/intraoperative diagnosis. Efforts to homogenize data among the numerous Transplant Centers are still ongoing together with the effort to improve the capture of donor cancers and to appropriately use donors with cancers. Similar limitations can partly apply also to other registries, keeping in mind that data of neoplastic transmission dating back to several decades ago could not be as precise as more recent recordings and data on donor transmitted malignancies are not always validated by a molecular analysis confirming donor origin. Moreover, different national protocols and guidelines are in use and are based mainly on the data of registries and on knowledge of the natural history of single cancer type, that has obviously evolved in the past decades with the refinement of prognostic and predictive markers. The intrinsic limitations of registries along with the updating of knowledge on cancer natural history indicate that there is an urgent need for standardization and harmonization of guidelines and protocols for risk assessment in the evaluation of donors with malignancy. These protocols have to be based not only on simple reporting experience but on evidence-based results from analysis of literature, bearing in mind that a more accurate refinement of risk for single tumoral entity could allow recovery of more suitable organs and thus reduce waiting lists for patients.

Highlights

- Transmission of a neoplastic disease is an undesirable consequence of organ transplantation.
- Guidelines have changed, considering neoplastic donors to expand the pool.
- In Italy, a Second Opinion consultation service was created in 2004 by the National Italian Transplant Centre.
- Classifying donors into definite risk category has been applied to stratify and manage donor's risk.
- Overall risk of transmission based on large series appears low, ranging from 0% to 0.06%

References

1. Goldfarb-Rumyantzev AS, Rout P. Characteristics of elderly patients with diabetes and end-stage renal disease. Semin Dial. 2010; 23(2):185–190.

2. Chapman J. Waiting for a liver transplant. Intern Med J. 2010 Sep;40(9):609–610.
3. European Committee (Partial Agreement) on Organ Transplantation. Guide to the quality and safety of organs for transplantation. 7th ed. Strasbourg, France: European Directorate for the Quality of Medicines & HealthCare of the Council of Europe (EDQM); 2018.
4. Kauffman HM, Cherikh WS, McBride MA, Cheng Y, Hanto DW. Deceased donors with a past history of malignancy: An organ procurement and transplantation network/united network for organ sharing update. Transplantation. 2007 Jul 27;84(2):272–274.
5. Kauffman HM, McBride MA, Delmonico FL. First report of the United Network for Organ Sharing Transplant Tumor Registry: Donors with a history of cancer. Transplantation. 2000 Dec;70(12):1747–1751.
6. Benkö T, Hoyer DP, Saner FH, Treckmann JW, Paul A, Radunz S. Liver transplantation from donors with a history of malignancy: A single-center experience. Transplant direct. 2017 Nov;3(11):e224.
7. Eccher A, Lombardini L, Girolami I, Puoti F, Zaza G, Gambaro G, et al. How safe are organs from deceased donors with neoplasia? The results of the Italian Transplantation Network. J Nephrol. 2019 Apr;32(2):323–330.
8. Ison MG, Nalesnik MA. An update on donor-derived disease transmission in organ transplantation. Am J Transplant. 2011 Jun;11(6):1123–1130.
9. Desai R, Collett D, Watson CJ, Johnson P, Evans T, Neuberger J. Cancer transmission from organ donors—Unavoidable but low risk. Transplant J. 2012;94(12):1200–1207.
10. Kauffman HM, McBride MA, Cherikh WS, Spain PC, Delmonico FL. Transplant tumor registry: Donors with central nervous system tumors. Transplantation. 2002 Feb 27;73(4):579–582.
11. Desai R, Collett D, Watson CJE, Johnson P, Evans T, Neuberger J. Estimated risk of cancer transmission from organ donor to graft recipient in a national transplantation registry. Br J Surg. 2014;101(7):768–774.
12. Engels EA, Castenson D, Pfeiffer RM, Kahn A, Pawlish K, Goodman MT, et al. Cancers among US organ donors: A comparison of transplant and cancer registry diagnoses. Am J Transplant. 2014;14(6):1376–1382.
13. Watson CJE, Roberts R, Wright KA, Greenberg DC, Rous BA, Brown CH, et al. How safe is it to transplant organs from deceased donors with primary intracranial malignancy? An analysis of UK registry data. Am J Transplant. 2010;10(6):1437–1444.
14. Moench K, Breidenbach T, Fischer-Fröhlich C-L, Barreiros AP, Kirste G, Samuel U. 6-year survey of organ donors with malignancies in Germany. Transplant J. 2012 Nov;94(10S):208.
15. Birkeland SA, Storm HH. Risk for tumor and other disease transmission by transplantation: A population-based study of unrecognized malignancies and other diseases in organ donors. Transplantation. 2002;74(10):1409–1413.
16. Ison MG, Hager J, Blumberg E, Burdick J, Carney K, Cutler J, et al. Donor-derived disease transmission events in the United States: Data reviewed by the OPTN/UNOS Disease Transmission Advisory Committee. Am J Transplant. 2009 Aug;9(8):1929–1935.

17. Buell JF, Trofe J, Hanaway MJ, Lo A, Rosengard B, Rilo H, et al. Transmission of donor cancer into cardiothoracic transplant recipients. Surgery. 2001;130(4):660–668.
18. Buell JF, Trofe J, Sethuraman G, Hanaway MJ, Beebe TM, Gross TG, et al. Donors with central nervous system malignancies: Are they truly safe? Transplantation. 2003 Jul 27;76(2):340–343.
19. Buell JF, Hanaway MJ, Thomas M, Munda R, Alloway RR, First MR, et al. Donor kidneys with small renal cell cancers: Can they be transplanted? Transplant Proc. 2005 Mar; 37(2):581–582.
20. Nalesnik MA, Woodle ES, Dimaio JM, Vasudev B, Teperman LW, Covington S, et al. Donor-transmitted malignancies in organ transplantation: assessment of clinical risk. Am J Transplant. 2011 Jun;11(6):1140–1147.
21. SaBTO (Advisory Committee on the Safety of Tissue and Organs). Transplantation of organs from deceased donors with cancer or a history of cancer. [Internet]. 2014. Available from: https://www.odt.nhs.uk/transplantation/
22. CNT. General criteria for evaluation of donor suitability adopted in Italy [Internet]. 2017. Available from: www.trapiantipiemonte.it/pdf/Linee/ProtocolloIdoneitaDonatore_dic2017.pdf
23. Doerfler A, Tillou X, Le Gal S, Desmonts A, Orczyk C, Bensadoun H. Prostate cancer in deceased organ donors: A review. Transplant Rev (Orlando). 2014 Jan;28(1):1–5.
24. Loh E, Couch FJ, Hendricksen C, Farid L, Kelly PF, Acker MA, et al. Development of donor-derived prostate cancer in a recipient following orthotopic heart transplantation. JAMA. 1997 Jan;277(2):133–137.
25. D'Errico-Grigioni A, Fiorentino M, Vasuri F, Corti B, Ridolfi L, Grigioni WF, et al. Expanding the criteria of organ procurement from donors with prostate cancer: The application of the new Italian guidelines. Am J Transplant. 2010 Aug;10(8):1907–1911.
26. Xiao D, Craig JC, Chapman JR, Dominguez-Gil B, Tong A, Wong G. Donor cancer transmission in kidney transplantation: A systematic review. Am J Transplant. 2013 Oct;13(10):2645–2652.
27. Sack FU, Lange R, Mehmanesh H, Amman K, Schnabel P, Zimmermann R, et al. Transferral of extrathoracic donor neoplasm by the cardiac allograft. J Heart Lung Transplant. 1997 Mar;16(3):298–301.
28. Barrou B, Bitker MO, Delcourt A, Ourahma S, Richard F. Fate of a renal tubulopapillary adenoma transmitted by an organ donor. Transplantation. 2001 Aug;72(3):540–541.
29. Llamas F, Gallego E, Salinas A, Virseda J, Pérez J, Ortega A, et al. Sarcomatoid renal cell carcinoma in a renal transplant recipient. Transplant Proc. 2009 Dec;41(10):4422–4424.
30. Gandhi MJ, Strong DM. Donor derived malignancy following transplantation: a review. Cell Tissue Bank. 2007;8(4):267–286.
31. Warrens AN, Birch R, Collett D, Daraktchiev M, Dark JH, Galea G, et al. Advising potential recipients on the use of organs from donors with primary central nervous system tumors RECOMMENDATIONS FOR CLINICAL PRACTICE. Transplantation. 2012;93:348–353.

32. Frank S, Müller J, Bonk C, Haroske G, Schackert HK, Schackert G. Transmission of glioblastoma multiforme through liver transplantation. Lancet (London, England). 1998 Jul;352(9121):31.
33. Penn I. Transmission of cancer from organ donors. Ann Transplant. 1997;2(4):7–12.
34. Górnicka B, Ziarkiewicz-Wróblewska B, Bogdańska M, Małkowski P, Wróblewski T, Krawczyk M, et al. Do all well-differentiated thyroid cancers constitute a definite contraindication to obtaining organs for transplantation? A case report. Transplant Proc. 2003;35(6):2160–2162.
35. Adler JT, Yeh H, Barbesino G, Lubitz CC. Reassessing risks and benefits of living kidney donors with a history of thyroid cancer. Clin Transplant. 2017 Sep;31(11):e13114. doi: 10.1111/ctr.13114.
36. Zwald FO, Christenson LJ, Billingsley EM, Zeitouni NC, Ratner D, Bordeaux J, et al. Melanoma in solid organ transplant recipients. Am J Transplant. 2010 May;10(5):1297–1304.
37. Bajaj NS, Watt C, Hadjiliadis D, Gillespie C, Haas AR, Pochettino A, et al. Donor transmission of malignant melanoma in a lung transplant recipient 32 years after curative resection. Transpl Int. 2010 Jul;23(7):e26–e31.
38. Morris-Stiff G, Steel A, Savage P, Devlin J, Griffiths D, Portman B, et al. Transmission of donor melanoma to multiple organ transplant recipients. Am J Transplant. 2004 Mar;4(3):444–446.
39. Matser YAH, Terpstra ML, Nadalin S, Nossent GD, de Boer J, van Bemmel BC, et al. Transmission of breast cancer by a single multiorgan donor to 4 transplant recipients. Am J Transplant. 2018 Jul;18(7):1810–1814.

38

Which tests in the potential multiple organ donor

Federico Genzano Besso

Introduction

The evaluation and risk assessment of a potential organ donor is an essential process to guarantee the safety and quality of the transplants to the recipients.[1] The safety of the transplant is assured by the evaluation and the consequent assessment of risk of transmitting diseases, fundamentally infections and malignancies, as discussed in Chapter 36 and 37 of this book. The quality of the transplant is assured by the evaluation of the anatomy, physiopathology, and functionality of the individual organs, and of the related apparatuses.

For organ allocation, it is important to determine blood group and genetic compatibility between donor and recipient by carrying out necessary laboratory and diagnostic tests.

Tests for infectious diseases

The risk of transmission of viral, bacterial, fungal, and parasitic infections is always present in transplants.[2] In addition, the ease with which people move around the world today has significantly increased the possibility of infections with non-endemic pathogens in the donor's region of origin.

It is generally accepted that it is necessary to perform tests for a basic set of systemic viral infections, irrespective of the donor origin: Hepatitis B Virus (HBV), Hepatitis C virus (HCV), and Human Immunodeficiency Virus (HIV) 1 and 2. To these, we can add Hepatitis D Virus (HDV) only in case of presence of HBV. Moreover, test is done for Human

T-lymphotropic virus (HTLV) 1 and 2 for donors living in, or originating from, high-incidence areas or with sexual partners originating from those areas or where the donor's parents originate from those areas.[3]

The determination of an actual or previous syphilis infection should happen prior to transplantation; both the risk of infection and any risky behaviour are investigated.[4] Table 38.1 summarizes tests to be performed in relation to determination results.

In specific situations, investigation for other pathogens, such as West Nile Virus, Zika Virus (ZIKAV), Trypanosoma cruzi (Chagas disease), malarial plasmodia, Flaviviridae (Dengue Fever, Chikungunya, Usutu, Japanese encephalitis, etc.), and others, has to be performed in donors who originate from areas endemic for these specific infections, or populations with increased risk for window or vertical transmission.[5] To identify the risks related to the region of origin, the governmental or supranational agencies of reference (e.g NIH, ECDC) can be helpful.[6,7]

The presence of pathogens including certain Herpes virus as Cytomegalovirus (CMV), Epstein-Barr Virus, Herpes Simplex Virus (HSV 1-2), Varicella Zoster Virus (VZV), and parasites like Toxoplasma gondii, has to be assessed in the donor. These pathogens may not

Table 38.1 HIV, hepatitis and syphilis test in relation to determination results

Infectious Agent	Standard	Particular Situations	If Positive
HBV	HBsAg	HBV-DNA	anti-HDV-Abs or Ag or RNA
	anti-HBc total Abs		anti-HBc Ab IgG + IgM
HCV	anti-HCV Abs	HCV-RNA	HCV-RNA
HIV 1,2	anti-HIV Abs	HIV-RNA	HIV-RNA
HTLV 1, 2	anti-HTLV Abs	HTLV-RNA	
HDV (in HBV + donors)			
Treponema pallidum	TPHA or anti-TP Abs		VDRL

Abs = Antibodies; DNA/RNA = molecular analysis; TPHA = Treponema pallidum haemagglutination

endanger the life of the patient, but must be assessed for their presence in the donor, as even after transplantation, possible infection should be managed.[8]

Local and systemic infections caused by bacteria and fungi have to be determined. In order to rule out the possible presence of infections, the evaluation of total WBC, subpopulations of leukocyte (leucocyte formula) and Procalcitonin may be useful. Culture methods are commonly utilized for identifying bacteria and fungi, although, often they do not produce the results before transplantation, and allow the screening for sensitivity or resistance to different antibiotics, which are useful to determine prophylaxis in transplanted patients.[9]

It is necessary to acquire any culture test performed during hospitalization, and to carry out culture tests for urine, tracheal suction or broncho-alveolar lavage (BAL) and blood before organ recovery, as well as a screening for multi drug resistant (MDR) bacteria, although the results will be available after transplantation.

Test for neoplastic diseases

The possibility of transmission of neoplasia with the transplant is always present. However, to overcome the shortage of organs for transplantation at a time when more and more patients are on the waiting list, organs derived from donors with past or current malignancy are accepted for selected patients.[10, 11]

It is, therefore, necessary to obtain, before transplantation, an adequate set of appropriate tests to exclude the presence of tumours and, if necessary, to characterize the malignancy.

For solid tumours, determination of markers is useful for cancers of the prostate (Prostate Specific Antigen, PSA) and for choriocarcinoma (human chorionic gonadotropin beta, βHCG). The determination of other tumour markers alone is not sufficient to establish the diagnosis of cancer. They must always be considered together with the results of other clinical and instrumental examinations.[12]

For all donors, every radiological test available in the hospital must be performed, including chest X-ray, abdominal ultrasonography, and Computerized Tomography (CT) or Magnetic Resonance Imaging

(MRI) scans of head, thorax, and abdomen, with or without contrast. Histological tests on biopsy or an excised sample are necessary for the diagnosis of any suspicious lesion, and the characterization of the neoplasm in the case of a neoplasm that allows transplantation.

For haematopoietic malignancies, laboratory test must always include Complete Blood Count (CBC) with differential leucocyte count. If there is a suspicion of leukaemia, lymphoma, myeloma, or myeloproliferative neoplasms, peripheral blood smear or bone marrow biopsy must be performed.

For Monoclonal Gammopathies of Undetermined Significance (MGUS), it is necessary to obtain serum protein electrophoresis, serum concentration of the monoclonal protein component, quantitative dosage of immunoglobulin subfractions (IgG, IgA, IgM), and possibly immunofixation.[12]

Test for organ quality for transplantation

A commonly applied basic data set is necessary for the assessment of the quality of organs to be transplanted, though the profile may vary among different centres. Laboratory tests must include data enabling an evaluation of the functionality of all organs destined for transplantation. It is also important to be able to gauge the progress of these data starting from admission to the hospital up to the organ recovery. If possible, it could be very useful to obtain data before the current admission.

The specific diagnostics test for the evaluation of organ quality must analyse its morphology and functionality. Instrumental tests as abdomen ultrasonography and/or CT scans with or without contrast and/or MRI are most frequently performed.

Lung

- Laboratory tests: pH, PaCO2, PaO2 and PaO2/FiO2 ratio.
- Diagnostic test: Chest X-ray, CT scan for the presence of fractures, pneumothorax, pleura and interstitial evaluation, infiltrates, bronchial thickening, and emphysema. Bronchoscopy for presence of inflammation, secretion before and suction, and bleeding.

Heart

- Laboratory tests: Creatine kinase MB isoenzyme (CPK-MB), troponin (either I or T), aspartate aminotransferase (AST);
- Diagnostic test: Electrocardiogram, echocardiography (contractility and function of ventricles and atriae, left ventricular ejection fraction, valves anatomy, wall motion disorders and function of both ventricles), and coronary angiography.

Kidney

- Laboratory tests: Creatinine, Urea, estimated Glomerular Filtration Rate (eGFR), Urine analysis (proteins, albumin, Hb, nitrite, sediment). Histological scoring on biopsy.
- Diagnostic test: Abdomen ultrasonography and/or CT scans for size measurements, evaluation of parenchymal thickness, presence of cysts, stones and possible anatomic variations.

Liver

- Laboratory tests: Alanine aminotransferase (ALT), aspartate aminotransferase (AST), gamma-Glutamyltransferase (γGT), Cholinesterase, Bilirubin total and direct, Lactate Dehydrogenase (LDH), Total Proteins and Albumin, Coagulation Tests (e.g. INR, aPTT), and Sodium. Biopsy for scoring (fibrosis and cirrhosis or steatosis).
- Diagnostic test: Abdomen ultrasonography and/or CT scans for size measurements, evaluation of echogenicity and fibrosis, liver edges, intrahepatic bile ducts, portal cava; evaluation of gall bladder and extrahepatic bile duct.

Pancreas

- Laboratory tests: Amylase, Lipase
- Diagnostic test: Abdomen ultrasonography and/or CT scans for size measurements, and parenchymal evaluation

Intestine

- Laboratory tests: Amylase, Lipase
- Diagnostic test: Abdomen ultrasonography and/or CT scans for size measurements and characterization.

Organ allocation

The importance of determining the blood group (antigens AB0 and Rhesus factor) and the genetics of the human leukocyte antigen (HLA) system responsible for regulating the immune system's reactions to transplant does not concern the evaluation of the donor or its organs, but is required for the allocation of organs. The success of the transplant depends on the blood group compatibility and on the immune reaction mediated by the patient's HLA system.

It is necessary to know typing for ABO and Rh to define the compatibility with transplant recipients. Although the ABO compatibility is almost mandatory, in selected programmes, for instance, in familiar living donor, it is possible to perform blood group incompatible transplants.

Likewise, HLA typing and crossmatching between donor serum and recipient cells is necessary to define organ recipients, rejection risk and immunosuppressive therapy to adopt before and after transplantation.

These tests must be carried out in qualified laboratories, certified by competent authorities, and the level of characterization must be adequate to the assignment rules agreed with the transplant centres.

Conclusion

The goal of organ transplantation is to make the best match between donor and patient, between organ and transplant, and between availability and need. The chapter summarizes the tests that can be helpful for this purpose. It is essential that we must obtain the tests in a short time, with resources that may not be optimal, in a multiphase, multicentre, and multidisciplinary context. The results should reveal the best possible detail, to relate them to clinical and anamnestic data, to allow correct information for the recipient and to allow the transplant that is needed at the right time.

Highlights

- Laboratory, clinical, and instrumental tests are necessary to characterize organ donors.

- Donor evaluation is a multiphase, multicentre, and multidisciplinary process.
- Time, situation, and logistics are critical variables, determining the achievable accuracy.
- Infectious and neoplastic diseases are a major risk to be assessed before organ transplantation.
- Quality of organs must be accurately evaluated for the best organ-patient match.
- A standard data set of tests should be stated, but specific situations or conditions must always be analysed.

References

1. Council of Europe. Guide to the quality and safety of organs for transplantation. 7th edition. Strasbourg: Council of Europe; 2018
2. Fischer SA. Is this organ donor safe? Donor-derived infections in solid organ transplantation. Infect Dis Clin North Am. 2018; 32: 495–506.
3. Seem DL, Lee I, Umscheid CA et al. PHS guideline for reducing transmission of human immunodeficiency virus (HIV), hepatitis B virus (HBV), and hepatitis C virus (HCV) through solid organ transplantation. Public Health Reports 2013; 128: 247–304.
4. Ison MG, Grossi P and the AST Infectious Diseases Community of Practice. Donor-derived infections in solid organ transplantation. Am J Transplant 2013; 23: 22–305.
5. Grossi P. Donor-derived infections, lessons learnt from the past, and what is the future going to bring us Curr Opin Organ Transplant. 2018; 23:4 17–422. PMID: 29916849 DOI: 10.1097/MOT.0000000000000551
6. https://www.ecdc.europa.eu/en/ 2021
7. https://www.nih.gov/ 2021
8. Fischer SA, Lub K. The AST Infectious Diseases Community of Practice Screening of Donor and Recipient in Solid Organ Transplantation. Am J Transplant. 2013 2013; 13: 9–21.
9. Len O, Garzoni C, Lumbreras C, et al. Recommendations for screening of donor and recipient prior to solid organ transplantation and to minimize transmission of donor-derived infections. Clin Microbiol Infect. 2014 Sep; 20 Suppl 7:10–8.
10. Nanni Costa A, Grossi P, Gianelli Castiglione A, Grigioni, W. Quality and safety in the Italian donor evaluation process. Transplantation 2008; 85: S52–S56.
11. Eccher A, Lombardini L, Girolami I et al. How safe are organs from deceased donors with neoplasia? The results of the Italian Transplantation. Network J Nephrol. 2019; 32(2) 323–330.
12. Centro Nazionale Trapianti Protocollo per la valutazione di idoneità del donatore di organi solidi Versione 1.0 approvata nella seduta CNT del 23 febbraio 2017. Centro Nazionale Trapianti, Roma; 2017.

39

Clinical risk management in transplantation

Tommaso Bellandi

Introduction

Patient safety is defined as the reduction of risk of unnecessary harm associated with health care to an acceptable minimum.[1] In many countries, patient safety is also recognized as a basic patient right,[2] that each health organization and professional must guarantee when delivering care. In 2002, the World Health Assembly (WHA) approved the first resolution on patient safety urging member states 'to establish and strengthen science-based systems, necessary for improving patients' safety and the quality of health care, including the monitoring of drugs, medical equipment and technology.[3] In 2019, a new resolution was released to launch the global action on patient safety,[4] integrated with the challenge to reach Universal Health Coverage within 2030. On reading these two documents along with the 2004 WHA resolution on transplantation,[5] it is understood that the goal of patient safety is hardwired in any clinical and managerial activities related to the donation and transplantations processes, that are probably the most complex components of a health system. Complexity can be defined in terms of quantity and quality of interactions between parts of a system; complexity increases with the number of interactions and the dependency of state and behaviour of a part with one another.[6] For instance, to accomplish a successful transplantation of a liver, up to one hundred professionals can be involved, interacting with different tokens (materials, information, relations) and mediated by rules and artefacts, where the success of the surgeon strongly depends on competencies and skills of individuals and organizations involved in organ procurement, retrieval, and allocation.

Clinical risk management (CRM) is the term commonly used to describe the activities performed to guarantee patient safety in any health service[1] and it is generally included in the institutional requirements for health organizations and professionals.

Since the publication of an international handbook[7] and relevant reports[8,9] in late 1990s and early 2000s, research and practices in CRM for patient safety quickly spread globally. The CRM has become one of the most important drivers of innovation and improvement in health systems.

Basic principles of CRM for patient safety

The key principles of CRM can be summarized as: (1) human fallibility is the norm; (2) delivery of health services is a complex human activity; (3) a systems' approach is needed to understand and prevent risks to humans (patients and workers) safety in health services.

Principle 1 has been widely demonstrated by a large number of studies on the epidemiology of patient safety incidents and analysis on the contribution of human error to unsafe practices.[10,11] Patient safety incident is a general term that includes all occurrences that lead (i.e. sentinel events, adverse events, or reactions) or may lead to harm (i.e. near misses, unsafe acts) to one or more patients. Despite differences in study design, unit of analysis and endpoints, WHO declares that one in ten patients admitted to a hospital is harmed as a consequence of a patient safety incident. Previously, experimental evidence and studies of accidents in other industries demonstrated that error is very frequent in human behaviour, or the price we have to pay to our flexibility and capacity of adaptation to changing conditions.[12] Therefore, any attempt to deny or hide human fallibility is a pre-condition to accept preventable risks and failures leading to unnecessary harm.

Principle 2 applies to health services because any interaction between humans dealing with health is complex, due to the numbers of variables involved and partially unpredictable effects that each action may produce on one patient. This is true for an individual consultation between a health worker and a patient, given the intrinsic complexity of any disease and the way it is perceived and communicated as an illness in patient's view, as well as in a patient pathway through a high-tech hospital, where multiple highly qualified professionals interact between them, using numerous devices in a highly regulated environment.

Principle 3 provides the lens to observe and possibly manage risks in health services. Drawing on experiences from other industrial sectors, CRM has been progressively installed in health organization to systematically identify, analyse, and prevent risks to patient safety. This is done by looking at incidents and processes with a systems' thinking, that encompasses the interactions between humans, technologies, and organizations as determinant of good or bad outcomes.(13) The systems' nature of patient safety is rooted in the International Classification for Patient Safety (ICPS), delivered and then validated by the WHO with the collaboration of a number of member states since 2009,(14,15) as well as in the Notify Library that is a global platform to share information and knowledge about adverse events and reactions in transplantation.(16)

Interventions for patient safety

In the next paragraphs, an overview of CRM through the lens of a human factors perspective is provided, where activities are associated to the profiles of actors involved in transplantations in health organizations. Three main categories of actors are considered: patients, clinicians, and managers of health systems. The interactions are considered at the micro- and meso-level of the system, without any consideration about macro-level factors such as the overall organization of health systems. Therefore, with a practical approach, a selection of CRM applications for patients, clinicians, and health managers is described, along with an expert review of strengths and weaknesses of each type of intervention, so as to provide the reader with an actionable set of basic resources for patient safety in transplantation. Table 39.1 summarizes interventions, classified by underlying theme and leading actor.

Table 39.1 Classification of interventions for patient safety

Actor \ Theme	Education on patient safety	Constructive interactions	Safe behaviours embedded in clinical practice	Structured reflection upon past experiences	Dealing with adverse outcomes and redesign systems
Patient	Participate in shared decision making	Be involved in diagnostic process	Contribute to the prevention of health-care associated infections (HAI)	Participate in medication reconciliation	Speak up
Clinician	Know guidelines and clinical recommendations	Be a team player	Do checklists	Learn from experience	Communicate openly and empathetically with patients
Healthcare Manager	Provide education and learning opportunities to clinicians and patients	Organize a reporting and learning system on patient safety incidents	Promote the application and monitoring of safe practices	Evaluate outcomes and provide feedback to patients and clinicians	Design, maintain and develop safe patient pathways

Patient's role for safety in transplantation

Patient centredness is an ethical and functional premise for each care process, because nothing can be done on them without patients' and families' engagement.

Participate in shared decision-making

Decision-making about a referral to a health professional or organization, treatment options, adherence to therapies and maintenance of a health regimen is a complex individual as well as a social-cognitive process. This process is based on personal experience of illness and well-being, interacting with expert knowledge collected from a history of consultations with health professionals, access to a formal and informal scientific base, and local traditions and habits. The concept of informed consent, that is, the aware expression of agreement to a treatment from a patient to a health professional, usually a doctor, emerged as a response to the risk of abuse of power on humans from health professionals. This consent has recently moved to a new definition of shared decision-making (SDM), that better encompass the communication process leading to an informed choice to perform or not to perform a treatment.[17,18] The SDM takes into account the risks and benefits of each option with an adequate communication for one individual patient, including meaningful data of performances on processes and outcomes at a specific health facility.[19] Evidence about compliance and effectiveness of SDM is still limited.[20] However, there is no doubt that a patient actively engaged in a decision about a transplantation is a powerful partner in the prevention of risks associated, for example, to the behaviours and health regimen needed to improve graft performance and life expectations.

Example: A patient enrolled for a non-life saving kidney transplantation has to comply with a rigid behavioural protocol in order to be kept in the waiting list, when she is supported and supervised by an expert counsellor. Compliance improves due to knowledge sharing about risks and benefits tailored to personal needs and expectations.

Be involved in diagnostic process

Diagnostic errors can undermine the donation and transplantation process, increasing the risk of transmission of infections and tumours, as well as risk of rejection or graft failure. Patients and their families play a fundamental role in the provision of medical history, description of symptoms and evolution of an illness, that are at the heart of a good diagnostic performance. Therefore, patients and families shall expect to be actively listened by professionals trained in the subject matter and in clinical communication, within an adequate environment, especially when the stake of the decision is very high like in organ donation or transplantation. To perform a good diagnostic process, communication skills and competencies of professionals are fundamental[21] and research has widely demonstrated their impact.[22] Unfortunately, in many countries, communication science is not included in health professionals academic curriculum or certification. However, health organizations involved in procurement and transplantation have invested significant resources in promoting education and training on communication skills and public campaigns to increase donation.

Example: The donation coordinator plays a crucial role in providing a safe psychological environment to the potential donor partner or relatives at the time of the communication about donation. Donor's risky behaviours can emerge through the dialogue and provide useful information to check risks of infection transmission during the donor evaluation process.

Contribute to the prevention of health-care-associated infections

Hand hygiene and correct use of antibiotics are two critical actions to prevent health-care-associated infections (HAI), where patient's behaviour and communication can help clinicians to reduce the risks and prevent the spread of HAI, when it is recognized.[23]

Given the characteristics of donation and transplantation processes, risk of HAI is high for both the frequency of exposure to contamination and severity of potential outcomes. At the same time, it is well known from research that bundled interventions to prevent HAI can eliminate, for example, the occurrence of Central Venous Catheter (CVC) related infections[24] and significantly reduce surgical wound infections.[25] Patients and families are fundamental partners of health organizations in following prevention and protection standards in acute settings. In particular, they are called to actively be watchful on professionals' compliance with hand hygiene and eventual isolation procedures.[23]

Example: When a patient or the family observe non-compliance to hand hygiene practices in any healthcare setting, especially after a transplant when a patient is more exposed to the risk of sepsis, they should be invited to speak up. Healthcare workers and clinical leaders should respond and be open to eventual explanation or excuse.

Participate in medication reconciliation

Medication reconciliation is the process of recognition of medication history and decisions about continuation or modification of therapies during clinical consultations and episodes of care.[26]

At the recognition stage, given the multiplicity of different specialities a patient encounters, it becomes the patient's responsibility to report or present a list of medications taken and eventual adverse effects experienced in the past. During reconciliation, a patient can ask the doctor to explain the meaning of discontinuation of a therapy, and the symptoms to monitor so as to evaluate effectiveness and eventual side effects of the therapy. When a patient is very sick, family members can help to assist and report vital information to doctors and nurses during treatment, especially when high-risk medications are on order list or the patient is in polypharmacy (more than four medications are administered).

Example: Non-compliance to medications after discharge is very common; therefore, the transplantation team should actively seek for eventual problems of compliance with a positive attitude and never blame patients.

Speak up

When things go wrong, a patient has the responsibility to speak up and express the preoccupations, doubts and can request an explanation of what happened during the process of care and what to do next, in order to restore or compensate either physical or emotional trauma.[27] Patients can also claim the professionals involved and the health system to make amend and to learn from what happened, in order to avoid recurrence of risks for patient safety.

Example: A patient suffering from a surgical wound infection due to poor post-surgical care may be discharged without any explanation, despite the prolongation of hospital stays, unnecessary pain and additional antibiotics. After discharge, due to the continuous pain and side effects of antibiotics, the patient may consult another doctor who observes the surgical wound and blames the earlier hospital doctors and nurses for the infection. The patient then reports a claim to the transplantation centre.

Role of healthcare professional in managing clinical risk

Scientific evidence about risk and benefit of a clinical treatment is at the core of modern medicine and, despite some criticism,[28] improvements in outcomes of health services are attributable to the capacity to translate the results of research into practice.[29] The healthcare professional can do the following to manage clinical risk.

Know guidelines and clinical recommendations

Guidelines and clinical recommendations are decision aids for clinicians, based on research evidence, developed according to a transparent methodology, generally from public institutions or scientific societies, to set a standard of practice. In transplantation, guidelines and recommendations are based on retrospective reviews and consensus, given the impossibility to perform clinical trials due to the shortage of substances of human origin and the ethical norms imposing to prevent the waste of any product of a donation. The reviews and consensus offer clinicians a safe harbour to perform under the umbrella of a standard recognized by the scientific community and health authorities, while they give patients the guarantee to delegate their care to professionals and health organizations whose operations are delivered following transparent scientific principles and protocols.

Example: Sound and clear criteria for donor evaluation are at the core of risks' anticipation and management. In Italy, a donor coordinator has to follow a detailed risk assessment process to evaluate donor, organs, and tissues suitability, including objective clinical assessment, clinical history, laboratory testing, and imaging.

Be a team player

Unfortunately, basic education in health science is still delivered as a matter for individual study and evaluation. In health organizations, work processes require reliable dynamics of cooperation between professionals to produce effective patient outcomes and prevent harm. Cooperation means the capacity to take shared decisions, to coordinate specialistic tasks distributed on a process, and to actively collaborate at the execution of complex activities; in other words, to perform like a team. Drawing on the experience of aviation, simulation-based training for teams and evaluation of clinical procedures have been transferred to healthcare in the past fifteen years,[30] with promising results that need to be further explored and systematically applied to the multiplicity of activities in donation and transplantation of organs, tissues, and cells.

Example: In some countries, licensing of transplant surgeons requires a number of simulation-based on scenarios designed to test individual and team performance on technical and non-technical skills.

Do checklists

A checklist is a structured set of controls, summarized in short sentences, usually printed on a sheet of paper, where each sentence represents an item that deserves to be under control and is associated with an empty box to be ticked in order to confirm check completion. Checklists help to prevent cognitive limitations of individuals and teams related to memory, attention, and situational awareness. Since the publication of WHO surgical safety checklist,[31] the flagship of the global campaign for safety in surgery, the tool has become very popular and sometimes considered like a 'silver bullet' to improve safety in healthcare. A wise approach to integrate checklist in clinical practice is needed, based on the integration of human factors and domain knowledge to analyse processes, envision critical steps, and eventually the need of explicit controls encoded in a checklist.[32]

Example: Before the allocation of an organ, the clinician in charge to perform donor evaluation at the procurement organization, systematically applies checklists to conduct a detailed analysis of all the requirements to confirm donor and organ suitability, select the recipient and deliver the organ on time.

Learn from experience

A complex system evolves with the capacity of its part to respond and adapt to the ongoing interactions and variations in the environment. In human systems, when the parts are individual subjects, teams or units of a formal organization, development can be guided through reflection and learning from practice. A doctor or a nurse is trained to perform diagnosis and treatment, while they sometimes lack an adequate preparation to reflect upon the reliability of a diagnosis and the effectiveness of a treatment. To learn about patient safety, reporting of incidents is one of the most recognized methods to raise awareness about risks and possibly learn from experience in order to prevent the recurrence of similar incidents.[33] Reporting and learning systems combine and integrate surveillance, because every worker is asked to report any unintended and undesired consequence of a decision or an action, besides the predefined list of event to surveille. For health professionals, reporting an incident shall be part of clinical practice, provided a safe space to avoid sanctions as a result of the report. The aim of the report is to enable individual and team learning, through a structured system analysis of the significant event, that can result in improvement of actions. The collective reflection on the event can also provide emotional restoration to the professionals involved.[34]

Example: With the help of the weekly mortality and morbidity meetings based on the retrospective analysis of their own clinical cases, young doctors and nurses are able to get in touch with individual and organizational knowledge created through experience, collective reflection, and feedback on clinical practice.

Communicate openly and empathetically with patients

When things go wrong, according to recommendations from high-level institutions,[35] a clinician has the duty to communicate the incident openly and empathetically by providing a clear explanation of the consequences and the possible actions to contain negative effects of the incident. The clinician can further restore any physical or emotional trauma, and describe what the healthcare organization and institutions can do to provide any further assistance, including economic compensation. Such a communication is different from routine clinical communication, because the professional is in the uncomfortable position to admit a failure where the individual or the team are personally involved. Therefore, specific skills are needed to make this difficult communication effective and the health institution must support the open disclosure of adverse events with a clear policy and procedure to provide support to patients and the involved professionals. Health care professionals may, in fact, suffer from the emotional trauma named 'second victim syndrome', as a consequence of the personal involvement in the incident.[36] Besides the ethical norm of open communication, evidence shows potential positive effects of disclosure in terms of mental health, both on the side of patients-families and clinicians, and on the prevention of litigation. However, the evidence is still limited to a small number of institutions that implemented such communication and compensation programmes.[37]

Example: A surgeon who openly communicates an object was retained in the surgical site, while offering fast track resolution and eventual compensation in case of clinical consequences, has more opportunity to maintain patient trust and prevent legal issues.

Healthcare manager's role in patient safety

The health manager can do the activities described below to guarantee patient safety.

Provide education and learning opportunities to clinicians and patients

CRM must be part of the academic curricula and continuous professional development (CPD) programmes. In 2009, the WHO published the multi-professional curriculum for patient safety, that is, a very rich compendium of basic theories and methods to prevent risks in all health-care settings.[1] The curriculum covers, especially, areas of knowledge not usually included in traditional education programmes for health professionals: human factors principles and techniques, methods and tools for CRM and quality improvement, how to improve patients engagement and priorities for patient safety related to the WHO global campaigns for the prevention of HAI, and surgical and medication safety. Health managers shall evaluate training needs and promote the integration of CRM and patient safety in CPD programmes, possibly in cooperation with academic institutions. Furthermore, an appropriate education on risk prevention shall reach individuals and communities with the communication campaign for the public, so as to create the conditions for patients' engagement for their safety.

Example: Significant event audits as well as mortality and morbidity meeting can become part of continuous professional development programmes, with the facilitation of risk managers and their staff, as a leverage to promote legitimate structured learning from mistakes and incidents.

Organize a reporting and learning system on patient safety incidents

The capacity to respond to a patient safety incident depends on the organization of a system for safety management. Reporting and learning from the incident are fundamental pillars of safety management. High-risk industries have developed their capacity to face hazards, prevent incidents, and eventually contain casualties due to the recognition of critical incidents as a source of information and knowledge about human, technical, and organizational failures and elements of good practice.[38] Health organizations that established and developed dedicated activities for reporting and learning about incidents have better process and outcome indicators.[34] The characteristic of a reporting and learning system is well described in institutional recommendations, for example, from the European Union[33] and WHO.[14,15] The basic elements of such a system are a clear definition of what and how to report, a confidential information flow and the capacity to conduct systems analysis and respond to the incidents with corrective and improvement actions. Each organization can adapt reporting and learning to its own resources and characteristics: strong local commitment and leadership are key success factors to facilitate learning and improvement from incidents, with a safe space to report and discuss what happens, free from blame to individuals, along with easy tools to register and analyse incidents under a system's perspective. On the other side, local reporting and learning systems shall be integrated with surveillance systems, so as to generalize learning and monitor eventual outbreaks of specific type of incidents, according to national and international regulations.

Example: thanks to the establishment of a reporting and learning system, guidelines for risk assessment and safety in transplantation are periodically updated by integrating evidence from research with practical knowledge built through the analysis of significant events.

Promote the application and monitoring of safe practices

Evidence on a number of interventions to improve patient safety is publicly available[40] and Ministries of Health have promoted their implementation. At the level of a health organization, a list of relevant interventions shall be embedded in daily clinical and managerial practices. The monitoring and measurement of these interventions may take the form of ongoing process control in terms of requirements and indicators, traditionally integrated in accreditation or certification schemes. Collaborative programmes to support the implementation and maintenance of safe practices, where clinicians actively participate in the collection of data about performance and their comparison with peers, represent a valid approach to speed up the translation of evidence into practice, that healthcare managers can facilitate through internal networking and external benchmarking.[41]

Example: Prevention of CVC related infections was accelerated by the bundled approach, where a number of simple actions are integrated to help doctors and nurses to take appropriate decisions for CVC application, perform the right actions in disinfection, insertion and monitoring of CVC.

Evaluate outcomes and provide feedback to patients and clinicians

An adverse event resulting in patient harm is the worse outcome any healthcare professional or organization may face. More in general, data about complications and risks associated with a clinical treatment or procedure are less likely to be published than good outcomes. Despite the human attitude to deny or minimize failures, health organizations and their managers have recently recognized the importance of outcome measures to improve performance, beyond the increasing pressure for transparency from patients and the general public. A close look at medical history reveals evaluation of morbidity and mortality is deeply rooted in the evolution of health professions and organizations. To remember two pioneers of quality and safety, we may refer to the work of Florence Nightingale in the 19th Century[42] and of Ernst Codman in the 1930s.[43] Nightingale, remembered as the founder of modern nursing, demonstrated the negative effect of a bad hospital organization on mortality and how to improve performing the presently called clinical audit. Codman, a surgeon, introduced the first systematic evaluation of surgical outcomes through morbidity and mortality reviews based on structured medical records and mortality registries analysis. Healthcare organization, nowadays, produce an incredible amount of data, to become information and actionable knowledge for patients and clinicians, clinical audit and morbidity and mortality reviews must be actively promoted and supported by management, investing on feedback to disseminate lessons learnt throughout the health system and to communities. In donation and transplantation of organs, tissues and cells, the evaluation of outcomes is often integrated in authorization or certification schemes.

Example: Countries with a public system to report transplantation outcomes developed a key driver for improvement through benchmark and public awareness.

Design, maintain, and develop safe patient pathways

Finally, the most important contribution of a health manager is about the design, maintenance, and development of safe patient pathways. A patient pathway is an organized sequence of clinical consultations and treatments to reach one or more health goals.[44] Provided a clear and updated understanding of the risks and benefits of medical treatments, healthcare organizations have the responsibility to guarantee the delivery of safe and quality care to those in need. The healthcare organizations should bring together professional and technological resources along a path that is easy to access for the patient, efficient to be sustained over time by payers and effective to produce the intended results for patients, professionals, and the organization itself. Interventions to improve safety should be hardwired in patient pathways, so as to become the default behaviour of professionals involved, from the front line to the bottom end of the organization. For the success of a transplantation, the donor and recipient needs have to be combined and all the steps fully integrated in traceable and transparent pathways, guided by clinical evidence, sound ethical principles, and proactive risk assessment.

Example: A clear design of donor and recipient pathways help clinicians to comply with standards on one side and health care managers on the other side to participate in accreditation programmes.

Highlights

- Patient safety is a human right and healthcare organizations/professionals have the duty to guarantee the same; it is hardwired in clinical practice.
- Transplantation is one of the more complex health activities, where risks for patient safety must be addressed from donation to follow-up on recipients.
- Evidence shows a number of actionable safe practices that each health organization/professional can apply to prevent and manage clinical risks.
- Patients' and families' role is fundamental to control and improve safety, their education and appropriate communication are the core of clinical and managerial accountability.
- A system for patient safety management includes all the evidence-based methods for risk management, in particular, incident reporting and learning, and integration of safe practices in clinical pathways.

References

1. World Health Organization. WHO Multi-professional Patient Safety Curriculum Guide. Geneva: WHO press; 2009. https://www.who.int/patientsafety/education/mp_curriculum_guide/en/ (accessed on 15 July 2019)
2. Bellandi T, Tartaglia R, Sheikh A, Donaldson L. Italy recognises patient safety as a fundamental right. BMJ. 2017: j2277.
3. WHA55, Resolution. 18. Quality of care: patient safety. Fifty-fifth World Health Assembly, Geneva, 2002, 18.
4. WHA72, Resolution. 26. Global action on patient safety. Seventy-second World Health Assembly, Geneva, 2019, 26.
5. WHA57, Resolution. 18. Human organ and tissue transplantation. Fifty-seventh World Health Assembly, Geneva, 2004, 18.

6. Perrow C. Normal accidents: Living with high risk technologies-Updated edition. Princeton: Princeton university press, 2011.
7. Vincent C (ed.). Clinical risk management: Enhancing patient safety. London: BMJ Publishing group, 2001.
8. Donaldson MS, Corrigan JM, Kohn LT (eds.). To err is human: building a safer health system. Washington DC: Vol. 6. National Academies Press, 2000.
9. Donaldson L. An organisation with a memory. Clinical Medicine. 2002; 2.5: 452–457.
10. de Vries EN, Ramrattan MA, Smorenburg SM, Gouma DJ, Boermeester MA. The incidence and nature of in-hospital adverse events: a systematic review. BMJ Qual Saf. 2008; 17(3): 216–223.
11. Jha AK, Larizgoitia I, Audera-Lopez C, Prasopa-Plaizier N, Waters H, Bates DW. The global burden of unsafe medical care: analytic modelling of observational studies. BMJ Qual Saf. 2013; 22(10): 809–815.
12. Reason, J. Human error. New York: Cambridge university press, 1990
13. Bellandi T, Tartaglia R, Albolino S. The tuscany's model for clinical risk management. In Healthcare systems Ergonomics and Patient Safety. London: Taylor and Francis, 2005: 94–100.
14. Runciman W, Hibbert P, Thomson R, Van Der Schaaf T, Sherman H, Lewalle P. Towards an International Classification for Patient Safety: Key concepts and terms. International journal for quality in health care. 2009; 21(1): 18–26.
15. WHO. Working paper: Preliminary version of minimal information model for patient safety. Geneva: WHO press; 2014.
16. Ison M, Strong D, Fehily D, Chatzixiros E, Costa A, Noel L. Project NOTIFY: A global database of serious adverse events and reactions in organs, tissues, and cells. Transplantation. 2012: 94(10S).
17. Coulter A. Partnerships with patients: The pros and cons of shared clinical decision-making. Journal of health services research & policy. 1997; 2.2: 112–121.
18. Elwyn G, Frosch D, Thomson R, Joseph-Williams N, et al. Shared decision making: A model for clinical practice. Journal of general internal medicine. 2012; 27(10): 1361–1367.
19. Elwyn G, Lloyd A, Joseph-Williams N, Cording E, Thomson R, Durand MA, Edwards A. Option Grids: Shared decision making made easier. Patient education and counseling. 2013; 90(2): 207–212.
20. Shay LA, Lafata JE. Where is the evidence? A systematic review of shared decision making and patient outcomes. Medical Decision Making. 2015; 35(1): 114–131.
21. National Academies of Sciences, Engineering, and Medicine. Improving diagnosis in health care. Washington DC: National Academies Press, 2016.
22. Silverman J, Kurtz S, Draper J. Skills for communicating with patients. London: CRC Press, 2016.
23. WHO campaign on infection prevention and control. https://www.who.int/infection-prevention/en/ (accessed on 15 July 2019)
24. Pronovost P, Needham D, Berenholtz S et al. An intervention to decrease catheter-related bloodstream infections in the ICU. NEJM. 2006; 355(26): 2725–2732.
25. WHO. Global guidelines on the prevention of surgical site infection. Geneva: WHO press, 2018.

26. WHO. Medication safety at the transition of care. Geneva: WHO press, 2019
27. WHO. World alliance for patient safety: forward programme 2005. Geneva: WHO press, 2004.
28. Wieringa S, Engebretsen E, Heggen K, Greenhalgh T. Rethinking bias and truth in evidence-based health care. Journal of evaluation in clinical practice. 2018; 24(5): 930–938.
29. Claridge JA, Fabian TC. History and development of evidence-based medicine. World journal of surgery. 2005; 29(5): 547–553.
30. Pucher P H, Tamblyn R, Boorman D et al. Simulation research to enhance patient safety and outcomes: Recommendations of the Simnovate Patient Safety Domain Group. BMJ Simulation and Technology Enhanced Learning. 2017; 3(Suppl 1): S3–S7.
31. Haynes A B, Weiser TG, Berry WR et al. A surgical safety checklist to reduce morbidity and mortality in a global population. NEJM. 2009; 360(5): 491–499.
32. Gawande A. Checklist manifesto. London: Penguin Books, 2010.
33. European Commission, Patient Safety and Quality of Care working group. Reporting and learning systems for patient safety incidents across Europe. 2014.: http://ec.europa.eu/health/patient_safety/policy/index_en.htm (accessed on 15th July 2019)
34. Howell AM, Burns EM, BourasG, Donaldson LJ, Athanasiou T, Darzi A. Can patient safety incident reports be used to compare hospital safety? results from a quantitative analysis of the english national reporting and learning system data. PloS one. 2015: 10(12); e0144107.
35. Wu AW, McCay L, Levinson W et al. Disclosing adverse events to patients: International norms and trends. Journal of patient safety. 2017: 13(1); 43–49.
36. Wu AW. Medical error: The second victim: the doctor who makes the mistake needs help too. *BMJ*. 2000; 320:726
37. Mello MM, Boothman RC, McDonald T et al. Communication-and-resolution programs: The challenges and lessons learned from six early adopters. Health affairs. 2014: 33(1); 20–29.
38. Woloshynowych M, Rogers S, Taylor-Adams S, Vincent C. The investigation and analysis of critical incidents and adverse events in healthcare. Health Technology Assessment. 2005; 9:19.
39. Vincent C, Amalberti R. Safer healthcare. Cham: Springer International Publishing, 2016.
40. Shekelle P G, Pronovost P J, Wachter RM et al. The top patient safety strategies that can be encouraged for adoption now. Annals of Internal Medicine. 2013; 158(5_Part_2): 365–368.
41. Øvretveit, J. Leading improvement effectively. London: The Health Foundation, 2009.
42. Neuhauser D. Florence Nightingale gets no respect: as a statistician that is. BMJ Quality & Safety. 2003; 12(4): 317–317.
43. Neuhauser D. Ernest Amory Codman MD (Heroes and Martyrs of Quality and Safety). Quality and Safety in Health Care. 2002; 11(1): 104–106.
44. Kinsman L, Rotter T, James E, Snow P, Willis J. What is a clinical pathway? Development of a definition to inform the debate. BMC medicine. 2010; 8(1): 31.

SECTION 4.

DONOR SELECTION, RECIPIENT SELECTION AND TRANSPLANTATION

40

Preparing for retrieval

The bag, the operating room, and the transport of the graft

Joseph Costa, Frank D'Ovidio

Introduction

Organ procurement teams going to evaluate donor organs are able to access commonly used surgical supplies and instruments at the donor hospital. However, there are specific supplies inherent to thoracic and abdominal procurements, which must be transported by the procurement team each time they are deployed. Required supplies may vary slightly, but in general are the similar and used in the same fashion.

A large bag is essential in all cases, to accommodate the necessary equipment. It should be portable enough for easy transportability and storage, especially when flying out. These bags can be in the form of large emergency medical bags or more conveniently, medical equipment roller bags (Figures 40.1a, b), which ease the burden of carrying a bag. Supplies such as delivery tubing, perfusion cannulas, and other required items should be conveniently stored and transported in these bags. Other supplies, such as preservation fluids, normal saline, and medications are transported in an ice-filled cooler. It is important to have an adequate number of supplies in the case of unforeseen events, such as inadvertently contaminating a sterile item while opening and passing onto the back table in the operating room.

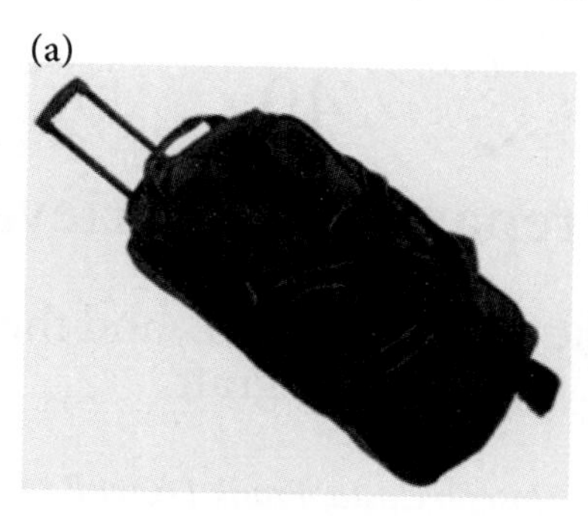

Figure 40.1a. Rolling medical equipment supply bag

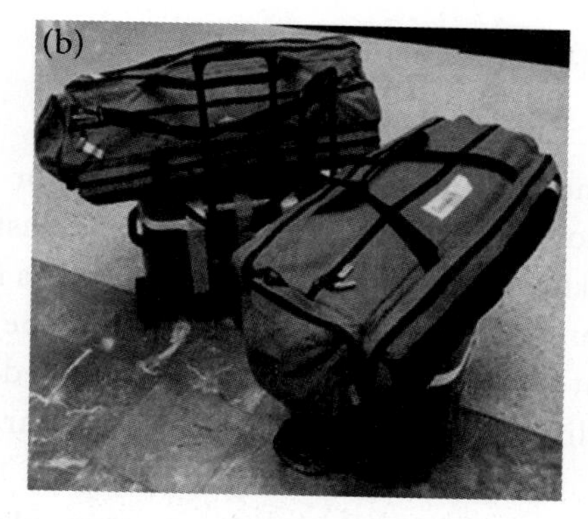

Figure 40.1b. Standard carry medical equipment supply bag

Overview of procurement supplies

There is some variation among transplant centres with regards to delivery of antegrade and retrograde perfusion solutions and the types of delivery tubing and cannulas used. While there are many choices of cannulas, most lung procurement teams will use either a wire reinforced dispersion cannula (Figure 40.2a, b) or a right-angle arterial cannula (Figure 40.2c), which can be either metal or plastic tipped. The type of cannula used is based on the preference of the transplant centre.

The diffusion-tipped cannula is commonly used to deliver antegrade pulmoplegia. This cannula is inserted in to the pulmonary artery (PA) and snared down using a purse stitch snare. The benefit of using a diffusion-tipped cannula is the avoidance of a 'jetting effect' normally encountered with single-lumen cannulas, resulting in a multidirectional

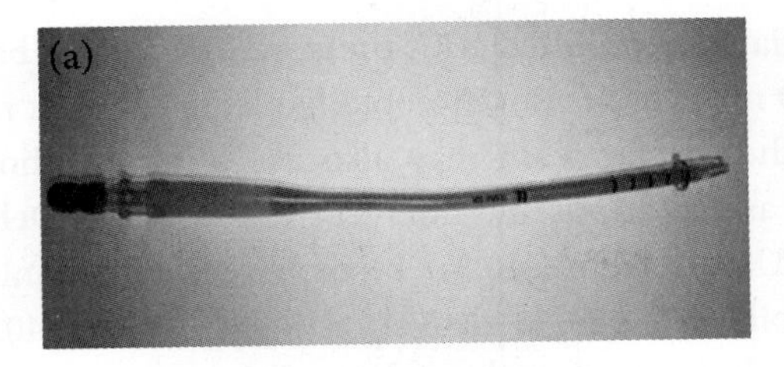

Figure 40.2a. Dispersion tip pulmonary artery cannula

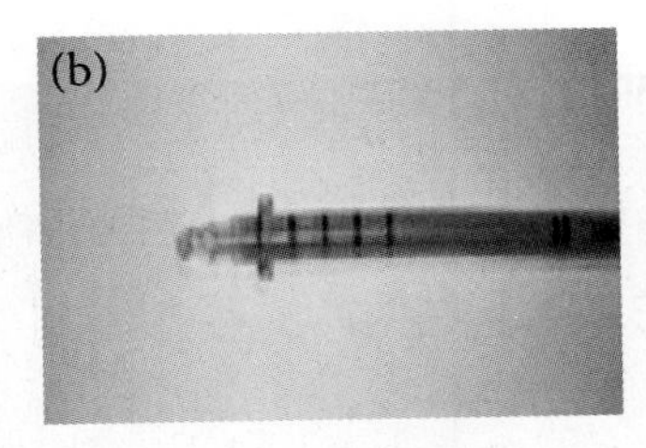

Figure 40.2b. Dispersion tip cannula with depth flange

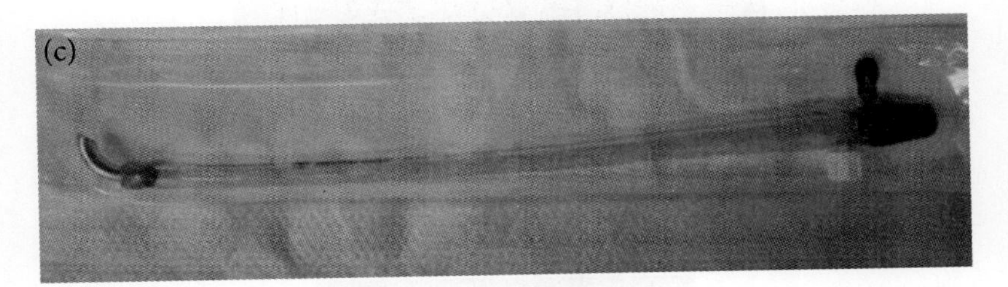

Figure 40.2c. Right angle pulmonary artery cannula

systemic flow into both pulmonary arteries. These diffusion cannulas may also be angled, however, do not need to be inserted with the tip facing the pulmonary valve, as in the case of single-lumen cannulas. When using a single flow right angle cannula, it is important that the tip of the cannula faces the pulmonary valve when inserted into the main PA. This allows for equal dispersion of antegrade preservation fluid into the right and left pulmonary arteries. If the right-angle cannula is inserted with the tip facing the PA raphe, it may result in preferential perfusion flow into the left PA and limiting flow into the right PA.

Cardiac teams will use a 14 French aortic cannula to deliver antegrade perfusion using simple dual spiked tubing with two 1 L bags of cardioplegia solution fitted with pressure monitoring bags for insufflation of 150 mm Hg pressure to obtain adequate aortic root pressure. Sometimes, the cardiac team may also use a more elaborate delivery system, such as the disposable Intercept Cardioplegia Delivery System (Medtronic, USA) (Figure 40.3a, b) or a reusable stainless steel hypothermic coil cardioplegia delivery system (Figure 40.4), allowing cardioplegia solution to flow through a coil system immersed in ice, assuring continuous hypothermic delivery of antegrade cardioplegia.

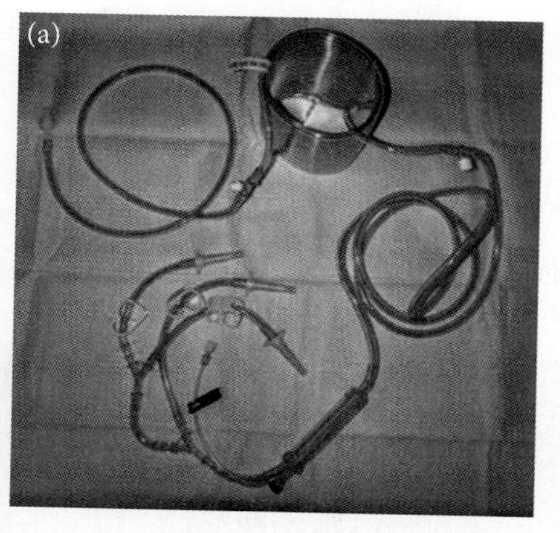

Figure 40.3a. Intercept cardioplegia delivery system (Medtronic, USA)

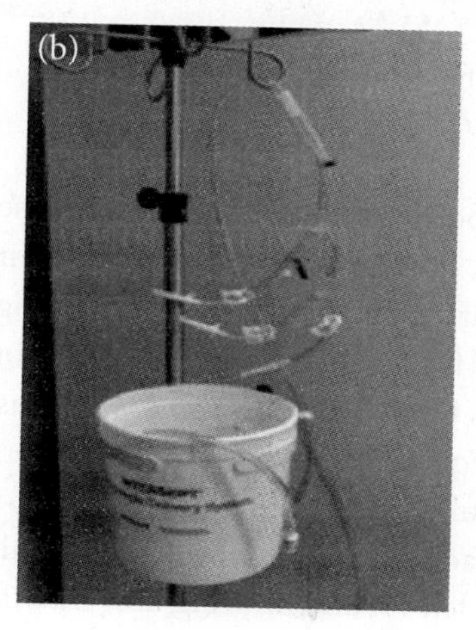

Figure 40.3b. Intercept cardioplegia delivery system (Medtronic, USA) set up

Abdominal procurement teams will typically use a soft tip cannula (Figure 40.5a) for the portal vein flush, and a 22–24 Fr aortic cannula (Figure 40.5a), which can differ based on aortic diameter connected to a high flow dual spiked organ perfusion set (Figure 40.5b).

The majority of lung and liver procurement teams use dual spiked tubing connecting two 3 L Perfadex Plus (Vitrolife AB, Göteborg, Sweden) bags to the PA cannula and four one-litre bags of University of Wisconsin Solution (UW) to the aortic cannula delivering antegrade lung and liver cold preservation fluids. At our centre, a cardiotomy reservoir is utilized, connected to two 3 L Perfadex Plus (Vitrolife AB, Göteborg, Sweden) bags, in which 3 litres of

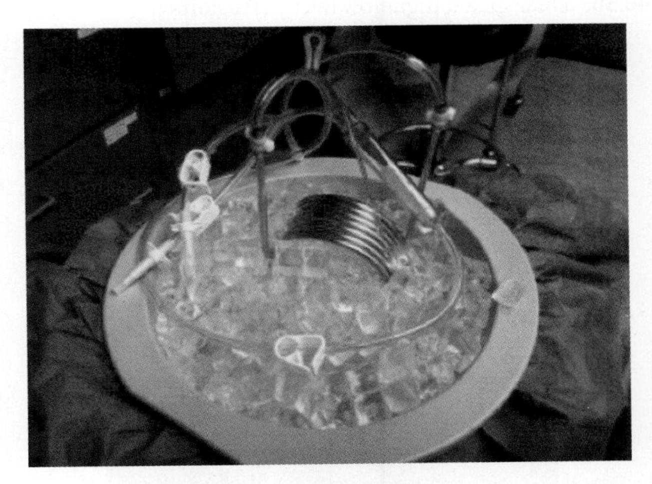

Figure 40.4. Stainless steel hypothermic coil cardioplegia delivery system

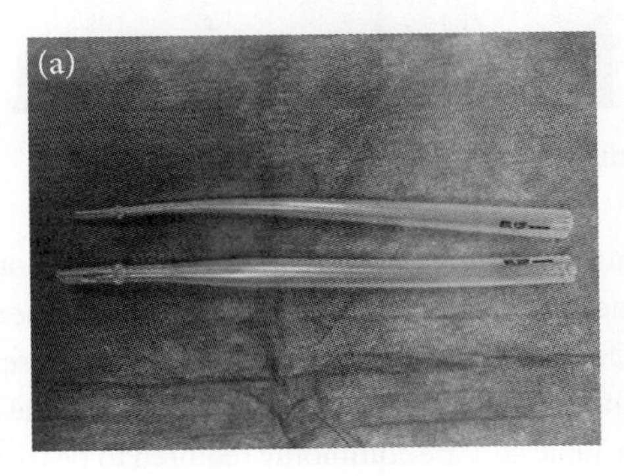

Figure 40.5a. Soft tip portal cannula 12 Fr & Abdominal aortic cannula 22 Fr

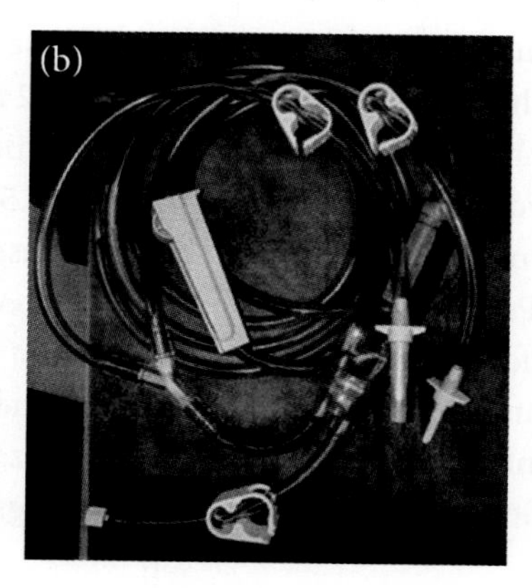

Figure 40.5b. Dual spiked high flow liver perfusion set

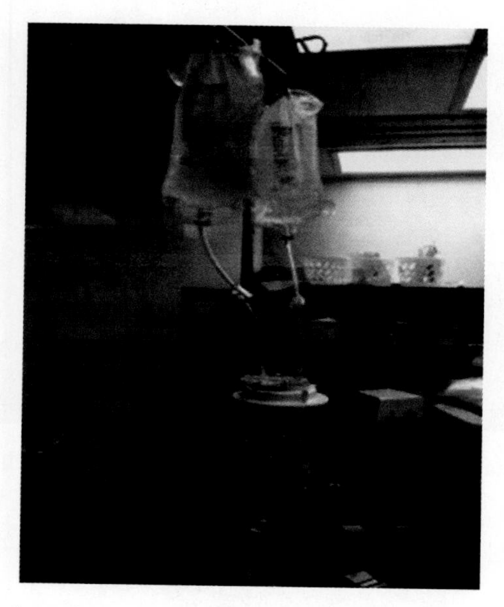

Figure 40.6. Pulmoplegia reservoir delivery system

solution are primed into the reservoir (Figure 40.6). A six-foot length of 3/8th inch tubing connects the reservoir to the PA cannula. The use of a cardiotomy reservoir allows for a precise and controlled amount of preservation fluid to be delivered in an antegrade fashion via low pressure into the PA. Remaining supplies listed in Table 40.1 are commonly required to be transported by the procurement teams or readily available at the donor hospital.

Table 40.1 Required transportable equipment/supplies for thoracic and abdominal organ procurements

Item	#	Purpose	Variations
Aortic root cannula—14 gauge	2	Delivery antegrade cardioplegia	1. 14 Ga. Dual Lumen Aortic Root Cannula with Vent Line
Aortic cannula—14 Fr	2	Delivery antegrade pulmoplegia	1. Right angle metal/plastic tip 2. Wire reinforced dispersion tip cannula
'Y' DLP adapter	2	Attachment between aortic cannula & cardioplegia line.	1. 2-Spike Y-Tubing
Delivery Tubing—Heart	2	Delivery antegrade cardioplegia	2. Interserpt Cardioplegia Delivery System (Medtronic, USA)[1] (Figure 40.3) 3. Stainless steel hypothermic coil cardioplegia delivery system (Figure 40.4)
Pressure Bags	2	Pressure (150 mmHg) delivery of cardioplegia solution	
Cardiotomy reservoir[1]	2	Measured delivery antegrade pulmoplegia	1. 2-Spike Y-Tubing—Perfadex to PA cannula connection
Rapid fire primes[1]	4	Perfedex to reservoir connection	
Delivery tubing 3/8" × 6'—Lung[1]	2	Reservoir to PA cannula connection—Antegrade pulmoplegia	1. 2-Spike Y-Tubing—Perfadex to PA cannula connection
C-Clamp[1]	1	Secure reservoir to IV pole	
2-Spike Y-tubing	2	Delivery of retrograde pulmoplegia	
Perfadex Plus adapter	4	Connection points for 3 L Perfadex Plus bags for spiking delivery tubing	
Stapler & reloads	2/6	Stapling trachea or left mainstem bronchus for single or twin single lungs	

(*continued*)

Table 40.1 *Continued*

Item	#	Purpose	Variations
Sterile Iso-bag	9	Allograft storage	
Snare packs	2	Securing aortic and PA cannula	
4-0 Prolene (cv-23)	4	Suture in aortic & PA cannula	
20 cc Syringe & needle	2	Delivery of vasodilator into PA	
Decanter	1	Siphoning 1 L cold Perfedex into iso-bag for lung storage	
Blood Tubes			
Yellow Top	6	Cross Match	
Gold Top	2	Toxoplasmosis	
Purple Top	4	HCV genotype, HCV quantitative RNA, NS3/4 and NS/5a Resistance analysis	1. Only for Hepatitis C donors
Dual spiked organ perfusion set—High flow. (Figure 40.5b)	2	Delivery antegrade liver perfusion	
Soft tip portal cannula 12 Fr. (Figure 40.5a)	2	Delivery antegrade portal vein perfusion	
Aortic cannula 22–24 Fr. (Figure 40.5a)	2	Delivery antegrade liver perfusion	

[1] Preservation supplies used only by Columbia University Medical Center

The operating room

The procurement teams arriving at the donor hospital operating rooms often meet with dynamic environments, varying personalities and engrained methodologies employed at that hospital. It is essential to remember that procurement team members are guests and they should always maintain an amicable and professional demeanour with the operating room staff, who are there for assistance, and in turn require friendly guidance, when it comes to particular team needs. The experience of the operating room staff will vary greatly and the guidance from procurement teams is always welcome and appreciated. Mutual respect and teamwork can be fostered with proper self-introduction of the procurement team members on entering the operating room in addition to thanking the staff for their help.

Chart review/essential paperwork

On arrival to the donor hospital operating room, the donor surgeon must go through relevant paperwork with the on-site transplant coordinator. Specifically, the donor chart review must include the signed brain death or donation after cardiac death consent for organ donation, brain death declaration, hospital and Organ procurement organization (OPO), ABO blood group confirmations, serologies, donor risk assessment interview form, and high-risk form, if applicable. It is a good practice for the donor surgeon to have a 'run sheet', containing match number, relevant donor and recipient information and donor clinical data, such as bronchoscopy, chest x-ray, CT chest and abdomen results, ABO, serologies, challenge gases, pertinent liver and renal lab test results and any prior liver biopsy results, if performed. It is important for the donor surgeon to review these reports and the actual films, and correlate findings with their subjective intraoperative assessment. During the review of paperwork with the OPO, the run sheet can be used to confirm relevant information, working as a checklist. In some cases where the heart is being procured for valves, the donor surgeon will have to sign a 'Processed Grafts' form, acknowledging vascular length critical for tissue graft production.

Often based on donor cause of death, the medical examiner will have specific restrictions, which are made aware to the donor surgeon by the on-site coordinator prior to starting the case. Multiple photographs of the donor by the OPO, required by the medical examiner office, prior to the donor being prepped and draped for incision. In some cases, the operative event may be video recorded in its entirety, as a matter of legal record. In the event of a medical examiners case, where circumstances of death are questionable and require further investigation following the retrieval of organs,[1] at the end of the case, the donor surgeon will be required to list and describe on a medical examiners form, any relevant intraoperative findings to the chest, and abdomen, which might have been encountered during the operation. This information will be corroborated by the medical examiner, as part of assessing the overall case based on cause of death.

Bronchoscope

Following the review of all relevant paperwork, the lung team must assure there is an adequate bronchoscope in the operating room. Donor surgeons must be facile when it comes to types of bronchoscopes provided. Bronchoscopes can vary between a standard Olympus bronchoscope connected to a video tower, and a monocular bronchoscope with a small light source. More commonly, a disposable bronchoscope attached to a small viewing screen can be used: the benefits of being immediate availability, portability, no potential for cross-contamination, no need for processing, and overall and cost effectiveness.[2–3] It is important to check on the bronchoscope, because in many instances an anaesthesia bronchoscope may be provided. This type of bronchoscope is mainly used for viewing purposes and in the case where the patient has secretions, the suction lumen will be too narrow and inadequate to suction out secretions. The bronchoscope should have a minimum external diameter of 5mm, in order to aspirate any airway secretions.

The required supplies such as endotracheal tube, bronchoscope adapter, silicon lubrication, sterile saline, leur-tip syringe and biopsy and suction port adapters are important and, in many cases, may or may not be readily available with the bronchoscope provided in the operating room. Inspecting the bronchoscope and ensuring the availability of all the accompanying supplies, will avoid any unnecessary delays and the bronchoscopy can be performed prior to prepping and draping, allowing for easy access to the donor.

Surgical instruments and supplies

Standard major chest, vascular, and laparotomy instrument trays are required for thoracic and abdominal procurement teams (Table 40.2). It is good practice to look over the instruments provided on the back table, such as the sternal retractor, sternal saw, and Balfour retractor. In some cases, the sternal retractor provided may be excessively large for a small donor and vice versa, however, thoracic procurement teams must adjust and make do, since often there is limited selection or none at all to choose from. The orientation of the sternal saw blade is based on donor surgeon's preference on whether they perform the sternotomy starting at the xiphoid process or the suprasternal notch. Based on this, the donor surgeon can direct the scrub nurse to insert the blade inserted in the saw and also test the battery, making sure it is fully charged. Additionally, making sure the scrub nurse has bone wax and 2-0 silk pop-off sutures is helpful along with a total of four suctions, two for the chest and two for the abdomen. This suction prevents any excessive pooling of pulmonary and liver preservation fluid draining into the chest and abdomen following venting and cross clamp.

The lung donor surgeon in many cases will elect to perform central aortic and selective pulmonary vein gas sampling,[4] and will require five arterial blood gas (ABG) syringes, which can be handed off to the scrub nurse prior to the case commencing. Following the intraoperative evaluation, our practice is to have our preservationist hand off one ABG syringe at a time in a sterile manner to the donor surgeon, who in turn draws the gas and hands the ABG syringe back identifying which pulmonary vein it was drawn from. The preservationist, in turn, labels each syringe with the specific PV sample and places them on ice for delivery to the lab or to be analysed using an i-STAT in the operating room.

Table 40.2 Surgical supplies checklist required for thoracoabdominal organ procurements

Supplies and Instruments	Thoracic Team (Heart & Lung)	Abdominal Team (Liver, Pancreas, & Kidney)
Bronchoscope and tower[1]	✓	✕
Major chest instrument tray	✓	✕
Major laparotomy tray	✕	✓
Vascular tray	✕	✓
Sterile ice slush machine (2)	✓	✓
Instrument tables	✓	✓
Sternal saw	✓	✓
Lebsche knife and mallet	✓	✓
Sternal retractor[2]	✓	✓
Balfour retractor[3]	✓	✓
Bone wax (2)	✓	✕
2-0 silk pop-off sutures	✓	✕
#15 blade on a handle	✕	✓
#11 blade on a handle	✓	✓
Electrocautery units (2)[4]	✓	✓
0, 3-0, and 4-0 silk ties	✓	✓
4-0 and 5-0 prolene sutures	✓	✓
Umbilical tape	✓	✓
Large and small hemoclips	✓	✓
Suction tubing (4)	✓	✓
Pool tip suction (4)	✓	✓
Yankauer tip suction (4)	✓	✓
Sterile basins (5)	✓	✓
GIA stapler(1)	✕	✓
GIA stapler reloads (4)	✕	✓
TA auto suture stapler (1)	✓	✕
TA auto suture stapler reload (3)	✓	✕

[1] Bronchoscope and tower is only required by lung team.

[2] Sternal retractor always required even in cases where heart and lung not being procured. Liver team will need to open chest to vent the inferior vena cava and place a cross clamp.

[3] Still required even in cases with no abdominal teams, thoracic team may be tasked with opening abdomen for lymph node samples and spleen, as required.

[4] Only required in brain dead donor cases. Not required for donation after circulatory death cases.

Table 40.3 Cold preservation fluids and medications

Item	#	Purpose
Perfadex Plus 3L	3 bags	Antegrade pulmoplegia solution
Perfadex Plus 1L	3 bags	Retrograde pulmoplegia solution
0.9% Normal Saline (500cc)	6 bottles	Iso-bag storage solution for lung allograft
Nitroglycerin (10mg/1cc) 10cc	1 bottle	Pulmonary vasodilator
Alprostadil (1cc/500mcg) 1cc	2 Ampules	Pulmonary vasodilator
UW solution 1L & 2 L	4/2 bags	Antegrade liver preservation solution
Custodial HTK solution 1 L[1]	3 bags	Antegrade cardioplegia solution

[1] Custodial HTK cardioplegia solution is currently used by our institution. Type of solution varies from centre to centre.

Back table preparation

In the operating room, multiple back tables are usually set up for each team, where they will perform back table assessment and delivery of preservation fluid to their respective organs (Table 40.3). It is a common practice for preservationists to pass off all their sterile supplies to the back table during the initial set up (Table 40.1). Along with these supplies, three medium DeBakey forceps, one metzenbaum scissor and one curved mayo scissor should be on the back table for each team.

In our standard setup, the back table will include two sterile basins, one basin with 3 iso-bags draped and the other basin with two lap pads covered with ice slurry and 500cc of cold saline. Having two separate basins allows for the en-bloc lung to be placed in one basin and each lung covered with a cold lap pad, allowing for continued topical hypothermia, while the anatomical structures are inspected and retrograde flush is administered. Following retrograde flush, the en-bloc lung allograft can be placed in three iso-bags in the other basin with 1 L of cold Perfadex Plus (Vitrolife AB, Göteborg, Sweden) solution in the first iso-bag containing the lung and 500 cc of cold 0.9% normal saline in the second and third iso-bag.

Transport of the graft

Cooling of donor lung allografts to 4–6° C is vital in order to reduce ischemia related cellular damage, by reducing cellular metabolism.[5–7] The premise of hypothermic preservation is made possible by delivery of cold antegrade and retrograde flush and storage of the lung allograft in a cooler at approximately 4° C. Lung and abdominal allografts are packed in a sterile three-layered bag configuration, with the first bag containing the lung filled with 1L of cold Perfadex or liver with 1 L of cold UW solution, followed by this bag being placed sequentially into two other sterile bags containing 500cc of cold saline for lungs and 1 L cold saline for abdominal organs.

Donor heart allografts are packaged in a similar fashion using a three-layer bag configuration. However, some centres are using advanced technology hypothermic organ transports systems, such as the Paragonix SherpaPak Cardiac Transport System (Braintree, MA) (Figure 40.7a–c),

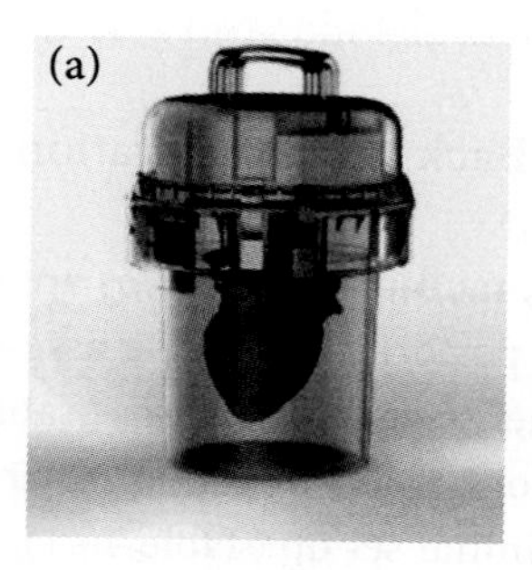

Figure 40.7a. SherpaPak organ container

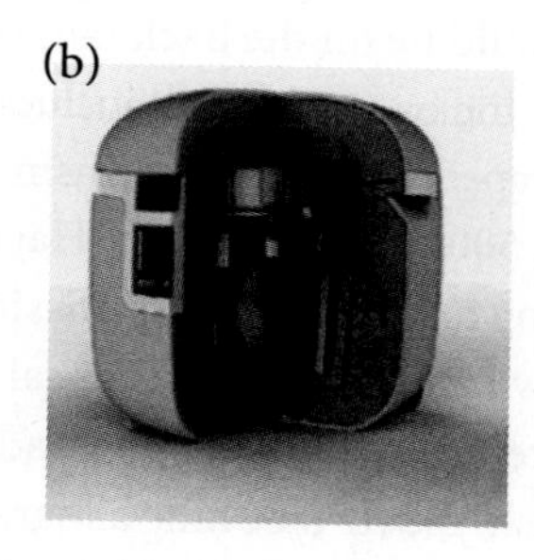

Figure 40.7b. SherpaPak configuration

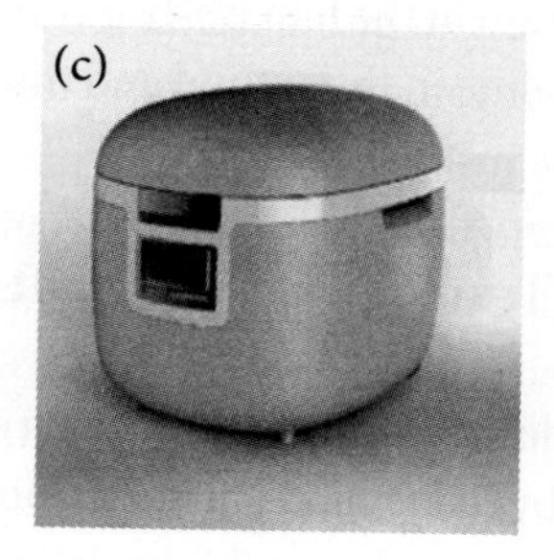

Figure 40.7c. SherpaPak transport pod

which allows for consistent temperature range between 4° C and 8° C during cold static preservation of the heart, preventing hypothermic injury, as well as real time data monitoring.[8] The SherpPak is approved for use in the United States, United Kingdom, France, Spain, Italy, Germany, Austria, and the Slovak Republic and in the future may likely be available for other donor organs.

The onsite OPO will complete package labelling of each organ using the Organ procurement and transplantation network (OPTN) organ tracking system,[9] prior to the transplant team leaving the donor hospital. In many cases, the donor surgeon will also be required to fill out and sign an operative report prior to leaving. The packaged allografts are placed in an ice cooler and covered with non-sterile ice for transport (Figure 40.8). It is good practice to secure the lid of the ice cooler with tape, preventing the lid from accidentally opening during transport or while being loaded in the aircraft.

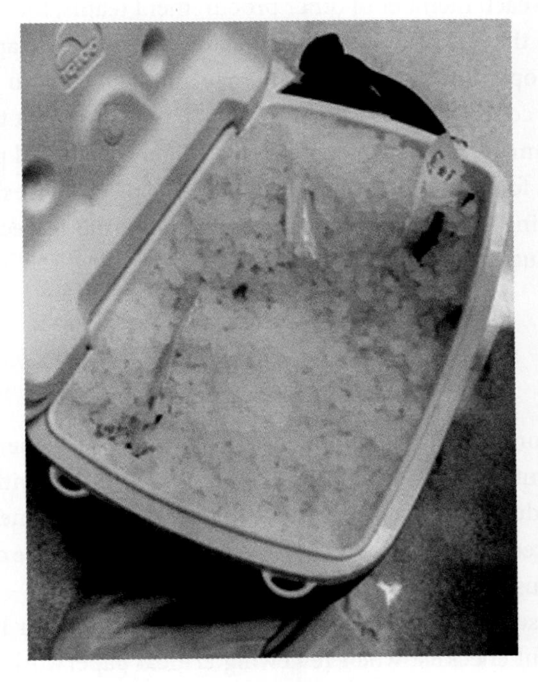

Figure 40.8. Hypothermic organ storage for transport

Conclusion

Preparation and forethought are especially important for the procurement teams going out to different geographical locations, with the necessity to work with other teams and operating room staff, who have engrained methods and protocols to follow. Specialized equipment required by each team, should never be assumed as available at the donor hospital. Basic surgical instruments, such as chest and vascular trays and general surgical supplies ubiquitous throughout all the operating rooms, are the standard armamentarium the procurement teams can confidently rely on. Redundancy of specific required items is necessary, given the dynamic atmosphere in the operating room and occasional accidental contamination of sterile supplies being passed on to the back table, thus avoiding any delays due to inadequate number of supplies.

Procurement teams are guests to the donor hospitals and it is of paramount importance that mutual respect, patience, and guidance be extended to each member of other procurement teams, the on-site coordinator and the operating room staff. Having an amicable approach and keeping an open mind, being considerate and adaptable to change, will foster more cohesive operative event, where all teams work together in a collegial manner. Having an experienced procurement and preservation team allows for continuity of expertise, checks and balances and assures success during organ procurements, which are vital to recipient post-transplant outcomes.

Highlights

- Transportability and redundancy of required equipment is important limiting any unintended obstacles and dealing with the unexpected during thoracic and abdominal organ procurements.
- Advanced preparation and having a plan allows for ease of execution and adjustment in the event of unintended events.
- Donor surgeon run sheet with detailed clinical donor information is helpful checklist when reviewing critical paperwork with onsite coordinator.

- Avoid complacency, utilize a mental checklist assuring necessary equipment and operating room set up is adequate.
- A bronchoscope with minimum external diameter of 5mm is required in the event aspiration of secretions is required.
- Communicate your needs to the scrub nurse and look over required surgical instruments, such as retractors and sternal saw, making sure they are proper sizes and configuration.

References

1. Nunnink L, Wallace-Dixon C. The impact of organ donation on coronial processes and forensic investigation: A literature review. J Forensic Leg Med. 2020;71:101940.
2. Mouritsen JM, Ehlers L, Kovaleva J, et al. A systematic review and cost effectiveness analysis of reusable vs. single-use flexible bronchoscopes. Anaesthesia. 2020;75(4):529–540.
3. Châteauvieux C, Farah L, Guérot E, et al. Single-use flexible bronchoscopes compared with reusable bronchoscopes: Positive organizational impact but a costly solution. J Eval Clin Pract. 2018;24(3):528–535.
4. Costa J, Sreekanth S, Kossar A, et al. Donor lung assessment using selective pulmonary vein gases. Eur J. Cardiothorac Surg. 2016;50(5):826–831.
5. von Dossow V, Costa J, D'Ovidio F, et al. Worldwide trends in heart and lung transplantation: Guarding the most precious gift ever. Best Pract Res Clin Anaesthesiol. 2017;31(2):141–152.
6. Latchana N, Peck JR, Whitson B, et al. Preservation solutions for cardiac and pulmonary donors grafts: A review of the current literature. J Thorac Dis. 2014;6(8):1143–1149.
7. Ishikawa J, Oshima M, Iwasaki F, et al. Hypothermic temperature effects on organ survival and restoration. Sci Rep. 2015;5:9563.
8. Michel SG, LaMuraglia II, GM, Madariaga MLL, et al. Innovative cold storage of donor organs using the Paragonix Sherpa Pak ™ devices. Heart Lung Vessel. 2015;7(3):246–255.
9. OPTN/Organ procurement and transplantation network Policies. Available https://optn.transplant.hrsa.gov. Accessed August 29, 2019.

41

The surgical phases of thoracic organ retrieval

Joseph Costa, Frank D'Ovidio

Introduction

Transplantation remains the treatment for end-stage heart and lung disease when medical therapy has been maximized and no longer offers patients the potential for a better quality of life. Pre-evaluation of heart and lung often determines the initial foundation for suitability; however intra-operative assessment performed by transplant donor surgeons is the final overall judgement in determining suitability for transplantation.

The organ procurement process is very dynamic, with multiple teams congregating at a donor hospital, often working with unfamiliar teams and operating room staff. Donor surgeons perform intraoperative evaluations using standards methodologies with minimal variation amongst transplant centres. The same complexity and dynamism hold true for the explantation phase, which is also standardized but varies slightly by the presence or absence of a heart or lung team. Maintaining a collegial and respectful operative environment among all teams, and openly communicating the needs will lead to a smooth operative event and the decreased incidence of surgical injury or disagreements during the explant phase.

Donor heart evaluation and *in-situ* preservation

Prior to starting the operative case, the heart team should carefully review the echocardiogram, chest x-ray, or computed tomography scan, as well as ascertain if the donor is currently requiring any hemodynamic support with pressors and/or inotropes.

The general procedure for cardiac dissection has been described under operative procedure and lung assessment. The pericardium should be inspected, especially in cases where the mechanism of brain death was trauma related to chest involvement. Once the pericardium has been opened and retracted with 0-silk pop off sutures, the amount and appearance of the pericardial fluid should be noted. The fluid should appear clear with slight yellowish hue; bloody (Traumatic) or cloudy fluid with increased viscosity potentially indicates infectious aetiology.

The heart is visually inspected for size, signs of trauma (contusions) and overall contractility, focusing on the right (RV) and left ventricles (LV). The donor surgeon should gently lift the heart in order to adequately inspect the contractility of the LV (Figure 41.1a), followed by gentle palpation of the left anterior descending and right coronary arteries, assessing for any signs of atherosclerosis (Figure 41.1b). This is, especially, important if the donor did not undergo coronary angiography. The right (RA) and left (LA) atria should not show any sign of distension, potentially indicating volume overload. If there is a concern, inserting a 20-gauge needle into the RA, connected to a pressure monitoring line will allow the donor surgeon to transduce the central venous pressure, helping to determine the volume status. The aorta and pulmonary artery (PA) should be palpated for any thrills, and visually inspected for any signs of dilation.

Specific to the cardiac dissection, on the inferior aspect of the superior vena cava (SVC), cephalad to the right pulmonary artery (RPA), the azygos vein should be identified, encircled, and tied down with two 0-silk ties. It is best not to transect the azygos vein until the cardiectomy is being performed. An inadvertent transection of one of the ties or improper ligations would result in significant bleeding, which would be extremely difficult to repair likely necessitating early heparinization and cross clamp.

Following systemic heparinization, a 'U' stitch is placed on the midpoint of the ascending aorta and an antegrade cardioplegia cannula is inserted (Figure 41.1c) and connected to two 1 L bags of cardioplegia solution fitted with pressure bags pumped to 150 mm Hg pressure. When all the teams are ready, the heart is gently lifted and the inferior vena cava (IVC) is partially transected, followed by transection of the left inferior pulmonary vein (PV). Cross clamp is applied, delivery of antegrade cardioplegia is started and ice slurry is placed on the heart, assuring global topical hypothermia. Aortic root pressure should be manually checked and pressure bag settings adjusted to necessary root pressure. The LV should be gently assessed for any distention. In case of LV distension, the aortic cross clamp is gently released until LV distension resolves and the aorta re-clamped.

Panel 1.

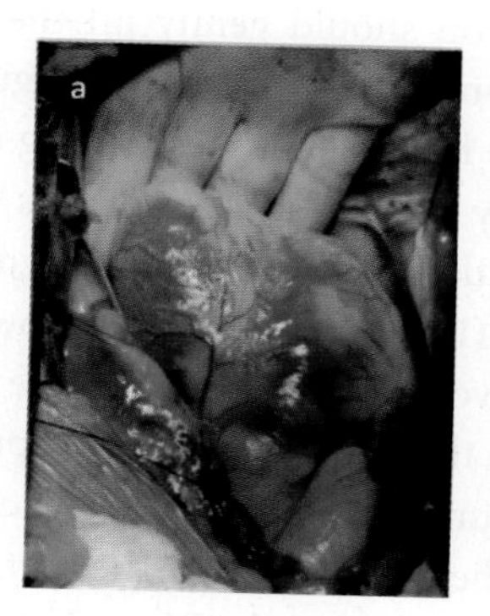

Figure 41.1a. Intraoperative assessment of the ventricular contractility

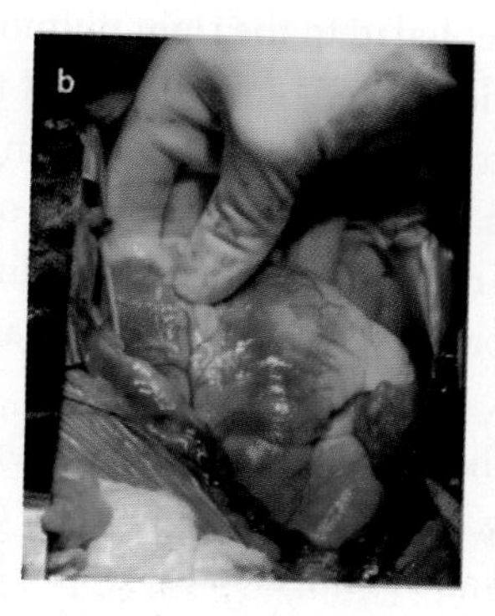

Figure 41.1b. Coronary artery assessment for atherosclerotic plaques

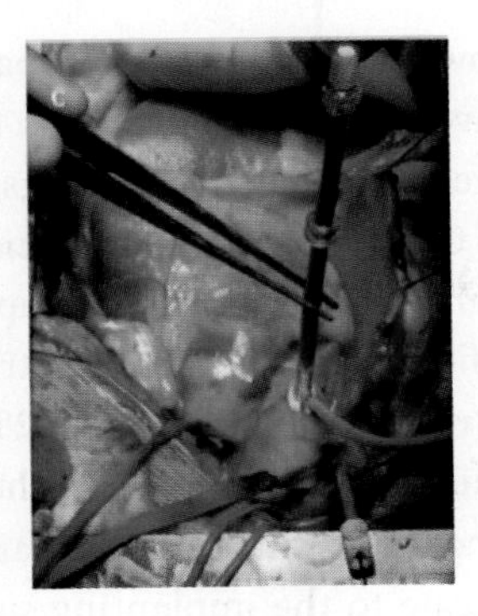

Figure 41.1c. Placement of anterograde aortic cardioplegia cannula

Cardiectomy

The antegrade cardioplegia cannula is disconnected from the circuit and may be entirely removed and tied down or left in place, secured by its snare. The heart is lifted and the IVC transection completed, allowing for adequate IVC length for both cardiac and liver transplantation teams. The four PVs are transected at the level of the posterior pericardial surface, assuring safe distance from the left atrium. Next, the azygos vein is transected, followed by the SVC, Aorta, and PA at the cannulation site. The heart is removed and taken to the back table and prepared for hypothermic storage and transport.

Pre-operative evaluation of donor lung

A flexible bronchoscopy is performed prior to incision to assess the airways for secretions, lesions, anatomical abnormalities, and the airway mucosa. The ventilator should be set to a FiO_2 of 100%, positive end expiratory pressure (PEEP) of 5 cm H_2O and a tidal volume of 5–7cc/kg. The airways should be thoroughly inspected and cleared of any secretions, noting the type and consistency of secretions possibly indicating infection (purulence), whether or not they re-accumulate and the mucosa of the airways inspected for any signs of pneumonitis, evident by oedema and hyperaemia. In cases where there are copious secretions or secretions appear purulent, it is recommended to repeat the bronchoscopy following recruitment and palpation of the lungs. If purulent secretions have re-accumulated, this finding is used to corroborate other objective and subjective findings, in order to determine suitability of the organ. One rare anatomical abnormality is a congenital anatomical variant of an aberrant bronchus supplying the right upper lobe, commonly identified at the supracarinal trachea, also known as a 'pig bronchus', having a reported incidence is 0.2% (Figure 41.2a). While there are many bronchial variants, a true tracheal bronchus will arise from the trachea ranging 2 to 6 cm above the carina.[1–3] This finding is important to communicate to the implanting surgeon, taking care not to transect this aberrant bronchus when splitting the lungs on the back table prior to implant.

Operative procedure and lung assessment

Following a 'time out' surgical pause and moment of silence, chest incision is made using a bovie, with dissection taken down to the anterior plate of the sternum. The interclavicular ligament is transected and any overlying tissue on the sternal notch is skeletonized using the bovie. Median sternotomy is performed using a sternal saw, or in some cases, a Lebsche knife after the anaesthesiologist holds ventilation. Following the sternotomy, ventilation is resumed and bleeding from the periosteal edges on each hemisternum is bovied and bone wax is applied to the marrow. In the event of sternotomy being performed using a Lebsche knife, bone wax is cautiously applied due to jagged and often splintered bone edges.

Sternal retractor is placed and the pericardium is divided from the level of the innominate vein to the diaphragm, where it is also divided laterally along the border of the diaphragm. Both pleural spaces are opened and 2–0 silk pop off sutures are placed to plicate the pericardium, each secured with a clamp, allowing access to each pleural space.

The FiO_2 of 100% is confirmed with the anaesthesiologist and advised about potentially causing minor compression to the heart during evaluation by the surgeon. Hemodynamics should be closely monitored during this phase. Initially, each pleural space should be inspected assuring there are no adhesions, which could potentially cause a tear in the lung parenchyma when eviscerating the lung for inspection. Each lung is gently eviscerated from the pleural space, and each lobe palpated, to assess for crepitations, contusions, and bogginess. Following palpation, a valsalva of 30 mmHg is administered to recruit any atelectasis (Figure 41.2b–2c). Once the atelectasis has been recruited, the anaesthesiologist should disconnect the ventilator directly from the endotracheal tube to assess lung deflation. In the event of lung deflation being poor, the procedure should be repeated with the lung in the pleural space, since the bronchus may have been kinked during the evisceration, leading to a false poor deflation.

Following the gross subjective assessment, selective PV gases should be drawn (Figure 41.2d). The evaluation of individual PV gases rests on the ability to isolate upper and lower lobe gas exchange assessment, in order to differentiate unilateral lung pathology, such as pneumonia. Selective gas results are then corroborated with the subjective assessment to determine suitability. Isolated ICU oxygen challenge gases are unable to differentiate between unilateral pathology, often presenting normal blood gas results, despite evolving isolated lower lobe pneumonia.[(4)] Using an arterial blood gas syringe, 1.5–2cc sample is drawn from each PV, and aorta, assuring each syringe is labelled accordingly. Challenge gases remain the focal point for assessing lung function, but are not fully representative of true lung function. Selective PV gases are a more accurate assessment of lung function, providing corroborative support to objective.

Cardiac dissection is performed in a standard fashion with the aorta dissected circumferentially, separating it from the PA and the branch of the RPA inferiorly. An umbilical tape is placed around the aorta and can also be used to retract it towards the left exposing the SVC (Figure 41.2e). The SVC is mobilized from its pericardial reflection and separated from the RPA, traversing inferiorly. Dissection may be done using a bovie or metzenbaum scissor. It's a good practice to use the metzenbaum scissor when dissecting the SVC laterally, in order to avoid contact with the phrenic, potentially disrupting the liver team during dissection. A 0-silk tie is placed around the SVC, to be used later to tie it down prior to cross clamp (Figure 41.2f). The PA is examined to assure adequate exposure for cannulation. In the event there is a heart team, a simple 'U' or purse stitch should be placed 1–1.5cm before the main PA bifurcation, allowing for adequate main PA length for the heart team and PA cuff for the lung team.[(5)] In case there is no heart team, the stitch may be placed lower in the main PA, making sure it is not too close to the pulmonary valve.

Panel 2.

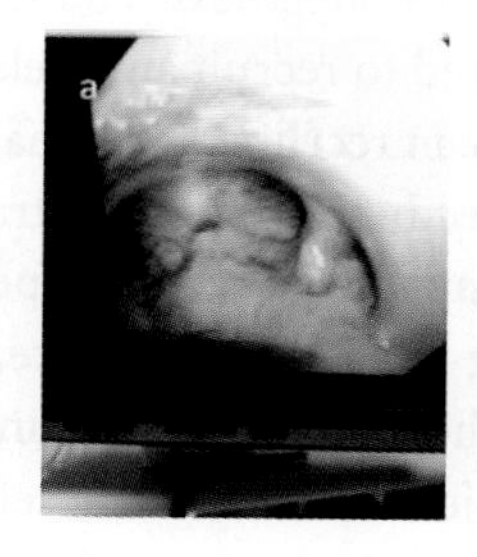

Figure 41.2a. Tracheal bronchus

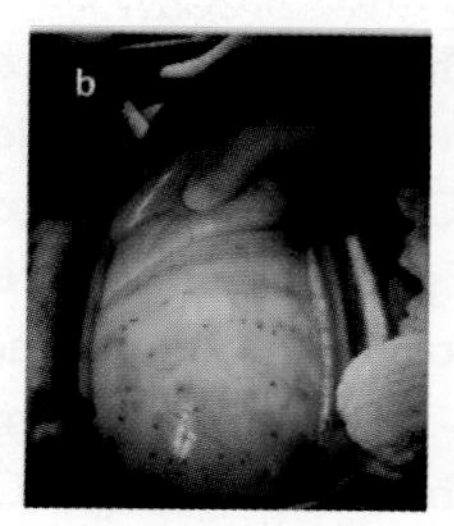

Figure 41.2b. Intraoperative recruitment of the left lung

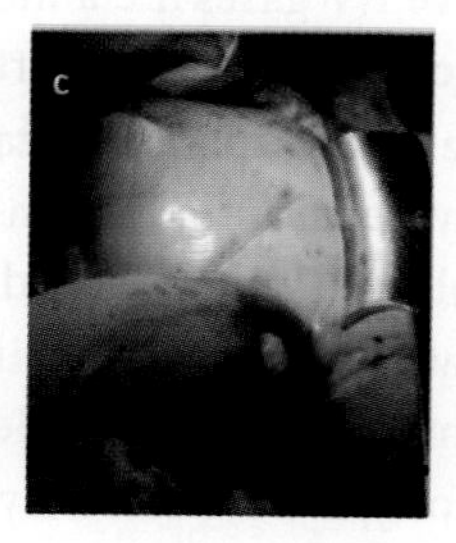

Figure 41.2c. Intraoperative recruitment of the right lung

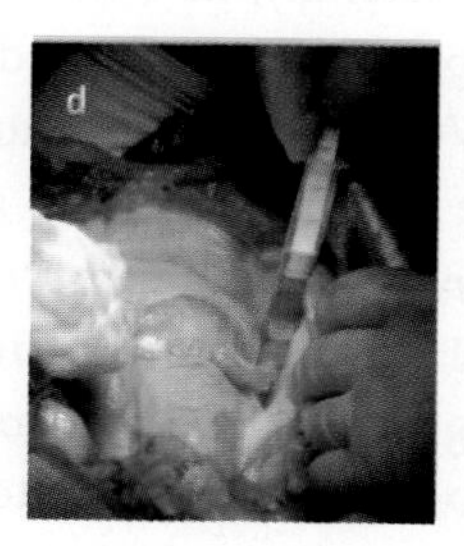

Figure 41.2d. Aspirating selective pulmonary vein blood sample

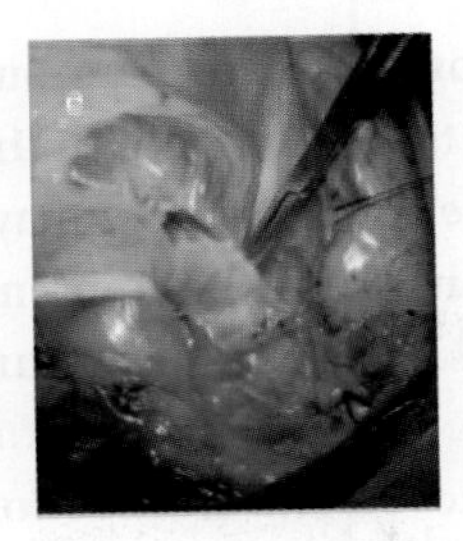

Figure 41.2e. Umbilical tape retraction of the Aorta for superior vena cava exposure

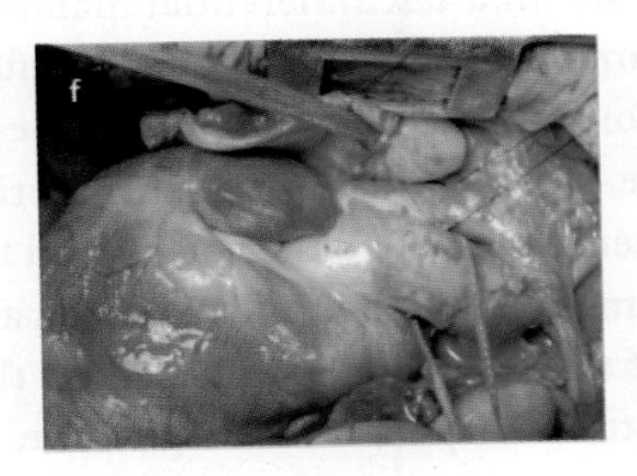

Figure 41.2f. Completed cardiac dissection

Heart explant and en-bloc pneumonectomy

When agreed upon by all teams, 30,000 Units of heparin is administered and allowed to circulate for 3 minutes. Using a #11 blade, a stab incision is made and the PA is cannulated using a right angle or dispersion cannula and snared down and secured. If a right-angle cannula is used, it must be inserted facing the PV, assuring equal distribution into the right and left PA. There should always be two independent suction lines, each with a pool tip for the chest. A pulmonary vasodilator, usually alprostadil and/or nitroglycerin,[5–8] is administered into the PA or the RA, if no heart team is present, followed by the SVC tied down (Figure 41.3a). The heart is lifted and the IVC transected, allowing adequate IVC length for the liver team, followed by amputation of the left atrial appendage. Cold antegrade flush with Perfadex Plus (Vitrolife AB, Göteborg, Sweden) at 60cc/kg is started and ice slurry is placed into each pleural space assuring topical hypothermia. One pool tip should be placed into the LA and the other in the IVC. If there is a heart team, they may choose to vent the left heart from Sondergaard's groove instead of amputating the left atrial appendage. It is important to place a pool tip into the LA, when vented from Sondergaard's grove, since outflow may be slightly reduced due to overlying compression of the LA, potentially causing increased back pressure. Anaesthesiologists should turn off all drips and continue ventilating.

The PA cannula is removed and transection of the IVC completed. The SVC is transected carefully to avoid any injury to the RPA, followed by the aorta and the PA. The PA transection should be started at the cannulation site in a circumferential manner remaining above the PA raphe (Figure 41.3b). Lastly, the heart is lifted and using a #11 blade, a stab incision is made in the middle of the LA below the coronary sinus (Figure 41.3c), at the level of the inferior PVs or midway between the confluence of the left inferior PV and the coronary sinus. Using a metzenbaum scissor, a circumferential left atrial cuff is started, towards the base of the LA, remaining just above the left inferior and superior PV. With the LA open, on the right side, each PV is visualized, and the atrial tissue remaining above each vein is divided, with the cuff being completed by dividing the roof of the LA towards the interatrial groove, leaving a rim of approximately 5mm of atrial muscle (Figure 41.3d).

Panel 3.

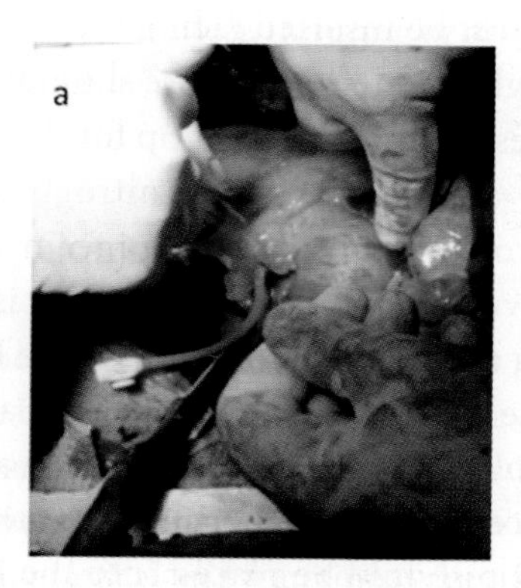

Figure 41.3a. Administration of pulmonary vasodilator

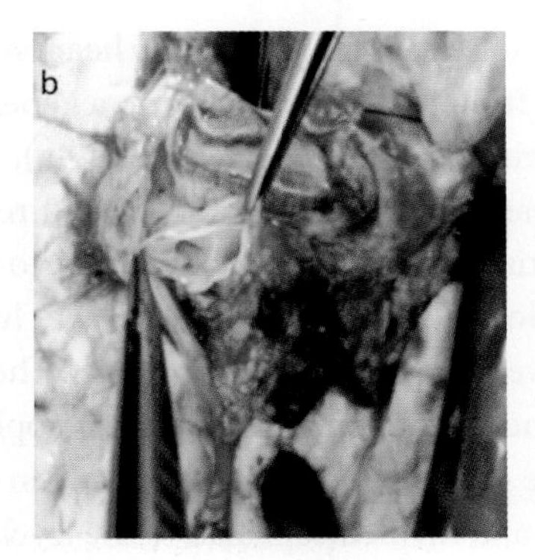

Figure 41.3b. Main pulmonary artery cuff

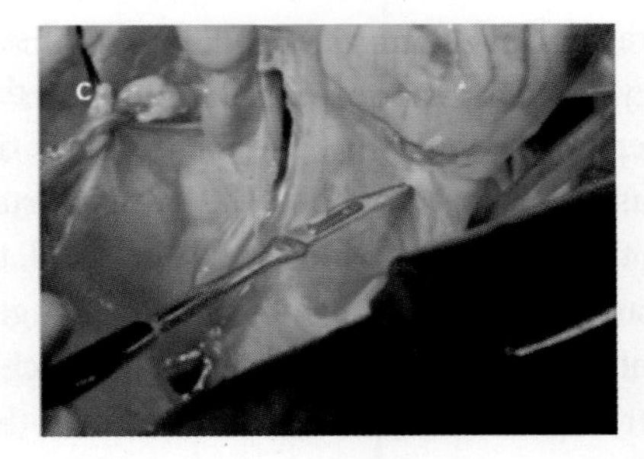

Figure 41.3c. Initial stab incision for creation left atrial cuff (No heart team)

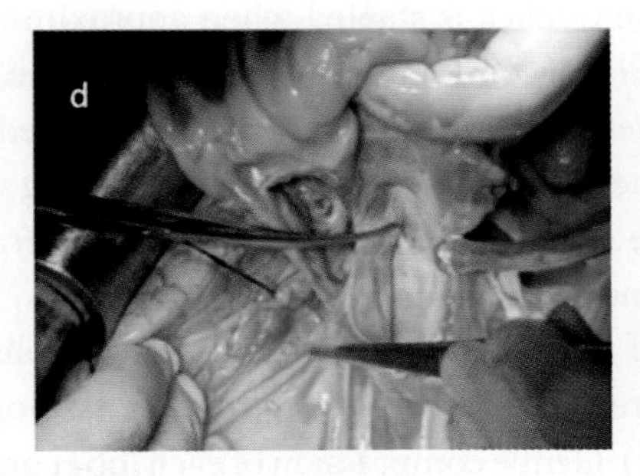

Figure 41.3d. Completion left atrial cuff

A note of caution, when there is a heart team and the heart is being stretched, despite the appearance of a mutually chosen area of where to divide the cuff, tissue retraction will occur leaving a very short, or in some cases, absent cuff, requiring reconstruction.[9–10] In these cases, the heart team may have to release tension on the heart and continue with the creation of the cuff. If there is no heart team, a generous LA cuff can be created and later trimmed, as needed (Figure 41.4a).

The inferior pericardium is divided and should remain above the oesophageal plane starting on the right, making sure to remain between the IVC and LA cuff, followed by the left side. The right lung is gently eviscerated and the right lower lobe is retracted superiorly. The inferior pulmonary ligament is divided and should remain above the oesophageal plane in order to avoid injury to the oesophagus; the tissue between the oesophagus and trachea is transected and divided cephalad to the level past the transection of the azygous vein. The lung is placed back in the chest, the right upper lobe is pulled down and all tissue adjacent to the trachea transected. On the left, the lung is eviscerated, the left lower lobe is displaced superiorly, and the inferior pulmonary ligament transected. Remaining at the level of the oesophageal plane, cephalad dividing is done and posterior tissue is transected to the level just past the transection of the thoracic aorta. Any remaining tissue posterior to the trachea is divided and transected, taking care not to injure the membranous trachea. The left upper lobe is gently displaced to transect all adjacent tissue towards the left side of the trachea.

A TA-30 stapler is placed around the trachea and the anaesthesiologist is asked to administer a gentle valsalva to 30 mmHg recruiting any remaining atelectasis. Once recruitment is completed, the vent is disconnected and the trachea is stapled when approximately 50% residual volume remains.[(5)] A second staple line is placed on the trachea and transected between them. The lungs are removed and placed in the basin with two lap pads immersed in an ice slurry, and each lung wrapped with the cold lap pads. The PA and LA cuff, as well as the general anatomy re-inspected to assure no surgical injury.

About 250cc of cold Perfadex Plus solution (Vitrolife AB, Göteborg, Sweden) is delivered into each PV in retrograde fashion, noting effluent flow (Figure 41.4b). Gentle compression of each lobe corresponding to the PV being perfused will help if there are small residual clots.[(11–13)] Following retrograde administration, the lungs are packed in a triple barrier, using three iso-bags, with the first bag containing one litre of cold Perfadex Plus (Vitrolife AB, Göteborg, Sweden) and the remaining two bags each with 500 cc of cold 0.9% saline. The lung is then placed in an ice cooler and surrounded by ice for hypothermic transport[(14–15)] (Figure 41.4c).

Panel 4.

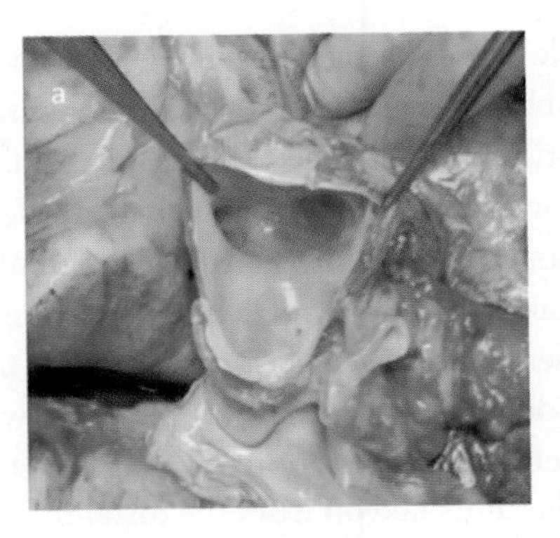

Figure 41.4a. Generous left atrial cuff (No heart team)

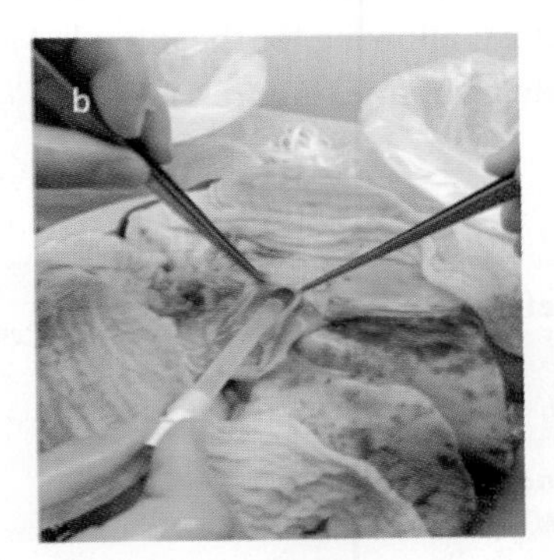

Figure 41.4b. Administration of back table retrograde pulmonary flush

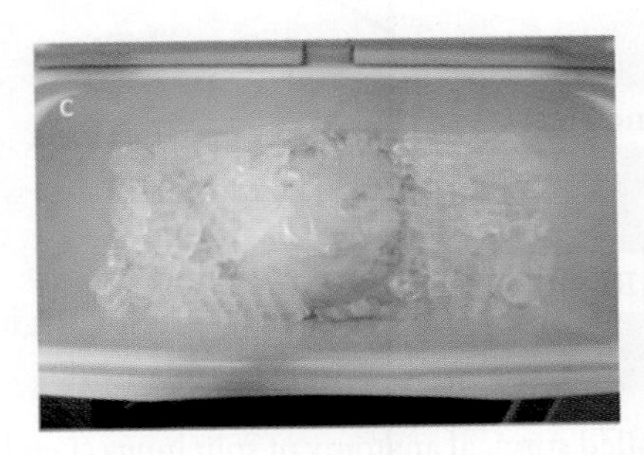

Figure 41.4c. Hypothermic storage and transport of lung allografts

Splitting lungs

In the event a single lung is deemed unsuitable for transplant, the lungs are split on the back table in a layered fashion. The remaining pericardium posterior to the left atrial cuff is divided towards the carina. In the case where twin single lung transplants are being performed, the left atrial cuff should be divided in half, assuring equal division of left atrial cuff tissue. When only one lung is being taken for transplant, a more generous division of the left atrial cuff may be performed in favour of the side being taken for transplant.

The PA is then divided at the raphe, at the point where the overlying tissue above the left main stem bronchus is dissected and divided, exposing the bronchus at its takeoff from the distal trachea. Using a TA-30 stapler, two staple lines are placed at the takeoff of the left main bronchus, if transplanting twin single lungs. If only transplanting a single lung, one staple line is satisfactory, allowing for the intended lung for transplant to maintain a 50% residual volume (Figure 41.5).

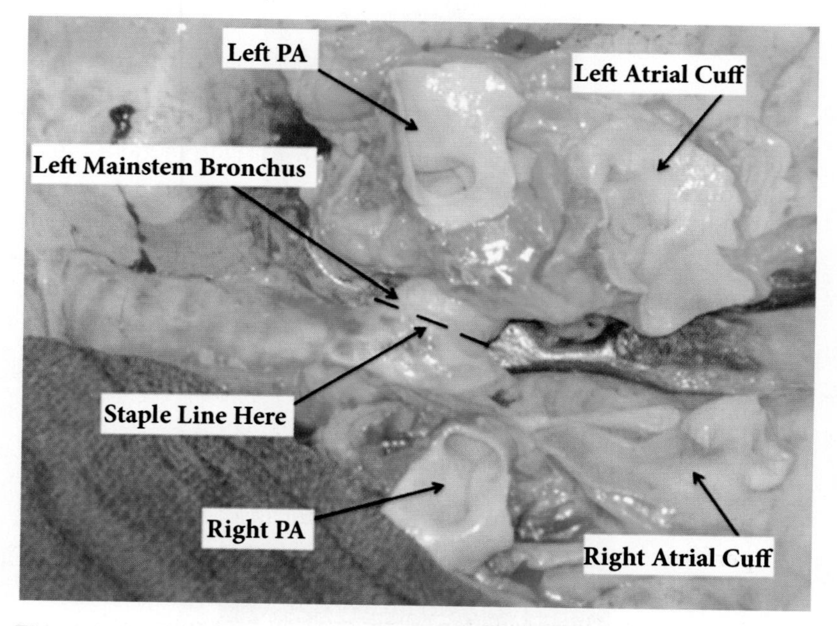

Figure 41.5. Detailed surgical anatomy of split lungs (Left lung only for transplant)

Conclusion

Proper subjective organ evaluation and successful operative phase of heart and/or lung procurement rely on adequate training and continued expertise of the donor surgeon. Continuity of expertise plays a major role in the judgement of organ suitability, as well as being a valuable and solvent source for training cardiothoracic surgical fellows tasked with organ procurements.[16] The foundation of organ suitability for transplantation relies on the intraoperative subjective judgement of the organ corroborated with objective data.

Donors' surgeons must always be flexible and understand that different centres may vary slightly with their methodologies; however, following baseline standard surgical and organ preservation procedures will allow for a positive overall outcome. While the incidence of surgical injury during procurement is low, ongoing communication between donor surgeons is the key, along with maintaining an amicable, professional, and respectful interaction among all personnel involved.

Highlights

- Echocardiogram, chest x-ray, and computed tomography of the chest should always be reviewed by the heart and lung donor surgeons respectively, prior to any operative intervention.
- Thorough assessment of cardiac function by means of corroborating echocardiogram findings along with coronary artery assessment in patients with no prior cardiac catheterization is critical to assessing suitability of the heart for transplant.
- The azygos vein should be ligated at two points and only transected during cardiectomy, due to the risk on significant bleeding, which is difficult to control and repair *in-situ*.
- Donor hospital provided flexible bronchoscope should have a minimum external diameter of 4.6 mm in order to adequately perform bronchoalveolar lavage and aspirate thick or copious secretions.
- Assessment of lung deflation *in-situ* requires the ventilator to be disconnected at the level of the endotracheal tube, due to resistance in ventilator tubing, potentially masking poor deflation.

- Given the inability of oxygen challenge gases to differentiate between unilateral lung pathology, selective PV gases are an important objective measure helping corroborate subjective findings.
- The trachea should be stapled at two points, preventing contamination of the surgical field and leaving approximately 50% residual volume in the lungs for hypothermic storage and transport, avoiding hyperinflation and potential barotrauma to the lung.
- During retrograde perfusion, gentle palpation of each lobe corresponding to the PV being flushed aids in the dislodging of any remaining residual clots.

References

1. Ghaye B, Szapiro D, Fanchamps JM, Dondelinger R. Congenital bronchial abnormalities revisited. Radiographics. 2001;21(1):105–119.
2. Chaddha U, Chang CF, Lee C. Congenital tracheobronchial branching anomalies. Ann Am Thorac Soc. 2018;15(8):995–997.
3. Chassagnon G, Morel B, Carpentier E, et al. Trancheobronchial branching abnormalities: Lobe-based classification scheme. Radiorgraphics. 2016;36(2):358–373.
4. Costa J, Sreekanth S, Kossar A, et al. Donor lung assessment using selective pulmonary vein gases. Eur J. Cardiothorac Surg. 2016;50(5):826–831.
5. von Dossow, Costa J, D'Ovidio F, Marczin N. Worldwide trends in heart and lung transplantation: Guarding the most precious gift ever. Best Pract Res Clin Anaesthesiol. 2017;31(2):141–152.
6. Chiang CH, Wu K, Yu, CP, et al. Hypothermia and prostaglandin E1 produce synergistic attenuation of ischemia-reperfusion lung injury. Am J Respir Crit Care Med. 1999;160(4):1319–1323.
7. DeCampos KN, Keshavjee S, Liu M, Slutsky S. Prevention of rapid reperfusion-induced lung injury with prostaglandin E1 during the initial period of reperfusion. J Heart Lung Transplant. 1998;17(11):1121–1128.
8. Yeung JCKS. Overview of clinical lung transplantation. Cold Spring Harbor Perspective Med. 2014;4(1):a015628.
9. Yarbrough WM, Bates MJ, Deuse T, et al. Alternative technique for salvage of donor lungs with insufficient atrial cuffs. Ann Thorac Surg. 2009;88(4):1374–1376.
10. Oto T, Rabinov M, Negri J, et al. Techniques of reconstruction for inadequate donor left atrial cuff in lung transplantation. Ann Thorac Surg. 2006;81(4):1199–1204.
11. Van De Wauwer C, Neyrinck Ap, Rega FR, et al. Retrograde flush is more protective than heparin in the uncontrolled donation after circulatory death lung donor. J Surg Res. 2014;187(1):316–323.
12. Van De Wauwer C, Neyrinck AP Geudens N, et al. Retrograde flush following topical cooling is superior to preserve the non-heart-beating-donor lung. Eur J Cardiothorac Surg. 2007;31(6):1125–32.

13. Venuta FRE, Bufi M, et al. Preimplantation retrograde pneumoplegia in clinical lung transplantation. J Thorac Cardiovasc Surg. 1999;63:625.
14. Vela MM, Saez DG, Simon AR. Current approaches in retrieval and heart preservation. Ann Cardiothorac Surg. 2018;7(1):67–74.
15. Jin Z, Hana Z, Alam A. et al. Review 1: Lung transplant—from donor selection to graft preservation. J Anesth. 2020;34(4):561–574.
16. Costa J, D'Ovidio F, Bacchetta M, et al. Physician assistant model for lung procurements: A paradigm worth considering. Ann Thorac Surg. 2013;96(6):2033–2037.

42

The surgical phases of abdominal organ retrieval

Damiano Patrono, Renato Romagnoli

Introduction

This chapter focuses on the technique of abdominal organs retrieval in the setting of donation after brain death (DBD). Albeit many of the concepts herein presented can be transferred to the setting of donation after circulatory death (DCD), specific aspects of organ retrieval in DCD donors will be treated in a separate chapter.

Organ preservation by static cold storage is based on the conjunct use of cold to slow down cell metabolism, and of preservation solutions to reduce cellular damage during preservation. Thus, one aim of donor operation is cooling down procured organs, wash out recipient blood and perfuse them with a preservation fluid. Although today this seems rather obvious, these concepts were established with the efforts of the Fathers of transplantation.[1–4]

Schematically, organ retrieval in a DBD donor can be divided into two phases. It should be noted that retrieval technique is highly variable across different countries and transplant centres. The main differences are relative to the degree of dissection carried out during each phase, handling of anatomic variants and vascular reconstruction techniques for each organ. The aim of this chapter is to provide a basic understanding of the steps, anatomy, and technique of abdominal organs retrieval.

Organ retrieval in DBD donor

During the first phase ('warm phase') or organ retrieval, after exposure and exploration of the abdominal and thoracic cavities, abdominal vessels are prepared for cannula placement, which will allow *in-situ* perfusion with the preservation solution. This phase ends when aorta is clamped, cold perfusion is started, and the abdomen and thorax are filled with ice slush. Once perfusion is over, ice is removed and organs are retrieved. The aim of this second phase ('cold phase') is procuring intact organs with undamaged vascular pedicles and exocrine drainage (liver and pancreas) or excretory duct (kidney), suitable for subsequent implant. After retrieval, attachments and unnecessary tissue will be removed ex-situ, during the so-called back table preparation.

First phase: Abdominal vessels preparation and organ perfusion

Access to the abdomen and thorax is gained through a wide median sternolaparotomy (Figure 42.1A). Pericardium and pleurae are opened. In case of high donor weight, a transverse laparotomy can be associated to enhance exposure. If thoracic organs are not retrieved, it is possible to retrieve abdominal organs without opening the thorax. In this case, however, the diaphragm will have to be sectioned during the second phase to allow thorax exploration.

An accurate exploration of both abdominal and thoracic cavities to rule out macroscopic signs of malignancy or infection is an unavoidable step of organ retrieval. Abnormal findings will have to be investigated by sending tissue samples for immediate frozen section examination.

In the absence of worrisome features and once organs have been deemed suitable for transplantation, abdominal vessels and retroperitoneum are exposed by an extended Cattel-Braasch manoeuvre. The right colon, along with the duodenum and pancreas head (Kocher manoeuvre), is fully mobilized. The mesenteric root is sectioned and viscera are lifted cephalad (Figure 42.1B). By gently pulling the sigmoid mesocolon root towards the left, the inferior mesenteric artery is ligated and sectioned (Figure 42.1C). Abdominal aorta and inferior vena cava

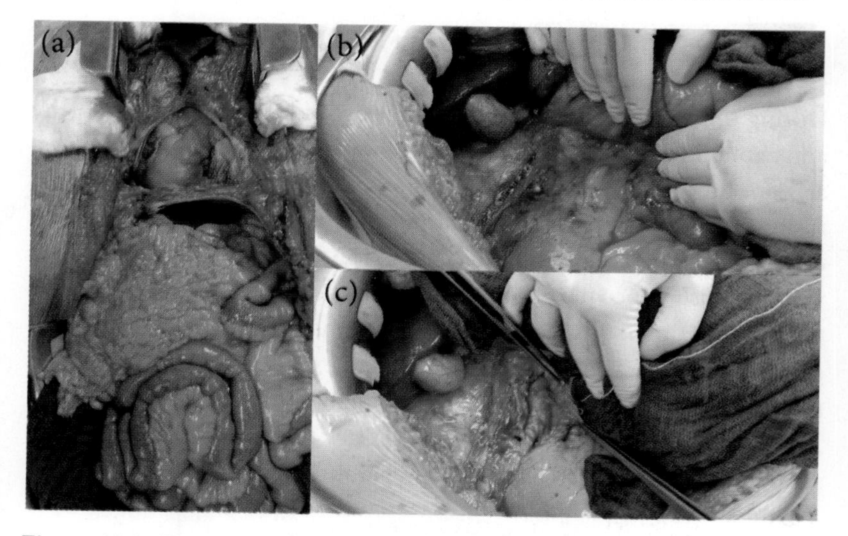

Figure 42.1. Exposure. Panel A. A wide median sterno-laparotomy usually allows good exposure. In difficult cases, median laparotomy can be extended by a transverse laparotomy to further enhance exposure. Panel B. Retroperitoneum is accessed by fully mobilizing right colon, duodenum, and by sectioning the mesenteric root. Abdominal viscera are lifted upwards, towards the head of the donor. Panel C. Infra-renal abdominal aorta is dissected. Inferior mesenteric artery is exposed by gently pulling the sigmoid colon root towards the left; this vessel can be tied to facilitate subsequent aortic cannulation and avoid unnecessary perfusion of the left colon, sigmoid and rectum

(IVC) are fully dissected up to the level of left renal vein and encircled for subsequent cannulation or ligation (Figure 42.2A). Celiac aorta is dissected and encircled through the right crus of the diaphragm, paying attention not to injure the oesophagus or the IVC (Figure 42.2B). Donor is then fully heparinized by 300 IU/kg of sodium heparin and a cannula having been purged from air is inserted into abdominal aorta (Figure 42.2C). IVC can be tied to avoid blood spillage from the inferior limbs.

At this point, chilled preservation solution bags are connected to the aortic cannula line and ice slush is set ready for use. Once everything is ready, the following actions must happen in rapid sequence: celiac aorta is clamped, cold perfusion is started, IVC is opened low in the abdomen

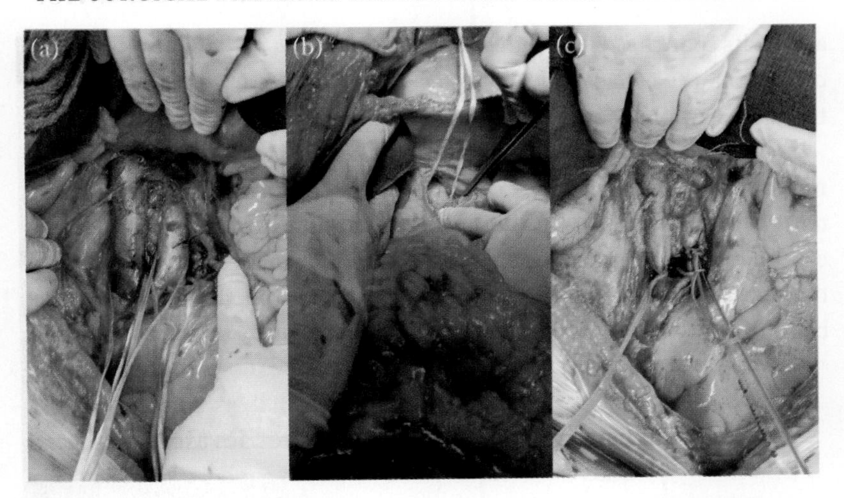

Figure 42.2. Abdominal vessels preparation during organ retrieval from a brain-dead donor: Panel A. Abdominal aorta and inferior vena cava have been dissected free and encircled with surgical tapes. Panel B. Coeliac aorta has been prepared and controlled for subsequent clamping, by opening right diaphragmatic crus. The assistant is pulling the oesophagus to the left, while the first operator is lifting upwards the left hepatic lobe. Inferior vena cava is visible under caudate lobe. Panel C. Aortic cannula has been placed and secured

and close to right atrium for venting, and abdomen is filled with ice slush. All previous manoeuvres have established a closed circuit in which abdominal organs are perfused through celiac trunk, superior mesenteric artery (SMA) and renal arteries, and vented through vena cava. By using this technique, portal vein is perfused by viscera effluent.

There are many technical variants to the reported technique, which can be applied according to centre practice or case peculiarities. For instance, celiac aorta is not the only site of clamping. In case of hemodynamic instability or difficult access to celiac region, aortic clamping in the thorax is a valuable alternative. Descending aorta can be easily accessed from the left thorax by sectioning mediastinal pleura above the diaphragm. Aortic pulsation can be easily located on the left side of the column and behind the oesophagus, which is identified with the presence of the naso-gastric tube in its lumen.

Regarding the cannulation site, iliac arteries can be used, in case, abdominal aorta is extensively calcified. If cannulation of abdominal aorta and of its branches is precluded, perfusion can be achieved by placing a cannula in the celiac or thoracic aorta, securing it by a purse string suture and clamping aorta above the cannula and at the iliac bifurcation.

Some studies have suggested that double aortic and portal perfusion might have some advantage over aortic-only perfusion, especially in extended criteria donors.[5,6] Portal perfusion is performed by placing a cannula in the inferior mesenteric vein below the Treitz ligament or in the portal vein through its posterior aspect at the hepatic pedicle, at the beginning of cold perfusion.

Second phase: Dissection and retrieval

Different techniques have been described to safely retrieve abdominal organs once they have been perfused, including en-bloc retrieval and subsequent back table separation.[7] Regardless of the chosen technique, the importance of quick organ retrieval cannot be overemphasized. Organ temperature persists far above the target 4°C value while organs are being dissected.[8,9] Together with the warm ischemia suffered during vascular anastomoses at implant, organ retrieval time has been associated with poorer outcome in liver and kidney transplantation, most likely due to the more severe damage determined by longer retrieval time.[10–13]

Liver and pancreas are usually retrieved first. The IVC is divided above renal veins outlet, leaving a suitable venous patch for kidney implant. Aorta is divided caudally to SMA orifice. As renal arteries are normally in close proximity, attention should be paid not to damage their aortic patch or accessory polar arteries. If pancreas is not retrieved for transplantation, it can partially or completely be retrieved together with the liver. In this case, pancreatic head is separated from the duodenum, ligating the bile duct distally close to the ampulla of Vater. The lesser omentum is dissected from the stomach and the mesenteric root sectioned distally to the pancreas. This technique is quick and, as any hepatic pedicle dissection is avoided, the risk of vascular injuries is particularly low. Furthermore, long vascular pedicles are retrieved, including spleno-mesenteric venous confluence and any possible aberrant hepatic artery. Obviously, it cannot be used if pancreas is to be transplanted. Liver dissection is completed by sectioning the diaphragm and the pericardium patch (including IVC outlet), sectioning the aorta above the clamp, and by dividing the liver from its posterior attachments following a plane that is posterior to IVC and aorta. Damage to the upper pole of the right kidney must be avoided during this phase.

Pancreas retrieval for whole organ transplantation increases substantially the degree of complexity of donor operation.[14] Due to its anatomy, pancreas is probably the most difficult organ to retrieve and the one that is most frequently damaged.[15] Systematic training has been associated with increased quality of procurement and increased utilization of pancreas grafts.[16] As pancreas is retrieved with a segment of duodenum, a povidone iodine solution can be injected through the nasogastric tube to decontaminate duodenum before the start of cold perfusion. The nasogastric tube is then retracted and the duodenum sectioned with two stapler charges next to the pylorus and at the Treitz angle. The pancreatic head and duodenum are freed from their attachments to the root of transverse mesocolon and hepatic colonic flexure. After section of the spleno-diaphragmatic ligament, the spleen and the pancreas body and tail are fully mobilized medially, following the avascular plane between Gerota's fascia and the pancreatic capsule. During this manoeuvre, injury to splenic vessels (especially, the splenic vein) must be carefully avoided.

From a vascular point of view, pancreas retrieval can be divided in three steps. The first step is the dissection of the hepatic pedicle, with identification of the bile duct, gastroduodenal artery, common and proper hepatic artery, splenic artery, and portal vein. The bile duct is divided close to the duodenum, to allow a maximum length for liver graft implant. Gastroduodenal and splenic arteries are divided close to their origin, leaving enough tissue to close their stumps. Splenic artery should be sectioned proximal to the outlet of dorsal pancreatic artery, in order to preserve arterial supply to pancreas body and neck. However, if dorsal pancreatic artery has to be sacrificed (as in the case of its origin from common hepatic artery), this does not preclude pancreas utilization, as intra-parenchymal anastomotic arcades normally provide collateral vascularization. Subsequently, portal vein is divided just above the level of the first pancreaticoduodenal vein. The second step is the section of middle colic vessels with ligatures or a stapler. The third and final step is the section of the mesenteric root distal to the origin of inferior pancreaticoduodenal vessels. Again, this can be achieved by ligatures or using a vascular stapler. Once all these steps have been completed, pancreas is separated from its posterior attachments and retrieved with the root of SMA and its aortic patch.

In case an aberrant right hepatic artery originating from the SMA is encountered, it is sectioned distal to the origin of the right hepatic artery. Depending on each centre practice, in a DBD donor, most of the aforementioned dissection can be carried out during the warm phase, which carries the advantage of a better haemostasis in the recipient at pancreas graft reperfusion. Once pancreas has been retrieved, a segment of iliac arteries, including internal-external iliac bifurcation, is also procured. It will be used for vascular inflow reconstruction during back table preparation, according to each centre revascularization technique.

Kidneys are usually the last organs to be retrieved. As supernumerary arteries and veins are very frequent, kidney retrieval technique should be adapted to avoid their accidental damage.[17] Polar arteries can originate from a wide area that goes from the level of SMA origin to the iliac arteries. They are terminal arteries and their damage determines an area of kidney hypoperfusion. Thus, they should ideally be retrieved with their aortic patch or with enough length to allow appropriate reconstruction. To do so, aorta is split medially and the trapezoid area between the medial aspect of the kidney, the ureter and aorta are retrieved en-bloc. This technique is also effective in preserving ureter blood supply. In presence of a normal anatomy, left renal vein is sectioned at its inlet into IVC and the segment of IVC is left with the right kidney, to allow lengthening of the right renal vein in case it is needed. Also supernumerary veins are very common, especially on the right side.[17] However, in contrast to renal arteries, intra-parenchymal collectors avoid venous congestion in case one vein is closed. This has to be evaluated on a case-per-case basis by the implanting surgeon. Finally, ureter is sectioned distally and each kidney is retrieved with its surrounding peri-renal fat, which will be removed after retrieval to rule out worrisome lesions having escaped in the pre-retrieval work-up. Ureter reduplication is also common.[17] Ureter anatomic variations include complete unilateral reduplication (two ureters draining separately into the bladder), incomplete unilateral reduplication (two ureters joining together in a common channel before draining into the bladder), and unilateral/bilateral crossed ureter (ureter draining on the opposite side of the bladder). Both ureters must be preserved; they

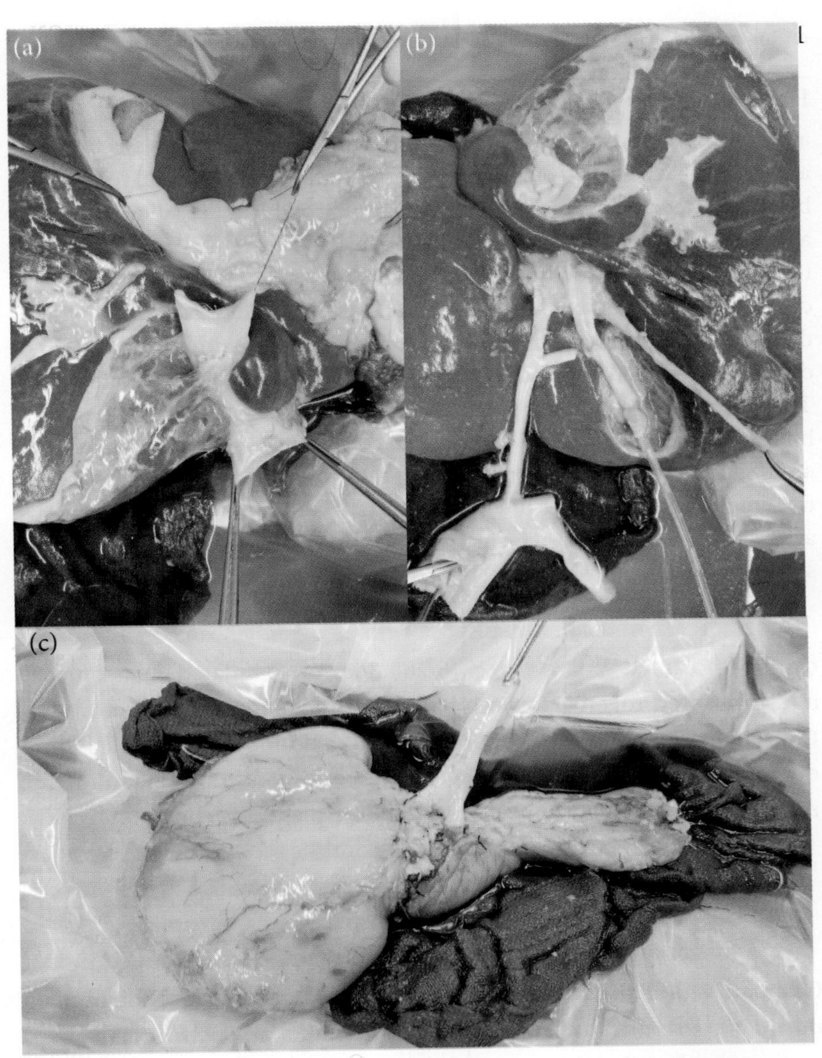

Figure 42.3. Liver and pancreas back-table preparation. Panel A. Retrohepatic inferior vena cava has been dissected free from diaphragm. Right adrenal, lumbar and diaphragmatic veins have been tied to avoid bleeding upon graft reperfusion. In this case, hepatocaval ligament (Makuuchi ligament) has been left intact, but it might be sectioned in case implantation by side-to-side cavo-cavostomy is going to be performed. Panel B. Elements of hepatic pedicle have been dissected. On the left side, celiac trunk and hepatic artery have been dissected up to hepatic artery bifurcation. Left gastric and splenic arteries have been tied, whereas the stump of gastroduodenal artery has been left open to allow flushing on backtable

(*continued*)

Figure 42.3 *Continued*

and before artery reperfusion on the recipient. During arterial dissection, attention must be paid to anatomic variants. In the middle, portal vein has been dissected and cannulated to allow flushing with chilled saline or 5% albumin solution before graft reperfusion. Splenic vein stump is left open to allow purging air from the circuit. On the right side, bile duct has been dissected, leaving its surrounding tissue close to the hilar plate intact to avoid damage to its frail blood supply. Gallbladder has been removed and cystic duct and artery tied. Panel C. Pancreas graft after back-table preparation. The spleen has been removed after selective ligation and section of splenic hilum vessels. Vascular inflow has been reconstructed using a Y donor iliac artery jump graft. Usually, external iliac artery is anastomosed to the superior mesenteric artery, whereas internal iliac artery is anastomosed to splenic artery. Gastroduodenal artery, inferior mesenteric vein and bile duct must be securely tied. During dissection, pancreatic capsule injury must be avoided.

can be implanted separately on the bladder or spatulated, anastomosed and implanted together on the bladder. Other kidney anatomic variations, like horseshoe kidney, pelvic (pancake) kidney and ectopic kidney do not necessarily preclude retrieval and subsequent transplantation, but requires careful evaluation by an expert transplant surgeon.

Back table preparation

Once arrived at the transplant centre, organs are prepared for implant during the so-called back table surgery. Liver and kidney back table preparation is rather straightforward and entails isolation of vascular pedicles, reconstruction of aberrant arteries, and preparation of bile duct and ureter. All collaterals that could cause bleeding upon reperfusion are identified and ligated (Figure 42.3 A and 3B). It is important to avoid excessive dissection of both bile duct and ureter, not to compromise their vascular supply.

Compared to liver and kidney, pancreas back table preparation is more demanding. Spleen is detached from pancreas tail by ligating all branches of splenic vessels. Duodenal stumps are oversewn. After having verified the integrity of inferior pancreaticoduodenal arteries by a perfusion test, gastroduodenal artery is ligated. Vascular inflow is created by anastomosis of donor iliac Y graft to splenic artery and SMA (Figure 42.3C). During pancreas preparation, it is of paramount importance to ligate all apparent arterial and venous branches (including inferior mesenteric vein) that could cause significant bleeding at graft reperfusion.

Conclusion

Organ retrieval in a donor after brain death is a surgical operation aimed at effectively perfusing organs with a preservation solution at low temperature, allowing their preservation until implantation into the recipient. Although several technical variants exist, basic principles remain constant across transplant units worldwide. Whichever the technique, frequent anatomical variations have to be taken into account to avoid retrieval-related injuries, possibly jeopardizing organ utilization and negatively impacting outcome in the recipient.

Highlights

- Standard organ preservation starts with *in situ* cooling and perfusion with preservation solution.
- Perfusion with preservation solution is most frequently achieved by cannulation of abdominal aorta.
- Aim of abdominal organs retrieval is the procurement of intact organs with preserved vascular pedicles and drainage, suitable for subsequent implant.
- Despite several technical variants, understanding of basic principles of ischemia-reperfusion injury and their implications is of paramount importance to achieve effective organ preservation.
- Detailed knowledge of anatomy, appropriate surgical technique and coordinated teamwork are the keys to effective organ retrieval.

References

1. Belzer FO, Ashby BS, Dunphy JE. 24-hour and 72-hour preservation of canine kidneys. Lancet. 1967;2(7515):536–538.

2. Calne RY, Pegg DE, Pryse-Davies J, Brown FL. Renal preservation by ice-cooling: An experimental study relating to kidney transplantation from cadavers. Br Med J. 1963;2(5358):651–655.
3. Collins GM, Bravo-Shugarman M, Terasaki PI, Braf Z, Sheil AG, Williams G. Kidney preservation for transportation. IV. Eight-thousand-mile international air transport. Aust N Z J Surg. 1970;40(2):195–197.
4. Rosenthal JT, Shaw BW, Jr., Hardesty RL, Griffith BP, Starzl TE, Hakala TR. Principles of multiple organ procurement from cadaver donors. Ann Surg. 1983;198(5):617–621.
5. D'Amico F, Vitale A, Gringeri E, Valmasoni M, Carraro A, Brolese A, et al. Liver transplantation using suboptimal grafts: Impact of donor harvesting technique. Liver Transpl. 2007;13(10):1444–1450.
6. Ghinolfi D, Tincani G, Rreka E, Roffi N, Coletti L, Balzano E, et al. Dual aortic and portal perfusion at procurement prevents ischaemic-type biliary lesions in liver transplantation when using octogenarian donors: A retrospective cohort study. Transpl Int. 2019;32(2):193–205.
7. Boggi U, Vistoli F, Del Chiaro M, Signori S, Pietrabissa A, Costa A, et al. A simplified technique for the en bloc procurement of abdominal organs that is suitable for pancreas and small-bowel transplantation. Surgery. 2004;135(6):629–641.
8. Hertl M, Howard TK, Lowell JA, Shenoy S, Robert P, Harvey C, et al. Changes in liver core temperature during preservation and rewarming in human and porcine liver allografts. Liver Transpl Surg. 1996;2(2):111–117.
9. Villa R, Fondevila C, Erill I, Guimera A, Bombuy E, Gomez-Suarez C, et al. Real-time direct measurement of human liver allograft temperature from recovery to transplantation. Transplantation. 2006;81(3):483–486.
10. Heylen L, Pirenne J, Samuel U, Tieken I, Naesens M, Sprangers B, et al. The impact of anastomosis time during kidney transplantation on graft loss: A Eurotransplant Cohort Study. Am J Transplant. 2017;17(3):724–732.
11. Jochmans I, Fieuws S, Tieken I, Samuel U, Pirenne J. The impact of implantation time during liver transplantation on outcome: A Eurotransplant Cohort Study. Transplant Direct. 2018;4(6):e356.
12. Jochmans I, Fieuws S, Tieken I, Samuel U, Pirenne J. The impact of hepatectomy time of the liver graft on post-transplant outcome: A Eurotransplant Cohort Study. Ann Surg. 2019;269(4):712–717.
13. Weissenbacher A, Oberhuber R, Cardini B, Weiss S, Ulmer H, Bosmuller C, et al. The faster the better: Anastomosis time influences patient survival after deceased donor kidney transplantation. Transpl Int. 2015;28(5):535–543.
14. Fridell JA, Powelson JA, Kubal CA, Burke GW, Sageshima J, Rogers J, et al. Retrieval of the pancreas allograft for whole-organ transplantation. Clin Transplant. 2014;28(12):1313–1330.
15. Ausania F, Drage M, Manas D, Callaghan CJ. A registry analysis of damage to the deceased donor pancreas during procurement. Am J Transplant. 2015;15(11):2955–2962.
16. Lam HD, Schaapherder AF, Kopp WH, Putter H, Braat AE, Baranski AG. Professionalization of surgical abdominal organ recovery leading to an increase in pancreatic allografts accepted for transplantation in the Netherlands: A serial analysis. Transpl Int. 2017;30(2):117–123.
17. Watson CJ, Harper SJ. Anatomical variation and its management in transplantation. Am J Transplant. 2015;15(6):1459–1471.

43

Anaesthesiological management of organ retrieval

Paolo Feltracco, Cristiana Carollo, Stefania Barbieri

Introduction

Organ retrieval from deceased donors began in the early 1960s, when a definition of brain death based on neurological criteria, improved organ preservation techniques, and the introduction of cyclosporine made solid organ transplantation feasible and the only effective therapy for end-stage organ failure—as is often still the case today. The first successful kidney transplant between siblings dates back to 1954, while the first successful kidney, lung, and liver transplants using organs retrieved from deceased donors were performed in 1963.(1) Apart from the now well-established practice of solid organ transplantation, composite tissue allotransplantation—or vascularized composite allotransplantation (VCA)—has been gaining acceptance in recent years as a solution for complex reconstructions.(2) Up to eleven organs (including the heart, lung, liver, kidneys, pancreas, intestine, face, upper extremities, musculoskeletal tissue, and saphenous veins from the lower extremities) have been recovered from a single deceased donor, as explained in the report on the largest procurement procedure completed to date.(3) However, even though much attention is paid to increasing the number of organs retrieved from a single donor, organ donation rates remain insufficient to cover the demand, as the number of patients requiring organ transplants continues to grow. The persistent shortage of grafts for transplantation has encouraged many countries to introduce (or reintroduce) organ donation after circulatory death (DCD), which has also been extended to organs with a lower tolerance of warm ischemia such as the liver, pancreas, and lungs. Given the importance of every donated organ, it is imperative for donors to be actively treated not only from the moment brain death is declared, but also throughout the organ retrieval procedure. Active management can optimize the donor's organ perfusion, maintain endocrine homeostasis, and protect weak organs. Poor management of brain-dead patients scheduled for organ donation reduces the number of organs that can be procured successfully and impairs their overall quality.(4) This is particularly true in a situation where organs from elderly donors, 'marginal or extended criteria' donors, and medically unstable donors with a suboptimal organ function are being recovered increasingly.(5) Because of the more or less recognized multiple comorbidities of some donors, ensuring proper 'anaesthesiological management' during organ retrieval becomes crucial to ensure the viability of all transplantable organs. One inadequately treated and dysfunctional organ can affect the functioning and outcome of other salvageable organs. For instance, the differences between the physiological issues involved in treating autonomic storms at the time of brain death at the intensive care unit (ICU) and those arising during the organ-harvesting procedure have to be considered.(6) When it is essential to optimally preserve multiple organs, we also have to bear in mind that some treatments to improve the functioning of one organ may damage the functioning of others. For instance, renal perfusion may require fluid loading while excessive hydration should be avoided for a lung transplant.(7) It is common knowledge that the quality of the donor patients' management during organ-harvesting surgery can greatly affect organ function and the recipient's prognosis.(8) In this setting, the main goal of the anaesthetist is not only to meet the specific hemodynamic and metabolic needs of the organs being retrieved (which is essential to the proper care of all organs), but also to manage the requests of different organ procurement teams. Most of the currently available literature on donor management focuses primarily on the action recommended during and after the declaration of brain death at the ICU, however, dwelling only marginally on the subsequent organ-harvesting procedure.

From the ICU to the operating room for organ retrieval

Before donors are moved from the ICU to the operating room (OR) for organ procurement, the ICU staff should try to give families as much time as possible at their loved one's bedside. In line with local hospital policies, and to comply with some families' wishes, relatives, and close friends are allowed to accompany brain-dead donors to the OR door. In the case of DCD, the family should be allowed to stay in the OR suite after the withdrawal of life support and up until cardiac death is declared. The family's comfort and end-of-life observances should be adequately facilitated.

Any clinical or ethical issues—such as those deriving from the stressful and emotional response of parents being separated from the paediatric donors, a lack of familiarity with the appropriate methods for communicating with donors' families, the need to transmit a positive attitude of the donation procedure to other members of staff, the awareness of the considerable workload involved in multiple organ harvesting, and the specific organizational requirements for donors after brain or cardiac death—should all be adequately managed prior to the donation procedure by the anaesthesiological staff involved.(9) Every effort should be made to preserve the function of perfusible organs after the donor's discharge from the ICU and until the moment of organ removal. Donors often depend on high doses of inotropes and/or vasopressors, in which case frank deterioration is likely, and even expected, making it urgent to proceed. Care should be taken to avoid interruptions or pauses in the infusion of fluids and drugs. In transit from the ICU to the OR, portable mechanical ventilators (on the same settings as in the ICU) are preferable to manual Ambu bag ventilation to guarantee a satisfactory gas exchange. In the case of donors with major lung disease or trauma, temporary disconnection from the ventilator may require adequate recruitment manoeuvres before or after re-starting with the previous ventilatory setting. The organ retrieval procedure can take hours to complete, and active donor management should continue until all organs have been procured.(10) Anaesthesiologists have an important role in ensuring a calm working atmosphere, where mutual cooperation among the various harvesting teams will ensure that all organs are considered equally important and receive the same amount of care to enhance their chances of survival outside the donor. Excellent communication is essential to coordinate manoeuvres such as vessel clamping, disconnecting ventilation, keeping the lung inflated, pulling out lines, administering fluids, heparin or cold preservative solutions, and so on. At the end of the harvesting procedure, proper care of the donor's body is also mandatory, as a sign of well-deserved respect for the patient's dignity.

Anaesthesia for organ procurement

The idea of providing anaesthesia for neurologically-deceased donors (NDDs) has been a matter of debate, as the common practice of using volatile agents and/or opioids for their 'anaesthetic' effect is theoretically based on the assumption that these substances are needed to prevent a patient from being aware of an unpleasant stimulus. The distinction between conscious awareness and reflex response should be perfectly clear to members of the medical profession. Before brain death can be diagnosed, all sedatives have to be stopped to ensure that their effects are not mimicking some of the signs of brain death. It consequently seems odd, after a doctor has stopped a patient's sedation to confirm that they are brain dead, that someone else should restore analgosedation again once the body is on the operating table. Having established that cerebral activity is irrelevant (i.e. absent) in a case of brainstem death, the concept of 'general anaesthesia' may be misleading, and potentially disturbing for the general public.[11] On the other hand, while there is a strong conviction that no analgesia or anaesthesia to prevent awareness or pain is needed to harvest organs from a brainstem-dead donor, it is advisable to routinely administer neuromuscular blocking agents and other drugs, so as to avoid excessive cardiovascular 'activation', and to prevent muscle contraction and hypertension/tachycardia.

Neuromuscular blocking drugs should be given only at the start of the organ retrieval procedure to avoid spinal reflex muscle movements being evoked by extensive surgical retraction. The neuromuscular activity observable may range from minimal muscle twitching to complex movements of the limbs and trunk. These spontaneous movements of the arms and hands towards the body are known as the Lazarus sign. Marked spinal reflexes, with reflex hemodynamic responses to nociceptive stimulation, have been observed in brain-dead patients, and some cardiovascular changes are known to be generated at spinal cord level alone. Spinal reflexes may increase plasma catecholamine concentrations, and hypertension and tachycardia may occur either spontaneously or on surgical stimulus.[11] Tachycardia and hypertension, and/or reflex body movements occurring during organ retrieval can be dangerous for the organs involved because, in a sense, they are the indirect sign of an organism in distress (albeit due to stimuli at spinal level alone), and they can also be distressing for OR personnel to witness. The intraoperative hyperdynamic response, manifesting with an initial rise in heart rate and blood pressure on surgical stimulation (mimicking a pain response), can be attenuated with short-acting opioids or a short-acting beta-blocker.

Reducing or stopping vasopressor infusions is obviously the first action taken to treat these episodes. A reasonable goal is to keep the mean arterial pressure (MAP) below 90 mmHg, but above 65–70 mmHg. Other drugs commonly used to prevent and treat intraoperative reflex tachycardia and hypertension include labetalol and esmolol, or nicardipine, nitroprusside, nitroglycerin, and urapidil in the event of hypertension alone. Volatile anaesthetic agents are also widely used to control any persistent autonomic or sympathetic storms (which raise blood pressure), or a 'dysregulated' hyperactivation of systemic vascular resistance.(12) All such gases share the side effect of causing dose-dependent hypotension via peripheral vasodilation. This phenomenon is easy to start, stop, and titrate; so anaesthetic gases are often the first-line agents used to control hypertension during organ harvesting procedures. It has been claimed that inhalational anaesthetics can reduce catecholamine release, which may occur with surgical stimulation. It has also been suggested that volatile anaesthetic exposure can elicit a delayed window of protection by virtue of an ischemic preconditioning mechanism.(13,14) Benefits of preconditioning with volatile anaesthetics have also been observed in terms of protecting the tissues against ischemia-reperfusion damage during various cardiac surgical procedures.(15,16) Beyond the myocardium, a clinically relevant protective effect of anaesthetic ischemic preconditioning has also reportedly involved a variety of non-cardiac tissues too.(17) Although published data on the use of volatile anaesthetic gases in organ donors is limited, many anaesthesiologists believe that these agents have a place among the pharmacological strategies for preconditioning donated organs.(18)

As for mechanical ventilation during organ retrieval procedures, the donor's lungs should be ventilated using the same settings as in the ICU.(19) To maintain tissue oxygenation and protect the lungs for transplantation, low tidal volume ventilation is recommended with a minimum FiO_2 to ensure Hb oxygen saturation >95%, and positive end expiratory pressure (PEEP) >5 cmH_2O. This is also known as lung protective ventilation. If necessary, PEEP can be raised to 8–10 cm H_2O to prevent lung unit de-recruitment. Limiting the tidal volume to 5–6 ml/kg of the ideal body weight, and the plateau pressure to 30 cm H_2O seems to reduce ventilator-induced lung injury.[20,21] Endotracheal suctioning may be needed to remove bronchial secretions, but intermittent disconnection of the ventilator necessitates re-recruitment manoeuvres. When lung harvesting is planned, careful attention to distal bronchial toilette, 'gentle' protective mechanical ventilation, frequent recruitment manoeuvres, maintenance of the plateau airway pressure below 25 cmH_2O, and use of the minimum FiO_2 sufficient to raise the donor's saturation to 98% can certainly help in preserving the lung. A PaO_2/FiO_2 of more than 300 is desirable. Asystole will occur after aortic cross clamping, but gentle ventilation should continue until the lungs have been explanted. A maximum tidal volume inspiration should be administered immediately before stapling across the trachea.

Severe intraoperative hypoxemia may occur as a consequence of previous infectious lung disease, acute respiratory distress syndrome, lung trauma, excessive fluid load, congestive heart failure, or pulmonary oedema. The persistence of neurogenic pulmonary oedema, which can occur after central nervous system insult with no underlying cardiovascular or respiratory disease, should also be considered among the various possible causes of intraoperative gas exchange derangement. Severe hypoxia can threaten organ preservation, and every effort should be made to prevent and treat it. Choosing 'more aggressive' mechanical ventilation may sometimes help to overcome a critical intraoperative period of severe oxygen desaturation. A very high FiO_2 and repeated recruitment manoeuvres may be needed, and higher levels of PEEP should be used immediately after these manoeuvres to prevent loss of alveolar recruitment. Nitric oxide insufflation has also been reported to improve severe hypoxia during organ harvesting.[22]

Intraoperative metabolic disturbances

Although treating brain-dead donors with thyroid hormone, glucocorticoids, vasopressin, and insulin may increase organ donation rates and improve graft and recipient survival, the need for combining various drugs with vasoactive medication may also be associated with metabolic disorders. The use of supportive measures to treat hyperglycaemia, electrolyte, and acid-base abnormalities in the same way as at the ICU is also recommended throughout the organ procurement procedure. Hypokalaemia and low calcium and magnesium levels need to be corrected. Preoperative hypernatremia is detrimental to the donor's organs (especially the liver), and should not be exacerbated during harvesting.

Hemodynamic changes associated with surgery

A multiple-organ donation involves extending a midline laparotomy with a sternotomy, even if no thoracic organs are to be retrieved. This is considered a major surgical procedure, carrying the possibility of substantial blood loss and physiological derangements. Surgical manipulations can cause cardiovascular instability, and great attention should be paid to potentially aggressive manipulations of the major organs (e.g. heart, liver, and lung), which can be associated with significant hypotension.[4] The aims of anaesthesiological management in this respect are to maintain cardiovascular stability and optimal oxygen delivery. This not only helps to ensure optimal organ perfusion and cellular oxygenation, but also allows an unhurried removal of organs in favourable, unharmed conditions. Administering appropriate fluids and vasoactive medication, as well as correcting acid-base and electrolyte disorders, will contribute to reducing early postoperative dysfunction due to ischemic injury.

Assessing the volemic status and fluid responsiveness can prove difficult, especially in donors with circulatory instability not submitted to advanced hemodynamic monitoring (as is often the case). Subclinical hypovolemia due to the trauma, or more commonly due to diabetes insipidus, often becomes apparent at the time of laparotomy, and may be aggravated by the fluid shifts that occur during thoracic and abdominal incisions. Evaporative losses while organs are exposed for lengthy periods of time also contribute to hypovolemia. If intravenous fluids are crucially important to avoid cardiovascular problems and maintain hemodynamic stability, anaesthesiologists should always bear in mind that while moderate amounts of fluids may be acceptable, or even necessary, to maintain a satisfactory liver and kidney perfusion, they may also be damaging to 'sensitive' organs such as the lungs and pancreas.[23,24] Avoiding excessive fluid loading in donor management and during harvesting has been found to increase the numbers of transplantable lungs obtained.[25,26] Vasopressors are generally needed to counteract the vasoplegic effects of brainstem death, but they have to be infused judiciously so as to improve organ perfusion without risking an excessive vasoconstriction and reduction of the blood flow to the organs.[27]

Donors are unlikely to have undergone pulmonary artery catheterization, oesophageal Doppler, continuous cardiac output measurement by pulse contour analysis, or other transpulmonary thermodilution measurements while in the ICU. To assess their heart and volemic status intraoperatively, transoesophageal echocardiography (TEE) is a valuable option, preferred by most heart transplant teams. In unstable donors, TEE enables an assessment of global and regional cardiac performance, and the condition of the valves. The TEE-guided fluid infusion and arterial waveform pulse pressure variation measurements, targeting a Central Venous Pressure of around 6–10 mm of Hg, and central venous oxygen saturation monitoring, are among the methods that may contribute to achieving the appropriate cardiovascular goals.[28,29] The 'rule of 100s' (systolic blood pressure >100 mmHg, urine output >100 ml/hr, PaO_2 >100 mmHg, haemoglobin>100 gm/L) was first proposed many years ago, but is still considered valid by many organ harvesting teams.[30]

There is no evidence to suggest that any specific fluid offers particular advantages in restoring intravascular volemia. The choice of fluid may depend on whether or not the lungs are to be harvested. Lung graft retrieval requires higher PaO_2 values, and an optimal management of myocardial function and intrathoracic volemia (a crucial strategy for preventing lung interstitial congestion). If the lungs are to be harvested, balanced crystalloids plus albumin solutions are preferred in an attempt to prevent lung interstitial fluid accumulation and keep the lung parenchyma intact. The rationale for administering albumin solutions is to promote fluid reabsorption from the interstitial space in an attempt to maintain the oncotic pressure in the capillaries and the fluids in the vascular system for a longer time. However, the protection offered by albumin solutions against interstitial overload can only be moderately effective following the administration of large volumes, and the high sodium content of albumin-based solutions should also be borne in mind.[31]

Crystalloids may be used, preferably in a balanced salt solution, for abdominal organ retrieval. Balanced solutions are recommended when large volumes are necessary. In fact, the infusion of large amounts of 0.9% sodium chloride can lead to the onset of hyperchloremic metabolic acidosis. Artificial colloids seem to offer few or no advantages, even in the case of severe hypovolemia, but one recent study found donor fluid therapy including colloids beneficial for the kidney graft.(32) In today's clinical practice, the use of starches has been abandoned due to concerns about the potential impairment of kidney function with starch-based colloids.(33,34) During fluid resuscitation, it is always important to avoid overhydration: in unstable donors, it can be associated with excessive cardiac chamber distension, pulmonary oedema, liver congestion, diffuse interstitial accumulation, and a possible decline in cell viability during cold storage.

Abdominal and thoracic organ retrieval is often associated with significant bleeding. Blood and blood products should be transfused according to the severity of anaemia and ongoing losses. An insufficient blood oxygen content and oxygen delivery may be detrimental to organ recovery. Hypotensive episodes are frequent during multiple-organ harvesting. They are related to surgical manipulations and can involve a reduced venous return, persistently impaired vasomotor control mechanisms, endocrine abnormalities, blood loss, and fluid shifts, diabetes insipidus, osmotic diuresis due to hyperglycaemia, and left ventricular dysfunction.

Treating hypotension is crucial to organ perfusion and can greatly affect the quality and success of transplants. Inotropes and vasopressors are the mainstay of treatment once a satisfactory volemia has been restored. Dopamine is usually regarded as the starting drug. At low doses (3–5 mcg/kg/min), dopamine improves myocardial function and causes a modest dilation of the renal, mesenteric, and coronary artery vascular beds. At higher infusion rates, it loses its vasodilatory effects and may cause vasoconstriction, and it may be pro-arrhythmogenic. One advantage of using dopamine during organ retrieval procedures derives from its capacity to stimulate the induction of heme-oxygenase-1 and other enzymes responsible for protecting organs against ischemia/reperfusion (I/R) and inflammatory injury.(35) Dobutamine is another potent inotrope. It has the effect of increasing cardiac output, possibly resulting in an increased organ blood flow. Dobutamine infusion alone may not suffice to raise blood pressure in the presence of hypovolemia, however, because its effect on peripheral vasodilation prevails over its effect on cardiac output.

A sustained increase in vascular tone is sometimes needed to treat hypotension and improve cardiovascular function in vasoplegic unresponsive brain-dead donors during organ harvesting surgery. The use of vasopressors during organ retrieval is always a debated issue because vasoconstriction may, theoretically, reduce blood flow to vital organs. As regards to organ function, however, even in the long term, it seems that the graft damage caused by insufficient organ perfusion and oxygen delivery may outweigh the risks associated with using vasoactive agents. If hypotension does not resolve with proper fluid resuscitation, vasopressor infusion is needed to achieve the recommended cardiovascular goals, i.e. a systolic blood pressure >100 mmHg, and a MAP >65–70 mmHg (higher values are preferable in elderly donors).[36] Vasopressin or norepinephrine infusion usually suffices to achieve a hemodynamic recovery and improve blood flow. Besides minimizing volume losses due to diabetes insipidus, vasopressin can also reduce the amount of catecholamines needed to achieve the target blood pressure.[37] Large doses of alpha-adrenergic agonists to improve oxygen delivery should be avoided because they can be associated with adverse effects on thoracic organ function. Previous and recent studies have demonstrated a close relationship between high doses of norepinephrine in donors and higher rates of initial cardiac dysfunction, a worse right ventricle performance, and higher early and late mortality in organ recipients.[38,39] In a report from Mukadam et al.,[40] using high doses of dopamine, epinephrine, or norepinephrine was associated with a worse gas exchange after lung transplantation.

Intraoperative arrhythmias

Many factors can be responsible for atrial, and ventricular arrhythmias and conduction defects in organ donors, including an increased intracranial pressure, blood gas disorders, electrolyte abnormalities, hypo- or hypertension, myocardial ischemia and injury, hypothermia, infusion of cardioactive drugs, and myocardial manipulations. Bradycardia in the brain dead is often resistant to atropine, and a direct-acting beta-agonist is the drug of choice. Lidocaine, amiodarone, and other antiarrhythmic drugs should be readily available in the OR, in addition to cardiac resuscitation devices and pacers. Serious arrhythmias proving resistant to therapy, and heavily affecting hemodynamics demand immediate cardiopulmonary resuscitation, especially if the donor is already in the OR and organ retrieval can be completed within a reasonably short period of time. Besides the heart, other organs may still be suitable for transplantation if organ perfusion can be achieved with open-chest cardiac massage.

Preventing hypothermia

Although cold preservation is an integral part of organ storage, and the active rapid cooling of organs prior to circulatory arrest seems to improve organ viability, manoeuvres to maintain a core temperature above 34°C need to be applied in the OR. This is because a significant drop in body temperature before and during organ retrieval can precipitate bradycardia and arrhythmic episodes, limit cardiac contractility, impair coagulation status, and induce electrolyte abnormalities. Disrupted hypothalamic thermoregulation (poikilothermia), combined with exposure of the abdominal and thoracic cavities, fluid shifts and blood loss, are usually responsible for the onset of hypothermia. Active warming with heating blankets, a gas heater/humidifier, and fluid warmers for all intravenous infusions, is usually recommended to attenuate the often-inexorable thermal loss.

Intraoperative oliguria/anuria

Although perioperative polyuria is quite common due to diabetes insipidus, a marked reduction in urinary output may also occur as a result of hemodynamic derangement, bleeding, fluid shift, evaporative losses, hypotension, and/or unrecognized hypovolemia. Renal dysfunction may also be due to previous trauma, myoglobinuria, renal ischemia, nephrotoxic substances, and antibiotics. Restoring an effective volemia and arterial pressure, combined with low-dose dopamine and/or diuretics, can usually facilitate an appropriate increase in diuresis.

Coagulopathy

Although frank coagulopathy is unusual, the occurrence of important intraoperative coagulation disorders can raise the risk of hemodynamic decompensation and seriously affect the stability of anaesthesia conduction.[41] Causes of coagulopathy include hypothermia, metabolic acidosis, adverse effects of multiple transfusions for trauma, the release of plasminogen activator and thromboplastin from injured tissues and brain death, and the effects of catecholamines on platelet function. These conditions can occasionally lead to a disseminated intravascular coagulopathy.[42,43] Active bleeding demands the prompt correction of coagulation defects with red blood cells, clotting factors, and platelets. The risk of irreversible hemodynamic derangement demands accelerated harvesting procedures in the event of coagulopathy-induced severe bleeding.

Conclusion

The organ retrieval process poses anaesthetists with the challenge of a complex and unusual surgical procedure in a donor with significant physiological derangements. The intensity of the anaesthetists' involvement depends essentially on the clinical conditions of the donor, the amount of cardiovascular support, and the bleeding diathesis. Appropriate donor management is essential to maximize the quality of the organs procured, and ultimately prevent early graft dysfunction in the recipient. Close cooperation between staff at the ICU and OR is extremely important to understand and deal with the pathophysiology of the changes that occur after brain death or circulatory death. Applying the most effective intraoperative management strategies to ensure a good perfusion to relevant organs can definitely influence transplant outcomes. Appropriate planning and a good coordination between all the organ procurement teams enable multiple organs and VCA transplants to be completed safely and successfully, with worthwhile long-term results. Donor management physicians, anaesthesiologists and other members of the organ retrieval team should aim not only to improve the use and survival of suitable organs, but also offer reassurance and show gratitude to donors' families, and demonstrate to the general public that donating the organs of a deceased loved one reduces the number of patients dying while on the waiting list, and the amount of time they have to wait for an organ transplant.

Highlights

- The procedure of organ retrieval poses anaesthetists with the challenge of a complex and 'unusual' surgical procedure in a donor with significant physiological derangements.
- Every effort should be made to preserve the function of perfusible organs after the donor's discharge from the ICU and until the moment of all organ removal.
- Active intraoperative donor management results are crucial to optimise donor's organ perfusion and viability, maintain metabolic homeostasis, and protect weak organs.
- It is advisable to routinely administer neuromuscular blocking agents and other drugs, in order to avoid excessive cardiovascular 'activation', and to prevent reflex muscle contraction.
- To maintain tissue oxygenation and protect the lungs for transplantation, protective ventilation and recruitment manoeuvres are recommended.
- Ensuring proper anaesthesia particularly benefits elderly donors, 'marginal or extended criteria' donors, and medically unstable donors with a suboptimal organ function.

References

1. Calner R. Essay: History of transplantation. The Lancet. December 2006;368(1): S51–S52.
2. Kueckelhaus M, Fischer S, Seyda M, et al. Vascularized composite allotransplantation: Current standards and novel approaches to prevent acute rejection and chronic allograft deterioration. Transpl Int. 2016;29(6):655–662.
3. Tullius SG, Pomahac B, Kim HB, et al. Successful recovery and transplantation of 11 organs including face, bilateral upper extremities, and thoracic and abdominal organs from a single deceased organ donor. Transplantation. 2016;100(10):2226–2229.
4. Anderson TA, Bekker P, Vagefi PA. Anesthetic considerations in organ procurement surgery: A narrative review. Can J Anaesth. 2015;62(5):529–539.
5. Feng S, Lai JC. Expanded criteria donors. Clin Liver Dis. 2014;18(3):633–649.

6. Smith M. Physiologic changes during brain stem death—lessons for management of the organ donor. J Heart Lung Transplant. 2004;23(9 Suppl):S217–S222.
7. Miñambres E, Rodrigo E, Ballesteros MA, et al. Impact of restrictive fluid balance focused to increase lung procurement on renal function after kidney transplantation. Nephrol Dial Transplant. 2010;25(7):2352–2356.
8. Boutin C, Vachiéry-Lahaye F, Alonso S, et al. Anaesthetic management of brain-dead for organ donation: Impact on delayed graft function after kidney transplantation. Ann Fr Anesth Reanim. 2012;31(5):427–436.
9. Van Norman GA. Another matter of life and death: What every anesthesiologist should know about the ethical, legal, and policy implications of the non-heart-beating cadaver organ donor. Anesthesiology. 2003;98(3):763–773.
10. Xia VW, Braunfeld M. Anesthesia management of organ donors. Anesthesiol Clin. 2017;35(3):395–406.
11. Young PJ, Matta BF. Anaesthesia for organ donation in the brainstem dead—why bother? Anaesthesia. 2000;55(2):105–106.
12. Karmanian, AL. 'Intraoperative blood pressure and effect of volatile anesthetic in brain dead organ donors. College of Science and Health Theses and Dissertations. 2017;216:1–48. https://via.library.depaul.edu/csh_etd/216
13. Beck-Schimmer B, Breitenstein S, Urech S, et al. A randomized controlled trial on pharmacological preconditioning in liver surgery using a volatile anesthetic. Ann Surg. 2008;248(6):909–918.
14. Minguet G, Joris J, Lamy M. Preconditioning and protection against ischaemia-reperfusion in non-cardiac organs: A place for volatile anaesthetics? Eur J Anaesthesiol. 2007;24(9):733–745.
15. Sergeev P, da Silva R, Lucchinetti E,et al. Trigger-dependent gene expression profiles in cardiac preconditioning: Evidence for distinct genetic programs in ischemic and anesthetic preconditioning. Anesthesiology. 2004;100(3):474–488.
16. Tanaka K, Ludwig LM, Krolikowski JG, et al. Isoflurane produces delayed preconditioning against myocardial ischemia and reperfusion injury: Role of cyclooxygenase-2. Anesthesiology. 2004;100(3):525–531.
17. Minguet G, Joris J, Lamy M. Preconditioning and protection against ischaemia-reperfusion in non-cardiac organs: A place for volatile anaesthetics? Eur J Anaesthesiol. 2007;24(9):733–745.
18. Minou AF, Dzyadzko AM, Shcherba AE, Rummo O. The influence of pharmacological preconditioning with sevoflurane on incidence of early allograft dysfunction in liver transplant recipients. Anesthesiol Res Pract. 2012; 2012:930487.
19. Bansal R, Esan A, Hess D, et al Mechanical ventilatory support in potential lung donor patients. Chest. 2014;146(1):220–227.
20. Mascia L, Pasero D, Slutsky AS, et al. Effect of a lung protective strategy for organ donors on eligibility and availability of lungs for transplantation: A randomized controlled trial. JAMA. 2010;304(23):2620–2627.
21. Wood KE, Becker BN, McCartney JG, D'Alessandro AM, Coursin DB. Care of the potential organ donor. N Engl J Med. 2004 Dec 23;351(26):2730–2739. PMID: 15616207.
22. Park ES, Son HW, Lee AR, et al. Inhaled nitric oxide for the brain dead donor with neurogenic pulmonary edema during anesthesia for organ donation: A case report. Korean J Anesthesiol. 2014;67(2):133–138.

23. Angel LF, Levine DJ, Restrepo MI, et al . Impact of a lung transplantation donor-management protocol on lung donation and recipient outcomes. Am J Respir Crit Care Med. 2006;174(6):710–716.
24. Pennefather SH, Bullock RE, Dark JH. The effect of fluid therapy on alveolar arterial oxygen gradient in brain-dead organ donors. Transplantation. 1993;56(6):1418–1422.
25. Fanelli V, Mascia L. Anesthetic optimization for nonheartbeating donors. Curr Opin Anaesthesiol. 2010;23(3):406–410.
26. Miñambres E, Rodrigo E, Ballesteros MA, et al. Impact of restrictive fluid balance focused to increase lung procurement on renal function after kidney transplantation. Nephrol Dial Transplant. 2010;25(7):2352–2356.
27. Belzberg H, Shoemaker WC, Wo CC, et al. Hemodynamic and oxygen transport patterns after head trauma and brain death: Implications for management of the organ donor. J Trauma. 2007;63(5):1032–1042.
28. Abdelnour T, Rieke S. Relationship of hormonal resuscitation therapy and central venous pressure on increasing organs for transplant. J Heart Lung Transplant. 2009;28(5):480–485.
29. Powner DJ, Doshi PB. Central venous oxygen saturation monitoring: Role in adult donor care? Prog Transplant. 2010;20(4):401–405.
30. Gelb AW, Robertson KM. Anaesthetic management of the brain dead for organ donation. Can J Anaesth. 1990;37(7):806–812.
31. Pandit RA, Zirpe KG, Gurav SK, et al. Management of potential organ donor: Indian Society of Critical Care Medicine: Position Statement. Indian J Crit Care Med. 2017;21(5):303–316.
32. Limnell N, Schramko AA. Is brain-dead donor fluid therapy with colloids associated with better kidney grafts? Exp Clin Transplant. 2018;16(1):55–60.
33. Mutter TC, Ruth CA, Dart AB. Hydroxyethyl starch (HES) versus other fluid therapies: Effects on kidney function. Cochrane Database Syst Rev. 2013; 23;(7):CD007594.
34. Blasco V, Leone M, Antonini F, Geissler A, Albanèse J, Martin C. Comparison of the novel hydroxyethylstarch 130/0.4 and hydroxyethylstarch 200/0.6 in brain-dead donor resuscitation on renal function after transplantation. Br J Anaesth. 2008;100(4):504–508.
35. Bugge JF. Brain death and its implications for management of the potential organ donor. Acta Anaesthesiol Scand. 2009;53(10):1239–1250.
36. Kotloff RM, Blosser S, Fulda GJ, et al. Society of Critical Care Medicine/ American College of Chest Physicians/Association of Organ Procurement Organizations Donor Management Task Force. Management of the Potential Organ Donor in the ICU: Society of Critical Care Medicine/American College of Chest Physicians/Association of Organ Procurement Organizations Consensus Statement. Crit Care Med. 2015;43(6):1291–1325.
37. Plurad DS, Bricker S, Neville A, Bongard F, Putnam B. Arginine vasopressin significantly increases the rate of successful organ procurement in potential donors. Am J Surg. 2012;204(6):856–860; discussion 860-1.
38. Stoica SC, Satchithananda DK, White PA, Parameshwar J, Redington AN, Large SR. Noradrenaline use in the human donor and relationship with load-independent right ventricular contractility. Transplantation. 2004;78(8):1193–1197.

39. Stehlik J, Feldman DS, Brown RN et al. Cardiac Transplant Research Database Group. Interactions among donor characteristics influence post-transplant survival: A multi-institutional analysis. J Heart Lung Transplant. 2010;29(3):291–298.
40. Mukadam ME, Harrington DK, Wilson IC, et al. Does donor catecholamine administration affect early lung function after transplantation? J Thorac Cardiovasc Surg. 2005;130(3):926–927.
41. Talving P, Benfield R, Hadjizacharia P, Inaba K, Chan LS, Demetriades D. Coagulopathy in severe traumatic brain injury: A prospective study. J Trauma. 2009;66(1):55–61; discussion 61-2.
42. de Oliveira Manoel AL, Neto AC, Veigas PV, Rizoli S. Traumatic brain injury associated coagulopathy. Neurocrit Care. 2015;22(1):34–44.
43. Hefty TR, Cotterell LW, Fraser SC, Goodnight SH, Hatch TR. Disseminated intravascular coagulation in cadaveric organ donors. Incidence and effect on renal transplantation. Transplantation. 1993;55(2):442–443.

44
Heart transplantation

Sahar Saddoughi, Vishal Khullar, Richard C. Daly

Introduction

Heart transplantation remains the gold standard for the treatment of end-stage heart failure. Median survival after adult heart transplantation presently exceeds twelve years, and exceeds fourteen years conditional on one-year survival.[1] The demand for heart transplantation continues to surpass the supply and there is an association with increased length of time on the transplant waitlist and mortality.[2] Advances in mechanical circulatory support have changed the landscape of patients undergoing heart transplantation; nearly half of the patients who receive heart transplantation are now bridged with a mechanical circulatory support device.[1]

The best single test to estimate prognosis related to heart failure, and the relative benefit of heart transplantation, is cardiopulmonary exercise testing.[3] Various heart failure prognostic scores take this as well as additional patient characteristics for consideration. Heart transplantation may also be indicated for life-threatening arrhythmias unresponsive to medical or surgical treatment, severe coronary artery disease not amenable to intervention, and refractory restrictive and hypertrophic cardiomyopathy. Selection of heart transplant candidates requires responsible assessment of potential to benefit from transplantation and awareness of the contraindications.[3–5]

Guidelines for recipient selection in heart transplantation

Patients identified as potential heart transplant recipients undergo extensive testing prior to being listed for transplantation. The consensus statement regarding listing potential cardiac transplant candidates was first published in 2006 by the International Society for Heart and Lung Transplantation,[5] and updated in 2016.[6]

Standard tests

Evaluation of a patient for heart transplant is done by a multidisciplinary team to select patients who have exhausted all conventional therapy and have a good chance to benefit from the limited resource of heart transplantation. Standard tests are listed in Table 44.1 and criteria for standard donors are listed in Table 44.2.

Cardiopulmonary stress testing

Cardiopulmonary stress testing is a critical part of the patient evaluation workup. In particular, the peak volume of oxygen consumption (peak VO2) is a major determinant to guide selection of heart transplant candidates. A peak oxygen consumption of <14mL/kg/min[3,6] is a general rule for listing (Class I, level B). However, if the patient is on beta blocker,

Table 44.1 Standard Evaluation Testing

1	Electrolytes, complete blood count, coagulation profile, liver function tests
2	Echocardiogram
3	Chest x ray and pulmonary function tests
4	Carotid Doppler and peripheral vascular studies for patients > 55 years, smoking history or other risks (hyperlipidaemia, hypertension)
5	CT scan of the chest, particularly for patients more than 65 years of age or those with any previous thoracic surgery
6	Abdominal ultrasound
7	Colonoscopy, mammogram and prostate specific antigen as indicated for standard cancer screening
8	Bone densitometry
9	Human leukocyte antigen (HLA) genotype
10	Anti-HLA antibodies
11	12-lead EKG, 24-hour Holter monitoring
13	Infectious Disease evaluation and serology
14	Dental, psychiatry, social worker, and dietician evaluation

Table 44.2 Selection criteria for standard donors

1	Age <55 years old
2	normal echocardiogram
3	normal coronary angiogram (if indicated)
4	Mean arterial pressure > 60 mm Hg, Central venous pressure 8 to 12 mmHg
5	Absence of chest trauma without evidence of cardiac injury or cardiac disease
6	Hemodynamic stability with inotropic support less than 10 micro gm/kg/min of dopamine
7	Negative Hepatitis B surface antigen, Hepatitis C and HIV serologies and nucleic acid testing
8	Normal ECG
9	Anticipate ischemic time more than 4 hours
10	Weight donor and recipient within 20% (some use 30%)

then this value changes to <12mL/kg/min. Patients require a respiratory exchange ratio > 1.05 and achievement of an anaerobic threshold to show maximum effort and be on optimal pharmacologic therapy.

Heart failure prognosis scores

The Heart Failure Survival Score can be helpful in making decisions about patients who have borderline cardiopulmonary test results. This score predicts survival based on presence of coronary artery disease, baseline heart rate, ejection fraction, blood pressure, serum sodium level, presence of intraventricular conduction delay on EKG and peak VO2. Based on the score, patients are stratified into high-risk, medium-risk, and low-risk groups. High-risk patients have a predicted one-year survival of 35% without a heart transplant.(7) Patients in the high/medium risk range should be considered for heart transplant waiting list.

Right heart catheterization

In preparation for heart transplantation, all adult patients should undergo right heart catheterization. The new cardiac allocation policy in the USA requires documentation of persistent hemodynamic parameters of advanced heart failure at fixed intervals for the higher United Network for Organ Sharing (UNOS) allocation statuses on the heart transplant waiting list. Elevated pulmonary vascular resistance puts recipients at risk for right ventricular failure or primary graft dysfunction in the donor heart. In patients with prohibitive elevation of pulmonary artery systolic pressures of > 50 mmHg, a transpulmonary gradient >15 mm Hg, or a pulmonary vascular resistance > 3 Wood units, a vasodilator challenge (such as nitroprusside or inhaled nitric oxide) should be performed during the catheterization while maintaining systolic blood pressure >85 mmHg.[5] If a vasodilator is unsuccessful in decreasing pulmonary vascular resistance, these patients should be admitted for monitoring, diuresis and inotropes followed by repeat right heart catheterization. Long-term support with a left ventricular assist device (LVAD) which lowers left heart filling pressure has been shown to decrease pulmonary vascular resistance over weeks or months of support.[8]

Assessment of co-morbidities

1. *Age:* Older patients require more careful assessment for comorbidities. Historically, patients over the age of seventy were not considered for heart transplantation. However, the most current guidelines suggest that in carefully selected patients, heart transplantation can be considered.[5–6]
2. *Weight:* High BMI is associated with worse outcomes after cardiac transplantation.[9] Current guidelines recommend that heart transplant recipients should have a BMI of <35 kg/m2 prior to listing.[9]
3. *Cancer:* Active cancer from sites other than skin is a contraindication to heart transplantation.[5–6] However, patients that have been treated and are in established remission can be considered for heart transplantation. There are no specific guidelines regarding time interval required prior to listing as this is dependent on tumour type. Input from oncology may be helpful to assist with decision making regarding long term outcomes and impact of immunosuppression.
4. *Diabetes*: Uncontrolled diabetes with end-organ dysfunction is a relative contraindication for transplantation.
5. *Renal Dysfunction*: Presence of irreversible renal dysfunction with a GFR < 40 ml/min as estimated by creatinine clearance is considered a relative contraindication to heart transplantation. In these patients, evaluation for heart/kidney transplantation may be

considered. It can be challenging to assess whether apparent renal dysfunction is reversible with heart transplantation and improved hemodynamics. Renal function should be re-evaluated after optimization on inotropes, or after mechanical support.

6. *Cerebral and Peripheral Vascular Disease:* Peripheral vascular disease is a contraindication when the disease limits post-operative rehabilitation. This recommendation has remained unchanged since the 2006 guidelines. Patients with cerebral vascular disease are at increased risk for stroke after heart transplantation.[10] Cerebral vascular disease that is clinically significant is a contraindication to transplantation.
7. *Assessment of Frailty:* Evaluation of frailty is a new assessment in the 2016 guidelines for heart transplantation.[11] Manifestations of frailty include unintentional weight loss (>10 pounds within one year), muscle loss, fatigue, slow walking speed and low physical activity. Patients who have three out of five of these symptoms are considered frail.[11] Currently, frailty is not a contraindication to heart transplantation, but a discussion point when considering listing.
8. *Psychosocial Assessment:* Medical care after heart transplantation is complex, particularly in the first few months and the patient should have a pre-established appropriate support system to assist in the care. A stable psychosocial environment and absence of severe psychiatric disturbances are important to ensure medical compliance, and evaluation for these is crucial prior to selecting a patient for transplantation. Absence of the appropriate support or advanced psychiatric disturbance is a contraindication for transplantation. Substance abuse is a contraindication to heart transplantation which includes active smoking in the previous six months.

Donor selection in heart transplantation

Patients who are identified as potential heart organ donors typically have had a devastating neurologic injury resulting in brain death. Donation after cardiac death has been described with various donor criteria and may become a significant source of donors as experience is gained.[12,13] Potential donors undergo an assessment which includes confirmation of brain death, consent, blood type, co-morbidities, ECG, troponin, history of cardiac or thoracic trauma, need for inotropic support, echocardiogram and, if indicated, cardiac catheterization with coronary angiogram. Coronary angiogram is indicated for male donors > 40 years of age and female donors > 45 years of age,[14] and younger donors at high risk for coronary artery disease including type 1 diabetes, prolonged exposure to cocaine, or other risk factors. Measuring the left ventricular end-diastolic pressure at the time of coronary angiogram is straightforward and may be useful especially in older donors or those with a history of hypertension.

Extended donor criteria are described in Table 44.3 and may decrease waitlist mortality.[15] Ideal donors are rare; donor selection involves considering the risks and co-morbid conditions of the recipient and donor. Combining multiple risk factors can lead to poor outcomes. For example, recipients with higher pulmonary vascular resistance may be able to be offered transplants provided the donors are vigorous, not undersized and anticipate a shorter ischemic time.

Some donor criteria that are concerning for an increased risk of graft failure after transplant have been recognized. Such situations include hearts with left ventricular hypertrophy which are more difficult to protect from ischemic injury and may have significant diastolic dysfunction. Poisoning by ethylene glycol (antifreeze) ingestion, methanol ingestion, carbon monoxide inhalation, cyanide, and other agents causes considerable cellular injury that may be masked by normal appearing echocardiogram, but the degree of systemic injury can be estimated by the magnitude of injury to other organ systems. Electrocution can also cause considerable myocyte injury. Drug intoxication may cause myocardial

Table 44.3 Selection criteria for extended donors

1	Donors with expected cold ischemic time 4–6 hours
2	Severe chest trauma with aortic hematoma/cardiac contusion
3	Donors with coronary artery disease that may require coronary artery bypass grafting
4	Donors from older age group > 50–55 years (13)
5	Left ventricular dysfunction with high dose inotropic support
6	Body weight difference > 20%
7	HCV-positive or HBV (core IgM-negative)—positive donors

injury, such as overdose with tricyclic antidepressants. Donors with late pregnancy can be associated with cardiomyopathy or left ventricular hypertrophy and warrants caution in interpreting the echocardiogram, though they can be suitable donors. Regional wall motion abnormalities on echocardiogram, prolonged cardiopulmonary resuscitation, and persistent tachycardia are potential warning signs. Caution is advised when the cause of death is unknown, particularly if there were central neurologic symptoms (headache, change of consciousness, etc.), due to potential for viral encephalitis. Transient cardiac dysfunction is not uncommon following brain death and frequently recovers over one to two days. Such potential donors will often recover normal cardiac function, particularly if younger and have normal size hearts; these donors warrant patience and re-evaluation if the donor family circumstances permit.

Heart transplant surgery

Before initiating the surgery, the procurement team confirms blood group compatibility and documentation of consent and brain death declaration of the donor. If possible, the echocardiogram and, when performed, coronary angiogram are reviewed. The current status of hemodynamics and any inotropic agents is reviewed.

Donor procurement

A median sternotomy is performed and the pericardium is opened. The heart is inspected visually for any anomalies or injuries. Contractility is carefully observed, the coronary arteries are inspected and the heart is palpated for any thrills. Observation of right ventricular contractility is particularly important as the echocardiogram may not have visualized this well. These findings are then communicated to the recipient implant team so that they can start the surgery in time to be ready for the anticipated arrival of the donor heart. The plane is developed between the aorta and the pulmonary artery. The position of the right pulmonary artery and the pulmonary veins is noted. The superior vena cava (SVC) is exposed to the innominate vein and the azygous vein is defined. The pericardium on the right side is incised down to the inferior vena cava (IVC) to allow flush solution and blood from the thoracic and abdominal teams to drain into the right pleural cavity freely after aortic cross-clamping, where it is easy to aspirate. Once the abdominal team is ready for the procurement, the patient is heparinized.

A cardioplegia needle is inserted into the ascending aorta and a cannula is inserted into the pulmonary artery if the lungs are also being procured. The SVC is either ligated or cross-clamped. After confirmation with the liver team, the IVC is divided near the diaphragm and the blood is allowed to drain into the right pleural cavity. With caval inflow interruption, the heartbeats to empty once or twice and become decompressed. The aorta is cross-clamped and the left atrium is vented with a generous incision in the left atrial appendage, pulmonary vein or the interatrial groove. Hypothermic antegrade cardioplegia is delivered into the aortic root. Copious amount of ice slush is poured into the pericardial cavity for topical cooling and the left ventricle (LV) is checked for distension. Efflux from the vented left atrium and IVC are checked periodically to ensure a free drainage. When cardioplegia is complete, the aortic cross-clamp and cardioplegia needle are removed. The IVC and SVC are completely transected. A quick retrieval of the donor heart is then performed by lifting its cephalad, dividing the pulmonary veins, transecting the aorta distal to the right innominate artery, and dividing the pulmonary arteries beyond the bifurcation. If the lungs are also being procured, then a careful coordination between the two teams can assure an adequate cuff of left atrial tissue around the pulmonary veins for the lung transplant and the pulmonary trunk is divided proximal to the bifurcation. To help protect the pulmonary veins for lung transplant, it is useful to open the interatrial groove and visualize the right pulmonary vein orifices.

Recipient procedure for heart transplantation

Induction of anaesthesia can be a dangerous time for patients with end-stage heart failure; severe hypotension and cardiac arrest can occur. The surgical team and cardiopulmonary bypass (CPB) should be immediately available. A pulmonary artery catheter, arterial line, CVP line, and urinary catheter are inserted. Preoperative antibiotics and immunosuppressive agents are given as per institutional protocols. External defibrillator pads are placed for redo sternotomies. Close communication between the harvest and the implant team can minimize the organ ischemic time. A skin incision is made once the procurement team confirms a good donor heart.

After median sternotomy and full heparinization, aortic, SVC, and IVC cannulation are performed distally. Immediately after CPB, the aorta is cross-clamped to avoid embolization of potential left atrial or left ventricular thrombus that may develop with end-stage heart failure. The right atrium is divided at the atrioventricular groove; superiorly this incision is extended towards the roof of the left atrium near the aorta, and inferiorly towards and into the coronary sinus (Figure 44.1). The great arteries are divided at the sinotubular junctions. The left atrium is divided at the atrioventricular groove following the coronary sinus and parallel to

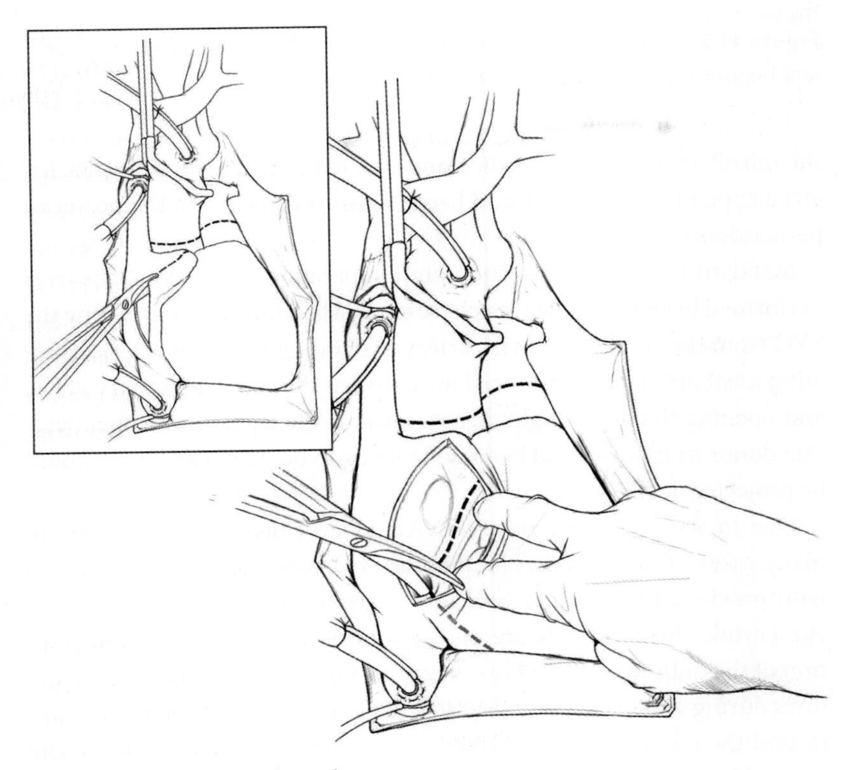

Figure 44.1. Recipient's cardiectomy

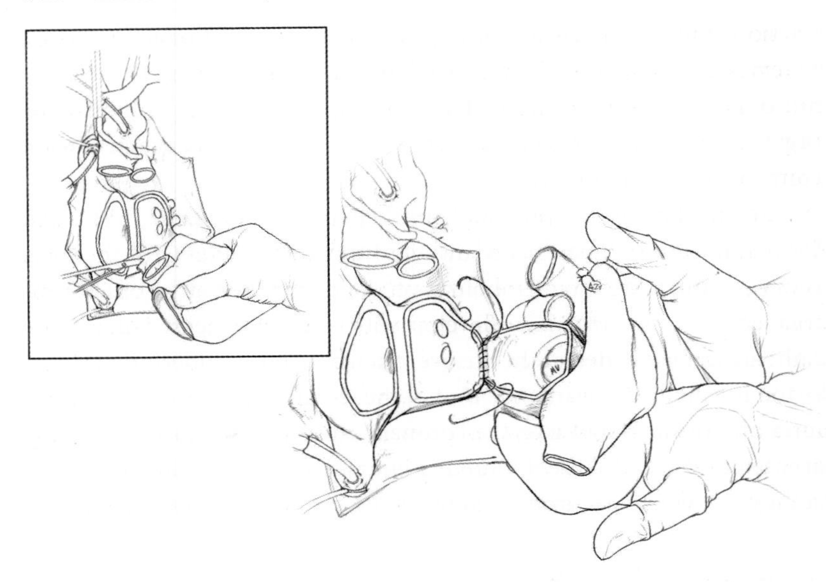

Figure 44.2. Completion cardiectomy for bi-atrial anastomosis technique and beginning of left atrial anastomosis

the mitral annulus. After cardiectomy, the left atrial cuff is trimmed, left atrial appendage is excised, and haemostasis is achieved in the posterior pericardium (Figure 44.2).

Standard back table dissection and preparation of the donor heart is performed by opening the transverse sinus which involves separating the SVC from the right pulmonary artery, separating the great arteries, creating a left atrial cuff with incisions between the four pulmonary veins, and opening the donor right atrium towards the right atrial appendage. The donor heart sinoatrial (SA) node tends to be vulnerable and should be protected at all times.

Due to the increasing use of LVAD as a bridge to transplantation, many cases of heart transplantation are redo-sternotomies. In patients with previous LVADs, it is very important to obtain a CT scan of the chest while these patients are on the waiting list to establish the position of the outflow graft and the driveline; injury of either of these structures during entry into the chest can be catastrophic. It is not uncommon to find the outflow graft and the driveline crossing the midline. At the time of LVAD implant, it is crucial to be aware that these structures be positioned and protected to allow a safe redo sternotomy. Echo should be reviewed to check for a persistent patent foramen ovale (PFO) and to rule out any clot on the aortic and mitral valves. Both the groins should be prepared for peripheral cannulation. Fresh frozen plasma or human prothrombin concentrate is started just before the skin incision to reverse the anticoagulation. During early dissection while the LVAD is still functioning, there should be awareness of the risk of air embolization with injury to the right atrium, persistent PFO, or injury to the inflow cannula, entry to the left side of the heart (left atrial appendage is a particular risk) due to a negative pressure in the left heart chambers created by the LVAD. Stopping the LVAD and immediate cross clamping of the aorta and/or the outflow graft is prudent when initiating cardiopulmonary bypass. Dissection of the cardiac apex and LVAD inflow cannula will be very close to the left phrenic nerve.

Bi-atrial anastomosis technique

The original bi-atrial technique for heart transplantation described by Lower and Shumway[16] is still prevalent today because of its simplicity and reproducibility; it avoids potential for SVC narrowing if this is a concern. A few studies have shown an increased incidence of tricuspid regurgitation, atrial arrhythmias, and sinus node dysfunction after bi-atrial technique, though chordal damage during endomyocardial biopsy is the most common cause of tricuspid regurgitation.[17]

The left atrial anastomosis is started adjacent to the left atrial appendage with a running suture, paying attention to the position of the fossa ovalis for every individual heart and the position of the donor IVC and SVC. A LV vent is placed either through the right superior pulmonary vein or through the completed left atrial anastomosis. The pulmonary trunks of donor and recipient are trimmed to the desired length to avoid kinking and are anastomosed end to end with a running polypropylene suture. The donor and recipient aorta are trimmed and the end-to-end anastomosis is performed with a running polypropylene stitch. A needle tack vent is placed in the ascending aorta and placed to suction. The cross-clamp is removed. The right atrial suture line can be completed during re-perfusion of the heart (Figure 44.3).

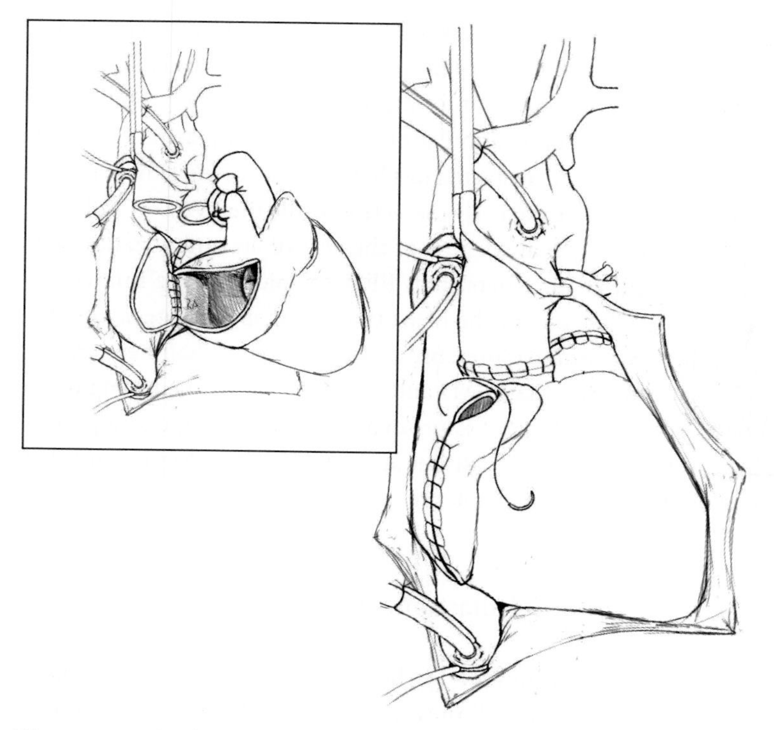

Figure 44.3. Right atrial anastomosis for bi-atrial anastomosis technique

Ventricular and atrial pacing wires are inserted. Removal of the implantable cardioverter defibrillator (ICD) lead can be performed during this time while the heart is being re-perfused. The heart is lifted cephalad out of the pericardial cavity and left atrial suture line is inspected for any potential bleeding as this area is extremely difficult to access once the cardiopulmonary bypass is terminated.

Bicaval anastomosis technique

In the bicaval anastomosis technique, the SVC is transected at the cavo-atrial junction and a cuff of right atrium is left with the recipient IVC. The remaining right atrial free wall and most of the atrial septum is excised (Figure 44.4). Injuring the right inferior pulmonary vein during

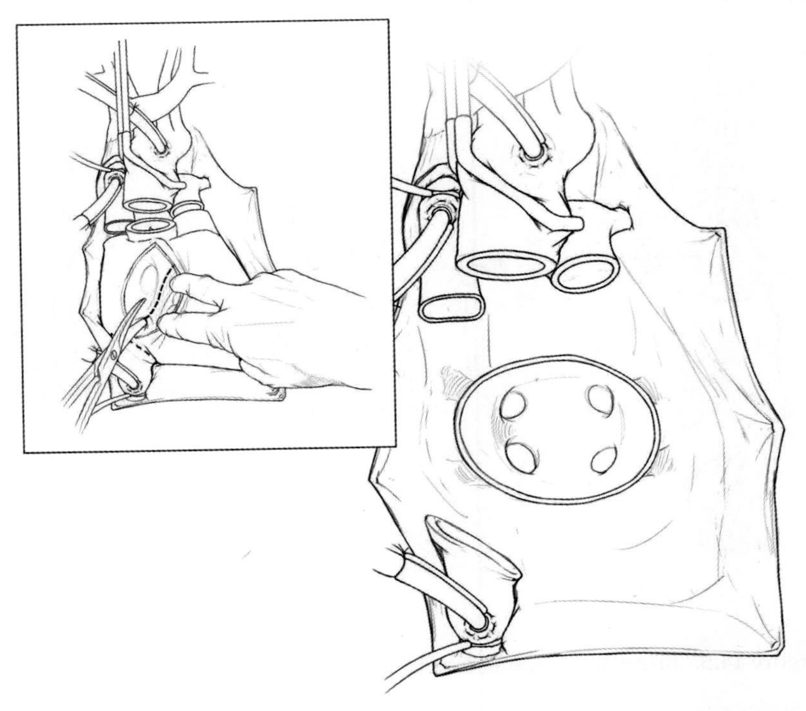

Figure 44.4. Completion cardiectomy for bi-caval anastomosis technique

dissection around the IVC should be avoided. After completing the left atrial anastomosis, the posterior aspect of the IVC anastomosis can be performed prior to removing the cross-clamp to improve visibility, if this is a concern. The anterior part of the suture line can be completed during the re-perfusion of the heart (Figure 44.5). The SVC anastomosis is performed during reperfusion taking care to avoid a purse-string so as not to narrow the SVC at the anastomosis; SVC access for biopsies will be required for life.

Immunosuppression

The primary aim of immunosuppressive therapy is to maintain a fine balance between the immune rejection in order to facilitate graft acceptance and to minimize the chances of toxic side effects in the postoperative

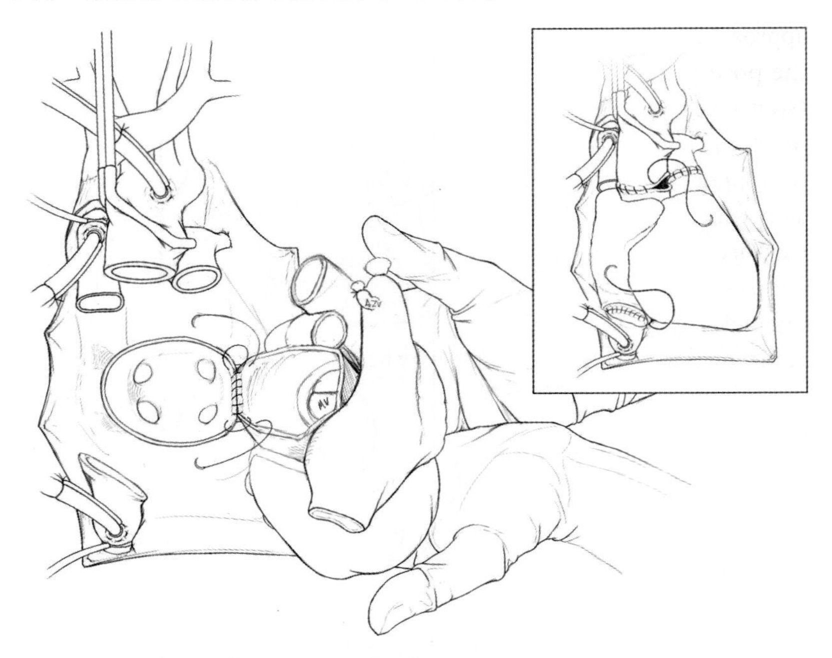

Figure 44.5. Bi-caval anastomosis technique

period. Pre and intraoperative high dose intravenous steroid therapy is universal. Induction therapy with polyclonal antibodies (antithymocyte globulin) depletes lymphocytes or monoclonal antibodies against cytokine receptors (basiliximab CD25, alemtuzumab CD52).[18]

Maintenance immunosuppression is generally a three-drug regimen including a steroid (prednisone), a calcineurin inhibitor (tacrolimus), and an antiproliferative agent (mycophenolate mofetil). We routinely transition from a calcineuron inhibitor to the proliferation signal inhibitor sirolimus when wound healing is complete. Sirolimus is less renal toxic and it has been shown to decrease the incidence of cardiac allograft vasculopathy and reduce late malignancy.[19]

Survival results

Between 1982 and June 2016, the median survival for adult recipients after heart transplantation was 10.8 years[20] with a one-year survival approaching 90%. In patients with LVADs used as a bridge to transplant, the postoperative survival does not appear to be adversely affected.[21] Graft failure and multi-organ dysfunction remain the leading cause of death in the first month. The right ventricle is the most vulnerable for postoperative dysfunction, particularly if there is pulmonary hypertension which can be aggravated by blood transfusion. Early mechanical support (with temporary VAD or extracorporeal membrane oxygenation—ECMO) for graft dysfunction is crucial to prevent peripheral organ dysfunction and allow the allograft to rest and recover. Recovery is common, but re-transplantation may be necessary.

Highlights

- Heart transplantation remains the gold standard for end-stage heart failure no longer responsive to medical treatment. Unfortunately, the waiting list for heart transplantation continues to outweigh the donor pool. The donor pool may be expanded with marginal donors, donation after cardiac death and allograft perfusion after procurement.
- The use of mechanical circulatory support, in particular LVADs, has been increasing as a bridge to transplantation. In fact, close to 50% of patients who undergo heart transplantation are bridged with a mechanical circulatory support device.
- Peak oxygen consumption is the best objective single predictor of heart failure prognosis. Recipient selection otherwise includes evaluation of pulmonary vascular resistance and co-morbid conditions with consensus statements published and updated by the International Society for Heart and Lung Transplantation and involves a multidisciplinary team.
- Most donors for heart transplantation are marginal and require careful consideration of the donor risk factors along with the recipient risk factors. Careful evaluation of all tests as well as the cause of death is important. Initial poor heart function may improve with time.
- There are two main techniques for heart transplantation: Biatrial anastomosis technique and Bicaval anastomosis technique. Many

heart transplants involve patients bridged with an LVAD, and the transplant surgery requires careful planning.

- One-year survival for heart transplantation is close to 90% with graft failure and multi-organ dysfunction being the leading causes of early death. Median long-term survival now exceeds twelve years.

References

1. Khush KK, Cherikh WS, Chambers DC et al. The International Thoracic Organ Transplant Registry: Thirty-fifth Adult Heart Transplantation Report-2018; Focus Theme: Multiorgan Transplantation. J Heart Lung Transplant. 2018; 37: 1155–1168.
2. Goldstein BA, Thomas L, Zaroff JG, Nguyen J, Menza R, Khush KK. Assessment of heart transplant waitlist time and pre- and post-transplant failure: A mixed methods approach. Epidemiology. 2016; 27: 469–476.
3. Mancini DM, Eisen H, Kussmaul W, Mull R, Edmunds LH, Jr., Wilson JR. Value of peak exercise oxygen consumption for optimal timing of cardiac transplantation in ambulatory patients with heart failure. Circulation. 1991; 83: 778–786.
4. Freeman R, Koerner E, Clark C, Halabicky K. The path from heart failure to cardiac transplant. Crit Care Nurs Q. 2016; 39: 207–213.
5. Mehra MR, Kobashigawa J, Starling R, et al. Listing criteria for heart transplantation: International Society for Heart and Lung Transplantation guidelines for the care of cardiac transplant candidates—2006. J Heart Lung Transplant. 2006; 25: 1024–1042.
6. Mehra MR, Canter CE, Hannan MM, et al. The 2016 International Society for Heart Lung Transplantation listing criteria for heart transplantation: A 10-year update. J Heart Lung Transplant. 2016; 35: 1–23.
7. Aaronson KD, Schwartz JS, Chen TM, Wong KL, Goin JE, Mancini DM. Development and prospective validation of a clinical index to predict survival in ambulatory patients referred for cardiac transplant evaluation. Circulation. 1997; 95: 2660–2667.
8. Guglin M, Khan H. Pulmonary hypertension in heart failure. J Card Fail. 2010;16(6):461–474.
9. Doumouras BS, Fan CS, Mueller B et. al. The effect of pre-heart transplant body mass index on posttransplant outcomes: An analysis of the ISHLT Registry Data.
10. Patlolla V, Mogulla V, DeNofrio D, Konstam MA, Krishnamani R. Outcomes in patients with symptomatic cerebrovascular disease undergoing heart transplantation. J Am Coll Cardiol. 2011; 58: 1036–1041.
11. Dunlay SM, Park SJ, Joyce LD et. al. Frailty and outcomes after implantation of left ventricular assist device as destination therapy. J Heart Lung Transplant. 2014: 33(4):359–365.
12. Messer S, Page A, Axell R, Berman M, Hernandez-Sanchez J, Colah S, et al. Outcome after heart transplantation from donation after circulatory-determined death donors. J Heart Lung Transplant. 2017; 36(2): 1311–1318.

13. Chew HC, Iyer A, Connellan M, Scheuer S, Villanueva J, Gao L, Hicks M, Harkness M, Soto C, et al. Outcomes after circulatory death heart transplantation in Australia. J Am Coll Cardiol. 2019; 73 (12): 1447–1459.
14. Kilic A, Emani S, Sai-Sudhakar CB, Higgins RS, Whitson BA. Donor selection in heart transplantation. J Thorac Dis. 2014; 6: 1097–1104.
15. Forni A, Luciani GB, Chiominto B, Pizzuti M, Mazzucco A, Faggian G. Results with expanded donor acceptance criteria in heart transplantation. Transplant Proc. 2011; 43: 953–959.
16. Stinson EB, Dong E, Jr., Iben AB, Shumway NE. Cardiac transplantation in man. 3. Surgical aspects. Am J Surg. 1969; 118: 182–187.
17. Chan MC, Giannetti N, Kato T, et al. Severe tricuspid regurgitation after heart transplantation. J Heart Lung Transplant. 2001; 20: 709–717.
18. Koch A, Daniel V, Dengler TJ, Schnabel PA, Hagl S, Sack FU. Effectivity of a T-cell-adapted induction therapy with anti-thymocyte globulin (Sangstat). J Heart Lung Transplant. 2005; 24: 708–713.
19. Asleh R, Briasoulis A, Kremers WK, et al. Long-term sirolimus for primary immunosuppression in heart transplant recipients. J Am Coll Cardiol. 2018; 71: 636–650.
20. Khush KK, Cherikh WS, Chambers DC, et al. The International Thoracic Organ Transplant Registry of the International Society for Heart and Lung Transplantation: Thirty-fifth Adult Heart Transplantation Report-2018; Focus Theme: Multiorgan Transplantation. J Heart Lung Transplant. 2018; 37: 1155–1168.
21. Takeda K, Takayama H, Kalesan B, et al. Outcome of cardiac transplantation in patients requiring prolonged continuous-flow left ventricular assist device support. J Heart Lung Transplant. 2015; 34: 89–99.

45

Lung transplantation

Massimo Boffini, Cristina Barbero, Davide Ricci, Erika Simonato, Mauro Rinaldi

Introduction

The appropriate selection of lung transplant recipients and the proper timing of listing are challenging processes and important determinants of the outcome.

There is a general agreement that referral to a lung transplant programme should occur early in patients who have an end-stage lung disease that might warrant transplant consideration. On the other hand, the decision to place the patient on the active waiting list and the timing of the decision are critical issues; the rationale should not expose the patient to the transplant surgery risk until all other viable treatments are exhausted.

Recipient selection

Lung transplantation should be considered in adults with chronic, end-stage lung disease who meet all the following general criteria in order to identify those patients with the most need and the greatest likelihood of survival:[1]

1. High (>50%) risk of death from lung disease within two years if lung transplantation is not performed.
2. High (>80%) likelihood of surviving at least ninety days after lung transplantation.
3. High (>80%) likelihood of five-year post-transplant survival.

Ideal candidates for lung transplantation are those with end-stage disease, limited life expectancy, and, at the same time, free of significant comorbidities that might negatively impact post-operative outcomes.

Exclusion criteria

According to the International Society for Heart and Lung Transplantation (ISHLT) guidelines, exclusion criteria could be major or minor:[(1)]

Major exclusion criteria are as follows:

- Untreatable significant dysfunction of another major organ system (heart, liver, kidney, or brain) unless combined organ transplantation can be performed.
- History of malignancy—In the case of low predicted risk of recurrence after lung transplantation, a two-year disease-free interval is requested; in the case of disease with a high degree malignancy (hematologic diseases, sarcoma, melanoma, or cancers of the breast, bladder, or kidney), a five-year disease-free interval is recommended.
- Coronary artery disease not suitable for percutaneous intervention or bypass grafting.
- Uncorrectable bleeding diathesis.
- Acute sepsis.
- Chronic infection with highly virulent and/or resistant microbes.
- Evidence of active Mycobacterium tuberculosis infection.
- Significant chest wall or spinal deformity expected to cause severe restriction after transplantation.
- Body mass index (BMI) >35.0 kg/m^2.
- Current non-adherence to medical therapy or a history of repeated or prolonged episodes of non-adherence to medical therapy.
- Psychiatric or psychologic conditions associated with the inability to cooperate with the medical team and/or comply with medical therapy.
- Absence of an adequate and reliable social support system.
- Severely limited functional status with poor rehabilitation potential.
- Active cigarette smoking, drug, or alcohol addiction or history of these habits within the last six months.

Minor exclusion criteria are as follows:

- Age older than sixty-five years.
- BMI between 30 and 34.9 kg/m^2.
- Progressive or severe malnutrition.
- Severe, symptomatic osteoporosis.
- Extensive prior chest surgery with lung resection.
- Colonization or infection with highly resistant bacteria, fungi, and mycobacteria. For patients infected with human immunodeficiency virus (HIV), a lung transplant can be considered in the case of controlled disease with undetectable HIV-RNA, and compliant on combined antiretroviral therapy.
- Peripheral atherosclerotic disease.
- Mechanical ventilation and/or extracorporeal life support (ECLS).

Recent improvements in lung transplant outcomes, likely related to better surgical techniques, improved post-transplant management, and better donor organ selection, have led centres to accept recipients with a higher profile of complexity (more acute illness and increasing numbers of comorbidities). Compared with earlier eras, there is an increasing trend in transplanting older-aged patients, as well as patients with systemic illnesses, patients with a previous lung transplant, and patients with a history of resistant organisms or malignancy.[2] Particularly, the age of a candidate for a lung transplant is considered exclusion criteria if higher than sixty-five years old only in the case of other important comorbidities or risk factors. Recent studies show encouraging results in older-aged patients as well, and it is uniformly accepted as allocation criteria to try to match older recipients with older donors.[3] Moreover, an increasing number of transplant centres have been utilizing extracorporeal membrane oxygenation (ECMO) in patients on the active waiting list. First indication is bridging to transplant in the case of a mechanical ventilation failure. However, evidences in the literature have demonstrated even better outcome using venous-venous ECMO as bridge to transplant to avoid the use of mechanical ventilation. These favourable results on supported patients are mainly due to availability of more reliable technologies such as poly-methylpentene oxygenators, heparin-coated circuits, double-lumen cannulas, pumpless technologies, and new generation centrifugal pumps.

Technological improvements allow a wider and an earlier application of extracorporeal support, reducing the need for mechanical ventilation that is considered a significant detrimental risk factor.[4–6]

Disease-specific considerations

The most common indications for lung transplant are chronic obstructive pulmonary disease (COPD), idiopathic pulmonary fibrosis (IPF), cystic fibrosis (CF), and pulmonary arterial hypertension (PAH) in the decreasing percentage order of transplant indication. There are a few other conditions requiring lung transplant as well.

Chronic Obstructive Lung Disease

Severe chronic obstructive lung disease (COPD) is the most common indication for lung transplantation representing 31% of all lung transplants performed.[7] The COPD is generally characterized by a slow progression, therefore candidate selection, in this case, requires careful consideration of mortality predictors, as many patients may not derive a survival benefit from transplant based on low forced expiratory volume in one second (FEV1) alone.[8] In the early days of lung transplantation, COPD patients were addressed to the active waiting list when their lung function showed a FEV1 of less than 30% of predicted without necessarily considering other disease-related factors that might impact survival; results on COPD patients transplanted in those years showed no benefit when compared with wait-list mortality.[9] More recent shreds of evidence claim that COPD patients should be stratified for the active waiting list according to BODE (body-mass index, airflow obstruction, dyspnoea, and exercise) index, number of exacerbations requiring hospitalization, hypercapnia, falling BMI, exercise tolerance, and pulmonary hypertension.[10,11]

To date, according to the ISHLT guidelines, it is recommended to refer patients to lung transplant centres in the following cases:

- In case of progressive disease despite maximal treatment,
- contraindication for lung volume reduction surgery,

- BODE index of 5–6,
- partial pressure of carbon dioxide ($PaCO_2$) > 50 mmHg and/or partial pressure of oxygen (PaO_2) < 60 mmHg, and/or FEV1 lower than 25% predicted.[1]

Criteria for listing patients are BODE Index ≥7, FEV1 lower than 20% predicted, three or more severe exacerbations in one year or one severe exacerbation with acute hypercapnic respiratory failure, and/or moderate to severe pulmonary hypertension.[1]

Idiopathic Pulmonary Fibrosis

IPF is characterized by a progressive parenchymal scaring and it is the second most common indication for a lung transplant. It has a three-year median survival from diagnosis, therefore, ISHLT guidelines recommend referral to transplant centres at the time of diagnosis and early listing. Particularly, IPF patients should be referred to transplant centres in the listed cases:

- histopathologic or radiographic evidence of usual interstitial pneumonia or fibrosing nonspecific interstitial pneumonitis,
- forced vital capacity (FVC) lower than 80% predicted
- diffusion capacity of the lung for carbon monoxide (DLCO) lower than 40% predicted,
- dyspnoea or functional limitation and/or oxygen requirement.

The IPF patients should be listed in the case of declines in FVC more than 10% during six months of follow-up, decline in DLCO more than 15% during six months of follow-up, desaturation to less than 88% or distance lower than 250 m on a 6-minute-walk test or more than 50 m decline in 6-minute-walk distance over six months, hospitalization because of respiratory decline, pneumothorax, or acute exacerbation, and/or moderate to severe pulmonary hypertension.[1,12]

Cystic Fibrosis

CF is the third most common indication for lung transplantation. It is a genetic disorder characterized by progressive bronchiectasis, chronic sinusitis, and pancreatic exocrine insufficiency, which eventually leads to end-stage lung disease and death.

It is well recognized that mortality in CF disease is dramatically increased when patients start to develop clinical decline characterized by increased frequency of hospitalization because of acute respiratory failure requiring non-invasive ventilation, increasing antibiotic resistance and poor clinical recovery from exacerbations, worsening nutritional status, pneumothorax, and severe haemoptysis despite embolization, when the FEV1 falls below 30% predicted or when there is a rapid decline in FEV1 despite optimal therapy, when the exercise tolerance (6-minute-walk distance) falls below 400 m, and/or when there are worsening hypoxemia, hypercapnia, and pulmonary hypertension. Criteria of listing for CF patients, according to the ISHLT guidelines, are:

- chronic respiratory failure with hypoxia alone (PaO_2 < 60 mm Hg) or hypercapnia ($PaCO_2$ > 50 mm Hg),
- long-term non-invasive ventilation therapy,
- FEV1 lower than 30% predicted or rapid decline in FEV1,
- World Health Organization functional class IV, rapid lung function decline requiring intensive care unit stay,
- frequent hospitalizations and/or pulmonary hypertension.[1]

Considerations on colonization with resistant bacteria and proper selection criteria are particularly important in this subgroup of patients due to recurrent pulmonary exacerbations with frequent exposures to antibiotics. These highly resistant organisms usually remain in the upper airways of the recipient, raising concerns about the risk for pulmonary infection with immunosuppression therapy after transplant. Studies show that while lung transplantation can be safely performed in the case of multidrug resistant (MDR) P. aeruginosa, and S. aureus, other organisms such as Burkholderia cenocepacia (genomovar III), Mycobacterium abscessus, and Scedosporium prolificans are associated with a significant decrease in survival after transplant.[13–15]

Pulmonary Arterial Hypertension

PAH is a progressive disease of the pulmonary vessels that leads to right heart failure and death. Patients should be addressed to a transplant centre in the following cases:

- when maximal disease-specific medical treatment for PAH has failed (New York Heart Association Functional Class III or IV with rapidly progressive disease),
- when there is no surgical indication for pulmonary endarterectomy in the case of chronic thromboembolic pulmonary hypertension,
- when there is persisting PAH after pulmonary endarterectomy or
- balloon pulmonary angioplasty and/or
- in the case of known or suspected pulmonary veno-occlusive disease or
- pulmonary capillary hemangiomatosis.

Patients should be listed in case of development of significant haemoptysis, pericardial effusion, and right heart failure (right atrial pressure >15 mmHg) with decreasing cardiac index (< 2 litres/min/m^2), pulmonary hypertension, and reduced exercise tolerance (6-minute walk test < 350 m).[1,16] During the last years, new therapies and surgical approaches have dramatically changed the course of the disease for these patients. New drugs such as prostanoids, endothelin receptor antagonists, and phosphodiesterase-5 inhibitors have significantly delayed the time of referral for lung transplant.

Good results have been reported in terms of survival and early right heart remodelling after bilateral lung transplant.[17,18] However, to date, among all indications for lung transplant, PAH-recipients still have the lowest reported one-year survival.[19] Along with endothelial ischemia-reperfusion injury, both right ventricular and left ventricular dysfunction may play a role in the development of primary graft dysfunction as a result of post-transplant acute hemodynamic changes in afterload and preload. Immediately after bilateral lung transplant, the hypertrophied right ventricle still ejects blood with high pressures into the new, low-resistance pulmonary vessels. This leads to pulmonary overflow and reperfusion injury. At the same time, the chronically volume-deprived left ventricle has to face an increased preload. Several groups have reported the use of prophylactic V-A ECMO during the first postoperative days intending to allow the left and right ventricles to adapt to the new hemodynamic changes.[20,21]

Other indications

Other less common indications for lung transplant are:

1. ***Lung re-transplantation.*** Re-transplantation candidates may be considered for bilateral or single-lung transplantation. If the initial transplant was a single-lung, consideration must be given to whether leaving the previous allograft *in situ*; the failed allograft may represent a source of ongoing immune stimulation or infections.
2. ***Sarcoidosis.*** Sarcoidosis is a systemic disease characterized by the presence of non-caseating granulomas in affected organs. Most aggressive cases develop pulmonary fibrosis and pulmonary hypertension. Patients with diagnosis of sarcoidosis are considered appropriate candidates for lung transplantation when they develop WHO functional class III to IV symptoms, hypoxemia at rest, pulmonary hypertension, and elevated right atrial pressure.
3. ***Lymphangioleiomyomatosis.*** It is a rare disorder characterized by smooth muscle proliferation within the airways of the lungs leading to cystic lesions of lung parenchyma and chronic respiratory failure. Patients with lymphangioleiomyomatosis are appropriate candidates for lung transplantation when there is a severe reduction in FEV1/FVC ratio, increased total lung capacity, and reduced oxygen consumption.

Donor selection

The gap between the number of potential recipients and the number of lung transplants performed widens each year: lung grafts are successfully addressed to transplant in only 15–20% of all multi-organ donors.[22] This is mainly related to lungs damage during the hours before retrieval due to resuscitation manoeuvres, neurogenic oedema, aspiration of gastric content and pneumonia, systemic pro-inflammatory response syndrome, and suboptimal mechanical ventilation.

To increase the rate of lungs procured per donor, it is of paramount importance:

1. To early identify possible donors. Any patient who meets specific clinical signs and criteria[23] should be referred to the donor coordinator for the evaluation process. Failure of early recognition and referral of donors is one of the most important reasons for organs shortage.[24]
2. To adopt a lung-protective strategy in intensive care unit to prevent atelectasis and infection. Active donor management includes proper ventilation with low tidal volume, recruitment manoeuvres, fluid restriction, and steroids administration.[25]
3. To get a targeted risk-benefit assessment with the aim to understand if the organ is suitable for the specific patient.

During the year 2019, viability lung donors' criteria changed towards an individual approach based on the knowledge that the specific graft may not be beneficial for one recipient while being life-saving for another.[26]

Standard and recognized general criteria for choosing the donor are as follows:[27]

- **Age < 55 years**. Older lungs may have increased probability to develop cancer, infections, emphysema, apical scars, or pleural adhesions with consequently reduced function. On the other hand, with the declining immune function in older lungs, they may be less vulnerable to rejection.[28] To address these issues and increase the number of organs available, units all over the world match the age of the donor with the age of the recipient.

- **Clear chest X-ray or minor CT scan abnormalities.** Multiple evidence in the literature shows that even with radiological abnormalities, lungs should be taken into consideration for transplantation, and available data show comparable results with standard lungs donors. In a retrospective analysis by McCowin MJ and colleagues, 30% of all donor chest X-rays had infiltrated, which resolved spontaneously or at least improved in the majority of cases.[29] Moreover, donors with significant unilateral abnormalities should not be excluded for donation of the contralateral lung.[30]
- **Normal gas exchange.** Particularly PaO_2> 300 mm Hg on FIO_2 1.0 and PEEP 5 cm H_2O. Several authors have shown that lower level of PaO_2/FiO_2 ratio after brain death diagnosis does not make the donors ineligible for lung donation. Gas exchange can be easily affected by reversible factors such as secretions, pulmonary oedema, and atelectasis and adequate treatment can increase the original PaO_2/FiO_2 by nearly 100 mmHg.[31] Ex vivo lung perfusion is a well-established technique used to evaluate high-risk donor organs characterized by a low PaO_2 level. Marginal lungs are explanted, reventilated, and re-perfused for functional assessment with measurement of gas exchange, haemodynamic, and lung dynamics parameters.[32,33]
- **Smoking history < 20 pack-years.** Major concern in the case of lung donors with a history of smoking is the risk of poor function due to a chronic obstructive pulmonary disease and the risk of an undetected cancer.[34] Smoking history in lung donors has been associated with decreased recipient survival,[7] but recipient survival is better than when remaining on the waiting list.[34]
- **No evidence of purulent aspirations at bronchoscopy or sepsis.** Post-transplantation pneumonia and sepsis are serious concerns and, along with graft failure, remain the leading causes of death in the first post-transplant year.[7] Systemic infections that are untreated or of unknown origin (such as viral encephalitis or febrile meningo-encephalitis), as well as ongoing sepsis, uncontrolled active infection, or infections without option of treatment are considered main exclusion criteria for organs donation. On the other hand, analysis of donor airway cultures revealed a very low (<1.5%) transmission rate of donor organ contamination.[35–37]

- **History of cancer.** Tumour transmission after solid organ transplant can lead to fatal consequences because of the rapid dissemination in a patient under immunosuppressive therapy. The risk of disease transmission has to be compared with the risk of death on the waiting list.[38]
- No history of primitive pulmonary disease.
- No evidence of significant chest trauma.
- No previous thoracic surgery.

The need to address the issue of lung donors' shortage has led to consider extended donor lung criteria and to consider different strategies to increase organ availability, including living donation, ex vivo lung perfusion, donation after cardiac death, and the use of organs from non-standard risk donors.

The transplant

Lung transplantation is the definitive treatment of end-stage respiratory failure. According to the Registry of the ISHLT, median survival after lung transplantation is 6 years in the adults and a conditional to 1-year median survival of 8.2 years.[19]

Single lung transplantation (SLTx) is usually indicated for older patients without pulmonary hypertension and lung colonization. The main indication for SLTx is, therefore, pulmonary fibrosis,[39] though it can be performed in COPD patients also. The SLTx has the potential advantage to increase the number of transplants because the lung block can be split and used on two different recipients. Another favourable aspect is that the surgical impact on the recipient is less severe and hence, it can be indicated in the most fragile patients. The main drawbacks are those related to the maintenance of the diseased lung that may cause complications. Another negative issue is that in the post-transplant follow-up, a ventilation-perfusion mismatch may occur, leading to recurrence of respiratory failure.

As a matter of fact, according to the ISHLT registry, SLTx provides poorer results in comparison with double lung transplantation (DLTx). For these reasons, DLTx is generally considered the strategy of choice for the majority of patients. The DLTx is mandatory for CF patients, it is highly recommended for COPD and pulmonary hypertension patients and it is also performed in patients with pulmonary fibrosis given the better results in comparison with SLTx. The DLTx is performed through a double thoracotomy in the fourth intercostal space. On selective contralateral ventilation, the first lung is explanted and the first graft is implanted without the use of extracorporeal circulation. In case of poor oxygenation, hemodynamic instability or pulmonary hypertension after pulmonary artery clamping, extracorporeal circulatory support may become necessary either with a standard extracorporeal circulation or veno-arterial ECMO. After the first graft is implanted, the selective ventilation is applied on the transplanted lung and the contralateral diseased lung is explanted followed by the implantation of the second graft. Particular attention is paid to the bronchial anastomosis that is at risk of ischemic complications. For this reason, bronchial stump on the graft is kept as short as possible to reduce the risk of dehiscence.

Conclusion

Early referral of patients with end-stage respiratory disease to a transplant centre is one of the most important determinants of good outcomes in lung transplant. This allows the transplant centre to identify the proper timing for the active waiting list. Second challenging point is the proper selection and matching between recipient and donor. DLTx is considered the strategy of choice for majority of patients on the active waiting list. However, the shortage of donors has led the transplant community to take into consideration single lung transplants in the case of older patients without pulmonary hypertension and lung colonization, and satisfactory results have been reported in the literature.

Highlights

- The appropriate selection of lung transplant recipients and the proper timing of listing are challenging processes and important determinants of outcomes.

- Lung graft suitability among the pool of multiorgan donors is about 20%; this organ shortage has led to considering marginal donors also.
- 3- DLTx is the surgical option applied in the majority of cases. SLTx remains a valid choice in older and more fragile patients without pulmonary hypertension and lung infection.
- Ideal candidates for lung transplantation are adults with end-stage lung disease, limited life expectancy, and, at the same time, free of significant comorbidities that might negatively impact post-operative outcomes.
- Venous-venous ECMO as bridge to transplant is a valid alternative to the use of mechanical ventilation in patients deteriorating during waiting list.

References

1. Weill D, Benden C, Corris PA, et al. A consensus document for the selection of lung transplant candidates: 2014—An update from the Pulmonary Transplantation Council of the International Society for Heart and Lung Transplantation. J Heart Lung Transplant. 2015;34:1–15.
2. Orens JB, Merlo CA. Selection of candidates for lung transplantation and controversial issues. Semin Respir Crit Care Med. 2018;39:117–125.
3. Hayes D, Black SM, Tobias JD, Higgins RS, Whitson BA. Influence of donor and recipient age in lung transplantation. J Heart Lung Transplant. 2015;34:43–49.
4. Biscotti M, Gannon WD, Agerstrand C, et al. Awake extracorporeal membrane oxygenation as bridge to lung transplantation: A 9-year experience. Ann Thorac Surg. 2017;104:412–419.
5. Fuehner T, Kuehn C, Hadem J, et al. Extracorporeal membrane oxygenation in awake patients as bridge to lung transplantation. Am J Respir Crit Care Med. 2012;185:763–768.
6. Boffini M, Ricci D, Ranieri VM, Rinaldi M. A bridge over troubled waters. Transpl Int. 2015;28:284–285.
7. Chambers DC, Yusen RD, Cherikh WS, et al. International Society for Heart and Lung Transplantation. The Registry of the International Society for Heart and Lung Transplantation: thirty-fourth adult lung and heart-lung transplantation report-2017; focus theme: allograft ischemic time. J Heart Lung Transplant. 2017;36:1047–1059.
8. Thabut G, Christie JD, Ravaud P, et al. Survival after bilateral versus single lung transplantation for patients with chronic obstructive pulmonary disease: A retrospective analysis of registry data. Lancet. 2008;371:744–751.
9. Hosenpud JD, Bennett LE, Keck BM, Edwards EB, Novick RJ. Effect of diagnosis on survival benefit of lung transplantation for end-stage lung disease. Lancet. 1998;351:24–27.

10. Charman SC, Sharples LD, McNeil KD, Wallwork J. Assessment of survival benefit after lung transplantation by patient diagnosis. J Heart Lung Transplant. 2002;21:226–232.
11. Celli BR, Cote CG, Marin JM, et al. The body-mass index, airflow obstruction, dyspnea, and exercise capacity index in chronic obstructive pulmonary disease. N Engl J Med. 2004;350:1005–1012.
12. Martinez FJ, Safrin S, Weycker D, et al. IPF Study Group. The clinical course of patients with idiopathic pulmonary fibrosis. Ann Intern Med. 2005;142:963–967.
13. Aris RM, Routh JC, LiPuma JJ, Heath DG, Gilligan PH. Lung transplantation for cystic fibrosis patients with Burkholderia cepacia complex. Survival linked to genomovar type. Am J Respir Crit Care Med. 2001;164:2102–2106.
14. Parize P, Boussaud V, Poinsignon V, et al. Clinical outcome of cystic fibrosis patients colonized by Scedosporium species following lung transplantation: A single-center 15-year experience. Transpl Infect Dis. 2017;19:5.
15. Dobbin C, Maley M, Harkness J, et al. The impact of panresistant bacterial pathogens on survival after lung transplantation in cystic fibrosis: Results from a single large referral centre. J Hosp Infect. 2004;56:277–282.
16. Miyamoto S, Nagaya N, Satoh T, et al. Clinical correlates and prognostic significance of six-minute walk test in patients with primary pulmonary hypertension. Comparison with cardiopulmonary exercise testing. Am J Respir Crit Care Med. 2000;161:487–492.
17. Mandich Crovetto D, Alonso Charterina S, Jiménez López-Guarch C, et al. Multidetector computed tomography shows reverse cardiac remodeling after double lung transplantation for pulmonary hypertension. Radiología. 2016;58:277.
18. Hill C, Maxwell B, Boulate D, et al. Heart-lung vs. double-lung transplantation for idiopathic pulmonary arterial hypertension. Clin Transplant. 2015;29:1067.
19. Chambers DC, Cherikh WS, Goldfarb SB, et al. The International Thoracic Organ Transplant Registry of the International Society for Heart and Lung Transplantation: Thirty-fifth adult lung and heart-lung transplant report-2018; Focus theme: Multiorgan Transplantation. *J* Heart Lung Transplant. 2018;37:1169–1183.
20. Moser B, Jaksch P, Taghavi S, et al. Lung transplantation for idiopathic pulmonary hypertension on intraoperative and postoperatively prolonged extracorporeal membrane oxygenation provides optimally controlled reperfusion and excellent outcome. Eur J Cardiothorac Surg. 2018;53:178.
21. Tudorache I, Sommer W, Kühn C, et al. Lung transplantation for severe pulmonary hypertension—awake extracorporeal membrane oxygenation for postoperative left ventricle remodelling. Transplantation. 2015;99:451.
22. Avlonitis VS, Fisher AJ, Kirby JA, Dark JH. Pulmonary transplantation: The role of brain death in donor lung injury. Transplantation. 2003;75:1928–1933.
23. Teasdale G, Jennet B. Assessment of coma and impaired consciousness. Lancet. 1974;304:81–84.
24. Achieving comprehensive coordination in organ donation throughout the European Union-ACCORD. Increasing the collaboration between donor transplant coordinators and intensive care professionals (www.accord-ja.eu/content/work-package-number-5-intensive-care-donor- transplant-coordination-collaboration, accessed 12 July 2019).

25. Sales G, Costamagna A, Fanelli V, et al. How to optimize the lung donor. Minerva Anestesiol. 2018;84:204–215.
26. Alliance-O (European Group for Co-ordination of National Research Programmes on Organ Donation and Transplantation) [http://ec.europa.eu/research/fp7/pdf/era-net/fact_sheets/fp6/alliance-o_en.pdf, accessed 12 July 2019].
27. Bhorade SM, Vigneswaran W, McCabe MA, et al. Liberalization of donor criteria may expand the donor pool without adverse consequence in lung transplantation. J Heart Lung Transplant. 2000;19:1199–1204.
28. Warnecke G, Moradiellos J, Tudorache I et al. Normothermic perfusion of donor lungs for preservation and assessment with the Organ Care System Lung before bilateral transplantation: A pilot study of 12 patients. Lancet. 2012;380:1851–1858.
29. McCowin MJ, Hall TS, Babcock WD et al. Changes in radiographic abnormalities in organ donors: Associations with lung transplantation. J Heart Lung Transplant. 2005;24:323–330.
30. Verleden GM, Martens A, Ordies S et al. Radiological analysis of unused donor lungs: a tool to improve donor acceptance for transplantation? Am J Transplant. 2017;17:1912–1921.
31. Miñambres E, Pérez-Villares JM, Chico-Fernández M et al. Lung donor treatment protocol in brain dead-donors: A multicenter study. J Heart Lung Transplant. 2015;34:773–780.
32. Boffini M, Ricci D, Barbero C, et al. Ex vivo lung perfusion increases the pool of lung grafts: analysis of its potential and real impact on a lung transplant program. Transplant Proc. 2013:45:2624–2626.
33. Cypel M, Keshavjee S. Strategies for safe donor expansion: Donor management, donation after cardiac death, ex-vivo lung perfusion. Curr Opin Organ Transplant. 2013;18:513–517.
34. Bonser RS, Taylor R, Collett D, et al. Effect of donor smoking on survival after lung transplantation: A cohort study of a prospective registry. Lancet. 2012;380:747–755.
35. Mattner F, Kola A, Fischer S et al. Impact of bacterial and fungal donor organ contamination in lung, heart-lung, heart and liver transplantation. Infection. 2008;36:207–212.
36. Campos S, Caramori M, Teixeira R et al. Bacterial and fungal pneumonias after lung transplantation. Transplant Proc. 2008;40:822–824.
37. Ciulli F, Tamm M, Dennis CM et al. Donor-transmitted bacterial infection in heart–lung transplantation. Transplant Proc. 1993;25:1155–1156.
38. Orens JB, Boehler A, de Perrot M, et al. A review of lung transplant donor acceptability criteria. The Journal of Heart and Lung Transplantation. 2003;22:1183–1200.
39. Rinaldi M, Sansone F, Boffini M, et al. Single versus double lung transplantation in pulmonary fibrosis: A debated topic. Transplant Proc. 2008;40:2010–2012.

46

Ex vivo lung perfusion

Aadil Ali, Marcelo Cypel

Introduction

Hypothermic static storage has been the gold standard for pulmonary graft preservation since the advent of lung transplantation. In this technique, the lungs are mildly inflated with a cold, low-potassium dextran solution flush and subsequent ice storage. While on ice, cellular processes within the organ are slowed down and the metabolic requirements of the lung are significantly reduced. The major limitation of cold static storage is the limited opportunity to assess and recondition the graft at such low temperature ranges. Therefore, there is a strong rationale for maintenance of the lungs under normothermic conditions.

The concept of normothermic ex vivo organ perfusion has been described as early as 1935 with cats and rabbits as research models. Ex vivo preservation of thyroid glands was achieved for one week using a glass-chambered perfusion pump.[1] This study served as an evidence for the possibility of ex vivo maintenance of organs. In 1987, the technique of normothermic ex vivo lung perfusion (EVLP) was proposed for extended pulmonary preservation during distant procurements. This concept was soon abandoned due to the development of circuit-induced lung injuries after prolonged perfusion periods.[2] In 2001, Steen and his colleagues proposed to perform EVLP for lung evaluation purposes, rather than preservation. Lungs obtained from non-heart beating donors were assessed within the ex vivo platform successfully; the recipient of such lung displayed exceptional post-transplant outcomes.[3] In 2008, the Toronto team published a modified protective approach to EVLP which enabled prolonged maintenance of lungs during extended perfusion periods.[4] In 2011, the same group performed a prospective non-randomized clinical trial demonstrating the safety and feasibility of EVLP to assess and recondition marginal donor lungs using their approach.(5) This was successively followed by rapid growth of literature involving EVLP within both clinical and experimental settings. Presently, the usage of EVLP is increasingly a part of clinical practices within North America, Europe, and Australia.(6–15)

Currently, four commercial devices are available to perform clinical EVLP. These include the Organ Care System™ Lung (OCS); the XPS™ (XVIVO Perfusion AB); the Lung Assist® (Organ Assist); and the Vivoline® LS1. Each system differs on the basis of individual components, design, and clinical usage. The OCS™ Lung is the only system which is used for transportation of the organ, while the primary usage of the other devices is organ assessment and treatment.

Although differences exist between individual components, the basic components of a standard EVLP system include: a solution to perfuse the lungs, a ventilator, a heater to control temperature, a pump to control flow, a reservoir to control circuit volume, a leukocyte filter to deplete immune cells, and a gas-exchange membrane. A schematic diagram of an EVLP circuit is shown in Figure 46.1. The ventilator parameters, type of pump, pressures, and flows may differ based on the technical protocol being used. In current clinical practice, the three major protocols are being performed, namely, the Toronto protocol, the Lund protocol, and the Organ Care System protocol; the approaches are summarized in Table 46.1.

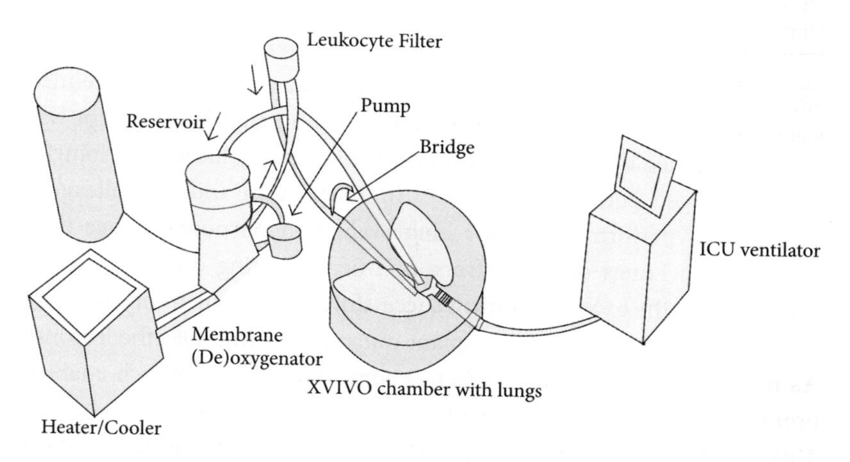

Figure 46.1. The Toronto Ex vivo lung perfusion system

Table 46.1 Comparison of different ex vivo lung perfusion systems used in clinical transplantation

	Protocol		
	Toronto	**Organ Care System (OCS)**	**Lund**
Flow			
Pump type	Centrifugal	Pulsatile	Roller
Target flow total	40% cardiac output	2.5 L/min	100% cardiac output
Ventilation			
Ventilator Mode	Volume control	Volume control	Volume control
Tidal volume	7 mL/kg BW	6 mL/kg BW	5–7 mL/kg BW
Frequency	7 bpm	10 bpm	20 bpm
PEEP	5 cmH_2O	5 cmH_2O	5 cmH_2O
FiO_2	21%	21%	50%
Pressure			
Pulmonary artery	< 15 mmHg	< 20 mmHg	< 20 mmHg
Left atrium	3–5 mmHg	Open atrium	Open atrium
Target Temperature	Normothermia	Normothermia	Normothermia
Perfusion solution	STEEN™ solution (buffered extracellular solution)	OCS™ solution + red cells (Hct 15–25%)	STEEN™ solution + red cells (Hct 14%)
Clinical Indication	Assessment	Transportation	Assessment
Clinical perfusion times	4–6 hours	Transport time	2 hours

PEEP = Positive-end Expiratory Pressure; bpm = breathes per minute; Hct = Hematocrit; FiO_2 = Fraction of inspired Oxygen; BW = Body Weight

Source: Reeb J et al., 2016

Evidence-based EVLP for organ reconditioning

As mentioned earlier, one of the greatest advantages of EVLP is the opportunity to assess and recondition the graft prior to transplant. This can be quite significant considering that the percentage of lungs used from multi-organ donors is between 15% and 20%; therefore, up

Table 46.2 A list of potential parameters which can be measured during EVLP

Means of Measurements	Parameter measured
Ventilator	Peak Airway Pressure
	Plateau Airway Pressure
	Dynamic Compliance
	Static Compliance
	Rate of Deflation
Perfusion	Oxygenation
	Glucose consumption
	Lactate Production
	STEEN loss (ml/hr)
	Pulmonary Vascular Resistance
Qualitative	Radiographic Infiltrations
	Bronchoscopic findings
	Gross anatomy

to 85% of lungs are rejected in some regions for transplantation.[16] During EVLP, graft function can be monitored by visualizing the trends in ventilator parameters, analysis of the perfusate, and qualitative inspection as seen in Table 46.2. Analysing these parameters help in monitoring the trends of organ function. Many reports have described the ability of EVLP to recondition the donor graft prior to transplantation. Reconditioning of the lung may occur through removal of airway secretions, lung recruitment, resolution of pulmonary oedema, washout of immunological components, and the activation of innate repair mechanisms within the lung. Certain key studies have described the concept of ex vivo lung reconditioning of marginal lungs within a clinical setting.

In 2007, Steen et al. described the first human transplantation of a nonacceptable donor lung after reconditioning with EVLP. The donor lung ratio of arterial oxygen partial pressure to fractional inspired oxygen (P/F ratio) was only 96.4 mmHg, even after ventilator treatment and attempts to clean the airways. The right lung was severely injured, while the left lung was oedematous with bleeding spots in the lower lobe, and the mediobasal segment was atelectatic. The left lung was reconditioned using EVLP, and the lungs were subjected to transplantation in a high-risk recipient.[17] The patient showed good recovery, and after three months, computed tomographic thoracic scan and transbronchial biopsies showed a normal left lung.[17]

In the 2011 study published by the Toronto group, twenty-three lungs considered to be high risk for transplantation were subjected to 4 hours of EVLP within a prospective nonrandomized trial.[5] High-risk donor lungs were defined by specific criteria, including pulmonary oedema, a P/F ratio of less than 300 mm Hg or other concerns.[5] Twenty of these lungs were used for transplant, in which no differences in Primary Graft Dysfunction (PGD) after 72 hours was found in comparison to contemporary donors, and no differences were seen in thirty-day mortality rate, bronchial complications, duration of mechanical ventilation, and length of stay in the intensive care unit and hospital.[5]

In 2012, the Vienna group published a prospective study which showed the utilization of a similar classification of high-risk donors within their centre. Of thirteen lungs which met the inclusion criteria of the study, nine lungs were successfully reconditioned and were deemed acceptable for transplantation. These lungs demonstrated a median donor PaO_2 of 216 mmHg which improved to a median PaO_2 of 466 mmHg at the final assessment of EVLP.[6] Of the patients who received these lungs, none developed grade 2 or 3 PGD, and patients showed no thirty-day mortality rate.[6]

Later that year, the Harefield group published a retrospective review of thirteen consecutive EVLPs over a span of less than two years. Ultimately, six lungs were deemed suitable for transplantation. The six transplanted patients showed similar early, three-month, and six-month survival rates and ICU and hospital length of stay to their contemporary transplant population.[13]

Two years later, Wallinder et al. published the EVLP experience from the Gothenburg group. In this case-control study, eleven donor lungs were proceeded to EVLP due to either inferior P/F ratio, bilateral infiltrate on chest X-ray or ongoing extra corporeal membrane oxygenation.[18] Donor grafts showed improved oxygenation with a median P/F ratio of 209 mmHg in the donor and to 447 mmHg at the end of EVLP.[18] The authors found a longer median time to extubation and median intensive care unit stay to be significantly higher in recipients receiving lungs from the EVLP group versus contemporary controls.[18] Despite this finding, no difference was seen in the length of hospital stay, and all recipients of EVLP lungs were discharged alive.[18]

In 2014, Sage et al. published the French EVLP experience. During EVLP, thirty-one out of thirty-two lungs initially rejected for transplant recovered from a median P/F ratio of 274 mmHg to 511 mm Hg.[8] There were no significant differences in PGD incidence after 72-hours, median extubation time, intensive care unit, and hospital lengths of stay, thirty-day mortality, and one-year survival rates among reconditioned lungs transplanted in comparison to lungs transplanted from standard criteria donors.[8]

In the same year, Henriksen et al. shared the first Danish experience using EVLP. In the study period, seven of thirty-three Danish lung transplantations were made possible due to EVLP. All lungs showed an improved median P/F ratio of 173.2 mmHg in the donor to 441 mmHg at the end of EVLP. No patients died due to EVLP-related causes by the end of the trial registration period (1 May 2012–13 April 2013).[14]

A lung transplant group from Italy evaluated the impact of reconditioning of lungs through EVLP in the post-transplant outcomes within their centre. The authors were able to recover eight out of eleven lungs, which would have otherwise been declined, by using EVLP.[12] The EVLP reconditioned lungs transplanted showed that the incidence of PGD3 at 72 hours was 0% in comparison to 25% for lungs from standard criteria (n = 28) which were transplanted during the study period.[12] Similar findings were observed in a recent international non-inferiority, randomized, controlled, open-label phase 3 trial. Normothermic machine preservation of lungs using the OCS system was compared to conventional cold storage techniques (n = 151 with OCS and n = 169 for control). Incidence of PGD3 within 72 hours was reported in 25 (17.7%) of 141 patients in the OCS group (95% CI 11.8 to 25.1) and 49 (29.7%) of 165 patients in the control group ($p = 0.015$).

There are upcoming single centre and multi-centre trials which are continuing to evaluate the reconditioning potential of EVLP within their respective transplant practices. The generation of such data will complement the existing literature and allow generalizing EVLP amongst different geographies.

EVLP for organ preservation

One of the futuristic indications of EVLP is optimizing pulmonary preservation lengths.[19] Using the current gold standard practice of cold ischemic preservation, the average preservation time is limited to approximately 6–8 hours. Delaying beyond the current preservation window may have several consequences, including overcoming geographical hurdles for organ donation, better donor-recipient matching, and optimizing transplant logistics. Within the setting of lung preservation, EVLP may have important implications. During prolonged cold ischemia, disruption of important cellular processes may subsequently lead to cell death and ultimately, inadequate function of the graft.[20] A large animal preclinical study published in 2015 demonstrated that the intervention of EVLP during cold ischemic preservation could effectively allow for an extension of total preservation time, which otherwise would not be possible using standard methods.[21] The exact mechanism by which this occurs still remains unanswered.

In 2014, the Leuven group published a successful case report of a combined liver–lung transplantation. In anticipation of a longer lung preservation time due to the liver transplantation, the authors subjected the donor lungs to preservation on the EVLP platform. The total normothermic perfusion time (total time on pump) was approximately 11 hours by which the lungs were transplanted. The total ex vivo preservation time (cold preservation + normothermic perfusion) of the lungs was 13 hours and 32 minutes for the first transplanted lung and 16 hours for the second.[22] The patient was extubated seven days after the surgery, and no rejection was reported until ten months.[22]

Recently, within a large cohort (n = 906), the Toronto group published a retrospective analysis comparing outcomes of transplant recipients who received lungs which were preserved for less than 12 hours versus those who received lungs which were preserved for more than 12 hours.[23] Preservation time greater than 12 hours was primarily achieved through the usage of EVLP for the assessment of extended criteria donor grafts. Interestingly, results of this analysis showed no differences in the hospital stay, intensive-unit length of stay, PGD grade, and overall survival amongst the two groups.[23]

Given this information, the thoughtful use of EVLP in the setting of lung preservation can be a feasible option to successfully extend total preservation periods. A prospective randomized trial and another multicentre international study, both, showed that EVLP can be used for standard criteria donor lungs without compromising lung quality.[7,24] Prospective trials evaluating the feasibility and efficacy of this approach are still required.

EVLP for targeted therapeutics

One of the major advantages of EVLP is that every individual lung can be diagnosed and assessed while being actively ventilated and perfused. Donor lungs may have a variety of complications which may include the presence of emboli, aspiration injury, and infection. Once these concerns are identified, they can be addressed by using intervening therapeutics during EVLP. Currently, the data generated using targeted therapeutics has mostly been pre-clinical. Data from clinical trials evaluating the feasibility and efficacy of these approaches are still required.

Immunomodulation

Studies have shown that the onset of ischemia-reperfusion injury is correlated with the rapid release of endogenous inflammatory mediators.[25,26] Therefore, promoting an anti-inflammatory environment prior to transplantation may have protective effects with regards to lung injury. In 2009, Cypel et al. investigated the functional repair of human donor lungs using Interleukin-10 (IL-10) gene therapy.[27] The IL-10 is an anti-inflammatory cytokine that has been shown to reduce the release of pro-inflammatory cytokines.[28] In this study, the authors delivered adenoviral vector encoding human IL-10 bronchoscopically within the EVLP platform. Throughout the course of perfusion, treated lungs showed significant improvement in pulmonary vascular resistance, alveoli oxygenation capabilities, and a favourable switch in cytokine expression.[27]

Another example of an immunomodulatory intervention attempted on the EVLP platform is Mesenchymal Stem Cell (MSC) based therapy. The MSCs are well known to play an immunomodulatory role by migrating to sites of inflammation, to participate in cell-to-cell interactions or secrete soluble factors.[29] By injecting these cells into the EVLP perfusate, lower levels of circulating pro-inflammatory Interleukin-8 (IL-8) were found within the EVLP circuit.[30]

Aspiration injury

Inci et al. put forth an aspiration-injury model by instilling a mixture of betaine-HCl/pepsin into the airways.[31] Surfactant lavage within these injured lungs during EVLP resulted in a higher P/F ratio, and lower pulmonary vascular resistance in comparison to the controls.[31] Likewise, Meers et al. described a model of aspiration-induced injury by instilling gastric juice into the airways, rather than an acidic substitute mixture.[32] Using a similar gastric-juice induced lung injury model, it was later shown that exogenous surfactant administered immediately before EVLP was able to improve PaO_2, lower pulmonary vascular resistance, and decrease the amount of apoptotic cell death.[33] With another similar model, the Toronto group attempted a strategy of performing a saline lavage immediately followed by the administration of exogenous surfactant for the treatment of an aspiration-induced injury.[34] The lungs were treated during EVLP, and were subsequently transplanted into a recipient animal.[34] Results of the study showed reduction of circulating inflammatory cytokines post-transplantation and superior lung function in comparison to controls, represented by a greater P/F ratio.[34]

Infection

In 2013, Lee et al. investigated the use of MSCs to recover endotoxin-induced acute lung injury within donor human lungs rejected for transplantation. The use of clinical-grade human MSCs restored alveolar fluid clearance to a normal level, decreased inflammation, and was associated with increased bacterial killing and reduced bacteraemia. This was achieved in part through increased alveolar macrophage phagocytosis and secretion of antimicrobial factors.[35]

In 2014, Andreasson et al. examined the effect of perfusing lungs, declined for transplantation, with a perfusate containing high-dose, empirical, broad-spectrum anti-microbial agents. Out of the eighteen lungs perfused, thirteen of them had positive bacteria cultures (72%), in which the bacterial load significantly decreased during EVLP.[36] Ultimately, six lungs were deemed suitable for transplantation, after which all the patients survived hospital discharge.[36]

In 2016, a study was published randomizing donor human lungs rejected for transplantation due to the clinical concern of infection; the infected lungs received 12 hours of conventional perfusion, or perfusion supplemented with high-dose antibiotics. Perfusate endotoxin levels at 12 hours were significantly lower in the antibiotic group compared with the control group.[37] In addition, the treatment group showed significant improvement in pulmonary oxygenation and compliance and reduced pulmonary vascular resistance during EVLP.[37]

In a recent publication, Zinne et al. put forth a *Pseudomonas aeruginosa* induced pneumonia pig model.[38] The authors investigated whether 2 hours of EVLP using circulating colistin followed by autotransplantation could be advantageous in comparison to conventional methods of daily intravenous colistin administration and controls. In the control and conventional treatment groups, the mortality rate related to infection after five days was 66.7%.[38] However, in the EVLP group, there was only one infection-related mortality and one procedure-related mortality, resulting in an overall mortality rate of 33.3%.[38] In addition, the authors found that lungs treated with EVLP displayed less clinical symptoms of infection.[38]

Pulmonary oedema

Studies have shown that the rate of alveolar epithelial ion and fluid transport can be upregulated through the use of β_2-adrenergic agonists.[39,40] Franck et al. showed that putting human lungs rejected for transplantation on the EVLP circuit, naturally led to alveolar fluid clearance and reduction in pulmonary oedema.[41] In addition, by adding a β_2-selective adrenergic agonist (terbutaline) to the EVLP perfusate, air space fluid clearance rates increased significantly by more than twofold.[41]

Along with the similar idea, another group tested whether a β-adrenergic receptor agonist (salbutamol) which is known to upregulate fluid transport in the lung would be effective in reducing pulmonary oedema.[42] Their primary indicator of oedema formation was lung glucose consumption during EVLP, which they validated within a previous study.[43] In the study, the authors randomized donor pig lungs to salbutamol infusion during EVLP, or a placebo. The results showed that glucose concentration in the perfusate was affected by salbutamol, and salbutamol infusion was associated with lower pulmonary pressures and better lung mechanics.[42]

Pulmonary emboli

The first case report treating pulmonary emboli (PE) during EVLP involved the administration of alteplase to the EVLP perfusate.[44] Improvements in pulmonary artery pressure and pulmonary vascular resistance during EVLP indicated successful thrombolysis, and the lungs proceeded to clinical transplantation.[44] These results were reconfirmed in 2015, when another case report was published showing alteplase as a successful adjunct for thrombolysis during EVLP, leading to subsequent clinical lung transplantation.[45] Urokinase, a known plasminogen activator, has also shown positive results in the treatment of PE.[46]

Virus inactivation

Currently, lungs offered from donors infected with hepatitis C virus are not routinely offered for transplantation. In a paper published in 2019, Galasso et al. examined whether targeted approaches on the EVLP platform could be used to inactivate and eliminate hepatitis C virus from Nucleic Acid Amplification Testing positive (NAT+) human donor lungs. In this paired study, the authors compared performing a complete circuit exchange, irradiating the perfusate with ultraviolet C light (UVC), and photodynamic therapy (PDT) to internal controls.[47] Exchange of the circuit and PDT resulted in a significant decrease in perfusate and tissue viral load examined by qPCR. Despite UVC showing no significant effects based on qPCR counts, further in vitro studies demonstrated that the virus was no longer infectious after UVC irradiation.[47]

Conclusion

The EVLP platform is a revolutionary technology which has many promising applications within the setting of lung transplantation. Currently, EVLP presents as an excellent platform for organ assessment and reconditioning. Indeed, in current clinical practice, lungs which were deemed initially unsuitable for transplantation have been transplanted with comparable outcomes to that of conventional lungs. Experimental models of EVLP have further shown its utility as a targeted platform, addressing common donor ailments such as infection, PE, and pulmonary oedema. Further clinical studies regarding its utility for targeted therapeutics are warranted. Lastly, EVLP has recently shown itself as an excellent platform for the extension of donor lung preservation times; future studies should be performed to validate this potential.

Highlights

- The usage of EVLP within clinical transplantation has been demonstrated to extend total organ preservation time.
- Clinical studies have shown that EVLP can recondition marginal donor lungs, allowing for the usage of lungs, which would have otherwise been discarded.
- The EVLP system has been demonstrated as an excellent platform to treat donor-specific issues such as infection, oedema, PE, and aspiration-injury.
- The EVLP platform serves as an ideal platform to perform isolated lung assessment.
- Studies have shown successful immunomodulation of the lung prior to transplantation using EVLP.

References

1. Carrel A, Lindbergh CA. The culture of whole organs. Science (80-). 1935;81 (2112):621–623.
2. Hardesty RL, Griffith BP. Autoperfusion of the heart and lungs for preservation during distant procurement. J Thorac Cardiovasc Surg. 1987;93 (1): 8–11.
3. Steen S, Sjöberg T, Pierre L, Liao Q, Eriksson L, Algotsson L. Transplantation of lungs from a non-heart-beating donor. Lancet. 2001;357(9259):825–829.
4. Cypel M, Yeung JC, Hirayama S, Rubacha M, Fischer S, Anraku M, et al. Technique for prolonged normothermic ex vivo lung perfusion. J Hear Lung Transplant. 2008;27(12):1319–1325.
5. Cypel M, Yeung JC, Liu M, Anraku M, Chen F, Karolak W, et al. Normothermic ex vivo lung perfusion in clinical lung transplantation. N Engl J Med [Internet]. 2011;364(15):1431–1440. Available from: http://www.ncbi.nlm.nih.gov/pubmed/21488765
6. Aigner C, Slama A, Hötzenecker K, Scheed A, Urbanek B, Schmid W, et al. Clinical ex vivo lung perfusion—Pushing the limits. Am J Transplant. 2012;12(7):1839–1847.
7. Slama A, Schillab L, Barta M, Benedek A, Mitterbauer A, Hoetzenecker K, et al. Standard donor lung procurement with normothermic ex vivo lung perfusion: A prospective randomized clinical trial. J Hear Lung Transplant. 2017;36 (7): 744–753.
8. Sage E, Mussot S, Trebbia G, Puyo P, Stern M, Dartevelle P, et al. Lung transplantation from initially rejected donors after ex vivo lung reconditioning: The French experience. Eur J Cardio-thoracic Surg. 2014;46(5):794–799.
9. Valenza F, Citerio G, Palleschi A, Vargiolu A, Fakhr BS, Confalonieri A, et al. Successful transplantation of lungs from an uncontrolled donor after circulatory death preserved in situ by alveolar recruitment maneuvers and assessed by ex vivo lung perfusion. Am J Transplant. 2016; 16 (4): 1312–1318.
10. Wallinder A, Riise GC, Ricksten SE, Silverborn M, Dellgren G. Transplantation after ex vivo lung perfusion: A midterm follow-up. J Hear Lung Transplant. 2016;35 (11): 1303–1310.
11. Warnecke G, Moradiellos J, Tudorache I, Kühn C, Avsar M, Wiegmann B, et al. Normothermic perfusion of donor lungs for preservation and assessment with the Organ Care System Lung before bilateral transplantation: A pilot study of 12 patients. Lancet. 2012;380(9856):1851–1858.
12. Boffini M, Ricci D, Bonato R, Fanelli V, Attisani M, Ribezzo M, et al. Incidence and severity of primary graft dysfunction after lung transplantation using rejected grafts reconditioned with ex vivo lung perfusion. Eur J Cardiothorac Surg [Internet]. 2014;46(5):789–793. Available from: http://ejcts.oxfordjournals.org/cgi/doi/10.1093/ejcts/ezu239
13. Zych B, Popov AF, Stavri G, Bashford A, Bahrami T, Amrani M, et al. Early outcomes of bilateral sequential single lung transplantation after ex-vivo lung evaluation and reconditioning. J Hear Lung Transplant. 2012;31(3):274–281.
14. Iversen Henriksen IS, Møller-Sørensen H, Holdflod Møller C, Zemtsovski M, Christian Nilsson J, Tobias Seidelin C, et al. First Danish experience with

ex vivo lung perfusion of donor lungs before transplantation. Dan Med J. 2014;61(3):A4809.

15. Zhang ZL, van Suylen V, van Zanden JE, Van De Wauwer C, Verschuuren EAM, van der Bij W, et al. First experience with ex vivo lung perfusion for initially discarded donor lungs in the Netherlands: a single-centre study. Eur J Cardio-Thoracic Surg. 2018;55(5): 920–926.
16. Punch JD, Hayes DH, Laporte FB, McBride V, Seely MS. Organ donation and utilization in the United States, 1996–2005. Vol. 7, American Journal of Transplantation. 2007: 7(5 Pt 2): 1327–1338.
17. Steen S, Ingemansson R, Eriksson L, Pierre L, Algotsson L, Wierup P, et al. First human transplantation of a nonacceptable donor lung after reconditioning ex vivo. Ann Thorac Surg. 2007;83(6):2191–2194.
18. Wallinder A, Ricksten SE, Silverborn M, Hansson C, Riisec GC, Liden H, et al. Early results in transplantation of initially rejected donor lungs after ex vivo lung perfusion: A case-control study. Eur J Cardio-thoracic Surg. 2014;45(1):40–45.
19. Ali A, Cypel M. Ex-vivo lung perfusion and ventilation. Curr Opin Organ Transplant [Internet]. 2019;24(3):297–304. Available from: http://insights.ovid.com/crossref?an=00075200-201906000-00015
20. de Perrot M, Liu M, Waddell TK, Keshavjee S. Ischemia-reperfusion-induced lung injury. Am J Respir Crit Care Med. 2003;167(4):490–511.
21. Hsin MKY, Iskender I, Nakajima D, Chen M, Kim H, Dos Santos PR, et al. Extension of donor lung preservation with hypothermic storage after normothermic ex vivo lung perfusion. J Hear Lung Transplant. 2016;35(1):130–136.
22. Ceulemans LJ, Monbaliu D, Verslype C, Van Der Merwe S, Laleman W, Vos R, et al. Combined liver and lung transplantation with extended normothermic lung preservation in a patient with end-stage emphysema complicated by drug-induced acute liver failure. Am J Transplant. 2014;14(10):2412–2416.
23. Yeung JC, Krueger T, Yasufuku K, de Perrot M, Pierre AF, Waddell TK, et al. Outcomes after transplantation of lungs preserved for more than 12 h: A retrospective study. Lancet Respir Med [Internet]. Elsevier Ltd; 2016;2600(16):1–6. Available from: http://linkinghub.elsevier.com/retrieve/pii/S221326001630323X
24. Warnecke G, Van Raemdonck D, Smith MA, Massard G, Kukreja J, Rea F, et al. Normothermic ex-vivo preservation with the portable Organ Care System Lung device for bilateral lung transplantation (INSPIRE): A randomised, open-label, non-inferiority, phase 3 study. Lancet Respir Med. 2018;6 (5): 357–367.
25. Kaneda H, Waddell TK, De Perrot M, Bai XH, Gutierrez C, Arenovich T, et al. Pre-implantation multiple cytokine mRNA expression analysis of donor lung grafts predicts survival after lung transplantation in humans. Am J Transplant. 2006;6(3):544–551.
26. De Perrot M, Sekine Y, Fischer S, Waddell TK, Mcrae K, Liu M, et al. Interleukin-8 release during early reperfusion predicts graft function in human lung transplantation. Am J Respir Crit Care Med. 2002;165(2):211–215.
27. Cypel M, Liu M, Rubacha M, Yeung JC, Hirayama S, Anraku M, et al. Functional repair of human donor lungs by IL-10 gene therapy. Sci Transl Med. 2009;1(4):4ra9.
28. Moore KW, De Waal Malefyt R, Coffman RL, O 'garra A. Interleukin-10 and the Interleukin-10 Receptor. Annu Rev Immunol. 2001;19:683–765.

29. Ryan JM, Barry FP, Murphy JM, Mahon BP. Mesenchymal stem cells avoid allogeneic rejection. J Inflamm (Lond). 2005;2:8.
30. Mordant P, Nakajima D, Kalaf R, Iskender I, Maahs L, Behrens P, et al. Mesenchymal stem cell treatment is associated with decreased perfusate concentration of interleukin-8 during ex vivo perfusion of donor lungs after 18-hour preservation. J Hear Lung Transplant. 2016;35(10):1245–1254.
31. Inci I, Ampollini L, Arni S, Jungraithmayr W, Inci D, Hillinger S, et al. Ex vivo reconditioning of marginal donor lungs injured by acid aspiration. J Hear Lung Transplant .2008. 27 (11): 1229–1236. I. Inci, Division of Thoracic Surgery, University Hospital, University of Zurich, Switzerland. E-mail: ilhan.inci@usz.ch: Elsevier USA (6277 Sea Harbor Drive, Orlando FL 32862 8239, United States); 2008;27(11):1229–36. Available from: http://ovidsp.ovid.com/ovidweb.cgi?T=JS&PAGE=reference&D=emed11&NEWS=N&AN=50287818
32. Meers CM, Tsagkaropoulos S, Wauters S, Verbeken E, Vanaudenaerde B, Scheers H, et al. A model of ex vivo perfusion of porcine donor lungs injured by gastric aspiration: A step towards pretransplant reconditioning. J Surg Res. 2011;170(1):e159–e167.
33. Khalife-Hocquemiller T, Sage E, Dorfmuller P, Mussot S, Le Houerou D, Eddahibi S, et al. Exogenous surfactant attenuates lung injury from gastric-acid aspiration during ex vivo reconditioning in pigs. Transplantation. 2014;97(4):413–418.
34. Nakajima D, Liu M, Ohsumi A, Kalaf R, Iskender I, Hsin M, et al. Lung lavage and surfactant replacement during ex vivo lung perfusion for treatment of gastric acid aspiration-induced donor lung injury. J Hear Lung Transplant [Internet]. S. Keshavjee, Division of Thoracic Surgery, Toronto General Hospital, 200 Elizabeth St. 9N-946, Toronto, ON M5G 2CS, Canada. E-mail: shaf.keshavjee@uhn.ca: Elsevier USA; 2017;36(5):577–85. Available from: http://www.elsevier.com/locate/healun
35. Lee JW, Krasnodembskaya A, McKenna DH, Song Y, Abbott J, Matthay MA. Therapeutic effects of human mesenchymal stem cells in ex vivo human lungs injured with live bacteria. Am J Respir Crit Care Med. 2013;187 (7): 751–760.
36. Andreasson A, Karamanou DM, Perry JD, Perry A, Özalp F, Butt T, et al. The effect of ex vivo lung perfusion on microbial load in human donor lungs. J Hear Lung Transplant. 2014;33(9):910–916.
37. Nakajima D, Cypel M, Bonato R, Machuca TN, Iskender I, Hashimoto K, et al. Ex vivo perfusion treatment of infection in human donor lungs. Am J Transplant. 2016;16(4):1229–1237.
38. Zinne N, Krueger M, Hoeltig D, Tuemmler B, Boyle EC, Biancosino C, et al. Treatment of infected lungs by ex vivo perfusion with high dose antibiotics and autotransplantation: A pilot study in pigs. PLoS One. 2018;13(3): e0193168.
39. Mutlu GM, Dumasius V, Burhop J, McShane PJ, Meng FJ, Welch L, et al. Upregulation of alveolar epithelial active Na + transport is dependent on beta2-adrenergic receptor signaling. Circ Res [Internet]. 2004;94(8):1091–1100. Available from: http://www.ncbi.nlm.nih.gov/pubmed/15016730
40. Lasnier JM, Wangensteen OD, Schmitz LS, Gross CR, Ingbar DH. Terbutaline stimulates alveolar fluid resorption in hyperoxic lung injury. J Appl Physiol [Internet]. 1996;81(4):1723–1729. Available from: http://www.ncbi.nlm.nih.gov/pubmed/8904592

41. Frank JA, Briot R, Lee JW, Ishizaka A, Uchida T, Matthay MA. Physiological and biochemical markers of alveolar epithelial barrier dysfunction in perfused human lungs. Am J Physiol Lung Cell Mol Physiol. 2007;293(1):L52–L59.
42. Valenza F, Rosso L, Coppola S, Froio S, Colombo J, Dossi R, et al. β-Adrenergic agonist infusion during extracorporeal lung perfusion: Effects on glucose concentration in the perfusion fluid and on lung function. J Hear Lung Transplant. 2012;31(5):524–530.
43. Valenza F, Rosso L, Pizzocri M, Salice V, Umbrello M, Conte G, et al. The consumption of glucose during ex vivo lung perfusion correlates with lung edema. In: Transplantation Proceedings. 2011:43 (4): 993–996.
44. Machuca TN, Hsin MK, Ott HC, Chen M, Hwang DM, Cypel M, et al. Injury-specific ex vivo treatment of the donor lung: Pulmonary thrombolysis followed by successful lung transplantation. Am J Respir Crit Care Med. 2013;188(7):878–880.
45. Luc JGY, Bozso SJ, Freed DH, Nagendran J. Successful repair of donation after circulatory death lungs with large pulmonary embolus using the lung organ care system for ex vivo thrombolysis and subsequent clinical transplantation. Vol. 99, Transplantation. 2015: 99 (1): e1–e2.
46. Inci I, Yamada Y, Hillinger S, Jungraithmayr W, Trinkwitz M, Weder W. Successful lung transplantation after donor lung reconditioning with urokinase in Ex vivo lung perfusion system. Ann Thorac Surg. 2014;98(5):1837–1838.
47. Galasso M, Feld JJ, Watanabe Y, Pipkin M, Summers C, Ali A, et al. Inactivating hepatitis C virus in donor lungs using light therapies during normothermic ex vivo lung perfusion. Nat Commun. 2019 10(1): 481.

47
Liver transplantation

Mauro Salizzoni, Renato Romagnoli, Francesco Tandoi, Damiano Patrono

History of liver transplantation

The first orthotopic (liver graft transplanted in the recipient into its natural site, after removing the native liver) liver transplant (LT) in the world was performed by T. Starzl at the North Western University of Denver on 1 March 1963, in a three-year-old child with biliary atresia who died during the operation due to uncontrollable bleeding. After the first failure and other animal experiments, in 1967, Starzl successfully carried out three LTs in children. In 1968, R. Calne (Cambridge) performed the first adult LT in Europe, while the first paediatric LT in Europe was performed in Belgium, at UCL of Brussels, on 17 March 1971 by J.B. Otte and P.J. Kestens, on a seventeen-month-old child with biliary atresia.(1,2)

The evolution of liver surgery allowed the development of the split-liver technique where the liver is divided into two functionally autonomous parts transplantable into two different recipients. The split liver technique was used for the first time in 1988 by Pichlmayr in Hannover to transplant a single liver graft into a paediatric and an adult recipient.(3) In the same year, Raia in Brazil performed the first paediatric LT from a living donor (from mother to her child).

Indications for liver transplantation

Liver transplantation is the therapeutic option for end-stage liver failure in both acute (fulminant or sub-fulminant) and chronic (cirrhosis) liver disease,(4) and is the gold standard therapy for early stage hepatocellular carcinoma (HCC) in the presence of liver cirrhosis(5) (Table 47.1). The

Table 47.1 Indications for liver transplantation

Adult Recipients		Pediatric Recipients	
Cirrhosis	• Viral (B, C, delta) • Alcoholic • Biliary • Autoimmune • Cryptogenic • Non-alcoholic steatohepatitis	**Cholestasic disease**	• Biliary atresia • Alagille syndrome • Progressive familiar intrahepatic cholestasis • Sclerosing cholangitis • Caroli disease • Langerhans' Cell Histiocytosis
Tumours	• HCC • Hepatic Haemangioendothelioma • Liver metastasis of neuroendocrine tumour • Cholangiocarcinoma (?) • Liver metastasis of colorectal tumour (?)	**Tumours**	• Hepatoblastoma • HCC / fibrolamellar HCC • Hepatic Haemangioendothelioma
Metabolic disease with chronic liver disease	• Alfa-1-antitripsin deficiency • Wilson disease • Hereditary hemochromatosis • Cystic fibrosis	**Metabolic disease with chronic liver disease**	• Alfa-1-antitripsin deficiency • Wilson disease • Tyrosinemia • Galactosemia • Neonatal hemochromatosis • Cystic fibrosis • Tipo IV glycogen storage disease • Niemann-Pick disease • Gaucher disease
Metabolic disease with enzymatic deficiency without liver disease	• Primary hyperoxaluria • Hereditary transthyretin amyloidosis	**Metabolic disease with enzymatic deficiency without liver disease**	• Primary hyperoxaluria • Crigler-Najiar syndrome • Urea cycle disorder • Familial hypercholesterolemia • Tipo IA glycogen storage disease • Type A and B haemophilia • Protein C deficiency
Others indications	• Budd-Chiari • Polycystic liver kidney disease	**Others indications**	• Budd-Chiari • Cryptogenic cirrhosis • Cholestasis related to total parenteral nutrition
Acute liver failure	• Viral • Acetaminophen • Mushroom	**Acute liver failure**	

treatment should be considered in all patients with end-stage liver failure when the life expectancy offered by the transplant is greater than that with the liver disease.

The MELD score (Model for End Stage of Liver Disease)[6] proposed by the Mayo Clinic is the tool to estimate the severity of the patient with liver disease: the higher the MELD, the more severe the patient's clinical conditions and consequently mortality. Likewise, PELD score is considered for paediatric patients.

The MELD score > 15 represents the indication for referral to LT centre, especially in the presence of liver cirrhosis and portal hypertension complications including decompensated ascites refractory to medical therapy, portosystemic encephalopathy, spontaneous bacterial peritonitis, bleeding from oesophageal varices. Indications for LT are alcoholic, viral, autoimmune, and cryptogenetic cirrhosis, biliary cirrhosis, and hepatocellular carcinoma (Table 47.1). In the last decade, there has been a progressive growth of indications for LT due to metabolic-based non-alcoholic steato-hepatitis (NASH).[7]

Hepatocellular carcinoma with cirrhotic liver

The international guidelines for the diagnosis and treatment of HCC identify LT as the therapy for patients with HCC at early stage on a cirrhotic liver where the liver resection is limited by the liver function and the size of the liver remnant. The main limitation of LT for HCC is the risk of recurrence influenced by the stage and the histological features of the tumour at transplant (size and number of nodules, histological grading and vascular invasion). In 1996, Mazzaferro et al. introduced the Milan Criteria to establish the eligibility for LT in patients with a single nodule <5cm or a maximum of three nodules the largest of which <3cm, in absence of vascular invasion and/or extra hepatic disease.[5] The Milan Criteria guaranteed a drastic improvement in post LT survival that exceeded 70% at five years. In the last decade, the need to expand these criteria while maintaining an adequate long-term survival has led to the proposal of new criteria. Yao et al proposed the UCSF criteria (single HCC <6.5 cm, or multifocal HCC with a major nodule of 4.5 cm, or the total sum of nodule <8 cm diameters) to obtain a disease-free survival comparable to that of patients transplanted within the Milan criteria.[8,9] In 2009, Mazzaferro et al elaborated up-to-seven criteria (HCC with seven as the sum of the size of the largest tumour [in cm] and the number of tumours) to achieve a five-year overall survival of 71.2% in the absence of microvascular invasion.[10] Recently, Toso et al., identified the prognostic value of total tumour volume and alfa feto protein (AFP) levels in predicting HCC recurrence after LT.[11,12] The HCC candidates for LT or those on the waiting list for LT can undergo bridging procedures to downstage the tumour to the transplant criteria or to avoid tumour progression and dropout from the waiting list.[13] The procedures for HCC downstaging/bridging are percutaneous ablative techniques (radiofrequency ablation, percutaneous ethanol injection)[14] and transarterial chemoembolization.[15] Liver resection as a downstaging procedure is limited by high mortality and morbidity in patients with end-stage liver disease. The concept of salvage LT was proposed as a recovery strategy in patients with recurrent HCC after the first treatment.[16,17]

Acute liver failure

Acute liver failure (ALF) is a rare but severe pathology with high mortality rate.[18] It is historically defined as a severe, but potentially reversible liver injury with the onset of hepatic encephalopathy within 8 weeks of the first appearance of the symptoms of liver injury, in the absence of pre-existing liver disease. The most frequent causes are viral, toxic drug, or autoimmune hepatitis, or hypoperfusion due to shock and sepsis.[19,20] In some cases (15%), the cause remains unknown. The ALF is defined by the presence of:

- **Coagulopathy**: tendency to bleeding, with INR≥1.5 or PT by 4–6 sec or <70% in the absence of other causes of coagulopathy or anticoagulant therapy.
- **Acute hepatic encephalopathy**: neuropsychic alterations that appear with a variable interval from the onset of jaundice and/or coagulopathy. It is commonly staged with West Haven criteria.

- **Liver disease**: known for less than 8 weeks and in the absence of cirrhosis. Presence of liver disease known for more than 8 weeks but less than 24 weeks is considered as sub-ALF.

The ALF is classified according to the onset of encephalopathy as:

- hyper-acute (0–7 days)
- acute (8–28 days)
- sub-acute (5–12 weeks)

The use of prognostic scores to select patients with low probability of overcoming the acute event with only medical and supportive therapy is crucial to identify patients to be referred to LT.[21,22] In this perspective, the correct timing for indicating LT is fundamental before the irreversible neurological damage is established due to the evolution of disease towards cerebral oedema.[23] The King's College Hospital criteria[24,25] are the most frequently used parameters to select patients with a high risk of mortality in the absence of LT.

1) Acetaminophen ALF:
    - pH <7.30 or arterial lactate> 3 mmol / L or simultaneously
    - INR> 6.5, creatinine> 3.4 mg / dL, grade III–IV encephalopathy
2) Other causes:
    - INR> 6.5 or 3 between:
        - Causes: halothane / hepatitis non-A non-B / drugs / idiopathic
        - Ages <10 to or> 40 years
        - Appearance of encephalopathy > 7 days from the onset of jaundice
        - INR > 3.5
        - Bilirubin > 17 mg/dL

The Clichy's criteria were developed in the 1980s as a prognostic assessment tool in patients with HBV hepatitis; they are based on encephalopathy and factor V activity.

According to the American Association for the Study of Liver Diseases (AASLD) guidelines, patients with ALF should be referred to an intensive care unit when the first symptom of encephalopathy (grade I and II) occurs. In case of high-grade encephalopathy (III–IV), the patient has a high risk of being not transportable and of having permanent neurological damage. For these patients, the work-up of LT should be started as soon as possible. The identification of the aetiology of ALF to begin adequate supportive therapy and to better guide the transplant indication is also fundamental.

Contraindications to liver transplantation

The contraindication for a LT can be absolute or relative.

Absolute contraindications:

- Extra hepatic malignancies and/or history of extra hepatic malignancies with follow-up<5 years
- Neoplastic portal vein thrombosis
- Sepsis (not biliary)
- Irreversible brain damage in patients with ALF
- Unacceptable cardiovascular risk
- Severe pulmonary hypertension with PAP>45 mmHg unresponsive to therapy
- Hepato-pulmonary syndrome with severe hypoxemia.
- Overt Acquired Immune-Deficiency Syndrome (AIDS)
- Serious psychiatric illnesses in the absence of adequate family support or access to Social Services in the area
- Low compliance

Relative:

- Age >70 years
- BMI>35 Kg/m^2
- Severe grade of non-neoplastic portal vein thrombosis

Surgical techniques

The aspects of LT procedures are discussed step-by-step in the following sections.

Laparotomy

LT can be performed through different types of laparotomy, including a bi-subcostal laparotomy with (Y inverted or 'Mercedes-shaped') or without an associated median subxiphoid incision, or a J-shaped laparotomy.[26–28] Patient habitus, severity of liver disease, and portal hypertension have to be taken into account to make the appropriate choice of laparotomy. A wide exposure of the operatory field is always of paramount importance.

Hepato-duodenal ligament dissection

This technique involves surgical dissection of common bile duct, hepatic artery, and portal vein. While the bile duct and hepatic artery are ligated and divided at the end of their dissection, the portal vein is skeletonized but clamped and divided at the end of the hepatectomy. Sometimes, a temporary T-L porto-caval shunt can be constructed; after clamping, the portal vein is divided at the bifurcation between right and left branch.[29,30] The inferior vena cava (IVC), in the subhepatic/suprarenal tract, is clamped tangentially and incised longitudinally for about 3 cm. The anastomosis between the portal vein and the IVC is then carried out.

Retrohepatic IVC dissection

After the section of the hepatic ligaments, the right side of the IVC is exposed. The right liver lobe is reflected to left in order to expose the right and anterior sides of the retrohepatic IVC. In the classic technique according to Starzl, the retrohepatic IVC is clamped and divided above and under the liver, removed with the native liver and replaced with the graft one. Starzl's originally described an extracorporeal circulation with an axillo-porto-femoral circuit. In the piggy-back technique, the retrohepatic IVC is dissected off the liver.[31] The division of the hepatocaval ligament is, as described by Makuuchi et al,[32] the key element in the dissection of the retrohepatic IVC, especially when the prominent part of the caudate lobe encircles the IVC. The small hepatic veins are ligated and sectioned, and IVC is completely preserved until the suprahepatic vein's ostium. In Tzakis's original description,[31] the three principal veins are joined by dividing the intervening septa, obtaining a single ostium. In the Belghiti's side-to-side technique, the right and common trunk of suprahepatic veins are stapled.[33] Piggy-back technique allows IVC flow, guarantees hemodynamic stability, and reduces renal venous congestion, a cause of post-operative renal failure.

Vena cava anastomosis

In the classic technique, anastomosis is performed between retrohepatic IVC of the graft and that of the recipient, above and under the liver. In the piggy-back technique, according to Tzakis, an end-to-side cavo-caval anastomosis is performed between the upper ostium of the graft IVC and the suprahepatic ostium of the recipient IVC.[34] The lower ostium of the IVC of the graft is closed by a stitch or by vascular stapler. In the Belghiti's technique, the upper and the lower ostium' of the graft IVC are closed and a side-to-side cavo-caval anastomosis is carried out between the retrohepatic IVC of the graft and the recipient.[33–36]

A technical variant is the piggy-back technique with caval triangulation; after completing the hepatectomy, a total caval clamping is performed (subdiaphragmatic and suprarenal). A longitudinal cavotomy of 3–5 cm is done starting from the ostium of the suprahepatic veins on the anterior wall of the recipient IVC; an analogous cavotomy is performed on the posterior wall of the IVC of the graft. The vena cava anastomosis is carried out with three sutures, one for each side of the triangle. A modification of this technique is the self-triangulating cavo-cavostomy performed with tangential clamping of the recipient's retrohepatic IVC, as in the Belghiti technique.[37] In adult recipients, the anastomosis is performed with a non-resorbable suture while in paediatric recipients with a resorbable suture.

Portal vein anastomosis

Anastomosis is performed between the portal vein of the recipient and that of the donor, with the so-called 'intima-to-intima' technique. The suture is knotted at about 1–1.5 cm from the anastomosis, to allow the expansion of the portal vein at the time of the graft reperfusion ('growth factor').

Portal vein thrombosis can substantially complicate portal vein reconstruction.[38,39] The thrombus can be mechanically removed with spatulas or surgical forceps. Eversion thrombectomy allows a satisfactory portal flow to be restored in most cases.

The portal thrombosis is classified, according to Yerdel, in four degrees[40]:

- Grade 1: Partial thrombosis <50% of the portal lumen with possible extension to the superior mesenteric vein
- Grade 2: Occlusion> 50% of the portal lumen with possible extension to the superior mesenteric vein
- Grade 3: Complete thrombosis of both portal vein and proximal superior mesenteric vein
- Grade 4: Complete thrombosis of both portal vein and superior mesenteric vein

Patients with portal vein thrombosis can be divided during LT into those with:

1. 'physiological' portal inflow: the portal-mesenteric circulation is physiologically re-established by:
   - Eversion thrombectomy
   - Venous patch interposition
   - Jump graft on superior mesenteric vein (Figure 47.1)
2. 'non-physiological' portal inflow: the native portal flow cannot be restored and the graft portal revascularization occurs through:
   - cavo-portal hemitransposition
   - reno-portal anastomosis
   - portal vein arterialization

When portal anastomosis is performed, in a rapid succession, the caval clamp is removed with retrograde reperfusion of the graft and then the portal clamp, thus obtaining the revascularization of the transplanted liver.

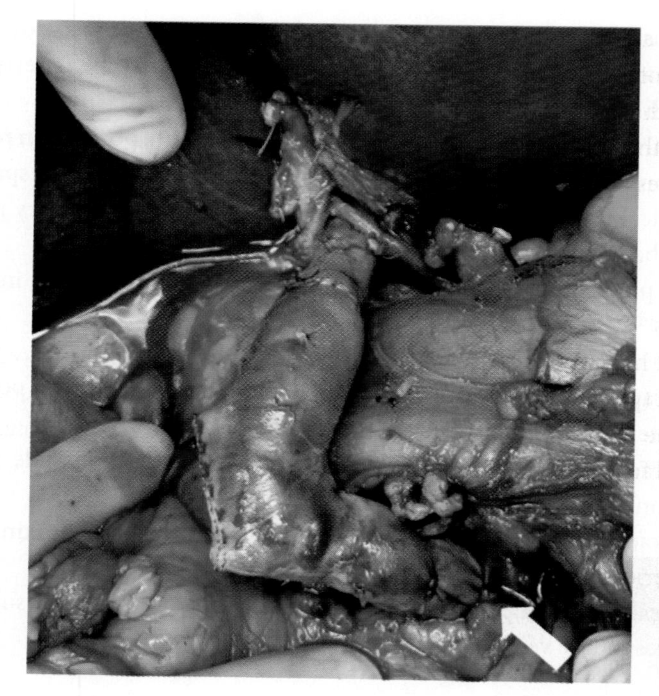

Figure 47.1. Portal vein reconstruction: donor iliac venous conduit on recipient superior mesenteric vein (white arrow) in the jump-graft technique

The graft reperfusion is a critical moment during transplantation, characterized by transient but sometimes, dramatic haemodynamic changes. Post-reperfusion syndrome (PRS)[41,42] is defined as a 30% reduction in mean arterial pressure which lasts at least one minute in the first 5 minutes after reperfusion. The PRS includes hypotension, bradycardia, arrhythmias, impaired cardiac output, reduction of systemic vascular resistance, and occasionally cardiac arrest. The syndrome is caused by a serious myocardial depression determined by an uncontrolled hyperkalaemia and a limited peripheral vasomotor sympathetic response, typical of patients with end-stage liver disease.[43] Clinical studies have also demonstrated the implication of mechanics of the left ventricle and the release of vasoactive mediators by the graft. The acute increase of the intravascular volume and, therefore, of the left ventricular preload that occurs at the time of graft revascularization, stimulates the reflex of the mechanoreceptors responsible for bradycardia and myocardial depression.

Arterial anastomosis

The graft hepatic artery can be anastomosed on the hepatic artery of the recipient (proper or common), or on the splenic artery, on the celiac axis, or on the supraceliac or sub-renal aorta interposing arterial conduits obtained from the same donor[44–47] (Figure 47.2).

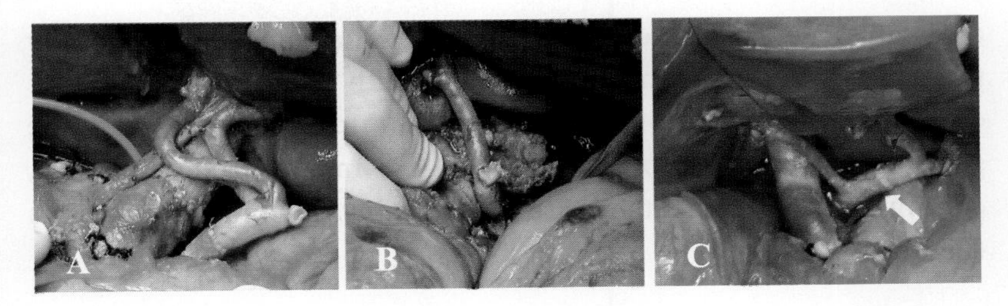

Figure 47.2. Hepatic artery reconstruction: (A) Donor celiac axis on the recipient splenic artery end-to-end. (B) Donor celiac axis on the supraceliac aorta end-to-side. (C) Pediatric liver transplantation: on back-table anastomosis between superior mesenteric artery and celiac axis (white arrow); during LT, donor superior mesenteric artery on recipient celiac axis (Gordon's technique)

Bile duct anastomosis

Anastomosis can be performed between the common hepatic duct or the common bile duct of the donor and recipient, always end-to-end and protected or not, by Kehr T-tube.[48] In some cases (primary sclerosing cholangitis, disparity in size between donor and recipient,

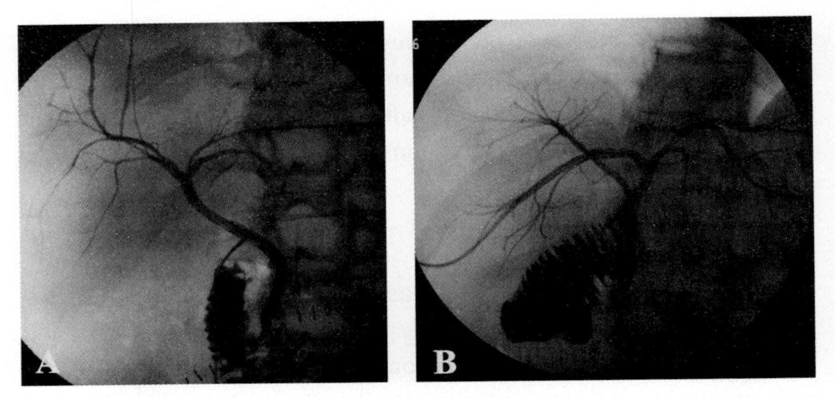

Figure 47.3. Biliary reconstruction. (A) End-to-end donor common hepatic duct and recipient common bile duct on T-tube. (B) End-to-side Roux-en-Y hepatico-jejunostomy

or as a rescue after an end-to-end biliary anastomosis), the biliary tract reconstruction can be carried out with an end-to-side Roux-en-Y hepatico-jejunostomy between the common hepatic duct of the graft and a jejunal loop of the recipient.[49,50] In both reconstructions, continuous or single stitches are associated with comparable results (Figure 47.3).

Split liver and living donor liver transplantation

The split liver is a technique of division of the liver into two functionally autonomous parts transplantable into two different recipients, both adults, or an adult and a paediatric recipient.[51,52] The split can be done at the back-table after harvesting (ex-situ)[53] or during the harvesting before the cross-clamp (*in-situ*).[54–56]

There are two split procedures in the donor:

1. *Left lateral segmentectomy*: This technique is useful for paediatric organ procurements. The liver section takes place along a line

immediately to the right of the falciform ligament and it allows to obtain a *right graft* (segments 4–5–6–7–8–1 equal to 75% of the donor's liver) suitable for an adult recipient, and a *left graft* (segments 2–3 equal to 25% of the hepatic parenchyma) suitable for a paediatric recipient. A variant of this technique consists of the trans-umbilical division.[57]

2. *Right hepatectomy*: This is useful for adult LT. The liver section takes place along the Cantlie line, according to right hepatectomy plane, and it allows to obtain a *right graft* (segments 5–6–7–8 equal to 60% of the donor's liver) and a *left graft* (segments 1–2–3–4 equal to 40% of the donor's liver), both suitable for two adult recipients.

At the end of the parenchymal transection and after the cross-clamp, the vascular section of the hepatic peduncles is carried out—generally, all the arterial axis and the left portal branch to the left graft, the right hepatic artery, and the portal trunk to the right graft. The presence of anatomical variations can require changes to the surgical technique.

In the living donation, the donor is a close relative. An accurate pre-operatory study of the liver anatomy in the donor and a psychological evaluation has to be performed before planning the surgery. The surgical procedure is similar to that used on a heart-beating donor during the *in-situ* split. Therefore, a left lateral segmentectomy (graft for paediatric recipient) or a right hepatectomy (graft for adult recipient) can be performed. These surgical procedures can be also carried out with minimally invasive techniques, both laparoscopic and robotic.

Complications of liver transplantation

Complications after liver transplantation can be divided into surgical and medical and are summarized in Tables 47.2, 47.3 and 47.4.

Table 47.2 Post-liver transplantation surgical complications (US = ultrasound; CT = computed tomography; MRI = magnetic resonance)

Complication	Type		Diagnosis
SURGICAL	**Abdominal bleeding**	Anastomosis	US – CT
		Hepatic site	US – CT
	Vascular	Hepatic artery thrombosis	US+doppler – CT – Angiography
		Hepatic artery stenosis	US+doppler – CT – Angiography
		Portal vein thrombosis	US+doppler – CT
		Portal vein stenosis	US+doppler – CT
		Inferior vena cava obstruction	US+doppler – CT – Angiography
		Veno-occlusive disease	US+doppler – CT – Angiography
	Biliary	Leakage	US – CT – Colangio MRI – Trans-T-tube cholangiography
		Stenosis	US – CT – Colangio MRI – Trans-T-tube cholangiography
		Biliary cast syndrome	US – CT – Colangio MRI
		Stenosis of the papilla of Vater	US – CT – Colangio MRI
	Not specific	Collections	US – CT
		Bowel obstruction	CT
		Injury to the abdominal organs	CT

Table 47.3 Post-liver transplantation medical complications graft related.

Complication	Type	Diagnosis
MEDICAL GRAFT RELATED	**Acute cellular rejection**	Blood chemistry – Liver biopsy
	Chronic rejection	Blood chemistry – Liver biopsy
	Immunosuppression-related toxicity	Blood chemistry
	B **or C Hepatitis recurrence**	Blood chemistry – Serological tests – Liver biopsy
	Autoimmune hepatitis recurrence and "de novo" autoimmune hepatitis	Blood chemistry – Autoantibody – Liver biopsy
	Cholestatic liver disease recurrence	Blood chemistry – Liver biopsy – MRI
	HCC recurrence	Blood chemistry – tumoral markers – TC

Table 47.4 Post-liver transplantation medical complications, not-graft related.

Complication	Type	
MEDICAL NOT GRAFT RELATED	**Infections (bacterial/viral/fungal)**	Pneumonia
		Cholangitis
		Urinary tract
		Abdominal
	Kidney failure	Acute
		Chronic
	Metabolic	Diabetes
		Hyperlipidaemia
		Obesity
		Osteoporosis
	Cardiovascular	'De novo' hypertension
		Acute myocardial infarction
		Atrial fibrillation and flutter
	Hematologic	
	Neuropsychiatric	
	'De novo' tumours	

Conclusion

Once identified as an 'impossible to perform operation', LT is nowadays a routine standard practice. However, proper surgical technique along with early recognition and management of anatomical variants and complications of portal hypertension remain are of paramount importance leading to success of the surgery. One fundamental principle is that surgical technique should be adapted on a case-by-case based on the recipient anatomy, aetiology and severity of liver disease, and graft features.

Highlights

- Liver transplantation is the substitution of the native diseased liver with a normal liver (or a part of it) from a deceased or living donor.
- In adult and paediatric patients, the indications for liver transplantation are end-stage liver failure, in both acute and chronic diseases.
- Liver transplantation is also indicated for primitive liver tumours; in adults, it is the gold standard therapy for early stage hepatocellular carcinoma (according with 'Milan Criteria') in the presence of liver cirrhosis. In paediatric recipients, for treatment of hepatoblastoma and, less frequently, hepatocellular carcinoma, evaluated with PRETEXT staging system. In some cases, liver transplantation may be indicated for treatment of metastatic liver tumours.
- Adult recipients are selected for transplantation on the basis of MELD score; paediatric recipients with PELD score.
- The native diseased liver is completely removed and replaced by the donor one (orthotopic position): the donor and recipient vena cava, the portal vein, the artery and the bile duct are anastomosed.
- The split liver is a technique of division of the liver into two functionally autonomous parts transplantable into two different recipients, both adults, or an adult and a paediatric. The split can be done in the donor during the harvesting before the cross-clamp (*in-situ*) or at the back-table after the harvesting (ex-situ). This technique is used also to obtain the liver graft from living donor.
- Many complications may occur after liver transplantation, some are surgical, other are medical, and these can be related or not to the graft.

References

1. Cinqualbre J. History of liver transplantation. Act I. 1963–1987. Ann Chir. 2003;128(3):195–201.
2. Cinqualbre J. History of liver transplantation. Act II: 1987–2002. Ann Chir. 2003;128(4):275–280.
3. Ringe B, Burdelski M, Rodeck B, Pichlmayr R. Experience with partial liver transplantation in Hannover. Clin Transpl. 1990;135–144.
4. European Association for the Study of the Liver. EASL clinical practice guidelines: Liver transplantation. J Hepatol. 2016;64(2):433–485.
5. Mazzaferro V, Regalia E, Doci R, Andreola S, Pulvirenti A, Bozzetti F, et al. Liver transplantation for the treatment of small hepatocellular carcinomas in patients with cirrhosis. N Engl J Med. 1996;334(11):693–699.
6. Kamath PS, Wiesner RH, Malinchoc M, Kremers W, Therneau TM, Kosberg CL, et al. A model to predict survival in patients with end-stage liver disease. Hepatology 2001;33(2):464–470.
7. Tsochatzis E, Coilly A, Nadalin S, Levistky J, Tokat Y, Ghobrial M, et al. International liver transplantation consensus statement on end-stage liver disease due to nonalcoholic steatohepatitis and liver transplantation. Transplantation. 2019;103(1):45–56.
8. Yao FY, Ferrell L, Bass NM, Watson JJ, Bacchetti P, Venook A, et al. Liver transplantation for hepatocellular carcinoma: Expansion of the tumor size limits does not adversely impact survival. Hepatology 2001;33(6):1394–1403.
9. Yao FY, Ferrell L, Bass NM, Bacchetti P, Ascher NL, Roberts JP. Liver transplantation for hepatocellular carcinoma: Comparison of the proposed UCSF criteria with the Milan criteria and the Pittsburgh modifiedTNM criteria. Liver Transplant 2002;8(9):765–774.
10. Mazzaferro V, Llovet JM, Miceli R, Bhoori S, Schiavo M, Mariani L, et al. Predicting survival after liver transplantation in patients with hepatocellular carcinoma beyond the Milan criteria: A retrospective, exploratory analysis. Lancet Oncol. 2009;10(1):35–43.
11. Toso C, Trotter J, Wei A, Bigam DL, Shah S, Lancaster J, et al. Total tumor volume predicts risk of recurrence following liver transplantation in patients with hepatocellular carcinoma. Liver Transplant 2008;14(8):1107–1115.
12. Toso C, Meeberg G, Hernandez-Alejandro R, Dufour J-F, Marotta P, Majno P, et al. Total tumor volume and alpha-fetoprotein for selection of transplant candidates with hepatocellular carcinoma: A prospective validation. Hepatology 2015;62(1):158–165.
13. Llovet JM, Mas X, Aponte JJ, Fuster J, Navasa M, Christensen E, et al. Cost effectiveness of adjuvant therapy for hepatocellular carcinoma during the waiting list for liver transplantation. Gut. 2002;50(1):123–128.
14. DuBay DA, Sandroussi C, Kachura JR, Ho CS, Beecroft JR, Vollmer CM, et al. Radiofrequency ablation of hepatocellular carcinoma as a bridge to liver transplantation. HPB 2011;13(1):24–32.
15. Lesurtel M, Müllhaupt B, Pestalozzi BC, Pfammatter T, Clavien P-A. Transarterial chemoembolization as a bridge to liver transplantation for hepatocellular carcinoma: an evidence-based analysis. Am J Transplant 2006;6(11):2644–2650.

16. Poon RT-P, Fan ST, Lo CM, Liu CL, Wong J. Long-term survival and pattern of recurrence after resection of small hepatocellular carcinoma in patients with preserved liver function: implications for a strategy of salvage transplantation. Ann Surg. 2002;235(3):373–382.
17. Roberts JP, Venook A, Kerlan R, Yao F. Hepatocellular carcinoma: Ablate and wait versus rapid transplantation. Liver Transplant 2010;16(8):925–929.
18. Bernal W, Wendon J. Acute liver failure. N Engl J Med. 2013;369(26):2525–2534.
19. Bernuau J, Rueff B, Benhamou JP. Fulminant and subfulminant liver failure: Definitions and causes. Semin Liver Dis. 1986;6(2):97–106.
20. Mochida S, Nakayama N, Ido A, Takikawa Y, Yokosuka O, Sakaida I, et al. Revised criteria for classification of the etiologies of acute liver failure and late-onset hepatic failure in Japan: A report by the Intractable Hepato-biliary Diseases Study Group of Japan in 2015. Hepatol Res 2016;46(5):369–371.
21. Lee WM, Stravitz RT, Larson AM. Introduction to the revised American Association for the Study of Liver Diseases Position Paper on acute liver failure 2011. Hepatology 2012;55(3):965–967.
22. Trey C, Davidson CS. The management of fulminant hepatic failure. Prog Liver Dis. 1970;3:282–298.
23. Simpson KJ, Bates CM, Henderson NC, Wigmore SJ, Garden OJ, Lee A, et al. The utilization of liver transplantation in the management of acute liver failure: comparison between acetaminophen and non-acetaminophen etiologies. Liver Transplant 2009;15(6):600–609.
24. O'Grady JG, Alexander GJ, Hayllar KM, Williams R. Early indicators of prognosis in fulminant hepatic failure. Gastroenterology 1989;97(2):439–445.
25. O'Grady JG, Schalm SW, Williams R. Acute liver failure: Redefining the syndromes. Lancet 1993;342(8866):273–275.
26. Starzl TE, Marchioro TL, Vonkaulla KN, Hermann G, Brittain RS, Waddell WR. Homotransplantation of the liver in humans. Surg Gynecol Obstet. 1963;117:659–676.
27. Starzl TE, Iwatsuki S, Esquivel CO, Todo S, Kam I, Lynch S, et al. Refinements in the surgical technique of liver transplantation. Semin Liver Dis. 1985;5(4):349–356.
28. Calne RY, Williams R. Liver transplantation in man. I. Observations on technique and organization in five cases. Br Med J. 1968;4(5630):535–540.
29. Belghiti J, Noun R, Sauvanet A. Temporary portocaval anastomosis with preservation of caval flow during orthotopic liver transplantation. Am J Surg. 1995;169(2):277–279.
30. Figueras J, Llado L, Ramos E, Jaurrieta E, Rafecas A, Fabregat J, et al. Temporary portocaval shunt during liver transplantation with vena cava preservation. Results of a prospective randomized study. Liver Transplant 2001;7(10):904–911.
31. Tzakis A, Todo S, Starzl TE. Orthotopic liver transplantation with preservation of the inferior vena cava. Ann Surg. 1989;210(5):649–652.
32. Makuuchi M, Yamamoto J, Takayama T, Kosuge T, Gunvén P, Yamazaki S, et al. Extrahepatic division of the right hepatic vein in hepatectomy. Hepatogastroenterology. 1991;38(2):176–179.
33. Belghiti J, Panis Y, Sauvanet A, Gayet B, Fékété F. A new technique of side to side caval anastomosis during orthotopic hepatic transplantation without inferior vena caval occlusion. Surg Gynecol Obstet. 1992;175(3):270–272.

34. Salizzoni M, Andorno E, Bossuto E, Cerutti E, Livigni S, Lupo F, et al. Piggyback techniques versus classical technique in orthotopic liver transplantation: A review of 75 cases. Transplant Proc. 1994;26(6):3552–3553.
35. Lerut J, Ciccarelli O, Roggen F, Laterre P-F, Danse E, Goffette P, et al. Cavocaval adult liver transplantation and retransplantation without venovenous bypass and without portocaval shunting: a prospective feasibility study in adult liver transplantation. Transplantation. 2003;75(10):1740–1745.
36. Lerut JP, Molle G, Donataccio M, De Kock M, Ciccarelli O, Laterre PF, et al. Cavocaval liver transplantation without venovenous bypass and without temporary portocaval shunting: the ideal technique for adult liver grafting? Transpl Int 1997;10(3):171–179.
37. Dasgupta D, Sharpe J, Prasad KR, Asthana S, Toogood GJ, Pollard SG, et al. Triangular and self-triangulating cavocavostomy for orthotopic liver transplantation without posterior suture lines: A modified surgical technique. Transpl Int 2006;19(2):117–121.
38. Hibi T, Nishida S, Levi DM, Selvaggi G, Tekin A, Fan J, et al. When and why portal vein thrombosis matters in liver transplantation: a critical audit of 174 cases. Ann Surg. 2014;259(4):760–766.
39. Stieber AC, Zetti G, Todo S, Tzakis AG, Fung JJ, Marino I, et al. The spectrum of portal vein thrombosis in liver transplantation. Ann Surg. 1991;213(3):199–206.
40. Yerdel MA, Gunson B, Mirza D, Karayalçin K, Olliff S, Buckels J, et al. Portal vein thrombosis in adults undergoing liver transplantation: Risk factors, screening, management, and outcome. Transplantation. 2000;69(9):1873–1881.
41. Aggarwal S, Kang Y, Freeman JA, Fortunato FL, Pinsky MR. Postreperfusion syndrome: Hypotension after reperfusion of the transplanted liver. J Crit Care. 1993;8(3):154–160.
42. Aggarwal S, Kang Y, Freeman JA, Fortunato FL, Pinsky MR. Postreperfusion syndrome: Cardiovascular collapse following hepatic reperfusion during liver transplantation. Transplant Proc. 1987;19(4 Suppl 3):54–55.
43. Nakasuji M, Bookallil MJ. Pathophysiological mechanisms of postrevascularization hyperkalemia in orthotopic liver transplantation. Anesth Analg. 2000;91(6):1351–1355.
44. Deshpande RR, Heaton ND, Rela M. Surgical anatomy of segmental liver transplantation. Br J Surg. 2002;89(9):1078–1088.
45. Abdullah SS, Mabrut J-Y, Garbit V, De La Roche E, Olagne E, Rode A, et al. Anatomical variations of the hepatic artery: Study of 932 cases in liver transplantation. Surg Radiol Anat 2006;28(5):468–473.
46. Brems JJ, Millis JM, Hiatt JR, Klein AS, Quinones-Baldrich WJ, Ramming KP, et al. Hepatic artery reconstruction during liver transplantation. Transplantation. 1989;47(2):403–406.
47. Takatsuki M, Chiang Y-C, Lin T-S, Wang C-C, Concejero A, Lin C-C, et al. Anatomical and technical aspects of hepatic artery reconstruction in living donor liver transplantation. Surgery. 2006;140(5):824–828; discussion 829.
48. Seiler CA. The bile duct anastomosis in liver transplantation. Dig Surg. 1999;16(2):102–106.
49. Scatton O, Meunier B, Cherqui D, Boillot O, Sauvanet A, Boudjema K, et al. Randomized trial of choledochocholedochostomy with or without a T tube in orthotopic liver transplantation. Ann Surg. 2001;233(3):432–437.

50. Shimoda M, Saab S, Morrisey M, Ghobrial RM, Farmer DG, Chen P, et al. A cost-effectiveness analysis of biliary anastomosis with or without T-tube after orthotopic liver transplantation. Am J Transplant 2001;1(2):157–161.
51. de Ville de Goyet J. Split liver transplantation in Europe—1988 to 1993. Transplantation. 1995;59(10):1371–1376.
52. Azoulay D, Castaing D, Adam R, Savier E, Delvart V, Karam V, et al. Split-liver transplantation for two adult recipients: Feasibility and long-term outcomes. Ann Surg. 2001;233(4):565–574.
53. Azoulay D, Marin-Hargreaves G, Castaing D, Bismuth H. Ex situ splitting of the liver: the versatile Paul Brousse technique. Arch Surg 2001;136(8):956–961.
54. Rogiers X, Malagó M, Gawad K, Jauch KW, Olausson M, Knoefel WT, et al. In situ splitting of cadaveric livers. The ultimate expansion of a limited donor pool. Ann Surg. 1996;224(3):331–339; discussion 339-341.
55. Malagó M, Rogiers X, Broelsch CE. Liver splitting and living donor techniques. Br Med Bull. 1997;53(4):860–867.
56. Otte JB, de Ville de Goyet J, Reding R, Van Obbergh L, Veyckemans F, Carlier MA, et al. Pediatric liver transplantation: From the full-size liver graft to reduced, split, and living related liver transplantation. Pediatr Surg Int. 1998;13(5–6):308–318.
57. de Ville de Goyet J, di Francesco F, Sottani V, Grimaldi C, Tozzi AE, Monti L, et al. Splitting livers: Trans-hilar or trans-umbilical division? Technical aspects and comparative outcomes. Pediatr Transplant. 2015;19(5):517–26.

48

Ex-vivo liver perfusion

Damiano Patrono, Renato Romagnoli

Historical perspective

History of liver transplantation is indissoluble from that of ex-vivo liver perfusion. From the pioneer era, several attempts were made at the preservation of abdominal organs for transplantation with continuous perfusion. In the 1960s, studies revealed that canine kidneys could be preserved for three or five days by continuous perfusion of cooled oxygenated blood or plasma.[1,2] In 1966, Lawrence Brettschneider conceived the hyperbaric oxygen chamber, which allowed preservation of canine and human livers using a combination of hypothermia, hyperbaric oxygenation, and perfusion with diluted homologous blood through the portal vein and hepatic artery.[3,4] Although it was successfully introduced in clinical transplantation, the hyperbaric chamber was bulky, cumbersome to utilize, and extremely heavy. During transport of procured graft to the recipient hospital, airplane pilots were worried the chamber could roll in the cabin, destabilizing their aircrafts.[5] As an alternative to ex-vivo perfusion, static cold storage (SCS) could represent a cheap, practical, and user-friendly method of organ preservation, but was initially limited by the lack of effective preservation solutions. With the advent of Collins[6] and subsequent preservation solutions, SCS progressively became the standard method for organ preservation, replacing ex-vivo perfusion.

In the following decades, clinical transplantation gained widespread acceptance and the number of indications and potential recipients grew exponentially, outweighing, by far, the number of available organs. This constantly increasing gap has urged the transplant community to push the boundaries of organ acceptance by utilizing organs from donors of advanced age, affected by several comorbidities or, more recently, after circulatory determination of death (DCD). Organs from these so-called 'extended criteria' or 'marginal' donors increase the donor pool, but are more subjected to ischemia-reperfusion injury. Prompted by favourable results in kidney transplantation,[7,8] a renewed interest in ex-vivo organ perfusion as a way to reduce ischemia-reperfusion injury, especially in organs from extended criteria donors emerged in liver transplantation.

As some kinds of apparatus are used for the ex-vivo liver perfusion, the term 'machine perfusion' is normally employed. Liver machine perfusion will be the subject of this chapter.

In clinical liver transplantation, machine perfusion encompasses a variety of techniques that differentiate in several aspects, including temperature, perfusate, device, and perfusion settings. Amongst them, temperature is probably the most important parameter and it can be considered the major discriminant between different techniques.

Hypothermic machine perfusion technique

Hypothermic machine perfusion (HMP) encompasses several techniques characterized by the low temperature (4°C–10°C) at which graft is perfused. After standard back table preparation, cannulas are placed in the portal vein only or in both the portal vein and hepatic artery; and the liver is perfused by a recirculating preservation solution, adapted for machine perfusion purpose. In the seminal studies by Guarrera et al.[9,10] perfusate was not actively oxygenated, but measured oxygen tension in the perfusate was ~ 140–230 mm Hg due to perfusate-air interchange at the organ chamber. As oxygen delivery to the perfused organ is accepted as the key of HMP mechanism of action,[11] vast majority of devices have been equipped to provide active perfusate oxygenation; hence liver HMP is also named as hypothermic oxygenated machine perfusion (HOPE). The effectiveness of HOPE performed by portal perfusion only or by simultaneous perfusion of both portal vein and hepatic artery (dual HOPE or DHOPE), especially with regards to bile duct protection, is still debated. Homogeneous and thorough liver perfusion, including peribiliary vascular plexus, can be achieved by portal perfusion only.[12,13] However, it has been questioned whether single portal perfusion also provides effective bile duct protection, including small intra-hepatic bile ducts.[14] To the best of our knowledge, a study comparing HOPE versus DHOPE has not been performed so far.

Regardless of the chosen technique, perfusion pressure should be kept lower that in the in-vivo setting to avoid endothelial injury.[11,15–17] Portal pressure is usually set at 3–5 mm Hg, whereas artery pressure is set at ~ 25 mm Hg; these values could be reduced in case very small grafts (for grafts from paediatric donors) are used.[18] From a logistic point of view, HOPE or DHOPE can be performed throughout preservation[19] or at the end of preservation.[17,20,21] The latter approach, also named end-ischemic HOPE, is logistically simple, does not require a transportable device, and is therefore, adopted most widely. Based on experimental evidence, retrieval and transplant logistics should be set up to allow a minimum perfusion time of 90 minutes.[11]

Mechanism of action of HMP

New concepts have recently been introduced concerning the common pathway of ischemia-reperfusion injury in different tissues.[22,23] Briefly, the initial burst of reactive oxygen species that characterizes the very early phase of ischemia-reperfusion injury after warm reperfusion is related to reverse electron transfer at mitochondrial complex I. This is caused by accumulation of negative potential across mitochondrial matrix during ischemia with succinate acting as an electron sink. This would lead to the disruption of mitochondrial electron transport chain, production of reactive oxygen species, and activation of the aspecific inflammatory response.

In a DCD rat model study by Schlegel et al, HOPE has been shown to downregulate mitochondrial respiration by putting mitochondria in a highly oxidized state. This resulted in the reduction of markers of mitochondrial, nuclear and cellular injury upon warm reperfusion.[11] In another study from the same group[24] HOPE treatment reduced tissue succinate content of fatty rat livers as compared to SCS. Overall, these results suggest a restoration of mitochondrial respiration during HOPE, which determines a reduction of inflammatory response and tissue damage after warm reperfusion. It is noteworthy that in both studies, perfusate oxygenation was required to achieve the aforementioned results, as replacement of oxygen by nitrogen largely suppressed the protective effect of machine perfusion.

The protective effect of HOPE is also related to reduced endothelial damage (an effect that would be independent from oxygen delivery), to washout of metabolites (e.g. inflammatory cytokines) produced during cold ischemia, and to HOPE-related downregulation of immune response.[25]

Clinical experience of HMP

Relevant clinical studies that explored the use of HMP or HOPE in liver transplantation are summarized in Table 48.1.[9,10,17,20,21,24,26,27] Other experiences have been reported in small case series or case reports.[18,28–33] In general, HMP use has been associated with reduced levels of markers of liver injury (AST, ALT, bilirubin), preserved renal function, lower rate of biliary complications and ischemic cholangiopathy, and improved graft survival. The superiority of HOPE over SCS appears rather clear in the DCD setting, whereas results are promising but less convincing in the setting of extended criteria DBD donors. In Italy, the association of normothermic regional perfusion with HMP has allowed the successful implementation of DCD Liver Transplant programs, despite the obstacle represented by the 20-minutes stand-off period prescribed by Italian law.[34] Future studies, including ongoing randomized trials, will hopefully confirm the benefits of HOPE and define the settings in which its use provides a significant advantage over SCS.

Table 48.1 Relevant clinical studies on hypothermic machine perfusion in liver transplantation

Author	Year	N	Technique	Perfusate	Design	Significant findings
Guarrera et al.	2010	20	HMP	Vasosol® 3 L	Cohort study	First feasibility study of HMP in standard human liver grafts. HMP reduced EAD rate (5% vs 25%; p=0.08), serum markers of hepatic and renal function (AST, ALT, Bilirubin, Creatinine), and time required for LFT's normalization. Perfusate AST and ALT correlated with recipient transaminase peak.
Dutkowski et al.	2014	8	HOPE	KPS-1®	Cohort study	In DCD recipients with median 38 minutes DWIT, HOPE allowed achieving similar results as in SCS-preserved DBD in terms of hepatic and renal function, ICU and hospital stay. No case of ischemic cholangiopathy was observed.
Guarrera et al.	2015	31	HMP	Vasosol® 3 L	Cohort study	In EC-DBD grafts recipients, HMP reduced serum markers of hepatic and renal function (AST, ALT, Bilirubin, Creatinine), 1-year biliary complications, biliary strictures (10% vs 33%; p=0.03) and length of stay
Dutkowski et al.	2015	25	HOPE	KPS-1®	Cohort study	As compared to a DWIT and BAR score-matched cohort, recipients of HOPE-treated DCD had lower ALT peak (1239 vs 2065 U/L; p=0.02), ischemic cholangiopathy (0% vs 22%; p=0.015) and biliary complications rate (20% vs 46%; p=0.042), and improved 1-year graft survival (90% vs 69%; p=0.035).

(*continued*)

Table 48.1 *Continued*

Author	Year	N	Technique	Perfusate	Design	Significant findings
Kron et al.	2017	6	HOPE	Belzer MPS® 3 L	Cohort study	Outcome in 6 recipients of grafts with ≥ 20% macrosteatosis (DCD n=5) was compared to 12 matched SCS-preserved grafts. HOPE was associated with improved patient and graft survival, reduced ALT peak, reduced dialysis requirement and PNF rate
Van Rijn et al.	2017	10	DHOPE	Belzer MPS® 4 L + glutathione 3 mmol/L	Cohort study	In recipients of DCD grafts, DHOPE increased hepatic ATP content, reduced median ALT (966 vs 1858 IU/L;p=0.006) and bilirubin level (1 vs 2.6 mg/dl; p=0.044) during first post-LT week, and improved 1-year graft survival (100% vs 67%;p=0.052).
Schlegel et al.	2019	50	HOPE	Belzer MPS® 3 L	Cohort study	In DCD recipients, HOPE treatment was associated with comparable results as those obtained in matched DBD-recipients, and, compared with SCS-preserved DCD, with a lower rate of ischemic cholangiopathy (8% vs 22%; p=0.09), non-tumour-related graft loss (8% vs 32%;p=0.005), and treated acute rejection (4% vs 22%;p=0.002).
Patrono et al.	2019	25	DHOPE	Belzer MPS® 3 L	Cohort study	Recipients of EC-DBD grafts treated with DHOPE had lower stage 2-3 AKI rate (16% versus 42%;p=0.046) and lower post-reperfusion syndrome rate (4% versus 20%, p = 0.13). DHOPE reduced transaminases peak and EAD rate.

Abbreviations: HMP, hypothermic machine perfusion; EAD, early allograft dysfunction; AST, aspartate aminotransferase; ALT, alanine aminotransferase; EC, extended criteria; DBD, donation after brain death; HOPE, hypothermic oxygenated machine perfusion; DWIT, donor warm ischemia time; SCS, static cold storage; ICU, intensive care unit; BAR, balance of risk score; DCD, donation after circulatory death; PNF, primary non-function; DHOPE, dual HOPE, ATP, adenosine triphosphate; AKI, acute kidney injury.

Normothermic machine perfusion technique

In contrast to HMP, Normothermic Machine Perfusion (NMP) aims at mimicking a near-physiologic environment in which liver graft is metabolically active, can restore its adenosine triphosphate (ATP) content and repair the damage suffered before and soon after retrieval. Thus, NMP separates the concepts of ischemia and preservation. Liver graft is perfused at 37°C with a recirculating oxygenated perfusate that is constituted by an oxygen carrier, colloids, electrolytes, antibiotics, heparin, and other optional components like vasodilators, bile salts, glucose, and other nutrients. Sodium bicarbonate can be added to adjust the pH. Perfusate composition varies according to different protocols, devices and especially depends on the time period of perfusion. Packed red blood cells are normally used as oxygen carrier, but NMP has been successfully performed using a synthetic haemoglobin-based oxygen carrier as well.[35–37]

NMP requires cannulation of both portal vein and hepatic artery; liver effluent can be collected by a cannula placed in inferior vena cava (close circuit) or from a reservoir draining liver effluent (open circuit). Depending on the device, perfusion can be pressure or flow-controlled and flow into hepatic artery circuit can be continuous or pulsatile.

From a logistic point of view, NMP can be started immediately at the donor hospital after initial cold perfusion and back table preparation, or later, once the liver has arrived at the recipient hospital (so-called 'back-to-base' approach). Although more logistically demanding and subject to the availability of a transportable device, immediate NMP has been preferred due to the concern that prolonged cold ischemia time could be particularly detrimental for severely damaged livers.[38] However, recent studies suggest that NMP after transient SCS could be equally effective.[39,40]

A minimum of 4 hours perfusion time should be allowed, which is the time necessary to restore ATP levels, evaluate liver viability, and complete recipient hepatectomy.[41]

Mechanism of action of NMP

By providing oxygen and nutrients at physiological temperature, NMP allows restoration of cellular ATP content, thereby reducing reactive oxygen species (ROS) production and ischemia-reperfusion injury at warm reperfusion. NMP, as compared to SCS, has been associated with reduced hepatocellular necrosis and apoptosis, lower liver injury marker levels and improved survival in experimental models of both DBD and DCD liver transplantation.(41,42) Recently, Jassem et al.(43) using gene microarray and immunoprofiling on hepatic lymphocytes and liver tissue samples, provided further insight into NMP effects by showing that NMP is associated with a downregulation of proinflammatory genes and an upregulations of genes involved in hepatic regeneration.

Clinical experience of NMP

More relevant studies on clinical NMP use are summarized in Table 48.2,(39,40,44–49) including two randomized controlled trials and six cohort studies. In the first clinical series reported by Ravikumar et al.,(46) NMP resulted as a safe and feasible technique, and was associated with a reduction of post-transplant AST peak. It is worth noting that preservation of up to 18 hours was reported. Therefore, NMP can safely extend preservation time and 24-hour preservation has been shown to be feasible.(50) In the landmark paper by Nasralla et al.,(45) which compared clinical outcome of 121 NMP versus 101 SCS preserved livers transplanted at seven European centres, NMP use determined a significant reduction of AST peak, early allograft dysfunction (EAD) rate, post-reperfusion syndrome, and post-reperfusion lactate. Furthermore, there was a 51.4% reduction of discard rate in the NMP arm. This latter important result points the finger at the possibility, during NMP, of assessing liver viability. Parameters drawn from perfusate (lactate clearance, glucose metabolism, pH trend, transaminase level) and bile analysis (quantity, pH, glucose, bicarbonate) can be used to predict liver function once transplanted and avoid potentially futile transplants.(48,51) This possibility has allowed recovering and successfully transplanting the liver that were previously deemed unsuitable for transplantation(52) and set the stage for an actual increase of donor pool.(53)

The randomized trial by Ghinolfi et al.,(44) which was focused on assessing benefits of NMP in ≥ 70-year-old DBD donors, failed to show a significant clinical advantage of NMP over SCS, but showed reduced

Table 48.2 Relevant clinical studies on normothermic machine perfusion in liver transplantation

Author	Year	N	Device	Design	Significant findings
Ravikumar et al.	2016	20	OrganOx metra®	Cohort study	The study confirmed safety and feasibility of NMP. Compared to matched controls, NMP resulted in reduced AST peak despite preservation times up to 18 hours
Selzner et al.	2016	10	OrganOx metra®	Cohort study	The study assessed feasibility of NMP using an albumin and dextran-based solution (Steen solution) with OrganOx metra® device. No adverse events were observed. Outcomes in NMP group were comparable to those in matched SCS group.
Watson et al.	2017	12	OrganAssist® LiverAssist®	Cohort study	In this study, 5 out of 6 recipients of grafts treated with NMP with high perfusate pO2 (621 – 671 mm Hg) experienced PRS and 4 had persistent refractory vasoplegia. No case of PRS was observed in the subsequent 6 cases with lower perfusate oxygen tensions (~ 150 mm Hg).
Watson et al.	2018	47 (22)*	OrganAssist® LiverAssist®	Cohort study	A deep insight into graft assessment during NMP, including kinetics of lactate clearance, glucose metabolism, perfusate pH and markers of bile quality. 22 out of 47 NMP-treated livers were transplanted. A patient with high perfusate transaminases developed PNF and 4 with bile pH < 7.4 developed graft cholangiopathy.
Nasralla et al.	2018	121	OrganOx metra®	Randomized controlled trial	Landmark study; NMP determined a significant reduction of discard rate (11.7% vs 24.1%;p=0.008) and of AST peak (– 49.4%;p<0.001), which was more pronounced for recipient of DCD (73.3%;p<0.001) than of DBD (40%;p=0.001) grafts. Recipients of NMP-preserved livers had also lower EAD rate (10.1% vs 29.9%;p<0.001), post-reperfusion syndrome rate (12.4% vs 33%;p<0.001) and post-reperfusion lactate (4.1 vs 3.6;p=0.018).

(continued)

Table 48.2 *Continued*

Author	Year	N	Device	Design	Significant findings
Ghinolfi et al.	2019	10	OrganAssist® LiverAssist®	Randomized controlled trial	The study compared SCS vs. NMP in ≥ 70-year-old DBD. NMP resulted in comparable clinical outcomes but improved histological features of ischemia-reperfusion injury, as mitochondrial swelling and activation of autophagy.
Bral et al.	2019	43	OrganOx metra®	Cohort study	The study compared immediate NMP (n=17) versus 'back-to-base' NMP (n=26) after transient SCS. Both approaches were safe and yielded comparable clinical outcome. NMP reduced AST peak as compared to SCS.
Ceresa et al.	2019	31	OrganOx metra®	Cohort study	The study assessed feasibility of NMP after a period of SCS. Clinical outcomes were compared with 104 patients receiving graft preserved by immediate NMP from the Nasralla study, confirming comparable results between two approaches.

Abbreviations: NMP, normothermic machine perfusion; AST, aspartate aminotransferase; SCS, static cold storage; PRS, post-reperfusion syndrome; PNF, primary non-function; DCD, donation after circulatory death; DBD, donation after brain death; EAD, early allograft dysfunction.

histological signs of endothelial and mitochondrial damage in the NMP group.

In contrast with these promising results, NMP has not been shown to determine a significant reduction of biliary complications. However, a study looking specifically at this outcome is still lacking.

As for hypothermic perfusion, further studies including a cost-benefit analysis are needed to identify scenarios in which NMP offers a substantial advantage over SCS.

Other approaches and research directions

The HMP and NMP techniques are not mutually exclusive approaches or the only methods that have been studied. The Bonn group explored the concept of controlled oxygenated rewarming (COR), in which liver graft temperature is progressively increased from 10°C to 20°C.[54] In their experience, this approach was superior to HMP or subnormothermic perfusion in terms of transaminase release and bile production upon warm reperfusion.

Sequential HOPE followed by NMP has also been explored, which combines the beneficial effects of HOPE in restoring mitochondrial respiration and cellular ATP reserves with the viability assessment allowed by NMP. This approach was pioneered by the Groningen group, which compared liver function parameters during NMP in two groups of discarded human livers preserved exclusively by SCS or by SCS followed by 2 hours of DHOPE.[55] ATP content increased 15-fold during DHOPE. Upon warm reperfusion, livers treated with DHOPE showed increased bile production, higher bile, bilirubin, and bicarbonate at 30 min, lower lactate and glucose levels during the first 4 hours of NMP, higher oxygen consumption and less bicarbonate requirement to maintain perfusate pH.[55] Mechanical stimulation of the endothelium during DHOPE resulted in improved endothelial function, as testified by the increased transcription of Krüppel-like-factor 2, thrombomodulin and endothelial nitric oxide synthase, which have anti-thrombotic and anti-inflammatory properties.[56]

Using a similar protocol, the Birmingham group recently confirmed these findings, showing that a 2-hour period of DHOPE prior to NMP resulted in decreased expression of markers of oxidative injury and inflammation upon warm reperfusion.[57] Furthermore, all livers in the DHOPE + NMP were deemed as potentially transplantable at the end of NMP, as compared to 60% in the NMP group.

The Groningen group recently took this approach one step further, by combining DHOPE + COR+NMP in 7 discarded human livers.[35] In this study, a perfusate based on a synthetic haemoglobin-base oxygen carrier was used that, having the advantage of a decreased viscosity, allowed its utilization at both low (~ 10°C) and physiologic (37°C) temperature. Briefly, discarded livers were subject to one-hour DHOPE, one-hour COR (during which temperature and perfusion pressures were gradually increased) and subsequent NMP. Livers were judged transplantable if they cleared lactate, normalized pH and produced ≥ 10 ml of bile with pH > 7.45 at 150 minutes of NMP. Remarkably, five out of seven livers were successfully transplanted with no early allograft dysfunction or ischemic cholangiopathy at a median follow-up of 6.5 months.[35] Overall, these findings suggest that HMP + NMP is a promising approach to rescue severely damaged livers and make them suitable for transplantation.

Apart from prolonged preservation, graft reconditioning and viability assessment, NMP allows a metabolically active liver in an extra-corporeal setting, paving the way for therapeutic interventions. This applies to both the transplantation and extra-transplantation milieu.

Hepatic steatosis is associated with an increased risk of graft dysfunction and non-function and is consequently one of the main factors leading to a graft being discarded. In this setting, the Birmingham group has demonstrated that liver macrosteatosis and triglyceride content can be significantly reduced after only 6 hours of NMP, by supplementing perfusate with defatting agents.[58]

NMP could also allow other therapeutic interventions. Stem cells and extra-cellular vesicles can be added to the perfusate during NMP. In a progressive hypoxic injury model induced by perfusate dilution during NMP, our group has shown that human liver stem cells derived extracellular vesicles are internalized into hepatocytes during NMP and reduce tissue damage, apoptosis, and transcription of hypoxia-inducible factor 1-α and transforming growth factor beta.[59] Also, antibiotics or antiviral agents could be administered during NMP to prevent donor-recipient transmission of known infections, thereby rescuing potentially good-quality grafts that would otherwise be discarded due to donor factors. With no concerns for a systemic toxicity, higher concentrations of these drugs could be achieved into perfusate, thereby increasing their efficacy.

With the same principle, NMP could serve as a platform to administer antineoplastic drugs at doses that are normally precluded due to their systemic toxicity, while the patient is temporarily put on a porto-caval shunt or a veno-venous by-pass. Similarly, NMP could be used to allow complex vascular reconstruction or ex-vivo tumour resection avoiding cold ischemia.

Conclusion

In conclusion, new technology has broadened the horizons of organ preservation and reconditioning, and opened new possibilities in the field of liver transplantation and hepatobiliary surgery. Nowadays, we are in the enthusiastic phase of adoption of these new strategies and machine perfusion is gaining widespread popularity in clinical practice. Several randomized studies on the subject are ongoing; they will hopefully better define the specific advantages of each technique and identify elective areas of application.

Highlights

- Ex-vivo liver perfusion, or machine perfusion, encompasses several techniques characterized by different principles and modalities.
- Regardless of the technique, dynamic preservation techniques have emerged as superior to cold storage in reducing ischemia-reperfusion injury in liver transplantation, especially in extended criteria donors.
- Hypothermic oxygenated machine perfusion has been associated with superior clinical outcome, especially in the setting of DCD liver transplantation.
- Normothermic machine perfusion allows extended preservation time and ex-vivo liver viability assessment, potentially increasing organ utilization rate.

- Apart from organ preservation and reconditioning, machine perfusion can be used as a platform for therapeutic interventions, also outside the transplantation setting.
- Several studies are ongoing, which will help assessing the benefits of liver machine perfusion and defining its indications.

References

1. Belzer FO, Ashby BS, Dunphy JE. 24-hour and 72-hour preservation of canine kidneys. Lancet. 1967;2(7515):536–538.
2. Humphries AL, Jr., Russell R, Stoddard LD, Moretz WH. Successful five-day kidney preservation. Perfusion with hypothermic, diluted plasma. Invest Urol. 1968;5(6):609–618.
3. Brettschneider L, Bell PR, Martin AJ, Jr., Tarr JS, Taylor PD, Starzl TE. Conservation of the liver. Transplant Proc. 1969;1(1):132–137.
4. Brettschneider L, Daloze PM, Huguet C, Porter KA, Groth CG, Kashiwagi N, et al. The use of combined preservation techniques for extended storage of orthotopic liver homografts. Surg Gynecol Obstet. 1968;126(2):263–274.
5. Starzl TE. The Puzzle People. University of Pittsburgh Press; 1992.
6. Collins GM, Bravo-Shugarman M, Terasaki PI. Kidney preservation for transportation. Initial perfusion and 30 hours' ice storage. Lancet. 1969;2(7632):1219–1222.
7. Moers C, Smits JM, Maathuis MH, Treckmann J, van Gelder F, Napieralski BP, et al. Machine perfusion or cold storage in deceased-donor kidney transplantation. N Engl J Med. 2009;360(1):7–19.
8. Jochmans I, Moers C, Smits JM, Leuvenink HG, Treckmann J, Paul A, et al. Machine perfusion versus cold storage for the preservation of kidneys donated after cardiac death: A multicenter, randomized, controlled trial. Ann Surg. 2010;252(5):756–764.
9. Guarrera JV, Henry SD, Samstein B, Odeh-Ramadan R, Kinkhabwala M, Goldstein MJ, et al. Hypothermic machine preservation in human liver transplantation: The first clinical series. Am J Transplant. 2010;10(2):372–381.
10. Guarrera JV, Henry SD, Samstein B, Reznik E, Musat C, Lukose TI, et al. Hypothermic machine preservation facilitates successful transplantation of 'orphan' extended criteria donor livers. Am J Transplant. 2015;15(1):161–169.
11. Schlegel A, de Rougemont O, Graf R, Clavien PA, Dutkowski P. Protective mechanisms of end-ischemic cold machine perfusion in DCD liver grafts. J Hepatol. 2013;58(2):278–286.
12. Schlegel A, Graf R, Clavien PA, Dutkowski P. Hypothermic oxygenated perfusion (HOPE) protects from biliary injury in a rodent model of DCD liver transplantation. J Hepatol. 2013;59(5):984–991.
13. Schlegel A, Kron P, De Oliveira ML, Clavien PA, Dutkowski P. Is single portal vein approach sufficient for hypothermic machine perfusion of DCD liver grafts? J Hepatol. 2016;64(1):239–241.

14. Bruggenwirth IMA, Burlage LC, Porte RJ, Martins PN. Is single portal vein perfusion the best approach for machine preservation of liver grafts? J Hepatol. 2016;64(5):1194–1195.
15. Schlegel A, Muller X, Dutkowski P. Hypothermic liver perfusion. Curr Opin Organ Transplant. 2017;22(6):563–570.
16. t Hart NA, der van Plaats A, Leuvenink HG, van Goor H, Wiersema-Buist J, Verkerke GJ, et al. Determination of an adequate perfusion pressure for continuous dual vessel hypothermic machine perfusion of the rat liver. Transpl Int. 2007;20(4):343–352.
17. van Rijn R, Karimian N, Matton APM, Burlage LC, Westerkamp AC, van den Berg AP, et al. Dual hypothermic oxygenated machine perfusion in liver transplants donated after circulatory death. Br J Surg. 2017;104(7):907–917.
18. Werner MJM, van Leeuwen OB, de Jong IEM, Bodewes F, Fujiyoshi M, Luhker OC, et al. First report of successful transplantation of a pediatric donor liver graft after hypothermic machine perfusion. Pediatr Transplant. 2019;23(3):e13362.
19. Compagnon P, Levesque E, Hentati H, Disabato M, Calderaro J, Feray C, et al. An oxygenated and transportable machine perfusion system fully rescues liver grafts exposed to lethal ischemic damage in a pig model of DCD liver transplantation. Transplantation. 2017;101(7):e205–e13.
20. Dutkowski P, Polak WG, Muiesan P, Schlegel A, Verhoeven CJ, Scalera I, et al. First comparison of hypothermic oxygenated perfusion versus static cold storage of human donation after cardiac death liver transplants: An international-matched case analysis. Ann Surg. 2015;262(5):764–770; discussion 70-1.
21. Schlegel A, Muller X, Kalisvaart M, Muellhaupt B, Perera M, Isaac JR, et al. Outcomes of DCD liver transplantation using organs treated by hypothermic oxygenated perfusion before implantation. J Hepatol. 2019;70(1):50–57.
22. Chouchani ET, Pell VR, Gaude E, Aksentijevic D, Sundier SY, Robb EL, et al. Ischaemic accumulation of succinate controls reperfusion injury through mitochondrial ROS. Nature. 2014;515(7527):431–435.
23. Chouchani ET, Pell VR, James AM, Work LM, Saeb-Parsy K, Frezza C, et al. A unifying mechanism for mitochondrial superoxide production during ischemia-reperfusion injury. Cell Metab. 2016;23(2):254–263.
24. Kron P, Schlegel A, Mancina L, Clavien PA, Dutkowski P. Hypothermic oxygenated perfusion (HOPE) for fatty liver grafts in rats and humans. J Hepatol. 2017 Sep 21;S0168–8278(17)32268–7. doi: 10.1016/j.jhep.2017.08.028. Online ahead of print.
25. Schlegel A, Kron P, Graf R, Clavien PA, Dutkowski P. Hypothermic Oxygenated Perfusion (HOPE) downregulates the immune response in a rat model of liver transplantation. Ann Surg. 2014;260(5):931–937; discussion 7-8.
26. Dutkowski P, Schlegel A, de Oliveira M, Mullhaupt B, Neff F, Clavien PA. HOPE for human liver grafts obtained from donors after cardiac death. J Hepatol. 2014;60(4):765–772.
27. Patrono D, Surra A, Catalano G, Rizza G, Berchialla P, Martini S, et al. Hypothermic oxygenated machine perfusion of liver grafts from brain-dead donors. Sci Rep. 2019;9(1):9337.
28. De Carlis L, Lauterio A, De Carlis R, Ferla F, Di Sandro S. Donation after cardiac death liver transplantation after more than 20 minutes of circulatory arrest and normothermic regional perfusion. Transplantation. 2016;100(4):e21–e22.

29. De Carlis R, Lauterio A, Ferla F, Di Sandro S, Sguinzi R, De Carlis L. Hypothermic machine perfusion of liver grafts can safely extend cold ischemia for up to 20 hours in cases of necessity. Transplantation. 2017;101(7):e223–e4.
30. Dondossola D, Lonati C, Zanella A, Maggioni M, Antonelli B, Reggiani P, et al. Preliminary experience with hypothermic oxygenated machine perfusion in an Italian liver transplant center. Transplant Proc. 2019;51(1):111–116.
31. Patrono D, Lavezzo B, Molinaro L, Rizza G, Catalano G, Gonella F, et al. Hypothermic oxygenated machine perfusion for liver transplantation: An initial experience. Exp Clin Transplant. 2018;16(2):172–176.
32. Ravaioli M, De Pace V, Pinna AD. From six thousand transaminases level to three hundred after liver transplantation: A new era seems to be open. Updates Surg. 2017;69(4):549–550.
33. Rayar M, Maillot B, Bergeat D, Camus C, Houssel-Debry P, Sulpice L, et al. A preliminary clinical experience using hypothermic oxygenated machine perfusion for rapid recovery of octogenarian liver grafts. Prog Transplant. 2019;29(1):97–98.
34. De Carlis R, Di Sandro S, Lauterio A, Botta F, Ferla F, Andorno E, et al. Liver grafts from donors after cardiac death on regional perfusion with extended warm ischemia compared with donors after brain death. Liver Transpl. 2018;24(11):1523–1535.
35. de Vries Y, Matton APM, Nijsten MWN, Werner MJM, van den Berg AP, de Boer MT, et al. Pretransplant sequential hypo- and normothermic machine perfusion of suboptimal livers donated after circulatory death using a hemoglobin-based oxygen carrier perfusion solution. Am J Transplant. 2019;19(4):1202–1211.
36. Laing RW, Bhogal RH, Wallace L, Boteon Y, Neil DAH, Smith A, et al. The use of an acellular oxygen carrier in a human liver model of normothermic machine perfusion. Transplantation. 2017;101(11):2746–2756.
37. Matton APM, Burlage LC, van Rijn R, de Vries Y, Karangwa SA, Nijsten MW, et al. Normothermic machine perfusion of donor livers without the need for human blood products. Liver Transpl. 2018;24(4):528–538.
38. Reddy SP, Bhattacharjya S, Maniakin N, Greenwood J, Guerreiro D, Hughes D, et al. Preservation of porcine non-heart-beating donor livers by sequential cold storage and warm perfusion. Transplantation. 2004;77(9):1328–1332.
39. Bral M, Dajani K, Leon Izquierdo D, Bigam D, Kneteman N, Ceresa CDL, et al. A back-to-base experience of human normothermic ex situ liver perfusion: Does the chill kill? Liver Transpl. 2019;25(6):848–858.
40. Ceresa CDL, Nasralla D, Watson CJE, Butler AJ, Coussios CC, Crick K, et al. Transient cold storage prior to normothermic liver perfusion may facilitate adoption of a novel technology. Liver Transpl. 2019;25(10):1503–1513.
41. Xu H, Berendsen T, Kim K, Soto-Gutierrez A, Bertheium F, Yarmush ML, et al. Excorporeal normothermic machine perfusion resuscitates pig DCD livers with extended warm ischemia. J Surg Res. 2012;173(2):e83–e88.
42. Brockmann J, Reddy S, Coussios C, Pigott D, Guirriero D, Hughes D, et al. Normothermic perfusion: a new paradigm for organ preservation. Ann Surg. 2009;250(1):1–6.
43. Jassem W, Xystrakis E, Ghnewa YG, Yuksel M, Pop O, Martinez-Llordella M, et al. Normothermic Machine Perfusion (NMP) inhibits proinflammatory responses in the liver and promotes regeneration. Hepatology. 2019 Aug;70(2):682–695. doi: 10.1002/hep.30475.

44. Ghinolfi D, Rreka E, De Tata V, Franzini M, Pezzati D, Fierabracci V, et al. Pilot, open, randomized, prospective trial for normothermic machine perfusion evaluation in liver transplantation from older donors. Liver Transpl 2019 Mar;25(3):436–449. doi: 10.1002/lt.25362.
45. Nasralla D, Coussios CC, Mergental H, Akhtar MZ, Butler AJ, Ceresa CDL, et al. A randomized trial of normothermic preservation in liver transplantation. Nature. 2018;557(7703):50–56.
46. Ravikumar R, Jassem W, Mergental H, Heaton N, Mirza D, Perera MT, et al. Liver transplantation after ex vivo normothermic machine preservation: A phase 1 (first-in-man) clinical trial. Am J Transplant. 2016;16(6):1779–1787.
47. Selzner M, Goldaracena N, Echeverri J, Kaths JM, Linares I, Selzner N, et al. Normothermic ex vivo liver perfusion using steen solution as perfusate for human liver transplantation: First North American results. Liver Transpl. 2016;22(11):1501–1508.
48. Watson CJE, Kosmoliaptsis V, Pley C, Randle L, Fear C, Crick K, et al. Observations on the ex situ perfusion of livers for transplantation. Am J Transplant. 2018;18(8):2005–2020.
49. Watson CJE, Kosmoliaptsis V, Randle LV, Gimson AE, Brais R, Klinck JR, et al. Normothermic perfusion in the assessment and preservation of declined livers before transplantation: Hyperoxia and vasoplegia-important lessons from the first 12 cases. Transplantation. 2017;101(5):1084–1098.
50. Vogel T, Brockmann JG, Quaglia A, Morovat A, Jassem W, Heaton ND, et al. The 24-hour normothermic machine perfusion of discarded human liver grafts. Liver Transpl. 2017;23(2):207–220.
51. Watson CJE, Jochmans I. From 'gut feeling' to objectivity: Machine preservation of the liver as a tool to assess organ viability. Curr Transplant Rep. 2018;5(1):72–81.
52. Perera T, Mergental H, Stephenson B, Roll GR, Cilliers H, Liang R, et al. First human liver transplantation using a marginal allograft resuscitated by normothermic machine perfusion. Liver Transpl. 2016;22(1):120–124.
53. Laing RW, Mergental H, Yap C, Kirkham A, Whilku M, Barton D, et al. Viability testing and transplantation of marginal livers (VITTAL) using normothermic machine perfusion: study protocol for an open-label, non-randomised, prospective, single-arm trial. BMJ Open. 2017;7(11):e017733.
54. Minor T, Efferz P, Fox M, Wohlschlaeger J, Luer B. Controlled oxygenated rewarming of cold stored liver grafts by thermally graduated machine perfusion prior to reperfusion. Am J Transplant. 2013;13(6):1450–1460.
55. Westerkamp AC, Karimian N, Matton AP, Mahboub P, van Rijn R, Wiersema-Buist J, et al. Oxygenated hypothermic machine perfusion after static cold storage improves hepatobiliary function of extended criteria donor livers. Transplantation. 2016;100(4):825–835.
56. Burlage LC, Karimian N, Westerkamp AC, Visser N, Matton APM, van Rijn R, et al. Oxygenated hypothermic machine perfusion after static cold storage improves endothelial function of extended criteria donor livers. HPB (Oxford). 2017;19(6):538–546.
57. Boteon YL, Laing RW, Schlegel A, Wallace L, Smith A, Attard J, et al. Combined hypothermic and normothermic machine perfusion improves functional recovery of extended criteria donor livers. Liver Transpl. 2018;24(12):1699–1715.

58. Boteon YL, Attard J, Boteon A, Wallace L, Reynolds G, Hubscher S, et al. Manipulation of lipid metabolism during normothermic machine perfusion: Effect of defatting therapies on donor liver functional recovery. Liver Transpl. 2019;25(7):1007–1022.
59. Rigo F, De Stefano N, Navarro-Tableros V, David E, Rizza G, Catalano G, et al. Extracellular vesicles from human liver stem cells reduce injury in an ex vivo normothermic hypoxic rat liver perfusion model. Transplantation. 2018;102(5):e205–e10.

49

Renal transplantation

Niraj Kumar, Anup Kumar

Historical overview

Renal replacement therapy (RRT) is one of the greatest innovations of the 20th-century medicine. The techniques of vascular suturing, transplantation experiments in animals, and immunological studies led to the ultimate success of renal transplantation among human beings. Significant contributors in the evolution of renal transplantation include Alexis Carrel, a French surgeon, who developed the technique of 'triangulation' for vascular suturing, where three stay-sutures were placed to minimize vascular wall damage during the suturing procedure. He received the Nobel Prize for his work in 1912; the technique is still being followed widely. Emerich Ullmann, an Austrian surgeon, performed the first successful renal auto-transplant in a dog. In 1906, Mathieu Jaboulay made the first attempt in human renal transplantation using pig and goat kidneys. Thereafter, various attempts with short-term success were made in human renal transplantation.[1,2] Ultimately, on 23 December 1954, Prof J E Murray, an American plastic surgeon, performed the first successful kidney transplant in identical twins. He was awarded Nobel Prize in 1990 for his pioneering work in the field of Medicine.[3,4]

Transplant Immunology was developed simultaneously to prevent transplant rejection. After successful kidney transplant among identical twins, the trials for allo-transplant were made with immunosuppression using whole body irradiation and cyclophosphamide followed by introduction of the corticosteroids and azathioprine, which remained the mainstay of immunosuppressive therapy to prevent graft rejection till 1978. Subsequent introduction of polyclonal anti-lymphocyte preparations by Starzl et al and addition of cyclosporine in the immunosuppressive regimen led to a considerable improvement in the outcome of renal transplantation.[2,4]

Renal transplant recipient

The prevalence of chronic kidney disease (CKD) among adults in the United States (US) is approximately 15%, mostly due to the increased risk factors. The common causes of end stage renal disease (ESRD) were diabetes (36%), hypertension (23%), glomerulonephritis (14%), cystic diseases (9%), and others (18%). The incidence of ESRD was 370.2 per million/year in the US population in 2017 and 86.9% of them started RRT with haemodialysis (HD), 10.1% with peritoneal dialysis (PD), and 2.9% had a pre-emptive kidney transplant. The prevalence of ESRD was 2204 per million in the US population in 2017 and among them, 62.7% were receiving HD therapy, 7.1% PD, and 29.9% living with a functioning kidney transplant. Overall, 20,945 kidney transplants were performed in the US in 2017, of which, 20476 were kidney-alone without liver or pancreas and 28% were from the living donors. Also, the respective adjusted mortality rates per 1000 patient-years for ESRD, dialysis, and transplant patients were 134, 165, and 29 respectively in 2017.[5]

Selection of recipient

With the goal of improved survival and quality of life, all prospective kidney transplant recipients need to be counselled regarding the cause of CKD and the risks associated with it, comorbidities, the pros and cons of different methods of RRT, different options of donors, and the need for immunosuppression. It is recommended that all CKD patients with glomerular function rate (GFR) < 30 ml/min/1.73 m^2, who are expected to reach ESRD, be informed of, educated about, and considered for renal transplantation, regardless of their socioeconomic status, sex, or race/ethnicity.[6–8]

Preliminary screening

Baseline evaluation in a prospective renal transplant recipient includes[6–9]:

1. Detailed clinical history, treatment history, immunization history.
2. Physical examination and dental examination.
3. Laboratory test including complete blood count, kidney, liver, and thyroid function test, coagulation profile, Infection serology (CMV, EBV, hepatitis B and C, HIV, syphilis) Tuberculin test, Stool occult blood, serum PSA in men≥40 years, urine analysis, Pap smear, Mammogram (≥40years), pregnancy test, if indicated.
4. Abdominal ultrasound.
5. Doppler ultrasound to assess symptomatic peripheral vascular disease.
6. Electrocardiogram and chest X-ray to identify high-risk cardiac patients.
   - Exercise tolerance test and cardiac ultrasound for asymptomatic high-risk patients.
   - In case of positive or inconclusive exercise tolerance test, non-invasive stress imaging (myocardial perfusion or dobutamine stress echocardiography) is indicated.
   - If test for cardiac ischaemia is positive, coronary angiography is indicated and treatment as per current cardiovascular guidelines.
7. Histocompatibility testing.
8. Any other test as indicated.

The specific evaluations are summarized in Table 49.1.[6–12]

Specific urological evaluation

Prospective recipients should be examined to ascertain optimal placement of graft kidney in the iliac fossa. The ESRD patients with low or minimal urine output may have abnormal bladder, which requires further evaluation. Additional urologic evaluation (Table 49.2) is required, if indicated, to assess the anatomy of urinary tract, bladder function, and risk of urological malignancy.[8,12,13]

Surgery for optimization of bladder or urinary outlet

Transplant team should aim to have an optimum urinary reservoir with at least 200 mL capacity, low storage pressure, and the ability to empty

Table 49.1[6–12] Specific evaluation of renal transplant recipient

	Parameter evaluated	Recommendations
1.	Age	• Not a contraindication per se
2.	Psychological assessment	• By a qualified health care professional • Treat active psychiatric disorder or ongoing substance abuse
3.	Compliance	• Educate the patient • Exclude if non-compliant
4.	Obesity	• Advise weight reduction, if BMI>30kg/m2
5.	Smoking	• Encourage to stop using tobacco products • Offer a tobacco cessation program
6.	ESRD and type I DM	• Simultaneous pancreas-kidney transplantation

7.	Cause of ESRD	• Try to establish cause, if possible, for counselling the patient regarding the risk of recurrence
		• Discuss risk of recurrence and perioperative management but do not exclude patient with Focal segmental glomerulosclerosis, Membranous glomerulopathy, IgA nephropathy, Immune-complex mediated membranoproliferative glomerulonephritis, C3 glomerulopathy, clinically silent lupus nephritis, antiphospholipid antibody syndrome, ANCA vasculitis, and anti-glomerular basement membrane disease
		• Hemolytic-Uremic syndrome:
		  • Secondary to *E. coli* infection: do not exclude
		  • Secondary to genetic or acquired defect in complement regulation: living related kidney transplant not recommended
		• Primary hyperoxaluria: Offer combined or sequential Liver-kidney transplant

8.	Infections	• Treat all active infections
		• Tuberculosis:
		  • Complete treatment prior to renal transplant
		  • Screen for latent TB on low TB prevalence area with chest X-ray, Tuberculin test or interferon gamma release assay
		  • Start antitubercular treatment in low TB prevalence area for latent TB immediately prior or after transplantation
		  • Screen for latent TB in intermediate and high TB prevalence area as per local guidelines
		• HIV infection: transplant only if
		  • compliant with treatment, particularly HAART therapy
		  • CD4+ T cell counts > 200/μL and stable for last 3–6 months
		  • undetectable HIV RNA for last 3 months
		  • no opportunistic infections in last 6 months
		  • no signs of progressive multifocal leukoencephalopathy, chronic intestinal cryptosporidiosis, or lymphoma

Table 49.1 *Continued*

	Parameter evaluated	Recommendations
9.	Malignancy	• Screen malignancy same as general population • USG to screen for renal malignancy • Do not delay transplant for in situ skin and cervical cancers, incidental detected and successfully treated kidney cancer and low risk prostate cancer • Delay for 1–3 years for localized cancer with good prognosis including intermediate and high-risk prostate cancer • Delay for 5 years for cancers with poor prognosis including high grade and invasive bladder malignancy • Avoid transplant in metastatic and disseminated cancers except testicular cancer and lymphoma

Table 49.2[8,12,13] Specific urological evaluation

	Investigation	Indication
1.	Cystoscopy	Suspected lower urinary tract cancer or to rule out outlet obstruction
2.	MCU	Vesico-ureteral reflux (VUR), voiding dysfunction
3.	Urodynamic study	Voiding dysfunction, Neurologic disease
4.	Abdominal computed tomography	Doubtful lesion on abdominal ultrasound, ADPKD
5.	Urine cytology	History of cyclophosphamide therapy, irritative voiding symptoms, hematuria
6.	Pouchogram/loopogram	History of intestinal urinary reservoir

completely. Potential kidney recipients with symptomatic benign prostatic enlargement should be treated with alpha-blockers, 5 alpha-reductase inhibitors, or trans urethral resection of prostate, as indicated. The ESRD patient with long history of low urinary output may have low urinary bladder capacity which may need augmentation preferably with urothelium lined tissue, to avoid interventions for mucus collection, or intestine. Timing of surgery should be decided such that the reconstructed bladder has adequate urine; otherwise risk of stricture, stone, infection, and loss of compliance may be anticipated. Adequacy of bladder emptying must be checked, if not adequate, clean intermittent catheterisation must be taught.[8,13]

Pre-transplant nephrectomy
Native kidney helps in maintenance of fluid and electrolyte balance, management of hypertension and also reduces the risk of cardiac complications. Therefore, the need for pre-transplant nephrectomy should be carefully assessed and should not be done unless benefit outweighs the risk involved. Indications include:

- Bilateral nephrectomy in symptomatic and unilateral nephrectomy in asymptomatic autosomal dominant polycystic kidney disease (ADPKD)
- Urinary disease predisposing to recurrent urinary tract infection (UTI) like grade 4/5 vesicoureteral reflex (VUR), recurrent pyelonephritis, or renal stone not cleared by minimal invasive technique
- Uncontrolled proteinuria
- Persistent anti-glomerular basement membrane antibody
- Renal tumour

The ideal time to perform the pre-transplant nephrectomy is still a matter of debate. While some surgeons prefer to do it at least 6 weeks prior to the scheduled transplant, others do it concurrent with the transplant surgery with the risk of increased morbidity.[8,12,13]

Graft nephrectomy:
It may be required prior to second or subsequent transplant in cases of:

- clinical rejection
- chronic systemic inflammation with no obvious cause
- recurrent infections

However, if residual graft urine output is >500ml/day with no sign of inflammation, graft nephrectomy can be avoided with low level of immunosuppression.[12]

Selection of donor

The advancement in the field of medicine, along with increasing awareness and society and government support, a huge number of living donors volunteer for the donation.

Living donor

There are important advantages of live donor renal transplantation including superior graft and patient survival, fewer immunologic complications, less need for dialysis, better quality of life along with greater cost-effectiveness when compared to deceased donor transplant; however, both the type of donors are immensely valuable in current scenario of RRT.(8,14–16)

Preliminary screening

The kidney donor should be subjected to AB0 blood grouping and Human leukocyte antigen (HLA) typing for major histocompatibility complex (MHC) Class I (A, B, C) and Class II (DP, DQ, DR) antigens with their intended recipients and the recipient should be assessed for donor-specific anti-HLA antibodies. Donors with ABO blood group mismatch or HLA incompatibility with their intended recipient should be counselled about the risks and benefits of the available treatment options, including paired kidney donation and transplant after incompatibility management. All eligible donors should be screened as per Table 49.3.(6,8,12,14–16)

Donors should be evaluated in detail with the aim to reduce the risks of perioperative surgery and anaesthesia related complications. Donor should be evaluated by a physician and a psychologist independent of the transplant team. The contraindications of living kidney donations are summarized in Table 49.4.(8,12–16)

GFR estimation

The initial assessment of GFR should be estimated from serum creatinine (estimated GFR (eGFR)). This eGFR should be confirmed using one or more of the following:(8,14,16)

- Measured GFR (mGFR) using preferably urinary or plasma clearance of inulin or iothalamate or 51Cr-EDTA or iohexol or urinary clearance of 99mTc-DTPA
- eGFR measured from the combination of serum creatinine and cystatin C
- Differential kidney GFR should be estimated using radionuclides or contrast agents that are excreted by glomerular filtration (eg,

Table 49.3[6,8,12,14–16] Screening investigations for the potential donor

1. Urine
   - Dipstick test for protein, blood and glucose
   - Urinalysis with microscopy,
   - Culture and sensitivity
   - Measurement of 24-hours protein excretion rate or protein/ creatinine ratio
2. Blood
   - Complete blood count
   - Coagulation profile including prothrombin time, international normalized ratio
   - Hemoglobinopathy screen, if indicated
   - Kidney function test
   - Liver function tests
   - Serum calcium, phosphate, and alkaline phosphatase
   - Fasting plasma glucose
   - Glucose tolerance test, if family history of diabetes or fasting plasma glucose100mg/dL
   - Fasting lipid profile
   - Thyroid function tests
   - Pregnancy test (if indicated)
3. Virology and infection serology
   - HIV
   - Hepatitis B and C
   - Cytomegalovirus
   - Epstein-Barr virus
   - Syphilis
   - Others, as per local guidelines
4. Imaging
   - Computed tomography angiogram or MRI abdomen to assess renal parenchyma, arterial and venous anatomy
   - Electrocardiogram
   - Chest X-ray
5. Renal function assessment using
   - 24-hour urine collection for calculation of creatinine clearance
   - Nuclear studies using radioactive isotope or iodinated tracer
6. Age specific cancer screening

99mTcDMSA, 99mTc-DTPA) in case there is parenchymal, vascular, or urological abnormalities or >10% kidney asymmetry on renal imaging.

- As per Kidney disease improving global outcomes (KDIGO) guidelines, donor is fit for a safe donation if GFR is ≥90 ml/min/1.73m^2. However, the decision to donate to donors with GFR between 60–89ml/min/1.73m^2 should be individualized. The British Transplant Society and UK renal association[15] recommend age and sex-based criteria for eligibility of kidney donation ranging from GFR of 90

Table 49.4[8,12–16] Contraindications of kidney donation

1. Live kidney donation[14]

1a. Absolute
- Age <18 and mentally incapable of making an informed decision
- Diabetes mellitus
- Active or incompletely treated malignancy
- HIV
- Evidence of acute symptomatic infection
- Active mental illness

Kidney specific
- Uncontrolled hypertension
- Hypertension with evidence of end-organ damage

1b. Relative contraindications
- History of certain prior malignancies or treatment with nephrotoxic therapy for malignancy
- Active substance abuse
- Disorders requiring anticoagulation, bleeding disorders
- Morbid obesity (BMI >35)
- Prediabetes

Kidney specific
- GFR <80 mL/min or <2 SD below the mean for donor age
- Proteinuria: Albumin/creatinine ratio >30 mg/mmol, protein/creatinine ratio>50 mg/mmol, albumin excretion >300 mg/day, or protein excretion >500 mg/day
- Persistent glomerular hematuria
- Renal collecting system or vasculature anomaly
- Kidney stones with high probability of recurrence
- Chronic, active viral infection (HBV, HCV)

2. Contraindication of kidney donation in DBD [24]
- Age >70years
- Age 50–69years with history of type 1 diabetes for more than 20 years
- Polycystic kidney disease
- Terminal serum creatinine >4.0 mg/dL
- ESRD or CKD stage 4 (eGFR 15–30 ml/min)
- Glomerulosclerosis ≥20% in kidney biopsy
- Acute cortical necrosis on pre-implantation kidney biopsy
- No urine output for 24 hours or longer

ml/min/1.73m^2 in 20–29 year age group to 58 and 49ml/min/1.73m^2 in 80 years male and female donor, respectively.

Surgical approach

The current surgical approaches for donor nephrectomy include:

1. Open nephrectomy
2. Minimal invasive donor nephrectomy:

- Pure or hand-assisted transperitoneal laparoscopy/ retroperitoneoscopic approach;
- Laparo-Endoscopic Single Site Surgery (LESS);
- Natural Orifice Transluminal Endoscopic Surgery-assisted (NOTES);
- Robotic-assisted transperitoneal or retroperitoneal approach

European association of urology guidelines strongly recommends pure or hand-assisted transperitoneal laparoscopy/retroperitoneoscopic approach for living donor nephrectomy. There is strong evidence in literature including systematic review and meta-analysis supporting laparoscopic living-donor nephrectomy over open donor nephrectomy; though the rates of graft outcome, urological complications, and patient and graft survival are same for both the methods; laparoscopic technique is significantly better in terms of pain, analgesic requirements, hospital stay, and time to return to work. Literature regarding LESS, NOTES, or robotic-assisted donor nephrectomy is not mature enough.(8,16)

Follow up of living donor must include annual check-up including blood pressure/BMI/Serum creatinine measurement with GFR estimation/albuminuria measurement/education and promotion of a healthy lifestyle and support for psychosocial health.(8,14,17,18)

Deceased donor evaluation

Deceased donor selection and allocation is usually governed by the Organ Transplant Act of the respective country, and is aimed to augment the effectiveness and efficiency of organ sharing and to ensure equity in organ allocation. Along with standard criteria donors, expanded criteria donors (ECD) (Table 49.5) are useful sources of organ procurement.

Table 49.5(8,13,19) Expanded criteria donors

- Elderly (≥60 years)
- Age between 50-59 with two of following risk factors:
  - history of hypertension
  - terminal serum creatinine over 1.5 mg/dl,
  - cerebrovascular accident as the cause of death.

Donors can be declared dead on the basis of neurological or cardiorespiratory criteria.[8,19]

Donation after brain death (DBD):

Brain death is irreversible loss of all functions of the brain, including the brainstem with coma, absence of brainstem reflexes, and apnoea being the essential findings. The process of declaration of brain death include:[8,20]

- Establishing the cause of irreversible coma
- Excluding confounding factors for brain death: Shock, Hypothermia, pharmacologic and metabolic intoxication, brain stem encephalitis, Guillain- Barre's syndrome
- Complete cessation of brainstem function including coma, absent brainstem reflexes, positive apnoea test
- At least 6-hour observation before second clinical examination in patients aged ≥1 year (24 hours for 2–12 months old child, 24 hours for child < 2 months of age)
    - Mandatory confirmatory tests, including but not limited to electroencephalogram, cerebral angiography, nuclear medicine brain scan, transcranial doppler ultrasonography, if any doubt exists.

Donation after cardiac death (DCD)

Death can be confirmed if there is 5 minutes of continuous cardio-respiratory arrest provided no subsequent attempt to restore artificial cerebral circulation.[21] DCD is classified by modified Maastricht classification (2013) into controlled and uncontrolled donors. In 2013, it was modified to include place of death (out-of-hospital or in-hospital) in category I and II whereas categories IV and V were merged into one and categorized as uncontrolled cardiac death.[22] The use of kidney from donors with functional warm ischaemic time >2 hr or 30 minutes of absent blood pressure should be limited to research protocols. The use of DCD kidney, whether controlled or uncontrolled, is associated with higher primary non-function and delayed graft function, but with satisfactory long-term outcome. Better outcome is reported with age of DCD donor <50 years and cold ischemia time <12 hours.[8,13,21,22]

Kidney preservation

The aim of organ preservation is maintenance of intracellular physiology. EAU guidelines[16] recommend perfusion with University of Wisconsin or HTK solution for cold storage. Celsior or Marshall's solution can be used in case of unavailability of University of Wisconsin or HTK solution.[8,16] It has been recommended to keep cold ischemia time as low as possible, preferably within 18–21 hours for DBD donors, less than 12 hours for DCD or ECD. Hypothermic-perfusion machine, if available, should be used for deceased donor kidney perfusion and should be controlled by pressure, and not by flow.[9]

Matching of donor and recipients

All potential kidney transplant donors and recipients must be tested for AB0 blood group and human leucocyte antigens A, B, and DR. Test for DQ, DP, and HLA C antigens should be done in sensitized patients. The HLA DR antigen compatibility should be given more value than HLA A and B.[8,9,11,16]

A complement-dependent cytotoxic (CDC) cross-match must be performed in HLA sensitized patients in order to prevent hyperacute rejection. However, a positive CDC cross-match should be accepted as truly positive only when donor-specific antibodies are present. Among ABO incompatible renal transplant candidates, inhibition of antibody production, and ABO antibody removal should be done earlier and transplant should be performed only if the ABO antibody titre can be kept lower than 1:8 after intervention. In incompatible transplant candidates, paired exchange should be considered, if allowed by local legal framework.[8,9,11,13]

Flow cytometry crossmatch is more sensitive in detection of HLA antibodies. The serum of potential recipient in waiting list should be subjected to CDC or flow cytometry crossmatch against a panel of cells comprising donor representative lymphocytes. The percentage of representative donors causing positive crossmatch is known as panel reactive antibody.[8,9,11,13,23]

Preparation of allograft

Once received from the donor, renal artery and vein should be identified and perfused with ice-cold solution. Once perfused properly, excess peri-renal fat should be excised, renal vein tributaries to be ligated if clipped during donor surgery and renal artery and vein to be reconstructed, if required before transplantation into the recipient. Shortness of renal vein can be compensated with saphenous vein (living donor) or with inferior vena cava (deceased donor). In case of multiple renal arteries, they can be reconstructed into one by side to side or end to side anastomosis.[8,13]

Recipient surgery

For adults and children weighing more than 20 kg, kidney should be transplanted into contralateral iliac fossa extraperitoneally by rectus preserving Gibson or Rutherford Morrison incision. During renal transplant bed preparation, care should be taken to minimize the damage to the lymphatic vessels and all the lymphatics dissected should be ligated on either end to minimise the risk of lymphocele. Renal artery is anastomosed preferably end to end to internal iliac artery or end to side to external iliac artery. Other options of arterial anastomosis include common iliac artery, aorta, splenic artery, or native renal artery. For arterial anastomosis in external iliac artery, common iliac artery or aorta, a vascular punch is useful for creating a round hole to prevent co-aptation or thrombosis of renal artery in case of occurrence of hypotension in post-operative period. Renal vein should be anastomosed end to side preferably to external iliac vein, with other options being common iliac vein, inferior vena cava, and splenic vein. It is more critical to anastomose the renal artery first, followed by venous one, except in cases where renal vein is short or access to recipient vein is limited. Venous occlusion should be avoided till arterial anastomosis is complete in order to reduce risk of iliofemoral venous thrombosis. Urinary tract reconstruction should be done with the technique of antireflux ureteroneocystostomy. Most surgeons prefer Lich-Gregoir like extravesical ureteroneocystostomy to prevent separate cystostomy incision, need for shorter length of ureter with better vascular supply. In case of short donor ureter or difficulty in reaching bladder or as per surgeon preference, pyeloureterostomy or ureteroureterostomy can be done. Modifications are required in cases of abnormal urinary tract like ileal conduit, continent pouch, or augmented bladder, with emphasis to prevent a redundant ureter and without disturbing the vascular supply of the reconstructed urinary tract. The use of ureteral stent is preferred in order to reduce the incidence of major post-operative ureteral complications. Incision should be over a closed suction drain.

During the surgery and in the immediate post-operative period, central venous pressure should be maintained in the range of 10–15 cm of H_2O with the help of intravenous crystalloids or colloids with or without additional inotropes.[8,11,13]

Though at an early stage of development, early publications found robot-assisted renal transplantation safe and reproducible in select cases with excellent graft function.[24]

Fluid and electrolyte management

The intravenous fluid for post-operative period should be 0.45% saline with or without dextrose in an amount equal to last hour of urine output with the monitoring of serum electrolyte 4–8 hourly and corrections as and when required. The oliguric patient needs urgent treatment of hyperkalaemia or dialysis. Ultrasonogram is required for oliguria, abdominal swelling, ipsilateral limb swelling, or falling haematocrit. In case oliguria persists, radioisotope renogram may be required twice weekly till serum creatinine start decreasing without dialysis. However, if renogram deteriorates, renal biopsy may be required to rule out graft rejection.[8]

Renal allograft function

The following parameters should be monitored to ascertain the normal functioning of the renal allograft[11]:

- Urine volume to be monitored every 1–2 hours for at least 24 hours and daily thereafter till stable graft function.

- Serum creatinine to be estimated (with estimated GFR calculation) daily for 7 days to the minimum or till discharge from hospital followed by 2–3 times per week for 1st month, weekly till 3 months, every 2 weeks till 6 months, monthly till 1 year and thereafter every 3 months.
- Urine protein excretion measured at least once in 1st month, then every 3 months and annually thereafter.
- Kidney allograft ultrasound to be performed for any allograft dysfunction.

Indications of kidney allograft biopsy

The indications for a kidney allograft biopsy are as follows:[8,11]

- An unexplained persistent rise in serum creatinine
- Failure of serum creatinine to reach baseline after acute rejection treatment
- In case of delayed graft function, biopsy to be taken every 7–10 days
- Failure of graft function to reach expected level within 1–2 months
- New onset of proteinuria or unexplained proteinuria ≥3.0 g/g creatinine or ≥3.0 g per 24 hours

Catheter, drain, and sutures

Catheter should be removed within first week after obtaining urine sample for culture just prior to removal. Drain should be removed once output is less than 50ml/24hours and ureteric stent should be removed between 1 and 3 weeks. Sutures can be removed in 8–10 days.[8,9,13]

Perioperative Immunosuppression

Induction therapy: The standard induction immunosuppression regimen with proven excellent efficacy and tolerability include[8,11,13,25]:

- Calcineurin inhibitors (CNI); tacrolimus as first line with cyclosporine as an alternative.

- Mycophenolate mofetil or enteric-coated mycophenolate sodium, with Azathioprine as alternative in mycophenolate intolerant patients
- Steroids including methylprednisolone or prednisolone
- Interleukin-2 receptor antibody basiliximab in low or normal risk patients and anti-thymocyte globulin in high-risk patients
- M-TOR receptor antagonist, Everolimus or Sirolimus, should be used in patients' intolerant to calcineurin inhibitors. If these drugs are to be used, it should be delayed till graft function is stable and wound healed.
- Balatacept may be used in EBV positive patients.

Maintenance therapy: The standard maintenance immunosuppression regimen should include a combination of:

- Calcineurin inhibitors, preferably tacrolimus
- Antiproliferative agent with mycophenolate as first-line
- Steroids should be withdrawn within first week in patients with low immunological risk

The blood level of calcineurin inhibitors (every alternate day in immediate post-operative period and whenever there is a change in patient status that may affect blood levels, and decline in kidney function), and m-TOR inhibitors (mTORi) should be monitored at regular intervals in order to allow for dose adjustment. Lowest possible dose of immunosuppression is targeted by 2–4 months of transplant, with continuation of low dose steroids if it could not be withdrawn within first week of transplant.[8,11,13,25]

Complications of transplantation

Complications from a renal transplantation can occur in the donor or the recipient. It can be short term or long term in nature.

Donor complications

1. Short-term: A recent review of laparoscopic donor nephrectomy reported overall peri-operative complication of 16.8% with mortality

of 0.007%; of these, 2.5% were Clavien grade IV or V complications. A favourable outcome was reported from centres with annual volume of >50 renal transplant. Obesity, pre-donation haematologic/psychiatric disease and robotic donor nephrectomy were associated with an adverse outcome.[26]

2. Long-term: The overall incidence (0.4–1.1%) of ESRD is similar to that of the general population with the risk being higher in obese donors. Donors are found to have higher health-related quality of life score compared to the general population.[13]

Recipient complications

- Haemorrhage (0.2–25%): Larger hematoma causing graft dysfunction require percutaneous ultrasound guided drainage and hemodynamic deterioration may need surgical exploration.[13]
- Renal arterial thrombosis (0.5–3.5%): The risk factor could be a technical error, donor and recipient's artery disease, acute rejection episodes, external compression, hypercoagulative state, severe hypotension, and immunosuppressive toxicity. The sudden drop in urine output and the rise in serum creatinine prompts colour Doppler for diagnosis. Surgical exploration is usually required to evaluate the graft status with a thrombectomy for a rarely salvageable graft or otherwise an allograft nephrectomy.[8,13]
- Venous thrombosis (0.5–4%): Being one of the most common causes of graft loss in 1st month with technical error or hypercoagulable state as the causative factor, venous thrombosis requires colour Doppler ultrasound for diagnosis. Once diagnosed, surgical exploration should be done with thrombectomy in viable graft or nephrectomy in unviable one.[8,13]
- Renal artery stenosis (1–25%): The causative factors are donor artery disease, trauma to donor artery, inappropriate suturing technique, and damage to the iliac artery during transplantation with the common site being the site of the anastomosis. Doppler ultrasound should be done in patients with arterial hypertension refractory to medical treatment and/or a rise in serum creatinine without urinary obstruction or infection. The diagnosis is confirmed with a peak

systolic velocity of > 200 cm/s in the graft renal artery and treatment requires transluminal angioplasty and surgical exploration for failed transluminal approach.[8,13]

- Lymphocele (1–26%): The risk factors are diabetes, m-TOR inhibitors, and acute rejection surgical approach. Percutaneous drainage is required to treat large lymphocele with laparoscopic or open fenestration in case of failure.[8,13]
- Urine leak (0–9.3%): It is usually a uretero-vesical anastomotic leak with avascular necrosis. Technical error is the aetiology and usually suspected by the low urine output and the higher creatinine level in the drain fluid. It should be managed with double-J stent, percutaneous drainage, or bladder catheter, with surgical exploration reserved for failure of conservative treatment.[8,13]
- Ureteral stricture (0.6–10.5%): The risk factors for early stenosis include technical error or ureteral ischemia and for late stenosis include infection, fibrosis, progressive vascular disease and/or rejection. Management includes percutaneous nephrostomy, antegrade nephrostogram, endoscopic reconstruction (stricture length <3cm), surgical reconstruction (recurrence or stricture length >3cm).[8,13]
- Reflux (1–86%) and acute pyelonephritis (13%): Endoscopic approach is the first line of treatment; surgical repair should be reserved for failed endoscopic treatment.[8,13]
- Urolithiasis (0.2–1.7%): The risk factors include hyperfiltration, renal tubular acidosis, recurrent UTIs, hypocitraturia, hyperoxaluria, hyperuricaemia, excessive alkaline urine, persistent tertiary hyperparathyroidism, and ureteral strictures. Treatment includes shockwave lithotripsy/flexible ureteroscopy for <15mm stone and percutaneous nephrolithotomy for stone >20mm.[8,13]
- Immunological complications: Recipients should be monitored closely for risk factors including graft dysfunction with infection, graft rejection, urinary obstruction, calcineurin inhibitor toxicity, dehydration, and hyperglycaemia. Once suspected, ultrasound of kidney should be performed to exclude the cause of graft dysfunction other than rejection. If rejection is suspected, ultrasound-guided renal biopsy with grading according to Banff criteria should be done prior to starting steroid pulse therapy.[8,11,13,25]

- Hyperacute rejection: It is a destructive immunological attack on the graft which can be prevented by adequate ABO and HLA matching between donor and recipients. Treatment is usually a graft nephrectomy.[8,13]
- Acute rejection: Risk factors for acute rejection include the number of HLA mismatches, younger age of recipient, older age of donor, panel reactive antibody >0%, presence of a donor-specific antibody, blood group incompatibility, delayed onset of graft function, and cold ischemia time >24 hours. Treatment of T-cell mediated acute rejection starts with steroid bolus therapy followed by lymphocyte-depleting antibodies or Muromonab-CD3 (traded as Orthoclone OKT3) in case of steroid nonresponsive rejection.

Antibody-mediated acute rejection requires antibody elimination by a combination of plasma exchange, intravenous immunoglobulin, anti-CD20 antibody, and lymphocyte-depleting antibody with or without steroids.[11,13,25]

- Chronic kidney rejection: One of the causes of delayed graft dysfunction includes chronic graft rejection, characterized by interstitial fibrosis and tubular atrophy on kidney biopsy. It usually presents with proteinuria, and hypertension, gradual rise in serum creatinine level. In case of chronic rejection with biopsy evidence suggestive of calcineurin inhibitor toxicity (arteriolar hyalinosis, striped fibrosis), CNI should be reduced, withdrawn, or replaced. In patients on CNI with eGFR >40 mL/min/1.73 m^2, and urine total protein excretion <500 mg/g creatinine, it should be replaced with an mTORi.[8,11,13,25] Patients with deteriorating renal function should be monitored and managed as per 2012 KDIGO CKD guidelines.[27]

Transplant outcome

Factors associated with adverse renal transplant outcome include higher age of donor or recipient, quality of kidney (deceased donor (standard vs ECD vs DCD) compared to living donor), multiple renal arteries, recurrence of native kidney disease, African-American race, HLA mismatch, anti-HLA immunization, longer time on dialysis, cardiovascular disease, lower GFR at one year post-transplant, proteinuria, chronic allograft dysfunction, and possibly delayed graft function.[8,26,28,29]

As per Organ procurement and transplantation network (OPTN)/ Scientific registry of transplant recipients (SRTR) 2017 Annual Data Report, the one-year graft survival and patient survival of kidney transplant from deceased donors and living donors were 93% and 96%, and 98% and 99%, respectively. The living donor kidney transplant recipients had continued graft and patient survival advantage at five and ten years post-transplant.[30]

Conclusion

Renal transplant is the best modality of RRT for ESRD. All patients with stages IV and V CKD should be counselled and considered for renal transplantation. A structured transplantation network is required to ensure legal, unbiased, and timely distribution of available organs. Transplant recipients should be carefully screened and prepared as per loco-regional protocol with the aim to utilize kidney graft to its maximum potential with minimum morbidity. The perioperative and structured follow up care should include multidisciplinary team to achieve a long-term success. The five and 10-year graft and patient survival has been reported to be better with the living donor kidney compared to that of the deceased donor kidney.

Highlights

- Renal transplant is the best mode of RRT for ESRD.
- Structured transplantation network is the need of the hour to ensure unbiased and timely distribution of available organs.
- All stage IV and V CKD patients should be counselled, evaluated, and considered for kidney transplants.
- Transplant recipients should be carefully screened and prepared with the aim to utilize kidney graft to its maximum potential with minimum morbidity.

- Pre-transplant nephrectomy is indicated only if benefit outweighs the risk involved.
- Multidisciplinary team approach is essential to closely monitor the perioperative and follow up care to achieve long term success.

References

1. Hatzinger M, Stastny M, Grützmacher P, Sohn M. The history of kidney transplantation. Urologe A. 2016 Oct;55(10):1353–1359.
2. Timsit MO, Kleinclauss F, Thuret R. History of kidney transplantation surgery. Prog Urol. 2016 Nov;26(15):874–881.
3. Murray JE, Merrill JP, Harrison JH. Kidney transplantation between seven pairs of identical twins. Ann Surg 1958;148:343–359.
4. Shrestha B, Haylor J, Raftery A. Historical perspectives in kidney transplantation: An updated review. Prog Transplant. 2015 Mar;25(1):64–9, 76.
5. United States Renal Data System. Annual data report; 2019. https://www.usrds.org/media/2371/2019-executive-summary.pdf [accessed 17.09.20].
6. Chadban SJ, Ahn C, Axelrod DA, et al. Summary of the kidney disease: Improving global outcomes (KDIGO) clinical practice guideline on the evaluation and management of candidates for kidney transplantation. Transplantation. 2020;104(4):708–714.
7. Dudley C, Harden P. Renal association clinical practice guideline on the assessment of the potential kidney transplant recipient. Nephron Clin Pract. 2011;118 Suppl 1:c209–c224.
8. Barry JM, Conlin JM. Renal transplantation. In: Wein AJ, Kavoussi LR, Novick AC, Partin AW, Peters CA. Campbell-Walsh Urology. 10th edition. Philadelphia: Elsevier; 2012. p1226–p1253.
9. Abramowicz D, Cochat P, Claas FH, et al. European Renal Best Practice Guideline on kidney donor and recipient evaluation and perioperative care. Nephrol Dial Transplant. 2015 Nov;30(11):1790–1797.
10. Malinis M, Boucher HW; AST Infectious Diseases Community of Practice. Screening of donor and candidate prior to solid organ transplantation-Guidelines from the American Society of Transplantation Infectious Diseases Community of Practice. Clin Transplant. 2019 Sep;33(9):e13548.
11. Kidney Disease: Improving Global Outcomes (KDIGO) Transplant Work Group. KDIGO clinical practice guideline for the care of kidney transplant recipients. Am J Transplant. 2009 Nov;9 Suppl 3:S1–S155.
12. European Renal Best Practice Transplantation Guideline Development Group. ERBP Guideline on the Management and Evaluation of the Kidney Donor and Recipient. Nephrol Dial Transplant. 2013 Aug;28 Suppl 2:ii1–ii71.
13. Breda A, Budde K, Figueiredo A, et al. EAU guidelines on Renal Transplantation. 2019. https://uroweb.org/wp-content/uploads/EAU-Guidelines-on-Renal-Transplantation-2019.pdf

14. Lentine KL, Kasiske BL, Levey AS, et al. KDIGO clinical practice guideline on the evaluation and care of living kidney donors. Transplantation. 2017 Aug;101(8S Suppl 1):S1–S109.
15. LaPointe Rudow D, Warburton KM. Selection and postoperative care of the living donor. Med Clin North Am. 2016 May;100(3):599–611.
16. Andrews PA, Burnapp L. British transplantation society/renal association UK guidelines for living donor kidney transplantation 2018: Summary of updated guidance. Transplantation. 2018 Jul;102(7):e307.
17. Wilson CH, Sanni A, Rix DA, Soomro NA. Laparoscopic versus open nephrectomy for live kidney donors. Cochrane Database Syst Rev. 2011 Nov 9;(11):CD006124
18. Serrano OK, Kirchner V, Bangdiwala A, et al. Evolution of living donor nephrectomy at a single center: Long-term outcomes with 4 different techniques in greater than 4000 donors over 50 years. Transplantation. 2016 Jun;100(6):1299–1305.
19. Akoh JA. Kidney donation after cardiac death. World J Nephrol. 2012;1(3):79–91.
20. Goila AK, Pawar M. The diagnosis of brain death. Indian J Crit Care Med. 2009 Jan-Mar;13(1):7–11.
21. Andrews PA, Burnapp L, Manas D; British Transplantation Society. Summary of the British Transplantation Society guidelines for transplantation from donors after deceased circulatory death. Transplantation. 2014;97(3):265–270.
22. Thuong M, Ruiz A, Evrard P, et al. New classification of donation after circulatory death donors definitions and terminology. Transpl Int. 2016 Jul;29(7):749–759.
23. Althaf MM, El Kossi M, Jin JK, Sharma A, Halawa AM. Human leukocyte antigen typing and crossmatch: A comprehensive review. World J Transplant. 2017;7(6):339–348.
24. Bruyère F, Doumerc N. Robotic kidney transplantation: Dream or future? Curr Opin Urol. 2018 Mar;28(2):139–142.
25. Baker RJ, Mark PB, Patel RK, Stevens KK, Palmer N. Renal association clinical practice guideline in post-operative care in the kidney transplant recipient. BMC Nephrol. 2017 Jun 2;18(1):174.
26. Lentine KL, Lam NN, Axelrod D, et al. Perioperative complications after living kidney donation: A national study. Am J Transplant. 2016;16(6):1848–1857.
27. Kidney Disease: Improving Global Outcomes (KDIGO) CKD Work Group. KDIGO 2012 clinical practice guideline for the evaluation and management of chronic kidney disease. Kidney Int Suppl 2013; 3: 1–150.
28. Zorgdrager M, Krikke C, Hofker SH, Leuvenink HG, Pol RA. Multiple renal arteries in kidney transplantation: A systematic review and meta-analysis. Ann Transplant. 2016 Jul 29;21:469–478.
29. Legendre C, Canaud G, Martinez F. Factors influencing long-term outcome after kidney transplantation. Transpl Int. 2014 Jan;27(1):19–27.
30. Hart A, Smith JM, Skeans MA, et al. OPTN/SRTR 2017 Annual Data Report: Kidney. Am J Transplant. 2019 Feb;19 Suppl 2:19–123.

50

Pancreas and intestinal transplantation

Mariya L. Samoylova, Samuel J. Kesseli, Deeplaxmi Borle, Kadiyala V. Ravindra

Introduction

Pancreas transplant increases survival and improves quality of life for patients with insulin-dependent diabetes with or without concurrent end-stage renal disease. It is currently the only long-term treatment that provides durable insulin independence for patients with severe and complicated diabetes, and may prevent or reverse many diabetic complications. Intestinal transplant is a life-saving procedure for patients with intestinal failure (due to short bowel syndrome, functional disorders, fistulae, mucosal defects, etc.) who develop life-threatening complications of total parenteral nutrition (TPN). The small intestine can be transplanted alone or in combination with the liver and other abdominal organs. Only a few centres offer pancreas or intestine transplants due to small case volume, technical complexity of the operations, and complex post-operative management. In the US, 700–900 pancreas transplants and 100–140 intestine and multivisceral transplants are performed per year (Figure 50.1).

The first human pancreas transplant was a simultaneous pancreas-kidney transplant (SPK), performed by Dr Lillehei and Dr Kelly in 1966 at the University of Minnesota.[1] This attempt was unfortunately complicated by a fatal pulmonary embolism. The same group went on to perform the first islet cell transplant in 1974,[2] and living donor segmental pancreas transplant in 1979.[3] Pancreas transplants suffered high rates of rejection until the development of modern immunosuppressants including tacrolimus, cyclosporine, and mycophenolate

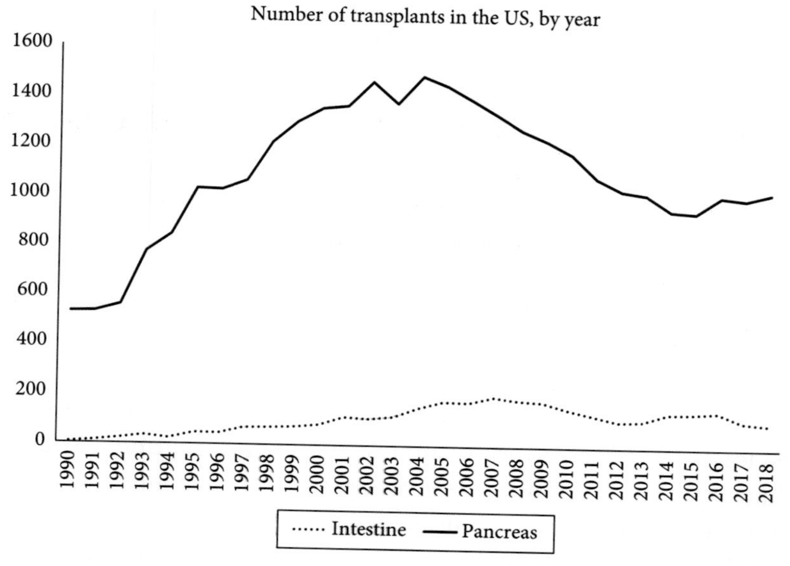

Figure 50.1. Transplants performed in the US since 1990, by year

mofetil in the 1980s.[4] Since then, the surgical technique, immunosuppression, and outcomes have continued to improve; three-year survival following SPK was 94% for transplants performed between 2009 and 2013.[5]

In 1967, Dr Lillehei's group also performed the first human intestinal transplantation.[6] Like early attempts in pancreas transplantation, intestinal transplantation was fraught with complications and high morbidity. In 1989, Starzl et al described two cases with one patient dying 30 minutes postoperatively due to shock, while the other survived six months before eventually succumbing to post-transplant lymphoproliferative disorder.[7] As this considerable morbidity outweighed that of parenteral nutrition at the time, intestinal transplant became a second line treatment for patients with intestinal failure, after they had failed TPN. Currently, the indications for intestinal transplantation remain largely unchanged, however long-term patient survival has dramatically improved, with 77%, 58%, and 47% of recipients alive at one, five, and ten years post-operatively.[8]

Essentials of pancreas transplantation

The pancreas may be transplanted simultaneously with a kidney (SPK), in sequence following a successful kidney transplant (pancreas-after-kidney, PAK), or alone (pancreas transplant alone, PTA). The SPK accounts for approximately 80% of pancreas transplanted in the US. As PAK is an attractive option for patients receiving a living donor kidney, it is offered to candidates with frequent, acute, and life-threatening complications of diabetes. Living donor pancreas grafts have been described, but are not common due to the high rate of donor complications.

Successful pancreas transplants result in insulin independence for up to fifteen years[9] (86% at one year, 54% at ten years for SPK), as well as improvement in glucose metabolism and stabilization or improvement of many microvascular complications of diabetes.[10–14] The recipients of SPK have better long-term survival than deceased donor kidney-alone recipients (72% vs 55% at eight years).[15] Islet cell transplantation (ICT) is an appealing alternative to whole organ transplant as it does not require a major operation for the recipient, but has not yet demonstrated comparable efficacy nor longevity.[16]

Donor selection

The ideal pancreas donor is a young, healthy, heart-beating donor weighing at least 30kg, with a normal BMI. Young children are rarely used due to small vessel calibre and donors with BMI >30 are avoided due to concern for fatty infiltrate increasing the risk of graft pancreatitis. Donors older than forty-five years are avoided due to risk of atherosclerosis and islet depletion. The use of donation after cardiac death (DCD) donors is controversial—while at higher risk of ischemic injury, the DCD pancreas may experience fewer metabolic insults.[17] The HbA1c value in the donor is often used to determine the presence of undiagnosed diabetes, though the use of pancreas from donors with HbA1c in the pre-diabetic range has not been associated with poor outcomes.[18]

Recipient selection

Patients are eligible for the pancreas transplant waiting list in the US if they have diabetes requiring insulin therapy with an absolute endogenous insulin deficiency as demonstrated by C-peptide < 2ng/mL, or diabetes requiring insulin therapy with C-peptide > 2ng/mL and BMI < 28 with significant complications of exogenous insulin administration. Historically, type 1 diabetes was necessary for pancreas transplant candidacy. As the prevalence of type 2 diabetes increased, an increasing proportion of pancreas transplants are now performed for type 2 diabetes. A few pancreas transplants are also performed for chronic pancreatitis and other conditions requiring total pancreatectomy.

Recipients should be < 50 years of age, have BMI < 30, and renal function adequate to sustain immunosuppression with calcineurin inhibitors (for pancreas transplant alone). Centres should pay particular attention to cardiovascular evaluation, as cardiovascular disease remains the most common cause of death following pancreas transplant. Candidates also undergo non-contrast computed tomography of the abdomen and pelvis for surgical planning, as well as the standard pre-transplant psychosocial evaluation.

Donor and recipient operations

Procurement of the pancreas graft is technically challenging due to delicate tissues and variable arterial anatomy. The liver graft is procured first, followed by the pancreas. The pancreas may also be retrieved together with the spleen and liver to prevent injury during handling, and separated on the back table. The superior mesenteric artery (SMA) and celiac artery are taken together on an aortic patch. If the right hepatic artery arises close to the SMA origin, the SMA is divided beyond the taken off the right hepatic artery. A cuff of duodenum and jejunum is taken with the pancreatic head. Arterial reconstruction is typically performed with donor iliac artery bifurcation, used as a Y-graft to provide a single inflow to the splenic artery and SMA (Figure 50.2).

Cold ischemic time is ideally kept < 12 hours; perfusion technology has not yet demonstrated a benefit.

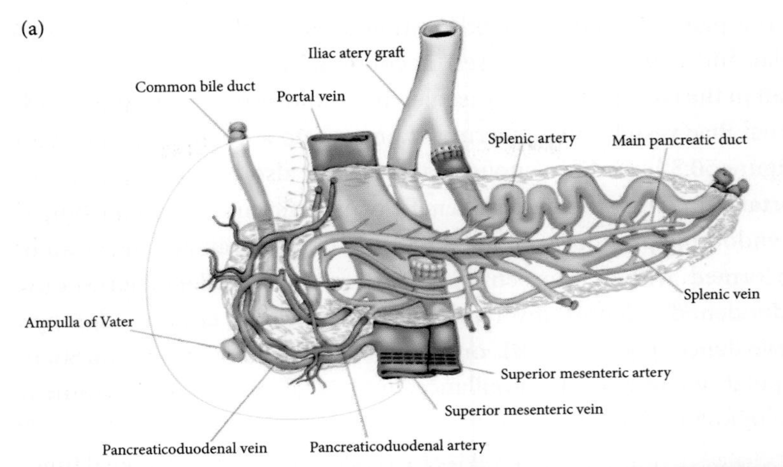

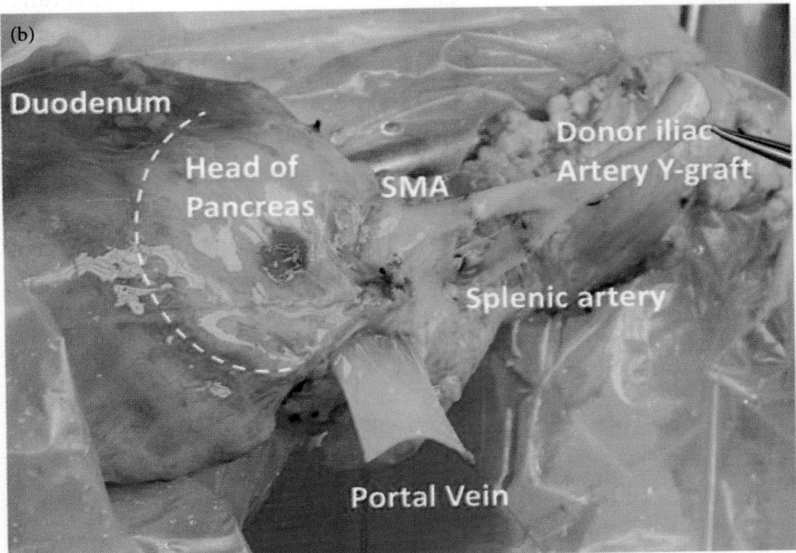

Figure 50.2. (A) Diagram of the pancreas allograft with iliac artery Y-graft. (B) Back table preparation of the pancreas allograft with iliac artery Y-graft. (*From* Samoylova M. et al. Pancreas transplantation: indication, techniques, and outcomes. Surg Clin North Am. 2019 Feb;99(1):87–101, with permission)

The pancreas graft implant location varies with the choice of vascular and enteric anastomoses. A common approach is to place the graft in the right pelvis with vascular anastomosis to the common or external iliac vessels, and exocrine drainage into a duodenojejunostomy (Figure 50.3A, C, D). Venous drainage may also be connected to the portal vein, with theoretical benefit of hepatic first-pass metabolism of endocrine products (Figure 50.3B). Exocrine drainage may also be performed with a roux-en-Y or side-to-side duodenojejunostomy, a duodenoduodenostomy (with the advantage of easier endoscopic surveillance, Figure 50.3B), or to the bladder. The latter was initially popular due to ease of surveillance, but has fallen out of favour due to urologic complications.

Immunosuppression

Higher levels of immunosuppression are used for pancreas transplants than for kidney transplants alone, due to high rates of rejection and greater difficulty in diagnosis. Antithymocyte globulin (ATG) induction has demonstrated advantage for graft and patient survival[(19)]; maintenance regimens are typically composed of a calcineurin inhibitor, mycophenolate, and a low-dose corticosteroid.

Complications

Early graft failure is frequently due to graft thrombosis, which is likely due to technical error or poor graft quality. Graft thrombosis accounts for 31% of graft losses and requires urgent pancreatectomy. Anastomotic leak is rare but challenging to treat due to contamination with pancreatic enzymes. Graft rejection occurs at a rate of 15–21% at one year and 27–30% at five years, and accounts for 36% of graft losses. Unfortunately, no biomarker is sensitive nor specific for pancreas graft rejection, biopsy is risky and frequently non-diagnostic, and there is only a 60% concordance with kidney graft rejection in SPK.[(20)] Thus, presumed rejection is treated aggressively with high-dose corticosteroids ± thymoglobulin.

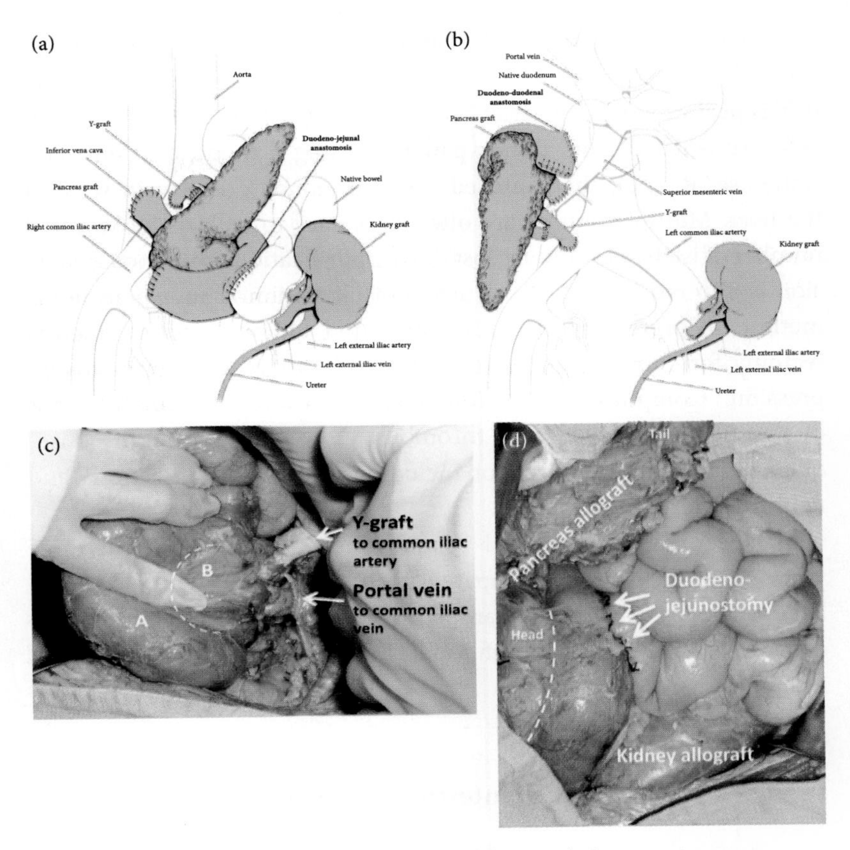

Figure 50.3. Diagram of pancreas allograft *in situ*: (A) systemic venous drainage via inferior vena cava, enteric exocrine drainage via duodeno-jejunostomy. Kidney allograft in left iliac fossa. (B) portal venous drainage via superior mesenteric vein, enteric exocrine drainage via duodeno-duodenostomy
Kidney allograft in left iliac fossa. (C) vascular anastomosis of pancreas graft to right common iliac artery and vein, using donor iliac artery Y-graft for arterial reconstruction. (a) allograft duodenum (b) allograft pancreatic head. (D) simultaneous pancreas and kidney allografts *in situ*; enteric exocrine drainage via duodeno-jejunostomy. (*From* Samoylova ML, Borle D, Ravindra KV. Pancreas transplantation: indication, techniques, and outcomes. Surg Clin North Am. 2019 Feb;99(1):87–101, with permission)

Islet cell transplantation

ICT is performed using variations of the Edmonton protocol[21]—islet cells are isolated from donor pancreas using a mixture of enzymes (Liberase, Roche), then infused into the donor portal vein to seed the liver. Multiple donors are often necessary to collect the required number of islets, as many are lost during purification; immunosuppression is also required. Islet cell autotransplantation is an experimental method of preserving pancreatic function following total pancreatectomy for chronic pancreatitis, and does not require immunosuppression. Complications of ICT include procedural complications of bleeding and portal vein thrombus, as well as long-term consequences of immunosuppression including neutropenia, infections, and nephrotoxicity.[22]

The ICT has demonstrated insulin independence of 44% at three years post-transplant,[16] compared to 69–85% at three years for isolated whole-organ pancreas transplant.[23] There is not yet sufficient evidence to confirm that the benefits of ICT outweigh the risks of long-term immunosuppression.

Essentials of intestine transplantation

The isolated small bowel graft is the most common, accounting for approximately half of the intestinal transplant grafts worldwide.[8] This graft consists of the donor jejunum and ileum supplied by the SMA and superior mesenteric vein (SMV). A combined liver-intestine graft may be used in patients with intestinal failure (IF) and IF-associated liver disease (IFALD); IFALD develops in approximately 50% of paediatric patients on TPN for >3 months and in 15–40% of adults.[9] Multivisceral transplantation with additional organs (such as the colon, pancreas, or stomach) may be performed for tumours involving the liver hilum, as well as for porto-mesenteric thrombosis and other intra-abdominal catastrophes. The reported survival from an international registry of intestinal transplants performed since 2000 was 77% at one year, 58% at five years, and 41% at ten years. Two-thirds of recipients had become independent of parenteral nutrition at six months post-transplant.[8] Recent advances in technique, donor-recipient matching, and immunosuppression have dramatically improved outcomes, with a recent series reporting 100% five-year patient survival and 85% graft survival in twenty-five patients transplanted since 2010.[24]

Donor selection

Heart-beating AB0-matched donors with normal intestines and requiring minimal pressor support are used as donors. The AB0 matching is necessary to avoid graft-versus-host disease, and crossmatch or virtual crossmatch[25] is performed to reduce rejection risk. Donor size is carefully considered as significant loss of abdominal domain is common in recipients who have undergone extensive intestinal resection. Cytomegalovirus (CMV) or Ebstein-Barr Virus (EBV) positive donors for seronegative recipients are occasionally avoided to decrease risk of severe CMV graft enteritis and post-transplantation lymphoproliferative disorder (PTLD), respectively.[26,27] The intestine is exquisitely sensitive to ischemia: a cold ischemia time of <8 hours is recommended, which limits the geographic range of recipient-donor pairs.

Recipient selection

Patients with intestinal failure who suffer life-threatening complications of parenteral nutrition, such as recurrent catheter-associated bloodstream infections, liver disease, loss of venous access, or frequent episodes of severe dehydration, are candidates for intestine transplants. Short gut syndrome is the most common indication for intestinal transplant. In children, this is most commonly due to gastroschisis, volvulus, and necrotizing enterocolitis; in adults, ischemia, Crohn's disease, volvulus, and trauma are more common.[16] In cases of short gut syndrome, autologous intestinal reconstruction techniques such as the serial transverse enteroplasty (STEP) and longitudinal intestinal lengthening and tapering (LILT) procedures[28,29] may be attempted prior to intestine transplant. After multidisciplinary evaluation at the transplant centre, the patient joins the transplant waiting list.

Donor and recipient operations

Initially, a total or partial (depending on the intended graft) colectomy is performed to facilitate removal of the intestinal graft. The root of the mesentery is mobilized until the graft is attached only by the SMA/SMV trunk, taking care to avoid injury to the inferior pancreatic vessels, if pancreas graft is also being procured. In contrast to procurement of liver without intestine or pancreas grafts, the use of portal venous system cold infusion is not recommended. The carotid artery may be harvested for use as arterial conduit. The spleen is typically removed on the back table.

The SMA and SMV are anastomosed to the infrarenal aorta and vena cava, and the proximal jejunum anastomosed to recipient jejunum. The SMV may be anastomosed to the portal system. The distal end of bowel may be anastomosed to the recipient colon and/or brought up as an ileostomy to allow for biopsies. Some surgeons prefer to include a segment of donor colon to preserve a functional ileocecal valve, which improves patient quality of life and continence.[30]

For multivisceral graft procurement, the organs are typically taken en bloc with a segment of thoracic and abdominal aorta including the celiac axis and the SMA. This preserves continuity of the extrahepatic biliary system (Figure 50.4A, D).

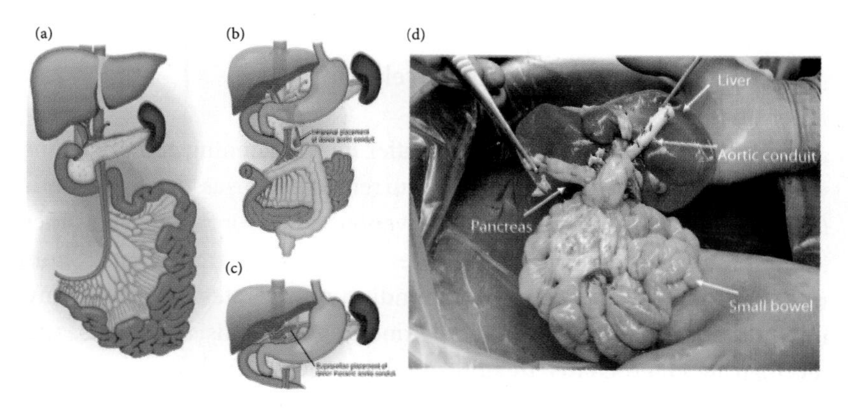

Figure 50.4. The combined liver-intestinal graft includes the pancreaticoduodenal complex with or without the spleen (A). The donor aorta may be anastomosed below the renal arteries (B) or to supraceliac aorta (C). (D) Back-table preparation of the multivisceral graft containing liver, pancreas, and small bowel from a paediatric donor. (*From* Sudan D. The current state of intestine transplantation: indications, techniques, outcomes and challenges. Am J Transplant 2014;14(9):1976–84; with permission)

The recipient operation begins with excision of the native liver, remnant small bowel, and additional abdominal organs as required by the recipient's pathology. The donor inferior vena cava (IVC) may be used to replace a segment of the recipient IVC, or in a piggyback technique with a single suprahepatic caval anastomosis. The donor aorta is anastomosed to the recipient aorta either below the renal arteries (Figure 50.4B) or above the celiac axis (Figure 50.4C). When the recipient foregut is retained (stomach, pancreas, spleen, duodenum), a portocaval or splenorenal shunt is performed to allow venous drainage.

The intestine and liver may also be taken separately, to allow the pancreas graft to be allocated to a different recipient. In this case, it is necessary to perform biliary reconstruction with a Roux-en-Y limb. While more technically complex, this procedure has the advantage of allowing for explantation of a failed intestine allograft without disrupting the liver allograft.

Immunosuppression

Up to 75% of intestine transplant recipients experience rejection, thought to be a consequence of bacterial colonization, a large amount of mucosal-associated lymphoid tissue, and high cell turnover.[31] Thus, these patients receive higher doses of immunosuppression than most other solid organ recipients. This begins with donor pre-treatment using anti-thymocyte globulin (ATG), followed by recipient leukodepletion with polyclonal antibody (ATG) or monoclonal antibody induction (alemtuzumab or basiliximab), and maintenance with a calcineurin inhibitor (tacrolimus or sirolimus), or mycophenolate mofetil and steroid. While there exists data to support the use of lymphocyte depletion induction therapy[8]; there is no consensus on the optimal maintenance regimen as yet.

Complications

Patients are frequently readmitted to the hospital during their early post-operative course for treatment of infection, rejection, diarrhoea, or dehydration. Sepsis is the most common cause of graft loss, followed by rejection and cardiovascular events. Intestinal allograft recipients are at higher risk of infections than other solid organ recipients. The most common technical complications are bowel anastomotic leak, bowel perforations, and wound complications. Vascular complications are rare, likely due to large vessel calibre, but are devastating when they occur. Biliary complications are rare if the extrahepatic biliary system is transplanted intact, though ischemic intrahepatic biliary strictures may occur. Graft-versus-host-disease occurs in 5–10% of patients due to mature donor lymphocytes present in the graft and carries a poor prognosis.[32] Post-transplant lymphoproliferative disorder (PTLD) is also more common than in other solid organ transplants, with an incidence of 10–20% vs 1% in kidney, 2–5% in liver, and 5–10% in lung-heart recipients.[33]

Rejection

Rejection occurs in up to 70% of intestinal graft recipients, though the percentage is now decreasing with improved donor-recipient matching and immunosuppression strategies.[34] Rejection presents with nonspecific signs and symptoms including fever, abdominal pain, and increased stool output. Diagnosis is challenging due to lack of distinctive features and biomarkers. Suspected rejection is treated aggressively with pulse-dose steroids and increased maintenance immunosuppression. Most centres will perform routine endoscopy and biopsy of the small bowel in the first week post-transplant, and continue weekly for 1–3 months. Further biopsies are generally done to investigate clinical symptoms such as diarrhoea.

Traditionally, intestinal allograft rejection has been regarded as a T-cell-mediated disease process. A growing body of evidence, however, suggests that humoral immunity plays an important role in intestinal graft acute and chronic rejection. Intestinal transplant recipients tend to be more sensitized than other solid organ recipients, most likely due to multiple prior operations, blood transfusions, and recurrent line infections that are common in their disease course. Antibodies directed against donor human leukocyte antigen (HLA), called donor-specific antibodies

(DSAs), may be present at the time of transplant (11–30%) or develop *de novo* following transplantation (18–25%). The presence of DSAs has been associated with chronic rejection and graft loss in solid organ transplantation including kidney, heart, lung, and liver. The DSAs have recently also been implicated in graft rejection and graft failure.[31] Several strategies have been proposed for preoperative desensitization and for treatment of post-operative DSA and refractory rejection, including high-dose steroids, intravenous immunoglobulin (IVIg), plasmapheresis, ATG, rituximab,[35,36] as well as novel uses of other anti-leukocyte antibodies. There is not yet consensus for optimal screening nor for management of pre- and post-operative DSA.

Conclusion

Though infrequent, pancreas and intestinal transplantation are lifesaving procedures. Pancreas transplantation offers the only durable cure for insulin-dependent diabetes and improves survival. Complicated type I and type II diabetes mellitus remain the most common indications for intestinal transplant. Careful donor and recipient selection are paramount for good outcomes. The pancreas may be transplanted alone or with a kidney. Several technical variations exist for the recipient operation. Rejection is challenging to diagnose and should be treated aggressively. Patient survival is excellent, and long-term insulin independence can be expected in the majority of recipients.

Intestinal transplant may be the only cure for patients with intestinal failure who have suffered life-threatening complications of parenteral nutrition. The intestine may be transplanted alone or together with the liver and other abdominal organs. The recipient operation is frequently complex due to surgical history and portal hypertension. The post-operative course is frequently complicated by rejection, which can be challenging to treat. Due to the low numbers of intestinal transplants performed worldwide, many aspects of perioperative care are not yet evidence-based. Recent series, however, demonstrate excellent patient and graft survival, and most patients can expect to achieve nutritional independence.

Highlights

- Pancreas transplant treats insulin-dependent diabetes, often together with kidney transplant for end stage renal disease.
- Benefits of pancreas transplant include increased survival, improved quality of life, and improvement or stabilization of diabetic microvascular complications.
- Intestinal transplant treats intestinal failure with life-threatening complications of parenteral nutrition.
- The intestine may be transplanted alone or in combination with the liver and other organs.
- Both organs are highly immunogenic; rejection is common and difficult to diagnose and treat.
- Recent intestinal transplant experience demonstrates excellent patient and graft survival, with high rates of nutritional independence.

References

1. Kelly WD, Lillehei RC, Merkel FK, Idezuki Y, Goetz FC. Allotransplantation of the pancreas and duodenum along with the kidney in diabetic nephropathy. Surgery. 1967 Jun;61(6):827–837.
2. Sutherland DE, Matas AJ, Najarian JS. Pancreatic islet cell transplantation. Surg Clin North Am. 1978 Apr;58(2):365–382.
3. Sutherland DE, Gruessner R, Dunn D, Moudry-Munns K, Gruessner A, Najarian JS. Pancreas transplants from living-related donors. Transplant Proc. 1994 Apr;26(2):443–445.
4. Sutherland DE, Gruessner RW, Dunn DL, Matas AJ, Humar A, Kandaswamy R, et al. Lessons learned from more than 1,000 pancreas transplants at a single institution. Ann Surg. 2001 Apr;233(4):463–501.
5. Stratta R. J., Gruessner A. C., Odorico J. S., Fridell J. A., Gruessner R. W. G. Pancreas transplantation: An alarming crisis in confidence. Am J Transplant. 2016 Aug 30;16(9):2556–2562.
6. Lillehei RC, Idezuki Y, Feemster JA, Dietzman RH, Kelly WD, Merkel FK, et al. Transplantation of stomach, intestine, and pancreas: Experimental and clinical observations. Surgery. 1967 Oct;62(4):721–741.
7. Starzl TE, Rowe MI, Todo S, Jaffe R, Tzakis A, Hoffman AL, et al. Transplantation of multiple abdominal viscera. JAMA. 1989 Mar 10;261(10):1449–1457.
8. Grant D, Abu-Elmagd K, Mazariegos G, Vianna R, Langnas A, Mangus R, et al. Intestinal transplant registry report: Global activity and trends. Am J Transplant Off J Am Soc Transplant Am Soc Transpl Surg. 2015 Jan;15(1):210–219.

9. Robertson RP, Sutherland DE, Lanz KJ. Normoglycemia and preserved insulin secretory reserve in diabetic patients 10-18 years after pancreas transplantation. Diabetes. 1999 Sep;48(9):1737–1740.
10. Aridge D, Reese J, Niehoff M, Carney K, Lindsey L, Chun HS, et al. Effect of successful renal and segmental pancreatic transplantation on peripheral and autonomic neuropathy. Transplant Proc. 1991 Feb;23(1 Pt 2):1670–1671.
11. Gaber AO, Cardoso S, Pearson S, Abell T, Gaber L, Hathaway D, et al. Improvement in autonomic function following combined pancreas-kidney transplantation. Transplant Proc. 1991 Feb;23(1 Pt 2):1660–1662.
12. Navarro X, Sutherland DE, Kennedy WR. Long-term effects of pancreatic transplantation on diabetic neuropathy. Ann Neurol. 1997 Nov;42(5):727–736.
13. Secchi A, Martinenghi S, Galardi G, Comi G, Canal N, Pozza G. Effects of pancreatic transplantation on diabetic polyneuropathy. Transplant Proc. 1991 Feb;23(1 Pt 2):1658–1659.
14. Pearce IA, Ilango B, Sells RA, Wong D. Stabilisation of diabetic retinopathy following simultaneous pancreas and kidney transplant. Br J Ophthalmol. 2000 Jul;84(7):736–740.
15. Reddy KS, Stablein D, Taranto S, Stratta RJ, Johnston TD, Waid TH, et al. Long-term survival following simultaneous kidney-pancreas transplantation versus kidney transplantation alone in patients with type 1 diabetes mellitus and renal failure. Am J Kidney Dis Off J Natl Kidney Found. 2003 Feb;41(2):464–470.
16. Barton FB, Rickels MR, Alejandro R, Hering BJ, Wease S, Naziruddin B, et al. Improvement in outcomes of clinical islet transplantation: 1999–2010. Diabetes Care. 2012 Jul 1;35(7):1436–1445.
17. Ridgway D, Manas D, Shaw J, White S. Preservation of the donor pancreas for whole pancreas and islet transplantation. Clin Transplant. 2010 Feb;24(1):1–19.
18. Arpali E, Scalea JR, Redfield RR, Berg L, Kaufman DB, Sollinger HW, et al. The importance and utility of hemoglobin A1c levels in the assessment of donor pancreas allografts. Transplantation. 2017;101(10):2508–2519.
19. Burke GW, Kaufman DB, Millis JM, Gaber AO, Johnson CP, Sutherland DER, et al. Prospective, randomized trial of the effect of antibody induction in simultaneous pancreas and kidney transplantation: Three-year results. Transplantation. 2004 Apr 27;77(8):1269–1275.
20. Shapiro R, Jordan ML, Scantlebury VP, Vivas CA, Jain A, McCauley J, et al. Renal allograft rejection with normal renal function in simultaneous kidney/pancreas recipients: does dissynchronous rejection really exist? Transplantation. 2000 Feb 15;69(3):440–441.
21. Shapiro AMJ, Ricordi C, Hering BJ, Auchincloss H, Lindblad R, Robertson RP, et al. International trial of the edmonton protocol for islet transplantation. N Engl J Med. 2006 Sep 28;355(13):1318–1330.
22. Hirshberg B, Rother KI, Digon BJ, Lee J, Gaglia JL, Hines K, et al. Benefits and risks of solitary islet transplantation for type 1 diabetes using steroid-sparing immunosuppression: The National Institutes of Health experience. Diabetes Care. 2003 Dec 1;26(12):3288–3295.
23. Gruessner RWG, Gruessner AC. Pancreas transplant alone: A procedure coming of age. Diabetes Care. 2013 Aug;36(8):2440–2447.

24. Beduschi T, Garcia J, Farag A, Selvaggi G, Tekin A, Fan J, et al. Breaking the 5 year mark with 100% survival for intestinal transplant—time to become protagonist in the management of intestinal failure?: Transplantation. 2017 Jun;101:S136.
25. Cheng E, DuBray B, Farmer D. The impact of antibodies and virtual cross-matching on intestinal transplant outcomes. Curr Opin Organ Transplant. 2017 Apr 1;22(2):149–154.
26. Ming YC. Post transplant lymphoproliferative disorders and intestinal transplant in children—single center experience: Transplantation. 2017 Jun;101:S36.
27. Nagai S, Mangus RS, Anderson E, Ekser B, Kubal CA, Fridell JA, et al. Cytomegalovirus infection after intestinal/multivisceral transplantation: A single-center experience with 210 cases. Transplantation. 2016 Feb;100(2):451–460.
28. Bianchi A. Intestinal loop lengthening—a technique for increasing small intestinal length. J Pediatr Surg. 1980 Apr;15(2):145–151.
29. Kim HB, Fauza D, Garza J, Oh J-T, Nurko S, Jaksic T. Serial transverse enteroplasty (STEP): A novel bowel lengthening procedure. J Pediatr Surg. 2003 Mar;38(3):425–429.
30. Matsumoto CS, Kaufman SS, Fishbein TM. Inclusion of the colon in intestinal transplantation. Curr Opin Organ Transplant. 2011 Jun;16(3):312–315.
31. Abu-Elmagd KM, Wu G, Costa G, Lunz J, Martin L, Koritsky DA, et al. Preformed and de novo donor specific antibodies in visceral transplantation: Long-term outcome with special reference to the liver. Am J Transplant. 2012;12(11):3047–3060.
32. Wu G, Selvaggi G, Nishida S, Moon J, Island E, Ruiz P, et al. Graft-versus-host disease after intestinal and multivisceral transplantation. Transplantation. 2011 Jan 27;91(2):219–224.
33. Allen UD, Preiksaitis JK, AST Infectious Diseases Community of Practice. Epstein-Barr virus and posttransplant lymphoproliferative disorder in solid organ transplantation. Am J Transplant Off J Am Soc Transplant Am Soc Transpl Surg. 2013 Mar;13 Suppl 4:107–120.
34. Abu-Elmagd KM, Costa G, Bond GJ, Wu T, Murase N, Zeevi A, et al. Evolution of the immunosuppressive strategies for the intestinal and multivisceral recipients with special reference to allograft immunity and achievement of partial tolerance. Transpl Int Off J Eur Soc Organ Transplant. 2009 Jan;22(1):96–109.
35. Kubal C, Mangus R, Saxena R, Lobashevsky A, Higgins N, Fridell J, et al. Prospective monitoring of donor-specific anti-HLA antibodies after intestine/multivisceral transplantation: Significance of de novo antibodies. Transplantation. 2015 Aug;99(8):e49–e56.
36. Garcia-Roca R, Tzvetanov IG, Jeon H, Hetterman E, Oberholzer J, Benedetti E. Successful living donor intestinal transplantation in cross-match positive recipients: Initial experience. World J Gastrointest Surg. 2016 Jan;8(1):101–105.

51

Ocular tissues: Recovery and processing issues

Alessandra Galeone, Stefano Ferrari,
Vincenzo Sarnicola, Diego Ponzin

Introduction

Corneal transplantation is the oldest and most common type of allogenic transplantation in the world.[1] In the US alone, more than 40,000 keratoplasties are performed each year[2] and other ocular tissues are used in a number of surgical procedures. Successful transplants depend on the availability of safe tissues, which are recovered, examined, stored, and processed by eye banks within the highest quality standards.

Ocular tissues for donation

The ocular tissues that can be transplanted and used in various other surgical procedures include the cornea, sclera, conjunctiva, and limbus.

Cornea

The cornea is a transparent and avascular tissue, measuring 11–12 mm horizontally and 10–11 mm vertically. It is approximately 550 μm thick and consists of six layers: epithelium, Bowman's layer, stroma, a pre-Descemet's (Dua's) layer, Descemet's membrane, and endothelium.[3] The corneal epithelium is a stable and impermeable barrier that includes five to seven cell layers. The deepest represents the mitotically active compartment which derives from adult stem cells located at the corneal limbus. The outermost stroma, the Bowman's layer, borders the epithelial basal membrane, and is an acellular zone, 10–15 μm thick. The lamellar stroma is composed of flattened bundles of parallel collagen fibrils of equal diameters, the regular arrangement of which is essential for corneal transparency. The pre-Descemet's (Dua's) layer is the innermost part of the stroma, in contact with the Descemet's membrane, the basal membrane of the corneal endothelium. The latter is a regular mosaic of hexagonal cells bordering the aqueous humour. The endothelium has virtually no mitotic activity and the cell number decreases with age. Endothelial density can be as high as 7.000 cell/mm^2 at birth, but decreases to approximately 3.000 cell/mm^2 in adolescence. A mean decrease of 0.5% per year is observed during adulthood, with large individual differences. The donor corneas are used in keratoplasty to replace a diseased cornea, which has irreversibly lost its transparency and physiologic curvature.

Sclera

The sclera is a fibrous, viscoelastic connective tissue, which contains the insertions of extraocular muscles.[(4)]

The donor sclera is used as allograft for a variety of procedures; most commonly to enclose orbital implants for reconstruction of anophthalmic cavities, reconstruction of eyelids, correction of cicatricial entropion, covering tubes in glaucoma surgery, and repairing scleral thinning. Any abnormalities such as discoloration, thinning or atypical vessels preclude the utilization of the tissue.

Conjunctiva and limbus

The conjunctiva is the thin, transparent tissue that covers the outer surface of the eye.[(5)] The bulbar conjunctiva covers the eyeball, the forniceal can be found in the superior and inferior fornices and the palpebral or tarsal conjunctiva covers the inner eyelid.

The limbus is an anatomical and functional area, located circumferentially along the periphery of the cornea. It acts as a barrier that prevents migration of conjunctival epithelial cells onto the transparent stroma. Epithelial stem cells, responsible for the homeostasis and wound repair of the corneal epithelium, are located at the limbus.[6] Keratolimbal allografts may be applied in cases of bilateral ocular surface diseases due to stem cell deficiency.

The establishment of the eye banks

Before the advent of corneal storage, corneal transplantation was performed using tissues from eyes enucleated for medical reasons from living donors. The first successful corneal transplant was done in 1905 by Eduard Zirm.[7] The living donor was an 11-year-old, who had lost one eye after a penetrating injury.[8] Zirm performed a bilateral penetrating keratoplasty using two grafts from the boy's single cornea. Although the graft in the right eye failed, the other remained clear, becoming the first successful corneal transplant. In the 1930s, Ramon Castroviejo developed instruments for keratoplasty.[9] The idea of using corneas from cadavers was initiated by Vladimir Filatov in 1935.[10] In 1974, the introduction of the McCarey-Kaufmann medium extended the storage time of donor corneas,[11] and corneal transplantation became a scheduled, rather than an emergency procedure.

During the same period, the organ culture technique was invented in the USA, mostly adopted in Europe,[12] and subsequently enhanced with methods for the evaluation of the corneal endothelium.

In 1944, Townley Paton established the first eye bank in New York[13,14] and nowadays, eye banks worldwide are responsible for graft procurement, evaluation, processing, and distribution of ocular tissues.

Ocular tissue retrieval—preliminary steps

Tissue donation depends on the development of a strong working relationship between a tissue bank and a hospital or other donor referral agency.

In order to delay the deterioration of the eyes prior to recovery, a physiologic solution is usually applied onto the surface of the cornea, thus moistening the corneal tissue. The donor's eyelids should be kept closed until retrieval, in order to reduce the risk of exposing the corneal epithelium to the air. Elevating the donor's head prevents pooling of blood in the head and decreases the incidence of bleeding and swelling in the periocular area following enucleation.

The enucleation or *in situ* excision should be performed as soon as possible after death, though a well-defined maximum time limit is not yet decided. A protracted *post mortem* interval induces eye dehydration and ocular hypotension, resulting in stromal and Descemet's folds, loss of transparency and further mortality. Many eye banks do not recover the ocular tissues after 24 hours of asystolia.

A physical inspection of the donor is aimed at evaluating potential signs of infectious diseases or high-risk behaviour such as intravenous drug use.

Before the recovery, the periorbital and orbital tissues, and the anterior segment of the eye are examined with the aid of a penlight for findings such as purulent material, corneal abnormalities, and intraocular surgery.

Ocular tissue recovery

The donor's head must be kept elevated during the retrieval, to prevent bleeding. A thorough irrigation of the cornea and conjunctival sac with sterile phosphate-buffered saline (PBS), followed by disinfection with iodine solution within 2 minutes after PBS are performed to prevent corneal toxicity. Subsequently, the eyelids and surrounding orbital area should be cleaned and disinfected. Finally, the donor is draped to create a sterile field at the operative site.

The upper eyelid of the donor's right eye is opened with a sterile gauze and the lid-speculum is inserted. All the operation must proceed without touching the corneal surface. The conjunctiva is grasped with the forceps, near the lateral edge of the cornea at the limbus. By using the microsurgery scissors, a continuing 360° cut is placed. Scissors are inserted under the conjunctiva, and a blunt dissection is performed by opening the blades to separate any adhesions.

In situ corneal sclera rim excision
Without perforating the choroid, a scleral incision is performed using a scalpel, approximately 4 mm from the limbus. The incision is extended 360°, avoiding the perforation of the underlying uvea. The tips of the scissor blades must not enter the anterior chamber and the corneas' normal curvature must be maintained.

The recovery is completed using one pair of small forceps to hold the scleral rim, and a second set of forceps, to push the ciliary body-choroid downward and away from the corneo-scleral button. The remaining adhesions can be gently separated, avoiding distortion of the cornea shape. The posterior chamber of the donor eye must be examined to check the presence of the natural crystalline lens.

Enucleation
Using a muscle hook, the rectus muscles are exposed and severed where they meet the sclera. The lateral rectus must be severed last, leaving a 5 mm stump on the sclera. The stump is grasped with a haemostat and the globe is lifted upwards with the aid of enucleation scissors. The optic nerve is identified and severed with the enucleation scissors, leaving a 5–10 mm stump. The globe is then lifted from the socket with the haemostat clamped to the lateral rectus muscle, while cutting away any remaining connective tissue. The globe is wrapped in sterile gauze with the cornea facing up and a small amount of PBS is poured over the cornea. The globe is then placed in an eye jar, and can be kept in position by inserting sterile, ophthalmologic tampons between the gauze and the sides of the jar.

Reconstruction
After enucleation, a moistened piece of gauze, rolled into a ball of approximate dimensions of the globe, can be placed in the socket and covered with a plastic eye cap or a plastic prosthesis. A plastic eye cap can be placed between the remains of the conjunctiva and the globe, covering part of the eye cap with the remains of the conjunctiva.

The eyelids are closed and gently manipulated to restore the donor's appearance. The donor's head should be left elevated, verifying the absence of bleeding. If the eyelids do not remain closed, they can be stitched on the posterior margins. It is recommended to ask the mortuary staff to check the conditions of the donor later. The process is illustrated in Figure 51.1.

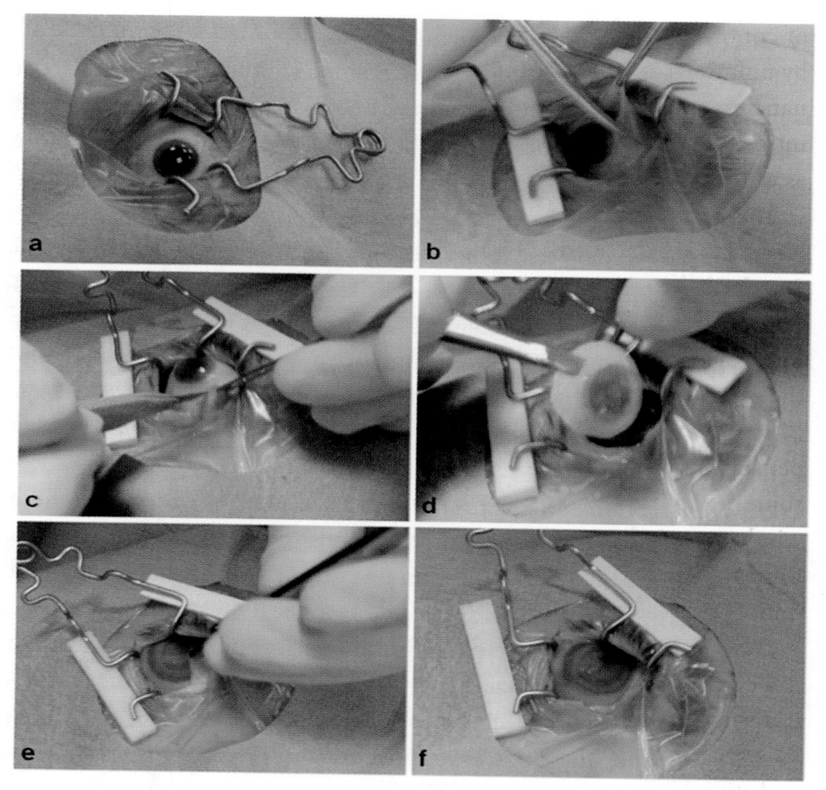

Figure 51.1. In situ corneo-scleral rim excision and donor reconstruction. (a) The globe is exposed using eye speculum to keep the eye lashes out of the field, (b) and (c) conjunctival remnants are cut, (d) the scleral incision is performed with a scalpel blade and extended to 360°, (e) the corneo-scleral rim is excised, (f) a plastic cap is placed back and the conjunctival remains are used for overall covering of the eye

After recovery, the tissue is placed in a storage medium. Post mortem blood for serological testing can be obtained directly after heart puncture or through accessible blood vessels.

Screening of donors

The screening of donors is aimed at minimizing the risk of donor-to-host transmission of systemic and local diseases. There is an established set of contraindications to ensure safety of corneal transplantation—death by unknown cause, local and/or systemic infections, hematologic malignancies, prion diseases, corneal disease, and intrinsic eye diseases. Prior intraocular or anterior segment surgery may not exclude from donation, as well as metastatic neoplasia.

The European Eye Bank Association (EEBA) and the Eye Bank Association of America (EBAA) have established Minimum Medical Standards[15] and Medical Standards,[16] respectively, available online. In Europe, the contraindication has been listed in the Directive 2004/23/EC that, together with Directive 2006/17/EC and Directive 2006/86/EC, set the standards for safety and quality of tissue transplantation.

The serological screening for HBV, HCV, HIV, and syphilis must be performed for every donor. Besides the search for antibodies of antigens, some nations require the nucleic acid (NAT) testing. Because of the window period (time between the infection and when a positive antibody/antigen can be revealed), the behaviours that may have put the donors at risk, such as intravenous drug use, must be evaluated.

Donor who died with neurological symptoms, or degenerative neurological conditions, must be excluded from donation. Despite low incidence, transmissible spongiform encephalopathies, such as Creutzfeldt-Jakob disease, have been transmitted via corneal transplantation.[17,18]

Active lymphoproliferative disorders including leukaemias, lymphomas, and lymphosarcomas pose a greatest risk of transfer from donor to host, because they may invade the cornea.

Transmission of local corneal disorders, a previously considered risk factor for corneal transplantation, is now minimized by the selective use of distinguished layers in corneal transplantation.

Tissue processing

Eye bank manipulations are carried out in sterility using a laminar flow cabinet, placed in a defined and monitored environment. For decontamination purposes, the eyes are rinsed with sterile PBS, then immersed in sterile polyvinylpyrrolidone-iodine for 2 minutes, sodium thiosulfate in PBS for 1 minute and rinsed again in PBS, where they are left until cornea excision. This procedure reduces the percentage of contaminated eyes.

Tissue evaluation

The corneas must be examined for the presence of biological characteristics that are required to ensure a good clinical outcome.[19,20] The morphological and functional status of the endothelium is the most important indicator of donor cornea quality. Corneas from eligible donors with local eye disease affecting the corneal endothelium, or previous ocular surgery that does not compromise the corneal stroma, can be used for lamellar (anterior, posterior) or patch grafts.

As shown in Figure 51.2, a cornea suitable for transplantation is required to display some essential biological characteristics:

- a non-interrupted epithelial layer;
- a stroma free of opacities in the optic centre and sufficient clear zone in case of an arcus lipoids;
- absence of folds in the stroma and the Descemet's membrane;
- a viable (absence of cell degenerations) and regular (absence of dystrophies, no substantial pleomorphism or polymegathism) endothelium, with a cell density above 2000 cells/mm^2.

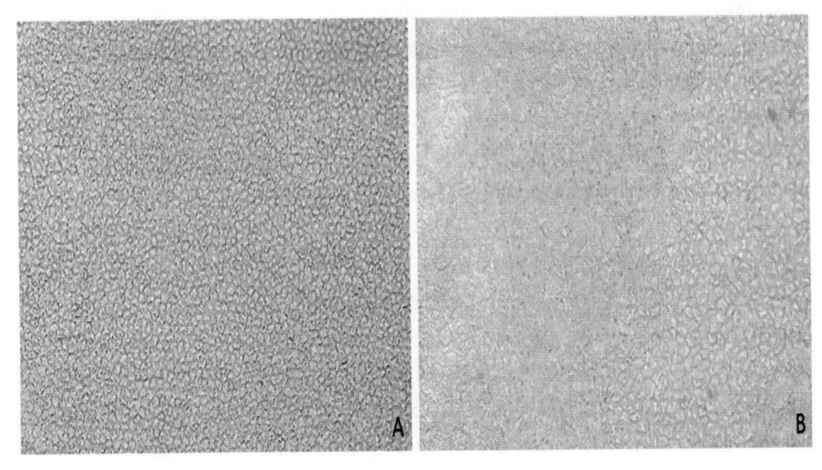

Figure 51.2. Human corneal endothelium. (a) Regular pattern, without any trypan blue positive cells and (b) damaged endothelium with large area of disorganized cells and presence of trypan blue positive cells

Storage of corneas

The aim of corneal storage is the maintenance of endothelial viability from the time of corneal excision to transplantation. Currently there are two storage practices for the cornea: the hypothermic storage at 2–6°C, adopted by many eye banks all over the world, and the organ culture at 30–37°C, the current method of choice for most eye banks in Europe.[12]

Few studies comparing the effect of the two storage methods demonstrate similar graft survival and post-operative decline in endothelial cell density.[21–24]

Hypothermic storage

Donor corneas are stored in serum-free tissue-culture medium at 2–6°C.[25] At this temperature, the metabolic activity of the endothelial cells is minimal. Corneal swelling may be prevented by the addition of water retentive compounds to the preservation medium. One of the most commonly used compounds is dextran, which is added to the storage medium either alone or in association with the glycosaminoglycan chondroitin sulphate. Furthermore, the storage media also contain antibiotics (gentamicin alone or with streptomycin) that, together with the low temperature, prevent or limit the bacterial growth. Certain commercially available solutions are also supplemented with additives (energy sources, antioxidants, membrane stabilizing components, growth factors), but their specific contributions have never been clarified.

During hypothermia, the cornea shows progressive degeneration of the epithelium and the endothelium and, eventually, cell death. Both apoptosis and necrosis occur during hypothermic storage, with apoptosis appearing to predominate.

The hypothermic storage method does not allow time for pre-operative microbiology controls before distribution of the tissue for transplant. However, ocular infections after penetrating keratoplasty are rare and, in most cases, related to the recipient eye condition or to the surgical procedure.

Overall, hypothermic storage seems to offer the donor tissues of good quality comparable to that obtained by organ culture, provided that the storage time is kept short.

Organ culture

The organ culture method consists of two phases—a storage period in culture medium at 30–37°C and a de-swelling and transportation phase at 30–37°C and room temperature in the same medium supplemented with 4–8% dextran. Organ culture solutions are based on cell culture media, such as a base of Eagle's MEM or its variant Dulbecco's MEM supplemented by penicillin, streptomycin and fungicide (amphotericin B or nystatin), and by 2-10% foetal calf serum as a source of growth factor. A storage period of thirty days can be achieved without significant loss of endothelial cells. The endothelium may exhibit reparative phenomena during storage.

Before distribution, the swelling is reversed by the dextran present in the transport medium. The final thickness is reached in about 24 hours, and is dependent on the dextran concentration.

Organ culture offers a longer storage time, corneal endothelium with a better-defined quality and a pre-operative sterility control.

Samples of the storage medium from cultured corneas are routinely tested for microbiology after 3–7 days in the first phase, and after 1 day in the second phase. A gradual change in colour of the medium is expected, but any cloudiness or significant colour change of the medium is indicative of bacterial or fungal contamination. A contaminated cornea is discarded regardless of whether the microbe is pathogenic or not. Identification helps to identify trends and opportunities for process improvement.(26,27)

Evolution in corneal transplantation

Traditionally, corneal transplantation refers to penetrating keratoplasty (PK), a full-thickness corneal replacement in which the diseased cornea is removed and substituted with a healthy donor cornea. Currently, lamellar keratoplasty has been adopted worldwide as an alternative to penetrating keratoplasy for anterior corneal diseases (e.g., keratoconus) and posterior corneal diseases (e.g., Fuchs' dystrophy). In the new partial corneal transplantations,(28,29) only diseased or scarred layers of the cornea are removed, sparing the healthy ones. A variety of Anterior

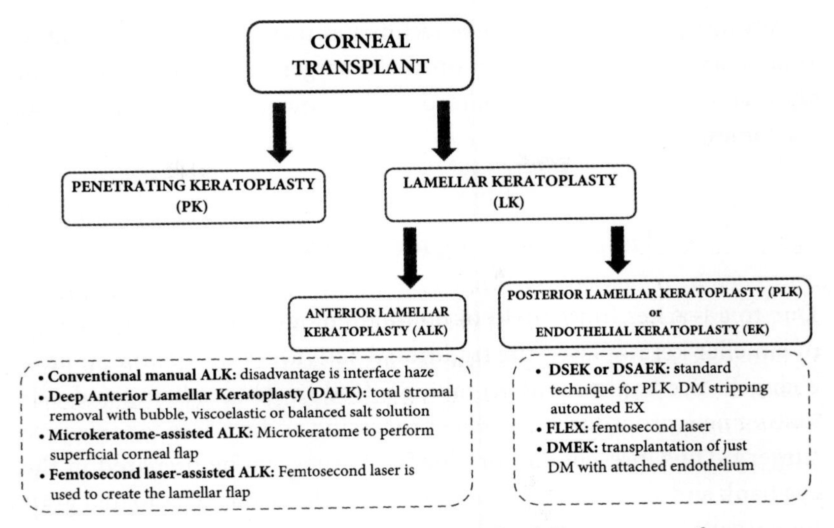

Figure 51.3. Schematic diagram illustrating the different types of keratoplasty procedures available

Lamellar Keratoplasty (ALK) procedures[30] have been described: conventional ALK surgery; deep anterior lamellar keratoplasty (DALK); microkeratome-assisted ALK and femtosecond laser-assisted ALK (Figure 51.3). The most used procedure is DALK, in which total corneal stroma is replaced, thus preserving host corneal endothelium and eliminating the risk of endothelium rejection.[31]

Endothelial keratoplasty (EK) or posterior lamellar keratoplasty is selective keratoplasty method used to replace the posterior part of the cornea. The most widely used EK procedures are DSAEK (Descemet Stripping Automated Endothelial Keratoplasty) and DMEK (Descemet's Membrane Endothelial Keratoplasty).[32]

In DSAEK, the donor endothelium, Descemet membrane, and a thin part of the posterior stroma are used to replace the host tissue.[33] In the standard DSAEK, posterior lamellar thickness is around 100 μm (Ultra-Thin DSAEK).[34]

In DMEK, surgeons replace only the host Descemet membrane and endothelium without the adherent corneal stroma. It is still not as common as other techniques due to the 'learning curve' required for tissue preparation and surgery.

Advantages of all the selective techniques include minimum surgical trauma and risks related to an open-sky surgery, reduced incidence of the graft rejection, faster visual recovery, and more predictable refractive outcomes.

Tissue processing for surgical purpose

Due to advances in the field of ophthalmology and the introduction of lamellar keratoplasty, the traditional activities of eye banking have changed. Eye banks focus on taking a lead in standardizing and validating new procedures of tissue processing and devices for selective surgery. Thus, pre-cut and pre-loaded tissues can be prepared in the eye bank and shipped to the surgical venue to ensure a validated graft for surgery.

Eye bank preparation of corneal tissue for lamellar keratoplasty

Corneas with prior laser photoablation surgery or non-infectious anterior stromal scars may be suitable for posterior keratoplasty.[35–37] After evaluation of the cornea by slit lamp biomicroscopy and specular microscopy, the lamellar keratectomy may be pre-formed using aseptic technique with an automated microkeratome under laminar flow. A 3–4 mm scleral rim is needed for corneas used in lamellar keratoplasty to ensure an adequate seal on the artificial chamber.

An automated microkeratome system may consist of a control unit, an artificial chamber, and microkeratome turbine and heads. Additional equipments required are a tank of nitrogen to power the system and a pachymeter to obtain corneal thickness measurements.

A sterile field is set up under the laminar flow cabinet with the artificial anterior chamber connected to an irrigation system and turbine connected to the control unit. The cornea is centred onto the artificial anterior chamber, and locked in place. The system must be watertight to ensure a smooth cut. The cornea is pressurized by infusing PBS through the irrigation system. A tonometer lens is placed on the corneal surface to confirm that a minimum of 65 mmHg pressure has been established inside the system. In case of anterior lenticules, the desired thickness of the graft is obtained by the correspondent microkeratome head. For posterior lenticules, a pachymetry reading is obtained after the removal of the epithelium to select the appropriate cutting head.

Resection of cornea with a swinging microkeratome

The corneal epithelium may be gently removed before the preparation. Two points are marked on the mid-periphery of the cornea using a sterile gentian violet or trypan blue marker to assist with re-aligning the cap back onto the remaining stromal bed after the cut.

The blade is inserted into the microkeratome head, which is secured into the turbine and lubricated with PBS. The power source is then activated and the microkeratome head is rotated manually across the cornea. Once the sectioning is completed, the free cap is removed from the microkeratome head and repositioned onto the corneal bed, taking care of re-aligning along the marks. The pre-cut cornea is removed from the artificial chamber.

Once lamellar keratectomy has been completed, the cornea should be re-evaluated by slit lamp biomicroscopy and specular/light microscopy to confirm that the tissue is suitable for the intended use.[38]

Storage of corneal lenticules for lamellar keratoplasty

Anterior corneal lenticules can be either dehydrated or freeze-dried, and stored at 2–6°C. Alternatively, for anterior/posterior lenticules, hypothermic storage or organ culture may be used.[39,40]

Pre-cut tissues for Descemet Stripping Automated Endothelial Keratoplasty

The donor tissue for DSAEK can be prepared by eye bank technicians through a microkeratome, thus allowing the entire tissue to be delivered to the surgeon as a pre-cut lenticule. The anterior cap of the cornea can be left in place for ease of transportation and to lower any potential endothelial cell damage.[41,42]

Tissues for Descemet Membrane Endothelial Keratoplasty

Current techniques for DMEK excision include stripping,[43–45] pneumatic dissection (Figure 51.4), and hydro-dissection.[46,47] The most commonly used technique is the stripping method performed by peeling the Descemet's membrane and the endothelium away from the stroma, and leaving a hinge at the end of the lenticule (Figure 51.5). This technique

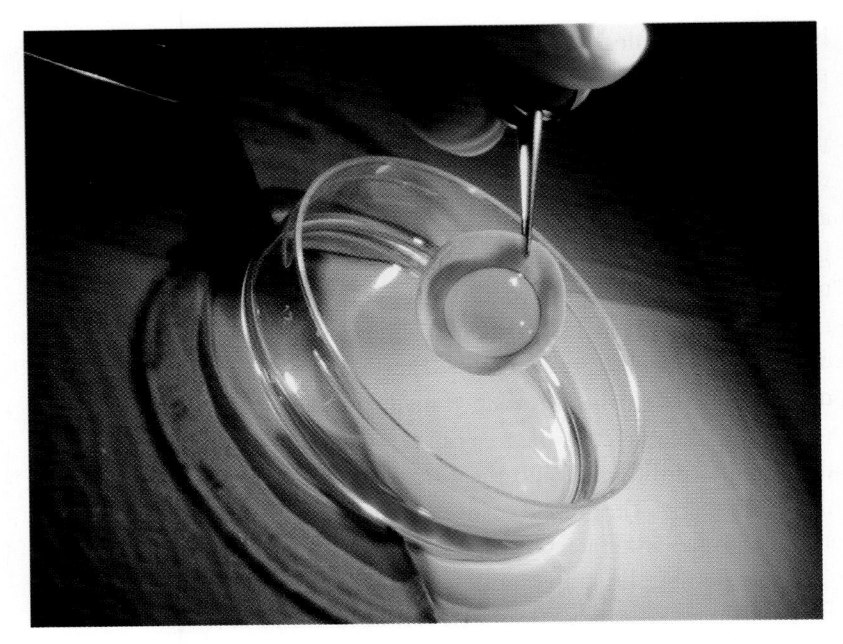

Figure 51.4. Pre-bubbled tissue prepared using submerged hydro-separation (SubHyS) method

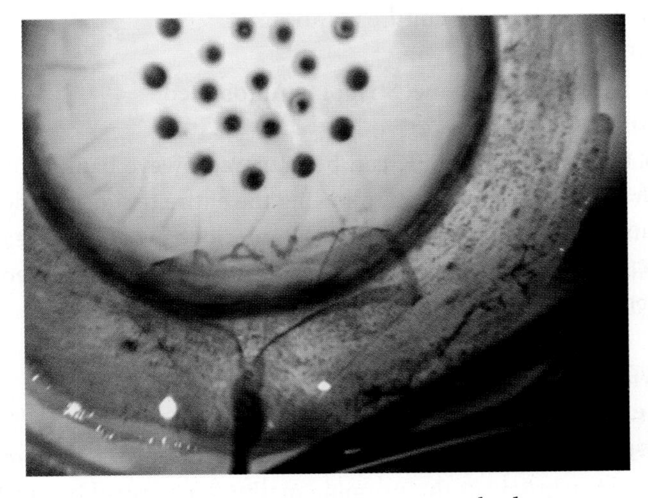

Figure 51.5. Pre-stripped tissue using stripping method

has shown minimum mortality rate as compared to the other currently performed techniques.

Pre-loaded tissues for EK

Commercially available devices give the opportunity to provide pre-cut and pre-loaded grafts ready to be transplanted.[48] They can be used to transport lenticules cut for DSAEK and UT-DSAEK. There are two types of pre-loaded DMEK membranes transporting protocols: endothelial cells facing out, which expose them to damages and make tissue handling difficult, or with the endothelial cells facing inwards. The latter might reduce unfolding time, which leads to quicker surgeries.[49–51]

Eye bank preparations have certain advantages, as tissues prepared by the surgeon in the operating theatre could be irregular, or perforated; the surgery must be postponed or an extra cornea has to be available in such cases.

Preparation of donor sclera

Donor sclera is prepared from the remaining ocular tissues following excision of the corneoscleral button or from donor globes which have been disqualified. Conjunctiva, remnants of muscles and the intraocular materials are removed, and the sclera is finally rinsed in PBS, reshaped to its original spherical form, and preserved dehydrated in ethanol (70% or higher concentration) or glycerol, fixed in formalin, and freeze dried, or frozen.[52]

Preparation of conjunctiva for keratolimbal allografts

In order to use the conjunctiva as a graft, conjunctival rim of 3–4 mm should be left during tissue recovery. The tissue, after thorough decontamination, can be dispatched as whole globes stored in a moist chamber or as corneoscleral rims in hypothermic storage medium, to be used as soon as possible.[53]

Human Corneal Endothelial Cell Culture

Corneal endothelial cell culture (HCEC) is the next challenge. Considering the requirement of donor corneal tissues for clinical purposes, *in vitro* cultured cells may help to meet the demand for EK. Challenges are represented by the requirement of clean room facilities and culture conditions, along with pre-defined scaffolds or a surgical technique.[54]

Conclusions

Each year, more than 100,000 corneal transplants are performed in the world, of which about 40,000 cases occur in the US. From the first successful corneal transplant in 1905 to the advent of lamellar keratoplasty, the role of eye banks has dramatically increased, in addition to the field of research and development. Without eye banks, corneal transplantation would not be as safe, as efficient and feasible as it is today.

Highlights

- Ocular tissues (cornea, sclera, conjunctiva, and limbus) are used in several surgical ocular procedures.
- Corneal transplantation is the oldest and most common type of allogenic transplantation in the world.
- Eye banks are responsible for collecting, evaluating, processing, and distributing donated ocular tissues.
- Penetrating keratoplasty is a full-thickness corneal replacement in which the diseased cornea is removed and substituted with a healthy donor cornea.
- Lamellar keratoplasty refers to a selective surgery aimed at replacing the anterior corneal stroma (anterior lamellar keratoplasty) or the posterior corneal stroma (posterior lamellar/EK).
- Pre-cut and pre-loaded tissues have led to increasing numbers of lamellar keratoplasty procedures being carried out.

References

1. Duman F, Kosker M, Suri K, Reddy JC, Ma JF, Hammersmith KM, et al. Indications and outcomes of corneal transplantation in geriatric patients. Am J Ophthalmol. 2013; 156:600–607.
2. Eye bank association of America. Penetrating keratoplasy. Available from: https://www.restoresight.org. 2015.
3. Nishida T. Cornea. In: Krachmer JH, Mannis MJ, Holland EJ, editors. Cornea. 2nd ed. Philadelphia, Elsevier Mosby Saunders publisher; 2005. Chapter 1, p.3–26.
4. Watson PG, Young RD. Scleral structure, organisation and disease. A review. Exp Eye Res 2004; 78:609–623.

5. Nelson JD, Cameron JD. The conjunctiva: anatomy and physiology. In: Krachmer JH, Mannis MJ, Holland EJ, editors. Cornea. 2nd ed. Philadelphia, Elsevier Mosby Saunders publisher; 2005. Chapter 3, p.37–43.
6. Dua HS, Shanmuganathan VA, Powell-Richards AO, Tighe PJ, Joseph A. Limbal epithelial crypts: A novel anatomical structure and a putative limbal stem cell niche. Br J Ophthalmol 2005; 89:529–532.
7. Zirm E. Eine erfolgreiche totale keratoplastik (A successful total keratoplasty). 1906 Archiv Ophthalmol 64, 580–593.
8. Armitage WJ, Tullo AB, Larkin DF. The first successful full-thickness corneal transplant: A commentary on Eduard Zirm's landmark paper of 1906. Br J Ophthalmol. 2006;90(10):1222–1223.
9. Castroviejo R. Keratoplasty. Am J Ophalmol. 1941;24:1–20.
10. Filatov VP, Sitchevska O. Transplantation of the cornea. Arch Ophthalmol 1935; 13(3):321–347.
11. McCarey BE, Kaufman HE. Improved corneal storage. Investigative Ophthalmol 13:165–173, 1974.
12. Pels L, Schuchard Y. Organ culture in the Netherlands. Preservation and endothelial evaluation. In: Brightbill FS, editor. Corneal Surgery. Theory, Technique and Tissue. 2nd ed. St. Louis, Mosby Elsevier publisher; 1993. Chapter 46, p.622–632.
13. Narayan RP. Development of tissue bank. Indian J Plast Surg. 2012;45(2):396–402.
14. Strong DM. The US Navy Tissue Bank: 50 years on the cutting edge. Cell Tissue Bank. 2000;1(1):9–16.
15. https://www.eeba.eu/files/pdf/EEBA%20Minimum%20Medical%20Standards%20Revision%205%20Final.pdf
16. https://restoresight.org/what-we-do/publications/medical-standards-procedures-manual/
17. Manuelidis EE, Angelo JN, Gorgacz EJ, Kim JH, Manuelidis L. Experimental creutzfeldt-jakob disease transmitted via the eye with infected cornea. N Engl J Med 1977; 296(23): 1334–1336.
18. Thiel HJ, Erb C, Heckmann J, Lang C, Neundorfer B. Manifestations of Creutzfeldt-Jakob disease 30 years after corneal transplantation. Klin Monbl Augenheilkd 2000; 217(5): 303–307.
19. Pels, E, Beele, H, Claerhout, I. Eye bank issues: II. Preservation techniques: Warm versus cold storage. Int Ophthalmol. 2008:28(3); 155–163.
20. Wiffen, SJ, Nelson, LR, Ali, AF, Bourne, WM. Morphologic assessment of corneal endothelium by specular microscopy in evaluation of donor corneas for transplantation. Cornea. 1995:14(6); 554–561.
21. Chu W. The past twenty-five years in eye banking. Cornea. 2000:19(5); 754–765.
22. Frueh, BE, Böhnke, M. Prospective, randomized clinical evaluation of Optisol vs organ culture corneal storage media. Arch Ophthalmol. 2000:118(6); 757–760.
23. Armitage, WJ, Easty, DL. Factors influencing the suitability of organ-cultured corneas for transplantation. Invest Ophthalmol Vis Sci. 1997:38(1); 16–24.
24. Rijneveld, WJ, Remeijer, L, van Rij, G, Beekhuis, H, Pels, E. Prospective clinical evaluation of McCarey–Kaufman and organ culture cornea preservation media: 14-Year Follow-up. Cornea. 2008:27(9); 996–1000.
25. Komuro, K, Hodge, DO, Gores, GJ, Bourne, WM. Cell death during corneal storage at 4°C. Inv Ophthalmol Vis Sci. 1999:40(12), 2827–2832.

26. Borderie, VM, Laroche, L. Microbiologic study of organ-cultured donor corneas. Transplantation. 1998:66(1);120–23.
27. Zanetti, E, Mucignat, G, Camposampiero, D, Frigo, AC, Bruni, A, Ponzin, D. Bacterial contamination of human organ-cultured corneas. Cornea. 2005:24(5), 603–607.
28. Melles GR, Wijdh RH, Nieuwendaal CP. A technique to excise the descemet membrane from a recipient cornea (descemetorhexis). Cornea. 2004;23(3):286–288.
29. Terry MA, Ousley PJ. Deep lamellar endothelial keratoplasty in the first United States patients: Early clinical results. Cornea. 2001;20(3):239–243.
30. Sarnicola E, Sarnicola V, Surgical corneal anatomy in deep anterior lamellar keratoplasty: Suggestion of new acronyms. Cornea 2019; 38:515–522.
31. Shimmura, S. Tsubota K. Deep anterior lamellar keratoplasty. Curr Opin Ophtalmol 2006; 17:349–355.
32. MM. Fernandez, NA. Afshari. Endothelial Keratoplasty: From DLEK to DMEK. Middle East Afr J Ophthalmol. 2010 Jan;17(1):5–8. DOI: 10.4103/0974-9233.61210.
33. FW Price Jr1, MO Price. Descemet's stripping with endothelial keratoplasty in 50 eyes: A refractive neutral corneal transplant. J Refract Surg. 2005 Jul-Aug;21(4):339–345.
34. M. Parekh, A. Ruzza, B. Steger, CE. Willoughby, S. Rehman, S. Ferrari, D. Ponzin, SB. Kaye, V. Romano. Cross-country transportation efficacy and clinical outcomes of preloaded large-diameter ultra-thin descemet stripping automated endothelial keratoplasty grafts. Cornea 2019;38:30–34. DOI: 10.1097/ICO.0000000000001777.
35. Wiffen, SJ, Weston, BC, Maguire, LJ, Bourne, WM. The value of routine donor corneal rim cultures in penetrating keratoplasty. Arch Ophthalmol. 1997:115(6); 719–24.
36. Wilhelmus, KR, Stulting, D, Sugar, J, Khan, MM. Primary corneal graft failure. A national reporting system. Arch Ophthalmol. 1995:113(12), 1497–1502.
37. Kim, T, Palay, DA, Michael, L. Donor factors associated with epithelial defects after penetrating keratoplasty. Cornea. 1996:15(5), 451–456.
38. Salvalaio, G, Fasolo, A, Bruni, A, Frigo, AC, Favaro, E, Ponzin D. Improved preparation and preservation of human keratoplasty lenticules. Ophthalmic Res. 2003:35(6); 301–358.
39. Sarnicola E, Sarnicola C, Cheung AY, Holland EJ, Sarnicola V. Surgical Corneal Anatomy in Deep Anterior Lamellar Keratoplasty: Suggestion of New Acronyms. Cornea. 2019;38:515–522.
40. Sarnicola E, Sarnicola C, Cheung AY, Holland EJ, Sarnicola V. Surgical Corneal Anatomy in Deep Anterior Lamellar Keratoplasty: Suggestion of New Acronyms. Cornea. 2019;38:515–522.
41. Ide, T, Yoo, SH, Kymionis, GD, et al. Descemet stripping automated endothelial keratoplasty. Effect of anterior lamellar corneal tissue-on/-off storage condition on Descemet-stripping automated endothelial keratoplasty donor tissue. Cornea. 2008:27(7); 754–757.
42. Terry, MA. Precut tissue for Descemet stripping automated endothelial keratoplasty: Complications are from technique, not tissue. Cornea. 2008:27(6); 627–629.
43. M. Parekh, M. Baruzzo, E. Favaro, D. Borroni, S. Ferrari, D. Ponzin, A. Ruzza. Standardizing Descemet Membrane Endothelial Keratoplasty Graft Preparation

Method in the Eye Bank—Experience of 527 Descemet Membrane Endothelial Keratoplasty Tissues. Cornea. 2017 Dec;36(12):1458–1466. DOI: 10.1097/ICO.0000000000001349.

44. M. Parekh, A. Ruzza, S. Ferrari, S. Ahmad, S. Kaye, D. Ponzin, V. Romano. Endothelium-in versus endothelium-out for Descemet membrane endothelial keratoplasty graft preparation and implantation Acta Ophthalmol. 2017 Mar;95(2):194–198. DOI: 10.1111/aos.13162.
45. M. Parekh, A. Ruzza, S. Ferrari, M. Busin, D. Ponzin. Preloaded Tissues for Descemet Membrane Endothelial Keratoplasty. Am J Ophthalmol. 2016 Jun;166:120–125. DOI: 10.1016/j.ajo.2016.03.048.
46. A. Ruzza, M Parekh, G. Salvalaio, S. Ferrari, D. Camposampiero, MC. Amoureux, M. Busin, D. Ponzin. Bubble technique for Descemet membrane endothelial keratoplasty tissue preparation in an eye bank: air or liquid? Acta Ophthalmol. 2015 Mar;93(2):e129–34. DOI: 10.1111/aos.12520.
47. M. Busin, V. Scorcia, AK. Patel, G. Salvalaio, D. Ponzin. Pneumatic dissection and storage of donor endothelial tissue for Descemet's membrane endothelial keratoplasty. Ophthalmology. 2010 Aug;117(8):1517–1520. DOI: 10.1016/j.ophtha.2009.12.040
48. Ruzza, M. Parekh, S. Ferrari, G. Salvalaio, Y. Nahum, C. Bovone, D. Ponzin, M. Busin. Preloaded donor corneal lenticules in a new validated 3D printed smart storage glide for Descemet stripping automated endothelial keratoplasty. Br J Ophthalmol. 2015 Oct;99(10):1388–1395. DOI: 10.1136/bjophthalmol-2014-306510.
49. V. Romano, M. Parekh, A. Ruzza, CE Willoughby, S. Ferrari, D. Ponzin, SB Kaye, HJ. Levis. Comparison of preservation and transportation protocols for preloaded Descemet membrane endothelial keratoplasty. Br J Ophthalmol. 2018 Apr;102(4):549–555. DOI: 10.1136/bjophthalmol-2017-310906.
50. M. Parekh, A. Ruzza, S. Ferrari, S. Ahmad, S. Kaye, D. Ponzin, V. Romano. Endothelium-in versus endothelium-out for Descemet membrane endothelial keratoplasty graft preparation and implantation Acta Ophthalmol. 2017 Mar;95(2):194–198. DOI: 10.1111/aos.13162.
51. K. Barnes, E. Chiang, C. Chen, J. Lohmeier, J. Christy, A. Chaurasia, A. Rosen, P. Vora, S. Cai, A. Subramanya, N. Durr, R. Allen, A.Omid Eghrari. Comparison of tri-folded and scroll-based graft viability in preloaded Descemet Membrane Endothelial Keratoplasty. Cornea. 2019 Mar;38(3):392–396. DOI: 10.1097/ICO.0000000000001831.
52. Enzenauer WR, Sieck EA, Vavra DE, Jacobs EP. Residual ethanol content of donor sclera after storage in 95% ethanol and saline rinse of various duration. Am J Ophthalmol 1999; 128(4):522–524.
53. Croasdale CR, Schwartz GS, Malling JV. Keratolimbal allograft: recommendations for tissue procurement and preparation by eye banks, and standard surgical technique. Cornea. 1999; 18(1):52–58.
54. Ferrari S, Barbaro V, Di Iorio E, Fasolo A, Ponzin D. Advances in corneal surgery and cell therapy: challenges and perspectives for the eye banks. Exp Rev Ophthalmol 2009; 4(3):317–329.

52

Skin banks: History, organization, and clinical role

Paola Franco, Carlotta Castagnoli, Maurizio Stella

Historical overview

The field of skin banking has its roots from the middle of 20th century. In 1949, the first proper skin bank, the US Navy Skin Bank,(1) was set up by Dr George Hyatt, as a result of innovative studies on freezing tissues for the purpose of preservation in the late 1930s and early 1940s documented by Luyet(2) and Webster.(3) The interest on skin banking grew together with the development of allografting and autografting procedures, to ensure the safety and efficacy of graft preservation. The first successful skin grafting procedure was described by Reverdin in 1869.(4) However, the first skin transplant attempt traces back to ancient India (sometime between 1000 and 800 BC) with the work of Sushruta, considered as the 'Father of Plastic Surgery'. In his manuscripts, he described many surgical instruments and procedures, including the reconstruction of the nose with a cheek flap, creating the so-called 'Indian method'.(5,6)

In Europe, the first tissue bank was established in the former Czechoslovakia (Hradec Kralove) in 1952, followed by the German Democratic Republic (1956), Great Britain (1955), and Poland (1962).(7)

In 1976, the Euro Skin Bank was established under the patronage of the Dutch Burns Foundation in order to supply allograft cadaver skin to the three main burn care centres in The Netherlands. This institution is, to this day, one of the main European research centres in the field of skin banking.(7)

Over the following decades, the variety of preserved and transplanted tissues and cells increased rapidly, including not only skin but also bone, heart valves, blood components, and so on. Simultaneously, preservation methods such as deep-freezing, cryopreservation, and freeze-drying were newly introduced or further refined.

The progress in science, together with the rising demand for allogenic tissues, led to the need of co-operation between tissue banks and relevant disciplines including ethics, biology, and technology. Therefore, during the first European Conference on Tissue Banking in Berlin in October 1991, 280 participants from eighteen European countries agreed to establish the European Association of Tissue Banks (EATB), for tissue bank professionals, scientists, and clinicians working in the fields of donation, processing, and transplantation of cells.[7] This association led to the definition of tissue banking standards and the regulation of provision of human materials for transplantation.

In Italy on 1 April 1999, the Law No.91 on transplant regulation was published as the starting point for the creation of the first laboratory. The centres for severe burns treatment were, later, organized into more complex structures (tissue establishments), including skin banks, to meet the growing demand for transplant tissues.[8]

Currently, the skin bank is described as an organization that, with its structure, equipment, laboratories, and expertise, can ensure safety and efficacy of the entire tissue banking process.

Today, there are five skin banks in Italy[9]:

- Cesena (Banca Regionale della Cute, Ospedale M. Bufalini)
- Milano (A.O Cà Granda Niguarda—CRR Innesti Cutanei)
- Torino (Banca Regionale della Cute—Tissue & Cell Factory Banca della Cute—A.O.U. Città della Salute e della Scienza di Torino, presidio C.T.O.)
- Siena (Centro conservazione cute—Banca Regionale Tessuti e Cellule—Policlinico S. Maria alle Scotte)
- Verona (Banca dei Tessuti di Verona—AOUI Ospedale Policlinico 'Borgo Roma')

Practice guidelines

The regulation of the skin banking is complex and involves many associations as well as the different national laws. For example, in the USA, the skin banks refer to the American Association of Tissue Banking guidelines and federal laws; in Europe, they comply with the European Association of Tissue Banks standards and with specific national guidelines and legislations. The most important European directives concerning the skin banking are the 2004/23/EC,[10] that sets the standards of quality and safety for the donation, procurement, testing, processing, preservation, storage, and distribution of human tissues and cells; this directive was later implemented by directives 2006/17/EC[11] and 2006/86/EC.[12]

Though skin banks aren't classified as pharmaceutical facilities, they comply with Good Manufacturing Practice (GMP) guidelines.[13] The GMP is worldwide recognized as the guide for describing the minimum standard process of medicine manufacturing. In Europe, the European Medicines Agency (EMA) plays a key role in harmonizing GMP activities at the European Union (EU) level, based on Regulation No. 1252/2014[14] and Directive 2003/94/EC,[15] concerning active substances and medicines for human use.[16]

The GMP guidelines prescribe the constant monitoring of environmental parameters (particulate and microbial contamination), and the control of structures and equipment, that are regularly calibrated, maintained, and validated according to written procedures.[17,18] If GMP guidelines are strictly followed, the aseptic processing takes place according to minimal particles criteria in Grade A conditions with Grade B background environment, according to the EU directives,[19] which require processing areas classified as Grade A with a surrounding environment of at least Grade D.

In Italy, the skin banks with their laboratories must be certified by the National Transplant Centre (CNT) that ensures their compliance with national and international directives. The CNT regulates and organizes the clinical use of the banked skin in transplant procedures,[20] other than the selection of the donors and the harvesting procedures (with dedicated guidelines), and complies with the Law 91/99.[21] The Regional

Transplant Centers, that are part of the CNT network, coordinate the work in their jurisdiction.

Skin bank structure

A section of the CNT guidelines[20] describes the general organizational requirements of a tissue bank as follows:

- The bank must have a documented purpose and the organization, the structure and the operational procedures must comply with it.
- The bank must have a qualified person in charge as well as trained and up to date staff.
- The bank must apply a documented management system, that is supervised by the person in charge and that complies with the guidelines and the laws.
- All documents must be accurate, complete, and confidential.
- The person in charge of the bank is responsible for the safety and the health of the staff and must ensure the application of the Legislative Decree 81/2008 obligations.
- The structure of the bank must be appropriate to its activity, in terms of access, cleaning, waste disposal, processing rooms, and storage units.
- If the tissues are exposed to the room without any microbial inactivation process, the quality of the room air must be of Grade A according to the GMP (Good Manufacturing Practice), the Legislative Decree 24/2006 and the Directive 2003/94/CE; the tissue that will undergo a microbial inactivation could be processed in a minimum Grade C room.

In the following paragraphs, the Tissue and Cell Factory (TCF) Skin Bank of Turin is taken as an example for the description of skin bank's structure, products, and operation processes in Italy.

The TCF Skin Bank of Turin is structured as shown in Figure 52.1. There are two main areas. The one on the right is the non-classified area that includes the administrative offices, the quality control laboratory and the research and development laboratory. On the left, there is a classified area, including 4 Clean Rooms, two for the handling of tissues and

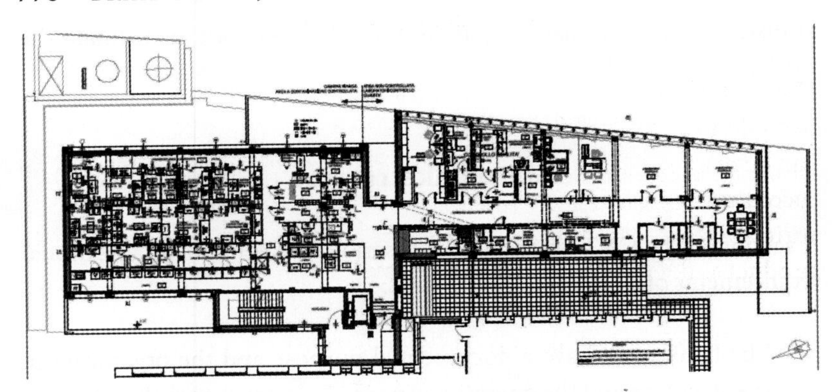

Figure 52.1. Planimetry of the Tissue and Cell Factory (TCF) Skin Bank of Turin

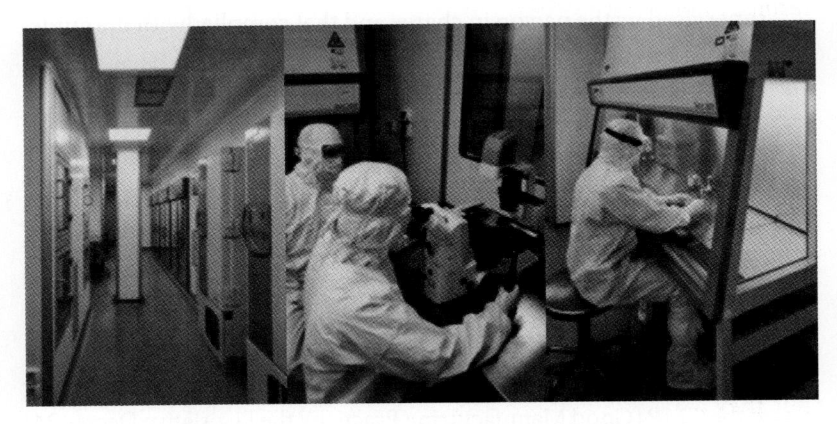

Figure 52.2. The classified area of the TCF Skin Bank of Turin

two for the handling of cells. These Clean Rooms are accessible only to trained staff, after proper dressing and qualified sterilization processes (Figure 52.2). Since the skin (and all other products) should be processed under aseptic conditions in a bacteriological- and climate-controlled environment, the Clean Rooms are under 24/7 control by a continuous monitoring system that surveys the environment sensitive parameters (contamination, air particles, air humidity, and temperature).

Skin bank products

The TCF Skin Bank of Turin receives skin and other tissues both from dead donors and living ones. There are two main types of products that can be manufactured, namely alloplastic and autologous products. Every incoming tissue undergoes an antibiotic treatment during the manufacturing process; however, quality and sterility tests are performed on every product as described in the next paragraph.

Alloplastic products

From a multiorgan or multitissue donor, both the skin and the reticular dermis can be harvested, according with the Law 91/99.[21] These tissues result in several products:

- Glycerol preserved skin
- Disepithelizated glycerol preserved skin
- Cryopreserved skin
- Decellularized reticular dermis

The difference between the first two products and the third one is the preservation method, the glycerol-preservation, and the cryopreservation; the main difference between the two methods is tissue viability. Glycerolized skin grafts maintain structural and mechanical properties but they are not viable, while cryopreserved skin grafts maintain cell viability.[22]

The glycerolizing process consists of three steps with progressive glycerol percentage increase in each step, until the skin graft preservation media composition reaches 85% of glycerol. At this stage, the skin graft is stored at 4°C. At any time, the skin graft can be de-glycerolized using 0.9% saline solution at 37°C. Disepithelizated glycerol preserved skin is where the epidermis has been mechanically removed.

The cryopreservation can be performed in two different ways; the skin grafts can either be deep freeze at –80°C (after a graduate cooling) or stocked in liquid nitrogen (temperature: −196°C) in cryoprotectant medium. Both methods allow the preservation of the cell viability.

Autologous products

Adipose tissue and skin can be harvested from patients during specific surgeries, for clinical or research purposes. Several products are obtained from these tissues:

- Cryopreserved adipose tissue
- Stromal Vascular Fraction (SVF, from the adipose tissue)
- Cryopreserved autologous skin (nipple-areola complex)

These cryopreserved products maintain their cell viability and could be used for specific clinical purposes as described in the Skin bank products application section of this chapter.

There isn't any evidence of a different result in terms of tissue structure, surface markers, and quality of tissue-derived SVF due to the use of either the −80°C or the liquid nitrogen for the adipose tissue preservation.[23]

Quality controls

All products of the TCF Skin Bank of Turin are strictly controlled and tested before their application; they undergo an evaluation for identifying anaerobic or aerobic bacterial and fungi contamination (as described in the European Pharmacopoeia, EuPh.2.6.27). With the absence of any contamination, the product can be certified as sterile and could be used for clinical application.

In addition, all the cryopreserved products undergo other tests to prove their cell viability:

- MTT test, that takes advantage of a specific compound (the 3-(4,5-dimethylthiazol-2-yl) -2,5-diphenyltetrazolium bromide) which is reduced by a mitochondrial enzyme (succinate dehydrogenase) only if viable cells are present. The test result depends on the number of the viable cells; therefore, the MTT test is a viability quantitative analysis.

- Histological analysis, that seeks to evaluate if the thermic stress (deep freezing or liquid nitrogen storage) affects the tissue quality in terms of structural tri-dimensional architecture.

Skin bank products application

The clinical application of all the products listed above as alloplastic and autologous is described as follows.

Alloplastic skin (glycerol- or cryo-preserved)

The CNT outlines the indications for alloplastic skin bank clinical applications in its guideline 'Indications for bank skin and bio-products use.[24]

The alloplastic skin can be used for the treatment of both acute and chronic injuries. Alloplastic skin grafts have a life-saving role not only in the extensive burns treatment, but also in other conditions[25] such as severe degloving injuries and amputations, Lyell syndrome[26] (toxic epidermal necrolysis) and congenital epidermolysis bullosa.[27]

The alloplastic skin grafts can also be used for treating smaller burns, surgical wounds, and chronic wounds, such as diabetic ulcers that are unresponsive to conventional treatment.[28]

However, the main indication for alloplastic skin grafts application is burn treatment; there are three methods of skin graft used for burns:

1. Temporary dressing: It is most frequently used and consists of the skin graft application on the burn areas to protect the exposed tissues. With such skin grafts, there is evidence of reduction of pain and infection rate, decrease in water, electrolytes and proteins loss, catabolism control and lower autograft need with the promotion of epithelialization.[29,30] Immunosuppression due to the burn and reduced immunoreactivity of the allograft permits successful engraftment, allowing it to protect the tissues until spontaneous healing

occurs or the wound bed gets prepared for the surgical treatment with autografts. This technique can be used not only as a life-saving treatment for extended burns (>40% total body surface area (TBSA)), but also as a supportive treatment for the other described conditions.

2. The Alexander technique: First described in 1981,[31] this technique consists of widely meshed autograft (6:1 or greater) covered by 1.5 or 3:1 expanded mesh allografts that provide more effective engraftment and reduced autograft need, along with higher survival rate at lower costs in comparison to alternative surgical procedures.[32]
3. The Cuono technique: This technique is adopted in 70–80% TBSA burns with two stages surgical procedure. First, excised burn wounds are resurfaced with allografts and keratinocyte cultures are initiated from a small skin biopsy performed on the patient. After three weeks, allogenic epidermis is removed and the dermal bed is resurfaced with keratinocytes culture. Further, the allogeneic dermis promotes rapid (less than seven days) stratification, maturation, and integration of the cultures and the synthesis of anchoring fibrils.[33]

Alloplastic decellularized reticular dermis

This tissue, after an appropriate manufacturing process,[34] provides a good cutaneous substitute for clinical application. It is an effective filler and support material for significant tissue losses, and it can be used, for example, in orthopaedic surgery procedures as a fascial or tendon substitute as well as in abdominal-wall, dermis or breast reconstruction. Moreover, the alloplastic dermis can serve as a scaffold for the production of complete skin substitute, together with autologous keratinocytes, fibroblasts, and mesenchymal stem cells. This biological substitute represents a promising research product in the future of tissue engineering future.

Autologous cryopreserved skin

The TCF Skin Bank has a storage unit for the cryopreservation of autologous skin. It may consist of skin taken during burn surgery but not employed for various complications. In other cases, it consists of nipple-areola complexes that come from oncological patients' mastectomy procedures and are completely healthy, so they can be preserved and stored. During the breast reconstruction process, they can be used, resulting in better aesthetic outcomes.[35]

Autologous cryopreserved adipose tissue

Along with the alloplastic dermis and the autologous skin, the autologous cryopreserved adipose tissue constitutes a useful tool for reconstructive surgery. Preserved adipose tissue can help in many clinical fields as plastic, cosmetic, orthopaedic, and general surgery.[36]

Autologous stromal vascular fraction (SVF)

The SVF is an adipose tissue-derived product that can be extracted from the lipoaspirate. It consists of a heterogeneous cell population that includes mesenchymal stem cells (MSCs), erythrocytes, endothelial cells, fibroblasts, lymphocytes, monocytes/macrophages, and pericytes. With its regenerative potential (typical of the multipotent stem cells) and its anti-inflammatory and immunomodulant proprieties, SVF can represent a promising future therapeutic instrument in many fields, such as orthopaedics, general and cosmetic surgery, and regenerative medicine.[37]

The role of skin banks in disasters

With the centralization of burns treatment, a well-rehearsed major incident plan for burns is critical to provide prompt treatment to potentially large numbers of patients simultaneously. Such situations can take place in several scenarios, such as terrorist attacks, natural disasters, or severe city fires.[38] Therefore, the cooperation between burn centres and skin banks is essential to be prepared for events of mass disaster.[39,40]

Future perspectives

In the present times, skin banks are no longer only storage structures, they are becoming very important research centres for innovative cell and tissue products manufacturing. With continuous technology development, the field of tissue engineering is gaining enormous significance and represents one of the most interesting branches of the future medical research.

Reconstructive surgery and regenerative medicine, in general, concern many fields including Orthopaedics, with increasing joint replacement requests due to population ageing; Gynaecology, for the post-oncological reconstructions; General Surgery, for several chronic and refractory wounds such as ulcers and fistulas; Paediatric Surgery, that includes various congenital defects rather difficult to treat; and so on.

Therefore, the production of fully functioning, safe, and effective biosubstitutes could drastically improve numerous clinical and surgical procedures. One example of this type of product is the popular complete human skin substitute; alloplastic dermis is combined with, among others, autologous mesenchymal stem cells to obtain an innovative and potentially very useful product.

This important form of innovation can take place in the skin banks, where decades of experience in tissue manipulation meet the latest cell physiology discoveries.

Highlights

- Skin banks were born as support structures for burn centres, but they have gained, over time, a crucial role in the cells and tissue study, leading to important development in this field.
- Skin banks organization and structure are strictly regulated by national and international guidelines and directives; in Italy, they follow the National Transplant Center (CNT).
- Skin banks receive skin and other tissue both from death donors and living ones; the main products are alloplastic skin (glycerol- or cryo-preserved), alloplastic decellularized reticular dermis, autologous cryopreserved nipple-areola complex, and autologous cryopreserved adipose tissue (that includes the Stromal Vascular Fraction).
- Skin bank products have several clinical applications, the main indication being burns (both extensive burns and smaller burns). Some products, such as the alloplastic dermis and the autologous adipose tissue, have key application in the reconstructive surgery field.

- Skin banks are gaining importance in one of the most innovative medicine field—the tissue engineering, for example, creating a fully functioning, safe and effective skin bio-substitute that could drastically improve numerous clinical and surgical procedures.

References

1. William Trier C, Kenneth Sell W. United States Navy Skin Bank. Plast Reconstr Surg. 1968;41(6):543–548.
2. Luyet BJ. Differential staining for living and dead cells. Science (80-). 1937. doi:10.1126/science.85.2195.106
3. Webster J. Refrigerated skin grafts. Ann Surg. 1944;120:431–448.
4. Klasen HJ, Klasen HJ. Skin Grafting by the Reverdin Method and Subsequent Developments. In: *History of Free Skin Grafting.*; 1981. doi:10.1007/978-3-642-81653-6_2
5. Champaneria MC, Workman AD, Gupta SC. Sushruta: Father of plastic surgery. Ann Plast Surg. 2014. doi:10.1097/SAP.0b013e31827ae9f5
6. Chakrovorty R. Surgical principles in the Sutrasthanam of Susruta samhita management of retained foreign bodies. Indian J Hist Sci. 1970;5:113–158.
7. Rudiger von Versen M. History of the European Association of Tissue Banks (EATB).
8. Tognetti L, Pianigiani E, Ierardi F, et al. Current insights into skin banking: storage, preservation and clinical importance of skin allografts. J Biorepository Sci Appl Med. 2017. doi:10.2147/bsam.s115187
9. Centro Nazionale Trapianti. http://www.trapianti.salute.gov.it/trapianti/dettaglioContenutiCnt.jsp?lingua=italiano&area=cnt&menu=chiSiamo&sottomenu=rete&id=237.
10. Directive 2004/23/EC of the European Parliament and Council on quality and safety standards for the donation, procurement, testing, processing, preservation, storage and distribution of human tissues and cells. Off J Eur Union. 2004.
11. Commission Directive 2006/17/EC implementing Directive 2004/23/ EC of the European Parliament and of the Council as regards certain technical requirements for the donation, procurement and testing of human tissues and cells. Off J Eur Union. 2006.
12. Commission Directive 2006/86/EC implementing Directive 2004/23/ EC of the European Parliament and of the Council as regards traceability requirements, notification of serious adverse reactions and events and certain technical requirements for the coding. Off J Eur Union. 2006.
13. European Commission. Good Manufacturing Practice (GMP) guidelines. 2010;4.
14. COMMISSION DELEGATED REGULATION (EU) No 1252/2014 of 28 May 2014 supplementing Directive 2001/83/EC of the European Parliament and of the Council with regard to principles and guidelines of good manufacturing practice for active substances for medicinal p. Off J Eur Union. 2014.

15. COMMISSION DIRECTIVE 2003/94/EC of 8 October 2003 laying down the principles and guidelines of good manufacturing practice in respect of medicinal products for human use and investigational medicinal products for human use. Off J Eur Union. 2003.
16. EMA. Good Manufacturing Practice.
17. European Directorate for the Quality of medicines & Health Care (EDQM). *Guide to the Quality and Safety of Tissues and Cells for Human Application*. France; 2015.
18. Vicentino W, Rodríguez G, Saldías M, Álvarez I. Guidelines to Implement Quality Management Systems in Microbiology Laboratories for Tissue Banking. Transplant Proc. 2009. doi:10.1016/j.transproceed.2009.09.012
19. Gaucher S, Elie C, Vérola O, Jarraya M. Viability of cryopreserved human skin allografts: Effects of transport media and cryoprotectant. Cell Tissue Bank. 2012. doi:10.1007/s10561-011-9239-3
20. CNT. Linee Guida per il prelievo, la processazione e la distribuzione di tessuti a scopo di trapianto. 2016.
21. L. 1 aprile 1999, n. 91, in materia di 'Prelievi e trapianti di organi e di tessuti.'
22. Kua EHJ, Goh CQ, Ting Y, Chua A, Song C. Comparing the use of glycerol preserved and cryopreserved allogenic skin for the treatment of severe burns: Differences in clinical outcomes and in vitro tissue viability. Cell Tissue Bank. 2012. doi:10.1007/s10561-011-9254-4
23. Roato I, Alotto D, Belisario DC, et al. Adipose Derived-Mesenchymal Stem Cells Viability and Differentiating Features for Orthopaedic Reparative Applications: Banking of Adipose Tissue. Stem Cells Int. 2016. doi:10.1155/2016/4968724
24. Centro Nazionale Trapianti (CNT). Indicazioni all'uso della cute e bioderivati da Banca. 2007.
25. M. F, E. P, F.C. DS, et al. Other uses of homologous skin grafts and skin bank bioproducts. Clin Dermatol. 2005.
26. Paquet P. Topical treatment options for drug-induced toxic epidermal necrolysis (TEN). Expert Opin Pharmacother. 2010;11(15):2447–2458.
27. Kiritsi D, Nyström A. Recent advances in understanding and managing epidermolysis bullosa. F1000Research. 2018. doi:10.12688/f1000research.14974.1
28. Maruccia M, Onesti MG, Sorvillo V, et al. An alternative treatment strategy for complicated chronic wounds: Negative pressure therapy over mesh skin graft. Biomed Res Int. 2017. doi:10.1155/2017/8395219
29. Blome-Eberwein S, Jester A, Kuentscher M, Raff T, Germann G, Pelzer M. Clinical practice of glycerol preserved allograft skin coverage. Burns. 2002. doi:10.1016/s0305-4179(02)00085-2
30. Khoo TL, Halim AS, Saad AZM, Dorai AA. The application of glycerol-preserved skin allograft in the treatment of burn injuries: An analysis based on indications. Burns. 2010. doi:10.1016/j.burns.2009.03.007
31. Alexander JW, MacMillan BG, Law E, Kittur DS. Treatment of severe burns with widely meshed skin autograft and meshed skin allograft overlay. J Trauma. 1981.
32. Gasperoni M, Neri R, Carboni A, Purpura V, Morselli PG, Melandri D. The alexander surgical technique for the treatment of severe burns. Ann Burns Fire Disasters. 2016.

33. Cuono CB, Langdon R, Birchall N, Barttelbort S, McGuire J. Composite autologous-allogeneic skin replacement: Development and clinical application. Plast Reconstr Surg. 1987. doi:10.1097/00006534-198710000-00029
34. Castagnoli C, Fumagalli M, Alotto D, et al. Preparation and Characterization of a Novel Skin Substitute. J Biomed Biotechnol. 2010. doi:10.1155/2010/840363
35. Nakagawa T, Yano K, Hosokawa K. Cryopreserved autologous nipple-areola complex transfer to the reconstructed breast. Plast Reconstr Surg. 2003. doi:10.1097/00006534-200301000-00023
36. Gutowski KA, Baker SB, Coleman SR, et al. Current applications and safety of autologous fat grafts: A report of the ASPS Fat Graft Task Force. Plast Reconstr Surg. 2009. doi:10.1097/PRS.0b013e3181a09506
37. Bora P, Majumdar AS. Adipose tissue-derived stromal vascular fraction in regenerative medicine: A brief review on biology and translation. Stem Cell Res Ther. 2017;8(1):1–10. doi:10.1186/s13287-017-0598-y
38. Mahoney EJ, Harrington DT, Biffl WL, Metzger J, Oka T, Cioffi WG. Lessons learned from a nightclub fire: Institutional disaster preparedness. J Trauma—Inj Infect Crit Care. 2005. doi:10.1097/01.TA.0000153939.17932.E7
39. Horner CWM, Crighton E, Dziewulski P. 30 Years of burn disasters within the UK: Guidance for UK emergency preparedness. Burns. 2012. doi:10.1016/j.burns.2011.10.007
40. Wilson D, Greenleaf G. The availability of allograft skin for large scale medical emergencies in the United States. Cell Tissue Bank. 2014. doi:10.1007/s10561-013-9367-z

53

Vascularized composite allotransplantation

Palmina Petruzzo, Emmanuel Morelon,
Pratick Metha, Giuliano Testa

Introduction

Vascularized Composite Allotransplantation (VCA) is a relatively new field of transplantation. The VCA refers to the transfer of a vascularized human body part containing multiple tissue types (such as skin, muscle, bone, bone marrow, tendons, nerves, and blood vessels) as an anatomical and/or structural unit from a human donor to a human recipient. The appropriate regulatory classification of VCA is among solid organ transplantations and a regulatory definition including nine criteria has been adopted[(1)] by the Department of Health and Human Service in the USA in 2011 as well as by Europe.[(2)]

It is interesting that almost every type of VCA is a unique field and every VCA recipient has a different tissue defect that must be reconstructed. In recent years, there has been a rapid growth in the application of VCA and upper extremities, face, abdominal wall, larynx, penis, uterus, and knee transplants have been performed worldwide. In the literature, 205 cases of VCAs[(3)] are reported and the most common types are upper extremities, face, and uterus transplantations.

After various historic attempts, upper extremity transplantation (UET) successfully began with the first-hand transplant in 1998 followed by the first face transplantation (FT) in 2005, both performed in France.[(4,5)] Both types of VCA include skin, bone, bone marrow, nerves, vessels, tendons, and muscles. Another crucial aspect is their visibility as they are exposed to the external environment.

Currently, the International Registry on Hand and Composite Tissue Transplantation (IRHCTT), supported by the International Society of VCA, includes seventy-three cases of UET performed in twenty-four centres and thirty-one cases of FT performed in ten centres.[6] To our knowledge, other twenty cases of UET (twelve recipients received UET in China and other eight recipients worldwide) and nine cases of FT (one recipient in China and other eight cases worldwide) have been performed and not reported to the IRHCTT.

Donor selection and harvesting procedure for UET and FT

Up to now, UET and FT have always concerned deceased donors.[7] Living donation was never used in UET and FT although it has been suggested to be possible when the recipients are children because less extensive transplants would be used to replace wide defects of tissues.

Careful donor selection is of utmost importance to prevent the transmission of any unwanted disease. A more detailed work-up of the donor is essential in VCA than in solid organ donation as VCA are not life-saving transplants. Donors have to be well characterized with radiomorphometric studies and detailed determination of the vessel status.

On the basis of the IRHCTT,[6] UET donors were heart beating donors in 91.7% of cases, the median age was thirty-three years; there were five cases of unmatched sex; skin colour was matched in 81.3% of cases, and size in 84.4% of them. There were no cases of positive crossmatch in UET.

In 78.2% of cases, donor limbs were procured prior to other solid organs while in the remaining cases, they were procured after solid organs. The procurement level was at the elbow or the shoulder in hand and forearm transplantation or arm transplantation respectively. About 85.5% of the procured upper extremities were perfused and 94.6% of them were preserved in cold solution; University of Wisconsin solution was used for cold flush and limb preservation in 78.8% of cases, while in few cases IGL-1 solution (5 cases) and HTK solution (4 cases) have been used. Warm ischemia time ranged from 0 to 1200 minutes (median time being 63 min) while cold ischemia time ranged from 30 to 750 minutes (median time being 356 min). The warm ischemia time associated to vascular anastomosis (the time between the end of cold ischemia and the first arterial anastomosis) ranged from 60 to 3720 minutes (median time being 742 min).

Faces were procured prior to other solid organs in 68% of cases; the donors were heart beating donors in 82.1% of cases, and in 21.4% cases only the face was recovered. Donors' median age was 42 years (17–65); skin was matched in 86.2% of cases. The cross-match was always negative but in one case.

Duration of the procurement procedure ranged from 145 min to 1560 min (median time being 454 min). The grafts were perfused in 88.9% of cases and preserved in cold perfusion solution in 96.3% (University of Wisconsin solution, IGL-1 solution, Scott Solution and Celsior solution were used). Median warm ischemia time was 82 min (0–270 min) and median cold ischaemia time was 132 min (20 min–540 min).

Classic multi-organ procurement should not be compromised by limb or face recovery; life-saving solid organs have priority over life-enhancing VCA during procurement. No case of compromised solid organ transplantation due to limb/face retrieval has been reported. To date no standardized protocol has been established for limbs or face procurement, but some experiences have been documented.[7–10] In 78.2% and 70.8% of cases, limbs and faces were retrieved prior to other solid organs, respectively.[6] Coordinated and detailed algorithm for each individual case, planning each team's function, operating room arrangements, and harvesting order are required before starting the procedure.[8,10]

The information about the intended donors should be summarized in a technical sheet provided by the VCA team and should contain information on expected donor criteria (mainly morphologic) for the best donor-recipient matching. This information should be available to the procurement centres in order to facilitate donor detection and selection. Requesting consent for the donation of a limb or face may be quite different from requesting a life-saving organ as these are external and highly sensitive body parts whose removal may naturally provoke some reluctance. This underlines the need for dedicated coordinators, who are trained and confident as much as in the communication with relatives of potential donors. Transplant coordinators begin the interview and secure consent by discussing the possibility of solid organ donation before approaching the subject of other body parts.(2)

Restoration of the donor's external appearance and physical integrity using cosmetic prostheses or masks is mandatory and this information must be provided during the interview.

Recipient selection for UET and FT

Unilateral or bilateral amputees at different levels (wrist, proximal, mid, and distal forearm level and at elbow, distal, mid, and proximal arm level) are the candidates of UET (Figure 53.1). There are no definitive indications for UET recipients. The evaluation process is similar to that used for screening recipients in solid organ transplantation. Proper selection

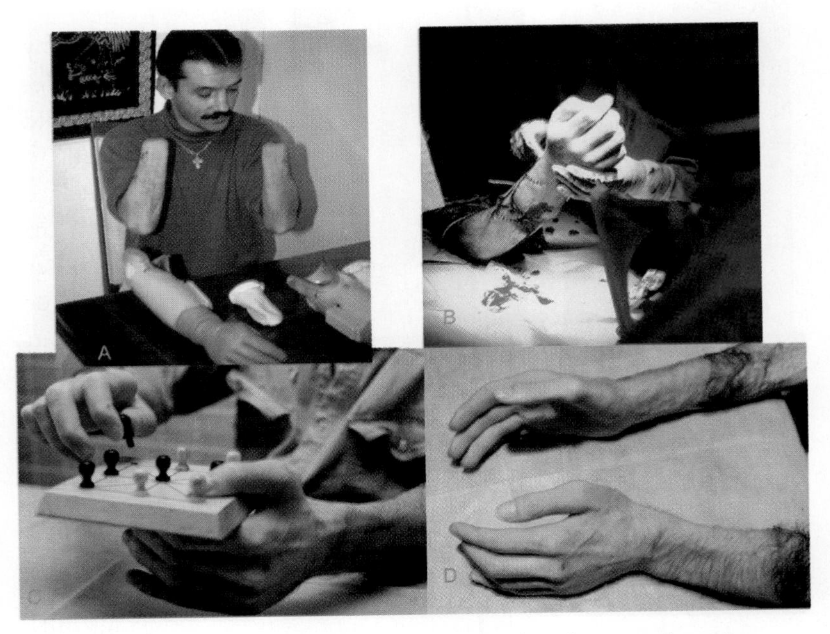

Figure 53.1A. The first case of bilateral UET before the transplantation; B. Transplantation of the UE; C. The recipient is performing a pinch grip with the grafted UE; D. Aspect of the grafted UE during the follow-up

is more critical in UET and in FT because they are not saving life transplants and are elective procedures.

Partial or total FT is considered when disfiguration affects more than two aesthetic units of the face or scalp[11] and other reconstructive procedures are not possible. Candidates to FT have severe disfiguration involving 'aesthetic' units, particularly those of the central part of the face (nose, upper and lower lips, chin, and tongue) as shown in Figure 53.2. The functional deficits are correlated with the units involved—blindness, impaired or impossible swallowing, oral eating and drinking difficulty, and slurred or unintelligible pronunciation. Many patients breathe through a tracheostomy and are fed via gastro- or jejuno-stomies.[12] The selection process must thoroughly examine the patient's overall physical health, emotional state, behavioural trends, and support structure eligibility before FT can be established. The complexity of this screening process requires a multidisciplinary team.

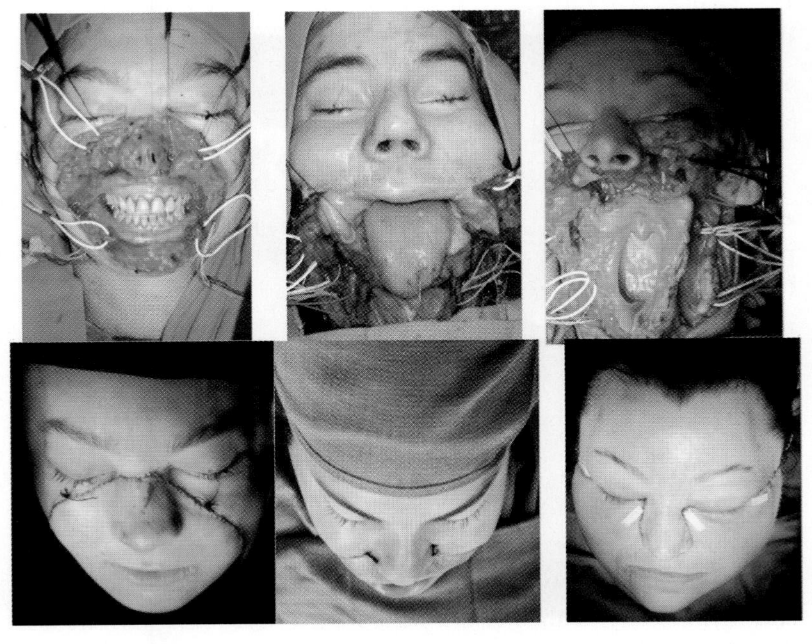

Figure 53.2. In the upper portion of the figure preparation of the recipients to the transplantation; in the lower portion the grafted faces immediately after the transplantation

Patients' compliance with the life-long immunosuppressive treatment and the long-lasting rehabilitation programme is the key to achieving a successful functional recovery in UET and in FT. Besides careful pre-transplant medical evaluation, including specific morphologic studies, and surgical and immunological evaluation, a pre-transplantation psychosocial assessment is considered crucial.[13] The patient's capacity to provide valid consent for VCA is a key element of the psychiatric evaluation. The patient must understand the risks of surgery, the risks of chronic immunosuppressive treatment, and the demand of rehabilitation during post-transplant life. It is important to know whether the candidate has realistic expectations about the transplant.[2]

Ongoing discussions with patients to ensure their understanding of the implications of proceeding with the surgery are needed during the pre-transplant visits. Candidates for UET should be offered rehabilitation treatment and alternative myoelectric prostheses before considering transplantation. Face transplant candidates should be thoroughly informed of all alternative surgical options for treating facial deformities or defects, as well as of psychological issues.

Upper extremities and face transplantations

As per the IRHCTT[6] seventy-three cases of UET have been reported, forty-three bilateral and thirty unilateral transplantations (twenty right and ten left cases). The majority of the recipients were men (80.8%), median age at the transplantation was thirty-five years. Three of them were quadruple amputees and two of them also required simultaneous FT. The level of amputation is usually distal (palmar, wrist, and distal forearm) but several arm transplants have also been performed.[14,15]

The principal causes of amputation are explosion, crush injury, electrocution, clean-cut lesions, and sepsis.[6,14,15]

In the large majority of patients, the induction therapy was based on anti-thymocyte globulins or alemtuzumab or basiliximab associated to tacrolimus, mycophenolate mofetil (MMF), and steroids; only 2% of the recipients received sirolimus in the first post-transplantation period.[6]

The maintenance therapy was based on tacrolimus (95.2%), MMF (91.9%), steroids (88.5%), and sirolimus (8.9%); during the follow-up there was steroid or/and MMF withdrawal in some cases and switch from tacrolimus to sirolimus in a group of patients to avoid anticalcineurin toxicity; while belatacept was introduced in few patients.[6]

Functional recovery was based on motion and sensitivity recovery (Figure 53.1). All transplanted patients reached protective sensation, 91% of them tactile sensation and 82% had a certain degree of discriminative sensation. Patients regained independence in daily activities, such as dressing, shaving, driving, riding motorcycles, writing, and some of them returned to work.[7,16]

The majority of UET recipients (87.8%) experienced acute rejection (AR) episodes (0 to 12; median 3) during the follow-up period ranging from four months to twenty years.[6] To date, 13.4% of the UET recipients have developed signs of chronic rejection and 6% of graft vasculopathy.[3,17]

Recipients of UET developed metabolic complications, opportunistic infections, and malignancies similarly to those reported after solid organ transplantation.[14,15,18] The IRHCTT reports a patient survival rate of 96.7% and a graft survival rate of 86.6% at ten years.[6]

On the basis of IRHCTT,[6,14] the majority of FT recipients were males; median age was 34 years (19–59). The causes of disfigurement were a trauma in 77.3% of cases with burn injury in 38.9%; congenital defect in 21.4% of cases, and tumour/malformation in 26.7% of cases. The majority of recipients (89.3%) experienced one or more surgical interventions before the transplantations.

The induction therapy included anti-thymocyte globulins (91.7%) or basiliximab (9.1%) associated to steroids in all patients (the intraoperative dose ranged from 70 to 2000 mg). The maintenance therapy included tacrolimus (100% of recipients), MMF (95.7%), and steroids (95.7%). In the follow-up, there was steroid withdrawal in several patients and switch from tacrolimus to sirolimus in few of them while in a patient the treatment also included belatacept.[6]

In FT[19,20] as well as in UET there was a high incidence of AR episodes, at least one episode of AR occurred in 72.7% of the recipients in the first post-transplant year. In this type of VCA, there was an involvement of skin and oral mucosa in the rejection process and the episodes, at first suspected by visual inspection, were later confirmed by histological evaluation of the skin and mucosal biopsies. The number of AR episodes experienced during the follow-up (from fifteen months to thirteen years) ranged from 0 to 9 (median number: 3). Banff VCA score was used to evaluate the severity of the rejection in UET and in FT.

Four cases of chronic rejection were reported to the IRHCTT[6] and one of the patients underwent face removal followed by re-transplantation. One transplant team reported signs of chronic rejection in seven face recipients.[21]

The aim of FT is to improve patient's quality of life, which is based on functional and aesthetic aspects of recovery. The functional recovery was based on recovery of discriminative sensibility, which was shown in 90% of recipients, and muscular tone with consequent motion recovery. Restoration of the expressive function was reported in all recipients after FT.[14,19,20,22] The daily activities, which were either difficult to be performed or not performed at all before transplantation, became possible or they were performed with less difficulty one year after FT. Activities included chewing, swallowing, eating, drinking, and speaking or smiling. Kissing and bowing showed more difficulty.[14,19,20,22]

The face transplant recipients were satisfied and the majority of them were 'very satisfied' with the new face which was considered 'new but own face'; the recipients improved the confidence in their personal appearance and felt well in a group. A total of 90% of recipients declared an improvement in their quality of life, although 50% required medical treatment for complications related to the transplantation.[6] The complications were similar to those reported in UET and in solid organ transplantation although the incidence of infectious complications and malignancies was higher in FT.[14]

The IRHCTT reports a patient survival rate of 89.9% at five years and 81.7% at ten years. Graft survival was 96,6% at five years and 80.5% at ten years.[6]

Uterus transplantation

Uterus transplant (UT) was first attempted in 2000 in Saudi Arabia with a living donor,[23] and in Turkey in 2011 with a deceased donor.[24] The first successful live birth following UT in 2014 from the Swedish group brought hope and renewed interest in the field.[25] The UT provides the only treatment for women suffering from absolute uterine factor infertility (AUFI). To date, more than fifty UT procedures have been performed worldwide.[26–29] These UT have resulted in more than ten newborns from living donors and recently, the first newborn after deceased donor uterine transplant.[25,29,30]

Presently, most of the clinical aspects relating to surgical techniques for both donor and recipient, monitoring of the recipient for acute cellular rejection and care during pregnancy are finding consistent answers in the ongoing controlled trials. The time of making UT clinical practice is approaching and the demand will depend on its cost and availability.

Recipient selection

The indication for UT is women who suffer from AUFI. The AUFI affects roughly 1/500 women and may be the result of congenital uterine agenesis (i.e. Mayer-Rokitansky-Kuster-Hauser syndrome) or from an acquired condition/surgically absent uterus.[31,32]

The AUFI was previously regarded as untreatable and surrogacy remained the only option for these women to have a genetically linked child. However, surrogacy is banned in many countries and raises its own set of ethical, legal, and financial dilemmas.[33] Publications have highlighted the considerable number of potential recipients seeking participation in UT clinical trials.[34,35] A deliberate, well-constructed screening and evaluation process needs to be implemented in any investigational study. A potential framework through pre-screening, screening, approval, in vitro fertilization, and ultimately uterine transplant for recipients are highlighted.

Pre-screening helps to inform interested recipients of the transplant process—existing alternatives, worldwide experience/outcomes, need for in-vitro fertilization, details of surgery, expectation for perioperative care, potential out of pocket expenses, and potential complications. Exclusion criteria will depend on institution/programme but will generally include an age cut off, BMI (limit 30–35), recent malignancy

(<5 years), or significant medical/obstetric comorbidities. Additional exclusion criteria may include single pelvic kidney, poor renal function and complicated vaginal reconstruction.

The screening process includes a complete medical workup. Existing work flows for living donor candidates and recipients of solid organ transplantation form the basis for the screening process in the UT. UT candidates meet with a multidisciplinary team of transplant surgeons, gynaecologists, obstetricians, psychologists, and transplant coordinators. Candidates undergo complete history and physical exams, blood tests, immunological testing, PAP smear, and viral/bacterial/fungal testing. A psychological evaluation focused on general psychological health, factors associated with infertility, and medication adherence is performed to identify and select the candidates.

Following the screening process candidates are presented at a multidisciplinary committee for approval. It is common practice to have the candidates undergo egg retrieval and fertilization prior to the transplant. The living donor uterus transplant can be then performed in a scheduled fashion or the candidate must await a suitable deceased donor.

Donor selection

The UT can utilize organs from both living and deceased donors. There is an ongoing ethical debate discussing whether living donor or deceased donor should be preferred.[36] From a donor supply point of view, if the demand for UT will grow as expected, it is foreseeable that neither donor type will suffice by itself and both will be required. From a clinical point of view, the living donor has the advantage of allowing a very meticulous work up while having the disadvantage of submitting a healthy person to surgery. On the other hand, still no clear consent pathways or listing practices are available for allowing uterus procurement from deceased organ donors.[37,38] Potential living donors are evaluated for age, BMI, PAP smear, HPV testing, complete history of physical, and HLA testing. Pelvic ultrasound is used to identify morphology of the uterus and to measure the uterus and endometrium. The Magnetic Resonance Angiography (MRA) and/or Computed tomography angiography (CTA) have been used to evaluate the pelvic vasculature, evaluate for atherosclerotic disease and map the arterial inflow and venous outflow. The MRA has been proven to be superior to the CTA in the visualization of the venous outflow, while CTA allows for a better visualization of the arteries.[26]

Living donors have been both, pre- and post-menopausal. The donors who are premenopausal must understand the consequences of undergoing the hysterectomy and must have decided to complete their family planning. The technique of the donor hysterectomy has been modified to preserve the ovaries in the donor avoiding any issues of early surgically induced menopause.[30]

Deceased donors unfortunately may suffer from a limited/incomplete obstetrical and gynaecological medical history. The evaluation of the vasculature is also limited due to timing and donor hospital capabilities. The logistics of the procurement operation may vary according to local practices and surgeon's preferences; the heart/lung/liver/pancreas/kidneys can be procured prior to the uterus or vice versa.[39] Further research is required to determine the tolerance of the uterus to cold ischemia and the answer to this question may facilitate the overall logistics of the transplant.[40,41]

Surgical considerations

Laparotomy is commonly used to perform the living donor operation but more recent attempts with laparoscopy and robotics have found favourable results.[42,43] For both deceased and living donor procurements, the key step is the proper dissection and retrieval of the vessels. The inflow given by the uterine arteries is secured by the dissection of the internal iliac artery. While in the deceased donor, the pedicle can comprise the entire main trunk of the internal iliac artery. In the living donor, care is taken to preserve the posterior trunk of the internal iliac artery. The venous outflow is represented by the uterine veins and the uterine segment of the ovarian veins. In the deceased donor, the entire ovarian vein can be dissected while in the pre-menopausal living donor the ovarian vein must be preserved. Another significant difference is the absolute need to avoid any injury to the ureter in the living donor, while in deceased donor it can be severed prior to its passage between the uterine vascular pedicle and the body of the uterus. When the uterus is procured after the other abdominal and thoracic organs, the preservation solution must be delivered either through the femoral vessels or in an ante grade fashion through the aortic cannula. When the uterus is procured prior to the other organs, it can be perfused in isolation on the back table as in the living donor operation.

The recipient operation begins with a lower midline laparotomy exposure of the bilateral external iliac arteries and veins and preparation of the vault of the vagina that needs to be dissected out from the bladder and rectum. The uterine artery is anastomosed in end to side fashion taking advantage of larger orifice offered by the donor internal iliac artery stump. The venous outflow is constructed on the best available vein, be it the uterine or the utero-ovarian vein. Following reperfusion, the vaginal cuff of the uterus graft is anastomosed to the recipient's vagina. The uterus is then fixated to the round/sacrouterine

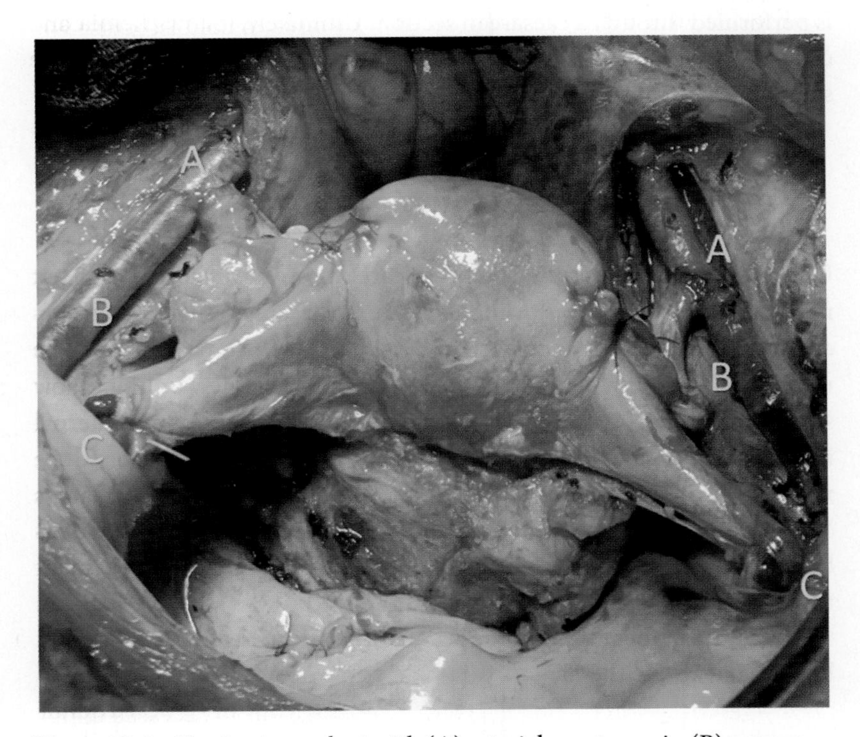

Figure 53.3. Uterine transplant with (A) arterial anastomosis, (B) venous anastomosis, and (C) pelvic fixation

ligament, paravaginal connective tissue, and the bladder peritoneum (Figure 53.3).

Follow-up and outcomes

Perioperative and postoperative care is focused on early recognition of vascular compromise and rejections. Ultrasounds are used in the perioperative period to monitor appropriate flow. Patients receive thymoglobulin for induction and are maintained on tacrolimus and either azathioprine or MMF. Monitoring for acute cellular rejection is done with protocol cervical biopsies. The timing of embryo implantation has been shortened to around 5–6 months after the transplantation with the aim of decreasing the time the recipient is exposed to the immunosuppressive therapy.[30] With successful implantation pregnancy, the delivery is performed through a caesarean section. Ultimately, following the conclusion of child bearing, the uterus is removed and the immunosuppressants are withdrawn.

Conclusion

UET can be considered as 'standard' care for strictly selected patients managed in expert centres. Although the encouraging results in aesthetic and functional recovery achieved in FT, the risk/benefit balance remains uncertain. The future for all types of VCA relies upon new immunologic strategies to limit the heavy burden of current immunosuppressive regimens. In addition, the paucity of donors contributes to the slow development of the programmes.

The great development of uterus transplantation in this last decade is based on the possibility to have living or deceased donors and to discontinue the immunosuppression following child's birth.

The future of these transplants is not only correlated to the risk/benefit balance but also to their cost.

Highlights

- VCA means transplantation of a vascularized human body part containing multiple tissue types as an anatomical and/or structural unit from a human donor to a human recipient.
- Up to now in upper extremity (UET) and in face (FT) transplantations, the donors were always deceased donors. Unilateral or bilateral amputees at different levels (wrist, proximal, mid, and distal forearm level; and at elbow, distal, mid, and proximal arm level) are the candidates of UET. Partial or total FT is considered when disfiguration affects more than two aesthetic units of the face or scalp and other reconstructive procedures are not possible.
- UET and in FT are not saving life transplants. Their aim is to improve the patient's quality of life, which is based on functional recovery in UET and on functional and aesthetic aspect recovery in FT.
- UT can utilize organs from both living and deceased donors. The indication for UT is women who suffer from AUFI.
- The final goal of UT is a successful live birth.

References

1. Organ Procurement and Transplantation Network. A Proposed Rule by the Health and Human Services Department on 12/16/2011. Federal Register 2011; 76(242). Available at: https://www.federalregister.gov/documents/2011/12/16/2011-32204/organ-procurement-and-transplantation-network.
2. Thuong M, Petruzzo P, Landin L, Mahillo B, Kay S, Testelin S, Jablecki J, Laouabdia-Sellami K, Lopez-Fraga M, Dominguez-Gil B. Vascularized composite allotransplantation—a Council of Europe position paper. Transpl Int. 2019 Mar;32(3):233–240.
3. Ng ZY, Lellouch AG, Rosales IA, Geoghegan L, Gama AR, Colvin RB, Lantieri LA, Randolph MA, Cetrulo CL Jr. Graft vasculopathy of vascularized composite allografts in humans: A literature review and retrospective study. Transpl Int. 2019; 32:831–838.
4. Dubernard JM, Owen ER, Herzberg G, Lanzetta M, Martin X, Kapila H, Dawahra M, Hakim N. Human hand allograft: Report on first 6 months. Lancet 1999; 353:1315–1320.
5. Devauchelle B, Badet L, Lengelé B, Morelon E, Testelin S, Michallet M, D'Hauthuille C, Dubernard JM. First human face allograft: Early report. Lancet. 2006 Jul 15;368(9531):203–209.

6. International Registry on Hand and Composite Tissue Transplantation – IRHCTT. www.handregistry.com [Accessed January 31, 2019]
Sosin M, Rodriguez ED. The Face Transplantation Update: 2016. Plast Reconstr Surg 2016; 137: 1841.
7. Pomahac B, Alhefzi M, Bueno EM, McDiarmid SV, Levin LS. Living Donation of Vascularized Composite Allografts. Plast Reconstr Surg. 2018 Sep;142(3):405e–411e.
8. Organ Procurement and Transplantation Network. *OPO guidance on VCA deceased donor authorization*. Available from: https://optn.transplant.hrsa.gov/resources/guidance/opo-guidance-on-vca-deceased-donor-authorization. [Accessed 15 June 2017].
9. Datta N, Yersiz H, Kaldas F, Azari K. Procurement strategies for combined multiorgan and composite tissues for transplantation. Curr Opin Organ Transplant 2015; 20: 121.
10. Brazio PS, Barth RN, Bojovic B, Dorafshar AH, Garcia JP, Brown EN et al. Algorithm for total face and multiorgan procurement from a brain-dead donor. Am J Transplant 2013; 13: 2743.
11. Siemionow MZ, Papay F, Djohan R, Bernard S, Gordon CR, Alam D et al. First U.S. near-total human face transplantation: a paradigm shift for massive complex injuries. Plast Reconstr Surg 2010; 125:111.
12. Cavadas PC, Landin L, Ibañez J, Thione A, Rodrigo J, Castro F et al. The Spanish Experience With Face Transplantation. In: Siemionow MZ, ed. The Know-How of Face Transplantation. London: Springer London; 2011:351.
13. Jowsey-Gregoire SG, Kumnig M, Morelon E, Moreno E, Petruzzo P, Seulin C. The Chauvet 2014 Meeting Report: Psychiatric and Psychosocial Evaluation and Outcomes of Upper Extremity Grafted Patients. Transplantation 2016; 100: 1453.
14. Petruzzo P, Sardu C, Lanzetta M, Dubernard JM. Report (2017) of the International Registry on Hand and Composite Allotransplantation (IRHCTT). Current transplantation Reports 2017; 4: 294–303.
15. Shores JT, Brandacher G, Lee WP. Hand and upper extremity transplantation: an update of outcomes in the worldwide experience. Plast Reconstr Surg 2015; 135: 351e.
16. Shores JT, Malek V, Andrew Lee WP and Brandacher G. Outcomes after hand and upper extremity transplantation. J Mater Sci Mater Med 2017; 28: 72.
17. Kanitakis J, Petruzzo P, Badet L, Gazarian A, Thaunat O, Testelin S et al. Chronic Rejection in Human Vascularized Composite Allotransplantation (Hand and Face Recipients): An Update. Transplantation 2016; 100: 2053.
18. Conrad A, Petruzzo P, Kanitakis J, Gazarian A, Badet L, Thaunat O, Vanhems P, Buron F, Morelon E, Sicard A; DIVAT consortium and the IRHCTT teams. Infections after upper extremity allotransplantation: a worldwide population cohort study, 1998–2017. Transpl Int. 2019 Jan 11.
19. Lantieri L, Grimbert P, Ortonne N, Suberbielle C, Bories D, Gil-Vernet S et al. Face transplant: long-term follow-up and results of a prospective open study. Lancet 2016; 388:1398.
20. Sosin M, Rodriguez ED. The Face Transplantation Update: 2016. Plast Reconstr Surg 2016; 137: 1841–1850.

21. Krezdorn N, Lian CG, Wells M, Wo L, Tasigiorgos S, Xu S, Borges TJ, Frierson RM, Stanek E, Riella LV, Pomahac B, Murphy GF. Chronic rejection of human face allografts. Am J Transplant. 2019 Apr;19(4):1168–1177.
22. Fischer S, Kueckelhaus M, Pauzenberger R, Bueno EM, Pomahac B. Functional outcomes of face transplantation. Am J Transplant 2015; 15:220.
23. Fageeh W, Raffa H, Jabbad H, Marzouki A. Transplantation of the human uterus. Int J Gynaecol Obstet 2002 Mar;76(3):245–251.
24. Ozkan O, Akar M, Ozkan O, Erdogan O, Hadimioglu N, Yilmaz M et al. Preliminary results of the first human uterus transplantation from a multiorgan donor. Fertility and Sterility. 2013;99(2):470–476.e5.
25. Brännström M, Johannesson L, Bokström H, Kvarnström N, Mölne J, Dahm-Kähler P et al. Livebirth after uterus transplantation. The Lancet. 2015;385(9968):607–616.
26. Testa G, Koon E, Johannesson L, McKenna G, Anthony T, Klintmalm G et al. Living Donor Uterus Transplantation: A Single Center's Observations and Lessons Learned From Early Setbacks to Technical Success. American Journal of Transplantation. 2017;17(11):2901–2910.
27. Brännström M, Johannesson L, Dahm-Kähler P, Enskog A, Mölne J, Kvarnström N et al. First clinical uterus transplantation trial: A six-month report. Fertility and Sterility. 2014;101(5):1228–1236.
28. Chmel R, Novackova M, Janousek L, Matecha J, Pastor Z, Maluskova J et al. Revaluation and lessons learned from the first 9 cases of a Czech uterus transplantation trial: Four deceased donor and 5 living donor uterus transplantations. American Journal of Transplantation. 2018;19(3):855–864.
29. Ejzenberg D, Andraus W, Baratelli Carelli Mendes L, Ducatti L, Song A, Tanigawa R et al. Livebirth after uterus transplantation from a deceased donor in a recipient with uterine infertility. The Lancet. 2018;392(10165):2697–2704.
30. Testa G, McKenna G, Gunby R, Anthony T, Koon E, Warren A et al. First live birth after uterus transplantation in the United States. American Journal of Transplantation. 2018;18(5):1270–1274.
31. Morcel K, Camborieux L, Guerrier D. Mayer-Rokitansky-Küster-Hauser (MRKH) syndrome. Orphanet Journal of Rare Diseases. 2007;2(1):13.
32. Hammer A, Rositch A, Kahlert J, Gravitt P, Blaakaer J, Søgaard M. Global epidemiology of hysterectomy: possible impact on gynecological cancer rates. American Journal of Obstetrics and Gynecology. 2015;213(1):23–29.
33. Robertson J. Other women's wombs: Uterus transplants and gestational surrogacy. Journal of Law and the Biosciences. 2016;3(1):68–86.
34. Johannesson L, Wallis K, Koon E, McKenna G, Anthony T, Leffingwell S et al. Living uterus donation and transplantation: Experience of interest and screening in a single center in the United States. American Journal of Obstetrics and Gynecology. 2018;218(3):331.e1–331.e7.
35. Taran F, Schöller D, Rall K, Nadalin S, Königsrainer A, Henes M et al. Screening and evaluation of potential recipients and donors for living donor uterus transplantation: Results from a single-center observational study. Fertility and Sterility. 2019;111(1):186–193.
36. Bruno B, Arora K. Uterus Transplantation: The Ethics of Using Deceased Versus Living Donors. The American Journal of Bioethics. 2018;18(7):6–15.

37. Wall A, Testa G. Living Donation, Listing, and Prioritization in Uterus Transplantation. The American Journal of Bioethics. 2018;18(7):20–22.
38. Lavoué V, Vigneau C, Duros S, Boudjema K, Levêque J, Piver P et al. Which Donor for Uterus Transplants. Transplantation. 2017;101(2):267–273.
39. Testa G, Anthony T, McKenna G, Koon E, Wallis K, Klintmalm G et al. Deceased donor uterus retrieval: A novel technique and workflow. American Journal of Transplantation. 2017;18(3):679–683.
40. Stega J, Smith J, Sieunarine K, Ungar L, Del Priore G. Human Uterus Retrieval From a Multiorgan Donor. Obstetrics & Gynecology. 2007;109(6):1459.
41. Tardieu A, Dion L, Lavoué V, Chazelas P, Marquet P, Piver P et al. The Key Role of Warm and Cold Ischemia in Uterus Transplantation: A Review. Journal of Clinical Medicine. 2019;8(6):760.
42. Puntambekar S, Puntambekar S, Nanda S, Parikh K, Zainab B. Laparoscopy Assisted Live-Donor Uterine Transplant. Journal of Minimally Invasive Gynecology. 2018;25(7):S178.
43. Wei L, Xue T, Tao K, Zhang G, Zhao G, Yu S et al. Modified human uterus transplantation using ovarian veins for venous drainage: the first report of surgically successful robotic-assisted uterus procurement and follow-up for 12 months. Fertility and Sterility. 2017;108(2):346–356.e1.

54

Extra-corporeal life support as a bridge to transplantation

Matteo Di Nardo, Edoardo Piervincenzi, Francesco Pugliese, Juglans Alvarez, Lorenzo Del Sorbo

Introduction

In the last five years, the thoracic organ transplant registry of the International Society of Heart and Lung Transplantation (ISHLT) recorded more than 4000 lung transplants (LTx) and more than 5500 heart transplants (HTx) per year.[1,2]

The availability of transplantable organs has been constantly increasing since the expansion of the donor pool including donation after cardiac death, transplantation across blood groups in children, and with the availability of new assessment technologies, such as ex-vivo perfusion. Simultaneously, the number of patients requiring lungs or heart transplantation has also grown over the years. Thus, there is always an unmet need of organs, leading to the progressive clinical deterioration of patients on the waiting list, which carries the risk of a high mortality rate ranging around 20% for both LTx and HTx patients.[2,3]

Extracorporeal life support (ECLS) as a bridge to transplant has been successfully used for patients waiting for lung as well as for heart transplantation. Due to the different pathophysiologic features associated with these conditions (chronic respiratory failure and chronic heart failure), bridging with extracorporeal membrane oxygenation (ECMO) is more common for LTx than for HTx. The bridge to HTX is mainly performed with the use of ventricular assist devices (VADs) and ECMO is considered as a 'bridge to decision' technique. Thus, these two ways of bridging will be treated separately.

ECLS as a bridge to lung transplantation

Several comprehensive strategies have been developed to decrease the high mortality rate on the LTx waiting list. These can be grouped as strategies to increase the lung donor pool and strategies of artificial life support as a 'bridge to LTx' (BTLT), including mechanical ventilation and ECLS, which will be reviewed and discussed in this chapter.

BTLT, therefore, refers to strategies to artificially support the vital functions of LTx candidates until a suitable organ becomes available.

Goals of bridge to transplant

Ideally, the two overall goals of strategies applied to bridge patients with end-stage lung disease and acute clinical deterioration to lung transplantation are (1) to prolong the pre-transplant life expectancy, thus increasing the chances to receive a lung transplant, and (2) to preserve the likelihood of a good post-transplant outcome by maintaining pre-transplant clinical stability.

Several techniques have been applied and evaluated as BTLT, including non-invasive mechanical (NIV), invasive mechanical ventilation (IMV), and ECLS. NIV has shown to be often not sufficient to support the respiratory function of patients with worsening end-stage lung disease.[4] IMV, although more efficacious in maintaining adequate gas exchange, carries considerable side effects, including sedation requirements, ventilator-associated pneumonia, ventilator-diaphragmatic dysfunction, and ventilator-induced lung injury. Pre-transplant patients treated with IMV have a considerably higher risk mortality than similar patients not ventilated.[5]

Thus, both NIV and IMV may not be appreciated as optimal BTLT strategies. Nevertheless, important limitations in the studies on this topic need to be recognized. First, most of the data are generated from case reports and observational investigations, as no randomized clinical trials have been performed on this issue. Second, the mortality of pre-transplant patients obviously increases with the level of respiratory support required. Third, the clinical application of NIV and IMV has remarkably improved over the past decades, and the clinical impact of the side effects of these strategies may have changed.

ECLS, conversely, can potentially provide an appropriate mode and intensity of cardio-pulmonary support tailored to the physiologic requirement of each patient, and theoretically allows patients to be less sedated, more mobile, and interactive. Hence, based on these features, and the considerable reduction in the potential mechanical, infective and bleeding complications due to substantial technological advancements, ECLS is regarded as the best current potential means to meet the goals of an optimal BTLT strategy.[6–11]

Ethical issues with ECLS as bridge to lung transplantation

The application of ECLS as BTLT remains ethically controversial. In addition to the historically poor outcomes, the main controversy stems from the fact that patients requiring BTLT are the ones with the largest perioperative resources utilization and the highest risk of perioperative mortality.

Due to the scarcity of donor lungs, it has been questioned whether it is ethically acceptable to utilize such a precious resource of a donor lung into a patient with the poorest prognosis among all candidates in the waiting list. Although the overall goal is to improve the prognosis of patients with end-stage respiratory failure, there is a dramatic risk of considerably worsening the outcome of lung transplantation by selecting the sickest recipients, without necessarily improving survival in the transplant waiting list.[5,12]

In clinical practice, these challenging concerns must be weighed for every single case, as the benefit from receiving LTx is likely higher in patients requiring advanced means of life support. Therefore, the good outcome of any clinical programme providing BTLT relies on the careful identification of inclusion and exclusion criteria, ECLS configuration, and issues in the daily clinical management, which will be discussed in the sections—Indications of ECLS as a bridge to lung transplantation, ECLS Circuit configurations, Patient management.[6,9] This process requires a multidisciplinary effort, involving surgeons, intensivists, and pulmonologists, and needs to be tailored to the specific features and capability of each centre. In addition, a continuous re-evaluation of risks, benefits, and outcomes of BTLT strategies is critical and must mirror the dynamic development of technology, improvement in critical care delivery, and LTx outcomes in each centre.

Another substantial ethical issue prompted in several patients bridged to LTx with ECLS is the end-of-life management, including potential discussion with patients and their family about withholding or withdrawal of life-sustaining treatments.[13,14] The process may particularly be challenging for this patient population, focused on the perspective of receiving LTx, for which they may become unsuitable due to progressive clinical deterioration and failure of the BTLT strategy. Transparency and consistency in the clinical decision-making process, granted by sharing the careful multidisciplinary definition of inclusion and exclusion criteria in each LTx centre, is one of the key factors in addressing this ethical challenge.

Indications of ECLS as bridge to lung transplantation

The decision to offer ECLS as BTLT results from the multidisciplinary evaluation of risks and benefits on a case-to-case basis. Clinical status, surgical and technical issues, risk of infection, bleeding diathesis, and functional status are some of the parameters considered during the evaluation.

Moreover, this evaluation needs to be clearly communicated to the patient, whenever possible, and the family to make them aware of the goals and potential complications, which may preclude the success of the BTLT strategy. Possibilities and methods of interruption of ECLS with the occurrence of irreversible exit conditions from the transplant list such as irreversible shock and neurological catastrophes may also be discussed with the patient. There are no high-grade evidence-based guidelines to help in this decision-making process; hence it is mainly based on consensus and expert opinion.

In 2015, the ISHLT, with a consensus document, proposed the general criteria to consider eligibility of patients with deteriorating gas exchange and/or severe pulmonary hypertension to be bridged to LTx with ECLS.

According to this document, ECLS is recommended as BTLT for candidates with:

- Young age
- Absence of multiple-organ dysfunction
- Good potential for rehabilitation

On the other hand, ECLS is not recommended as BTLT for candidates with:

- Septic shock
- Multi-organ dysfunction
- Severe arterial occlusive disease
- Heparin-induced thrombocytopenia
- Prior prolonged mechanical ventilation
- Advanced age.
- Obesity.

Specific criteria for the evaluation of risks and benefits of ECLS as BTLT may vary in each centre, as many different factors, including number of patients on the waiting list and volume of lung transplants, which may change outcome of BTLT strategies.[5–9] Indeed, appropriate patient selection and timing for ECLS initiation remain the crucial aspects to optimize its outcome as BTLT.[6–11]

ECLS Circuit configurations

The ECLS system is composed of the assembly of a membrane oxygenator, a pump, and tubing circuits. Considerable technological advancements have become available in the last two decades and contributed to the reduction of ECLS related complications, and hence to the broad clinical application of this advanced means of life support. These technological innovations include the development of more efficient membrane oxygenators, centrifugal pumps, and heparin-coated circuits.

The ECLS systems can be configured in different ways based on the site of blood drainage, the site of blood return, the blood flow, and the presence or absence of a pump. The possible ECLS configurations as BTLT are described in Table 54.1. The choice of the ECLS configuration as BTLT

Table 54.1 ECLS configuration characteristics for BTLT

	ECLS configuration characteristics for BTLT						
	ECCO2R	**VV**	**VV+AS**	**VA femoral**	**VA Subclavian**	**V-VA**	**PA-LA**
Effect on gas exchange	efficient for CO_2 removal no effect on oxygenation	good	good	lower body: good upper body: variable	Good	good	good
Effect on RV function	very modest	modest	partial	good	Good	good	good
Effect on pulmonary arterial pressure	very modest	modest	partial	good	Good	good	good
Possibility of mobilization	good	good	good	modest	Good	modest	good
Other limitations	/	/	AS requires surgical repair	potential reduction of lower limb perfusion	limited durability		requires thoracotomy

Abbreviations: ECCO2R: extracorporeal carbon dioxide removal; VV: veno-venous ECMO; AS: atrial septostomy; VA: veno-arterial; PA-LA: Pulmonary artery-Left atrium shunt.

must be carefully evaluated and tailored according to the patient`s physiologic needs and clinical goals. Moreover, the configuration can change according to the patient clinical evolution.

Hypercapnic respiratory failure

Patients with refractory hypercapnic respiratory failure and respiratory acidosis awaiting LTx, usually diagnosed with cystic fibrosis or chronic obstructive pulmonary disease, without clinically significant hypoxemia or pulmonary hypertension can be managed with extracorporeal CO_2 removal ($ECCO_2R$).[6,9,15,16] Due to the high solubility of CO_2 and the high permeability of the ECLS membrane to CO_2, the blood flow required for clinical effective $ECCO_2R$ is below 1 L/min.[6,9] This flow rate is achieved in systems with veno-venous configuration through the action of a pump and delivered through a relatively small double lumen catheter, usually inserted in the internal jugular or subclavian vein to allow for active mobilization.

Alternatively, artero-venous pumpless circuits, providing blood flow through the blood pressure gradient between femoral artery and femoral vein have been used. This specific system has been progressively less applied for $ECCO_2R$, given the rate of complications secondary to the femoral artery cannulation.[6] The development of hypoxemia during $ECCO_2R$, due to derecruitment or change in the respiratory quotient, has been described[6,9] and, warrant in specific cases, the switch to veno-venous extracorporeal membrane oxygenation (VV-ECMO).

Hypoxemic respiratory failure

Lung transplant candidates who develop severe hypoxemia without substantial hemodynamic instability can be managed with VV-ECMO.[6–11] Improvement of oxygenation during ECLS depends on extracorporeal blood flow rate, therefore high blood flow is usually required in hypoxemic pre-transplant patients to maintain adequate gas exchange. High blood flow can be achieved with VV-ECMO, which can be deployed cannulating the femoral vein for blood drainage (generally 22–25 Fr cannula) and the internal jugular vein for reinfusion (generally 17–22 Fr cannula). Alternately, both femoral veins can be cannulated.[17] Although this cannulation can be done without radiologic guidance in an emergent situation, generally it prevents patients from being ambulatory.

A more effective strategy to facilitate early mobilization is the use of single site insertion of a bicaval dual lumen cannula. Even though these cannulas have been traditionally used to cannulate the right internal jugular vein, the left internal jugular or right subclavian vein cannulation has been successfully performed when the right internal jugular vein was not accessible.[18]

Respiratory failure and hemodynamic compromise

For patients with respiratory failure and hemodynamic compromise due to RV failure, ECMO in veno-arterial configuration (VA-ECMO) is the recommended option because it provides both cardiac and lung support. The initial experience with ECLS as BTLT employed this mode.[9] Usually a femoral vein is cannulated for drainage and a femoral artery is cannulated for blood return.

Recently, Chichotka et al.[19] reported their experience of ECMO as a BTLT in patients with interstitial lung disease and pulmonary hypertension. The VA-ECMO showed a higher survival rate compared to VV-ECMO. The same authors also reported that the conversion rate of VV-ECMO to VA-ECMO was higher especially when patients deteriorate (e.g. intolerance to physical exercise, increasing in the pulmonary pressure or worsening of the right heart function). The development of right heart dysfunction leads to an insufficient oxygen delivery and multiorgan failure, which if not managed properly, can increase the mortality.

During VA-ECMO with femo-femoral configuration, the fully oxygenated blood from the ECMO circuit is delivered in the distal aorta in retrograde direction and mixes with the forward blood flow ejected from the heart. The portion of the aorta where this admixture occurs depends on the heart function and ECMO settings. The fully oxygenated blood from the ECMO circuit preferentially perfuses the lower extremities and the abdominal viscera, whereas the blood flow generated by the heart may perfuse the coronaries, the brain and the upper extremities, as the blood supply to these areas is from the aortic arch. Therefore, if the lung function is severely compromised, cardiac and cerebral hypoxia may develop and remain unrecognized if oxygenation is not properly monitored on the right upper extremity of the patient. Cerebral tissue hypoxia should be promptly reversed by means of IMV or by increasing the blood flow through the ECLS circuit. Another option to improve oxygenation of the blood ejected by the heart is to convert the circuit into a hybrid V (femoral vein for blood drainage)-VA (jugular vein and femoral artery for blood return) ECLS, by inserting an additional cannula into the internal jugular vein.[6,9,20]

Thus, it is important to choose adequate size cannulas and a versatile ECMO configuration to guarantee adequate life support according to the physiologic need, which may change over time. Unfortunately, this cannot always be adequately performed in the paediatric population due to small vessels size.

Pulmonary hypertension and right ventricular failure

In patients with severe pulmonary hypertension with right heart impairment, VA-ECMO is used to unload the right ventricle and improve organ perfusion.[9]

In addition to the VA-ECMO configuration, there are other ECLS strategies to manage patients with severe pulmonary hypertension. Camboni et al.[23] and Kon et al.[24] used an atrial septostomy in combination with VV-ECMO performed with a dual lumen cannula to overcome the desaturation resulting from the artificial right-to-left shunt. This strategy, however, presents some limits, including the maintenance of an adequate cannula position, and the creation of a large atrial septostomy, which needs to be surgically reversed during the LTx surgery.[11]

Strueber et al.[21] developed an alternative approach for these patients with the connection of a low-resistance gas exchange device (Novalung; Novalung, Heilbronn, Germany) between the main trunk of the pulmonary artery and the left atrium, the so-called PA-LA ECLS, which creates an effective oxygenating shunt that unloads the right ventricle much like an atrial septostomy. The elevated pressure in the pulmonary arteries serves as the driving force for the device and obviates the need for a pump. The advantage of this approach is that the membrane oxygenates the blood and thus the central hypoxemia seen with a simple septostomy is avoided. More importantly, PA-LA ECLS easily allows extubation, rehabilitation, and ambulation. Eight successful cases have been reported using this technique to bridge patients with pulmonary hypertension to LTx.[22] Of note, in most cases, heart-lung transplantation is not required because the unloaded right ventricle recovers on this ECLS configuration, and bilateral LTx provides ongoing remodelling and recovery of the right heart. Recently, the Vienna Lung Transplant programme has introduced the implantation of the PA-LA ECLS through a muscle-sparing left-sided anterolateral thoracotomy. This approach seems to favour the awake ambulatory setting.[7–11]

Patient management

The management of patients with end-stage respiratory disease awaiting LTx and experiencing an acute deterioration warranting ECLS is very complex.

While the immediate goal after ECLS deployment is recovery from the acute decompensation, the ultimate purpose of ECLS as a BTLT is to maintain suitability for transplantation. The management of each patient should, therefore, be personalized and based on each individual's physiologic needs, while preventing the potential ECLS related complications. In selected rare cases, ECLS can also be applied to recondition and improve the clinical conditions of transplant candidates rather than to only maintain clinical stability preventing further clinical deterioration.[6–11]

Team effort is required to optimize the management of patients on ECLS awaiting transplant. All the personnel involved in the care of BTLT patients require specific expertise and training in both LTx and ECLS. The personnel generally include surgeons, pulmonologists, intensivists, palliative care physicians, psychiatrists, nurses, physiotherapists, nutritionists, pharmacists, social workers, and spiritual care providers.

The complexity of these patients requires their management to be performed in the intensive care unit for feasibility and safety issues. Parameters of organ function need to be frequently monitored as the clinical conditions and the efficiency of the ECLS equipment may rapidly change. Adequate position and functioning of the ECLS circuit need to be regularly confirmed. The skin at the ECLS cannula insertion sites and the limbs need careful monitoring for potential complications, especially bleeding, infection, and inadequate perfusion.

In order to avoid a critical deterioration in neuromuscular and functional condition and prevent the occurrence of ICU acquired weakness, which may compromise the outcome of these patients, particular attention has been given to the management of mechanical ventilation during ECLS as a BTLT. Given the capability of effectively replacing pulmonary function, in BTLT patients ECLS and ECMO in particular is often considered as an alternative strategy rather than an adjunct to IMV. Safe removal of mechanical ventilation allows the potential avoidance of its side effects, including sedation requirement, poor mobility, ventilator-associated pneumonia, and ventilator-induced lung injury.[6,9,10,17,25,26] This approach has been recently defined as 'awake ECMO', which is nevertheless incomplete and it would be better defined as 'active ECMO'. Without the need of sedation, not only the patients are alert and able to interact and communicate their needs, but also they tolerate physical conditioning exercises and meet their caloric needs in a better way.

However, the 'awake ECMO' is not the ideal option for all patients. Some patients, in fact, have uncomfortable respiratory distress despite full ECMO support, related to the severity of lung injury and the abundance of secretions, cough, and anxiety. In these patients, requiring IMV in addition to ECLS, an early tracheostomy is a good option to ensure optimal airway clearance and reduce the sedation requirements. The 'awake ECMO' also requires adequate spaces and healthcare personnel dedicated to the patient's nursing, rehabilitation, and psychological support.[9,11]

Anticoagulation requires a protocolized management to prevent bleeding or thrombotic complications, whose incidence varies according to the ECLS configuration, blood flow rate and patient characteristics. The use of low level of anticoagulation is generally maintained in patients with VV-ECMO to avoid the risk of bleeding events. However, for ECLS configurations with arterial cannulation is mandatory to increase the level of anticoagulation to reduce the risk of thromboembolic complications.[25]

A conservative transfusion policy is generally used. High lung transplant volume centres suggest to transfuse packed red blood cells only if the haemoglobin level is lower than 7 g/dl or if the patient remains severely hypoxemic ($SpO2<92\%$) despite maximal ECLS support. Unless anaemia impacts on hemodynamics, organs function, or physical therapy, the transfusions are restricted to reduce the risk of generating donor-specific antibodies that may ultimately affect the outcome of the transplant severely.[9–25]

Appropriate nutritional support and physical active rehabilitation are one of the highest priorities, as a poor pre-transplant functional status is associated with worse post-transplant outcomes.[6,9,25]

Outcomes of ECLS as bridge to lung transplantation

The outcome of patients bridged to LTx using ECLS has improved in the recent years and can be regarded as satisfactory considering the severity of their diseases and the overall survival of LTx recipients.[6]

Survival during BTLT is affected by several complications related to the use of ECLS. The most common complications during BTLT are: haemolysis, bleeding at cannulation site, sepsis (typically from pneumonia or catheter site infection), disseminated intravascular coagulation, acute renal failure, and neurological injuries.[6,27,28]

A review from the United Network for Organ Sharing (UNOS) experience totalling fifty-one subjects bridged to LTx from 1987 to 2008 using ECLS showed a 1-, 6-, 12-, and 24-month survival of 72%, 53%, 50%, and 45%, compared with 93%, 85%, 79%, and 70% for unsupported patients, respectively.[29]

However, the most recent reports in 2018–2019 from experienced centres in both LTx and ECLS have shown that approximately 80% of patients can be successfully bridged to LTx, and the outcomes after LTx in the BTLT patients are close to the ones who received LTx without BTLT.[6,9,11,30–32]

Extra-corporeal life support as a bridge to heart transplantation

Heart transplantation still holds the seat as a gold standard therapy for end-stage heart failure refractory to medical management.[33] It relies on careful selection of recipients and donors, as the worldwide reality is the scarce availability of donated hearts suitable for transplantation.

Although cardiac ECLS has an important role in the management of acute cardiogenic shock, bridging patients from this modality directly to heart transplantation has not been the prevalent strategy.[34] More frequently, VA-ECMO has been used as a rescue therapy in scenarios of acute cardiogenic shock or acute severely decompensated heart failure (Intermacs 1 and 2 group of patients). After achieving the goal of stabilization on support, usually, these patients will undergo additional evaluation regarding transplant eligibility, which integrates clinical, social, and psychological assessments. If they are deemed acceptable for transplant, most frequently a subsequent bridge to transplantation with more prolonged support via paracorporeal or implantable VADs is pursued.

However, there is a niche where heart transplants directly from VA-ECMO support can be implemented as a safe option. In high volume/high performance centres, where teams are familiar with the ECLS therapy, fast track eligibility for transplant is available, and a short time in the waiting list can be expected; ECLS bridging to heart transplant can be an alternative. For instance, patients already listed becoming acutely decompensated, with low level or no sensitization, average size and weight, blood groups A, B, AB characterize a specific subgroup where ECLS could be the bridge for a transplant. Another example would be a newcomer patient with the before mentioned matching profile that fully recovered from a cardiogenic shock, has the work up done on support within a few days and gets listed on a high status; if an offer does not materialize in a short time, bridging with more permanent devices would be the next step.

As centres gain experience and familiarity with rehabilitation strategies (e.g. ambulating patients on VA ECMO)[35] while maintaining safe and excellent results with this therapy, more frequent utilization of VA-ECMO as modality of bridging is anticipated. In addition, as prolonged VA-ECMO runs of few weeks become safer with improvement in technology and management, keeping the chest virgin of any open surgical intervention, will circumvent bridging patients with other devices, decreasing the risk of sequential multiple interventions (ECLS—VAD—transplant). That is an important element to add to the equation as recent analysis has shown increased early mortality and worst outcomes for those recipients bridged with a permanent LVAD compared to virgin chest patients.[36]

Historical data associate cardiac ECLS with poor outcomes in heart transplantation. However, it is likely that this association is more related to the fact that these patients are sicker at the baseline (lower INTERMACS status) than to the isolated fact of being on mechanical support.

Conclusion

The technique of ECLS can be successfully applied to bridge patients with rapidly worsening lung or heart failure. The ECLS as BTLT performed in experienced centres with stringent inclusion criteria and protocols has shown good survival outcomes. Bridging cardiac ECLS patients to heart transplantation, instead, represents a challenging scenario, which is rarely used given the acuity and severity of patients when this therapy is applied.

Considerable ethical and clinical issues need to be addressed in future studies to fully optimize the application of this extremely complex salvage therapeutic strategy for patients with cardio-respiratory failure.

Highlights

- ECLS is increasingly used to 'bridge' patients to lung and heart transplantation.
- ECLS can potentially provide appropriate mode and intensity of cardio-pulmonary support tailored to the physiologic requirement of each patient.
- The outcome of patients bridged to LTx using ECLS has improved in the recent years and can be regarded satisfactory considering the severity of their diseases and the overall survival of LTx recipients.
- In high volume/high performance centres, where teams are familiar with the ECLS therapy, fast track eligibility for transplant is available, and a short time in the waiting list can be expected; ECLS bridging to heart transplant can be an alternative to VA-ECMO in HTx.
- Considerable ethical and clinical issues need to be addressed in future studies to fully optimize the application of this extremely complex salvage therapeutic strategy for patients with end-stage cardio-respiratory failure waiting for transplantation.

References

1) Khush KK, Cherikh WS, Chambers DC, Harhay MO, Hayes D Jr, Hsich E, Meiser B, Potena L, Robinson A, Rossano JW, Sadavarte A, Singh TP, Zuckermann A, Stehlik J. International Society for Heart and Lung Transplantation. The International Thoracic Organ Transplant Registry of the International Society for Heart and Lung Transplantation: Thirty-sixth adult heart transplantation report—2019; focus theme: Donor and recipient size match. J Heart Lung Transplant. 2019 Oct;38(10):1056–1066. doi: 10.1016/j.healun.2019.08.004. Epub 2019 Aug 10.
2) Valapour M, Lehr CJ, Skeans MA, et al. OPTN/SRTR 2016 annual data report: Lung. Am J Transplant 2018;18(Suppl 1):363–433.
3) Colvin M, Smith JM, Hadley N, Skeans MA, Uccellini K, Lehman R, Robinson AM, Israni AK, Snyder JJ, Kasiske BL. OPTN/SRTR 2017 Annual Data Report: Heart. Am J Transplant. 2019 Feb;19 Suppl 2:323–403.
4) Hodson ME, Madden BP, Steven MH, Tsang VT, Yacoub MH. Non-invasive mechanical ventilation for cystic fibrosis patients--a potential bridge to transplantation. Eur Respir J. 1991 May;4(5):524–527.
5) Mason DP, Thuita L, Nowicki ER, Murthy SC, Pettersson GB, Blackstone EH. Should lung transplantation be performed for patients on mechanical respiratory support? The US experience. J Thorac Cardiovasc Surg. 2010 Mar;139(3):765–773.
6) Cypel M, Keshavjee S. Extracorporeal life support as a bridge to lung transplantation. Clin Chest Med. 2011 Jun;32(2):245–251.
7) Benazzo A, Schwarz S, Frommlet F, Schweiger T, Jaksch P, Schellongowski P, Staudinger T, Klepetko W, Lang G, Hoetzenecker K. Vienna ECLS Program. Twenty-year experience with extracorporeal life support as bridge to lung transplantation. J Thorac Cardiovasc Surg. 2019 Jun;157(6):2515–2252.
8) Tipograf Y, Salna M, Minko E, Grogan EL, Agerstrand C, Sonett J, Brodie D, Bacchetta M. Outcomes of Extracorporeal Membrane Oxygenation as a Bridge to Lung Transplantation. Ann Thorac Surg. 2019 May;107(5):1456–1463.
9) Biscotti M, Sonett J, Bacchetta M. ECMO as bridge to lung transplant. Thorac Surg Clin. 2015;25(1):17–25.
10) Biscotti M, Gannon WD, Agerstrand C, Abrams D, Sonett J, Brodie D, Bacchetta M. Awake Extracorporeal Membrane Oxygenation as Bridge to Lung Transplantation: A 9-Year Experience. Ann Thorac Surg. 2017 Aug;104(2):412–419.
11) Hoetzenecker K, Donahoe L, Yeung JC, Azad S, Fan E, Ferguson ND, Del Sorbo L, de Perrot M, Pierre A, Yasufuku K, Singer L, Waddell TK, Keshavjee S, Cypel M. Extracorporeal life support as a bridge to lung transplantation-experience of a high-volume transplant center. J Thorac Cardiovasc Surg. 2018 Mar;155(3):1316–1328.
12) Russo MJ, Davies RR, Hong KN, Iribarne A, Kawut S, Bacchetta M, D'Ovidio F, Arcasoy S, Sonett JR. Who is the high-risk recipient? Predicting mortality after lung transplantation using pretransplant risk factors. J Thorac Cardiovasc Surg 2009; 138:1234–1238.

13) Lin J Extracorporeal membrane oxygenation support bridge to transplant: Avoiding a bridge to nowhere. Thorac Cardiovasc Surg. 2017 Nov;154(5):1796–1797. doi: 10.1016/j.jtcvs.2017.07.051. Epub 2017 Aug 12.
14) Lansink-Hartgring AO, van der Bij W, Verschuuren EA, Erasmus ME, de Vries AJ, Vermeulen K, van den Bergh W. Extracorporeal life support as a bridge to lung transplantation: A single-center experience with an emphasis on health-related quality of life. Respir Care. 2017 May;62(5):588–594.
15) Fischer S, Hoeper MM, Bein T, Simon AR, Gottlieb J, Wisser W, Frey L, Van Raemdonck D, Welte T, Haverich A, Strueber M. Interventional lung assist: A new concept of protective ventilation in bridge to lung transplantation. ASAIO J. 2008 Jan-Feb;54(1):3–10.
16) Schellongowski P, Riss K, Staudinger T, Ullrich R, Krenn CG, Sitzwohl C, Bojic A, Wohlfarth P, Sperr WR, Rabitsch W, Aigner C, Taghavi S, Jaksch P, Klepetko W, Lang G. Extracorporeal CO2 removal as bridge to lung transplantation in life-threatening hypercapnia. Transpl Int. 2015 Mar;28(3):297–304.
17) Crotti S, Bottino N, Ruggeri GM, Spinelli E, Tubiolo D, Lissoni A, Protti A, Gattinoni L. Spontaneous Breathing during Extracorporeal Membrane Oxygenation in Acute Respiratory Failure. Anesthesiology. 2017 Apr;126(4):678–687.
18) Abrams D, Brodie D, Javidfar J, Brenner K, Wang D, Zwischenberger J, Sonett J, Bacchetta Insertion of bicaval dual-lumen cannula via the left internal jugular vein for extracorporeal membrane oxygenation. ASAIO J. 2012 Nov-Dec; 58(6):636–637.
19) Chicotka S, Pedroso FE, Agerstrand CL, Rosenzweig EB, Abrams D, Benson T, Layton A, Burkhoff D, Brodie D, Bacchetta MD. Increasing opportunity for lung transplant in interstitial lung disease with pulmonary hypertension. Ann Thorac Surg. 2018 Dec;106(6):1812–1819.
20) Chicotka S, Rosenzweig EB, Brodie D, Bacchetta M. The 'Central Sport Model': Extracorporeal Membrane Oxygenation Using the Innominate Artery for Smaller Patients as Bridge to Lung Transplantation. ASAIO J. 2017 Jul/Aug;63(4):e39–e44.
21) Strueber M, Hoeper MM, Fischer S, Cypel M, Warnecke G, Gottlieb J, Pierre A, Welte T, Haverich A, Simon AR, Keshavjee S. Bridge to thoracic organ transplantation in patients with pulmonary arterial hypertension using a pumpless lung assist device. Am J Transplant. 2009 Apr;9(4):853–857.
22) de Perrot M, Granton JT, McRae K, Cypel M, Pierre A, Waddell TK, Yasufuku K, Hutcheon M, Chaparro C, Singer L, Keshavjee S. Impact of extracorporeal life support on outcome in patients with idiopathic pulmonary arterial hypertension awaiting lung transplantation. J Heart Lung Transplant. 2011 Sep;30(9):997–1002.
23) Camboni D, Akay B, Sassalos P, Toomasian JM, Haft JW, Bartlett RH, Cook KE. Use of venovenous extracorporeal membrane oxygenation and an atrial septostomy for pulmonary and right ventricular failure. Ann Thorac Surg. 2011 Jan;91(1):144–149.

24) Kon ZN, Pasrija C, Shah A, Griffith BP, Garcia JP. Venovenous Extracorporeal Membrane Oxygenation With Atrial Septostomy as a Bridge to Lung Transplantation. Ann Thorac Surg. 2016 Mar;101(3):1166–1169.
25) Abrams D, Brodie D, Arcasoy S. Extracorporeal Life Support in Lung Transplantation. Clin Chest Med 2017: 38(4):655–666.
26) Fuehner T, Kuehn C, Hadem J, Wiesner O, Gottlieb J, Tudorache I, Olsson KM, Greer M, Sommer W, Welte T, Haverich A, Hoeper MM, Warnecke G. Extracorporeal membrane oxygenation in awake patients as bridge to lung transplantation. Am J Respir Crit Care Med. 2012 Apr 1;185(7):763–768.
27) Fischer S, Bohn D, Rycus P, Pierre AF, de Perrot M, Waddell TK, Keshavjee S. Extracorporeal membrane oxygenation for primary graft dysfunction after lung transplantation: analysis of the Extracorporeal Life Support Organization (ELSO) registry. J Heart Lung Transplant. 2007 May;26(5):472–477.
28) Nosotti M, Rosso L, Tosi D, Palleschi A, Mendogni P, Nataloni IF, Crotti S, Tarsia P. Extracorporeal membrane oxygenation with spontaneous breathing as a bridge to lung transplantation. Interact Cardiovasc Thorac Surg. 2012;16(1):55–59.
29) Mason DP, Thuita L, Nowicki ER, Murthy SC, Pettersson GB, Blackstone EH. Should lung transplantation be performed for patients on mechanical respiratory support? The US experience. J Thorac Cardiovasc Surg. 2010 Mar;139(3):765–773.
30) Abdelnour-Berchtold E, Federici S, Wurlod DA, Bellier J, Zellweger M, Kirsch M, Nicod L, Marcucci C, Baeriswyl M, Liaudet L, Soccal PM, Gonzalez M, Perentes JY, Ris HB, Krueger T, Aubert JD. Outcome after extracorporeal membrane oxygenation-bridged lung retransplants: a single-centre experience. Interact Cardiovasc Thorac Surg. 2019 Jun 1;28(6):922–928.
31) Hakim AH, Ahmad U, McCurry KR, Johnston DR, Pettersson GB, Budev M, Murthy S, Blackstone EH, Tong MZ. Contemporary Outcomes of Extracorporeal Membrane Oxygenation Used as Bridge to Lung Transplantation. Ann Thorac Surg. 2018 Jul;106(1):192–198.
32) Bellier J, Lhommet P, Bonnette P, Puyo P, Le Guen M, Roux A, Parquin F, Chapelier A, Sage E; Foch Lung Transplantation Group. Extracorporeal membrane oxygenation for grade 3 primary graft dysfunction after lung transplantation: Long-term outcomes. Clin Transplant. 2019 Mar;33(3):e13480.
33) Lund LH, Khush KK, Cherikh WS, Goldfarb S, Kucheryavaya AY, Levvey BJ, Meiser B, Rossano JW, Chambers DC, Yusen RD, Stehlik J; International Society for Heart and Lung Transplantation. The registry of the International Society for Heart and Lung Transplantation: thirty-fourth adult heart transplantation report—2017; focus theme: allograft ischemic time. J Heart Lung Transplant 2017;36: 1037–1046.
34) Fukuhara S, Takeda K, Kurlansky PA, Naka Y, Takayama H. Extracorporeal membrane oxygenation as a direct bridge to heart transplantation in adults. J Thorac Cardiovasc Surg. 2018;155:1607–1618.
35) Chetan Pasrija, Kristen M. Mackowick, Maxwell Raithel, Douglas Tran, Francesca M. Boulos, Kristopher B. Deatrick, Michael A. Mazzeffi, Raymond Rector, Si M. Pham, Bartley P. Griffith, Daniel L. Herr, Zachary N. Kon.

Ambulation With Femoral Arterial Cannulation Can Be Safely Performed on Venoarterial Extracorporeal Membrane Oxygenation. The Annals of Thoracic Surgery, Volume 107, Issue 5, May 2019, Pages 1389–1394.
36) Urban M, Booth K, Jungschleger J, Netuka I, Schueler S, MacGowan G. Impact of donor variables on heart transplantation outcomes in mechanically bridged versus standard recipients. Interact CardioVasc Thorac Surg 2019;28:455–464.

55

Donation after circulatory death

Marinella Zanierato, Sara Tardivo, Luca Brazzi

Introduction

In the last twenty-five years Donation after Circulatory Death (DCD) has become one of the growing strategies to overcome the problem of organ shortage, offering the possibility to realize various organ procurements including kidney, liver, and lung transplants with good results.[1]

The DCD takes place after declaration of death based on cardiorespiratory criteria in contrast to donation after brain death in which neurological criteria are applied. Originally called non-heart-beating donation (NHBD), the current terminology (DCD) more precisely reflects the concept of the cessation of peripheral blood flow due to the absence of cardiac activity and blood pressure.[2] Furthermore, the criteria of death determination and the period of death declaration (no touch period) vary around the world according to different national laws.[3] The determination of death is based on evaluation of circulatory arrest (absent heart sounds, asystole, absent blood pressure, absent breathing), but the majority of guidelines require specific diagnostic procedures.[4] The no touch period, described as the time between the cessation of circulation and respiration and the determination of death, varies among countries, between 2 and 10 minutes. Most centres use 5 minutes and only in Italy, the time interval required by law to death diagnosis is 20 minutes of continuous flat EKG recording.[5]

Maastricht classification

The 1995 Maastricht's classification[6] defines DCD categories according to the circumstances of donor's death[7,8]:

Type I: Donors who are declared dead outside the hospital and are brought into the hospital without any attempt at resuscitation;
Type II: Donors in whom cardiac arrest occurs unexpectedly, and for whom resuscitation attempts are unsuccessful;
Type III: Donors for whom cardiac arrest is expected after withdrawal of treatment;
Type IV: Donors in whom cardiac arrest occurs during or after brain death diagnostic procedures.

Legislation in some countries allows euthanasia (medically assisted cardiac arrest) and subsequent organ donation is described as an additional category.[8]

The original Maastricht Classification has been modified during the International DCD Conference in Paris in 2013 (Table 55.1), to better define the exact circumstances of the circulatory arrest and consequent warm ischemic organ damage (in or out of hospital). Donors are classified as controlled (cDCD) or uncontrolled (uDCD) according to whether the cardiac arrest is planned or unexpected. Types I and II are defined as uncontrolled donors (uDCD) on the basis of unexpected cardiac arrest and unsuccessful resuscitation. Subjects with witnessed refractory in or out-of-hospital cardiac arrest (CA) are considered eligible for donation. Uncontrolled DCD should be considered only when available therapeutic options are unsuccessful or not clinically indicated, to avoid precluding some potentially recoverable patients from receiving optimum treatment. Death declaration is performed after decision to stop cardiopulmonary resuscitation (CPR). Simultaneous efforts are made to obtain family consent or document first-person consent by the newly deceased to preserve organs (heparin administration and vessel cannulation). The process of donation in this setting should be designed to minimize the duration of warm ischemia time (WIT) and its impact on organ viability, while ensuring the highest possible safety on the donated organ. In these donors, the exact length of the warm ischemic period is often known.

Table 55.1 Modified Maastricht classification

Category	Scenario	Location	Specific consideration
Ia	Dead on arrival	Ia. Out-of-hospital	Sudden unexpected cardiac arrest, with no attempt at resuscitation by a medical team. Only tissue can be considered from these donors
Ib		II b. In-hospital	
IIa	Unsuccessful resuscitation	Out-of-hospital	Sudden unexpected refractory cardiac arrest, with unsuccessful resuscitation by a medical team
IIb		In-hospital	
III	Withdrawal from life support: controlled	ICU	Planned, expected cardiac arrest, following the withdrawal of life-sustaining treatment in subject with end-stage neuro or cardiac/respiratory failure
IV	Cardiac arrest after brain death diagnosis: controlled/uncontrolled	ICU	Sudden or planned cardiac arrest occurs during or after brain death diagnostic procedures

In contrast, type III donors are defined as controlled donors, when death occurs after a planned withdrawal of life-sustaining therapies (WSLT), mainly cardiorespiratory support. As cardiac arrest is expected, the medical decision of WLST is taken in a defined and multidisciplinary approach, consistent with local/national legal requirements, by the clinical team together with the family, whenever further treatment is considered futile.[9] The WLST decision (disconnection of cardiovascular support and mechanical ventilation) must be completely independent from the option of organ donation. During the end-of-life care and the withdrawal phase, adequate comfort should be guaranteed to the dying patient and at the same time, organ protective measures should be taken, respecting the 'Dead Donor Rule'.

Although the majority of actual cDCD donors die from catastrophic, non-recoverable brain injury, data from the Netherlands, Spain, United Kingdom, and the USA suggest that up to 15% of cDCD die from other conditions such as end-stage respiratory failure or neuromuscular disease.[10] The majority of DCD are type III.

Type IV may be controlled or uncontrolled, depending on whether the circulatory arrest in a suspected or confirmed brain death condition was sudden or planned.

Countries practising DCD

The DCD is currently practised in twelve out of twenty-seven European Union nations as well as in the United States, Canada, Australia, Japan, China, the Far East, and a few South American nations.[11] The different approaches may be related to different legislations, ethical concerns, practices at the end of life, and organizational approaches to the treatment of out-of-hospital cardiac arrest. Some countries perform donations only from selected categories of DCD donors. In China, a donor who is declared dead by neurological criteria must undergo cDCD before organ donation and informed consent is obtained from family for WLST and organ donation.[12]

WIT in DCD organs

The main impediment to DCD is the increased incidence of impaired graft function after transplantation as a result of extended periods of warm ischemia. WIT is defined as the time from cardiac arrest to organ *in situ* perfusion (cold flush or regional perfusion). Ischaemia causes a rapid accumulation of toxic products such as lactate and hypoxanthine, deriving from anaerobic metabolism. These processes are exacerbated by reperfusion, resulting in inflammatory response with subsequent release of free radicals, expression of endothelial adhesion factors, and leucocytes activation. Furthermore, inflammatory response plays a pivotal role in the development of graft dysfunction.

In uncontrolled DCD, WIT can impact more significantly on organ viability, since the exact period of circulatory arrest is usually prolonged. Furthermore, between cardiac arrest and the initiation of organ perfusion, there is a period of CPR of variable duration and efficacy (low-flow

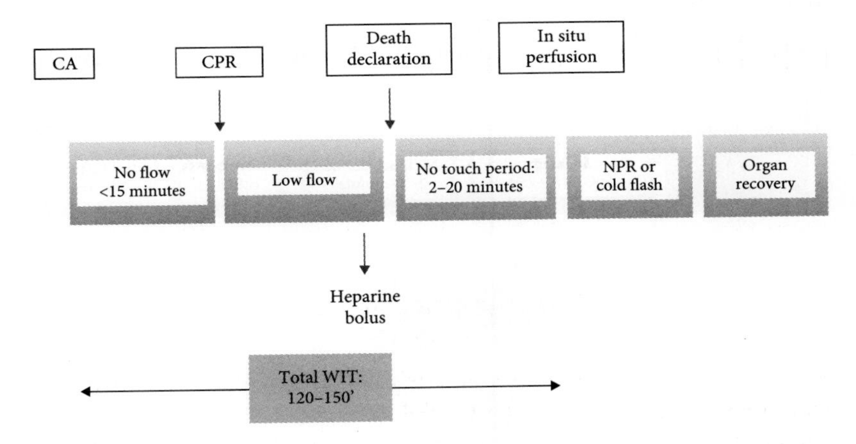

Figure 55.1. Uncontrolled DCD process
No-flow is defined as time from cardiac arrest (CA) to the start of resuscitation maneuvers. Low-flow is defined as the length of cardiopulmonary resuscitation. The total WIT is defined as the time from CA to start organ *in situ* preservation

period). Usually, automated chest compression can be used until *in situ* organ perfusion is started. The total WIT (time from CA to start organ *in situ* preservation) should be lower than 150 minutes.[13] The timeline of DCD II programme is showed in Figure 55.1.

The criteria for donation in the uDCD setting include: witnessed arrest, no-flow period without CPR limited to a maximum 15–20 minutes, total WIT less than 150 minutes, age below 65 years for kidneys and livers, and between 50 and 55 years for lungs, cause of death known or presumed, and non-bleeding abdominal injuries.

In cDCD, WIT can be defined as the interval between WLST and the beginning of *in situ* perfusions.[14] Nevertheless, controlled donors suffer from hypoxia, hypotension, and inadequate organ perfusion during the progression towards circulatory arrest (agonic time). Currently,[15] there is a tendency to consider warm ischemia, starting from the onset of hemodynamic instability (referred to as 'functional WIT' or FWIT) (Figure 55.2). The definition of FWIT is yet to be universally agreed, but in general, a sustained fall in systolic blood pressure ≤ 50 mmHg and SpO_2 < 75% is accepted in both Europe and the United States. Controlled DCD will only occur if the cardio-respiratory arrest follows soon after WLST (less than 2 hours) and most transplant programmes will limit

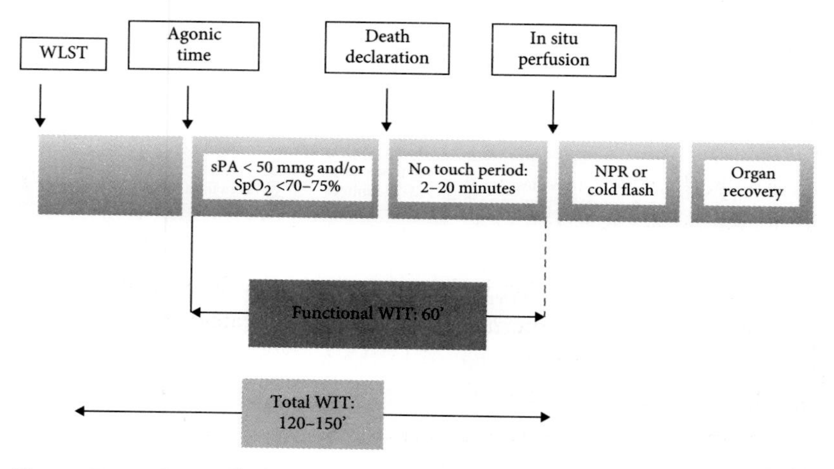

Figure 55.2. Controlled DCD process
Agonic time is defined as the period from treatment withdrawal to circulatory arrest
Functional WIT is defined as time from drop in systolic arterial pressure below 50 mmHg and/or SpO2 below 70-75% to start organ *in situ* perfusion. The total WIT is defined as the time from WSTL to start organ *in situ* preservation

the agonal phase to 60 minutes to exclude potential harmful effects. The University of Wisconsin score may be used to predict the probability of death occurring after the discontinuation of life support. This index is computed based on vital parameters, level of spontaneous respiration, and requirement for vasopressors, all of which indicate the likelihood of death within 1 hour after extubation.

Preservation and procurement techniques

Traditional methods of preservation based on static, hypothermic storage may not be the most appropriate for DCD grafts. Organs from DCD have already suffered tissue damage secondary to hypoxia and hypoperfusion, and cold storage would certainly exacerbate the damage. The key to the recovery of a great portion of these grafts is the modification of preservation techniques in order to stop or even reverse, through cytoprotective mechanisms, the cellular injury.

In many centres, the method of choice for uDCD is *in situ* preservation with a double-balloon triple-lumen (DBTL) catheter.[16] This technique allows only kidney preservation. This is a minimally invasive, relatively simple procedure that can be performed by personnel with limited technical experience. The DBTL is usually performed in the Emergency Room after failed resuscitation.

The use of extracorporeal membrane oxygenation (ECMO) technology exclusively for abdominal organs perfusion (abdominal Regional Perfusion, ARP) is an alternative preservation strategy to restore the circulation with oxygenated blood to the abdominal organs in the *in situ* donors. The use of ECMO to facilitate organ donation was first described in 1997.[17] The ARP may be performed at either hypothermic or normothermic temperatures. In hypothermic regional perfusion (HPR), the temperature of the diluted blood solution is actively cooled to anywhere from 4 to around 20° C. Theoretical benefits for its use include more efficient cooling and reduced warm ischemia.[18]

Normothermic regional perfusion technique

Normothermic Regional Perfusion (nRP) has emerged as a procurement technique to overcome unpredictable effects of prolonged WIT, following pioneering work on DCD II in Spain.[19] The nRP allows organs to recover *in situ* from warm ischemic damage. It provides oxygen and nutrients to restore metabolic processes, which in turn, enables repair of damaged cells, correction of acidosis, restoration of depleted ATP, regulation of calcium homeostasis, and removal of free radicals. It is possible that nRP plays an important role in the preconditioning of organs before cold storage. This observation suggests that nRP has a protective role following a severe ischemic insult. Another key benefit of nRP is dynamic organ assessment during perfusion prior to recovery which permits better grafts selection. This may lead to superior outcomes compared to standard preservation strategy (cold storage). nRP also turns an urgent procedure into an elective organ recovery procedure, a means to potentially reduce organ damage and organ losses because of surgical events[20]; this is particularly relevant for liver procurement.[20]

Following the Spanish experience in uDCD,[21,22] several countries have explored the feasibility of nRP in cDCD using similar technology (heat exchanger, oxygenator, and pump). Few studies describe the use of regional perfusion in controlled DCD donation in normothermic conditions, reporting an increase in organ recovery rates compared with standard preservation procedures.[23]

The nRP system includes an extra-corporeal oxygenator, a heat exchanger, and a centrifugal pump[24] (Figure 55.3). Femoral vessels are cannulated (surgically or percutaneously) to establish nRP to reperfuse and reoxygenate abdominal organs while donor evaluation and preparations for organ recovery are undertaken. The contralateral femoral artery is cannulated with a Fogarty balloon catheter, which is advanced into the supraceliac aorta. The balloon is inflated to prevent cardiac and brain perfusion. Proper positioning of the balloon is confirmed by chest radiography. In the cases of post-mortem cannulation, the surgical team

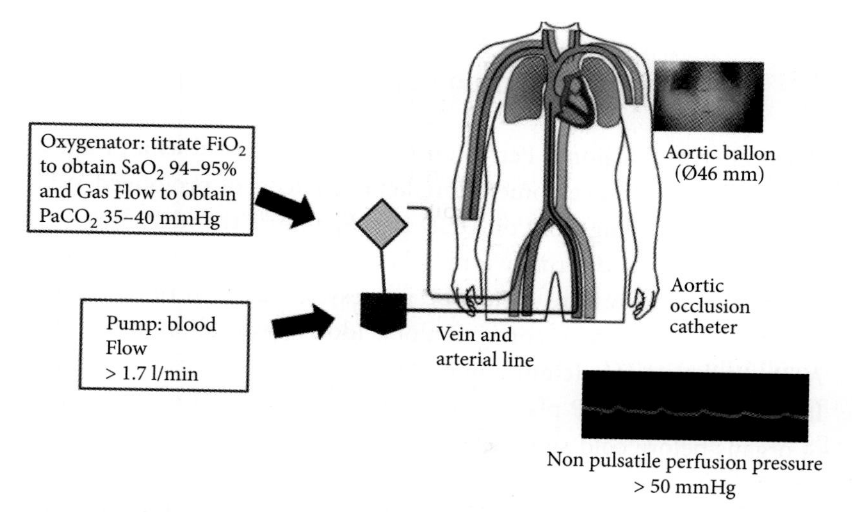

Figure 55.3. Normothermic Regional extracorporeal membrane circuit. Femoral cannulae are connected to an ECMO circuit. Fogarty balloon catheter is advanced into the supraceliac aorta and inflated to prevent cardiac and brain perfusion. Proper positioning of balloon is confirmed by chest radiography. Once NRP is started, abdominal perfusion pressure is monitored from the femoral arterial cannula or from occlusion catheter introducer

performs a midline laparotomy to cannulate the abdominal aorta and inferior vena cava. The descending thoracic aorta is clamped, and nRP is started.

Pump flow is maintained over 1.7 l/min, temperature at 35.5–37.5°C and pH at 7.0–7.4.[17,18] The circuit sweep gas levels (FiO_2 and air flow) are adjusted to keep $PaCO_2$ between 35 and 45 mmHg and SaO_2 about 98–100%. Post-oxygenator arterial blood gas is sampled at baseline and throughout NRP to determine oxygenation parameters and acid-base status. Sodium bicarbonate should be added to the circuit to correct metabolic acidosis. Red blood cells transfusion may be required to maintain the haematocrit over 20%. Anticoagulation is obtained by full heparinization (3 mg/kg) prior to cannulation and is subsequently maintained by heparin bolus, in accordance with activated coagulation time (ACT) values. The optimal duration of nRP is yet to be determined. Although in the uncontrolled setting in Spain and France, nRP is maintained for up to 4 hours. This duration may not be required in cDCD and may be logistically difficult in smaller referring hospitals. Recently, data appear to suggest that even a shorter nRP duration may reverse ischemic damage and provide a good outcome.

Ethical issues in pre- and post-mortem intervention

Legal and ethical permissibility of pre- or post-mortem intervention to organ preservation remains controversial in many countries[25] and there are several key differences related to heparin administration and timing of vascular cannulation. Pre-mortem *measures* (heparin administration) are intended to optimize organ viability and they should be consistent with the wish of the patient to become a donor. On the other end, *interventions* to preserve and improve organ quality *in situ* can be taken post-mortem, after death has been declared. In uDCD setting, in Spain, France, Italy,[26] Russia, and Portugal,[27] vascular cannulation and heparinization occur during a period of mechanical chest compression post-death declaration,[24,28] even in cases where first-person donation consent has not yet been obtained. Subsequently, next-of-kin can decide, whether or not to proceed with donation, taking into consideration the potential donor's wishes. A similar protocol has been developed in USA.[29]

The timing of heparin administration and vascular cannulation in cDCD is still debated and varies by country. Several authors do not recommend using pre-mortem intervention because of ethical problems and lack of evidence of improved outcomes. Pre-mortem heparin administration and cannulation are permitted in Spain[23] and France[28] to reduce functional WIT and to start NRP immediately after the death declaration. In Italy,[17] national recommendations permit pre-mortem heparin administration and vascular wires positioning, but not cannulation. In contrast, the UK approach establishes post-mortem nRP cannulation, without pre-mortem heparinization.[30] The use of shunts to bypass the oxygenator in the ECMO circuit is empirical to avoid intra-circuit thrombus.[31]

In uDCD, the nRP is the preferred recovery option, especially if liver retrieval is involved. It has been reported that DCD Type II kidneys undergoing nRP showed a lower rate of delayed graft function (DGF) and Primary Graft Non Function (PGNF) than did kidneys used after hypothermic preservation. In kidneys from DCD undergoing nRP, the 1-year graft survival rate has been reported to be as high as 87.4%. The use of liver from these donors is somewhat problematic and an increased incidence of ischemic cholangiopathy and subsequent primary graft non-function was observed.[21] The use of nRP in cDCD is associated with increased organ recovery rates compared with standard DCD retrieval [32]. In cDCD liver transplantation, the application of nRP reduces post-operative biliary strictures and ischemic type biliary lesions (ITBL) and improves graft survival compared with rapid recovery. The use of nRP in DCD does not preclude retrieval of lungs, as dual temperature multiorgan retrieval is possible using abdominal nRP and concomitant cold lung flushing, allowing both rapid removal of the lungs and normothermic preservation of the abdominal organs.

Given the encouraging organ utilization rates and clinical outcomes,[33] the extension of nRP to include cardio-thoracic organs was a logical step to facilitate heart and lung retrieval and to reduce the rate of primary graft dysfunction.[34]

Very recently, international statements and algorithms have been published as a reference guide for expanding, all around the world, controlled donation after the circulatory determination of death, providing evidence-based recommendations on the use of nRP in uncontrolled and controlled DCDs.[38,39]

Conclusion

The use of *in situ* nRP is a significant advancement in organ retrieval and has the potential to increase organ recovery rates due to its applicability in both controlled and uncontrolled DCD donors. Furthermore, the ability to restore the ATP supplies and the dynamic assessment of organ function prior to transplantation may allow a better selection of grafts and provide a superior long-term outcome.

Highlights

- Donation after circulatory death is an accepted strategy to expand the potential donor pool.
- The outcome of transplantation with organs from DCD donors is significantly influenced by the length of WIT.
- The unpredictable consequences of the warm ischemic injury results in an extensive damage due to ischemia-reperfusion injury (IRI).
- nRP may restore the flow of oxygen and other metabolic substrates to improve the cellular energy charge.
- nRP enables a dynamic *in-situ* functional assessment of abdominal grafts.
- Ante mortem interventions (heparin and vessels cannulation) can be justified, both ethically and legally, on the grounds of best interests if they facilitate the wishes of a patient to donate.

References

1. Manyalich M, Nelson H, Delmonico F. The need and opportunity for donation after circulatory death worldwide. Curr Opin Organ Transplant. 2018 Feb; 23(1): 136–141.
2. Thuong M, Ruiz A, Evard P, et al. New classification of donation after circulatory death donors definitions and terminology. Transpl Int. 2016; 29(7): 749–759.
3. Dominiguez-Gil B, Haase-Kromwijk B, Van Leiden H, et al. Current situation of donation after circulatory death in European countries. Transpl Int. 2011 Jul; 24(7): 676–686.
4. Dhanani S, Ward R, Hornby L, et al. Survey of determination of death after cardiac arrest by intensive care physicians. Crit Care Med. 2012 May; 40(5): 1449–1455.

5. Nanni Costa A, Procaccio F. Organ donation after circulatory death in Italy? Yes we can! Minerva Anestesiol. Transplant Proc. 2016 Mar; 82(3): 271–273.
6. Kootstra G, Daemen J, Oomen A. Categories of non-heart-beating donors. 1995 Oct; 27(5): 2893–2894.
7. Morrissey P, Monaco A. Donation after circulatory death: current practices, ongoing challenges, and potential improvements. Transplantation. 2014 Feb; 97(3): 258–264.
8. Ysebaert D, Van Beeumen G, De Greef K, et al. Organ procurement after euthanasia: Belgian experience. Transplant Proc. 2009 Mar; 41(2): 585–586.
9. Manara A, Murphy P, O'Callaghan G. Donation after circulatory death. Br J Anaesth. 2012 Jan; 108(Suppl 1): 108–121.
10. Neyrinck A, Van Raemdonck D, Monbaliu D. Donation after circulatory death: current status. Curr Opin Anaesthesiol. 2013 Jun; 26(3): 382–390.
11. Ortega-Deballon I, Hornby L, Shemie S. Protocols for uncontrolled donation after circulatory death: a systematic review of international guidelines, practices and transplant outcomes. Crit Care. 2015 Jun; 19: 268.
12. Hattori R, Ono Y, Yoshimura N, et al. Long-term outcome of kidney transplant using non-heart-beating donor: multicenter analysis of factors affecting graft survival. Clin Transplant. 2003 Dec; 17(6): 518–521.
13. Domingez-Gil B, Duranteau J, Mateos A, et al. Uncontrolled donation after circulatory death: European practices and recommendations for the development and optimization of an effective programme. Tranpl Int. 2016 Aug; 29(8): 842–859.
14. Algahim M, Love R. Donation after circulatory death: the current state and technical approaches to organ procurement. Curr Opin Organ Transplant. 2015 Apr; 20(2): 127–132.
15. Coffey J, Wanis K, Monbaliu D, et al. The influence of functional warm ischemia time on DCD liver transplant recipients' outcomes. Clin Transplant. 2017 Oct; 31(10). doi: 10.1111/ctr.13068. Epub 2017 Aug 29.
16. Wind J, Hoogland ER, van Heurn LW. Preservation techniques for donors after cardiac death kidneys. Curr Opin in Organ Transplant. 2011 Apr; 16(2): 157–161.
17. Hoshino T, Maley, Stump K, Tuttle T, Burdick, Williams G. Evaluation of core cooling technique for liver and kidney procurement. Transplant Proc. 1987 Oct; 19(5): 4123–4128.
18. García-Valdecasas, Fondevila C. In-vivo normothermic recirculation: an update. Curr Opin Organ Transplant. 2010 Apr; 15(2): 173–176.
19. Valero R, Cabrer C, Oppenheimer F, et al. Normothermic recirculation reduces primary graft dysfunction of kidneys obtained from non-heart-beating donors. Transpl Int. 2000; 13(4): 303–310.
20. Oniscu J, Randle L, Muiesan P, Butler A, Currie I, Perera M, et al. In situ normothermic regional perfusion for controlled donation after circulatory death—the United Kingdom experience. Am J Transplant. 2014 Dec; 14(12): 2846–2854.
21. Hessheimer A, García-Valdecasas J, Fondevila C. Abdominal regional in-situ perfusion in donation after circulatory determination of death donors. Curr Opin Organ Transplant. 2016 Jun; 21(3): 322–328.
22. Shapey I, Muiesan P. Regional perfusion by extracorporeal membrane oxygenation of abdominal organs from donors after circulatory death: a systematic review. Liver Transpl. 2013 Dec; 19(12): 1292–1303.

23. Miñambres E, Suberviola B, Dominguez-Gil B, et al. Improving the Outcomes of Organs Obtained From Controlled Donation After Circulatory Death Donors Using Abdominal Normothermic Regional Perfusion. Am J Transplant. 2017 Aug; 17(8): 2165–2172.
24. Fondevila C, Hessheimer A, Ruiz A, et al. Liver transplant using donors after unexpected cardiac death: novel preservation protocol and acceptance criteria. Am J Transplant. 2007 Jul; 7(7): 1849–1855.
25. Haase B, Bos M, Boffa C, et al. Ethical, legal, and societal issues and recommendations for controlled and uncontrolled DCD. Transpl Int. 2016 Jul; 29(7): 771–779.
26. Giannini A, Abelli M, Biancofiore G, et al. 'Why can't I give you my organs after my heart has stopped beating?' An overview of the main clinical, organisational, ethical and legal issues concerning organ donation after circulatory death in Italy. Minerva Anestesiol. 2016 Mar; 82(3): 359–368.
27. Roncon-Albuquerque Rj, Gaião S, Figueiredo P, et al. An integrated program of extracorporeal membrane oxygenation (ECMO) assisted cardiopulmonary resuscitation and uncontrolled donation after circulatory determination of death in refractory cardiac arrest. Resuscitation. 2018 Dec; 133: 88–94.
28. Antoine C, Mourey F, Prada-Bordenave E. How France launched its donation after cardiac death program. Ann Fr Anesth Reanim. 2014 Feb; 33(2): 138–143.
29. Reznik O, Skvortsov A, Loginov I, Ananyev A, Bagnenko S, Moysyuk Y. Kidney from uncontrolled donors after cardiac death with one hour warm ischemic time: resuscitation by extracorporal normothermic abdominal perfusion 'in situ' by leukocytes-free oxygenated blood. Clin Transplant. 2011 Jul-Aug; 25(4): 511–516.
30. Oniscu G, Randle L, Muiesan P, et al. In situ normothermic regional perfusion for controlled donation after circulatory death--the United Kingdom experience. Am J Transplant. 2014 Dec; 14(12): 2846–2854.
31. Butler AJ, Randle VL, Watson CJ. Normothermic regional perfusion for donation after circulatory death without prior heparinization. Transplantation. 2014 Jun; 97(12): 1272–1278.
32. Watson C, Hunt F, Messer F, et al. In situ normothermic perfusion of livers in controlled circulatory death donation may prevent ischemic cholangiopathy and improve graft survival. Am J Transplant. 2019 Jun; 19(6): 1745–1758.
33. Tsui S, Oniscu G. Extending normothermic regional perfusion to the thorax in donors after circulatory death. Curr Opin Organ Transplant. 2017 Jun; 22(3): 245–250.
34. Dhital K, Chew H, Macdonald P. Donation after circulatory death heart transplantation. Curr Opin Organ Transplant. 2017 Jun; 22(3): 89–197.
35. Vergano M, Magavern E, Baroncelli F, et al. Making a case for controlled organ donation after cardiac death: the story of Italy's first experience. J Crit Care. 2017 Apr; 38: 129–131.
36. Hessheimer A, García-Valdecasas J, Fondevila C. Abdominal regional in-situ perfusion in donation after circulatory determination of death donors. Curr Opin Organ Transplant. 2016 Jun; 21(3): 322–328.
37. Ysebaert D, Van Beeumen G, De Greef K, et al. Organ procurement after euthanasia: Belgian experience. Transplant Proc. 2009 Mar; 41(2): 585–586.

38. Domínguez-Gil B, Ascher N, Capron AM, et al. Correction to: Expanding controlled donation after the circulatory determination of death: statement from an international collaborative. Intensive Care Med. 2021 Sep;47(9):1059–1060.
39. Jochmans I, Hessheimer AJ, Neyrinck AP et al. Consensus statement on normothermic regional perfusion in donation after circulatory death: report from the European Society for Organ Transplantation's Transplant Learning Journey. Transplant International 2021 Nov;34(11):2019–2030.

56

Lung donation after circulatory death

Bronwyn Levvey, Gregory Snell

Introduction

Lung transplantation (LTx) has been successfully utilized as a life-saving, therapeutic strategy for severe end-stage lung disease. The challenge has been to identify a suitable number of quality donor lungs for transplant. Various potential sources have been actively pursued, including medically 'extended' lungs (e.g. localized infection or fluid laden), older lungs (>75 years), or donation after circulatory death (DCD) lungs.[1–3] Outcomes for all these lungs have proved perfectly acceptable.

The DCD concept of a definition of death based on irreversible loss of the circulation is well understood by the general public and legal system. Indeed, the average person incorrectly believes most donors have died by such a process, rather than appreciating the reality that donation after brain death (DBD) has actually been the most common donation pathway. This chapter will focus on the DCD lung donation evolving from humble beginnings to becoming a major successful lung donation strategy in 2019.

On the coat-tails of twenty years of excellent short- and long-term outcomes following DCD kidney transplantation, controlled DCD LTx was initially described as a small case series by Love et al from the USA in 1995.[4] In 2001, Steen et al from Sweden reported a successful lung transplant from a DCD donor using a novel topical preservation technique and ex-vivo lung perfusion (EVLP) rig to assess functionality.[5] Simultaneously, other countries, including Belgium[6] and Spain,[7] were also evaluating the benefits of DCD lung donation and transplantation.

Table 56.1 Traditionally recognized Categories of DCD donors[10]:

1 Death outside hospital
2 Unsuccessful resuscitation in hospital
3 Awaiting cardiac arrest after planned withdrawal of life-sustaining therapies
4 Awaiting cardiac arrest in a known brain-dead donor

The Alfred Hospital's DCD LTx journey

Starting in 2003, with the aim of developing clinical DCD LTx protocols, a team from The Alfred Hospital (Melbourne, Australia) consisting of LTx physicians, surgeons, perfusionists and a DCD project coordinator spent two years completing large-animal experiments evaluating and optimizing potential methods of DCD lung preservation and retrieval timing.[8,9] International experience had described DCD lung donation from both 'uncontrolled- Maastricht Category 1 and 2', and 'controlled- Maastricht Category 3 and 4' donors (as defined by Koostra,[10] Table 56.1). Experimental models evaluated these different scenarios to determine which was most clinically applicable and practically acceptable within the existing organ donation and transplantation system in Australia.

Alfred DCD LTx guideline development

On completion of the background feasibility research in 2005, the first draft of a clinical protocol for controlled (Category 3 and 4) DCD lung donation and transplantation was devised by the LTx DCD project team, in consultation with the various stakeholders involved in organ donation and transplantation within The Alfred Hospital. Presentations of the proposed protocol were subsequently made to Intensive Care Unit (ICU) physicians, nursing staff, surgeons and operating theatre (OT) staff, transplant physicians, and transplant clinic staff, as well as the local state Victorian DonateLife organ donation organization, the Victorian Transplant Immunology Service (VTIS) and the Victorian State

Coroner's Office, with any areas of concerns identified and negotiated or clarified at this time.

The DCD project team also met with the Alfred Hospital Research and Ethics Unit and the Alfred Hospital Legal Service,[11] who ultimately granted approval for the project, with a request for ongoing audit of all DCD donations and subsequent transplants. A separate consent for recipients receiving DCD donor organs was deemed unnecessary. However, the already extensive consent process for all patients on the lung transplant waiting list was modified to include discussion about DCD donation, on the understanding that any lung transplant recipient may potentially receive DCD donor lungs if and when they become available.

It is important to acknowledge that some donation ICU consultants were initially concerned about the perceived 'conflict of interest', particularly as the DCD lung protocols had been initially developed by the LTx 'recipient' team. However, with extensive ICU consultant input, the protocol was designed to very clearly outline the responsibilities of the ICU physicians in the management of a potential DCD donor in the ICU, and specifically designates in the pathway when the local (Victorian) donation team and recipient LTx team should be contacted. The process of consent for DCD donation prompted intense discussion amongst the ICU consultants, and the resulting section in the guidelines regarding consent is extremely detailed to ensure that decisions of withdrawal of active treatment based on futility are completely separate, and made prior, to any discussions about DCD donation. Indeed, a second independent ICU consultant is brought in to undertake DCD donation discussions.

Some ICU and OT nurses were also challenged by this new direction in organ donation, primarily due to the differences in the care of a brain-dead donor compared to the care of patient where withdrawal of treatment occurs.[12] An extensive education programme was undertaken in these areas to ensure all the staff are given the opportunity to voice any concerns and also contribute to the protocol development.

After further six months of consultation, education, and refinement, the Alfred DCD Guidelines[13] (Box 56.1) were officially endorsed in May 2006, for controlled DCD lung-only procurement at that stage.

Box 56.1 Principles of Alfred DCD Lung Donation Guidelines

- Facilitates organ donation of Category 3 and 4 DCD donor lungs (10)
- Consent for DCD donation must be obtained as specifically outlined in guidelines.
- Management of withdrawal of life sustaining treatment occurs in ICU as per institutional standard practice.
- Death after withdrawal should be likely to occur within 90 minutes.
- The organ donation agency coordinates the donation process.
- No pre-mortem interventions related to organ procurement permitted except standard blood tests obtained for cross-matching, arterial blood gas measurements and bronchoscopy.
- A 'team meeting' at least 30 minutes prior to the planned withdrawal of treatment allows surgical teams and OT staff to meet with the donor coordinators, the ICU physician in charge and ICU nurse caring for the potential donor, and go through the proposed plan, clarifying when and where withdrawal will occur (for example in the ICU or in the OT), details of the local clinical DCD guidelines and the order of planned surgical procedures (in a multiorgan retrieval scenario).
- The mechanism of withdrawal is typically patient extubation and the withdrawal of inotropic support.
- Death is certified 5 minutes after the onset of asystole by an ICU doctor who is not a member of the procurement or transplant team.
- The donor is transferred to a ready and waiting OT as soon as practicable after death and the retrieval procedure starts immediately.
- Re-intubation occurs immediately on arrival in the OT prior to transfer on to the operating table.
- If death does not occur within 90 minutes after withdrawal of support, the OT team is stood down.
- In early cases, a post-case de-briefing meeting was held with OT and ICU nursing staff and other relevant team members to discuss any issues/challenges and concerns.

General acceptance criteria and contra-indications for DCD lung donation and retrieval have always been identical to those around the potential retrieval of DBD donor lungs.[1]

- *Specific DCD LTx donor acceptance criteria:* Sufficient time is required for the cardiothoracic retrieval team to be onsite by the time of withdrawal of treatment (typically> 2 hrs).
- *Specific DCD LTx donor contra-indication:* A history of prior significant cardiothoracic surgery in the potential DCD donor which could considerably delay access to the major pulmonary arteries for the preservation flush (prior chest tube for simple fluid removal or pneumothorax management is usually acceptable).

DCD lung procurement, preservation, and transplantation technique

A DBD donor lung retrieval technique has been described in detail in Chapter 41, 'The Surgical Phases of Thoracic Organ Retrieval'.[14,15] In brief, every effort is made to prevent aspiration of gastric contents post-withdrawal of life-sustaining treatment (WLST) (e.g. aspiration of nasogastric tube immediately prior to WLST, head of bed of donor elevated 30 degrees), donor re-intubation (if extubated) occurs only after the locally mandated 2–5 minute stand-off time following documented cessation of circulation and a rapid sternotomy and pulmonary arterial cannulation is then performed for delivery of preservation solution (Perfadex®, XVIVO, Goteborg, Sweden). In order to avoid inadvertent cardiac reanimation,[16] post-mortem donor ventilation is reinitiated at least15 minutes after asystole. Explant surgery of donor lungs and LTx surgery follows standard practice and does not vary according to the donor type.[17,18] No Alfred lung donor assessments have been undertaken using EVLP.

Specific DCD LTx recipient acceptance criteria

The only specific recipient criteria for DCD lungs are the selected recipient needs to live <300 km from the centre to reduce the risks and cost associated with transporting a sick recipient over a long distance for a potential DCD donor that may not die within the required time frame.

DCD lung donation and transplant outcomes

In the thirteen years since the DCD lung donation protocol was initiated at The Alfred, 220 DCD LTx have been performed, representing 25% of the overall LTx donor pool over this time period (Figure 56.1). The outcomes are essentially equivalent to those reported from DBD donors with both donor types having a 50% thirteen-year survival and a similar profile of early and later causes of mortality. Multiorgan DCD retrieval is now common, with lungs, kidneys, and occasionally livers and hearts,[19] recovered simultaneously for transplantation.

Early Alfred success with DCD LTx saw other Australian LTx centres follow and collectively evolve as a national endeavour in the form of the Australian DCD Lung Transplant Collaborative. The Collaborative provided agreement on standardized guidelines, definitions, audit processes, and a single interface with national Donation Services and Government agencies. The DCD LTx Collaborative

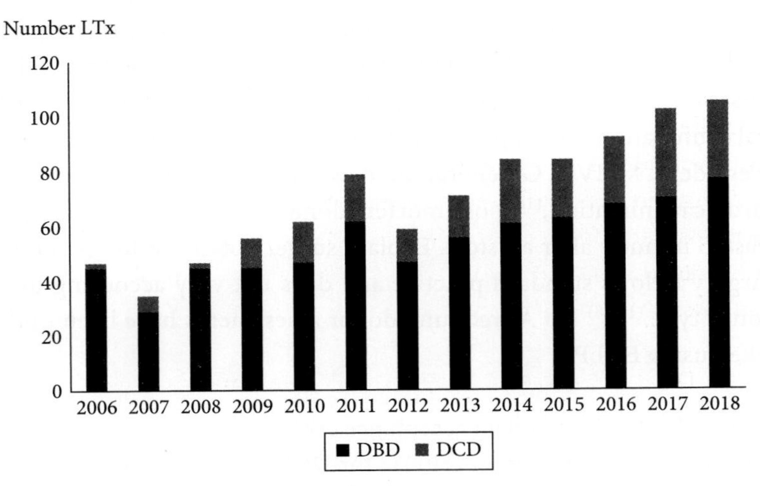

Figure 56.1. The number and proportion of Alfred Hospital DCD and DBD LTx performed each year since DCD LTx started in 2006

proved to be a very successful endeavour producing some significant presentations, contributions, and publications both nationally and internationally.

In 2011, with increasing DCD lung donor utilization in Australia, Europe, and Canada, the multi-national International Society for Heart and Lung Transplantation (ISHLT) DCD LTx Registry was conceived, based on the format of the Australian DCD LTx Collaborative. The first ISHLT DCD Registry Report published in 2015[20] was the largest multi-centre international report evaluating survival of LTx recipients receiving DCD donors at that time. Analyses comparing DCD to DBD LTx cohort survival rates over the same time period concluded that there was no differences in short (one year) and long-term (five year) survival, which is an extremely reassuring result. The recently completed 2019 ISHLT DCD Registry Report confirms these survival outcomes in the 1090 DCD versus 10,426 DBD donor lung transplants entered into this Registry, with a five-year survival of 63% versus 61% respectively (p = ns).[21] A more recent 2019 ISHLT DCD Registry Report notes no significant effect of DCD donor agonal or warm graft ischemic time on thirty day or one-year mortality.[22]

Clinical considerations in DCD LTx

The set-up of a DCD lung retrieval process requires clear advance planning, collaboration, protocolization, and extensive education that must include all of the ICU, OT, donation, and transplantation staff who will be involved in the various steps in the DCD process. Real-time problem solving and staff feedback are important to smoothen the way through any institution's first few DCD donor lung retrievals and subsequent transplants. Important points to note in the DCD LTx procedure are as follows:

1) DCD donors are a significant quality source of transplantable donor lungs.[1,3,20,23,24]
2) Not all potential DCD donors actually become donors; 25–30% of intended donors will not reach asystole within the subsequent 90–120 minutes after withdrawal of life-sustaining treatment (the

typical institutionally acceptable time to have a donor OT and retrieval team waiting on stand-by). This must be considered when developing a DCD protocol: if the potential DCD donor does not die within the required time frame, particularly if WLST is not occurring in ICU, there needs to be a plan of where the patient and family/next of kin will be located until the patient has eventually passed away.

3) There continues to be no accurate tool(s) to predict the time interval from withdraw of life-sustaining treatment to asystole.[25]
4) There were initial questions raised about how to characterize the inherent ischemic insult that follows cessation of the donor circulation prior to donor lung retrieval. Accurate, consistent recording of specific DCD time points has enabled the creation of DCD time intervals, which have subsequently been used to determine their impact on DCD LTx recipient outcomes.[20] In the DCD pathway, the warm ischemic time (WIT) will always be significantly longer than in the DBD setting and can actually be defined in several ways.[26] The WIT for DCD donation is most consistently and practically defined as the time interval from when the donor's systemic blood pressure falls below 50mmHg to attainment of a graft temperature of less than 10 degrees Celsius via the pulmonary arterial flush, and is generally around 45 minutes.[20,26]
5) Primary Graft Dysfunction (PGD) and early or intermediate graft failure were specific concerns as a potential consequence of the prolonged warm ischemic time intrinsic to DCD LTx.[24,27] As a result, some centres have advocated a role for EVLP as a protective tool for DCD donor lungs.[24,28] However, when undertaking controlled DCD LTx, the addition of EVLP as an anti-ischemic injury tool or therapy adds significant challenges, being complex, expensive, and not of proven efficacy.[29] Analyses from the ISHLT DCD LTx Registry has recently noted 85% of DCD LTx have been done without EVLP and, within the limitations of current controlled DCD LTx practice, warm ischemic time itself is not associated with early or late mortality.[22]
6) Relatively few uncontrolled DCD LTx have been performed in comparison to controlled DCD LTx, however it is in this type of DCD donor that EVLP may play a greater role in the assessment

of lungs to determine if they can be used for LTx. Although useful, EVLP still has not provided proven efficacy in preventing or ameliorating ischemic injury in uncontrolled DCD lungs at this time either. Consistent with this, a recent small cases series demonstrates good outcomes in an uncontrolled DCD LTx population without universally using EVLP.[30]

7) It is very important to consider the interplay of DBD and DCD organ donation practices within the donor ICU. The process of DCD organ donation has the potential to 'steal' DBD heart, liver, and pancreas donors from the donor pool. This would result in the unintended consequences of decreasing heart, liver, and pancreas transplant opportunities, as for the foreseeable future, these will be more commonly associated with DBD donation. If a potential organ donor is likely to be brain dead, then the DBD pathway should be used rather than the less efficient, but potentially quicker, DCD pathway. In an Australian context, this theoretical conflict has not arisen, with a simultaneous, although subtler, rise in the overall number of DBD LTx, as well as DCD LTx in the recent years (Figure 56.1). Indeed, studies suggest that the extra ICU focus on donation and potential choice of a DCD pathway in some cases has actually allowed time for late progression to brain death. This has subsequently enabled identification of useable DBD donors, initially only recognized as DCD donors.[31,32]

Future directions for DCD LTx

In contrast to DBD LTx, a recent large audit of potential DCD LTx donors suggests a large pool of currently unrecognised controlled Category 3 donors.[33] This pool included both quality and extended lungs. In many cases, the DCD pathway was simply not considered when only the potential donor's lungs, and no other organs, were suitable for transplantation. Potentially, in an Australian context (where DCD lungs are already commonly used), this unrecognized DCD pool could result in a further doubling of activity in terms of ideal donors, extending to tripling of activity if extended donors are considered as well.[33] In a North American context,

Box 56.2 Sub-categorization and modifications to the traditional Categories of DCD donors[35,36]

1 (a) Death outside hospital, no witness
  (b) Death outside hospital, witnessed and attempted resuscitation
2 (a) Unsuccessful resuscitation in the ICU, Emergency Room or OT
  (b) Unsuccessful resuscitation in a hospital ward
3 (a) Awaiting cardiac arrest after planned withdrawal of life-sustaining therapies in the ICU, Emergency Room or OT
  (b) Awaiting cardiac arrest after planned withdrawal of life-sustaining therapies in a hospital ward
  (c) Spontaneous cardiac arrest occurring before planned withdrawal of life-sustaining therapies
4 (a) Spontaneous cardiac arrest in known brain-dead donor
  (b) Awaiting cardiac arrest in known brain-dead donor
5 Medically assisted death (i.e. Euthanasia, Assisted dying)

where the use of DCD lungs is less common, the potential for DCD LTx is as much 20–30 times above what is currently being achieved.[34]

Lungs from DCD donors for transplant are not just available from the current Category 3 and 4 scenarios described in Table 56.1, rather there are other situations that could be considered and these are expanded upon in Box 56.2.[35,36] Lung transplant from DCD donors can be undertaken utilizing donors whose history is known and who have an expected, or even unexpected, cardiac arrest in a hospital Emergency Room, ICU or ward. The use of specifically trained staff (ICU staff or the ward Medical Emergency Treatment (MET) on-call team) and robust protocols are mandated to successfully use these approaches. Use of EVLP may be appropriate in this uncontrolled Box 56.2 Category 2b, 3b, or 3c cases to provide an assessment tool for lungs where lung quality is not necessarily clinically known or characterized at the time of asystole.[28]

Additionally, with little in the way of metabolic activity and associated with air or oxygen as an energy source in adjacent alveoli, there is evidence that inflated DCD lungs (particularly if ventilated) may actually be perfectly useable for several hours after asystole; given the fact, the true clinical limits of lung ischemic time are not actually known.[22,37] When combined with the possibility of simple in-vivo topical cooling of the lungs post-mortem for 4–6 hours, there is definite potential for consideration of allowing time for the subsequent arrival of an off-site retrieval team and/or a delayed OT setup[37–39] in the Box 56.2 Category 1–5 situations.

Conclusion

DCD lung donors are a realistic source of quality lungs for LTx, with excellent long-term clinical outcomes, now clearly comparable to those of traditional DBD LTx. Lung transplant after circulatory death has been successfully applied to both 'extended' donors as well as 'extended' recipients. It is absolutely clear that EVLP is not an essential or required tool to start a lifesaving, successful, DCD LTx programme. We should continue expanding DCD LTx donor opportunities, referrals, retrievals, and innovation.

Highlights

- Sustainable DCD transplantation requires a collaborative protocol.
- DCD LTx techniques are essentially same as those applied to donation after brain death (DBD) LTx.
- EVLP is not required for routine controlled DCD LTx.
- The outcomes of controlled DCD and DBD LTx are essentially identical.
- The pool of non-utilized potential DCD lung donors is large.
- Novel strategies are emerging to expand the use of uncontrolled DCD LTx.

References

1. Kotecha S, Hobson J, Fuller J, Paul E, Levvey BJ, Whitford H, et al. Continued successful evolution of extended criteria donor lungs for transplantation. Ann Thorac Surg. 2017;104(5):1702–1709.

2. Snell GI, Westall GP, Oto T. Donor risk prediction: How 'extended' is safe? Curr Opin Organ Transplant. 2013;18(5):507–512.
3. Cypel M, Levvey B, Van Raemdonck D, Erasmus M, Dark J, Mason D, et al. Lung transplantation using controlled donation after circulatory death donors: Trials and tribulations. J Heart Lung Transplant. 2016;35(1):146–147.
4. Love RB SJ, Chorniak PN. First successful lung transplant using a non-heart beating donor. J Heart Lung Transplant. 1995;14:S88.
5. Steen S, Sjoberg T, Pierre L, Liao Q, Eriksson L, Algotsson L. Transplantation of lungs from a non-heart-beating donor. Lancet. 2001;357(9259):825–829.
6. Van Raemdonck DE, Rega FR, Neyrinck AP, Jannis N, Verleden GM, Lerut TE. Non-heart-beating donors. Semin Thorac Cardiovasc Surg. 2004;16(4):309–321.
7. Nunez JR, Del Rio F, Lopez E, Moreno MA, Soria A, Parra D. Non-heart-beating donors: An excellent choice to increase the donor pool. Transplant Proc. 2005;37(9):3651–3654.
8. Snell GI, Levvey B, Oto T, McEgan R, Mennan M, Eriksson L, et al. Effect of multiorgan donation after cardiac death retrieval on lung performance. ANZ J Surg. 2008;78(4):262–265.
9. Snell GI, Oto T, Levvey B, McEgan R, Mennan M, Higuchi T, et al. Evaluation of techniques for lung transplantation following donation after cardiac death. Ann Thorac Surg. 2006;81(6):2014–2019.
10. Kootstra G, Daemen JH, Oomen AP. Categories of non-heart-beating donors. Transplant Proc. 1995;27(5):2893–4.
11. Snell GI, Levvey BJ, Williams TJ. Non-heart beating organ donation. Intern Med J. 2004;34(8):501–503.
12. Levvey B. Nursing challenges associated with non-heart beating organ donation Aust Nursing J. 2006;13:43.
13. https://alfredhealthconnect.sharepoint.com/Dept/ICU/Pages/Organ-and-Tissue-Donation-Guidelines.aspx. 2018 Alfred Hospital DCD Guidelines. accessed 25/4/2019.
14. Snell GI, Levvey BJ, Oto T, McEgan R, Pilcher D, Davies A, et al. Early lung transplantation success utilizing controlled donation after cardiac death donors. American Journal of Transplantation. 2008;8(6):1282–1289.
15. Saxena P, Zimmet AD, Snell G, Levvey B, Marasco SF, McGiffin DC. Procurement of lungs for transplantation following donation after circulatory death: The Alfred technique. J Surg Res. 2014;192(2):642–646.
16. Edwards J, Mulvania P, Robertson V, George G, Hasz R, Nathan H, et al. Maximizing organ donation opportunities through donation after cardiac death. Crit Care Nurse. 2006;26(2):101–115.
17. Esmore DS, Brown R, Buckland M, Briganti EM, Fetherston GJ, Rabinov M, et al. Techniques and results in bilateral sequential single lung transplantation. The National Heart & Lung Replacement Service. J Card Surg. 1994;9(1):1–14.
18. Snell GI, Levvey BJ, Oto T, McEgan R, Pilcher D, Davies A, et al. Early lung transplantation success utilizing controlled donation after cardiac death donors. Am J Transplant. 2008;8(6):1282–1289.
19. Dhital KK, Iyer A, Connellan M, Chew HC, Gao L, Doyle A, et al. Adult heart transplantation with distant procurement and ex-vivo preservation of donor hearts after circulatory death: A case series. Lancet. 2015;385(9987):2585–2591.

20. Cypel M, Levvey B, Van Raemdonck D, Erasmus M, Dark J, Love R, et al. International Society for Heart and Lung Transplantation Donation After Circulatory Death Registry Report. J Heart Lung Transplant. 2015;34(10):1278–1282.
21. Van Raemdonck D, Keshavjee S, Levvey B, Cherikh WS, Snell G, Erasmus ME et al. 5 year results from the ISHLT DCD Lung Transplant Registry confirm excellent recipient survival from donation after circulatory death donors. J Heart Lung Transplant. 2019;38:S103.
22. Levvey B, Keshavjee S, Cypel M, Robinson A, Erasmus M, Glanville A, et al. Influence of lung donor agonal and warm ischemic times on early mortality: Analyses from the ISHLT DCD Lung Transplant Registry. J Heart Lung Transplant. 2019;38(1):26–34.
23. Levvey BJ, Harkess M, Hopkins P, Chambers D, Merry C, Glanville AR, et al. Excellent clinical outcomes from a national donation-after-determination-of-cardiac-death lung transplant collaborative. Am J Transplant. 2012;12(9):2406–2413.
24. Machuca TN, Mercier O, Collaud S, Tikkanen J, Krueger T, Yeung JC, et al. Lung transplantation with donation after circulatory determination of death donors and the impact of ex vivo lung perfusion. Am J Transplant. 2015;15(4):993–1002.
25. He X, Xu G, Liang W, Liu B, Xu Y, Luan Z, et al. Nomogram for predicting time to death after withdrawal of life-sustaining treatment in patients with devastating neurological injury. Am J Transplant. 2015;15(8):2136–2142.
26. Levvey BJ, Westall GP, Kotsimbos T, Williams TJ, Snell GI. Definitions of warm ischemic time when using controlled donation after cardiac death lung donors. Transplantation. 2008;86(12):1702–1706.
27. Cypel M, Yeung JC, Machuca T, Chen M, Singer LG, Yasufuku K, et al. Experience with the first 50 ex vivo lung perfusions in clinical transplantation. J Thorac Cardiovasc Surg. 2012;144(5):1200–1206.
28. Cypel M, Keshavjee S. Extracorporeal lung perfusion (ex-vivo lung perfusion). Curr Opin Organ Transplant. 2016;21(3):329–335.
29. Snell GI, Levvey BJ, Westall GP. The changing landscape of lung donation for transplantation. Am J Transplant. 2015;15(4):859–860.
30. Suberviola B, Mons R, Ballesteros MA, Mora V, Delgado M, Naranjo S, et al. Excellent long-term outcome with lungs obtained from uncontrolled donation after circulatory death. Am J Transplant. 2019;19(4):1195–1201.
31. Opdam H. Intensive care solely to facilitate organ donation—new challenges. Transplantation. 2017;101(8):1746–1747.
32. Sidiropoulos S, Treasure E, Silvester W, Opdam H, Warrillow SJ, Jones D. Organ donation after circulatory death in a university teaching hospital. Anaesth Intensive Care. 2016;44(4):477–483.
33. Rakhra S GL, Arcia B, Fink M, Kanellis J, MacDonald P, et al. Untapped potential for donation after circulatory death in Australian hospitals. Med J Aust. 2017; In press.
34. OPTN Registry. https://optntransplanthrsagov/data/view-data-reports. 2018; Accessed 11/9/18.
35. Snell GI, Paraskeva M, Westall GP. Donor selection and management. Semin Respir Crit Care Med. 2013;34(3):361–370.

36. Detry O, Le Dinh H, Noterdaeme T, De Roover A, Honore P, Squifflet JP, et al. Categories of donation after cardiocirculatory death. Transplant Proc. 2012;44(5):1189–1195.
37. Reeb J, Keshavjee S, Cypel M. Successful lung transplantation from a donation after cardiocirculatory death donor taking more than 120 minutes to cardiac arrest after withdrawal of life support therapies. J Heart Lung Transplant. 2016;35(2):258–259.
38. Snell GI, Levvey BJ, Levin K, Paraskeva M, Westall G. Donation after brain death versus donation after circulatory death: Lung donor management issues. Semin Respir Crit Care Med. 2018;39(2):138–147.
39. Rega FR, Neyrinck AP, Verleden GM, Lerut TE, Van Raemdonck DE. How long can we preserve the pulmonary graft inside the nonheart-beating donor? Ann Thorac Surg. 2004;77(2):438–444; discussion 44.

57

Heart donation after circulatory death

Simon Messer, Stephen Large, Steven Tsui

Historical overview

The world's first successful heart transplant performed by Christiaan Barnard at the Groote Schuur Hospital, Cape Town, in 1967, was from a donation after circulatory death (DCD) donor.[1] Twenty-four-year-old Denise Darvall had suffered a severe traumatic brain injury following a road traffic accident. However, since brain death was not legally recognized at the time, cadaveric organ donation could only proceed after death had been confirmed by 'conventional' means, i.e. loss of heartbeat and spontaneous respiration, and absence of reflexes. When death was imminent despite therapy, Darvall was taken to the operating room where life-sustaining therapy was withdrawn by stopping the ventilator. Hypoxic cardiac arrest ensued and death was declared when the electrocardiogram showed no activity for 5 minutes. Following intravenous heparinisation, a rapid sternotomy was undertaken by Marius Barnard, the younger brother of Christiaan Barnard. Right atrial and ascending aorta cannulae were inserted for cardiopulmonary bypass (CPB) in order to rapidly cool the donor. At 26°C, CPB flow was reduced to 0.5 $L.min^{-1}$ and the donor aorta was clamped distal to the aortic cannula so that only the donor heart was perfused. The heart was further cooled to 16°C while the kidneys were retrieved. The heart recipient, Louis Washkansky, was a fifty-four-year-old man with end-stage ischemic cardiomyopathy. He was brought to the adjacent operating room and placed on CPB for explant of his diseased heart. At this point, the *in-situ* cooled donor heart was retrieved and placed in a bowl of Ringer's lactate solution at 10°C, transferred to the neighbouring operating room and immediately connected to the recipient's CPB machine for oxygenated blood reperfusion. The donor heart was continually perfused during implantation thus avoiding any further ischaemia. The recipient was weaned off CPB on the third attempt and extubated on day one post-transplant. He progressed well for the first ten days but thereafter developed exhaustion, fever, and dyspnoea. As he was assumed to be suffering from rejection at that time, immunosuppression was intensified with steroid boluses. In reality, the recipient was actually suffering from Klebsiella pneumonia and continued to deteriorate until death on day 18 from overwhelming sepsis.

This first human heart transplant had already indicated that DCD heart transplantation following hypoxic cardiac arrest was possible by using strategies including rapid reperfusion and cooling in combination with continuous perfusion during implantation.

The second DCD human heart transplant was performed three days later by Adrian Kantrowitz in the Maimonides Medical Centre in New York.[(2)] The donor was an anencephalic male infant. The recipient suffered from Ebstein's malformation and right ventricular outflow obstruction. The retrieval team did not wait for mechanical or electrical asystole. Instead, after an irregular cardiac rhythm was observed, topical cooling of the donor in ice cold water was commenced. The donor heart was then removed and placed in ice cold solution. Fifty-five minutes following donor asystole, the recipient aortic cross-clamp was released and the transplanted heart was reperfused. Unfortunately, the heart was unable to support the circulation and the recipient died 6 hours later.

Following Barnard's success, there was a flurry of heart transplant activities across the world but the initial excitement and enthusiasm were short lived. On the 17 September 1971, Life magazine published the article *The Tragic Record of Heart Transplants* detailing the failure of heart transplantation and cited a report from the American Heart Association which stated that on the third anniversary of Barnard's first attempt, a total of 166 heart transplants had been performed worldwide with only twenty-three survivors, giving the procedure an overall survival rate of 13%.[(3)] Following this disclosure, heart transplantation was more or less abandoned with the exception of a few teams: Christian Cabrol in Paris, Norman Shumway in Stanford, (whose survival rate was 34%) and Christiaan Barnard in Cape Town, whose second heart transplant recipient had survived for nineteen months.

Over the next decade, important progresses were made including the introduction of endomyocardial biopsy of the transplanted heart by Philip Caves in 1973 allowing rejection to be detected before clinically evident[4] and Margaret Billingham's work classifying histological rejection.[5]

Although an Adhoc Committee of the Harvard Medical School first proposed irreversible coma as a criterion of death in 1968, adoption of this into practice was slow.[6] It was not until 1976 that the diagnostic criteria of brain death became clarified at a conference of the Medical Royal Colleges in the United Kingdom.[7] Thereafter, transplant teams abandoned DCD organs in favour of DBD as the latter organs do not have the penalty of a warm ischaemic insult before organ preservation.

In 1980, Cyclosporin was introduced as an immunosuppressant for heart transplantation and the one-year post-transplant survival rate increased to a readily acceptable 83%.[8] Thereafter, global heart transplant activity soared leaving DCD heart transplantation to the past.

DCD heart transplantation in infants

In 2004, Boucek and Campbell (Denver, Colorado, US) were the first to re-explore clinical DCD heart transplantation in the modern era.[9] With a 25% mortality for paediatric patients on their heart transplant waiting list, they set up a programme of clinical DCD heart transplantation for potential recipients <18 months old. This was based upon evidence from prior large animal experiments performed by Gundry et al (Loma Linda University Hospital, California) which reported that DCD heart transplantation could be performed on juvenile animals safely if the warm ischaemic period was kept below 30 minutes.[10] Therefore, the Denver team simply relied on cold preservation for DCD heart preservation.

In their protocol, after treatment futility was established and consent obtained, the dying patient was heparinized and the femoral vessels cannulated under local anaesthesia. Comfort measures including sedation and analgesia were given before the dying patient was extubated. For their first DCD donor, death was declared 3 minutes after asystole. However, the observation period after asystole was reduced to 75 seconds for the next two donors.

Following the declaration of death, cold preservation fluid was infused through a balloon catheter into the ascending aorta while a rapid sternotomy was performed. The heart was topically cooled and vented, and then removed for cold storage until transplantation.

Three paediatric DCD hearts were successfully transplanted using this technique in recipients with a mean age of 2.2 months old, two of them suffering with congenital heart disease and one with dilated cardiomyopathy.

The cause of death of all three donors was birth asphyxia. The mean donor age was 3.7 days and the mean donor weight was 3.2 kg. The mean time to death following extubation was 18 minutes with a mean total cold ischaemic time of 162 minutes. Following transplantation, one recipient required extra corporeal membrane oxygenation (ECMO) support for primary graft dysfunction in the early post-transplant period. All recipients survived to hospital discharge after a mean hospital stay of twenty days. At six months follow-up, all three heart recipients were alive with good ventricular function.[9]

Although this effort from the Denver group was pivotal in renewing interests in DCD heart transplantation, reducing the observation period after asystole from 3 minutes to 75 seconds attracted much criticism as this came within the window during which auto resuscitation had previously been reported.[9]

A registry study of the International Society of Heart and Lung Transplantation (ISHLT) database reported 21 DCD paediatric heart transplants between 2005 and 2014 with seventeen cases in the first half of the period and only four cases in the second half (0.5% of overall paediatric heart transplants). The study reported a one-year survival of only 61% with paediatric DCD heart transplants compared with 91% for paediatric DBD heart transplants.[11]

Adult DCD heart transplantation

Two techniques are currently used successfully for retrieval of the donor heart in a DCD setting, namely, Direct Procurement and Perfusion (DPP) and Thoraco-abdominal Normothermic Regional Perfusion (TANRP). The latter can be followed by machine perfusion for distant procurement or cold preservation for local procurement.

Direct Procurement and Perfusion (DPP)

In 2015, Dhital and MacDonald (St Vincent's Hospital, Sydney) reported three successful cases of adult DCD heart transplants following distant procurement.[(12)] This accomplishment was the result of a combination of their large animal research investigating adjuncts to cardioplegia to limit reperfusion injury, and their experience of transporting DBD hearts on the Organ Care System Heart (OCS Heart, TransMedics Inc., MA) across the vast distances of Australia.[(13)]

Inclusion criteria were Maastricht category III donors, <40 years old with preserved biventricular function prior to WLST and donation withdrawal ischaemic time (DWIT) <30 minutes (i.e. the time from WLST to administration of cardioplegia to the heart). In Australia, the required observation period after asystole before death is certified varies between States and ranges from 2 to 5 minutes.[(13)]

Following asystole and declaration of death, a sternotomy was undertaken and the donor was heparinized. A cannula was placed in the right atrium to collect heparinized donor blood which was passed through a leucocyte filter and added to the OCS Heart module pre-primed with 500mls of TransMedics proprietary solution and methyl prednisolone. The donor heart was flushed with 1 L of cold St Thomas' cardioplegic solution supplemented with 5,000 IU of erythropoietin and 100mg of glycerine trinitrate. The heart was then explanted. The donor aorta and pulmonary artery were cannulated for connection onto the OCS organ chamber.

The TransMedics OCS Heart comprises a portable console with a disposable module encompassing a diaphragmatic pump, an in-line heat exchanger, an oxygenator, and an organ chamber (Figure 57.1).

The device pumps warm, oxygenated blood through the donor ascending aorta to the coronary arteries. The superior and inferior vena cavae are sutured closed and blood draining from the coronary sinus into the right atrium and right ventricle is ejected through the cannulated pulmonary artery where coronary flow can be monitored. Coronary blood flow is regulated by either varying the OCS pump flow or the infusion rate of the maintenance solution which contains adenosine.[(14)]

The donor heart being perfused in the OCS is beating but the left ventricle is vented and unloaded. Therefore, it is not possible to assess the

(a)

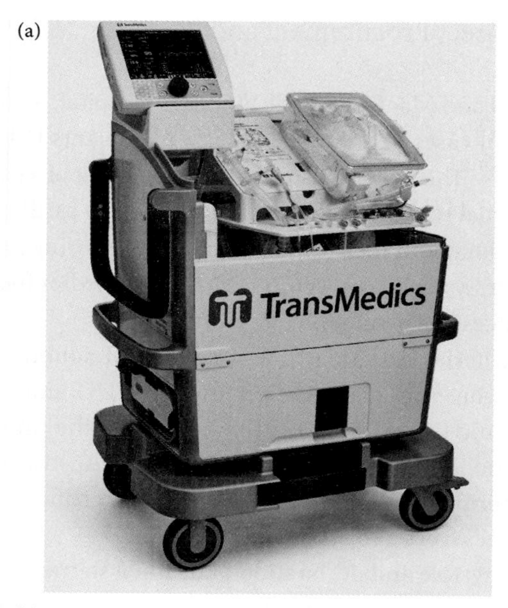

(b)

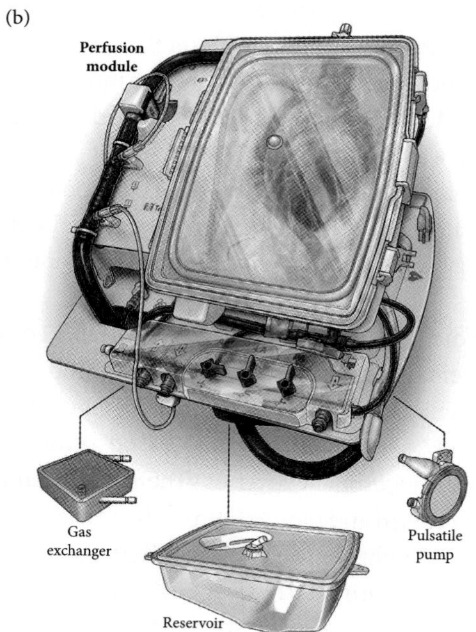

Figure 57.1. The TransMedics Organ Care System and Single-use Heart Module

mechanical function of the donor heart with the OCS. To assess the acceptability of a DBD heart perfused by the OCS, the manufacturer recommends using serial paired arterial and venous lactate concentrations to ensure a falling trend and an end lactate below 5 mmol/L.

Of the first three DCD heart transplants reported using the DPP technique, the mean donor age was twenty-six years and the mean WLST to cardioplegia time of 25 minutes. The donor hearts were perfused on the OCS Heart for an average of 254 minutes. Of the three recipients, one required ECMO support for primary graft dysfunction which was weaned four days later. All three recipients were discharged home alive with a mean hospital length of stay of twenty-five days.

Thoraco-abdominal normothermic regional perfusion

In 2016, Messer and Large (Royal Papworth Hospital, Cambridge, UK) reported the first series of adult DCD heart transplants using the NRP technique.[15] The cornerstone of this technique pivoted around *in-situ* reperfusion and reanimation of the heart within the DCD donor followed by functional assessment of the heart prior to retrieval and transplantation.

Following extensive laboratory research and prolonged deliberations by the UK transplant regulatory body, the Papworth team was given approval for a clinical programme of DCD heart transplantation in early 2015. The technique involved restoring perfusion to the DCD heart within the donor with exclusion of the cerebral circulation. After reanimation of the asystolic DCD heart, it was volume loaded to allow full functional assessment. With this approach, the Papworth team was able to extend the margins of DCD donor acceptability criteria, increasing donor age up to fifty-seven years and a DWIT of up to 4 hours.

In the UK, no antemortem interventions or drugs are permitted and the legally defined observation period following mechanical asystole is 5 minutes. In the TANRP protocol, following asystole and declaration of death, the donor was taken to the operating room where a rapid sternotomy and laparotomy were performed simultaneously. The pericardium was opened and heparin was injected into the right atrium (30,000IU) and the pulmonary artery (20,000IU). The three aortic arch branches were clamped, the right atrium was cannulated for venous return, and the proximal aortic arch cannulated for arterial inflow TANRP was commenced at a flow rate of 5 $l.min^{-1}$. Exclusion of the cerebral circulation was confirmed with carotid Doppler. Following re-establishment of circulation, dopamine was commended at 5 $mcg.kg^{-1}.min^{-1}$ and vasopressin at 4 $units.hr^{-1}$. The donor was re-intubated and ventilated before weaning from NRP support. Thereafter, a trans-oesophageal echocardiogram was undertaken and thermodilution cardiac outputs assessed with a pulmonary artery catheter. The acceptance criteria of DCD hearts following TANRP and functional assessment are shown in Table 57.1.

TANRP followed by machine perfusion for distant procurement.
For distant procurement at donor hospitals >30 minute travel from Papworth Hospital, DCD hearts accepted after TANRP and functional assessment will have to be retrieved and transported back to Papworth Hospital while continually perfused in the OCS Heart to minimise further ischaemia.[15]

In the first report, nine adult DCD hearts were retrieved after TANRP and *in-situ* functional assessment. The mean donor age was thirty-six years and the mean duration from WLST to aortic perfusion was 41 minutes. After weaning from TANRP, functional assessment of the DCD hearts demonstrated a mean cardiac index of 3.4 $L.min^{-1}.m^{-2}$ and a left ventricular ejection fraction of 65%. The mean recipient age was fifty-two years. One recipient required seven days of post-transplant ECMO (11%) support for primary graft dysfunction. On an average, recipients spent eight days in intensive care and were discharged after a total hospital stay of twenty-nine days. All remained alive at five-year follow-up.

Table 57.1 Acceptance criteria for DCD hearts following TANRP and functional assessment

Left Ventricular Ejection Fraction	>50%
Central venous pressure	<12 mmHg
Pulmonary capillary wedge pressure (PCWP)	<12 mmHg
Cardiac Index	>2.5 $l.min^{-1}.m^{-2}$

TANRP followed by cold preservation for local procurement of DCD hearts

One of the main limitations of expanding adult DCD heart transplantation is the cost of using the OCS Heart. For DCD donors co-located with the heart recipient, a DCD heart reanimated with TANRP with satisfactory functional assessment could be transplanted directly with a brief period of cold preservation, thus avoiding the cost of using the OCS Heart. Three such DCD heart transplants have been performed by the Papworth team,[16] and a further two have been described by a team at Liege in Belgium.[17] All recipients survived to hospital discharge.

Clinical results of DCD heart transplantation

Although there have been several published case reports, only Sydney,[18] Royal Papworth,[19] and Manchester, UK[20] have published their case series of adult DCD heart transplants (Table 57.2). While the Sydney and Manchester teams used the DPP technique only, the Papworth team practice all three retrieval techniques, namely DPP, TANRP followed by machine perfusion, and TANRP followed by cold storage. The one-year survival for DCD heart transplantation of 85% is comparable with that of DBD heart transplants.

Potential of DCD heart transplantation

There have been four published studies postulating on the potential of DCD heart transplantation with varying predictions. The study by Singhal et al in 2005 using data from the Pennsylvania Gift of Life Donor programme suggested that overall heart transplant activity in the USA could be increased by 4–6% if DCD heart transplantation were adopted (assuming donor age < 45 years and a DWIT of < 30 mins).[21] Another study from Wisconsin in 2010 suggested that overall heart transplant activity could increase by 17% if DCD were to be introduced.[22] A Belgian study in 2013 estimated that DCD had the potential to increase overall heart transplant activity by 11%.[23]

Table 57.2 Published DCD Donor Heart Transplant Programme Outcomes

Features of comparison	Sydney n=23	Papworth n=26		Manchester n=7
	DPP	NRP=12	DPP=14	DPP
Donor				
Age (years)	29 (24–33)	37 (33–42)	35 (26–36)	28 (25–37)
Sex: Male n (%)	19 (86%)	9 (75%)	13 (93%)	7 (100%)
Donor Cause of Death				
Hypoxic Brain Injury n (%)	8 (35%)	13 (50%)	10 (71%)	4 (57%)
Intracerebral Haemorrhage n (%)	2 (7%)	7 (27%)	2 (14%)	2 (29%)
Traumatic Brain Injury n (%)	10 (44%)	5 (19%)	2 (14%)	1 (4%)
Other n (%)	3 (13)	1 (4%)	0 (0%)	0 (0%)
Donor Warm Ischaemic Time * mins	24 (20–27)	24 (21–28)	37 (33–42)	34 (31–39)
Recipient				
Age (years)	57 (44–62)	58 (49–60)	55 (44–61)	57 (39–59)
Sex: Male n (%)	17 (74%)	10 (83%)	12 (86%)	6 (86%)
Pre transplant VAD	8 (23%)	1 (8%)	5 (36%)	2 (29%)
Outcomes				
Intra-aortic balloon pump	7%	17%	36%	29%
ECMO	30%	8%	14%	43%
ICU Stay (Days)	7	5 (4–5)	6 (3–10)	14 (9–16)
Hospital Stay (Days)	24	19 (17–27)	20 (19–27)	31 (26–32)
30 day survival	95%	100%	100%	100%
90 day survival	95%	100%	86%	85%
1 year survival	95%	100%	86%	NR

[Continuous values are presented with medians and interquartile ranges. Categorical data are summarized with counts and percentages. * Donor warm ischaemic time—time from withdrawal of life supportive therapy to the onset of cardioplegia or reperfusion. VAD—ventricular assist device; ECMO—extra corporeal membrane oxygenation; ICU Intensive Care Unit Duration; NR-not reported]

WORLDWIDE ACTUAL DONORS AFTER CIRCULATORY DEATH 2018 (pmp)
SPAIN 13,50
BELGIUM 10,40
UNITED KINGDOM 9,37
NETHERLANDS* 8,59
USA 6,62
AUSTRALIA 6,16
CANADA* 5,49
SWITZERLAND 3,80
PORTUGAL 2,73
NEW ZEALAND* 2,50
FRANCE* 2,11
AUSTRIA 1,80
CZECH REPUBLIC* 1,23
ITALY 1,20
LEBANON* 1,10
LATVIA* 1,03
SWEDEN 0,98
IRELAND 0,85
ISRAEL 0,50
RUSSIA* 0,35
SAUDI ARABIA* 0,18
POLAND 0,10
* Data from 2017

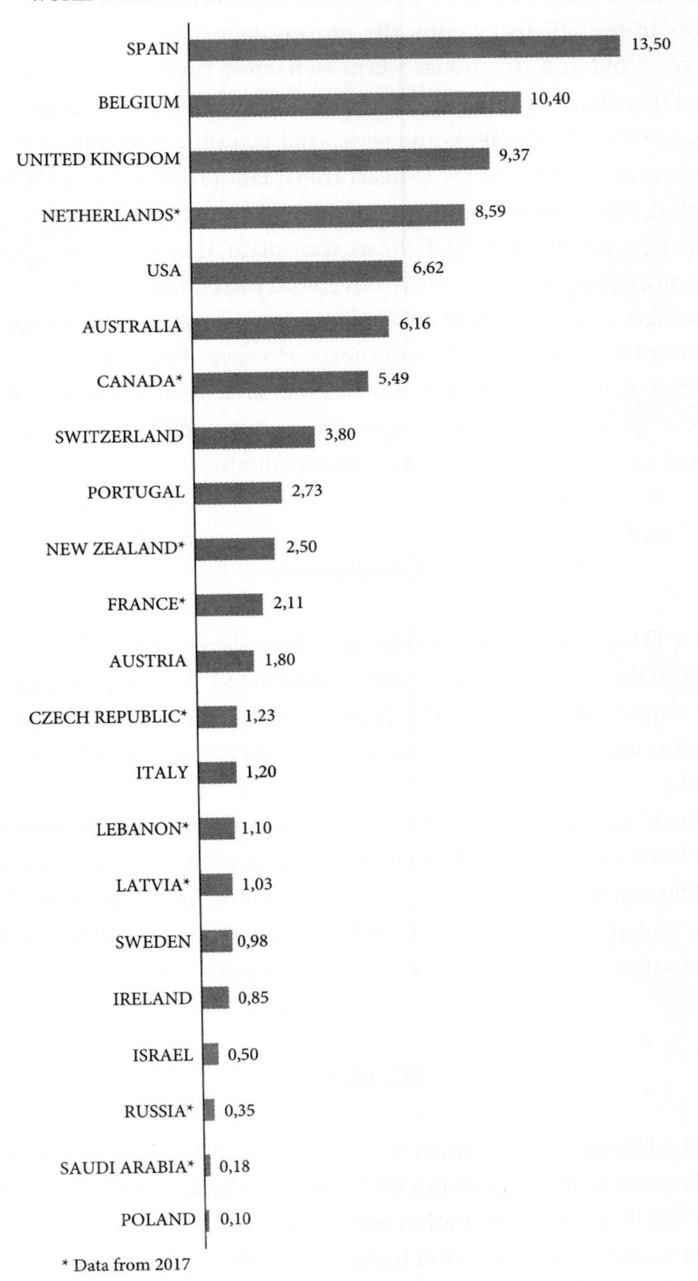

Figure 57.2. Worldwide actual donors after circulatory death per million population in 2017[25]

The most recent study in 2019 screening over 6,000 potential DCD donors in the UK using clinically proven inclusion criteria (donor age <50 years old and functional warm ischaemic time <30 minutes) suggested that DCD has the potential to increase overall heart transplant activity by 56%.[24] This is in line with what was observed during the first five years of the clinical DCD heart transplant programme at Papworth Hospital, where overall heart transplant activity increased by 47%.

The true potential of DCD heart transplantation will depend on the incidence of DCD which varies from country to country (Figure 57.2),[25] the relative contribution of DCD donors to overall deceased donors in that country and the acceptance criteria. However, the incidence of DCD has been increasing in many countries year after year; if a historical incidence of DCD was used for the calculation, it would likely underestimate the true potential of DCD on heart transplantation.

Conclusion

The DCD heart transplantation has now been shown to be safe and reproducible if the warm ischaemic period is respected. Early outcomes appear to be comparable to that of DBD heart transplants. Although longer-term outcomes are as yet unknown, these are not expected to be inferior to that of DBD.

Several techniques now exist for procuring and reconditioning the DCD heart in order to facilitate its recovery from the warm ischaemic insult after asystole. The DCD heart transplantation has the potential to increase global heart transplant activities significantly and offer new hope to thousands of more patients with advanced heart failure.

Highlights

- The first successful human heart transplant performed by Christiaan Barnard in 1967 was from a DCD donor co-located with the recipient.
- DCD heart transplantation was abandoned following poor results in favour of donation after brain death (DBD) donation after the acceptance of brain death criteria in the mid-1970s.

- DCD heart transplantation was reintroduced in 2008 when a group from Denver, Colorado successfully transplanted three paediatric DCD hearts using cold static storage.
- In 2015, St Vincent's Hospital, Sydney, reported three successful adult heart DCD transplants following distant procurement using normothermic *ex-situ* machine perfusion during transportation.
- In 2016, Royal Papworth Hospital, Cambridge, reported the first series of nine DCD heart transplants where the donor heart underwent functional assessment within the donor after reconditioning with thoraco-abdominal normothermic regional perfusion.
- Early outcomes following DCD and DBD heart transplantation are comparable and the use of DCD donor hearts has the potential to increase overall heart transplantation by up to 56%.

References

1. Barnard CN. The operation. A human cardiac transplant: An interim report of a successful operation performed at Groote Schuur Hospital, Cape Town. S Afr Med J. 1967;41:1271–1274.
2. Kantrowitz A, Haller JD, Joos H, Cerruti MM, Carstensen HE. Transplantation of the heart in an infant and an adult. Am J Cardiol. 1968;22:782–790.
3. Thompson T. The tragic record of heart transplantation. Graves R, editor. Life Magazine. September 17, 1971(12):56.
4. Caves PK, Stinson EB, Graham AF, Billingham ME, Grehl TM, Shumway NE. Percutaneous transvenous endomyocardial biopsy. JAMA. 1973;225:288–291.
5. Caves PK, Stinson EB, Billingham ME, Shumway NE. Serial transvenous biopsy of the transplanted human heart. Improved management of acute rejection episodes. Lancet. 1974;1:821–826.
6. Landmark article Aug 5, 1968: A definition of irreversible coma. Report of the Ad Hoc Committee of the Harvard Medical School to examine the definition of brain death. JAMA. 1984;252:677–679.
7. Diagnosis of brain death. Statement issued by the honorary secretary of the Conference of Medical Royal Colleges and their Faculties in the United Kingdom on 11 October 1976. Br Med J. 1976;2:1187–1188.
8. McGregor CG, Oyer PE, Shumway NE. Heart and heart-lung transplantation. Prog Allergy. 1986;38:346–365.
9. Boucek MM, Mashburn C, Dunn SM, Frizell R, Edwards L, Pietra B, et al. Pediatric heart transplantation after declaration of cardiocirculatory death. N Engl J Med. 2008;359:709–714.
10. SR Gundry, M Kawauchi., H Liu, A Raziouk, LL Bailey. Successful heart transplantation in lambs using asystolic, pulseless, dead donors. J Am Coll Surg. 1990;15:224A.

11. Kleinmahon JA, Patel SS, Auerbach SR, Rossano J, Everitt MD. Hearts transplanted after circulatory death in children: Analysis of the International Society for Heart and Lung Transplantation registry. Paediatr Transplant 201;21:e13064
12. Dhital KK, Iyer A, Connellan M, Chew HC, Gao L, Doyle A, et al. Adult heart transplantation with distant procurement and ex-vivo preservation of donor hearts after circulatory death: A case series. Lancet. 2015;385:2585–2591.
13. Iyer A, Gao L, Doyle A, Rao P, Cropper JR, Soto C, et al. Normothermic ex vivo perfusion provides superior organ preservation and enables viability assessment of hearts from DCD donors. Am J Transplant. 2015;15:371–380.
14. Messer S, Ardehali A, Tsui S. Normothermic donor heart perfusion: current clinical experience and the future. Transpl Int. 2015;28:634–642.
15. Messer SJ, Axell RG, Colah S, White PA, Ryan M, Page AA, et al. Functional assessment and transplantation of the donor heart after circulatory death. J Heart Lung 2016: 35: 1443–1452.
16. Messer S, Page a, Colah C, Axell R, Parizkova B, Tsui S, Large S. Human heart transplantation from donation after circulatory-determined death donors using normothermic regional perfusion and cold storage. J Heart Lung Transplant. 2018;37:865.
17. V Tchana-Sato, D Ledoux,O Detry, G Hans, A Ancion, VD'Orio et al. Successful clinical transplantation of hearts donated after circulatory death using normothermic regional perfusion. J Heart Lung Tran 2019;38:593–598.
18. Chew H, Iyer A, Connellan M, Scheuer S, Villaneuva J, Gao L et al. Outcomes of donation after circulatory death heart transplantation in Australia. JACC. 2019:73; 1447–1458.
19. Messer S, Page A, Axell R, Berman M, Hermandez-Sanchez J, Colah S, et al. Outcome after heart transplantation from donation after circulatory-determined death donors. J Heart Lung Transplant 2017:36:1311–1318.
20. Mehta V, Taylor M, Hasan J, Dimarakis I, Barnard J, Callan P et al. Establishing a heart transplant programme using donation after circulatory determined death donors: a United Kingdom based single centre experience. Interact CardioVasc Thorac Surg 2019; 29:422–429.
21. Singhal AK, Abrams JD, Mohara J, Hasz RD, Nathan HM, Fisher CA, et al. Potential suitability for transplantation of hearts from human non-heart-beating donors: Data review from the Gift of Life Donor Program. J Heart Lung Transplant. 2005;24:1657–1664.
22. Osaki S, Anderson JE, Johnson MR, Edwards NM, Kohmoto T. The potential of cardiac allografts from donors after cardiac death at the University of Wisconsin Organ Procurement Organization. Eur J Cardiothorac Surg. 2010;37:74–79.
23. Noterdaeme T, Detry O, Hans M-F, Nellessen E, Ledoux D, Joris J, et al. What is the potential increase in the heart graft pool by cardiac donation after circulatory death? Transpl Int. 2013;26:61–6.
24. Messer S, Page A, Rushton S, Berman M, Tsui S, Catarino P, Large S. The potential of heart transplantation from donation after circulatory death donors within the United Kingdom. J Heart Lung Transplant 2019:38:872–874.
25. International Registry in Organ Donation and Transplantation. Preliminary Numbers 2017. Last accessed 29/09/2019 Available at http://www.irodat.org/img/database/pdf/NEWSLETTER2018_June.pdf

58

Organ donation after circulatory death: Abdominal organs with particular reference to liver transplantation

Paolo Muiesan, Chiara Lazzeri and Andrea Schlegel

Introduction

Donation after circulatory death (DCD) emerged in the past twenty years as the greatest approach to provide potential additional organs for transplantation. The majority of people die of causes that do not lead to brain death and, therefore, DCD could help meet the growing requirements of organ transplantation.[1]

There are several challenges to successful DCD programs. Despite large numbers of potential donors, DCD cannot be the definitive remedy to the shortage of organs for transplantation due to hurdles, mainly related to ischaemia reperfusion injury (IRI), which may be responsible for graft dysfunction or failure. The liver displays an exceptional sensitivity to IRI and presents organ-specific injury in terms of ischaemic damage to the biliary tree.

The rate of DCD donation can be limited by ethical concerns and religious beliefs, which vary between countries and have a vast impact upon organ donation. For example, controlled DCD donation is not possible in some countries, where withdrawal of life-sustaining treatment is prohibited. Ethical issues are greater in uncontrolled compared to controlled DCD donation and are associated mainly with the efforts of resuscitation and the non-invasive and invasive procedures required. Logistic issues surrounding organ donation are also greater for uncontrolled DCD donors, where a network of mobile intensive care units is an essential requirement. Thus, the process of DCD organ donation and associated transplant programs is presented with strong challenges from individuals, society, and the technical and logistical process of the organ procurement strategy.

Donor warm ischaemia time and liver procurement

The hypoxia and cardiovascular instability (agonal phase), that follow treatment withdrawal in a donor (WLST) and the mandatory stand-off period in the DCD donation process are responsible for the additional period of warm ischaemia time and aggravation of hepatic IRI, compared to donation after brain death (DBD).

At this time, there is no consensus regarding the definition of donor warm ischaemia time (DWIT) and various definitions are being used. Overall DWIT (or total DWIT) can be divided into two periods: the agonal phase from WLST until circulatory arrest and the asystolic phase from circulatory arrest until the start of cold perfusion. For the graft to be considered for liver transplantation, the maximum length of the full period of DWIT cannot extend over 60 minutes in most countries including the Netherlands and the United Kingdom (UK). [(2)] On average, the time for a potential DCD donor to die of circulatory arrest is 36 minutes.[(3)] However, DWIT is a dynamic period, and some donors have a longer period of a hypoxia or hypotension during the agonal phase with a potential major impact on the severity of later hepatic IRI. The impact of DWIT on post-operative outcomes after DCD liver transplantation has been studied by many, with however various definitions and durations of DWIT, accepted by national protocols. Such cofounders led to highly variable studies and difficulties to interpret and compare risk and outcomes in DCD transplantation.[(4)] Donor warm ischaemia time is frequently reported as the functional DWIT (fDWIT). The latter is counted from the start of the agonal phase with a deterioration of oxygen saturation (pO_2<70% or 80% in Spain) or blood pressure (MAP or SBP < 50 mm Hg or 60mmHg in Spain), until the start of cold perfusion (Figure 58.1). In the UK and other countries, the threshold for discarding a DCD liver is 30 minutes of fDWIT.[(5)]

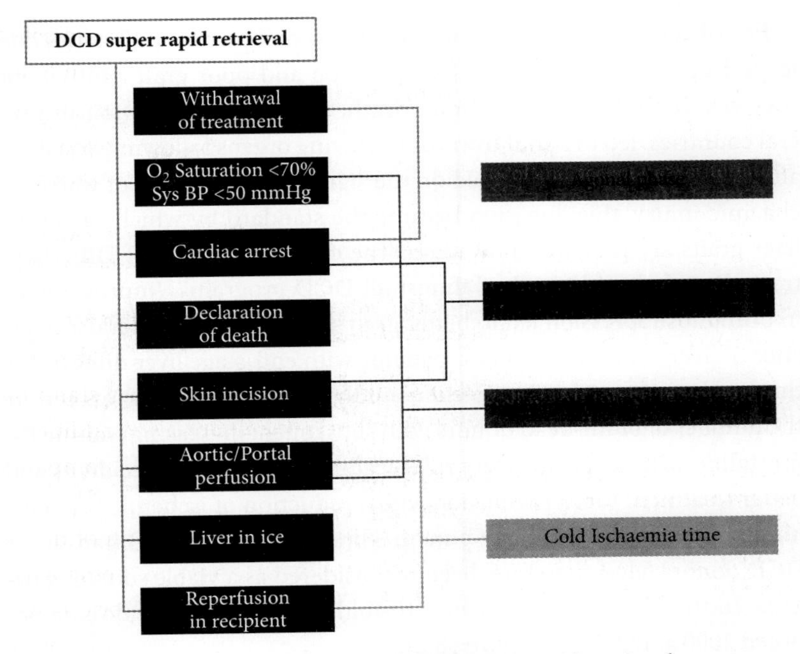

Figure 58.1. Time periods of the modified super rapid retrieval technique in DCD

History of DCD liver transplantation

The very first organ transplants were from donors after circulatory death. In 1936, six patients in Kiev received kidney transplants for mercury poisoning.[6] All patients died, presumably due to ischaemic injury of the graft as organ procurement occurred hours after death.

The first human liver transplants were associated with no survivors beyond two months and utilized solely DCD. Starzl recognized the role of ischaemic injury related to DCD and described, at this early stage, biochemical evidence of hepatocellular damage, postoperative coagulopathy, and biliary necrosis in transplanted grafts at autopsy.[7] The importance of limiting ischaemic injury by slowing down the metabolism by hypothermic perfusion (cold organ flush) and reducing the time from donor death to revascularization was emphasized in these early experiments. Calne, also utilizing DCD donor organs, suggested to limit the time from death to cold perfusion to 15 min.[8]

Early liver transplant programs experienced numerous difficulties due to peri-operative care, immunosuppression and poor graft and patient survival. The recognition of brain death, and its legal adoption in several countries, led to a shift towards retrieving organs following donation after brain death (DBD). Based on the significant reduction of warm ischaemic injury, this donation became the standard by which cadaveric liver grafts are procured nowadays. The clear superiority of DBD liver transplants led to the end of almost all DCD programs. Improvements in immunosuppression led to better graft survival and to general acceptance of liver transplantation for patients with end-stage liver disease. So, the number of potential recipients rapidly increased at a rate exceeding the number of brain-dead donors with subsequent increasing waiting list mortalities. Stricter road safety rules leading to fewer fatal accidents and better treatment for hypertension with a reduction of ischemic brain injuries and a further decline of potential brain-dead donors. Organs from DCD donors have, therefore, been reconsidered as a viable source of organs. In the UK, there has been a 10-fold increase in DCD donors between 2000 and 2010[9] (Figure 58.2).

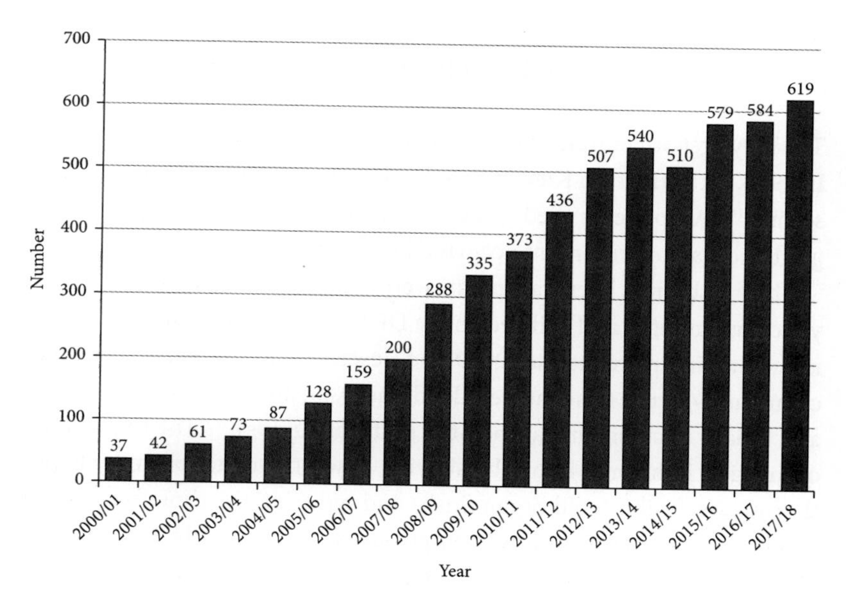

Figure 58.2. DCD donors in the UK

Early enthusiasm with DCD renal transplantation was justified by the similar long-term renal function when compared to DBD renal grafts.[10,11] In contrast, early liver DCD programs, showed a high incidence of allograft dysfunction and failure in addition to an almost doubled rate of biliary complications.[12] The Pittsburgh group published an early small experience of both controlled and uncontrolled DCD liver transplants. Only one of six uncontrolled DCD liver grafts survived longer than a month, whereas controlled DCD grafts had better initial function but a high rate of vascular complications.[13] The group of the University of Wisconsin (UW) revealed a comparable 1-year patient survival of recipients of DBD or DCD liver grafts but at the expense of high rates of re-transplantation in the DCD group due to primary nonfunction (PNF). One-year DCD graft survival was 54% versus 81% for DBD grafts.[14] The reduction of warm and cold ischaemic times in addition to a careful donor and recipient selection became important tools to achieve equivalent graft and patient survival comparing DBD and DCD liver recipients.[15] A distinctive problem of DCD liver transplantation is the high risk of postoperative biliary complications and of ischaemic-type biliary lesions (ITBL) in particular. This was first described in 1995[13] and subsequently recognized to be associated with an increased duration of DWIT.[16,17]

Current scenario of DCD liver donation and transplantation in practice

Due to logistical reasons and the associated risk of ischaemic injury in uncontrolled DCD, only deaths occurring at a centre with established organ retrieval pathways and teams are appropriate for donation of solid organs. An answer to some logistical challenges may be the deployment of healthcare resources outside the hospital. In order to maximize rates of uncontrolled DCD and optimize donor management, mobile medical teams are tasked to manage patients in out-of-hospital cardio-circulatory arrest.

In contrast, controlled DCD donation occurs with the attendance of the organ procurement surgical team to limit the ischaemic injury associated with the process of deterioration and circulatory death, which usually entails an agonal premortem period of hypotension and hypoxia. The ischaemic injury, that follows may preclude organ donation or be accountable for graft dysfunction or nonfunction of the transplanted organ.[18]

Considering the logistic constraints among others, the main challenges that face DCD liver transplantation include the preservation of organ function and the achievement of outcomes similar to those of DBD grafts. Meticulous selection of donor and recipient is a key to lower the incidence of the major complications, that arise from DCD liver utilization, including delayed or absent graft function, ITBL and acute kidney injury (AKI). These are all closely related to the added injury suffered solely by DCD organs during the DWIT.

Ethical and legal considerations are also intrinsically associated with DCD procedures. DCD donation allows deceased patients and their relatives the possibility of proceeding to organ donation even if, at the time of dying, brain death criteria are not met.[19] It also benefits those individuals, who do not recognize brain death and in whom death can only be accepted following the cessation of the cardiac activity and circulation of blood. However, some of the processes associated with DCD donation may raise ethical and legal concerns.[20] The change of culture towards a return to DCD has been challenging particularly for healthcare professionals in regard to a potential conflict of interest when faced with patients in whom ongoing treatment is futile and who may be suitable DCD donors. Ambiguity also exists on what are acceptable interventions pre- and post-mortem during the process of DCD donation, particularly in the case of uncontrolled DCD of the liver, and what conditions must be met in order to confirm death in DCD donors.

Controlled DCD donation

The current challenge in DCD donation is to achieve equivalent graft and patient survivals compared to recipients of DBD grafts, while expanding the DCD donor pool and decreasing the rate of ITBL, which is the main cause of graft loss in DCD liver transplantation. An active cDCD program, which may diminish the DBD activity was a big concern in the past. A review of organ donation within twenty-three European countries identified that eighteen had demonstrated an increase in DBD rates between 2000 and 2009,[21] Three of the five countries with stagnant rates of DBD were those with expanding controlled donation after circulatory death (cDCD) programs (Belgium, the Netherlands, and the United Kingdom). More recently these issues have been addressed and for example Spain has piloted cDCD programmes without an impact on DBD rates.[22]

Ethical perspectives of controlled DCD

It is essential from an ethical perspective, that the decision to undertake WLST is made prior to and independently from the decision to donate. Once withdrawal of treatment is agreed and decided, a separate team, which is independent and not involved in the treatment of the patient, will assess the suitability of donation to avoid any conflict of interest.

When donation is considered possible, the family or next of kin are approached and consent for DCD is sought. Organ retrieval teams are organized to be available at the donor hospital in a timely manner so that the WLST can be performed without delay. In the UK, medical care to patients diagnosed with an unrecoverable illness is limited to what is thought to be in the best interests of the patient. Thus, any procedure or intervention deemed unnecessary for that patient's ongoing medical care could be considered unethical. However, in controlled DCD a broader approach to assessing the best interest of an individual has been upheld by the courts and is fundamental in UK law.[19] A person's wish with regard to organ donation can be assessed by discussion with family and by checking the national organ donor registry. When organ donation is considered to have been a dying patient's wish, then interventions may be appropriate, including discussing donation with family, reviewing a patient's past medical history for the purposes of donation, taking blood and serum, maintenance of life-sustaining treatment, and delaying WLST until the surgical team is on site.

Controversial interventions include those that may place the person at risk of harm or distress, including the systemic heparinization which might hasten death, placement of femoral catheters or cannula, and cardiopulmonary resuscitation prior to the commencement of organ recovery processes.[23]

Both the procedure and the location of WLST are controversial. During WLST in cDCD, the process of extubation has been perceived as *uncomfortable* by some health professionals.[24] In terms of logistics, the operating theatre would be ideal to keep the fDWIT to a minimum for the purposes of organ donation and successful organ transplantation. However, choosing the best site of WLST is usually a compromise between providing the final treatment to the patient, respecting the dying patient's right to dignity and privacy, offering access to family and loved ones and the benefit for the prospective recipient. This plan must also take into consideration the outcome if donation does not proceed.

Donor selection in controlled DCD

The increased incidence of graft dysfunction and non-function associated with DCD organs have resulted in great attention being placed upon donor selection. A very strict selection policy of the very best controlled DCD grafts has achieved excellent results so that some of these liver grafts were even reduced to allow transplantation in children.[25,,26] This selection process is dynamic and is influenced by several events following WLST. The key component that is considered is the fDWIT. The latter was originally defined in the United Kingdom as the duration of time from either when a patient's systolic blood pressure falls below 50 mm Hg or, when the arterial oxygen saturation falls below 70%, whichever comes first, to the commencement of cold perfusion in aorta.[27] Similar definitions have been proposed in the United States and make a distinction between the total DWIT (time from WLST and cold perfusion) and the true DWIT (another term for functional DWIT, from when systolic blood pressure falls below 50 mm Hg and cold perfusion). In Spain, the threshold in systolic blood pressure is 60 mmHg.

The tolerance to warm ischaemic injury appears organ specific. Therefore, the maximum fDWIT ranges between 30 min for liver and pancreas, to 60min for lungs and 120min for kidneys. Such timings

Table 58.1 Extended criteria for DCD liver donation

Age >50 years
Weight >100kg
Intensive care stay >5 days
Functional warm ischaemic time >20 minutes, < 30 minutes
Cold ischaemia time >8 hours (up to 12 hours)
Steatosis >15%

are not absolute but represent, on average, the maximum duration that could be tolerated by the organs. Other factors that may affect DCD liver quality include donor age, body mass index, comorbidities, and premortem events. Characteristics associated with 'standard' and 'extended criteria' donors of liver grafts and other organs are shown in Table 58.1.

The prediction of the time required for a donor to proceed to circulatory death following WLST, would help to identify donors likely to provide organs with minimal ischaemic injury, optimized resource allocation, and limit the family distress. A United network of Organ sharing (UNOS) committee presented five criteria to accurately predict death within 60 or 120 min from WLST.(28) An external validation showed a less accurate prediction power.(29) Other authors have studied neurological criteria to predict death in DCD patients.(30) However, none of these scores have been validated outside of the United States or were able to adequately predict which DCD will have a fDWIT of 30 min or less. A project from the UK focused upon predicting death in Maastricht-type 3 donors and liver graft usage.(31) Independent predictors of death in this study included age under forty years, the use of inotropes, and the absence of a cough/gag reflex.

An external validation by a European group revealed that four previously published models had a good discrimination, but modest calibration, with an overoptimistic predicted probabilities of death within 60 minutes.(32) It also showed that the absence of brainstem reflexes, persistent ventilatory failure, and aspects of WLST practices should be incorporated as the basis for future validation studies. These criteria are summarized in Table 58.2.

Table 58.2 Criteria for predicting death within 60 minutes from WLST in cDCD

Factors	Odds ratio	95% CI		P
		Lower	Upper	
Absent cough reflex	8.04	5.51	11.7	< .001
Absent corneal reflex	3.76	2.65	5.32	< .001
Dosage Morphine at WLST	0.88	0.82	0.95	0.002
Midazolam use after WLST	1.15	0.097	0.023	< .001
Oxygenation index	1.18	1.17	2.8	0.008

Surgical procedure for controlled DCD procurement

Casavilla et al. originally described the super-rapid organ retrieval technique for DCD.[13] This procedure has been modified at King's College Hospital to allow for decongestion of abdominal organs and aortic cannulation within 2 to 3 minutes from skin incision.[25] A midline thoraco-laparotomy is followed by opening of the supra-diaphragmatic inferior vena cava and venting of the blood, relieving congestion of the vena cava due to cardiac failure and arrest. Then a rapid cannulation of one of the iliac arteries or distal abdominal aorta is performed and immediately followed by perfusion with preservation fluid and clamping of the descending thoracic aorta. In order to improve further the liver perfusion, the portal system is also cannulated either via the inferior or superior mesenteric veins or directly. In case of pancreas retrieval, the cannula is directly inserted in the main portal vein, thus allowing for the pancreas to vent preservation fluid via the portal vein stump. This is followed by packing of the abdominal cavity with ice cold slush. In the UK, heparin is added to both aortic and portal perfusion fluid as it is prohibited to administer heparin prior to declaration of death. Aortic perfusion by gravity produces insufficient perfusion pressure at the level of the hepatic artery. Hence, to produce a peripheral liver flush, preservation fluids are pressurized at 200 mm Hg. The portal system is flushed by gravity as, at higher pressure and cold temperature, it may cause severe endothelial damage. A careful surgical technique is required to avoid iatrogenic vascular damage of the liver, which appears more challenging due to the absence of arterial pulse and the more difficult recognition of non-standard hepatic arterial anatomy at the porta hepatis, which occurs in nearly 50% of the cases. When available, surgeons should review premortem computerized tomographic imaging to identify the type of hepatic vascular anatomy prior to organ procurement.

An alternative technique of donor organ recovery consists of en-bloc removal of the abdominal viscera. The dissection time is shorter, even in the presence of aberrant hepatic arterial anatomy.[33] However, en-bloc retrieval has little, if no advantage, in terms of overall and particular cold ischaemia time, as it requires prolonged times of dissection on the bench at the transplant centre with a significant risk of rewarming of the organs.

Following *in situ* hypothermic perfusion, the retrieval procedure continues with similar steps of dissection performed during DBD organ retrieval. The adoption in the Netherlands and in the UK of National Organ Retrieval Systems seems to have increased the length of extraction of abdominal organs, including the liver. It has, however, been shown that slight liver extraction time variations among the retrieval teams in the UK did not affect the quality of the liver grafts.[34]

The selection of preservation solution

Flushing the blood from the hepatic vasculature and rapid cooling of the liver is essential to minimize the effects of warm ischaemia. The preservation fluids play a significant role. UW solution is preferred for perfusion during DCD organ retrieval procedures as it is associated with improved liver graft function compared to histidine-tryptophan-ketoglutarate (HTK) solution according to data from the UNOS database of over 17,000 liver transplants. In controlled DCD, HTK was linked with early graft loss with an odd ratio of 1.63 compared to UW solution.[35] The UW solution, however, due to its high viscosity, may prove slow in flushing the microcirculation and its high content of potassium may worsen the already difficult reperfusion syndrome typical of DCD livers.

Recipient selection and procedure

In order to better understand the overall donor and recipient risk, new tools were defined to suggest thresholds when to decline a certain donor-recipient combination in context of a predicted impaired outcome.[36–38] However, the acceptance of survival and complication rates depends also on the number of available organs and the risk a centre or country is willing to take.[39,40] In order to identify unfavourable donor-recipient risk combinations, the group from the University of California, Los Angeles, was the first to suggest a prognostic scoring system with the aim to define cut-off values for risk factors to enable clinicians to decide whether to accept a certain donor and recipient combination.[36] Further scores were developed in the UK, for example, based on the King's College Hospital DCD transplant cohort or the UK-DCD-risk-score, developed by the Birmingham team, and based on the national DCD liver transplant cohort in the UK.[37,38] Such models identified low risk or 'good quality' DCD livers, which led to excellent graft survival rates of more than 80% after five years, when respecting a balance between donor and recipient risk factors.[31,41,42]

Specialized, large volume centres for example achieved excellent outcomes with a five-year graft survival of almost 80% already in earlier years.[15,26] The limitation of donor risk factors and a standardized organ retrieval practice with for example a short donor hepatectomy time and cold storage have contributed to such good outcomes.[26,34,37,43,44]

An early assessment of the donor graft for its suitability for transplantation is essential to reduce cold ischaemia. This may not be without risk. A reassuring opinion on the DCD liver graft by the donor surgeon may drive the recipient team to start the transplant early with the aim of reducing cold ischaemia time (CIT). In case of inaccurate assessment, the implantation of a marginal DCD may lead to potentially adverse consequences. That is why many surgeons prefer to compromise slightly on CIT in order to personally inspect the graft at its arrival before sending the recipient to the operating room. In case a protracted recipient hepatectomy is a possibility, the expected duration of CIT must be known. Should the hepatectomy be more challenging than anticipated, there is a substantial risk of prolonging CIT in excess of 8 hours. Accordingly, patients with extensive previous upper abdominal surgery, previous spontaneous bacterial peritonitis or pre-transplant portal vein thrombosis and those requiring a late liver re-transplant are considered unfavourable recipients of a DCD liver. Furthermore, following the implantation of DCD grafts, recipients predictably display more severe IRI compared to DBD grafts. This physiological stress can manifest itself as cardiovascular instability at reperfusion of the graft, followed by coagulopathy in the latter part of the transplant procedure. Therefore, patients with significant cardiovascular comorbidity are also not considered good recipients of DCD grafts. Postoperative organ dysfunction is often present affecting the liver as well as other organs. The requirement for renal support is higher following DCD liver implantation compared to DBD liver grafts.[45]

Uncontrolled DCD

Given the steady growth of the number of patients being added to the waitlist annually, in addition to the somewhat stagnant number of DBD donors and ageing donor population, novel ways to increase the organ donor pool must be sought. It has been reported that the number of potential donors in the United States and UK[46] could be increased by many thousands per year if uncontrolled DCD (uDCD) donors were used. Combined with the current advancements in liver preservation and organ resuscitation, namely *ex vivo* organ perfusion, successful clinical acceptance could become reality in a not-too-distant future.

However, despite the potential to dramatically increase the organ donor pool, uDCD donors (category Maastricht category II), have not yet gained broad acceptance. This is due to multiple important factors. Uncontrolled donors present logistical challenges but, more importantly, require a supportive legal structure and widespread community acceptance. Additional issues include higher rates of primary graft nonfunction and lower rates of graft survival. Transplant teams in Spain have been at the forefront of the utilization of uDCD donors to expand the organ donor pool.[47,48]

Unique challenges of uncontrolled DCD

As mentioned, distinctive challenges are associated with uDCD. As the timing of death is uncontrolled, skilled resources must be directed rapidly to potential donors to limit DWIT and preserve organ function. This process is resource heavy and is directly responsible for most ethical issues inherent with uDCD. It is usual for a potential donor's family not to be present when procedures to preserve organ function are required. These must, therefore, be performed with presumed consent. There are also issues with obtaining consent from the coroner for organ donation.

Apart from Spain, protocols for uDCD have already been implemented in other European countries including France, Italy, the UK, and The Netherlands.(49) Further protocols have also been developed in other countries, such as Belgium, Switzerland, and Austria, and Saint Petersburg (Russia), and New York City.(50) Although uDCD seems to be promising in terms of potential expansion of the donor pool, it raises a number of ethical, medical, legal, financial, and logistic challenges in regards of cardiac arrest, resuscitation measures, organ donation, and preservation.(51) Little is still known regarding the comparative outcomes with the implementation of the various existing protocols.(52) With regard to uDCD donor selection and management, the impact of innovative preservation strategies, such as normothermic regional perfusion and its influence on liver transplant outcomes should be understood. One of the more challenging aspects of DCD liver transplants is the increased incidence and extent of postreperfusion coagulopathy. The proactive approach of the anaesthetic team includes monitoring, prophylaxis, and treatment of the anticipated coagulopathy associated with uDCD livers. When compared with a matched control group of liver transplants from DBD donors, uDCD liver transplants had higher transfusion requirements, rates of re-operation, early allograft dysfunction and renal replacement therapy, and more hours of mechanical ventilation, intensive care unit, and hospital stay. Despite a significant decrease in graft survival, remarkably, patients' survival remains similar due to a high rate of re-transplantation. Despite reports suggesting that flushing the hepatic artery with tissue plasminogen activator (tPA) during DCD liver transplantation reduces the incidence of ITBL and improves graft and patient survival without increasing the risk for bleeding,(53,54) recent research has shown coagulopathy and excessive endogenous fibrinolysis at the moment of death in uDCD donors,(55) obviating the need for fibrinolytic therapy in this setting. While uDCD may be different from cDCD, the group from Rotterdam evaluated biopsy specimens from discarded cDCD liver grafts stained specifically to detect the presence of microthrombi with fibrin, though none were found in any of the 288 sections evaluated.[56] It should be noted that donors in this study did not receive heparin before withdrawal. These findings may be explained by the fact that endogenous fibrinolytic systems are activated in response to systemic hypoperfusion and ischaemia and, therefore, the debated strategy to flush DCD liver grafts with fibrinolytic agents is unlikely to be useful. Early experience of uncontrolled DCD demonstrated very poor outcomes. All the early patients of Starzl transplanted with uDCD died within thirty days of transplantation.[7] Recognition of warm ischaemic injury during organ recovery prevented further efforts at uDCD at that time. In 1995, Casavilla et al. reported on the outcome of fourteen uDCD subjects, all of whom suffered in-hospital cardiac arrest.[57] Six organs were transplanted but outcomes were poor and only one graft survived past two months. Spain produced most subsequent series of uDCD. The legal framework in Spain supports uncontrolled DCD programs. Contemporary uDCD includes the concurrence of advanced cardiorespiratory support, femoral cannulas placement, normothermic regional perfusion (NRP), and organ retrieval. Even with these processes and careful donor selection, PNF still affects 10% of grafts and graft and patient survival at one year is 49% and 62%, respectively.[58] In the largest published series, there is evidence of improving outcomes; six-month graft survival was 53% in the first half of the series compared to 88% in the second cohort.[59] An evolution of technical processes and a better understanding of recipient selection appear responsible for this improvement.

There are also potential advantages to the use of uncontrolled DCD compared to controlled DCD. Selected uDCD donors may be younger and healthier at the time of donation compared to cDCD donors who have experienced intensive care unit hospital stay up to the point of donation. Uncontrolled donors will never become cDCD or DBD donors and therefore, they represent a true expansion of the donor pool.

From certain ethical perspectives, uDCD presents somewhat different challenges than controlled DCD. The process of dying in uDCD is a spontaneous event and it does not follow a WLST. In countries where the WLST is not legal, uDCD may be the only viable method of DCD. Certain aspects of uDCD do raise issues of ethical concern. Post-mortem procedures, such as systemic heparinization and cannulation, are required typically without specific consent. In Spanish law, following declaration of death steps to ensure organ viability for the purpose of donation should be performed without the need of specific consent. In other countries, the law is less clear.

Due to the risks of PNF and graft dysfunction, careful selection of donors is key and resource intensive in uncontrolled liver DCD. The Barcelona experience over eight years yielded 400 uDCD protocol activations. A total of 110 patients were excluded during the process of cardio-respiratory support, then 145 further during Extra corporeal membrane oxygenation to leave 145 organ donors from which 34 liver transplants were performed.

Donor procedure for uncontrolled DCD

With uDCD, it is essential that the cardiac arrest is witnessed so that the DWIT is known. Bystander basic life support is provided until advanced life support by medical/paramedical professionals. The duration of resuscitation required before death is certified varies according to local protocols; in centres with established programmes, this is 20 min.[59] Once the resuscitation procedure has occurred and the donor fulfils basic criteria, including age limits and cause of death, a no touch period of 5 min of absent cardiac and respiratory functions is required before death can be certified. After the donor is pronounced dead, chest compressions are restarted only for the purpose of donation. This may be provided by mechanical external thoraco-abdominal compression devices. Donor coordinators activate the process of organ donation; blood samples are obtained, heparin is given, and the organ recovery team mobilized.

Normothermic regional perfusion and ex-situ machine perfusion

The aim of NRP is to restore circulation to the abdominal organs for 1.5 to 4 hours before *in situ* perfusion with cold preservation solution.

The circuit includes an oxygenator, heat exchanger, pump, and when available, a leucocyte filter. A standard cardiopulmonary bypass equipment can be used or purpose to fit devices are also commercially available including the Donor Assist (Organ Assist, Groningen, Netherlands), which is a dedicated NRP System.

The target for abdominal NRP flow is 2.5–3 L/min, with higher flow rates (4–6 L/min) for thoraco-abdominal NRP.[60]

The prime solution usually includes compound sodium late and succinylated gelatine and antimicrobials, sodium bicarbonate and heparin with additional mannitol and heparin for thoraco-abdominal NRP.

There are several ways to undertake NRP, depending on whether the donor is a uDCD or cDCD and on the local protocols and regulations.[61]

In case of a uDCD or cDCD, NRP may be initiated before arrival in theatre if the perfusion guidewires/catheters can be placed premortem in the femoral artery and vein. A large bore balloon catheter is introduced via the contralateral femoral artery and inserted so that the aorta above the origin of the coeliac axis or the thoracic aorta is effectively occluded. Once the radiopaque balloon correct position is confirmed on X-ray the balloon can then be inflated to exclude the cerebral circulation from warm perfusion.

In countries where ante-mortem cannulation and heparinisation are not permitted in cDCD, as for example in the UK, abdominal NRP is performed in the operating theatre after a laparotomy by cannulating the aorta and the inferior vena cava. When the heart is also retrieved in a DCD, a thoraco-abdominal NRP may be performed, usually cannulating the abdominal aorta, since that affords better access for clamping the arch vessels to prevent cerebral perfusion.[62]

After establishment of adequate flows and monitoring of transaminases and lactate levels in the perfusate every 30 minutes, a full abdominal exploration is performed in the warm phase during NRP prior to cold portal and aortic perfusion and final organ retrieval. This latter process is similar to that of DBD organ recovery.

NRP is a mandatory part of the multiorgan retrieval process in uDCD and in all DCD in countries with a prolonged *no-touch* period like Italy. Otherwise, NRP has been used in cDCD, in a systematic way, under the umbrella of a national protocol in France and also in several units in Spain, given their experience acquired with uDCD. In other countries it has been used very selectively and, despite early favourable results, particularly in terms of low rates of ITBL, NRP has not yet shown yet to be a tool to significantly increase utilisation of cDCD liver grafts. A novel technique, which aims to decrease the incidence of ITBL following DCD liver transplantation, is the sequential arterial followed by portal reperfusion of the graft during implantation. It is possible that standard staged portal perfusion followed by arterial perfusion prolongs the duration of warm ischaemia of the biliary tissue. In theory, this strategy would limit a second warm hypoxic injury specific to the hepatic arterial circulation of the biliary tree. Though, there is no evidence at this time of a reduced incidence of ITBL, the strategy of initial hepatic artery reperfusion with a temporary portocaval shunt has shown an improvement in reduced blood loss.(63) There is clear potential, however, to review this strategy in future studies of recipients of DCD grafts looking at severity of IRI and incidence of ITBL. A randomised trial is ongoing at the Liver Unit in Birmingham.

Ex-situ liver perfusion strategies are currently tested in the setting of DCD transplantation. A recent multicentre, randomized controlled trial (RCT) has demonstrated a significant reduction of ITBL after DCD liver transplantation with hypothermic oxygenated perfusion (HOPE).(64) This technique is therefore currently introduced as new standard of DCD liver preservation in an increasing number of countries in Europe, including the Netherlands and Switzerland, being also commissioned in Italy, where HOPE treatment is combined with NRP in the donor. (65)

Conclusion

Liver transplantation using DCD grafts increases the donor pool. However, due to concerns over graft dysfunction and ischaemic biliary injury, careful donor and recipient selection is essential to maintain outcomes as close as possible to DBD liver transplantation. Uncontrolled DCD may expand the donor pool further, but it is likely at the expense of reduced graft survival. Still most outcome reports rely on retrospective analyses from single centre or national cohort studies, with either specific risk profiles or large volumes of missing data. In this context, future analyses should aim for international data collection with inclusion of most relevant outcomes and the comprehensive complication index. A benchmarking-type analysis with DCD liver transplants is, therefore, currently prepared, where results from most cases transplanted in all Western countries are included. Such benchmarking concept is not new; but has previously defined valid reference values for most outcome measures in standard and primary DBD liver transplantation, where the impact of new technology and the results from large randomized controlled trials can be compared with.[66]

The overall donor and recipient risk a specific country, centre or surgeon is willing to accept depends also on national regulations and the internal and external support a centre receives. A more uniform donor and recipient risk factor application with subsequent development of general thresholds would be of importance to compare results and develop guidelines.

Novel machine perfusion technology is currently improved and tested in the clinical setting of liver transplantation and in other solid organ transplantations. Results expected from various randomized controlled trials are awaited and will possibly impact future outcomes. Importantly, viability criteria are currently developed for various types of cold and warm *in-situ* and ex-situ perfusion strategies to increase the generally poor utilization rate and safety of DCD donor liver transplants. Future prediction models will, therefore, retain not only donor and recipient risk factors but will also capture a metabolic liver assessment to more accurately predict outcomes, and the risk for certain complications prior to decision making of utilising a graft.

Highlights

- DCD is effective in increasing the number of organs transplanted.
- There are two main DCD types discussed in this chapter—uncontrolled and controlled.
- There are ethical and logistical issues related to setting up a DCD program.
- Outcomes for kidney donation from DCD are similar to those from DBD.
- DCD livergraft survival is inferior to that of DBD due to a higher incidence of ITBL, particularly in donors with prolonged warm and cold ischemia times.

- Initial experience with NRP and ex vivo machine perfusion is promising in terms of reducing specific complications associated with transplantation of DCD organs.

References

1. Miniño AM, AE., Kochanek KD, Murphy SL, Smith BL., Deaths: Final Data for 2000., in National Vital Statistics Reports. 2002.
2. Bradley, J. A., Pettigrew, G. J., & Watson, C. J. (2013). Time to death after withdrawal of treatment in donation after circulatory death (DCD) donors. Current Opinion in Organ Transplantation, 18(2), 133–139.
3. Suntharalingam C, Sharples L, Dudley C, Bradley JA, Watson CJE. Time to cardiac death after withdrawal of life-sustaining treatment in potential organ donors. Am J Transplant. 2009 Sep;9(9):2157–2165.
4. Arne N, Dirk Van R, Diethard M. Donation after circulatory death: current status. Curr Opin Anaesthesiol. 2013 Jun;26(3):382–390.
5. Transplantation from deceased donors after circulatory death. Compiled by a Working Party of The British Transplantation Society. July 2013 https://bts.org.uk/wp-content/uploads/2016/09/15_BTS_Donors_DCD-1.pdf
6. Hamilton, D.N. and W.A. Reid, Yu. Yu. Voronoy and the first human kidney allograft. Surg Gynecol Obstet, 1984. **159**(3): p. 289–94.
7. Starzl, T.E., et al., Experimental and Clinical Homotransplantation of the Liver. Ann N Y Acad Sci, 1964. **120**: p. 739–65.
8. Calne, R.Y. and R. Williams, Liver transplantation in man. I. Observations on technique and organization in five cases. Br Med J, 1968. **4**(5630): p. 535–40.
9. Manara, A.R., P.G. Murphy, and G. O'Callaghan, Donation after circulatory death. Br J Anaesth, 2012. **108 Suppl 1**: p. i108–21.
10. Weber, M., et al., Kidney transplantation from donors without a heartbeat. N Engl J Med, 2002. **347**(4): p. 248–55.
11. Summers, D.M., et al., Analysis of factors that affect outcome after transplantation of kidneys donated after cardiac death in the UK: a cohort study. Lancet, 2010. **376**(9749): p. 1303–11.
12. Abt, P.L., et al., Survival following liver transplantation from non-heart-beating donors. Ann Surg, 2004. **239**(1): p. 87–92.
13. Casavilla, A., et al., Experience with liver and kidney allografts from non-heart-beating donors. Transplantation, 1995. **59**(2): p. 197–203.
14. D'Alessandro A, M., et al., Liver transplantation from controlled non-heart-beating donors. Surgery, 2000. **128**(4): p. 579–88.
15. Muiesan, P., et al., Single-center experience with liver transplantation from controlled non-heartbeating donors: a viable source of grafts. Ann Surg, 2005. **242**(5): p. 732–8.
16. Abt, P., et al., Liver transplantation from controlled non-heart-beating donors: an increased incidence of biliary complications. Transplantation, 2003. **75**(10): p. 1659–63.

17. Kaczmarek, B., et al., Ischemic cholangiopathy after liver transplantation from controlled non-heart-beating donors-a single-center experience. Transplant Proc, 2007. **39**(9): p. 2793–5.
18. Hernandez-Alejandro, R., et al., Kidney and liver transplants from donors after cardiac death: initial experience at the London Health Sciences Centre. Can J Surg, 2010. **53**(2): p. 93–102.
19. Coggon, J., et al., Best interests and potential organ donors. BMJ, 2008. **336**(7657): p. 1346–7.
20. Bell, M.D., Non-heart beating organ donation: in urgent need of intensive care. Br J Anaesth, 2008. **100**(6): p. 738–41.
21. Dominguez-Gil, B., et al., Current situation of donation after circulatory death in European countries. Transpl Int, 2011. **24**(7): p. 676–86.
22. Cascales-Campos, P.A., et al., Controlled donation after circulatory death up to 80 years for liver transplantation: Pushing the limit again. Am J Transplant, 2020. **20**(1): p. 204–212.
23. Murphy, P., et al., Controlled non-heart beating organ donation: neither the whole solution nor a step too far. Anaesthesia, 2008. **63**(5): p. 526–30.
24. Mandell, M.S., et al., National evaluation of healthcare provider attitudes toward organ donation after cardiac death. Crit Care Med, 2006. **34**(12): p. 2952–8.
25. Muiesan, P., et al., Segmental liver transplantation from non-heart beating donors--an early experience with implications for the future. Am J Transplant, 2006. **6**(5 Pt 1): p. 1012–6.
26. DeOliveira, M.L., et al., Biliary complications after liver transplantation using grafts from donors after cardiac death: results from a matched control study in a single large volume center. Ann Surg, 2011. **254**(5): p. 716–22; discussion 722-3.
27. Gunning, K.R., K.; Murphy, P.; Martineau, A.; Rudge, C., Organ Donation after Circulatory Death. Report of a consensus meeting. Intensive Care Society, NHS Blood and Transplant, and British Transplantation Society. 2010: ODT.
28. Lewis, J., et al., Development of the University of Wisconsin donation After Cardiac Death Evaluation Tool. Prog Transplant, 2003. **13**(4): p. 265–73.
29. DeVita, M.A., et al., Donors after cardiac death: validation of identification criteria (DVIC) study for predictors of rapid death. Am J Transplant, 2008. **8**(2): p. 432–41.
30. Rabinstein, A.A., et al., Prediction of potential for organ donation after cardiac death in patients in neurocritical state: a prospective observational study. Lancet Neurol, 2012. **11**(5): p. 414–9.
31. Davila, D., et al., Prediction models of donor arrest and graft utilization in liver transplantation from maastricht-3 donors after circulatory death. Am J Transplant, 2012. **12**(12): p. 3414–24.
32. Kotsopoulos, A.M.M., et al., External validation of prediction models for time to death in potential donors after circulatory death. Am J Transplant, 2018. **18**(4): p. 890–896.
33. Jeon, H., et al., Combined liver and pancreas procurement from a controlled non-heart-beating donor with aberrant hepatic arterial anatomy. Transplantation, 2002. **74**(11): p. 1636–9.
34. Boteon, A., et al., Retrieval Practice or Overall Donor and Recipient Risk: What Impacts on Outcomes After Donation After Circulatory Death Liver Transplantation in the United Kingdom? Liver Transpl, 2019. **25**(4): p. 545–558.

35. Stewart, Z.A., et al., Histidine-Tryptophan-Ketoglutarate (HTK) is associated with reduced graft survival in deceased donor livers, especially those donated after cardiac death. Am J Transplant, 2009. **9**(2): p. 286–93.
36. Hong, J.C., et al., Liver transplantation using organ donation after cardiac death: a clinical predictive index for graft failure-free survival. Arch Surg, 2011. **146**(9): p. 1017–23.
37. Khorsandi, S.E., et al., Developing a donation after cardiac death risk index for adult and pediatric liver transplantation. World J Transplant, 2017. 7(3): p. 203–212.
38. Schlegel, A., et al., The UK DCD Risk Score: A new proposal to define futility in donation-after-circulatory-death liver transplantation. J Hepatol, 2018. **68**(3): p. 456–464.
39. Marcon, F., et al., Utilization of Declined Liver Grafts Yields Comparable Transplant Outcomes and Previous Decline Should Not Be a Deterrent to Graft Use. Transplantation, 2018. **102**(5): p. e211–e218.
40. Croome, K.P., et al., Improving National Results in Liver Transplantation Using Grafts From Donation After Cardiac Death Donors. Transplantation, 2016. **100**(12): p. 2640–2647.
41. Nemes, B., et al., Extended criteria donors in liver transplantation Part I: reviewing the impact of determining factors. Expert Rev Gastroenterol Hepatol, 2016. **10**(7): p. 827–39.
42. Nemes, B., et al., Extended-criteria donors in liver transplantation Part II: reviewing the impact of extended-criteria donors on the complications and outcomes of liver transplantation. Expert Rev Gastroenterol Hepatol, 2016. **10**(7): p. 841–59.
43. Farid, S.G., et al., Impact of Donor Hepatectomy Time During Organ Procurement in Donation After Circulatory Death Liver Transplantation: The United Kingdom Experience. Transplantation, 2019. **103**(4): p. e79–e88.
44. Kollmann, D., et al., Expanding the donor pool: Donation after circulatory death and living liver donation do not compromise the results of liver transplantation. Liver Transpl, 2018. **24**(6): p. 779–789.
45. Leithead, J.A., et al., Donation after cardiac death liver transplant recipients have an increased frequency of acute kidney injury. Am J Transplant, 2012. **12**(4): p. 965–75.
46. Roberts, K.J., et al., Uncontrolled organ donation following prehospital cardiac arrest: a potential solution to the shortage of organ donors in the United Kingdom? Transpl Int, 2011. **24**(5): p. 477–81.
47. Fondevila, C., et al., Liver transplant using donors after unexpected cardiac death: novel preservation protocol and acceptance criteria. Am J Transplant, 2007. **7**(7): p. 1849–55.
48. Blasi, A., et al., Liver Transplant From Unexpected Donation After Circulatory Determination of Death Donors: A Challenge in Perioperative Management. Am J Transplant, 2016. **16**(6): p. 1901–8.
49. Borry, P., et al., Donation after uncontrolled cardiac death (uDCD): a review of the debate from a European perspective. J Law Med Ethics, 2008. **36**(4): p. 752–9, 610.
50. Wall, S.P., et al., Derivation of the uncontrolled donation after circulatory determination of death protocol for New York city. Am J Transplant, 2011. **11**(7): p. 1417–26.

51. Rodriguez-Arias, D. and I.O. Deballon, Protocols for uncontrolled donation after circulatory death. Lancet, 2012. **379**(9823): p. 1275–6.
52. Lazzeri, C., et al., Uncontrolled donation after circulatory death and liver transplantation: evidence and unresolved issues. Minerva Anestesiol, 2019.
53. Hashimoto, K., et al., Use of tissue plasminogen activator in liver transplantation from donation after cardiac death donors. Am J Transplant, 2010. **10**(12): p. 2665–72.
54. Bohorquez, H., et al., Safety and Outcomes in 100 Consecutive Donation After Circulatory Death Liver Transplants Using a Protocol That Includes Thrombolytic Therapy. Am J Transplant, 2017. **17**(8): p. 2155–2164.
55. Vendrell, M., et al., Coagulation profiles of unexpected DCDD donors do not indicate a role for exogenous fibrinolysis. Am J Transplant, 2015. **15**(3): p. 764–71.
56. Verhoeven, C.J., et al., Liver grafts procured from donors after circulatory death have no increased risk of microthrombi formation. Liver Transpl, 2016. **22**(12): p. 1676–1687.
57. Casavilla, A., et al., Experience with liver and kidney allografts from non-heart-beating donors. Transplant Proc, 1995. **27**(5): p. 2898.
58. Jimenez-Galanes, S., et al., Liver transplantation using uncontrolled non-heart-beating donors under normothermic extracorporeal membrane oxygenation. Liver Transpl, 2009. **15**(9): p. 1110–8.
59. Fondevila, C., et al., Applicability and results of Maastricht type 2 donation after cardiac death liver transplantation. Am J Transplant, 2012. **12**(1): p. 162–70.
60. Oniscu, G.C., et al., In situ normothermic regional perfusion for controlled donation after circulatory death--the United Kingdom experience. Am J Transplant, 2014. **14**(12): p. 2846–54.
61. Shapey, I.M. and P. Muiesan, Regional perfusion by extracorporeal membrane oxygenation of abdominal organs from donors after circulatory death: a systematic review. Liver Transpl, 2013. **19**(12): p. 1292–303.
62. Watson, C.J.E., et al., In situ normothermic perfusion of livers in controlled circulatory death donation may prevent ischemic cholangiopathy and improve graft survival. Am J Transplant, 2019. **19**(6): p. 1745–1758.
63. Pietersen, L.C., et al., Impact of Temporary Portocaval Shunting and Initial Arterial Reperfusion in Orthotopic Liver Transplantation. Liver Transpl, 2019. **25**(11): p. 1690–1699.
64. Van Rijn et al. Hypothermic machine perfusion in liver transplantation—A Randomized Trial, N Engl J Med. 2021 Apr 15;384(15):1391–1401. doi: 10.1056/NEJMoa2031532. Epub 2021 Feb 24.
65. De Carlis R et al. How to preserve liver grafts from circulatory death with long warm ischemia? A retrospective Italian cohort study with Normothermic Regional Perfusion and Hypothermic Oxygenated Perfusion—Transplantation. 2021 Nov 1;105(11):2385–2396.doi: 10.1097/TP.0000000000003595.
66. Muller, X., et al., Defining Benchmarks in Liver Transplantation: A Multicenter Outcome Analysis Determining Best Achievable Results. Ann Surg, 2018. **267**(3): p. 419–425.

59

Indications and outcome of emergency organ transplantation

Massimo Boffini, Cristina Barbero, Davide Ricci, Erika Simonato, Damiano Patrono, Renato Romagnoli, Mauro Rinaldi

Introduction

End-stage solid organ failure requiring transplantation may have a dramatic worsening and patients on the active waiting list may not survive. A national programme has, to date, the role to consider these patients for transplant on urgent basis. Strict criteria have the role to avoid wasting of time for the patients and wasting of organs for the country. This chapter will discuss indications and outcomes related to urgent heart, lung, and liver transplantation.

Urgent heart transplantation

In the current era, the rate of patients on the active heart transplant (HTx) list with progressive deterioration and, therefore, deemed at imminent risk of death is continuously growing. This is mainly due to an increasing number of patients with end-stage heart diseases, a persistent scarcity of donors, and long waiting list times. Moreover, transplant centres have to face frequently unknown patients (not previously referred for HTx) with a profile of advanced heart failure at first presentation. Therefore, a proper clinical evaluation and identification of patients real eligibility for HTx is a major concern in order to optimize the risk/benefit ratio of the surgical procedure and to avoid futile transplants.[1]

INTERMACS profile

Though HTx is the gold standard for end-stage heart failure, data in the literature have shown worse outcomes when procedures are performed on urgent basis.[2–4] Barge-Caballero and colleagues reviewed 704 adult patients listed for high-urgent HTx in fifteen Spanish Institutions and found an overall 2-fold increase in postoperative mortality (29%) in-hospital in comparison with the historical cohort of elective HTx procedures.[2,3] Stratifying for Interagency Registry for Mechanically Assisted Circulatory Support (INTERMACS) profiles, in-hospital postoperative mortality rates were 43%, 26.8%, and 18% in patients with profiles 1 (critical cardiogenic shock), 2 (progressive decline, sliding on inotropes), and 3 (stable but inotrope dependent) to 4 (resting symptoms) ($p<0.001$), respectively. The INTERMACS 1 patients also presented the highest incidence of primary graft failure and postoperative need for dialysis; this may be explained considering that patients with profile 1 had higher chances to receive marginal donor organs and to be transplanted 'too early' before complete recovery of organ function could be achieved. However, post-transplant long-term survival curves of patients who survived the early postoperative period did not differ significantly across INTERMACS groups.[2] Comparable results on patients with advanced heart failure, INTERMACS level 1 or 2, undergoing urgent HTx were also reported by the University of Turin (in-hospital mortality 42.3%).[4]

These evidences, along with the scarcity of donor organs, have motivated many centres to take into consideration an early implantation of temporary mechanical circulatory support (MCS) like venous-arterial extracorporeal membrane oxygenation (va-ECMO) or temporary left ventricular assist device (T-LVAD) as a first step for further evaluation before long-term therapies including HTx or durable ventricular assist device (VAD). According to data from the ISHLT registry, the use of MCS, particularly durable VAD, as bridge to HTx has constantly grown during the recent years.[5] The MCS results in hemodynamic improvement and end-stage organ function's recovery; therefore, the aim of MCS is not only to keep patients alive while awaiting for an organ, but also to improve their clinical condition so as to undergo transplantation with a higher probability of survival.

Outcome of bridge to HTx

Experiences of HTx in patients bridged with short-term MCSs are controversial. Chung et al. reported that only 44% (31 out of 70) of patients on va-ECMO were successfully bridged to HTx.(6) More recently, higher rate of success was reported in a multicentric Spanish study (76.3%).(7) Poptsov et al. reviewed 182 patients supported with va-ECMO between the period 2013–2017; 166 (91.2%) patients were successfully bridged to HTx. However, hospital mortality and early cardiac allograft dysfunction were significantly higher in these subgroups of patients when compared with recipients without pre-transplant MCS (respectively 13.9% vs 6.1%, $p = 0.003$ and 91.3% vs 65.4%, $p = 0.068$).(8) Risk factors for post-HTx mortality were impaired kidney and liver function, high procalcitonin, pre-existing cardio-embolic stroke, and the need for left ventricle drainage for heart decompression. Poor outcomes regarding early cardiac allograft dysfunction can be explained bearing in mind that donors in the cohort of pre-transplant ECMO recipients were older, had significantly higher vasoactive-inotropic support and lower left ventricular ejection fraction. Moreover, patients supported with va-ECMO showed the shortest time from device implantation to HTx; this data highlights the impact of the presumed durability of the pre-HTx device on the timing of clinical decisions (i.e. some va-ECMO patients were transplanted before proper recovery of organ function). Similar results with worst outcome in recipients bridged to HTx with va-ECMO were also reported by Lechiancole et al.(9)

In this context, the use of T-LVAD as a bridge strategy in patients with refractory cariogenic shock has increased. It is still a point of debate if, in patients without contraindication for both HTx and durable VAD, the T-LVAD bridge strategy should be considered towards a high urgent listing priority or towards a durable device. Published experiences are limited, and with concerning results. In Europe, Spain yields one of the broad experiences regarding high urgent HTx in patients supported by T-LVAD. Due to severe economic restrictions on long-term VADs and due to an efficient donor allocation system, T-LVAD is the most common setting of bridging critically ill candidates directly to HTx. According to the national protocol, the highest level of waiting list priority is reserved to HTx candidates not weanable from T-LVADs, or to those who develop complications related to durable VADs. Data from the Spanish registry during the period 2010–2015 showed that T-LVAD was independently associated with a lower risk of death over the first year after listing (hazard ratio 0.52, 95% confidence interval 0.30–0.92) when compared with va-ECMO and temporary biventricular assist devices. Age, vasoactive-inotropic score, serum lactate levels, active infection, and renal replacement therapy at the time of listing were independent predictors of mortality. Isolated T-LVAD support was independently associated with higher survival.(7) Shah and colleagues reported data from five American Institutions on 804 patients with INTERMACS profiles 1 to 3 that underwent durable VAD after or not T-LVAD and concluded that T-LVAD restores hemodynamics and reverses end-stage organ dysfunction. However, patients undergoing durable VAD after T-LVAD had higher morbidity and mortality than parallel INTERMACS 1 patients without mechanical support.(10) Yoshioka and colleagues reviewed data of 382 patients that underwent durable VAD implantation in a ten-year study period; 45 out of 382 patients were bridged to durable VAD by means of T-LVAD. Multivariable analysis did not recognize T-LVAD as a risk factor for death.(11) A six-year study on 49 patients with INTERMACS level 1 or 2 from the University of Turin showed better results in patients undergoing T-LVAD and subsequently durable VAD than in patients undergoing urgent HTx. In-hospital mortality was significantly higher in the latter group (42.3% vs 4.3%; P = 0.002); survival at six and twelve months of VAD-implanted patients was significantly higher than in patients who underwent urgent HTx.(4)

Urgent lung transplantation

Organs supply is grossly inadequate when compared to the large number of patients awaiting a lung transplant (LTx). The scarcity in organ supply is responsible for a long waiting time and the high risk of clinical deterioration while on the waiting list till the need of supportive strategies, such as mechanical ventilation (MV), and extracorporeal support (i.e. venous-venous extracorporeal membrane oxygenation, vv-ECMO).(12) However, these strategies allow only a short period of assistance; therefore, LTx remains the definitive therapy. In this context, priority graft allocation strategies are of paramount importance to increase the chances of receiving suitable organs.[13,14] It is well known in the literature that transplantation of the severely ill patients may impair short- and long-term outcomes. Moreover, ethical concerns arise when organs are used on an urgent basis because it may have a significant impact on the 'elective' patients.

Outcomes of LTx in patients on supportive therapy

It is known that MV is associated with a higher risk of pulmonary infections, sepsis, ventilator-induced lung injuries, diaphragmatic weakness, and muscle atrophy; all these may lead to prolonged and troublesome weaning after LTx with poor post-operative outcome. Mechanical ventilation is a recognized risk factor for one-year mortality with a relative risk of 1.53%.[15–17]

On the other hand, vv-ECMO could likely provide a proper respiratory and hemodynamic support with less side effects than MV.[18,19] One of the points of strength of this strategy is definitely the chance to maintain the awakened state so that patients could preserve their muscle tone with greater probability of mobilization and participation in the intensive physical therapy while on the waiting list.[20,21]

However, given the mixed outcomes in patients transplanted from ECMO, it has been considered as a contraindication in many LTx centres for many years, and, to date, concerns still remain on its effective role.[22,23] Recent reports have shown encouraging results in patients bridged to transplant with vv-ECMO.[24] This is attributed, in part, to improvements in technology, safety profile, and manageability of extracorporeal life support strategies and, in part, to the experience gained through the years in the transplant centres all over the world.[17,24–26] Fuehner et al comparing patients bridged to transplant with ECMO and patients bridged to transplant with MV found significantly better six-month survival in the former group (62% vs 35%). The authors concluded that preserving spontaneous breathing may keep patients in a better condition, with fewer drawbacks in comparison with MV.[27] Good results with the vv-ECMO support as bridge to LTx were confirmed in a systematic review by Chiumello et al. also.[28]

Proper patient selection is clearly essential to get reliable and good long-term outcomes. Sepsis, neurologic impairment, and severe malnutrition are considered contraindication for vv-ECMO support in patients awaiting a lung graft.[28,29] Moreover, different factors can affect post-transplant outcomes in patients bridged with this support. The most important is definitely the duration of the bridge. Crotti et al. showed that each day on ECMO increases the risk of death (mortality hazard ratio of 1.06) and that patients receiving a lung transplant after fourteen days of support have significantly higher rates of mortality and morbidity.[30] Therefore ECMO-bridged patients should be routinely re-assessed in order to confirm the transplantability.[25]

Global experience in urgent LTx

In 2005, the lung allocation score system (LAS) was introduced in the United States with the aim of prioritizing candidates on the basis of predictors of disease severity and of post-transplant survival at one year.[31] Germany was the first country in Europe to adopt the LAS in 2011 with a significant impact on results: a 26% reduction in waiting list mortality and an improved one-year post-transplant survival rate from 76% to 81%.[32] This system has definitely shifted the allocation of organs towards the sicker patients and has dramatically reduced the waiting list mortality. However, all over the world, transplant authorities have set up different dedicated emergency programmes, regardless of the adoption of LAS for organ allocation.

To date, reports of urgent LTx results are scarce. Román et al. described the urgent LTx programme in Spain in the early 2000. During a five-year study period, 109 patients waiting for lung transplant were considered for priority graft allocation and seventy-three were transplanted after a median of 7.7 days. Peri-operative mortality was significantly higher (about four times) than that expected for elective LTx. Survival rates at one, three, and five years were similar to that of 'elective patients'.[33] These results may be explained with reference to an early era and that indication for urgent listing in this protocol included only patients on MV or with end-stage primary pulmonary hypertension.

Better results were reported by the French experience. Saeressig et al. compared urgent and elective transplant on a single-centre cystic fibrosis population. No differences were reported in terms of intensive care unit length of stay, primary graft dysfunction, 1- and 2.5-year survival rates.[(34)] A broader report on the French experience considering 101 candidates with all the indications for LTx showed that the French high emergency LTx protocol was substantially able to decrease death on the standard waiting list (from 8.6% in 2006 to 3.5% in 2011) and to successfully bridge to LTx 87.5% of the patients. Overall, 30-day, 1-year, and 3-year survival rates were 81%, 67.5%, and 59.4%, respectively. According to the French protocol, MV and ECMO were not essential requirements for priority patients and only 32% of patients enrolled in the French high emergency program were supported by ECMO. As a matter of fact, the ECMO subgroup showed a 3-fold increased risk of death after LTx and ECMO resulted as a significant independent risk factor of death (HR = 2.77; 95% CI [1.26–6.11]).[(35)] Donor organ allocation in the United Kingdom has been historically based on local zones and only from 2017, two national urgency tiers (urgent and super-urgent) preceded over zonal allocation for LTx candidates in whom survival without transplantation was expected to be less than ninety days.[(36)]

In Italy, urgent transplants are reserved for patients younger than fifty years of age, on MV and/or extracorporeal oxygenation. Data on the Italian early experience showed that the urgent lung transplant programme was allowed in a significant percentage of prioritized patients (78.6%) with acceptable thirty-day mortality rates and one-year survival rate (respectively 18% and 71.4%).[13]

Urgent liver transplantation

In orthotopic liver transplantation (OLT), current allocation systems strive to achieve optimal balance between ensuring equal access to transplant, prioritizing sicker patients, and maximizing the benefit from a limited resource, as available liver allografts are scarce.[(37)] In many systems, patients suffering from a more severe degree of hepatic insufficiency and shorter life expectancy are given priority. In the majority of cases, these systems are based on model for end-stage liver disease (MELD) score[38] and adjusted according to particular indications or conditions (hepatocellular carcinoma, hepato-pulmonary syndrome, refractory ascites, concomitant renal failure, polycystic disease, etc.). To overcome potentially limited local donor availability, patients with a particularly high MELD score can be given priority outside the procurement area of their centre, in a setting of an urgent OLT. This is the case of United States of America Share 35 and Italian MELD 30 programs, in which MELD 35 and 30 cut off, respectively, are used to identify patients who can benefit from a macro area allocation, being prioritized over regional candidates.[37,39] Implementation of Share 35 policy in the USA in 2013 resulted in a greater proportion of patients with MELD ≥ 35 being transplanted, with a trend towards decreased waitlist mortality.[40] In Italy, regional disparities in donor availability have created an imbalance in the possibility to access a timely transplant across different macro areas and a formal analysis of MELD 30 results is still lacking.[41]

Acute liver failure

The highest level of priority (super urgent OLT) is granted to patients with acute liver failure (ALF). This condition is defined as an acute disturbance of liver function tests in a patient without previous liver disease, which is associated with coagulopathy and clinically altered mental status due to hepatic encephalopathy (HE).[42] Most common causes of ALF are viral hepatitis (especially A, B, and E), drugs, toxins, and vascular (Budd-Chiari syndrome and hypoxic liver injury), pre-eclamptic liver rupture and HELLP (hemolysis, elevated liver enzymes, and low platelet count) syndrome. In contrast with the aforementioned definition, also patients with acute presentation of autoimmune hepatitis, Wilson disease and Budd-Chiari syndrome, despite pre-existing liver disease, are considered as having ALF due to their poor prognosis. ALF has been further subclassified into hyperacute, acute, and subacute based on the delay between the appearance of first symptoms and the onset of HE.[43,44] Subacute liver failure may be insidious to diagnose, as these patients usually present with milder increase in serum transaminases and coagulopathy and deep jaundice, associated with signs of chronic liver disease as shrinking liver, ascites, and splenomegaly. In this population, timely diagnosis is of paramount importance as spontaneous survival is very low after HE develops. Once the diagnosis is established, timely referral to a specialized unit with OLT availability for thorough assessment, and search for an aetiology and multi-organ clinical management is mandatory.

The indication of approximately 8% of OLT performed in Europe is ALF and is associated with ~80% one-year survival[45] but the proportion of ALF patients who are actually transplanted might be difficult to evaluate and depend upon region and ALF aetiologies.[43] The dilemma of OLT for ALF is accurately differentiating those patients with a poor prognosis and with an indication for OLT from those who will likely recover without OLT. Criteria have been developed based on retrospective series from the eighty patients managed with and without OLT, taking into account factors like candidate age, aetiology, HE, and coagulopathy.[46,47] To overcome limitations due to recent improvements in patient management, several new criteria taking into account other factors like serum phosphate and lactate level, Factor VIII/V ratio, Acute Physiology And Chronic Health Evaluation II (APACHE II), and MELD score have been developed.[48–51] However, none of these criteria have been clinically validated so far.

Another issue of the ALF setting is the limited time for thorough patient work-up, especially with regards to psychological evaluation. Many patients with ALF could be at risk of post-transplant non-adherence to treatment. The decision as to whether or not to proceed with OLT should be taken after gathering all the available data about medical and psychosocial history, ensuring that post-transplant support will be available.

Auxillary partial OLT

The absolute contraindication for OLT is represented by irreversible brain injury, whereas severe vasoplegia, acute respiratory distress syndrome, and haemorrhagic pancreatitis are relative contraindications.

Timely OLT is the treatment of choice in appropriately selected patients. Factors determining reduced survival are older recipient age, male sex, high vasopressor requirement, and use of suboptimal grafts, i.e. those from donors aged ≥ 60 years, ABO-incompatible or partial/reduced size grafts. From a technical point of view, preservation of portal vein and inferior vena cava flow by temporary porto-caval shunt and piggyback technique has been shown to be feasible in ALF patients and may be preferable in patients with vasoplegic shock and high inotropes requirement.[52]

One drawback of OLT is the need for life-long immunosuppression. To obviate this constraint, the concept of auxiliary partial orthotopic liver transplantation (APOLT) has been proposed. The rationale for APOLT is that liver will eventually regenerate in a significant proportion of patients if enough time is allowed for this to take place.[53] Unfortunately, liver support devices have failed showing a consistent survival advantage in ALF and heterotopic auxiliary liver transplantation has been abandoned due to poor results.[54] Thus, the only option to bridge ALF patients towards native liver regeneration is APOLT. In this procedure, a portion of the native liver is resected and a partial graft is implanted orthotopically, allowing reversal of hepatic insufficiency and patient stabilization. Immunosuppression is then progressively tapered to allow regeneration of the native liver and shrinkage of the transplanted graft, which can be eventually resected or left in place. The APOLT is a technically more demanding procedure as compared to standard OLT and initial results were somewhat disappointing.[55] However, with technical refinements and better recipient and donor selection, recent results, especially in children, were more encouraging, achieving survival comparable to standard OLT and in about two-thirds of patients immunosuppression could be successfully weaned off.[56] Thus, although regular OLT represents the standard of care in ALF patients with poor prognosis, APOLT is a valuable alternative in selected cases.

Finally, a rare and peculiar indication for urgent OLT is represented by liver trauma. In this setting, OLT might be indicated for uncontrollable haemorrhage, secondary liver failure, or long-term injury sequelae.[57] It can be performed either as a standard single-stage procedure, in which hepatectomy and graft implantation are performed at the same time, or as a two-stage procedure, i.e. total hepatectomy associated with porto-caval shunt, followed by delayed graft implantation as soon as a graft becomes available.[58] A study from the European Liver Transplant Registry evidenced inferior results as compared to other indications, with 42.5% and

46.6% 90-days patient mortality and graft loss, respectively.[59] Thus, indication for OLT in this setting needs careful evaluation.

Conclusion

Urgent organ transplantation poses unique challenges due to the severity of baseline patient conditions and stringent time constraints. Where available, bridging interventions like use of a ventricular assistance device or ECMO can help buying time and stabilizing patients awaiting transplant, but their use is still controversial. Although results of urgent transplantation are generally inferior to those of elective transplantation, this represents the only chance of survival. Careful recipient evaluation and selection is of paramount importance to maintain acceptable survival results.

Highlights

- Heart transplant is the gold standard for end-stage heart failure; however, data in the literature have shown worse outcome in procedures performed on urgent basis.
- The use of MCS, particularly durable VAD, as bridge to heart transplant has constantly grown during the last years.
- Mechanical ventilation is a recognized risk factor for 1-year mortality after lung transplant.
- vv-ECMO could likely provide a proper respiratory and hemodynamic support with less side effects than mechanical ventilation in patients waiting for lung transplant.
- Most frequent indications for urgent liver transplantation are severe hepatic insufficiency and ALF.
- Careful recipient and donor selection are key to achieve good outcome.
- Orthotopic liver transplantation is the standard of care in patients with poor prognosis. Other technical options, like APOLT, may be valuable alternatives in selected cases.

- Urgent liver transplantation can be a life-saving procedure in carefully selected cases of traumatic liver injury.

References

1. McMurray JJ, Adamopoulos S, Anker SD, et al. ESC Committee for Practice Guidelines. ESC Guidelines for the diagnosis and treatment of acute and chronic heart failure 2012: The Task Force for the Diagnosis and Treatment of Acute and Chronic Heart Failure 2012 of the European Society of Cardiology. Developed in collaboration with the Heart Failure Association (HFA) of the ESC. Eur Heart J. 2012;33:1787–1847.
2. Barge-Caballero E, Segovia-Cubero J, Almenar-Bonet L, et al. Preoperative INTERMACS profiles determine postoperative outcomes in critically ill patients undergoing emergency heart transplantation: analysis of the Spanish National Heart Transplant Registry. Circ Heart Fail. 2013;6:763–772.
3. Almenar L, Segovia J, Crespo-Leiro MG, et al. Spanish Registry on Heart - Transplantation. 23rd Official Report of the Spanish Society of Cardiology Working Group on Heart Failure and Heart Transplantation (1984–2011). Rev Esp Cardiol. 2012;65:1030–1038.
4. Attisani M, Centofanti P, La Torre M, et al. Advanced heart failure in critical patients (INTERMACS 1 and 2 levels): ventricular assist devices or emergency transplantation? Interact Cardiovasc Thorac Surg. 2012;15:678–684.
5. Lund LH, Edwards LB, Kucheryavaya AY, et al. The registry of the international society for heart and lung transplantation: thirty-second official adult heart transplantation; focus theme: early graft failure. J Heart Lung Transplant. 2015;34:1244–1254.
6. Chung JC, Tsai PR, Chou NK, et al. Extracorporeal membrane oxygenation bridge to adult heart transplantation. Clin Transplant. 2010;24:375–180
7. Barge-Caballero E, Almenar-Bonet L, Gonzales- Vilchez F, et al. Clinical outcomes of temporary mechanical circulatory support as a direct bridge to heart transplantation: a nationwide Spanish registry. Eur J Fail. 2018;20:178–186.
8. Poptsov, Spirina E, Dogonasheva A, Zolotova E. Five years' experience with a peripheral veno-arterial ECMO for mechanical bridge to heart transplantation. Vitaly J Thorac Dis. 2019;11:889–901.
9. Lechiancole A, Sponga S, Isola M, et al. Heart transplantation in patients supported by ECMO: is the APCHE IV score a predictor of survival? Artif Organs. 2018;42:670–673.
10. Shah P, Pagani FD, Desai SS, et al. Mechanical Circulatory Support Research Network. Outcomes of patients receiving temporary circulatory support before durable ventricular assist device. Ann Thorac Surg 2017;103:106–111.
11. Yoshioka D, Takayama H, Garan A, et al. Bridge to durable left ventricular assist device for refractory cardiogenic shock. J Thorac Cardiovasc Surg. 2017;153:752–762.

12. Mason DP, Thuita L, Nowicki ER, et al. Should lung transplantation be performed for patients on mechanical respiratory support? The US experience. J Thorac Cardiovasc Surg. 2010;139:765–773.
13. Boffini M, Venuta F, Rea F, et al. Urgent lung transplant programme in Italy: analysis of the first 14 months. Interact Cardiovasc Thorac Surg. 2014;19:795–800.
14. Del Sorbo L, Boffini M, Rinaldi M, Ranieri VM. Bridging to lung transplantation by extracorporeal support. Minerva Anestesiol. 2012;78:243–250.
15. Christie JD, Edwards LB, Kucheryavaya AY, et al. The Registry of the International Society for Heart and Lung Transplantation: 29th adult lung and heart-lung transplant report-2012. J Heart Lung Transplant. 2012;31:1073–1086.
16. Singer JP, Blanc PD, Hoopes C, et al. The impact of pretransplant mechanical ventilation on short- and long-term survival after lung transplantation. Am J Transplant. 2011;11:2197–2204.
17. George TJ, Beaty CA, Kilic A, et al. Outcomes and temporal trends among high-risk patients after lung transplantation in the United States. J Heart Lung Transplant. 2012;31:1182–1191.
18. Del Sorbo L, Ranieri VM, Keshavjee S. Extracorporeal membrane oxygenation as 'bridge' to lung transplantation: what remains in order to make it standard of care? Am J Respir Crit Care Med. 2012;185:699–701.
19. Javidfar J, Brodie D, Iribarne A, et al. Extracorporeal membrane oxygenation as a bridge to lung transplantation and recovery. J Thorac Cardiovasc Surg. 2012;144:716–721.
20. Schechter MA, Ganapathi AM, Englum BR, et al. Spontaneously breathing extracorporeal membrane oxygenation support provides the optimal bridge to lung transplantation. Transplantation. 2016;100:2699–2704.
21. Mohite PN, Sabashnikov A, Reed A, et al. Extracorporeal life support in 'awake' patients as a bridge to lung transplant. Thorac Cardiovasc Surg. 2015;63:699–705.
22. Zapol WM, Snider MT, Hill JD, et al. Extracorporeal membrane oxygenation in severe acute respiratory failure. A randomized prospective study. JAMA. 1979;242:2193–2196.
23. Orens JB, Estenne M, Arcasoy S, et al. Pulmonary Scientific Council of the International Society for Heart and Lung Transplantation: International guidelines for the selection of lung transplant candidates: 2006 update–a consensus report from the Pulmonary Scientific Council of the International Society for Heart and Lung Transplantation. J Heart Lung Transplant. 2006;25:745–755.
24. Diaz-Guzman E, Hoopes CW, Zwischenberger JB. The evolution of extracorporeal life support as a bridge to lung transplantation. ASAIO J. 2013;59:3–10.
25. Javidfar J, Bacchetta M. Bridge to lung transplantation with extracorporeal membrane oxygenation support. Curr Opin Organ Transplant. 2012,17:496–502;
26. Riley JB, Scott PD, Schears GJ. Update on safety equipment for extracorporeal life support (ECLS) circuits. Semin Cardiothorac Vasc Anesth. 2009;13:138–145.
27. Fuehner T, Kuehn C, Hadem J, et al. Extracorporeal membrane oxygenation in awake patients as bridge to lung transplantation. Am J Respir Crit Care Med. 2012;185:763–768.
28. Chiumello D, Coppola S, Froio S, et al. Extracorporeal life support as bridge to lung transplantation: a systematic review. Critical Care. 2015;19:19.

29. Shafii AE, Mason DP, Brown CR, et al. Growing experience with extracorporeal membrane oxygenation as a bridge to lung transplantation. ASAIO J. 2012,58:526–59.
30. Crotti S, Iotti GA, Lissoni A, et al. The organ allocation waiting time during extracorporeal bridge to lung transplantation affects outcomes. Chest. 2013;144:1018–1025.
31. Egan TM, Murray S, Bustami RT, et al. Development of the new lung allocation system in the United States. Am J Transplant. 2006;6:1212–1227.
32. Gottlieb J, Smits J, Schramm R, et al. Lung transplantation in Germany since the introduction of the lung allocation score: a retrospective analysis. Dtsch Arztebl Int. 2017;114:179.
33. Román A, Calvo V, Ussetti P, et al. Urgent lung transplantation in Spain. Transplant Proc. 2005;37:3987–3990.
34. Saeressig MG, Pellau S, Sermet I, Souilamas R. Urgent lung transplantation in cystic fibrosis patients: experience of a French center. Eur J Cardiothorac Surg. 2011;40:101–106.
35. Orsinia B, Sageb E, Ollandc A, et al. High-emergency waiting list for lung transplantation: early results of a nation-based study. Eur J Cardiothorac Surg. 2014;46:41–7.
36. Rushton S, Al-Aloul M, Carby M, et al. The Introduction of Urgent and Super-Urgent Lung Allocation Schemes in the United Kingdom. JHLT. 2018;37:185.
37. Cillo U, Burra P, Mazzaferro V, et al. A Multistep, Consensus-Based Approach to Organ Allocation in Liver Transplantation: Toward a "Blended Principle Model". Am J Transplant. 2015;15(10):2552–2561.
38. Kamath PS, Wiesner RH, Malinchoc M, et al. A model to predict survival in patients with end-stage liver disease. Hepatology. 2001;33(2):464–470.
39. Nicolas CT, Nyberg SL, Heimbach JK, et al. Liver transplantation after share 35: Impact on pretransplant and posttransplant costs and mortality. Liver Transpl. 2017;23(1):11–18.
40. Edwards EB, Harper AM, Hirose R, Mulligan DC. The impact of broader regional sharing of livers: 2-year results of "Share 35". Liver Transpl. 2016;22(4):399–409.
41. Trapani S, Morabito V, Oliveti A, et al. Liver Allocation in Urgent MELD Score >/=30: The Italian Experience. Transplant Proc. 2016;48(2):299–303.
42. European Association for the Study of the Liver. Electronic address eee, Clinical practice guidelines p, Wendon J, et al. EASL Clinical Practical Guidelines on the management of acute (fulminant) liver failure. J Hepatol. 2017;66(5):1047–1081.
43. O'Grady JG, Schalm SW, Williams R. Acute liver failure: redefining the syndromes. Lancet. 1993;342(8866):273–275.
44. Tandon BN, Bernauau J, O'Grady J, et al. Recommendations of the International Association for the Study of the Liver Subcommittee on nomenclature of acute and subacute liver failure. J Gastroenterol Hepatol. 1999;14(5):403–404.
45. Germani G, Theocharidou E, Adam R, et al. Liver transplantation for acute liver failure in Europe: outcomes over 20 years from the ELTR database. J Hepatol. 2012;57(2):288–296.
46. O'Grady JG, Alexander GJ, Hayllar KM, Williams R. Early indicators of prognosis in fulminant hepatic failure. Gastroenterology. 1989;97(2):439–445.

47. Bernuau J SD, Durand F, Saliba F, Bourlière M, Adam R, Gugenheim J. Criteria for emergency liver transplantation in patients with acute viral hepatitis and factor V (FV) below 50% of normal: a prospective study. Hepatology. 1991;14(S4) S48–S290.
48. Bernal W, Hyyrylainen A, Gera A, et al. Lessons from look-back in acute liver failure? A single centre experience of 3300 patients. J Hepatol. 2013;59(1):74–80.
49. Hadem J, Stiefel P, Bahr MJ, et al. Prognostic implications of lactate, bilirubin, and etiology in German patients with acute liver failure. Clin Gastroenterol Hepatol. 2008;6(3):339–345.
50. Rutherford A, King LY, Hynan LS, et al. Development of an accurate index for predicting outcomes of patients with acute liver failure. Gastroenterology. 2012;143(5):1237–1243.
51. Schmidt LE, Dalhoff K. Serum phosphate is an early predictor of outcome in severe acetaminophen-induced hepatotoxicity. Hepatology. 2002;36(3):659–665.
52. Belghiti J, Noun R, Sauvanet A, et al. Transplantation for fulminant and subfulminant hepatic failure with preservation of portal and caval flow. Br J Surg. 1995;82(7):986–989.
53. Quaglia A, Portmann BC, Knisely AS, et al. Auxiliary transplantation for acute liver failure: Histopathological study of native liver regeneration. Liver Transpl. 2008;14(10):1437–1448.
54. Kribben A, Gerken G, Haag S, et al. Effects of fractionated plasma separation and adsorption on survival in patients with acute-on-chronic liver failure. Gastroenterology. 2012;142(4):782–789 e783.
55. Bismuth H, Azoulay D, Samuel D, et al. Auxiliary partial orthotopic liver transplantation for fulminant hepatitis. The Paul Brousse experience. Ann Surg. 1996;224(6):712–724; discussion 724-716.
56. Rela M, Kaliamoorthy I, Reddy MS. Current status of auxiliary partial orthotopic liver transplantation for acute liver failure. Liver Transpl. 2016;22(9):1265–1274.
57. Patrono D, Brunati A, Romagnoli R, Salizzoni M. Liver transplantation after severe hepatic trauma: a sustainable practice. A single-center experience and review of the literature. Clin Transplant. 2013;27(4):E528–E537.
58. Ringe B, Lubbe N, Kuse E, Frei U, Pichlmayr R. Total hepatectomy and liver transplantation as two-stage procedure. Ann Surg. 1993;218(1):3–9.
59. Krawczyk M, Grat M, Adam R, et al. Liver Transplantation for Hepatic Trauma: A Study From the European Liver Transplant Registry. Transplantation. 2016;100(11):2372–2381.

60

Immunosuppression in solid organ transplantation

Francesco Lupo

Introduction

As globally accepted, solid organ transplantation (SOT) is a galaxy of surgical and medical procedures aiming to successfully treat single or multiple end-stage diseases, that may possibly lead to death if untreated. The continuously evolving immunosuppressive therapy is one of the main branches of this galaxy. During the last four decades, a series of new drug discoveries have changed the protocols and clinical outcomes. Currently, clinicians are focused on obtaining further improvements on the use of such drugs.

Mechanism of graft rejection

The good use of immunosuppressive drugs cannot disregard the knowledge of the graft rejection mechanism. During allograft rejection, the non-specific innate response could predominate in the early phase of the immunologic activity, while donor-specific adaptive response resulting from host T cells alloantigen recognition account for later reactions.[1]

Hyperacute rejection (HR) occurs early following graft vascularization. This rejection is caused by the presence of pre-existing anti-donor antibodies in the recipient. The result of these antibodies' action is the complement activation and stimulation of endothelial cells to secrete pro-coagulant factor, resulting in intravascular thrombosis and subsequent graft loss.[2]

Acute rejection (AR) is caused by an immune response directed against the graft and occurs between the first week and several months after transplantation. It is histologically diagnosed on a graft biopsy. The AR results from two immunological mechanisms that may act alone or in combination: (1) a T-cell-dependent process that corresponds to acute cellular rejection, and (2) a B-cell-dependent process that generates the acute humoral rejection. In the former, host's T cells interact with foreign HLA presented by antigen-presenting cells (APC) of the donor (direct allorecognition) or foreign HLA molecules are first processed and then presented in peptide form by patient's APCs to his own helper T-cells (indirect allorecognition). After APC activation, naïve alloreactive CD4 + T cells can differentiate into T-helper cells, including Th1, Th17, Th2, or into regulatory T cells (Tregs, see the section 'tolerance concept'). In a proinflammatory environment, naïve CD4 + T cells differentiate mainly into Th1 and Th17 cells. Th1 cells produce IFNg and IL-2 and are involved in cytotoxic T lymphocyte priming, stimulation of the humoral response, and activation of other cell.[1,3]

The presence of pre-formed donor specific antibodies affects graft survival, inducing an antibody mediated rejection (AMR). This is particularly evident with pre-sensitized patients and in patients with sub-optimal levels of immunosuppression. It has been reported that following kidney transplantation, AMR component may be found in over 60% of patients who experience an episode of biopsy-proven acute rejection (BPAR).[4] In heart transplantation, there is evidence for significantly increased graft loss and mortality in patients with Donor Specific Antigens (DSA). Cumulative survival of DSA-positive patients after five, ten, and fifteen years was 89.3%, 80.3% and 53.6% respectively compared with 98.4% after five and 97.3% after ten and fifteen years for DSA-negative controls.[5]

Chronic rejection (CR), on the other hand, accounts for the late graft rejection. CR can be mediated by either humoral or cellular mechanisms linked to memory/plasma cells and antibodies.

The tolerance concept

Central tolerance refers to the deletion of reactive clones within the thymus during negative selection. In contrast, peripheral T cell tolerance encompasses several mechanisms that take place outside the thymus, including peripheral deletion, anergy/exhaustion, and the suppressive function of regulatory T cells (Tregs).[6] Clinical Operational Tolerance (COT) in SOT is defined as spontaneous graft acceptance without histological evidence of rejection, for at least one year after cessation of immunosuppression. Immunosuppressive medication has some cost in terms of side effects, but non-adherence to therapy is one of the major risk factors for graft rejection and loss.[7,8,9]

COT is so named as a result of the following circumstances:

- recipients who, despite non-adherence with medications, exhibit long-term graft survival with good graft function;
- recipients who are weaned off or have discontinued their immunosuppressive medications as advised by their transplant physician because of severe toxicity or life-threatening complications;
- clinically stable long-term survivors who follow protocols for planned immunosuppression weaning with eventual discontinuation of immunosuppressive medications;
- patients who follow protocols combining haematopoietic cell and kidney transplant from the same donor with nonmyeloablative conditioning, to establish temporary or persistent mixed chimerism aimed to the discontinuation of immunosuppressive therapy.[10]

Haematopoietic cell chimerism is defined as the presence of donor haematopoietic cells in the blood circulation of the recipient. Complete chimerism is present when all the cells are of donor origin. Mixed chimerism is the presence in the recipient of a variable number of donor cells of multiple lineages. Microchimerism is present when the donor cells in the recipient are below the level of detection by flow cytometry or by DNA based methods.[11]

There are organ specific differences to be taken into consideration. Liver grafts bear some inherent immunological privilege (i.e. irrelevance of HLA matching, independency of a positive cross match), which renders these grafts somewhat more capable of developing tolerance.[12] Starzl described COT in five liver transplant recipients in 1993. The recipients were 12.5 to 18.6 years post-transplant and had been off immunosuppression for 5 to 11 years at the time of the report.[13,14]

Kidney transplanted tolerant patients exhibited higher frequencies of circulating naive and transitional B cells and Tregs and a lower frequency of plasma cells.[15,16,17]

Tregs (expressing CD4 + Foxp3+) are essential in maintaining immune homeostasis as well as promoting allograft tolerance.[18] Moreover, suppressive role of Treg has even been demonstrated in mixed chimerism recipients, which exhibit robust tolerance to donor antigens.[19] Tregs originate in the thymus and then populate the secondary lymphoid as well as non-lymphoid organs. They could act by expressing high levels of CD25, which depletes IL-2 from the microenvironment, limiting its availability for T-cell functions,[20] or releasing immunosuppressive cytokines such as IL-10, IL-35, and TGF-b, to prevent T-cell proliferation and maturation of APC.[21] They could secrete granzymes and perforins that cause apoptosis of target cells[22] or they can express CTLA-4 which binds CD80/CD86, limiting T-cell activation.[23] Finally, Treg-derived exosomes inhibited T-cell proliferation in vitro and in vivo.[24,25]

Prophylactic and therapeutic immunosuppressive molecules

The most frequently used immunosuppressive agents include calcineurin inhibitors such as cyclosporine and tacrolimus; the rest are antimetabolites, corticosteroids, mTOR inhibitors, and biological drugs.

Calcineurin Inhibitors (CNI)

Belongs to this family are two 'old' drugs, Cyclosporine (CyA) and Tacrolimus (TAC). CyA was introduced in the early 1980s and suddenly changed the outcomes of SOT improving patient and graft survival rates from 30–50% to 80% at one year.[26] Tacrolimus, ten times more powerful than CyA, was introduced in 1990s, and is nowadays, the reference drug. Both original formulations have undergone changes in structure in the last years, maintaining the functional role. About mechanism of action, CyA (as cyclosporine-cyclophilin complex) and TAC (as tacrolimus-FKBP12 complex) inhibit calcineurin and suppress synthesis of IL-2, which is responsible for lymphocyte activation. The CNIs are toxic because of overexposure, interactions with other drugs, genotypes of cytochrome P450 enzymes 3A4, 3A5, 3A5*1, and their polymorphisms.[27]

Original CyA formulation absorption was strictly related to bile acids, causing a relevant inter and intra-patient variability.[28] In the late 1990s, a modified formulation (microemulsioned, Neoral®, Novartis Pharma) was introduced, improving, but not eliminating discrepancy between patients.[29]

The TAC is extensively used in every transplant setting. Since its introduction, compared to CyA, TAC has demonstrated lower AR rates and higher patient and graft survival rates.[30,31] However, TAC was affected by higher rates of *de-novo* post-transplant diabetes mellitus and neurological disorders.[32,33] Moreover, hypertension, electrolyte imbalance, and hyperlipidaemia are among the common adverse effects of TAC, shared with other CNIs. In 2007, a new extended-release formulation of Tacrolimus (IR-TAC, Advagraf®/Astagraf®, Astellas Pharma), with a once-daily dosing was introduced,[34] with the aim of better therapy adherence,[35,36] showing besides some significant improvement in kidney function and overall survival.[37,38] More recently, was presented a new TAC formulation (Envarsus®-Veloxis®, Chiesi Pharma), based on the Meltdose® technique, which allows single daily dosing. Results from registered clinical studies show better bioavailability, significantly higher exposure, lower intraday fluctuation and prolonged time (Tmax) to peak concentration (Cmax) versus IR-TAC or immediate release TAC.[39]

Both CNIs showed a narrow therapeutic window requiring close monitoring. The pharmacokinetic data shows that TAC through blood level (sample taken before TAC administration), well correlates with the area under the curve (AUC) between doses,[40] i.e. the drug exposure, while the best AUC surrogate for CyA is the C2 level (level at the second hour post drug administration).[41] Therapeutic drug monitoring (TDM) is based on the principle of maintaining immunosuppressive blood and plasma levels within their respective desirable ranges.[42] Furthermore, characteristics such as age, race, type of graft received, pre-existing renal and liver function, diet, and genetic polymorphisms can also affect the effectiveness of the immunosuppressive regimen.[43,44] Aiming to a more precise determination, high performance liquid chromatography (HPLC) test allows the best estimation of the amount of drug exposure.[45,46]

Antimetabolites

These are immunosuppressive drugs with a strong anti-proliferative activity. Azathioprine, a 6-mercaptopurine derivate, was introduced in transplantation in 1960. It inhibits both the *de novo* DNA and RNA synthesis, resulting in nonspecific cell-cycle arrest at the G2-M phase and preventing cell proliferation. Its use, in combination with CNI and steroids, although limited, is still debated.

Mycophenolate mofetil (MMF), and the enteric formulation of mycophenolate sodium, delivers the active moiety mycophenolic acid (MPA), which acts on inosine monophosphate dehydrogenase (IMPDH), inhibiting the *de novo* pathway of guanosine nucleotide synthesis, without incorporation to DNA. The most common side effects are bone marrow suppression with leucopoenia and thrombocytopenia. Diarrhoea and abdominal discomfort are common GI complaints. The MMF has conventionally been administered at a fixed dose without routinely monitoring blood levels of MPA, the active metabolite. The contribution of TDM during MMF therapy remains controversial. With regard to MPA toxicity, most studies showed no correlation between MPA pharmacokinetics and adverse effects.[47] The drug was introduced in SOT during the 1990s and suddenly allowed the implementation of CNI sparing regimen and steroid free protocols.[48,49]

Corticosteroids

'Avoid steroids' is the most common mantra since side effects due to long-term use were focused in transplant population.[50] But steroids have been the mainstay for induction of immunosuppression since the first successful case of SOT.[51,52]

They inhibit the expression and the production of cytokines including IL-1, IL-2, IFN-g, TNF-a, and colony-stimulating factors, which causes profound inhibition of T-cell effector function, suppression of T-cell proliferation, and inhibition of migration of immune cells into inflammatory sites. Steroids are administered in high doses intravenously during surgery as a bolus and usually up to the third day. Corticosteroids are rapidly tapered over the first week to relatively low doses and then discontinued, unless the autoimmune disease is present.

The main side effects are neurotoxicity (headache, mood disturbance up to psychosis), electrolyte disturbances and fluid retention, glucose intolerance, and leukocytosis. The severity of these adverse effects will diminish as the dose is reduced. Long-term use of corticosteroids can lead to Cushingoid-type effects such as growth suppression, osteoporosis, and loss of muscle mass, fragile skin, impaired wound healing, glaucoma and lipodystrophy.

Steroid withdrawal or steroid free regimens have been applied in selected patients with good outcomes.[53,54,55,56]

mTOR inhibitors (mammalian target of rapamicine)

The mammalian target of rapamycin (mTOR) is a serine/threonine kinase that regulates multiple cellular functions: responds to amino acids, stress, oxygen, energy, and growth factors. It promotes cell growth by inducing and inhibiting anabolic and catabolic processes, respectively, and also drives cell cycle progression.[57] Sirolimus (SRL, Rapamune®, Pfizer Pharma) and Everolimus (EVE, Certican®, Astellas Pharma) are the mainstays of mTOR inhibition in transplantation, as they interfere with T-cell activation by blocking the cytokine signal during the G1 build-up, preventing the progression of cytokine-stimulated T cells from G1 phase to the S phase of DNA synthesis and suppressing T-cell proliferation. The European and U.S. Drug Agencies have approved SRL and EVE for solid organ transplant immunosuppression between 2003 and 2010. Both have been used as immunosuppressive agents in SOT as valid alternatives to CNI mainly in patients with chronic renal dysfunction[58,59,60] or those at high risk of malignancies.[61,62] Nevertheless, recent studies show that a certain danger of hypoimmunosuppression after mTORi conversion could be suspected In the ZEUS trial, the conversion from CNI to Everolimus® increased the risk for *de novo* donor-specific antibodies production.[63] The Symphony study showed a higher rejection rate and dropout frequency in renal transplant recipients under mTORi based regimen without CNI, compared with a standard CNI-based therapy.[64] The use of mTORi could be associated with renal (e.g. proteinuria) and systemic side effects, including pulmonary toxicity, haematological and metabolic disorders, lymphedema, and stomatitis.[65,66]

Biological drugs

Polyclonal antibodies are directed against a variety of cell-surface molecules expressed on T lymphocytes, B cells, NK cells, and macrophages which are responsible for T-cell activation and proliferation, finally resulting in lymphocytes depletion. Monoclonal antibodies (mAb), instead, have a single well-defined specificity and target a specific CD (cluster of differentiation) protein present on the T-cell or B-cell surface wielding their immunomodulatory effects.

Polyclonal antithymocyte globulin (ATG)

Therapeutic antibodies directed against human lymphocyte antigens (i.e. Thymoglobuline®, Genzyme Pharma), are created by immunizing rabbits or horses with human thymocytes. The primary mechanism of action of ATGs is lymphocyte depletion, predominantly by complement-dependent lysis and T cell activation–induced apoptosis.[67] In addition, these agents have recently demonstrated the ability to induce regulatory cell phenotypes, i.e. Tregs.[68] The main side effects are related to cytokine release (fever, chills, hypotension, and pulmonary oedema) as well as cellular cytotoxicity.[69]

IL-2 receptor [CD25] antagonist (Basiliximab)

Activated T cells produce IL-2 and express the a-subunit of the IL-2 receptor, making it fully functional. Humanized antibodies directed against the a-subunit of the IL-2 receptor (basiliximab, Simulect®, Novartis Pharma), limit proliferation of activated T cells. Acting on the same pathway of CNI allows CNI sparing protocols.

Costimulation blockade by CD80/86:CD28 targeting

After the antigen stimulation, the T cell expresses the Cytotoxic T lymphocyte–Associated protein 4 (CTLA4), which competitively binds to CD80/86, downregulating the T-cell response. Human IgG heavy chains were linked with CTLA4 to create a fusion protein for clinical use, with high affinity for CD80/86 (Belatacept, Nulojix®, Bristol-Myers Pharma).[70] This agent is now a good substitute of CNI in kidney transplant protocols.[71]

B Cell and plasma cell targeting

The CD20 is a trans-membrane protein present on pre-B and mature B lymphocytes. It regulates the activation for cell cycling and B cell differentiation. Rituximab (Mab Thera®, Roche Pharma) is a chimeric anti-CD20 mAb that leads to B cell depletion through a number of mechanisms, including complement-dependent cytotoxicity, growth arrest, and apoptosis.[72] Efficacy data pertinent to nephrology practice include the treatment of Anti-Neutrophil Cytoplasmic Antibodies (ANCA)—associated vasculitis, with supportive data in antibody-mediated rejection and forms of nephrotic syndrome.[73,74] In diseases in which plasma cell maturation and antibody production are the pathogenic mechanism, the inhibition of the proteasome leads to inhibition of cell cycling and induction of cell apoptosis.[75] Eculizumab (Bortezomib®, Sandoz Pharma) is a proteasome inhibitor that was found to be particularly effective in treatment of the plasma cell dyscrasia, multiple myeloma and showed clinical benefit in the treatment of the antibody-mediated rejection of kidney allografts by targeting antibody-producing plasma cells.[76,77,78]

Panlymphocyte depleting agents

CD52 is an antigen that is present on both B and T cells. Anti-CD52 (campath-1H, alemtuzumab, MabCampath®, Genzyme Pharma) is a humanized mAb that binds to this target, resulting in depletion of both lymphoid cell lines. It can induce significant lymphopenia for up to 6–12 months. Its use as an induction agent was introduced in kidney transplantation,[79] but long-term effect as risk for infection or post-transplant lymphoproliferative disorder is not well established.[80]

Need for immunosuppressive strategies: Standardization and customization

The aim of immunosuppressive therapies is to facilitate the tolerance to the graft and to achieve the absence of clinically relevant episodes of rejection. On the other hand, a number of diseases are more common in SOT patients than in the general population and many of these are closely linked to the side effects of the immunosuppressive drugs, such as infection and cancer. The reduction of dose-dependent toxicities, with relatively low dosing strategies in synergistic combinations, could result in better tolerability and efficacy.[81] Immunosuppressive regimens employed for SOT are generally classified as induction and maintenance therapy (early post-operative and mid or long term or rescue therapies).

Induction

Induction immunosuppression involves intense prophylactic therapy administered before or at the time of transplantation, with the goal of preventing AR and ultimately facilitating a tolerogenic state. The need of an immunosuppressive boost in the very early phases of organ transplantation is well known in kidney transplantation, where the percentage of patients with treated rejection episodes within one-year post-transplant were significantly higher in sensitized patients (PRA = 50–100 14.3%, and PRA = 1–49 13.9%) than in non-sensitized patients (12.4%). Rabbit ATG (Thymoglobulin®) was the most commonly used induction agent in the last ten years while the use of Alemtuzumab (Campath-1H®) and Rituximab (Mabthera® or Rituxan®) reached 16% and 11% respectively.[82] Induction protocols are introduced in other transplant settings and are commonly employed in heart and lung transplantation,[83] but its use in liver transplantation remains controversial[84] and aimed to improve the post-transplant renal function in a perspective of CNI sparing and decreased corticosteroid dependence.[85] The use of ATG as induction therapy has been described as a possible treatment for reducing the prevalence of Delayed Graft Function (DGF) on the basis of ATG related control of ischemia reperfusion injury.[86,87] Moreover, in adults, ATG induces peripheral expansion and new thymic migration of T cells with a Treg phenotype.[88] Lighter protocols which contemplate a single dose of ATG are more favourable in terms of rejection rate, infection, and renal function at three years.[89] More selective induction with anti-CD25 (basiliximab, Simulect®) are less impacting, allowing either CNI effect enhancement or CNI sparing protocols.[90,91,92,93]

Early post-operative period

In the early post-operative period, a triple therapy approach is usually adopted; CNI, steroids and anti-metabolite are given. Nowadays, Tacrolimus represents the mostly used CNI in every transplant setting, while microemulsioned Cyclosporine accounts for the minor part of the prescriptions.

There are some favourable reports of mTORi *de-novo* or early-conversion use,[94,95,96] although, during the first month, MMF is usually preferred as anti-metabolite medication, because of the remarkable anti-proliferative activity of mTORi leading to incisional site infection and dehiscence.[97]

Steroids are usually quickly tapered and discontinued as soon as possible, following local rules. The use of belatacept as first-line immunosuppression in kidney transplants was published in a phase III study.[98] At twelve months, the mean eGFR was significantly higher in the belatacept arms as compared to the control group (on CyA), despite higher rejection rates, with significant advantages in terms of antibody-mediated rejection, development of *de novo* anti-HLA DSA, prevalence of biopsy-proven chronic allograft nephropathy at twelfth month, better cardiovascular and metabolic outcome, and without statistical difference in patient and graft survival.[86]

Rejection treatment

Episodes of rejection, usually biopsy-proven, are treated initially with steroid bolus (500mg to 1000 mg of methylprednisolone, up to 10–12 mg/kg), eventually tapered. Steroid resistant rejections require a rescue treatment, usually with polyclonal ATG.[99,100] In this case, a T-Cell strict monitoring is needed.

Maintenance and long-term: CNI sparing

The maintenance regimen results from a delicate balance between the continuous need of immunosuppression and the necessity to limit the severe drug-related side effects. During the early phase (usually up to the third year), gradual CNI reduction, steroids tapering and discontinuation and switch between drugs are the commonly adopted strategies in the whole SOT scenario. The most concerning adverse side effect of CNIs is their nephrotoxicity, due to renal arteriolar vasoconstriction, which is dose-dependent and reversible.[101] As described earlier, CNIs can cause hypertension, neurotoxicity, metabolic abnormalities, including hyperglycaemia and *de novo* diabetes, electrolyte imbalance, and hyperlipidaemia. The diabetogenic effect of tacrolimus is greater than cyclosporine and this could be a good reason to consider CyA as an alternative in patients with metabolic disorders, with a significant HbA1c improvement after the CyA switch.[102] Cyclosporine can cause hirsutism and gingival hyperplasia.[103] All CNIs are associated with an increased risk of infection.[104]

The 'kidney sparing' axiom and the need to expose the patient to the lowest achievable neoplastic risk (including recurrence of neoplasm in case of tumoral indication, i.e. hepatocellular carcinoma), steer the switch to the mTORi medications (sirolimus and everolimus).

Since the clinical introduction, mTORi was investigated in a CNI sparing view. Till date the results are controversial. Some large pharmaceutical industry RCTs have tested the hypothesis that *de novo* CNI-free immunosuppression based on an mTOR is safe and advantageous to CNI reduction, including the Symphony Study,[64] the Orion study,[105] and the 318 Study.[106] In each trial instead, the *de novo* SRL group (with MMF/P) demonstrated a statistically significant increased incidence of biopsy confirmed AR (37%, 31%, 21%, respectfully) compared to CNI (CsA or tacrolimus [TAC]) and control arms (with MMF/P) at one year (12%, 8%, 6%, respectively). However, in none of these trials, *de novo* mTOR-treated patients experienced significantly increased delayed graft function rate and they had better estimated GFR of 5 to 10 mL/min. Having said that, to overcome early mTORi issues, seem to be preferable than the late switch. The CONVERT trial has shown the advantages of early CNI antirejection prophylaxis and then conversion to an mTORi before six months. There was a substantial increase in GFR at two years for recipients with an entry GFR greater than 40 mL/min. Those recipients that entered with a GFR less than 40mL/min or proteinuria did not have an advantage.[107] In the

ZEUS trial, Basiliximab induction and CsA-mycophenolate sodium were randomized 1:1 to continue or convert to EVL at four to five months post-transplant with a significant improvement in GFR at five years and a slight, but not significant loss in AR rate.[108]

As previously described, mTORi is supposed to have some anti-tumoral activity and therefore protect against *de-novo* malignancies. A planned, proactive switch from a CNI to sirolimus at 3–6 months post-transplantation is an appropriate alternative strategy when long term, CNI-free immunosuppression is possible, including for standard-risk patients and those with extended criteria kidneys donors, with high immunologic risk.[109] Post-transplant kidney recipients have a lower incidence of malignancy when treated with an mTORi, whether it is used in combination with CNIs or not. This beneficial effect remains significant even when non-melanoma skin cancers are excluded. Despite this, with currently used mTORi based regimen, patient and graft survival is not different compared to CNI therapies.[110] As mTOR is the main proliferation pathway in approximately half of the patients with hepatocellular carcinoma (HCC) and increased expression of mTOR is associated with larger, poorly differentiated and more advanced tumours, mTORi was advocated as the best immunosuppressive treatment in liver transplanted patients with HCC. Up to date, there is no strong evidence of such effect (see results of SiLVER trial[111]), although a great number of small local studies report positive influence of mTOR use on HCC recurrence.[112]

In kidney transplants, under standard therapy with TAC and MMF, the late maintenance phase (after the third-year post-transplant) is characterized by an extremely low risk of acute cellular rejection (<2%).[113] Because of this decreasing time-dependent immunological risk, the immunosuppression is reduced over time, tapering steroids and lowering CNI levels gradually.[114,115] Regarding the long-term results of BENEFIT study, the Belatacept® groups had a sustained yearly improvement in eGFR while the CsA group had a persistent decline.[116] A Cochrane database review published in 2016 mirrored and summarized the findings of BENEFIT.[117] To avoid prolonged exposure to CNIs, in a phase 2 RCT, six months post-transplant kidney recipients with stable graft function were switched from a CNI-based to a Belatacept®-based regimen with a significant GFR improvement with an acceptable rate of rejection. Cardiovascular and metabolic outcomes did not differ clinically between the two groups.[118] Two and three year results from the same study population confirm the sustained improvement in GFR in the Belatacept® group.[119,120]

In liver transplant, some matters can be related to the indication or to the co-morbidities. The hepatitis C virus recurrence no longer acts as the pitfall in the post-operative period, because of the new antiviral therapies' efficacy. Patients transplanted for Non Alcoholic Fatty Liver Disease (NAFLD) with its corollary of metabolic complications (renal dysfunction secondary to the diabetes, hypertension, and atherosclerotic disease) represent the new line of challenge for immunosuppressive protocols,[121] with the need of CNI reduction or withdrawal and the steroids avoidance.[122] On the other hand, are the so-called liver eaters, patients with a significant need of re-transplantation because the extremely high levels of recurrent autoimmunity, with the need to maintain long-term steroids and high levels of CNI.[123,124,125]

De novo uses of Belatacept® was explored in a phase 2 RCT in liver transplant recipients, which are more immunocompromised at baseline, with the CD28 pathway critical to their protective immunity. That's probably the reason for study failure, with a higher incidence of death, primarily related to infections, in investigational arm. Nevertheless, GFR was better in the study group as compared with controls.[126]

Furthermore, there was a higher incidence of post-transplant lymphoproliferative disease (PTLD) with Belatacept® in the first year after transplantation and Epstein–Barr virus (EBV) seronegative status was the strongest associated risk factor.[127,128]

In heart transplantation, there are two large randomized trials on CNI-reduction and CNI-withdrawal, NOCTET study[129] and the SCHEDULE study[130] respectively. In the former, a CNI-reduction with a concurrent mTORi introduction was made ≥1 year in Heart Transplant patients with moderate chronic kidney disease (CKD) and compared with a control group on standard CNI-doses. In the latter, an m-TORi introduction within 5 days, and CNI-withdrawal at weeks 7–11 was scheduled in patients with moderate CKD and compared with a control group on standard CNI-doses. In both trials, glomerular filtration rate was better in the study group compared with the control group, while maintaining the same rejection rate.

Steroid free protocols

Literature review on the safety of low dose glucocorticoid treatment in rheumatoid arthritis suggested that the toxicity of steroids is overestimated, because adverse effects of chronic low dose treatment (≤ 10 mg/d prednisolone) were found to be modest and rarely, statistically, significantly different from placebo.[131] Steroids show several adverse effects as previously described, but steroid avoidance and withdrawal potentially increase the risk of AR, which is associated with late graft loss. In kidney transplantation, a comprehensive meta-analysis on 48 RCT studies and 7457 patients, showed that steroid avoidance or withdrawal after kidney transplantation significantly increased the risk of AR but without difference in patient and graft survival up to five years after transplantation.[132]

In liver transplantation, several authors report beneficial effects for steroid-free regimens.[34,133,134,135,136] On the other hand, in a recent systematic review, 16 RCT studies with 1347 patients were analysed to assess steroid avoidance or withdrawal versus steroid-containing immunosuppression for liver transplanted people. Many of the benefits and harms of steroid avoidance or withdrawal remain uncertain, because of the limited number of published RCTs and high risk of bias. Steroid sparing could be of benefit in selected patients, especially those at low risk of rejection and high risk of hypertension or diabetes mellitus. The optimal duration of steroid administration remains unclear.[137] Guidelines reported by the International Society of Heart and Lung Transplantation certify that steroid avoidance, early weaning, or very low-dose maintenance therapy, are acceptable therapeutic approaches with level of evidence B.[138] Steroid free therapy should be advisable in paediatric age and in cases of related co-morbidities (i.e. severe diabetes, infections). In all heart transplant patients, withdrawal is feasible with a success rate of 50–80% and safe (does not increase rejection-related mortality and has no adverse impact on survival). But due to lack of evidence due to some bias in RCTs, further focused randomized trials are mandatory.[139]

Operational tolerance

There are three active protocols aimed to achieve COT through chimerism in USA, namely, the Massachusset General Hospital (MGH),[140] the Standford and the Northwestern (NW) protocol. They differ in conditioning regimen and timing, nature of the Hematopoietic Cell Transplantation (HCT) and timing of infusion and goal of type of chimerism. Both the MGH and NW protocols employ a combination of chemotherapy and thymic (MGH) or total body (NW) irradiation. Both initiate the conditioning days prior to transplantation of the kidney, which restricts these protocols to living donation. The Stanford protocol uses a conditioning regimen of rATG and total lymphoid irradiation (TLI) following kidney transplantation, allowing its use in deceased donor as well. In the MGH protocol, the HCT is unselected marrow, whereas in both the Stanford and NW protocols, the HCT is selected subsets of donor cells. In NW protocol, 'facilitator' cells are added to the HCT. The HCT is given on the day of kidney transplantation in the MGH protocol and given one day following kidney transplantation in the NW protocol. In the Stanford protocol, the conditioning regimen ends the eleventh day following kidney transplantation, and the HCT is given that day. Transient mixed chimerism was the goal of the MGH protocol. Permanent chimerism was the goal of the NW protocol. Mixed chimerism, ideally persistent, was the goal of the Stanford protocol.[141] Nowadays, the best results are obtained with the NW protocol; among the first thirty-one subjects who have reached >12 months, durable donor chimerism was established in twenty-three subjects and immunosuppression was successfully discontinued in twenty-two subjects with immunosuppression-free survival ranging from eight to eighty-one months. Full donor chimerism (>98% whole blood and T cell lineage) was observed in nineteen of these twenty-two subjects. The Stanford group is continuing to elevate the dose of donor T cells, with the aim to increase the levels and duration of mixed chimerism.

Authors conclude that persistence of chimerism is necessary to achieve tolerance in HLA-mismatched kidney transplant recipients.[142] In liver transplantation, IS withdrawal has been successful for about 20–30% of patients (range 6–63%).[143,144,145] Differences in patient populations, clinical approaches, and assessments account for this large variation. Simple weaning success increases with selection of recipients who are older in age, far off from the transplant, and with 'normal' pre-weaning liver biopsies.[146] There is an independent association between tolerance and male gender, older age, and time since transplant.[145] Several studies have shown an association between weaning success and lower portal inflammation (lymphoplasmacytic) and C4d staining scores on pre-weaning biopsies.[147] There is poor literature about induced chimerism in LT. A recent study demonstrated the effectiveness of Treg-based therapy in the development of operational tolerance in ten living donations. Approximately six months after LT, patients with stable graft function on TAC monotherapy started withdrawal over twelve months. A total of 70% of them were successfully weaned from TAC and met both biochemical and histological criteria of tolerance.[148]

Use of biomarkers

To date, there has not been an established 'signature' of tolerance. The microarray technology has been widely employed to evaluate the whole transcriptome of blood and/or organ tissue samples from solid-organ transplant patients. The reproducibility of some of these studies is still an open question. Tolerance in liver and kidney transplantation demonstrates an increase in both the peripheral T regulatory population and associated peripheral transcripts.[149] Peripheral markers provide a more convenient platform for frequent monitoring of allo-immunity, avoiding the need of an invasive biopsy. In tolerant kidney transplant recipients, there is an increased B cell percentage, increase in transitional and naïve B cell population, and increased B cell transcripts.[150] In tolerant liver transplants, NK cells remain important. In both kidney and liver transplant recipients, the T regulatory cell population appears to be the driver of tolerance.[151] With the wide variability in gene transcripts found among tolerance biomarker studies, it is difficult to identify one specific signature that will encompass all organ transplants. The most accurate fingerprint will likely consist of the detection of an expansion of a particular cellular subset with an enrichment of its accompanying transcripts.[152]

Conclusion

During the editing of this chapter, a new and dramatic health emergency occurred: the SARS-CoV2 pandemic is putting a strain on the world's health systems. Transplantation medicine promptly reacted by finding new approaches to the available immunosuppressive drugs.[153] In a recent multi-centre cohort study, mortality among the SOT recipients hospitalized for COVID-19 was found to be 20.5%. Age and underlying comorbidities, rather than immunosuppression intensity-related measures, were major drivers of this mortality.[154] The study reveals that the well-based pharmacological platform of immunosuppressive treatment and its proper management can ensure good results, even in the presence of new issues potentially affecting clinical course.

Highlights

- SOT is a clinical practice that includes the use of immunosuppressive therapies, aimed to cut down the risk of graft rejection.
- The risk of rejection must be balanced with the severe side effects of these drugs.
- There are different transplantation settings which mean different rules. Good clinical practice in immunosuppressive therapy is like 'to sail in a sea of different protocols'.
- Not all the immunosuppressive drugs are 'young'. The clinician philosophy must be 'using old drugs, get new and cheering results'.
- Special attention must be dedicated to the new frontiers of transplantation, as the immunological tolerance to the graft, otherwise intended as induced operational tolerance. This could be related to particular clinical situation (optimal donor/recipient HLA match) or pursued with new pharmacological approaches or protocols facilitating chimerism.

References

1. Moureau A et al. Effector mechanism of rejection. Cold Spring Harb Perspect Med 2013;3:a015461.

2. Wasowska BA. Mechanisms involved in antibody and complement-mediated allograft rejection. Immunol Res. 2010 Jul;47(1-3):25–44.
3. Becker LE et al. Immune mechanisms of acute and chronic rejection. Clin Biochem. 2016;49:320–323.
4. Lefaucheur C et al. Determinants of poor graft outcome in patients with antibody-mediated acute rejection. Am J Transplant. 2007;7:832–841.
5. Smith JD et al. De novo donor HLA-specific antibodies after heart transplantation are an independent predictor of poor patient survival. Am J Transplant. 2011;11:312–319.
6. Zuber J et al. Mechanisms of mixed Chimerism-based transplant tolerance. Trends Immunol. 2017 November;38(11):829–843.
7. Scheel et al. Patient-reported non-adherence and immunosuppressant trough levels are associated with rejection after renal transplantation. BMC Nephrol. 2017;18:107.
8. Shneider C et al. Assessment and treatment of nonadherence in transplant recipients. Gastroenterol Clin North Am. 2018 Dec;47(4):939–948.
9. Burra P et al. Quality of life and adherence in liver transplant recipients. Minerva Gastroenterol Dietol. 2018 Jun;64(2):180–186.
10. Fine RN Tolerance in Solid-Organ Transplant. Exp Clin Transpl. 2016;Suppl 3:1–5.
11. Scandling JD et al. Macrochimerism and clinical transplant tolerance. Human Immunol. 2018;79:266–271.
12. Demetris AJ et al. Monitoring of human liver and kidney allograft tolerance: a tissue/histopathology perspective. Transpl Int. 2009;22(1):120–141.
13. Starzl TE et al. Cell migration and chimerism after whole organ transplantation: the basis of graft acceptance. Hepatology. 1993;17(6):1127–1152.
14. Mazariegos GV et al. Weaning of immunosuppression in liver transplant recipients. Transplantation. 1997;63(2):243–249.
15. Louis S et al. Contrasting CD25hiCD4þT cells/FOXP3 patterns in chronic rejection and operational drug-free tolerance. Transplantation. 2006;81:398–407.
16. Baron D et al. A common gene signature across multiple studies relate biomarkers and functional regulation in tolerance to renal allograft. Kidney Int. 2015;87:984–995.
17. Chesneau M et al. Tolerant kidney transplant patients produce B cells with regulatory properties. J Am Soc Nephrol. 2015;26:2588–2598.
18. Sakaguchi Set al. Regulatory T cells and immune tolerance. Cell. 2008;133:775–787.
19. Sachs DH et al. Induction of tolerance through mixed chimerism. Cold Spring Harb Perspect Med. 2014;4: a015529.
20. Sakaguchi S et al. Immunologic self-tolerance maintained by activated T cells expressing IL-2 receptor alpha-chains (CD25). Breakdown of a single mechanism of selftolerance causes various autoimmune diseases. J Immunol. 1995;155:1151.
21. Chaudhry A et al. Interleukin-10 signaling in regulatory T cells is required for suppression of Th17 cell-mediated inflammation. Immunity. 2011;34:566.
22. Vignali D et al. How regulatory T cells work. Nat Rev Immunol. 2008;8:523.
23. Qureshi OS et al. Trans-endocytosis of CD80 and CD86: a molecular basis for the cellextrinsic function of CTLA-4. Science 2011;332:600.

24. Okoye IS et al. MicroRNA-containing T-regulatory-cellderived exosomes suppress pathogenic T helper 1 cells. Immunity. 2014;41:89.
25. Yu X et al. CD4 + CD25+ regulatory T cells-derived exosomes prolonged kidney allograft survival in a rat model. Cell Immunol. 2013;285:62.
26. Starzl TE et al. The use of cyclosporine A and prednisolone on cadaver kidney transplantation. Surg Gynecol Obstet. 1980;151:17–26.
27. Vanhove T et al. Clinical determinants of calcineurin inhibitor disposition: a mechanistic review. Drug Metab Rev. 2016;48(1):88–112.
28. Yee GC Recent advances in cyclosporine pharmacokinetics. Pharmacotherapy. 1991;11(5):130S–134S.
29. Levy GA. Neoral/cyclosporine-based immunosuppression. Liver Transpl Surg. 1999 Jul;5(4 Suppl 1):S37–S47.
30. Krämer BK et al. Efficacy and safety of tacrolimus compared with ciclosporin-A in renal transplantation: 7-year observational results. Transpl Int. 2016.
31. Levy G et al. 12-month follow-up analysis of a multicenter, randomized, prospective trial in de novo liver transplant recipients (LIS2T) comparing cyclosporine microemulsion (C2 monitoring) and tacrolimus. Liver Transpl. 2006 Oct;12(10):1464–1472.
32. Song JL et al. Minimizing tacrolimus decreases the risk of new-onset diabetes mellitus after liver transplantation. World J Gastroenterol. 2016 Feb 14;22(6):2133–2141.
33. Mueller AR et al. Neurotoxicity after orthotopic liver transplantation in cyclosporin A- and FK 506-treated patients. Transpl Int. 1994;7 Suppl 1:S37–S42.
34. https://www.ema.europa.eu/en/documents/scientific-discussion/advagraf-epar-scientific-discussion_en.pdf
35. De Geest S et al. Incidence, determinants, and consequences of subclinical noncompliance with immunosuppressive therapy in renal transplant recipients. Transplantation. 1995;59:340.
36. Krämer BK et al. Tacrolimus once daily (ADVAGRAF) versus twice daily (PROGRAF) in de novo renal transplantation: a randomized phase III study. Am J Transplant. 2010;10:2632.
37. Trunečka P et al. Renal Function in De Novo Liver Transplant Recipients Receiving Different Prolonged-Release Tacrolimus Regimens—The DIAMOND Study. Am J Transplant. 2015;15:1843–1854.
38. Adam R et al. Improved survival in liver transplant patients receiving prolonged-release tacrolimus-based immunosuppression in the European Liver Transplant Registry (ELTR): an extension study. Transplantation. 2019 May 7. doi: 10.1097/TP.0000000000002700. [Epub ahead of print]
39. Tremblay S et al. A steady-state head-to-head pharmacokinetic comparison of all FK-506 (Tacrolimus) formulations (ASTCOFF): An open-label, prospective, randomized, two-arm, three-period crossover study. Am J Transplant. 2016; XX:1–11. doi: 10.1111/ajt.13935.
40. Takeuchi H et al. Evidence of different pharmacokinetics including relationship among AUC, peak, and trough levels between cyclosporine and tacrolimus in renal transplant recipients using new pharmacokinetic parameter--why cyclosporine is monitored by C(2) level and tacrolimus by trough level. Biol Pharm Bull. 2008 Jan;31(1):90–94.

41. Levy G et al. Improved clinical outcomes for liver transplant recipients using cyclosporine monitoring based on 2-hr post-dose levels (C2). Transplantation. 2002 Mar 27;73(6):953–959.
42. de Jonge H et al. New insights into the pharmacokinetics and pharmacodynamics of the calcineurin inhibitors and mycophenolic acid: possible consequences for therapeutic drug monitoring in solid organ transplantation. Ther Drug Monit. 2009 Aug;31(4):416–435.
43. Legendre C1 et al. Factors influencing long-term outcome after kidney transplantation. Transpl Int. 2014 Jan;27(1):19–27.
44. Wallemacq PE1, Verbeeck RK. Comparative clinical pharmacokinetics of tacrolimus in paediatric and adult patients. Clin Pharmacokinet. 2001;40(4):283–295.
45. Wallemacq P et al. Opportunities to optimize tacrolimus therapy in solid organ transplantation: report of the European consensus conference. Ther Drug Monit. 2009 Apr;31(2):139–152.
46. Yang Z, Wang S. Recent development in application of high performance liquid chromatography-tandem mass spectrometry in therapeutic drug monitoring of immunosuppressants. J Immunol Methods. 2008 Jul 31;336(2):98–103.
47. Arns W et al. Therapeutic drug monitoring of mycophenolic acid in solid organ transplant patients treated with mycophenolate mofetil: review of the literature. Transplantation. 2006 Oct 27;82(8):1004–1012.
48. Schnitzbauer AA et al. Study protocol: a pilot study to determine the safety and efficacy of induction-therapy, de novo MPA and delayed mTOR-inhibition in liver transplant recipients with impaired renal function. PATRON-study. BMC Nephrol. 2010 Sep 14;11:24.
49. Birkeland SA. Steroid-free immunosuppression after kidney transplantation with antithymocyte globulin induction and cyclosporine and mycophenolate mofetil maintenance therapy. Transplantation. 1998 Nov 15;66(9):1207–1210.
50. Lerut JP. Avoiding steroids in solid organ transplantation. Transpl Int. 2003 Apr;16(4):213–224.
51. Starzl TE et al. Homotransplantation of the liver in humans. Surg Gynecol Obstet. 1963;117:659–676.
52. Starzl TE et al. The reversal of rejection in human renal homografts with subsequent development of homograft tolerance. Surg Gynecol Obstet. 1963;117:385–395.
53. Pirenne J et al. Steroid-free immunosuppression during and after liver transplantation—A 3-yr follow-up report. Clin Transplant. 2003 Jun;17(3):177–182.
54. Haller MC et al. Steroid avoidance or withdrawal for kidney transplant recipients. Cochrane Database Syst Rev. 2016 Aug 22;(8):CD005632.
55. Baraldo M et al. Steroid-free and steroid withdrawal protocols in heart transplantation: the review of literature. Transpl Int. 2014 Jun;27(6):515–529.
56. Lerut JP et al. Is minimal, [almost] steroid-free immunosuppression a safe approach in adult liver transplantation? Long-term outcome of a prospective, double blind, placebocontrolled, randomized, investigator-driven study. Ann Surg. 2014;260:886–891.
57. Laplante M et al. mTOR signaling in growth control and disease. Cell. 2012;149:274–293.

58. Schena FP et al. Conversion from calcineurin inhibitors to sirolimus maintenance therapy in renal allograft recipients: 24-month efficacy and safety results from the CONVERT trial. Transplantation. 2009;87:233–242.
59. Lebranchu Y et al. Efficacy on renal function of early conversion from cyclosporine to sirolimus 3 months after renal transplantation: Concept study. Am J Transplant. 2009;9:1115–1123.
60. Paoletti E et al. Effect of early conversion from CNI to sirolimus on outcomes in kidney transplant recipients with allograft dysfunction. J Nephrol. 2012;25:709–718.
61. Stallone G et al. Sirolimus for Kaposi's sarcoma in renal-transplant recipients. N Engl J Med. 2005;352:1317–1323.
62. Monaco AP. The role of mTOR inhibitors in the management of posttransplant malignancy. Transplantation. 2009;87:157–163.
63. Liefeldt L et al. Donor-specific HLA antibodies in a cohort comparing everolimus with cyclosporine after kidney transplantation. Am J Transplant. 2012;12:1192–1198.
64. Ekberg H et al. Reduced exposure to calcineurin inhibitors in renal transplantation. N Engl J Med. 2007;357:2562–2575.
65. Zaza G et al. Systemic and nonrenal adverse effects occurring in renal transplant patients treated with mTOR inhibitors. Clin Dev Immunol. 2013;2013:403280.
66. Stallone G et al. Management of side effects of sirolimus therapy. Transplantation. 2009;87(S8):S23–S26.
67. Zand MS et al. Polyclonal rabbit antithymocyte globulin triggers B-cell and plasma cell apoptosis by multiple pathways. Transplantation. 2005;79:1507–1515.
68. Lopez M et al. A novel mechanism of action for anti-thymocyte globulin: induction of CD4 + CD25+ Foxp3 + regulatory T cells. J Am Soc Nephrol. 2006;17:2844–2853.
69. Buchler M et al. French Thymoglobuline Pharmacovigilance Study Group: Induction therapy by anti-thymocyte globulin (rabbit) in renal transplantation: A 1-yr follow-up of safety and efficacy. Clin Transplant. 2003;17:539–545.
70. Larsen CP et al. Rational development of LEA29Y (belatacept), a high-affinity variant of CTLA4-Ig with potent immunosuppressive properties. Am J Transplant. 2005:(5):443–453.
71. Vincenti F et al. Costimulation blockade with belatacept in renal transplantation. N Engl J Med. 2005;353(8):770–781.
72. Pescovitz MD et al. Rituximab, an anti-cd20 monoclonal antibody: History and mechanism of action. Am J Transplant. 2006;6:859–866.
73. Burton SA et al. Treatment of antibody-mediated rejection in renal transplant patients: a clinical practice survey. Clin Transplant. 2015 Feb;29(2):118–123.
74. Zhao YG et al. Clinical efficacy of rituximab for acute rejection in kidney transplantation: a meta-analysis. Int Urol Nephrol. 2014 Jun;46(6):1225–1230.
75. Cenci S. The proteasome in terminal plasma cell differentiation. Semin Hematol. 2012;49:215–222.
76. Walsh RC et al. Proteasome inhibitor-based therapy for antibody-mediated rejection. Kidney Int. 2012;81:1067–1074..
77. Wan SS et al. The treatment of antibody-mediated rejection in kidney transplantation: An updated systematic review and meta-analysis. Transplantation. 2018 Apr;102(4):557–568.

78. Tan EK et al. Use of Eculizumab for active antibody-mediated rejection that occurs early post-kidney transplantation: A consecutive series of 15 cases. Transplantation. 2019;(2):19. doi: 10.1097/TP.0000000000002639.
79. Hanaway MJ et al. INTACStudyGroup: Alemtuzumab induction in renal transplantation. N Engl J Med. 2011;364:1909–1919.
80. Kirk AD et al. Dissociation of depletional induction and posttransplant lymphoproliferative disease in kidney recipients treated with alemtuzumab. Am J Transplant. 2007;7:2619–2625.
81. Jamal Bamoulid et al. The need for minimization strategies: current problems of immunosuppression. Transplant Int. 2015;28:891–900.
82. Cai J, Terasaki PI. The current trend of induction and maintenance treatment in patient of different PRA levels: A report on OPTN/UNOS Kidney Transplant Registry data. Clin Transpl. 2010:45–52.
83. Ruan V et al. Use of anti-thymocyte globulin for induction therapy in cardiac transplantation: A review. Transplant Proc. 2017 Mar;49(2):253–259.
84. Bittermann T et al. The use of induction therapy in liver transplantation is highly variable and is associated with post transplant outcomes. Am J Transplant. 2019 Jun 27. doi: 10.1111/ajt.15513. [Epub ahead of print]
85. Petite SE et al. Antithymocyte globulin induction therapy in liver transplant: old drug, new uses. Ann Pharmacother. 2016;50(7):592–598.
86. Halldorson JB. Differential rates of ischemic cholangiopathy and graft survival associated with induction therapy in DCD liver transplantation. Am J Transplant. 2015 Jan;15(1):251–258.
87. Guirado L. Does Rabbit Antithymocyte Globulin (Thymoglobuline®) Have a Role in Avoiding Delayed Graft Function in the Modern Era of Kidney Transplantation? J Transplant. 2018; doi: 10.1155/2018/4524837.
88. Gurkan S. Immune reconstitution following rabbit antithymocyte globulin. Am J Transplant. 2010 September;10(9):2132–2141.
89. Stevens RB et al. A randomized 2×2 factorial trial, part 1: single-dose rabbit antithymocyte globulin induction may improve renal transplantation outcomes. Transplantation. 2015 Jan;99(1):197–209.
90. Wang K et al. Induction therapy of basiliximab versus antithymocyte globulin in renal allograft: a systematic review and meta-analysis. Clin Exp Nephrol. 2018 Jun;22(3):684–693.
91. Thomusch O et al. Rabbit-ATG or basiliximab induction for rapid steroid withdrawal after renal transplantation (Harmony): an open-label, multicentre, randomised controlled trial. Lancet. 2016 Dec 17;388:3006–3016 Erratum in: Lancet. 2017 Feb 25;389(10071):804.
92. Penninga L et al. Antibody induction therapy for lung transplant recipients. Cochrane Database Syst Rev. 2013 Nov 27;(11):CD008927.
93. Butts RJ et al. Comparison of basiliximab vs antithymocyte globulin for induction in pediatric heart transplant recipients: An analysis of the International Society for Heart and Lung Transplantation database. Pediatr Transplant. 2018 Jun;22(4):e13190. doi: 10.1111/petr.13190.
94. Qazi Y et al. Efficacy and safety of everolimus plus low-dose tacrolimus versus mycophenolate mofetil plus standard-dose tacrolimus in de novo renal transplant recipients: 12-month data. Am J Transpl. 2017 May;17(5):1358–1369.

95. de Fijter JW et al. Early conversion from calcineurin inhibitor- to everolimus-based therapy following kidney transplantation: Results of the randomized ELEVATE trial. Am J Transplant. 2017 Jul;17(7):1853–1867.
96. Cillo U et al. Very Early introduction of everolimus in de novo liver transplantation: Results of a multicenter, prospective, randomized trial. Liver Transpl. 2019 Feb;25(2):242–251.
97. Fine NM et al. Recent advances in mammalian target of rapamycin inhibitor use in heart and lung transplantation. Transplantation. 2016;100(12):2558–2568.
98. Vincenti F et al. A phase III study of belatacept-based immunosuppression regimens versus cyclosporine in renal transplant recipients (BENEFIT study). Am J Transplant. (2008);10(3):535–546.
99. Lee JG. Efficacy of rabbit anti-thymocyte globulin for steroid-resistant acute rejection after liver transplantation. Medicine (Baltimore). 2016 Jun;95(23):e3711. doi: 10.1097/MD.0000000000003711.
100. Webster AC. Polyclonal and monoclonal antibodies for treating acute rejection episodes in kidney transplant recipients. Cochrane Database Syst Rev. 2017 Jul 20;7:CD004756. doi: 10.1002/14651858.CD004756.pub4.
101. Issa N et al. Calcineurin inhibitor nephrotoxicity: A review and perspective of the evidence. Am J Nephrol. 2013;37:602–612 [PMID: 23796509 DOI: 10.1159/000351648].
102. Rathi M et al. Conversion from tacrolimus to cyclosporine in patients with new-onset diabetes after renal transplant: an open-label randomized prospective pilot study. Transplant Proc. 2015 May;47(4):1158–1161.
103. Hatahira H et al. Drug-induced gingival hyperplasia: A retrospective study using spontaneous reporting system databases. J Pharm Health Care Sci. 2017 Jul 19;3:19. doi: 10.1186/s40780-017-0088-5.
104. Haddad EM et al. Cyclosporin versus tacrolimus for liver transplanted patients. Cochrane Database Syst Rev. 2006;(4):CD005161 [PMID: 17054241 DOI: 10.1002/14651858.CD005161.pub2]
105. Flechner SM et al. The ORION study: Comparison of two sirolimus-based regimens versus tacrolimus and mycophenolate mofetil in renal allograft recipients. Am J Transplant. 2011;11:1633–1644.
106. Flechner SM et al. A randomized, open-label study of sirolimus versus cyclosporine in primary de novo renal allograft recipients. Transplantation. 2013;95:1233–1241.
107. Schena FP et al. Conversion from calcineurin inhibitors to sirolimus maintenance therapy in renal allograft recipients: 24-month efficacy and safety results from the CONVERT trial. Transplantation. 2009 Jan 27;87(2):233–242.
108. Budde K et al. Five-year outcomes in kidney transplant patients converted from cyclosporine to everolimus: the randomized ZEUS study. Am J Transplant. 2015 Jan;15(1):119–128.
109. Tedesco-Silva H et al. Optimizing the clinical utility of sirolimus-based immunosuppression for kidney transplantation. Clin Transplant. 2019 Feb;33(2):e13464. doi: 10.1111/ctr.13464.
110. Wolf S et al. Effects of mTOR-Is on malignancy and survival following renal transplantation: A systematic review and meta-analysis of randomized trials with a

minimum follow-up of 24 months. PLoS One. 2018 Apr 16;13(4):e0194975. doi: 10.1371/journal.pone.0194975.
111. Geissler EK et al. Sirolimus use in liver transplant recipients with hepatocellular carcinoma: A randomized, multicenter, open-label Phase 3 trial. Transplantation. 2016;100:116–125.
112. Nashan B. mTOR Inhibition and Clinical Transplantation. Liver Transpl. 2018;102:S19–S26.
113. Nankivell BJ et al. The natural history of chronic allograft nephropathy. N Engl J Med 2003;349:2326.
114. Flechner SM et al. Calcineurin inhibitor-sparing regimens in solid organ transplantation: focus on improving renal function and nephrotoxicity. Clin Transplant. 2008 Jan-Feb;22(1):1–15.
115. Stevens RB et al. A randomized 2x2 factorial clinical trial of renal transplantation: Steroid-free maintenance immunosuppression with calcineurin inhibitor withdrawal after six months associates with improved renal function and reduced chronic histopathology. PLoS One. 2015 Oct 14;10(10):e0139247. doi: 10.1371.
116. Vincenti F et al. Belatacept and long-term outcomes in kidney transplantation. N Engl J Med (2016);374(4):333–343.
117. Masson P et al. Belatacept for kidney transplant recipients. Cochrane Database Syst Rev 2014;11:CD010699. doi:10.1002/14651858.
118. Rostaing L et al. Switching from calcineurin inhibitor-based regimens to a belatacept-based regimen in renal transplant recipients: a randomized phase II study. Clin J Am Soc Nephrol (2011);6(2):430–439.
119. Grinyo J et al. Improvement in renal function in kidney transplant recipients switched from cyclosporine or tacrolimus to belatacept: 2-year results from the long-term extension of a phase II study. Transpl Int (2012) 25(10):1059–1064.
120. Grinyó JM et al. Safety and efficacy outcomes 3 years after switching to belatacept from a calcineurin inhibitor in kidney transplant recipients: results from a phase 2 randomized trial. Am J Kidney Dis (2017) 69(5):587–594.
121. Yuval A et al. Nonalcoholic Fatty Liver Disease: Key Considerations Before and After Liver Transplantation. Dig Dis Sci. 2016 May;61(5):1406–1416.
122. Moini M et al. Review on immunosuppression in liver transplantation. World J Hepatol. 2015 June 8;7(10):1355–1368.
123. Stirnimann G et al. Recurrent and De Novo Autoimmune Hepatitis. Liver Transpl. 2019 Jan;25(1):152–166.
124. Hanouneh M et al. A review of the utility of tacrolimus in the management of adults with autoimmune hepatitis. Scand J Gastroenterol. 2019 Jan;54(1):76–80.
125. Beal EW et al. Autoimmune Hepatitis in the Liver Transplant Graft. Clin Liver Dis. 2017 May;21(2):381–401.
126. Klintmalm GB et al. Belatacept-based immunosuppression in de novo liver transplant recipients: 1-year experience from a phase II randomized study. Am J Transplant. 2014;14(8):1817–1827.
127. Grinyó J et al. An integrated safety profile analysis of belatacept in kidney transplant recipients. Transplantation. (2010) 90(12):1521–1527.
128. Belatacept-NULOJIX. Prescribing information. Princeton, NJ: Bristol-Myers Squibb Company; revised April 2018.

129. Gullestad L et al. Everolimus with reduced calcineurin inhibitor in thoracic transplant recipients with renal dysfunction: a multicenter, randomized trial. Transplantation. 2010;89:864–872.
130. Andreassen AK et al. Everolimus initiation and early calcineurin inhibitor withdrawal in heart transplant recipients: a randomized trial. Am J Transplant. 2014;14:1828–1838.
131. Da Silva JA et al. Safety of low dose glucocorticoid treatment in rheumatoid arthritis: published evidence and prospective trial data. Ann Rheum Dis. 2006;65(3):285–293.
132. Haller MC et al. Steroid avoidance or withdrawal for kidney transplant recipients. Cochrane Database Syst Rev. 2016 Aug 22;(8):CD005632.
133. Tisone G et al. A pilot study on the safety and effectiveness of immunosuppression without prednisone after liver transplantation. Transplantation. 1999 May 27;67(10):1308–1313.
134. Lladó L and Thosin Study Group. Immunosuppression without steroids in liver transplantation is safe and reduces infection and metabolic complications: results from a prospective multicenter randomized study. J Hepatol. 2006 Apr;44(4):710–716 Erratum in: J Hepatol. 2006 Jul;45(1):166.
135. Washburn K et al. Steroid elimination 24 hours after liver transplantation using daclizumab, tacrolimus, and mycophenolate mofetil. Speeg KV et al.. Transplantation. 2001 Nov 27;72(10):1675–1679.
136. Saliba F et al. Corticosteroid-sparing and optimization of mycophenolic acid exposure in liver transplant recipients receiving mycophenolate Mofetil and Tacrolimus: A randomized, multicenter study. Transplantation. 2016;100:1705–1713.
137. Fairfield C et al. Glucocorticosteroid-free versus glucocorticosteroid-containing immunosuppression for liver transplanted patients. Cochrane Database Syst Rev. 2018 Apr 9;4:CD007606.
138. Costanzo MR et al. Guidelines for the care of heart transplant recipients. J Heart Lung Transplant. 2010;29:914.
139. Baraldo M et al. Steroid-free and steroid withdrawal protocols in heart transplantation: the review of literature. Transpl Int. 2014 Jun;27(6):515–529.
140. Kawai T et al. Long-term results in recipients of combined HLA-mismatched kidney and bone marrow transplantation without maintenance immunosuppression. Am J Transplant. 2014 Jul;14(7):1599–1611.
141. Scandling JD et al. Macrochimerism and clinical transplant tolerance. Human Immunol. 2018;79:266–271.
142. Kawai T et al. Summary of the Third International Workshop on Clinical Tolerance. Am J Transplant. 2019;19:324–330.
143. Tisone G et al. Complete weaning off immunosuppression in HCV liver transplant recipients is feasible and favourably impacts on the progression of disease recurrence. J Hepatol. 2006;44(4):702–709.
144. Feng S et al. Complete immunosuppression withdrawal and subsequent allograft function among pediatric recipients of parental living donor liver transplants. JAMA. 2012;307(3):283–293.
145. Benitez C et al. Prospective multicenter clinical trial of immunosuppressive drug withdrawal in stable adult liver transplant recipients. Hepatology. 2013;58(5):1824–1835.

146. Shaked A et al. Gradual Withdrawal of Immune System Suppressing Drugs in Patients Receiving a Liver Transplant (AWISH) National Institute of Allergy and Infectious Diseases, Immune Tolerance Network, NCT00135694 (clinicaltrialsgov).
147. Banff Working Group on Liver Allograft P. Importance of liver biopsy findings in immunosuppression management: Biopsy monitoring and working criteria for patients with operational tolerance. Liver Transpl. 2012;18(10):1154–1170.
148. Todo S et al. A pilot study of operational tolerance with a regulatory T-cell-based cell therapy in living donor liver transplantation. Hepatology. 2016;64(2):632–643.
149. Roedder S et al. The pits and pearls in translating operational tolerance biomarkers into clinical practice. Curr Opin Organ Transplant. 2012;17(6):655–662.
150. Li Y et al. The presence of Foxp3 expressing T cells within grafts of tolerant human liver transplant recipients. Transplantation. 2008;86(12):1837–1843.
151. Vionneta J et al. Biomarkers of immune tolerance in liver transplantation. Human Immunol. 2018;79:388–394.
152. Sarwal MM. Fingerprints of transplant tolerance suggest opportunities for immunosuppression minimization. Clin Biochem. 2016;49:404–410.
153. Miarons M et al. COVID-19 in solid organ transplantation: A matched retrospective cohort study and evaluation of immunosuppression management. Transplantation. 2021;105(1):138–150. doi: 10.1097/TP.0000000000003460.
154. Kates OS et al. COVID-19 in solid organ transplant: A multi-center cohort study. Clin Infect Dis. 2021;73(11):e4090–e4099. doi: 10.1093/cid/ciaa1097.

61
Common infectious diseases in the recipient

Francesco Giuseppe De Rosa, Michele Bartoletti, Silvia Corcione

Introduction

Infections may be associated with solid organ transplant (SOT) procedures for reasons including pre-existing diseases, complex surgeries, anaesthesiology and intensive care, immunosuppression, epidemiology of infectious diseases in the community or inside the hospital, or even when the recipient gets back to life and travel. Infections are classified according to the period of hospitalization or immunosuppression, the aetiology (bacterial, fungal, viral, and parasitic), the site of infection, and the type of transplanted organ. Such infections may be in the range of diagnostic clinical routine to a devastating syndrome, for example, in the setting of central nervous system infections, invasive diseases, multi-drug resistant (MDR) bacteria, bloodstream infection (BSI).(1)

In this chapter, we will briefly review the common infectious diseases in the recipient, briefly illustrating the most common aetiologies (Figure 61.1). The infectious risk of SOT recipients is strictly related to the intensity of immunosuppression and the time period that elapses between the transplant and the onset of symptoms. Typically, in the early post-transplant period (<30 days), infections are hospital- or ICU-acquired and are related to surgery or presence of devices.(2) Accordingly, in this period the prevalence of MDR pathogens is high, especially in certain geographical areas.(3) Beyond 6–12 months post-transplant, infections occurring in patients with acceptable graft function are related to community exposures or, less frequently, reactivation of latent infections. Thus, the majority of infection in this period are community-acquired

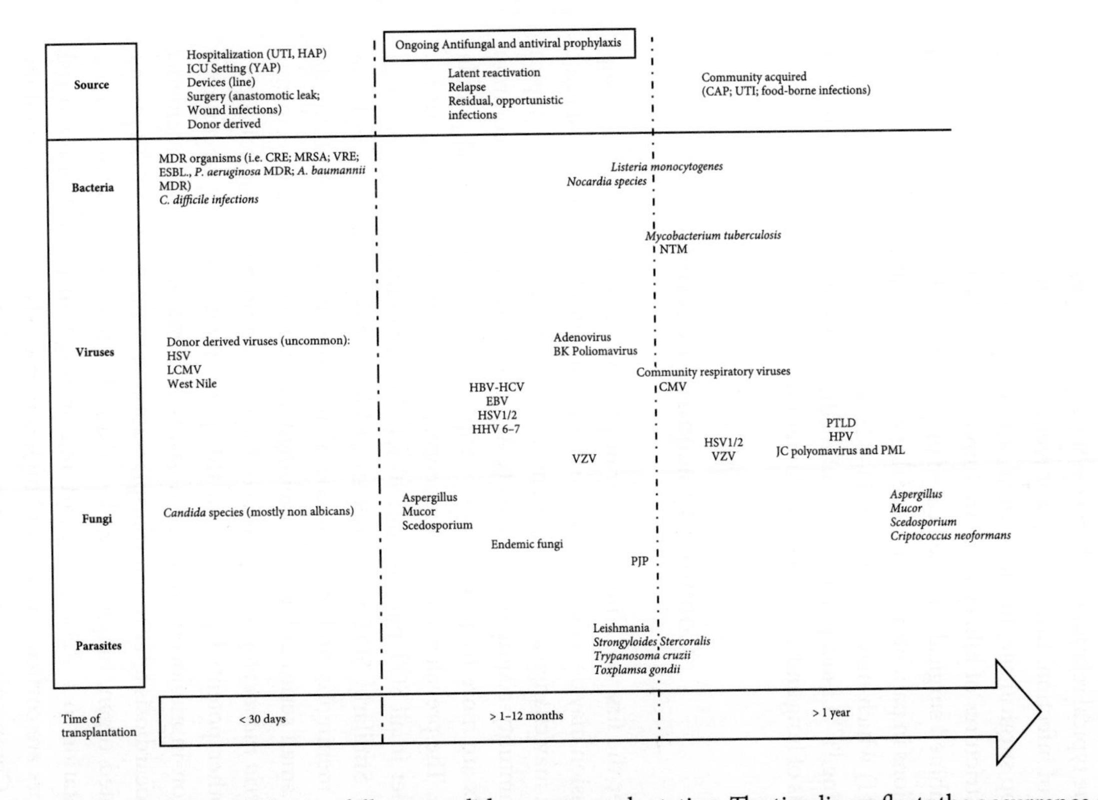

Figure 61.1. Common patterns of infection following solid organ transplantation. The timeline reflects the occurrence of opportunistic infections according with the 'net state of immunosuppression' based on time lapse between surgery and infection onset or intensity of immunosuppression. (Adapted form Fishman 2017).[(4)]

pneumonia, urinary tract, and food-borne infections (gastroenteritis or *Listeria monocytogenes* infection).[4]

Another important characteristic of bacterial infections in this setting is the typical relationship between the type of organ transplanted and the site of infection. Liver transplant recipients are particularly prone to develop surgical site, intrabdominal, and BSIs. In this case, biliary leakage or strictures of biliary tract are important risk factors that may require combined surgical and medical management.[5] The most important infections in patients receiving renal transplants are urinary tract infection (UTI) which may account for 56–82% of all bacterial infections in this setting.[6,7] Lastly, pneumonia and mediastinitis are common complications of lung and/or heart transplantation.[8,9]

Community-acquired infections

After the first 6–12 months of transplant the intensity of immunosuppression may be reduced. Thus, in this period the characteristics of infection may change and most patients are likely to experience more typical community-acquired infections (CAI). It is worth noting that common CAIs are more frequent in SOT recipients than in the general population. The prevalence of pneumococcal invasive disease (PID) is 10-fold higher in all SOT patients and 40-fold higher in lung transplant recipients. Similarly, SOT recipients are at higher risk for developing bacterial meningitis and meningococcal invasive disease.[10] Additionally, in a small series of bacterial meningitis in kidney transplant recipients, *Listeria monocytogenes* was one of the most common etiological agents. Another potential pathogen in this population, relatively uncommon in non-immunocompromised hosts, is *Nocardia* spp.[11] The incidence of nocardiosis after organ transplantation varies according to the transplanted organ, ranging from less than 1% after kidney or liver transplantation to 1–3.5% after heart and/or lung transplant. Common risk factors are corticosteroids, and high serum levels of calcineurin inhibitors. Commonly, nocardiosis occurs after the first year of transplantation and disseminated disease may be as high as 40% with a reported mortality of 16% of cases.[12,13] Nocardia is an important pathogen in immunosuppressed patients and is associated with skin and soft tissue, lung, central nervous system, or disseminated disease. A review of thirteen studies over the last five years dealing with Nocardia skin and soft tissue infections (SSTIs) has been recently published in SOT recipients.[14] The most common underlying type of transplant was kidney and the time from transplantation to infection varied from six months to sixteen years. Misdiagnosis was frequent. Available identified species included *N. brasiliensis* (2 isolates), *N. farcinica* (2), *N. flavorosea* (1), *N. abscessus* (1), *N. anaemiae* (1), *N. asteroides* (1), *N. nova* (1), and *N. vinacea* (1).

Epidemiology of MDR pathogens among SOT recipients

The prevalence, risk factors, and mortality of infection caused by MDR pathogens in the setting of organ transplant are summarized in Table 61.1. Significant differences are present between different pathogens. Furthermore, the prevalence and incidence of infections may vary among different centres located in different countries and between American and European centres.

Methicillin-resistant Staphylococcus aureus and Vancomycin Resistant Enterococci

Staphylococcus aureus is a major cause of invasive infection in the general population, being the second most common bacterial species.[15] Among all *S. aureus* infections, those due to Methicillin Resistant Staphylococcus Aureus (MRSA) represent 21–24% of cases in Europe and 31–39% in the U.S.[16,17]

The incidence of MRSA infection appears higher in lung and liver transplant recipients (0.2–5.7 cases per 100 transplant-years for the former, 0.1 cases per 100 transplant-years for the latter) with respect to other kinds of transplants. Most MRSA infections occur in the early post-transplant period, after a median of 7–29 days following liver and lung transplantation.[18–20] The most frequent sources of infection are pneumonia, BSI, vascular catheters, and the surgical site itself, the latter found mostly in heart and lung transplants. Risk factors for infection found in previous

Table 61.1 Summary of prevalence, risk factors and outcome of infection caused by multidrug-resistant pathogens in solid organ transplant recipients

Micro-organism or group	Organ transplanted	Prevalence	Risk factors	Mortality
All MDR pathogens[24,58,72–75]	Liver	15%	Abdominal infection episodes, reoperation acute rejection, use of pre-transplant broad-spectrum antibiotics and prolonged (≧72h) endotracheal intubation	6-month mortality 39%
	Kidney	14%	Age > 50 years, HCV infection, double kidney-pancreas transplantation, post-transplant RRT, surgical reoperation, nephrostomy	19%
	Lung	37–51%*	ICU stay >14 days, presence of a tracheostomy, previous exposure to broad-spectrum antibiotics	14%
	Heart	25%	NA	NA
MRSA[19–21,76–79]	Liver	1.4–23%	ICU stay, CMV primary co-infection	30-day mortality 21-25%
	Kidney	0.8–2%	NA	In-hospital mortality 0-10%
	Lung	10–60%	Mechanical ventilation > 5 days MRSA nasal carriage MRSA in recipient sterile cultures	30-day mortality 17%
	Heart	30%	NA	NA
VRE[27,29]	Liver	2–11%	Biliary leak, reoperation	In hospital 9-48% 54% 1-year mortality 56-80%
	Kidney	0%*		

Table 61.1 *Continued*

Micro-organism or group	Organ transplanted	Prevalence	Risk factors	Mortality
ESBL[37,40,80]	Liver	7%	Pre-transplant ESBL fecal carriage, MELD >25, Re-operation	30-day mortality 15-41%
	Kidney	3–11%	Double kidney/pancreas transplantation, previous use of antibiotics, post-transplant dialysis requirement, post-transplant urinary obstruction	30-day mortality 14%
	Lung	2%	NA	30-day mortality 15-41%
	Heart	5%	NA	30-day mortality 14%
CRE[43,44,48,50,81,82]	Liver	5–19%	RRT; mechanical ventilation >48 h; HCV recurrence, colonization at any time with CR-KP	In hospital mortality 18%
	Kidney	2–26%	multi-organ transplantation, the use of a uretheral stent	In-hospital mortality 33-41%
	Lung	0.4–20%	NA	30-day mortality 26- 1-year mortality 53%
	Heart	5–17%	NA	50%
Carbapenem-resistant Acinetobacter baumannii[52–54]	Liver	8–29%	prolonged cold ischemia, post-LT dialysis, LT due to fulminant hepatitis	60-day mortality 42%
	Kidney	3%	NA	30-day mortality 39%
	Lung	21%	NA	30-day mortality 62%
	Heart	7%	NA	NA

(*continued*)

Table 61.1 *Continued*

Micro-organism or group	Organ transplanted	Prevalence	Risk factors	Mortality
MDR-Pseudomonas aeruginosa[56,59,60,72,73]	Liver	4%	Previous transplantation	37-38%
	Kidney	6–9%	Hospital-acquired BSI	NA
	Lung	14%	ICU admission in the previous year	1-year mortality 27%
	Heart	19%	Septic shock	NA

Abbreviations: MDR multidrug-resistant; RRT renal replacement therapy, ICU intensive care unit, HCV hepatitis C virus, MRSA methicillin resistant Staphylococcus aureus, CRE carbapenem-resistant Enterobacteriaceae, ESBL-E extended spectrum β-lactamase-producing Enterobacteriaceae, NA not available, LT liver transplantation, CMV cytomegalovirus, MELD model for end-stage liver disease, VRE vancomycin resistant Enterobacteriaceae studies are pre-transplant and post-transplant nasal colonization, ICU stay, mechanical ventilation for more than five days and cytomegalovirus (CMV) primary infection in CMV-seronegative recipients. Mortality for infection caused by MRSA ranges between 14% and 36%.[20–22]

Enterococcus spp infection is common after abdominal SOT. Prevalence of *Enterococcus* spp infection is reported in up to 15% of SOT recipients, mainly liver transplant recipients.[23] *Enterococcus* spp is the causative pathogen of 6–15% of BSIs in SOT recipients. This rate can reach 20% in hospital-acquired BSI.[24–26] Among all enterococcal infections, the impact of Vancomycin Resistant Enterococcus (VRE) is extremely variable between countries. Centres in North America reported a prevalence of 2–11% of VRE infection in liver transplant recipients,[27–29] whereas nearly no infections were reported in studies conducted in Europe.[23,24] The VRE infections occur mainly in liver transplant recipients, probably as a consequence of high prevalence of colonized or infected patients before transplantation.[30,31] The main types of infection are bacteraemia, peritonitis, surgical site infection (SSI), urinary and biliary tract infections.[30,32,33] Lastly, VRE in heart transplant recipients has been described mostly in patients with a left ventricular assist device (LVAD) infection in the pre-transplant period.[34] Overall, crude mortality for VRE infection represents 9–48% of cases, but can reach 56–80% during the one-year of follow-up period.[28,29,32,33]

Extended spectrum beta-lactamase producing enterobacteriaceae

The prevalence of extended spectrum beta-lactamase (ESBL) producing strains among transplant patients has increased dramatically in recent years. In a study analysing the aetiology of BSI occurring among transplant recipients in a centre in Spain in the first-year post-transplant, an increasing rate of ESBL-producing strains was found, principally *Klebsiella pneumoniae*, from 7% in 2007–2008 to 34% in 2015–2016.[35]

Most infections in patients receiving liver, lung, and heart transplants occur early in the post-transplant period.[36–38] However, longer delays between transplant and infection have been observed in kidney transplant recipients (28–864 days).[36,39] Mortality associated with infection due to ESBL-producing strains may vary from 8% to 26% of cases.[36,37] In addition, a significant rate of recurrent infection has been observed (21–41% of cases). In particular, recurrent UTI in kidney transplant recipients is frequently reported.(37,39,40)

Carbapenem-resistant Enterobacteriales

Nowadays the global emergence of carbapenem-resistant Enterobacteriales (CRE) is a major health challenge. Studies analysing CRE BSI episodes in the general patient population have revealed SOT patients are involved in 14–37% of cases.(41,42) In addition, a multicentre study conducted in SOT recipients in Italy shows that the prevalence of carbapenem resistance was 26% among all isolated Enterobacteriaceae and 49% among all isolated *Klebsiella* spp.(43)

Overall, in endemic areas, the incidence of CRE infection following SOT is approximately 5%, CRE infection commonly occurs in the initial post-transplant period (on average 11–36 days).(44–46) Infections associated with CRE are usually BSI, including catheter-related BSI, pneumonia, UTI, intraabdominal infection, and SSI. Post-transplantation renal replacement therapy, CRE rectal colonization, Hepatitis C Virus (HCV) recurrence in liver transplant recipients, bile leak, and prolonged mechanical ventilation are risk factors for CRE during the early post-transplant period.(44,47) CRE associated crude mortality rates vary from 25% to 71%.(46,48–51)

Carbapenem-resistant Acinetobacter baumannii

Carbapenem-resistant *Acinetobacter baumannii* (CR-AB) is commonly reported to affect 9–29% of SOT patients. This variability is primarily related to the distinctive propensity of CR-AB to generate outbreaks.(52–54) Epidemiological studies of BSI in SOT patients report a rate of CR-AB of 2–6%.(24) Most infections occur in liver and lung transplant recipients, commonly during the ICU stay in the early post-transplant period. The most common infections are SSI, pneumonia, and BSI, with a mortality rate after thirty days of 57–62%.

MDR Pseudomonas aeruginosa

Pseudomonas aeruginosa is involved in 6–13% of BSI after SOT, being a leading pathogen in lung transplant patients.(26,35,55) Prevalence of drug resistance among *P. aeruginosa* strains may vary significantly between centres. There are also concerns regarding *P. aeruginosa* infections and colonization among lung transplant candidates, especially those affected by cystic fibrosis. Studies conducted in this population showed close to 50% of lung transplant candidates harbouring pan-drug-resistant *P. aeruginosa* in the airways.(56) Colonization and/or infection by *P. aeruginosa* after lung transplantation is associated with higher risk of developing bronchiolitis obliterans syndrome and death.(57) Finally, MDR *P. aeruginosa* is frequently found among recurrent cases of UTI among kidney transplant recipients.(58) Outside the lung transplantation setting, the most common sources of MDR/extensively drug-resistant (XDR) *P. aeruginosa* BSI are the urinary tract, central venous catheters, and the abdomen.(59,60)(61)

Fungal infections

Amongst yeast infections, invasive candidiasis is the most common, with timing, clinical manifestations and risk factors continuously changing according to the complex scenario of SOT: organ, surgery, nosocomial complications, and immunosuppression.(62) Further complicating the epidemiology, prophylaxis, empiric, and *pre-emptive* antifungal administration strategies may delay or profoundly affect the clinical suspect of such complications. Antifungal resistance, such as in *Candida glabrata* or in the worldwide emergence of *Candida auris*, and biofilm production is as important as effective source control. Cryptococci are also important and *Cryptococcus gattii*, amongst Cryptococci, add other complexities: the site of infection (central nervous system vs lung, disseminated disease or cutaneous involvement), differential diagnosis, reduced *in vitro* activity of some antifungals and the possibility of Immune Reconstitution Inflammatory Syndrome (IRIS).(62)

Mould infections are associated with significant increase in healthcare expenses also due to the variable clinical presentation, often but not completely dependent on the immune system activity; these infections include Aspergillus, Zygomycetes, Fusarium, Scedosporium/Pseudoallescheria, dematiaceous (dark) moulds(63) (Table 61.2). Invasive Aspergillosis is the most common fungal infection after invasive candidiasis. Invasive mould infections emphasize the need of a multidisciplinary

Table 61.2 Mould Infections and aetiology in solid organ transplantation (SOT) (Adapted from Lemonovich et al. 2018)[63]

Aetiology	Predominant Species	Risk Factors/Type of SOT	Clinical Manifestations
Aspergillus	A. *fumigatus*, A. *flavus*, A. *niger*, A. *terreus*	Neutropenia Lung, Liver, Heart	Invasive pulmonary TBA (lung transplant) Disseminated
Zygomycetes	*Rhizopus, Mucor, Rhizomucor, Absidia, Cunninghamella, Apophysomyces, Myocladus*	Diabetes mellitus Steroids Neutropenia Renal failure Immunomodulating viruses Malnutrition Prior voriconazole or caspofungin use Liver, lung, kidney	Most commonly pulmonary Rhino-sino-orbital Disseminated Primary cutaneous Gastrointestinal Bronchial anastomosis (LT)
Fusarium	F. *solani*, F. *oxysporum*, F. *verticillioides*	Lung, liver	Pulmonary Primary cutaneous Disseminated (often with skin involvement) Sinusitis Osteomyelitis/septic arthritis Endophthalmitis Brain abscess
Scedosporium/ pseudallescheria	S. *apiospermum*, P. *boydii*, *Lomentospora prolificans*	Lung	Pulmonary Sinusitis Surgical site Skin Disseminated
Dematiaceous fungi (dark moulds)	Alternaria, Exophiala, Curvularia, Cladosporium, Ochroconis, Bipolaris	All solid organ transplant	Skin (nodules, abscesses, ulcers) Pulmonary Disseminated
Paecilomyces		Heart Lung	Skin and soft tissue Peritonitis Sternal wound infection

TBA: Tracheobronchial aspergillosis

LT: lung transplant SOT: Solid organ transplantation

stewardship approach to correctly use all diagnostic (including molecular and biomarkers) and treatment strategies, including surgery, also to reduce healthcare expenses and optimize the use of definitions. The management includes a high degree of suspicion and a multidisciplinary approach, sometimes with combined medical and surgical approaches.(64) Mould infections are usually acquired via the respiratory tract and invasive aspergillosis is diagnosed in 1–15% of SOT, with 12-week mortality exceeding 20%.(65,66) Rare forms are associated with surgical site infection or organ-space infection after surgery. Invasive mucormycosis caused by Zygomycetes (order Mucorales) is responsible for up to 2% of fungal infections in SOT.(67) *Scedosporium* species and *Lomentospora prolificans* are second only to Aspergillus as mould aetiology in lung transplant recipients, according to a recent international survey, 2016–2017.(68)

The diagnosis is based on a combination of conventional cultural tests, biomarkers, molecular biology with invasive techniques, and tissue biopsies. Endemic mycoses are caused by endemic, geographically restricted, dimorphic fungi; such as histoplasmosis, coccidioidomycosis, and blastomycosis in North America. Such infections are important because of the variety of settings of invasive infections including primary infection, reactivation of latent disease or donor-derived infection.(69)

Viral infections

SOT recipients are uniquely predisposed to develop clinical illness, often with increased severity, due to a variety of common and opportunistic viruses. Patients may acquire viral infections from the donor (donor-derived infections), from reactivation of the endogenous latent virus, or from the community. Herpes viruses, most notably cytomegalovirus, and Epstein Barr virus, are the commonest among opportunistic viral pathogens that cause infection after solid organ transplantation.

CMV infections in SOT

Cytomegalovirus (CMV) is still an expected problem in SOT. Latency of CMV-infected lymphoid cells, organ transmission, and immunosuppression all contribute to the special setting of CMV diagnostic, preventive, and treatment strategies. Primary, secondary, and reactivation strategies require specific interventions with antivirals to limit the extension of disease and reduce the morbidity and mortality.[70]

BK polyomavirus (BKV) infection in kidney and kidney-pancreas transplant recipients

With effective strategies, BKV is associated with graft failure in <5% of kidney recipients. The BKV associated nephropathy probably emerged as a complication of complex immunosuppression regimens and was previously associated with graft failure in up to 70% of patients.[71]

Conclusion

Immunocompromised patients may also develop all other types of infections where the balance between immune system activity and the exposure may result in complex, severe, and early or precocious clinical manifestations, such as respiratory infections, viral hepatitis, infections by *Mycobacterium tuberculosis*, Mycobacteria other than tuberculosis, *C. difficile* infection and diarrhoea and Strongyloides hyperinfection syndromes. Such a variety of infections will continuously need complex diagnostic and treatment strategies and up-to-date epidemiological data as well as extreme attention to the underlying degree of immunosuppression.

Highlights

- Infection in SOT is a major cause of morbidity and mortality
- Infectious risk is different according to type of surgery, timing of infection after transplantation and geographic areas
- Antimicrobial resistance is common in SOT recipients. Among others, extended spectrum beta-lactamase or carbapenem-resistant

Enterobacteriales and MDR non-fermenting bacilli are important threats in this setting

- Invasive fungal infections are common, especially in bowel, lung, and liver transplants. Prevention, early diagnosis, and prompt treatment are pivotal keys of management of these complications.
- Cytomegalovirus is a main viral pathogen in SOT recipients. Several factors may contribute to CMV disease including type of organ transplanted (thoracic and bowel transplant are at higher risk than liver and kidney transplant), type and intensity of immunosuppression, donor/recipient CMV serostatus.

References

1. Fischer SA. Is This Organ Donor Safe?: Donor-Derived Infections in Solid Organ Transplantation. Infectious disease clinics of North America. 2018;32(3):495–506.
2. Fishman JA. Infection in solid-organ transplant recipients. The New England journal of medicine. 2007;357(25):2601–14.
3. Bartoletti M, Giannella M, Tedeschi S, Viale P. Multidrug-Resistant Bacterial Infections in Solid Organ Transplant Candidates and Recipients. Infectious disease clinics of North America. 2018;32(3):551–580.
4. Fishman JA. Infection in Organ Transplantation. American journal of transplantation: official journal of the American Society of Transplantation and the American Society of Transplant Surgeons. 2017;17(4):856–879.
5. Patel G, Huprikar S. Infectious complications after orthotopic liver transplantation. Seminars in respiratory and critical care medicine. 2012;33(1):111–124.
6. Adamska Z, Karczewski M, Cichanska L, Wieckowska B, Malkiewicz T, Mahadea D, et al. Bacterial Infections in Renal Transplant Recipients. Transplantation proceedings. 2015;47(6):1808–1812.
7. Shendi AM, Wallis G, Painter H, Harber M, Collier S. Epidemiology and impact of bloodstream infections among kidney transplant recipients: A retrospective single-center experience. Transplant infectious disease: an official journal of the Transplantation Society. 2018;20(1). doi: 10.1111/tid.12815.
8. Miller LW, Naftel DC, Bourge RC, Kirklin JK, Brozena SC, Jarcho J, et al. Infection after heart transplantation: A multiinstitutional study. Cardiac Transplant Research Database Group. The Journal of heart and lung transplantation: the official publication of the International Society for Heart Transplantation. 1994;13(3):381–392; discussion 93.
9. Kotloff RM, Ahya VN. Medical complications of lung transplantation. The European respiratory journal. 2004;23(2):334–342.
10. van Veen KE, Brouwer MC, van der Ende A, van de Beek D. Bacterial meningitis in solid organ transplant recipients: A population-based prospective study. Transplant infectious disease: an official journal of the Transplantation Society. 2016;18(5):674–680. Epub 2016/07/08.

11. Coussement J, Lebeaux D, Rouzaud C, Lortholary O. Nocardia infections in solid organ and hematopoietic stem cell transplant recipients. Current opinion in infectious diseases. 2017;30(6):545–551.
12. Coussement J, Lebeaux D, van Delden C, Guillot H, Freund R, Marbus S, et al. Nocardia Infection in Solid Organ Transplant Recipients: A Multicenter European Case-control Study. Clinical infectious diseases: an official publication of the Infectious Diseases Society of America. 2016;63(3):338–345.
13. Lebeaux D, Freund R, van Delden C, Guillot H, Marbus SD, Matignon M, et al. Outcome and Treatment of Nocardiosis After Solid Organ Transplantation: New Insights From a European Study. Clinical infectious diseases: an official publication of the Infectious Diseases Society of America. 2017;64(10):1396–1405.
14. Hemmersbach-Miller M, Catania J, Saullo JL. Updates on Nocardia Skin and Soft Tissue Infections in Solid Organ Transplantation. Current infectious disease reports. 2019;21(8):27.
15. Laupland KB, Gregson DB, Flemons WW, Hawkins D, Ross T, Church DL. Burden of community-onset bloodstream infection: a population-based assessment. Epidemiology and infection. 2007;135(6):1037–1042.
16. Landrum ML, Neumann C, Cook C, Chukwuma U, Ellis MW, Hospenthal DR, et al. Epidemiology of Staphylococcus aureus blood and skin and soft tissue infections in the US military health system, 2005–2010. Jama. 2012;308(1):50–59.
17. de Kraker ME, Jarlier V, Monen JC, Heuer OE, van de Sande N, Grundmann H. The changing epidemiology of bacteraemias in Europe: trends from the European Antimicrobial Resistance Surveillance System. Clinical microbiology and infection: the official publication of the European Society of Clinical Microbiology and Infectious Diseases. 2013;19(9):860–868.
18. Bert F, Larroque B, Paugam-Burtz C, Janny S, Durand F, Dondero F, et al. Microbial epidemiology and outcome of bloodstream infections in liver transplant recipients: an analysis of 259 episodes. Liver transplantation: official publication of the American Association for the Study of Liver Diseases and the International Liver Transplantation Society. 2010;16(3):393–401.
19. Florescu DF, McCartney AM, Qiu F, Langnas AN, Botha J, Mercer DF, et al. Staphylococcus aureus infections after liver transplantation. Infection. 2012;40(3):263–269.
20. Shields RK, Clancy CJ, Minces LR, Kwak EJ, Silveira FP, Abdel Massih RC, et al. Staphylococcus aureus infections in the early period after lung transplantation: epidemiology, risk factors, and outcomes. The Journal of heart and lung transplantation: the official publication of the International Society for Heart Transplantation. 2012;31(11):1199–1206.
21. Singh N, Paterson DL, Chang FY, Gayowski T, Squier C, Wagener MM, et al. Methicillin-resistant Staphylococcus aureus: the other emerging resistant gram-positive coccus among liver transplant recipients. Clinical infectious diseases: an official publication of the Infectious Diseases Society of America. 2000;30(2):322–327.
22. Garzoni C, Vergidis P. Methicillin-resistant, vancomycin-intermediate and vancomycin-resistant Staphylococcus aureus infections in solid organ transplantation. American journal of transplantation: official journal of the American Society of Transplantation and the American Society of Transplant Surgeons. 2013;13 Suppl 4:50–58.

23. Bucheli E, Kralidis G, Boggian K, Cusini A, Garzoni C, Manuel O, et al. Impact of enterococcal colonization and infection in solid organ transplantation recipients from the Swiss transplant cohort study. Transplant infectious disease: an official journal of the Transplantation Society. 2014;16(1):26–36.
24. Bodro M, Sabe N, Tubau F, Llado L, Baliellas C, Roca J, et al. Risk factors and outcomes of bacteremia caused by drug-resistant ESKAPE pathogens in solid-organ transplant recipients. Transplantation. 2013;96(9):843–849.
25. Berenger BM, Doucette K, Smith SW. Epidemiology and risk factors for nosocomial bloodstream infections in solid organ transplants over a 10-year period. Transplant infectious disease: an official journal of the Transplantation Society. 2016;18(2):183–190.
26. Moreno A, Cervera C, Gavalda J, Rovira M, de la Camara R, Jarque I, et al. Bloodstream infections among transplant recipients: results of a nationwide surveillance in Spain. American journal of transplantation: official journal of the American Society of Transplantation and the American Society of Transplant Surgeons. 2007;7(11):2579–2586.
27. Russell DL, Flood A, Zaroda TE, Acosta C, Riley MM, Busuttil RW, et al. Outcomes of colonization with MRSA and VRE among liver transplant candidates and recipients. American journal of transplantation: official journal of the American Society of Transplantation and the American Society of Transplant Surgeons. 2008;8(8):1737–1743.
28. Newell KA, Millis JM, Arnow PM, Bruce DS, Woodle ES, Cronin DC, et al. Incidence and outcome of infection by vancomycin-resistant Enterococcus following orthotopic liver transplantation. Transplantation. 1998;65(3):439–442.
29. McNeil SA, Malani PN, Chenoweth CE, Fontana RJ, Magee JC, Punch JD, et al. Vancomycin-resistant enterococcal colonization and infection in liver transplant candidates and recipients: a prospective surveillance study. Clinical infectious diseases: an official publication of the Infectious Diseases Society of America. 2006;42(2):195–203.
30. Banach DB, Peaper DR, Fortune BE, Emre S, Dembry LM. The clinical and molecular epidemiology of pre-transplant vancomycin-resistant enterococci colonization among liver transplant recipients. Clinical transplantation. 2016;30(3):306–311.
31. Tandon P, Delisle A, Topal JE, Garcia-Tsao G. High prevalence of antibiotic-resistant bacterial infections among patients with cirrhosis at a US liver center. Clinical gastroenterology and hepatology: the official clinical practice journal of the American Gastroenterological Association. 2012;10(11):1291–1298.
32. Gearhart M, Martin J, Rudich S, Thomas M, Wetzel D, Solomkin J, et al. Consequences of vancomycin-resistant Enterococcus in liver transplant recipients: a matched control study. Clinical transplantation. 2005;19(6):711–716.
33. Orloff SL, Busch AM, Olyaei AJ, Corless CL, Benner KG, Flora KD, et al. Vancomycin-resistant Enterococcus in liver transplant patients. Am J Surg 1999;177(5):418–422.
34. Simon D, Fischer S, Grossman A, Downer C, Hota B, Heroux A, et al. Left ventricular assist device-related infection: treatment and outcome. Clinical infectious diseases: an official publication of the Infectious Diseases Society of America. 2005;40(8):1108–1115.

35. Oriol I, Sabe N, Simonetti AF, Llado L, Manonelles A, Gonzalez J, et al. Changing trends in the aetiology, treatment and outcomes of bloodstream infection occurring in the first year after solid organ transplantation: a single-centre prospective cohort study. Transplant international: official journal of the European Society for Organ Transplantation. 2017;30(9):903–913.
36. Aguiar EB, Maciel LC, Halpern M, de Lemos AS, Ferreira AL, Basto ST, et al. Outcome of bacteremia caused by extended-spectrum beta-lactamase-producing Enterobacteriaceae after solid organ transplantation. Transplantation proceedings. 2014;46(6):1753–1756.
37. Bui KT, Mehta S, Khuu TH, Ross D, Carlson M, Leibowitz MR, et al. Extended spectrum beta-lactamase-producing Enterobacteriaceae infection in heart and lung transplant recipients and in mechanical circulatory support recipients. Transplantation. 2014;97(5):590–594.
38. Bert F, Larroque B, Paugam-Burtz C, Dondero F, Durand F, Marcon E, et al. Pretransplant fecal carriage of extended-spectrum beta-lactamase-producing Enterobacteriaceae and infection after liver transplant, France. Emerging infectious diseases. 2012;18(6):908–916.
39. Espinar MJ, Miranda IM, Costa-de-Oliveira S, Rocha R, Rodrigues AG, Pina-Vaz C. Urinary Tract Infections in Kidney Transplant Patients Due to Escherichia coli and Klebsiella pneumoniae-Producing Extended-Spectrum beta-Lactamases: Risk Factors and Molecular Epidemiology. PloS one. 2015;10(8):e0134737.
40. Pilmis B, Scemla A, Join-Lambert O, Mamzer MF, Lortholary O, Legendre C, et al. ESBL-producing enterobacteriaceae-related urinary tract infections in kidney transplant recipients: incidence and risk factors for recurrence. Infect Dis (Lond). 2015;47(10):714–718.
41. Giannella M, Graziano E, Marconi L, Girometti N, Bartoletti M, Tedeschi S, et al. Risk factors for recurrent carbapenem resistant Klebsiella pneumoniae bloodstream infection: a prospective cohort study. European journal of clinical microbiology & infectious diseases: official publication of the European Society of Clinical Microbiology. 2017;36(10):1965–1970.
42. Shields RK, Nguyen MH, Chen L, Press EG, Potoski BA, Marini RV, et al. Ceftazidime-Avibactam Is Superior to Other Treatment Regimens against Carbapenem-Resistant Klebsiella pneumoniae Bacteremia. Antimicrobial agents and chemotherapy. 2017;61(8): e00883–17. doi: 10.1128/AAC.00883-17.
43. Lanini S, Costa AN, Puro V, Procaccio F, Grossi PA, Vespasiano F, et al. Incidence of carbapenem-resistant gram negatives in Italian transplant recipients: a nationwide surveillance study. PloS one. 2015;10(4):e0123706.
44. Giannella M, Bartoletti M, Morelli MC, Tedeschi S, Cristini F, Tumietto F, et al. Risk factors for infection with carbapenem-resistant Klebsiella pneumoniae after liver transplantation: the importance of pre- and posttransplant colonization. American journal of transplantation: official journal of the American Society of Transplantation and the American Society of Transplant Surgeons. 2015;15(6):1708–1715.
45. Cicora F, Mos F, Paz M, Allende NG, Roberti J. Infections with blaKPC-2-producing Klebsiella pneumoniae in renal transplant patients: a retrospective study. Transplantation proceedings. 2013;45(9):3389–3393.

46. Freire MP, Oshiro IC, Pierrotti LC, Bonazzi PR, de Oliveira LM, Song AT, et al. Carbapenem-Resistant Enterobacteriaceae Acquired Before Liver Transplantation: Impact on Recipient Outcomes. Transplantation. 2017;101(4):811–820.
47. Harris PN, Tambyah PA, Paterson DL. beta-lactam and beta-lactamase inhibitor combinations in the treatment of extended-spectrum beta-lactamase producing Enterobacteriaceae: time for a reappraisal in the era of few antibiotic options? The Lancet Infectious diseases. 2015;15(4):475–485.
48. Kalpoe JS, Sonnenberg E, Factor SH, del Rio Martin J, Schiano T, Patel G, et al. Mortality associated with carbapenem-resistant Klebsiella pneumoniae infections in liver transplant recipients. Liver transplantation: official publication of the American Association for the Study of Liver Diseases and the International Liver Transplantation Society. 2012;18(4):468–474.
49. Lubbert C, Becker-Rux D, Rodloff AC, Laudi S, Busch T, Bartels M, et al. Colonization of liver transplant recipients with KPC-producing Klebsiella pneumoniae is associated with high infection rates and excess mortality: a case-control analysis. Infection. 2014;42(2):309–316.
50. Bergamasco MD, Barroso Barbosa M, de Oliveira Garcia D, Cipullo R, Moreira JC, Baia C, et al. Infection with Klebsiella pneumoniae carbapenemase (KPC)-producing K. pneumoniae in solid organ transplantation. Transplant infectious disease: an official journal of the Transplantation Society. 2012;14(2):198–205.
51. Clancy CJ, Chen L, Shields RK, Zhao Y, Cheng S, Chavda KD, et al. Epidemiology and molecular characterization of bacteremia due to carbapenem-resistant Klebsiella pneumoniae in transplant recipients. American journal of transplantation: official journal of the American Society of Transplantation and the American Society of Transplant Surgeons. 2013;13(10):2619–2633.
52. Freire MP, Pierrotti LC, Oshiro IC, Bonazzi PR, Oliveira LM, Machado AS, et al. Carbapenem-resistant Acinetobacter baumannii acquired before liver transplantation: Impact on recipient outcomes. Liver transplantation: official publication of the American Association for the Study of Liver Diseases and the International Liver Transplantation Society. 2016;22(5):615–626.
53. Liu H, Ye Q, Wan Q, Zhou J. Predictors of mortality in solid-organ transplant recipients with infections caused by Acinetobacter baumannii. Therapeutics and clinical risk management. 2015;11:1251–1257.
54. Biderman P, Bugaevsky Y, Ben-Zvi H, Bishara J, Goldberg E. Multidrug-resistant Acinetobacter baumannii infections in lung transplant patients in the cardiothoracic intensive care unit. Clinical transplantation. 2015;29(9):756–762.
55. Husain S, Chan KM, Palmer SM, Hadjiliadis D, Humar A, McCurry KR, et al. Bacteremia in lung transplant recipients in the current era. American journal of transplantation: official journal of the American Society of Transplantation and the American Society of Transplant Surgeons. 2006;6(12):3000–3007.
56. Hadjiliadis D, Steele MP, Chaparro C, Singer LG, Waddell TK, Hutcheon MA, et al. Survival of lung transplant patients with cystic fibrosis harboring panresistant bacteria other than Burkholderia cepacia, compared with patients harboring sensitive bacteria. The Journal of heart and lung transplantation: the official publication of the International Society for Heart Transplantation. 2007;26(8):834–838.

57. Gregson AL, Wang X, Weigt SS, Palchevskiy V, Lynch JP, 3rd, Ross DJ, et al. Interaction between Pseudomonas and CXC chemokines increases risk of bronchiolitis obliterans syndrome and death in lung transplantation. American journal of respiratory and critical care medicine. 2013;187(5):518–526.
58. Linares L, Cervera C, Cofan F, Ricart MJ, Esforzado N, Torregrosa V, et al. Epidemiology and outcomes of multiple antibiotic-resistant bacterial infection in renal transplantation. Transplantation proceedings. 2007;39(7):2222–2224.
59. Johnson LE, D'Agata EM, Paterson DL, Clarke L, Qureshi ZA, Potoski BA, et al. Pseudomonas aeruginosa bacteremia over a 10-year period: multidrug resistance and outcomes in transplant recipients. Transplant infectious disease: an official journal of the Transplantation Society. 2009;11(3):227–234.
60. Bodro M, Sabe N, Tubau F, Llado L, Baliellas C, Gonzalez-Costello J, et al. Extensively drug-resistant Pseudomonas aeruginosa bacteremia in solid organ transplant recipients. Transplantation. 2015;99(3):616–622.
61. Humphries RM, Hindler JA, Wong-Beringer A, Miller SA. Activity of Ceftolozane-Tazobactam and Ceftazidime-Avibactam against Beta-Lactam-Resistant Pseudomonas aeruginosa Isolates. Antimicrobial agents and chemotherapy. 2017;61(12). :e01858-17. doi: 10.1128/AAC.01858-17.
62. Taimur S. Yeast Infections in Solid Organ Transplantation. Infectious disease clinics of North America. 2018;32(3):651–666.
63. Lemonovich TL. Mold Infections in Solid Organ Transplant Recipients. Infectious disease clinics of North America. 2018;32(3):687–701.
64. Hand J. Strategies for Antimicrobial Stewardship in Solid Organ Transplant Recipients. Infectious disease clinics of North America. 2018;32(3):535–550.
65. Singh N, Husain S. Aspergillosis in solid organ transplantation. American journal of transplantation: official journal of the American Society of Transplantation and the American Society of Transplant Surgeons. 2013;13 Suppl 4:228–241.
66. Husain S, Camargo JF. Invasive Aspergillosis in solid-organ transplant recipients: Guidelines from the American Society of Transplantation Infectious Diseases Community of Practice. Clinical transplantation. 2019:Sep;33(9):e13544. doi: 10.1111/ctr.13544.
67. Park BJ, Pappas PG, Wannemuehler KA, Alexander BD, Anaissie EJ, Andes DR, et al. Invasive non-Aspergillus mold infections in transplant recipients, United States, 2001-2006. Emerging infectious diseases. 2011;17(10):1855–1864.
68. Rammaert B, Puyade M, Cornely OA, Seidel D, Grossi P, Husain S, et al. Perspectives on Scedosporium species and Lomentospora prolificans in lung transplantation: Results of an international practice survey from ESCMID fungal infection study group and study group for infections in compromised hosts, and European Confederation of Medical Mycology. Transpl Infect Dis. 2019;21(5):e13141.
69. Nel JS, Bartelt LA, van Duin D, Lachiewicz AM. Endemic Mycoses in Solid Organ Transplant Recipients. Infectious disease clinics of North America. 2018;32(3):667–685.
70. Koval CE. Prevention and Treatment of Cytomegalovirus Infections in Solid Organ Transplant Recipients. Infectious disease clinics of North America. 2018;32(3):581–597.

71. Elfadawy N, Yamada M, Sarabu N. Management of BK Polyomavirus Infection in Kidney and Kidney-Pancreas Transplant Recipients: A Review Article. Infectious disease clinics of North America. 2018;32(3):599–613.
72. Tebano G, Geneve C, Tanaka S, Grall N, Atchade E, Augustin P, et al. Epidemiology and risk factors of multidrug-resistant bacteria in respiratory samples after lung transplantation. Transplant infectious disease: an official journal of the Transplantation Society. 2016;18(1):22–30.
73. Shi SH, Kong HS, Xu J, Zhang WJ, Jia CK, Wang WL, et al. Multidrug resistant gram-negative bacilli as predominant bacteremic pathogens in liver transplant recipients. Transplant infectious disease: an official journal of the Transplantation Society. 2009;11(5):405–412.
74. Dudau D, Camous J, Marchand S, Pilorge C, Rezaiguia-Delclaux S, Libert JM, et al. Incidence of nosocomial pneumonia and risk of recurrence after antimicrobial therapy in critically ill lung and heart-lung transplant patients. Clinical transplantation. 2014;28(1):27–36.
75. Zhong L, Men TY, Li H, Peng ZH, Gu Y, Ding X, et al. Multidrug-resistant gram-negative bacterial infections after liver transplantation - spectrum and risk factors. The Journal of infection. 2012;64(3):299–310.
76. Schneider CR, Buell JF, Gearhart M, Thomas M, Hanaway MJ, Rudich SM, et al. Methicillin-resistant Staphylococcus aureus infection in liver transplantation: a matched controlled study. Transplantation proceedings. 2005;37(2):1243–1244.
77. Hsu RB, Fang CT, Chang SC, Chou NK, Ko WJ, Wang SS, et al. Infectious complications after heart transplantation in Chinese recipients. American journal of transplantation: official journal of the American Society of Transplantation and the American Society of Transplant Surgeons. 2005;5(8):2011–2016.
78. Oliveira-Cunha M, Bowman V, di Benedetto G, Mitu-Pretorian MO, Armstrong S, Forgacs B, et al. Outcomes of methicillin-resistant Staphylococcus aureus infection after kidney and/or pancreas transplantation. Transplantation proceedings. 2013;45(6):2207–2210.
79. Gupta MR, Valentine VG, Walker JE, Jr., Lombard GA, LaPlace SG, Seoane L, et al. Clinical spectrum of gram-positive infections in lung transplantation. Transplant infectious disease: an official journal of the Transplantation Society. 2009;11(5):424–431.
80. Linares L, Cervera C, Cofan F, Lizaso D, Marco F, Ricart MJ, et al. Risk factors for infection with extended-spectrum and AmpC beta-lactamase-producing gram-negative rods in renal transplantation. American journal of transplantation: official journal of the American Society of Transplantation and the American Society of Transplant Surgeons. 2008;8(5):1000–1005.
81. Freire MP, Abdala E, Moura ML, de Paula FJ, Spadao F, Caiaffa-Filho HH, et al. Risk factors and outcome of infections with Klebsiella pneumoniae carbapenemase-producing K. pneumoniae in kidney transplant recipients. Infection. 2015;43(3):315–323.
82. Raviv Y, Shitrit D, Amital A, Fox B, Bakal I, Tauber R, et al. Multidrug-resistant Klebsiella pneumoniae acquisition in lung transplant recipients. Clinical transplantation. 2012;26(4):E388–E394.

62

Psychological support and rehabilitation after transplantation

Gabriella Biffa, Lucia Golfieri, Silvana Grandi, Nicola Girtler

'The thing is, we didn't open up,
wide open, to replace my heart,
but that this opening cannot be closed....
.... I am open closed.
There is in me an opening through which it passes
an incessant flow of strangeness.'

Jean-Luc-Nancy

Introduction

The organ transplantation differs from any other surgery due to the deep psychological implications induced by the replacement of the diseased part in the patient's body by 'a foreign part', belonging to another person; a part that must be integrated not only in the body but also in the body image.(1)

The transplant can be seen as a process consisting of several phases ranging from the diagnosis of organ failure, the evaluation for eligibility, and inclusion in waiting list, to transplantation and follow-up.

The phases of the transplant process are defined by psychological phases characterized by:

- uncertainty and fear of death
- concerns about the risks of intervention
- emotional ambivalence

- hope, trust, and risk awareness
- unrealistic illusions and expectations
- psychological distress for the long therapeutic and diagnostic process

Therefore, it is necessary to consider the transplant as a long and articulated process of adaptation involving the patient, the family, and the caring system.

Chronic illnesses are accompanied not only by somatic changes and functional limitations but also by emotional, cognitive, and social changes requiring a long adaptation process and coping skills.[(2)]

The transplantation can also be defined as a form of chronicity due to the need for lifelong care, ensuring a good quality of life until the psychophysical adaptation process is successful.

Depression and coping

The prognosis of organ transplantation can be influenced by social, psychological, and psychiatric factors. It has been reported that pre-transplant psychiatric and psychological variables such as treatment adherence, social support, and coping (defined as the attitude to invest own conscious effort to answer to some difficulty, in order to try to control, minimize or tolerate conflict and psychological distress), might influence the post-transplant morbidity and mortality of heart and bone marrow transplant recipients.[(3–5)]

In the context of organ transplantation, depression is surely the most studied mental disease. In the general population, depression (major depressive disorder or dysthymia) is not only a significant determinant of quality of life impairment[(6)] but also a relevant predictor of increased medical burden, health costs, and poor treatment adherence.[(7)]

Also depression and hopelessness, anxiety, aggression, hope can be considered as experiences of the gradual process of adaptation that needs various coping strategies. The internal adaptation process is accompanied by an increasing loss of autonomy, social roles (family and occupational), contacts, and activities. Furthermore, occupational and financial problems might cause existential worries. While in the waiting list, fear of death, inner conflicts, and the uncertainty of a timely transplantation are prevailing emotional stressors of the illness.[2]

Some patients experience problems accepting the new organ and suffer feelings of guilt towards the donor which, in turn, can increase psychological stress and non-adherence.[8]

In a clinical context, life-long immunosuppressant therapy represents the backbone of this medical therapy; hence, adherence is a key issue requiring particular attention. Moreover, inter-specialist cooperation is an essential therapeutic element in the transplantation surgery framework.[9]

Also, the transplant and intensive care unit experience may cause symptoms of post-traumatic stress disorder or reactivate pre-existing traumata.[10]

After transplantation, the psychosocial burden is usually less severe than during the preoperative period because the feeling of having survived is strong. Nevertheless, patients must still be regarded as chronically ill and have to demonstrate considerable coping skills. Transplant patients learn to adapt to their new situation, often by re-evaluating life goals and by focusing on more positive consequences, for example, personal growth.[11] An unsuccessful adaptation is associated with lower quality of life and psychiatric morbidity.[12–14] The most common psychological disorders among patients before and after transplantation are affective and anxiety disorders.[10,12]

The extent of the perceived psychosocial burden depends on personal and social resources defined as resilience factors, that is favourable coping skills, self-efficacy, sense of coherence, optimism, and social support.[15,11,16,17–21]. Furthermore, associations of psychosocial variables with medical outcome and even mortality in transplant patients could be demonstrated.[12,13,22–28]

According to the above, we can speak of post-transplant rehabilitation from the initial stages of this process, that is, the evaluation for the inclusion in the waiting list.

Psychological evaluation of transplant patient

The psychological evaluation of the patient should be able to represent the initiation of a treatment relationship which continues throughout the waiting period with the aim of identifying early factors of psychological vulnerability, protective factors such as patient and family resources, motivation and awareness and to prevent the onset of psychological discomfort and post-transplant psychopathology. Also the goal of a thorough psychological evaluation is to identify recipients with psychological stress, psychiatric disorder, or potential risk for medication non-adherence.[29]

Somatization and symptoms of the depressive anxious spectrum, when present, may improve during the first year after the transplant, but tend to get worse again after the first- and second-year post-surgery. In the early post-operative period, the patient can benefit from a 'new-life perception' effect. However, over the years, the consequences of uninterrupted medicalization, which consists particularly of the anti-rejection therapy, may lead to resurgence in the psychopathological framework.[30]

Psychological consultation can be helpful in all disease stages enabling patients to better cope with their extraordinarily stressful situation.[2] A need for psychological care was found in up to 50% of transplant patients.[31,32] In this regard of particular importance are educational and supportive therapy elements, cognitive-behavioural interventions including relaxation techniques.[33–35]

The basic requirement for establishing a reliable therapeutic relationship is the correctness, completeness, and neutrality of the information provided to the patient. These become necessary in order to be able to elaborate an informed decision on the clinical reality and the extent of the transplant, the probability of the risks and possible post-operative limitations and the alternative possibilities (e.g. dialysis, living transplant, etc.).

Psychological-clinical and/or psychiatric evaluation should include assessment of cognitive functions, psychiatric distress, addiction and abuse, personality profile, psycho-affective resources, coping strategies, and psychosocial support.

As a result of the diagnostic action, the treatment plan is defined, as a pathway of qualification and rehabilitation, and includes all activities aimed at promoting well-being, development and maintenance of individual health.

Psychological well-being of patient and family

Psychological well-being is understood as a state of balance between the person—with his needs and resources—and the demands of the environment in which he lives.

Dew and DiMartini[36] advise a multicomponent interventional approach focused on risk factor reduction and the enhancement of personal coping resources. However, interventional studies are still rare, and further research is necessary regarding the effectiveness of interventions in order to develop evidence-based therapy strategies.

It is important to remember that family members and/or caregivers are involved in the long transplant process and report psychological distress before and after transplantation.[37] Family counselling, and if necessary, psychotherapeutic support can help reduce psychological distress, thus also maintaining the valuable social support provided by caregiving family members of the transplant patient. In this context, the issue of possible conflicts due to changing family roles may also be addressed.[2]

Relationships between patients, family members, and medical staff can change throughout the transplant process because of the lengthy chronic disease and the transplant surgery, experienced as a ritual of death and rebirth of a new life.[38] Returning to physical activity, social relationships, and work after transplant surgery may also be associated with psychopathological distress.[39,40]

Psychosocial studies, in the framework of organ transplant, mostly focused on quality of life[41–44] report that the psychosocial factors contribute to the improvement,[45,46] of the coping strategies.[47] Very few studies took into consideration the possibility for the transplant patients to get some positive changes, rather than only negative consequences.[48]

Moreover psychological rehabilitation, including cognitive-functional rehabilitation, includes all those activities aimed at reintegration and recovery of skills or competencies that have undergone modification, deterioration, or loss or compensation, in cases where recovery is not possible.

A careful psychological-clinical follow-up finally allows monitoring the effective adherence to care, to activate any corrective actions, and to facilitate the rehabilitation process and social reintegration.

Integration to new body image

A large part of the adaptation process concerns the integration of the new body image; in fact, regaining bodily integrity is often complex because people have difficulty in accepting the new organ as part of the own body and not as a separate identity.[1]

In transplant recipients, body image can be influenced by several factors including underlying chronic organ disease[49–51] treatment received before transplantation,[52] many surgical interventions[53] or multiple effects of immunosuppressant medications.[54–56] So, the body image can alter the psychological status of the patients: negative body image in patients with chronic medical illness has been associated with anxiety, depression, and post-traumatic stress disorder (PTSD)-like symptoms.[57,58]

The process of psychic integration of the transplanted organ is often long and difficult but indispensable for the recovery of the unity of one's bodily image and for preserving the sense of personal identity.

Studies about psychological aspects of organ integration overlap often with descriptions of personality changes or of post-transplant psychosis. About fourteen studies describe the preoccupation with body image or organ integration using a psychoanalytic approach.[59] In a report about kidney recipients, the graft is interpreted as good/bad object in the line of Melanie Klein's theory; the organ is 'good', a promise for life, a motherly nurturing presence and 'bad'—carrying the recipient's hostile impulses, which are unacceptable to the patient.[60] Other authors consider that the role of the transplanted organ is of a transitional object, allowing an ongoing relationship with the donor as imagined by the recipient.[61]

An important goal of transplantation and a result of a good psychological rehabilitation is to enable patients return to work, and improving employment outcomes for transplant recipients can positively contribute to a patient's identity, self-esteem, and quality of life (QoL).[62] Detailed information on the working lives of transplanted patients is limited, mainly because employment after transplantation is generally considered among the QoL aspects evaluating social relationships. The return-to-work rates reported in the literature vary widely, moreover, from as low as 20% to as high as 80%.[63]

A very important area of post-transplant psychological adaptation is sexuality. Sexual dysfunction is highly prevalent among people with end-stage organ disease, with a strong impact on their QoL and a multifactorial pathogenesis, due to both disease-related and psychological factors.[1] Contributing factors to these sexual difficulties were fear of death during coitus, effects of medication on interest and ability to function, body-image concerns, depression, and uncertainty about the sexuality of the donor, and altered roles and responsibilities within the family.[64]

Special attention should be given to paediatric transplantation. Paediatric psychology and consultation-liaison child psychiatry have emerged as subspecialty fields in response to the psychosocial needs of children, adolescents, and young adults with medical conditions such as solid organ transplantation. Given the medical and psychosocial complexities of organ transplantation, including the crucial need for lifelong medication adherence, it is important that behavioural health providers develop a high level of clinical skill as well as necessary scientific knowledge specific to paediatric transplantation.[65]

Psychological interventions

It is important to underline that rehabilitation optics place the patient at the centre of his or her treatment path. The psychological intervention has to be fully integrated in a multidisciplinary clinical approach with the involvement of all the main professional figures of the transplant process (primarily surgeons, internists, and psychologists) collaborating, interchanging information and face together the main clinical events of the transplant process, from the pre-listing evaluation until the post-transplant period. Members of multidisciplinary team might perform joint visits and ward round to reinforce the clinical exchange. In fact, only a global intervention results to be effective as diagnostic and therapeutic tool.[66] The psychological support and care can be instruments for early diagnosis and quick treatment but also elements of empathy towards the entire clinical transplant team. The medical approach alone might favour the onset of negative psychological patient's reactions such as depression as a sign of somatization.[67] One of the main aims of the transplant psychologist should be the achievement of active coping strategy. As reported, coping can be defined as all abilities used to face stressful situations. Notably, the psychological concept of coping has been already applied in the field of transplant psychology. The assessment of coping strategies should be explored during the transplant process encouraging patients to use action-oriented methods and discourage the passive reactions that definitely can negatively impact the prognosis.[68,48]

Remarkably, multidisciplinary team and transplant psychologist should help patients to develop a positive attitude towards transplant process. In particular, transplant recipients should get a post-traumatic growth that represents a positive psychological change consequent to an adverse life experience. Notably, Pérez-San-Gregorio et al.[68] analysed the predictors of post-traumatic growth (assessed with Posttraumatic Growth Inventory) in liver transplant recipients demonstrating that active coping, instrumental support, emotional support, and acceptance, were associated to a major growth.

Conclusion

Transplant surely is a stressful event, but at the same time it can lead to major confidence in own capacities particularly regarding the management of difficulties. Organ transplantation can favour the aptitude to organize and plan the everyday activities and facilitate new adaptive strategies.[69]

Seeing the relationship between psychosocial patterns and clinical outcome, the multidisciplinary approach and the development of biopsychosocial model represent the only reasonable ways to obtain a global benefit for patients and put them at the centre of the care process, paying attention to a doctor-patient relationship of mutual trust.[70]

Highlights

- Organ transplantation is a dynamic process composed of phases requiring psychological adaptation.
- The prognosis of organ transplantation can be influenced by many social, psychological, and psychiatric factors.
- As a result of the diagnostic action, the treatment plan is defined as a pathway of qualification and rehabilitation, and includes all activities aimed at promoting well-being, development, and maintenance of individual health.
- A large part of the adaptation process concerns the integration of the new body image; regaining bodily integrity is often complex because

people have difficulty in accepting the new organ as part of their own body and not as a separate identity.

- It is important to underline that rehabilitation optics place the patient at the centre of his or her treatment path.
- The multidisciplinary approach and the development of biopsychosocial model represent the only reasonable ways to obtain a global benefit for patients and put them at the centre of the care process, paying attention to a doctor-patient relationship of mutual trust.

References

1. Burra P., De Bone M. quality of life after organ transplantation. Transpl Int. 2007 May;20(5):397–409. Review.
2. Schulz KH., Kroencke S. Psychosocial challenges before and after organ transplantation. Transplant Research and Risk Management 2015:7 45–48.
3. Sirri L, Potena L, Masetti M, Tossani E, Magelli C, Grandi S. Psychological predictors of mortality in heart transplanted patients: A prospective, 6-years follow-up study. Transplantation 2010; 89: 879–86.
4. Tschuschke V, Hertenstein B, Arnold R, Bunjes D, Denzinger R, Kaechele H. Associations between coping and survival time of adult leukemia patients receiving allogeneic bone marrow transplantation Results of a prospective study. J Psychosom Res 2001; 50: 277–85.
5. Dew MA, Roth LH, Thompson ME, Kormos RL, Griffith BP. Medical compliance and its predictors in the first year after heart transplantation. J Heart Lung Transplant 1996; 15: 631–45.
6. Pirkola S, Saarni S, Suvisaari J, Elovainio M, Partonen T, Aalto AM, Perälä J, et al. General health and quality of life measures in active, recent, and comorbid mental disorders: a population-based health 2000 study. Compr Psychiatry 2009; 50: 108–14.
7. Lavretsky H, Zheng L, Weiner MW, Mungas D, Reed B, Kramer JH, Jagust W, et al. Association of depressed mood and mortality in older adults with and without cognitive impairment in a prospective naturalistic study. Am J Psychiatr 2010; 167: 589–97.
8. Goetzmann L, Irani S, Moser KS, et al. Psychological processing of transplantation in lung recipients: a quantitative study of organ integration and the relationship to the donor. Br J Health Psychol. 2009; 14(pt 4):667–680.
9. De Bona M, Ponton P, Ermani M, Iemmolo RM, Feltrin A, Boccagni P et al. The impact of liver disease and medical complication on quality of life and psychological distress before and after liver transplantation. J Hepatol 2000; 33: 609–615.
10. DiMartini A, Crone C, Fireman M, Dew MA. Psychiatric aspects of organ transplantation in critical care. Crit Care Clin. 2008;24(4):949–981.
11. Goetzmann L, Lieberherr M, Krombholz L, et al. Subjektives Erleben nach einer Organtransplantation – eine qualitative Studie mit 120 Herz-, Lungen-,

Leber- und Nierenempfängern. [Subjective experiences following organ transplantation – a qualitative study of 120 heart, lung, liver, and kidney recipients]. Z Psychosom Med Psychother. 2010; 56(3):268–282. German.

12. Heinrich TW, Marcangelo M. Psychiatric issues in solid organ transplantation. Harv Rev Psychiatry. 2009;17(6):398–406.
13. Butt Z, Parikh ND, Skaro AI, Ladner D, Cella D. Quality of life, risk assessment, and safety research in liver transplantation: new frontiers in health services and outcomes research. Curr Opin Organ Transplant. 2012;17(3):241–247.
14. Goetzmann L, Ruegg L, Stamm M, et al. Psychosocial profiles after transplantation: a 24-month follow-up of heart, lung, liver, kidney and allogeneic bone-marrow patients. Transplantation. 2008; 86(5):662–668.
15. Grady KL, Wang E, White-Williams C, et al. Factors associated with stress and coping at 5 and 10 years after heart transplantation. J Heart Lung Transplant. 2013;32(4):437–446.
16. Dew MA, DiMartini AF, DeVito Dabbs AJ, et al. Onset and risk factors for anxiety and depression during the first 2 years after lung transplantation. Gen Hosp Psychiatry. 2012;34(2):127–138.
17. Goetzmann L, Klaghofer R, Wagner-Huber R, et al. Psychosocial vulnerability predicts psychosocial outcome after an organ transplant: results of a prospective study with lung, liver, and bone-marrow patients. J Psychosom Res. 2007;62(1):93–100.
18. Archonti C, D'Amelio R, Klein T, Schäfers HJ, Sybrecht GW, Wilkens H. Gesundheitsbezogene Lebensqualität und soziale Unterstützung bei Patienten auf der Warteliste und nach einer Lungentransplantation. [Physical quality of life and social support in patients on the waiting list and after a lung transplantation]. Psychother Psychosom Med Psychol. 2004;54(1):17–22. German.
19. Milaniak I, Wilczek-Rużyczka E, Przybyłowski P, Wierzbicki K, Siwińska J, Sadowski J. Psychological predictors (personal recourses) of quality of life for heart transplant recipients. Transplant Proc. 2014;46(8):2839–2843.
20. Weng LC, Dai YT, Huang HL, Chiang YJ. Self-efficacy, self-care behaviours and quality of life of kidney transplant recipients. J Adv Nurs. 2010;66(4):828–838.
21. White-Williams C, Grady KL, Myers S, et al. The relationships among satisfaction with social support, quality of life, and survival 5 to 10 years after heart transplantation. J Cardiovasc Nurs. 2013;28(5):407–416.
22. Chilcot J, Spencer BW, Maple H, Mamode N. Depression and kidney transplantation. Transplantation. 2014;97(7):717–721.
23. Corruble E, Barry C, Varescon I, Falissard B, Castaing D, Samuel D. Depressive symptoms predict long-term mortality after liver transplantation. J Psychosom Res. 2011;71(1):32–37.
24. Dew MA, Switzer GE, DiMartini AF, Matukaitis J, Fitzgerald MG, Kormos RL. Psychosocial assessments and outcomes in organ transplantation. Prog Transplant. 2000;10(4):239–259; quiz 260–261.
25. Psychosocial Outcomes Workgroup of the Nursing and Social Sciences Council of the International Society for Heart and Lung Transplantation; Cupples S, Dew MA, et al. Report of the Psychosocial Outcomes Workgroup of the Nursing and Social Sciences Council of the International Society for Heart and Lung Transplantation: present status of research on psychosocial outcomes in

cardiothoracic transplantation: review and recommendations for the field. J Heart Lung Transplant. 2006;25(6):716–725.

26. Rosenberger EM, Dew MA, Crone C, DiMartini AF. Psychiatric disorders as risk factors for adverse medical outcomes after solid organ transplantation. Curr Opin Organ Transplant. 2012;17(2):188–192.
27. Griva K, Davenport A, Newman SP. Health-related quality of life and long-term survival and graft failure in kidney transplantation: a 12-year follow-up study. Transplantation. 2013;95(5):740–749.
28. DiMartini A, Dew MA, Chaiffetz D, Fitzgerald MG, Devera ME, Fontes P. Early trajectories of depressive symptoms after liver transplantation for alcoholic liver disease predicts long-term survival. Am J Transplant. 2011;11(6):1287–1295.
29. Dieplinger G, Mokhaberi N, Wahba R, Peltzer S, Buchner D, Schlösser HA, Ditt V, von Borstel A, Bauerfeind U, Lange U, Arns W, Kurschat C, Stippel DL, Vitinius F. Correlation Between the Transplant Evaluation Rating Scale (TERS) and Medical Outcomes in Living-Donor Kidney Transplant Recipients: A Retrospective Analysis. Transplant Proc. 2018 Jun;50(5):1276–1280.
30. Telles-Correia D, Barbosa A, Mega I, Barroso E, Monteiro E. Psychiatric and Psychosocial predictors of medical outcome after liver transplantation: a prospective, single-center study. Transpl Proceed 2011; 43:155–157
31. Goetzmann L, Klaghofer R, Wagner-Huber R, et al. Psychosozialer Beratungsbedarf vor und nach einer Lungen-, Leber- oder allogenen Knochenmarkstransplantation – Ergebnisse einer prospektiven Studie. [Psychosocial need for counselling before and after a lung, liver or allogenic bone marrow transplant – results of a prospective study]. Z Psychosom Med Psychother. 2006;52(3):230–242. German.
32. Schulz KH, Ewers H, Rogiers X, Koch U. Bedarf und Inanspruchnahme psychosozialer Betreuung nach Lebertransplantation. [Need and utilization of psychosocial care after liver transplantation]. Psychother Psychosom Med Psychol. 2007;57(5):221–230. German.
33. Engle D. Psychosocial aspects of the organ transplant experience: what has been established and what we need for the future. J Clin Psychol. 2001;57(4):521–549.
34. Heilmann C, Kuijpers N, Beyersdorf F, et al. Supportive psychotherapy for patients with heart transplantation or ventricular assist devices. Eur J Cardiothorac Surg. 2011;39(4):e44–e50.
35. Köllner V, Archonti C. Psychotherapeutische Interventionen vor und nach Organtransplantation. [Psychotherapeutic interventions before and after organ transplantation]. Verhaltenstherapie. 2003;13(1):47–60. German.
36. Dew MA, DiMartini AF. Psychological disorders and distress after adult cardiothoracic transplantation. J Cardiovasc Nurs. 2005; 20(5 Suppl):S51–S66.
37. Rodrigue JR, Dimitri N, Reed A, Antonellis T, Hanto DW, Curry M. Quality of life and psychosocial functioning of spouse/partner caregivers before and after liver transplantation. Clin Transplant. 2011;25(2): 239–247.
38. Rauch JB, Kneen KK. Accepting the gift of life: heart transplantation recipients' post-operative adaptive tasks. Soc Work Health Care 1989; 14: 47.
39. Dew MA, Myaskovsky L, Switzer GE, DiMartini AF, Schulberg HC, Kormos RL. Profiles and predictors of the course of psychological distress across four years after heart transplantation. Psychol Med 2005; 35: 1215.

40. Muehrer RJ, Becker BN. Life after transplantation: new transitions in quality of life and psychological distress. Semin Dial 2005; 18: 124.
41. Tedeschi RG, Calhoun LG. Posttraumatic growth: conceptual foundations and empirical evidence. Psychological Inquiry 2004; 15
42. Sainz-Barriga, M., Baccarani, U., Scudeller, L., Risaliti, A., Toniutto, P. L., Costa, M. G., Ballestrieri, M., Adani, G. L., Lorenzin, D., Bresadola, V., Ramacciatto, G., & Bresadola, F. Quality-of-Life Assessment Before and After Liver Transplantation. Transplantation Proceedings 2005; 37: 2601–2604
43. Fredericks, E. M., Lopez, M. J., Magee, J. C., Shieck, V., & Opipari-Arrigan, L. Psychological Functioning, Non-adherence and Health Outcomes After Pediatric Liver Transplantation. American Journal of Transplantation 2007; 7: 1974–1983
44. Goetzmann L, Sarac N, Ambühl P, Boehler A, Irani S, Muellhaupt B, Noll G, Schleuniger M, Schwegler K, Buddeberg C, Klaghofer R. Psychological response and quality of life after transplantation: a comparion between heart, lung, liver and kidney recipients. Swiss Med Wkly. 2008; 23;138(33-34):477–83
45. Golfieri, L., Lauro, A., Tossani, E., Sirri, L., Venturoli, A., Dazzi, A., Zanfi, C., Zanello, M., Vetrone, G., Cucchetti, A., Ercolani, G., Vivarelli, M., Del Gaudio, M., Ravaioli, M., Cescon, M., Grazi, GL., Faenza, S., Grandi, S., Pinna, A. D.. Psychological adaptation and quality of life of adult intestinal transplant recipients: University of Bologna experience. Transplantation Proceeding 2010; 42: 42–44
46. Broersa, S., Kapteina, A. A., Le Cessieb, S., Fibbec, W., & Hengeveld. M. W. Psychological functioning and quality of life following bone marrow transplantation: A 3-year follow-up study. Journal of Psychosomatic Research 2000; 48:11–21
47. Grady, K. L., Naftel, D. C., Kobashigawa, J., Chait, J., Young, J. B., Pelegrin, D., Czerr, J., Heroux, A., Higgins, R., Rybarczyk, B., McLeod, M., White-Williams, C., & Kirklin, J. K.. Patterns and Predictors of Quality of Life at 5 to 10 Years After Heart Transplantation. The Journal of Heart and Lung Transplantation 2010; 26:535–543
48. Golfieri, L., Lauro, A., Tossani, E., Sirri, L., Dazzi, A., Zanfi, C., Vignudelli, A., Amaduzzi, A., Cucchetti, A., La Barba, G., Pezzoli, F., Ercolani, G., Vivarelli, M., Del Gaudio, M., Ravaioli, M., Cescon, M., Grazi, G. L., Grandi, S., Pinna, A. D. Coping strategies in intestinal transplantation. Transplantation Proceeding 2007; 39: 1992–1994
49. Galpin C. Body image in end-stage renal failure. Br J Nurs 1992; 1:21–23.
50. Furr LA, Wiggins O, Cunningham M, Vasilic D, Brown CS, Banis JC Jr, et al. Psychosocial implications of disfigurement and the future of human face transplantation. Plast Reconstr Surg 2007; 120:559–565.
51. Eshuis EJ, Polle SW, Slors JF, Hommes DW, Sprangers MAG, Gouma DJ, Bemelman WA. Long-term surgical recurrence, morbidity, quality of life, and body image of laparoscopic-assisted vs. open ileocolic resection for Crohn's disease: a comparative study. Dis Colon Rectum 2008; 51:858–867.
52. Morales LC, Castillo E. Lived experiences of adolescents in dialysis: Life with multiple loses [in Spanish]. Colombia Medica 2007; 4(Suppl 2):44–53.
53. Klop KWJ, Hussain F, Karatepe O, Kok NF, Ijzermans JN, Dor FJ. Incisional hernias after laparoscopic donor nephrectomy: a single center experience. Transplantation 2012; 94:188.
54. Buturovic Ponikvar J, Novljan G, Ponikvar R. Cosmetic side effects of immunosuppressive therapy in children and adolescents with renal grafts. Transplant Proc 2002; 34:3009–3011.

55. Cansick JC, Hulton SA. Lip hypertrophy secondary to cyclosporin treatment. Pediatr Nephrol 2003; 18:710–711.
56. Stiefel P, Malehsa D, Stru¨ ber M, Bara C, Haverich A, Kugler C. Gender specific symptom experiences in patients after heart transplantation. Thorac Cardiovasc Surg 2011; 59:MO15.
57. Hellgren EM, Lagergren P, Larsson AC, Schandl AR, Sackey PV. Body image and psychological outcome after severe skin and soft tissue infection requiring intensive care. Acta Anaesthesiol Scand 2013; 57:220–228.
58. Lichtenberger CM, Ginis KAM, MacKenzie CL,McCartney N. Body image and depressive symptoms as correlates of self-reported versus clinician-reporte physiologic function. J Cardiopul Rehab 2003; 23:53–59.
59. Zimbrean PC. Body image in transplant recipients and living organ donors. Curr Opin Organ Transplant. 2015 Apr;20(2):198–210.
60. Tabbane K, Ben Rejeb R, Ghodhbane T, Douki S. The body image of patients under hemodialysis or having had renal transplantation [in French]. Ann Med Psychol (Paris) 1989; 147:325–328.
61. Goetzmann L. 'Is it me, or isn't it?' Transplanted organs and their donors as transitional objects. Am J Psychoanal 2004; 64:279–289.
62. Callahan MB. Dollars and sense of successful rehabilitation. Prog Transplant 2005; 15: 331.
63. Slapak M. Sport and transplantation. Ann Transplant 2005; 10: 62.
64. Tabler JB, Frierson RL. Sexual concerns after heart transplantation. J Heart Transplant 1990; 9: 397.
65. Eaton C, Gutierrez-Colina AM, Fredericks EM, et al. Organ Transplantation. In: Roberts M, Steele RG, eds. Handbook of Pediatric Psychology, 5th edn. New York, NY: The Guilford Press; 2017:364-374.
66. Bunzel B, Laederach-Hofman K. Solid organ transplantation: are the predictors for posttransplant noncompliance? A literature overview. Transplantation 2000; 70: 711–6.
67. Santos GG, Gonçalves LC, Buzzo N, Mendes TA, Dias TP, da Silva RC, da Silva RF, et al. Quality of life, depression, and psychosocial characteristics of patients awaiting liver transplants. Transplant Proc 2012; 44: 2413–5.
68. Pérez-San-Gregorio MÁ, Martín-Rodríguez A, Borda-Mas M, Avargues-Navarro ML, Pérez-Bernal J, Gómez-Bravo MÁ. Coping Strategies in Liver Transplant Recipients and Caregivers According to Patient Posttraumatic Growth. Front Psychol 2017; 8: 18. doi: 10.3389/fpsyg.2017.00018.
69. Park CL, Lechner SC, Antoni MH, Santon AL. Medical illness and positive life change: can crisis lead to personal transformation? Washington DC: American Psychological Association 2009. https://doi.org/10.1037/11854-000.
70. De Geest S, Burkhalter H, Berben L, Bogert LJ, Denhaerynck K, Glass TR, Goetzmann L, et al. The Swiss Transplant Cohort Study's framework for assessing lifelong psychosocial factors in solid-organ transplants. Prog Transplant 2013; 23: 235–246.

SECTION 5.

ORGANIZATIONAL ASPECTS IN ORGAN DONATION

63

The role of donation and transplantation network

Massimo Cardillo, Francesco Procaccio, Letizia Lombardini, Paola Di Ciaccio, Alessandro Nanni Costa

Brief historical overview

Organ donation and transplantation is one of the most complex processes in modern medicine. In each country, activities depend as well on international standards as national laws and guidelines, but efficiency and quality of results are strictly linked with rapid and uniform exchange of information, shared rules, and controlled medical actions. Moreover, citizens need continuous, complete, and reliable information about deceased and living organ donation, transplant waiting list, and clinical criteria. Only a well-structured national network can achieve these targets.

Internationally, dedicated networks exist in single states (i.e. Spain, France, Croatia, Portugal, Italy, etc. in Europe), multi-state countries (i.e. in the United States) and multi-countries (i.e. Eurotransplant) with different aims, structures, and operative roles.[1]

In the US, the United Network for Organ Sharing (UNOS) is a private, non-profit organization that manages the nation's organ transplant system under contract with the federal government. The UNOS brings together hundreds of transplant and organ procurement professionals and thousands of volunteers.[2]

In Europe, Eurotransplant (ET) is a non-profit organization that facilitates patient-oriented allocation and cross-border exchange of deceased donor organs. The ET is active in donor hospitals, transplant centres, and tissue-typing laboratories across eight European countries and it is responsible for the allocation of donated organs.[3]

The Italian donation and transplantation network

A good example of dealing with the challenge of structuring a national donation and transplant network can be found in Italy, where a dedicated public national network was created in 1999 (following the Law 91/1999 and the previous experience of multiregional organizations) (Figure 63.1). The network is made of three levels: a National Transplant Center (CNT) headed by a general director appointed by the Health Minister and supported by a National Technical Transplant Council; 19 Regional Transplant Coordinating Centers; and the in-hospital procurement coordination units (mainly part-time intensivists and full-time intensive care unit (ICU) nurses) directed by an experienced physician depending from the hospital medical direction.[4]

All the donation centres (at least one organ donation has been performed in 222 hospitals in 2019), transplant departments, and different specialists including second opinion experts for oncological, legal, and infective problems (around 25% of potential donation after brain death (DBD) donors per year) participate in the network, their activities are supported by a dedicated information system (SIT), managed by the CNT.[5]

The dedicated information system gathers the declared will for consent or opposition to donation (if the potential donor has not had his/her will registered, the family is informed in ICU and can veto donation), all relevant donor data, wait-listed patients, and transplant outcomes, thus ensuring equity, traceability, transparency, safety, and quality (Table 63.1)

Coordination of organ donation

Since 1999, the Spanish model based on in-hospital transplant (procurement) coordinators and regional transplant coordination centres have been implemented in each hospital with ICU. In areas where acute patients are managed following the hub and spoke model, coordination teams have been tailored to the local donation potentiality, enhancing the strict cooperation between procurement coordinators and donation champions in ICUs.

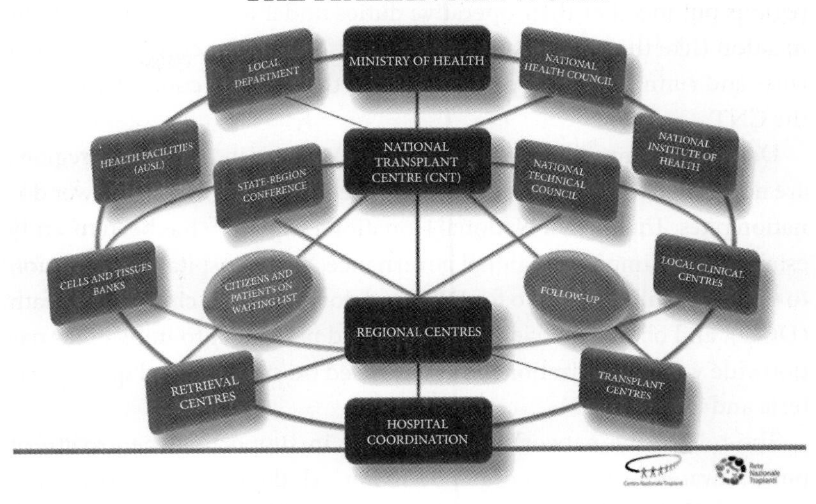

Figure 63.1. The Italian Donation and Transplantation Network

Table 63.1 Databases in the National Donation and Transplantation Information System

National Transplant Information System (SIT)

	DATA COLLECTED	REGISTRED BY
Declaration of will	*Statement of will signed by citizens (consent/opposition)*	Local health units, Municipality office, National donor association (AIDO)
Waiting list	*Enrollment in waiting list of Transplant Centres (regional based) and in National transplant programs*	Regional Tx Centers Operative National Coordination (CNTo)
Possible organ donors	*National Registry of deaths with acute cerebral injury in ICU*	Hospital coordinators Regional Coordination centers
Donation process *(cadaveric and living donors)*	• *All brain death declarations* • *Donor clinical data* • *Organs and tissues recovered from cadaveric donors* • *Organ and tissues recovered from living donors*	ICUs Regional Tx Centers Tissue banks
Severe organ dysfunction* *work in progress	*Registries of patients with severe organ dysfunction*	Treating clinical centers
Transplants	*All organ transplants performed in italy from cadaveric or living donors*	Regional Tx Centers
Follow-up of the recipient	*At least one follow-up per year for each transplant performed*	Transplant Centers

Regional centres perform donor evaluation and organ allocation in the region. To improve the efficiency of the coordination activities, some regions put together their operative duties under a multi-regional organization (like the North Italian Transplant Network) acting with shared rules and running quality programmes in the national context driven by the CNT.

Despite 28 per million population (pmp) donors in 2017, some regions are not adequately structured and organized, resulting in much lower donation rates. Thus, a new National Donation Program[6] has been recently established to improve regional governance, tailor hospital coordination to the new clinical scenario for DBD and donation after circulatory death (DCD), and obtain sufficient resources and personnel to implement nationwide valid organizational models based on standardized quality criteria and indicators.

The role of the network is also pivotal in supporting the growth of public awareness towards organ donation. All the different network actors, together with donor associations, should commit to make the general public aware of the importance of declaring its willingness to become an organ donor. In Italy, a devoted project in town council offices has allowed to collect 11 million donation living will statements, out of which 70% registered as organ donors.[7] This activity includes training of town council staff as well as communication events in schools and universities; carried out by a joint effort of regional transplant centres and patients' associations.

Another important field that can benefit from the setting up of a transplant network is the living donation and transplantation. On one hand, it can guarantee the identification of adequate shared protocols and support their proper application, and on the other, it can foster the development of more complex programmes, such as the crossover transplant, which requires the involvement of several transplant centres and can supply difficult-to-transplant patients with additional therapeutic opportunities. In this same framework, due to the existence of the Italian national transplant network, the chains of crossover couples have had the possibility to be triggered not only from samaritan donors, but also from cadaveric donors, thus giving a further option to these patients. Recently, a new plan for improving kidney transplantation programme from living donor has been developed: It foresees the appointment of a physician and a nurse inside nephrology departments located at hospitals devoid of transplant centre, who would be in charge of identifying potential compatible donors, before the end-stage kidney failure patient starts dialysis treatment. This devoted expertise would allow to offer the patient and his/her relatives a further therapeutical opportunity and organize the suitability assessment of donor-recipient couples to be referred to transplant centres.

Organ allocation and transplantation

Since 2014, the CNT has also implemented a new centralized operative coordination centre with the aim of running national programs (urgencies, paediatric, DCD, and split liver transplantations, international organ exchange, etc.) and cooperating with regional centres to offer organs not regionally allocated to every other centre nationwide, following defined algorithms for every different clinical situation and specific programme. The operative CNT is driven 24/7 hours by physicians and specialized nurses and is located, as the CNT office, inside the National Health Institute in Rome.(5)

The CNT also manages directly national programmes of critical subgroups of waitlisted patients and national re-allocation of suboptimal organs.

More than 8.500 patients are waitlisted in Italy and about 3500 transplants are performed yearly. Standard waiting lists are managed regionally but controlled by the CNT. Organ transplantation is performed in more than forty hospitals, (forty-one kidneys, twenty-two livers, eleven lungs, sixteen heart programmes) with sizable differences in the number of transplants per centre.(8)

Procured organs are first considered for national programmes run by CNT that utilize around 20% of total organs; the remaining organs are allocated in the region where the donation occurred based on the agreed national, shared criteria. When an organ cannot be used in the donor region, it is offered by the CNT to all the other Italian centres to minimize organ discarding. The median age of organ donors in Italy ranges from 60–65 years; and donors up to 99 years of age have been utilized for liver transplantation. The utilization of most recovered organs has been improved through nationwide organ reallocation; moreover, an intense exchange of organs based on international cooperation in Europe is routinely performed. In order to cope with remarkable variety in procurement rates and centre distribution, allocation criteria for kidney transplantation have been nationally agreed, whereas liver surgeons have developed an algorithm that takes into account the quick evolution of indications for transplant. Such criteria have been defined by the network professionals organized in the committees driven by the CNT.[9,10]

Last, but not least, the territorial morphology, the increasingly widespread use of ex-situ perfusion machines for DCDs or extended criteria donors, the necessity to improve packaging and transport procedures require an effective network of professional, safe, and traceable transport managers, that can be ensured by the different coordinating actors, namely local, regional, and national coordinating centres.

Over the last few years, referral of controlled DCDs has substantially increased and the number of regions and hospitals taking part in the programme has been steadily growing.

Safety and quality of organ donation and transplantation

As part of the network main activities, CNT and national committees issue guidelines and carry out a safety and quality surveillance activity, and safety of transplants has stood high on CNT agenda from the very start (Figure 63.2). The adopted strategies have allowed a safe use of many organs that would have been previously discarded, since changes in epidemiology and frequent donation in elderly patients requested a dedicated round-the-clock available organization, at national and regional level, to detect and evaluate potential donor-recipient transmittable diseases. This approach has been ensured through the development of steadily updated guidelines[11] and expert second opinion[12] when necessary. The operative CNT supports and coordinates the screening process and the correct dissemination of relevant data to the centres. This network effort is rewarded by making it possible to utilize organs with non-standard risk profiles (40% of total utilized organs in Italy).

Transplant programmes can only be run in public hospitals based on a formal authorization that is issued every two years by the regional authority upon fulfilment of CNT- and Health Ministry-defined criteria in terms of transplant volumes and outcomes.[5] All transplant activities and follow-up data of the Italian centres are published yearly and per centre on the CNT website. Additionally, ad hoc registries gathering data on severe organ dysfunctions are presently been set up.[8] They will be run by CNT, which will be able to monitor and measure the need for transplant and evaluate the criteria used for patient addition to waiting lists. Finally, special transplant programmes[13] and innovative strategies of organ preservation based on *ex situ* organ perfusion can be better supported, controlled, and audited within a structured network system with shared criteria and results. A dedicated national programme for new techniques of organ perfusion in DCD and DBD donation has been recently implemented, including an ad hoc dataset with all the clinical data and utilized organ outcomes.[14,15]

Education and research

National and regional educational programmes are promoted and coordinated by the CNT in cooperation with the regional centres; for specific issues a partnership with the scientific societies is realized and courses, workshops and simulations are centrally and regionally conducted. In particular, education is addressed to intensivists to improve deceased DBD and DCD[16] procedures and donor treatment, including the innovative techniques aimed to maximize the number and quality of transplantable organs.

Finally, the national network can promote and support multicentre clinical trials, suggest and fund strategic national research based on centres cooperation and synergy, including new methods for organ function preservation and experimental transplant programmes.

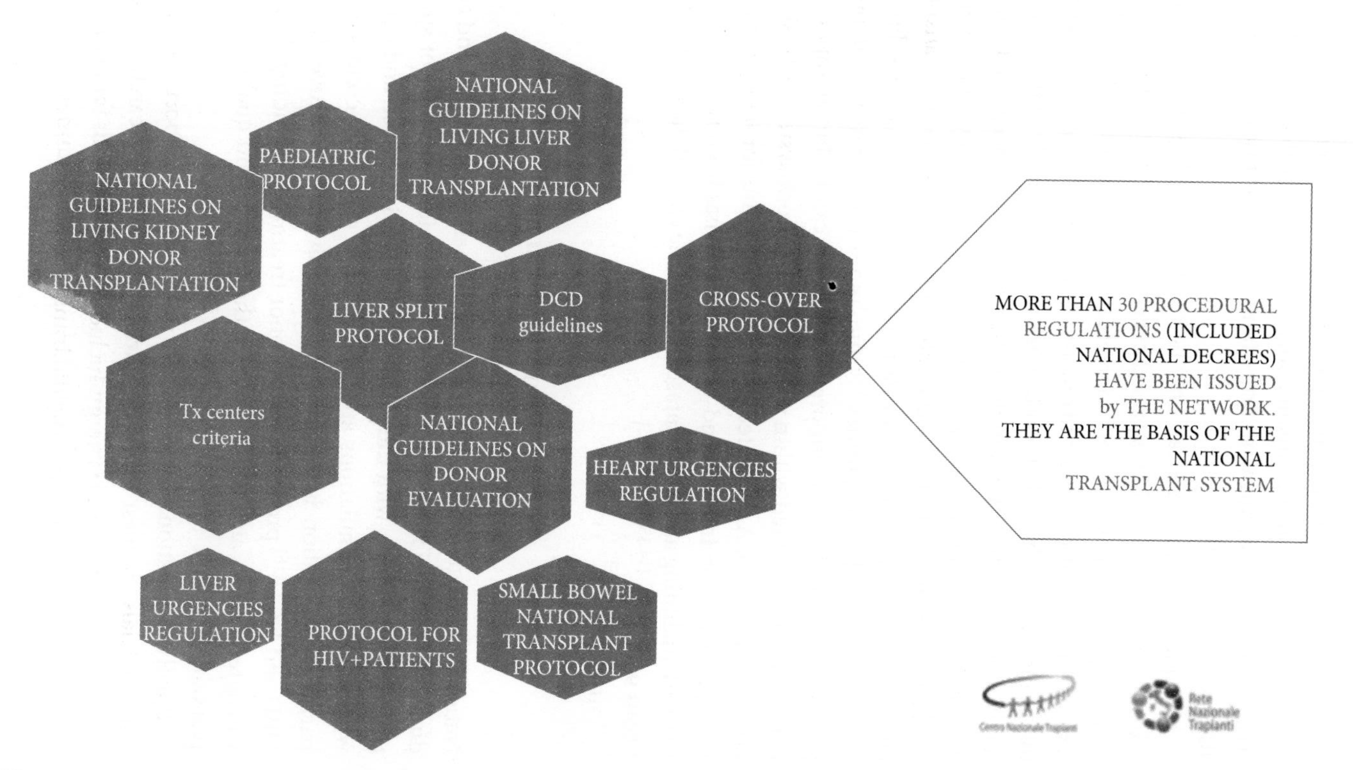

Figure 63.2. Protocols and guidelines in the National Network

The network value

The real value of the national network is represented by the continuous operative support to donation and transplantation activities, including shared judgement of suitability, checking of donation living will, organ recipient matching, and transport organization.

Coordination of personnel from different hospitals and services (more than 150–200 physicians and nurses, logistics, airports, etc.) is needed for the transplants from each donor.[17] All these activities occur with continuous interaction between the three levels of the network: national centre, regional, and hospital coordination.

The national network has a double function. One is the 24/7 clinical operative control of organ donation and organ allocation procedures with periodic auditing of results at hospital, regional, and national levels.[18,19,20] The other function is the definition, revision, and updating of guiding principles and clinical and organization guidelines within the national health system. In the future along, two pivotal organizational responsibilities will be defined. Firstly, each hospital director will be directly responsible for the efficiency of the donation activity under continuous support and control carried out by a local ad hoc hospital donation committee. Secondly, transplant activities will be driven under a single clinical director by regional programmes for different organs based on hub and spoke model, thus decreasing waiting lists as well as improving and harmonizing centres' capacities and skills. In this framework, transplant programmes should always be part of the pathways for patients with severe organ dysfunction, including diagnostic-therapeutic procedures before and after transplant and long-term follow-up.

The continuous monitoring and recording of all the relevant data in a single centralized informative system can also play a pivotal role. In Italy, this common collection of data on donation processes, waiting lists, living will statements from citizens, adverse events, and transplant outcomes (published yearly, by single centre, on Ministry of Health website) have spurred network's growth, while allowing improvement of national and regional clinical governance, policy-making and even triggering scientific collaborations. In the near future, the network will also benefit of the soon-to-be national registries on end-stage organ failure disease, which are presently being set up by CNT.

In a region-based healthcare system, like the Italian one, the transplant network has allowed defining and updating common standards, through the periodic meeting of working groups and transplant councils, but, admittedly the essential value of a dedicated national transplant network goes beyond the harmonization and coordination of clinical and operative experiences. Overall, it is a precious tool to foster innovative ideas and projects nationwide, to reach a consensus on several pivotal ethical aspects, to ensure a unique interface internationally and with policymakers, thus supporting the entire transplant system growth.

The Italian Transplant Network and COVID-19 pandemic

The Italian National Transplant Network has coped quite well with the impact of Covid-19 pandemic. From the beginning of the first wave, CNT has developed measures to safeguard donation and transplantation, setting up dedicated pathways for donor and patient evaluation[(21)]. In 2020 the number of transplants dropped by 10% as to previous year, less than in other European countries (Spain -18%, France -25%, United Kingdom -26%). Despite the pandemic, in Italy the first transplant of uterus was performed in 2020 and first transplant programme at global level from Covid-19 positive donors for patients in urgent, life-saving conditions was launched.[(22)] In this purview, twenty liver transplants and two heart transplants have been carried out so far, all of them successfully, with no disease transmission to recipients.

CNT has also set up a platform to monitor Covid-19 infections in waitlisted and transplanted patients, this has highlighted an increased frailty of transplanted patients versus the general population, as well as an increased infection risk for waitlisted patients.[(23)]

Eventually, transplanted patients were given a priority access during the Covid-19 vaccination campaign and, presently, more than 80% of transplanted patients have received two doses and about 50% the third dose.

Conclusions

Only a well-defined network of dedicated structures and professionals can support and lead, at high level of quality and safety, the complex activity of organ donation and transplantation in advanced health systems. This is a priority task in most of the countries where a huge number of patients crowd the waiting lists and may die before organs for transplantation are available. Different models of national or supra-national networks exist; during the author's twenty-year experience in Italy, the national public network defined by law and based on shared clinical, ethical, operative procedures has allowed to double the number of organ donors and transplants. Quality standards shared in the country continuously improve transplant results, test new criteria and methods, implement more effective rules and procedures for zeroing the waste of organs, and increasing the citizens' trust in a well-organized, homogeneous and controlled system, eventually facilitating new strategies and clinical research. An important target achieved by the national network is to ensure that thousands of citizens can benefit from this precious, unfortunately limited, life-saving resource. The ethical principles of accessibility and transparency are always fulfilled in every donation and transplantation activity in the country, finally maximizing the beneficial effects of transplants.

Highlights

- Organ donation and transplantation process needs attentive governance.
- Dedicated networks are national competent authorities, supra-national/supra-state organizations.
- Hub and spoke model brings together local, regional, and national actors and stakeholders.
- A network can foster harmonization of clinical and organizational activities, safety and quality, education, and research.
- A network can maximize the results of donation and transplantation activities at national and international levels.

References

1. European Commission. 'HUMAN ORGAN TRANSPLANTATION IN EUROPE: AN OVERVIEW' 2003. Available at: https://ec.europa.eu/health/ph_threats/human_substance/documents/organ_survey.pdf Accessed October 2020

2. UNOS website. Available at: https://unos.org/about/ Accessed: July 2019
3. EUROTRANSPLANT website. Available at: https://www.eurotransplant.org Accessed: November 2021
4. Nanni Costa A, Lombardini L. Storani D, CNT working group. Organ procurement and transplantation in Italy. Transplantation 2019; 103: 1065–1069.
5. Law April 1 1999 n.99 'Rules for organ and tissue procurement and transplantation'. 1999. Available at: http://www.parlamento.it/parlam/leggi/99091l.htm. Accessed: October 2020
6. AA. Piano nazionale donazione 2018 -2020 (Editoriale). Trapianti 2017;21:80–94.
7. Italian Health Ministry. Guidelines for registering organ donation will of statement on ID paper. Available at: https://www.interno.gov.it/sites/default/files/allegati/linee_guida_donazione_organi.pdf Accessed: October 2020.
8. Italian Health Ministry, National Transplant Centre. Italian data. Available at: http://www.trapianti.salute.gov.it/trapianti/archivioDatiCnt.jsp. Accessed: October 2020.
9. Cillo U, Burra P, Mazzaferro V, Belli L, Pinna AD, Spada M, Nanni Costa A, Toniutto P; I-BELT (Italian Board of Experts in the Field of Liver Transplantation). A Multistep, Consensus-Based Approach to Organ Allocation in Liver Transplantation: Toward a Blended Principle Model. Am J Transplant. 2015 Oct;15(10):2552–2561.
10. Amoroso A, Magistroni P, Biancone L. Long-Term Outcomes and Discard Rate of Kidneys by Decade of Extended Criteria Donor Age. Clin J Am Soc Nephrol. 2017 Feb 7;12(2):323–331. Epub 2016 Dec 15.
11. AA. Protocollo per la valutazione di idoneità del donatore di organi solidi. Available at: https://www.trapiantipiemonte.it/pdf/Linee/ProtocolloIdoneitaDonatore_dic2017.pdf Accessed November 2021
12. Nanni Costa A, Grossi P, Gianelli Castiglione A, Grigioni WF. Quality and safety in the Italian donor evaluation process. Transplantation 2008; 85:S52–S56.
13. Dello Strologo L, Murer L, Guzzo I, Morolli F, Pipicelli AM, Benetti E, Longo G, Testa S, Ricci A, Ginevri F, Ghio L, Cardillo M, Piazza A, Nanni Costa A. Renal transplantation in sensitized children and young adults: A nationwide approach. Nephrol Dial Transplant. 2017 Jan 1;32(1):191–195.
14. National Transplant Centre. National Program. 'Organ perfusion techniques in transplant activities' Available at:. https://www.trapianti.salute.gov.it/trapianti/dettaglioComunicatiNotizieCnt.jsp?lingua=italiano&area=cnt&menu=media&sottomenu=news&id=590 Accessed: November 2021
15. De Carlis R, Schlegel A, Frassoni S, Olivieri T, Ravaioli M, Camagni S, Patrono D, Bassi D, Pagano D, Di Sandro S, Lauterio A, Bagnardi V, Gruttadauria S, Cillo U, Romagnoli R, Colledan M, Cescon M, Di Benedetto F, Muiesan P, De Carlis L. How to preserve liver grafts from circulatory death with long warm ischemia? A retrospective Italian cohort study with Normothermic Regional Perfusion and Hypothermic Oxygenated Perfusion. Transplantation. 2021 Nov 1;105(11):2385–2396.
16. Nanni Costa A, Procaccio F. Organ donation after neurological or circulatory death? Two is better than one. Minerva Anestesiol 2018;84:1337–1339.
17. AA.VV.Transplant Coordination Manual, University of Barcelona, 2015.

18. Cannavò A, Passamonti SM, Vincenti D, Aurelio MT, Torelli R, Poli F, Piccolo G, Cardillo M; North Italy Transplant program. Quality of Life Before and After Transplantation in Solid Organ Recipients Referred to the North Italy Transplant program (NITp): A Cross-sectional Study. Transplant Proc. 2019;Jul 10.pii:S0041-1345(18)313812.
19. Gagliotti C, Morsillo F, Moro ML, Masiero L, Procaccio F, Vespasiano F, Pantosti A, Monaco M, Errico G, Ricci A, Grossi P, Nanni Costa A; SInT Collaborative Study Group. Infections in liver and lung transplant recipients: a national prospective cohort. Eur J Clin Microbiol Infect Dis. 2018;37:399–407. Epub 2018 Jan 29.
20. Eccher A, Lombardini L, Girolami I, Puoti F, Zaza G, Gambaro G, Carraro A, Valotto G, Cima L, Novelli L, Neil D, Montin U, Scarpa A, Brunelli M, Nanni Costa A, D'Errico A. How safe are organs from deceased donors with neoplasia? The results of the Italian Transplantation Network. J Nephrol 2019;32:323–330. Epub 2019 Jan 2.
21. Vistoli F, Furian L, Maggiore U, Caldara R, Cantaluppi V, Ferraresso M, Zaza G, Cardillo M, Biancofiore G, Menichetti F, Russo A, Turillazzi E, Di Paolo M, Grandaliano G, Boggi U; Italian National Kidney Transplantation Network; the Joint Committee of the Italian Society of Organ Transplantation and the Italian Society of Nephrology. COVID-19 and kidney transplantation: an Italian Survey and Consensus. J Nephrol. 2020 Aug;33(4):667–680. Epub 2020 Jun 3.
22. Romagnoli R, Gruttadauria S, Tisone G, Maria Ettorre G, De Carlis L, Martini S, Tandoi F, Trapani S, Saracco M, Luca A, Manzia TM, Visco Comandini U, De Carlis R, Ghisetti V, Cavallo R, Cardillo M, Grossi PA. Liver transplantation from active COVID-19 donors: A lifesaving opportunity worth grasping? Am J Transplant. 2021;21(12):3919–3925. doi: 10.1111/ajt.16823.
23. Trapani S, Masiero L, Puoti F, Rota MC, Del Manso M, Lombardini L, Riccardo F, Amoroso A, Pezzotti P, Grossi PA, Brusaferro S, Cardillo M; Italian Network of Regional Transplant Coordinating Centers Collaborating group; Italian Surveillance System of Covid-19, Italian Society for Organ Transplantation (SITO), The Italian Board of Experts in Liver Transplantation (I-BELT) Study Group, Italian Association for the Study of the Liver (AISF), Italian Society of Nephrology (SIN), SIN-SITO Study Group. Incidence and outcome of SARS-CoV-2 infection on solid organ transplantation recipients: A nationwide population-based study. Am J Transplant. 2021 Jul;21(7):2509–2252. Epub 2021 Jan 20.

64

The role of the transplant coordinator

María Paula Gómez, Ricard Valero Castell, Marti Manyalich Vidal, Ramon Adalia Bartolomé

Introduction

The success of a transplant programme lies in the professionalization of the donation process and in the setting up of well-defined responsibilities for all the professionals involved in the deceased organ donation pathway. The Pittsburg Syndrome clearly describes the issue when specialists go abroad to receive training. They learn transplant techniques, but discover, on returning to their own countries that their centres cannot put all this into practice, or have a low level of activity, due to the lack of organs.[1]

Without an organ donor there is no transplant. The current problems are the lack of organs to meet the growing demand, greater transplant indications, and increasingly lengthy waiting lists. Implementing strategies to reduce the lack of organs available for transplant is perhaps one of the priorities for the transplant authorities and transplant centres.

In 1985, the first Spanish Transplant Coordination team was created in Hospital Clinic de Barcelona. This progressed to become a medical speciality, necessary for the development and growth of organ and tissue transplant programmes in the hospital. This model gradually spread to other centres, regions, and countries with the creation of a Transplant Coordination Department or hospital-based Organ Procurement Unit (H-OPU). The role of the transplant coordinator or Transplant Procurement Management coordinator (TPM coordinator) proved to increase the activity of organ and tissue transplant programmes.[2,3,4]

The TPM coordinator is a clinical specialist and manager in charge of transforming the greatest possible number of deceased patients, in any centre, region, or country, into real donors and channelling the distribution of organs and tissues to the most suitable recipient in accordance with the existing distribution rules. The TPM coordinator's mission is to obtain and distribute organs and tissues for transplantation.[1]

Well-known best practices in organ donation leading to increase the deceased organ donation refer to the positive impact of having healthcare professionals specialized in organ donation ideally belonging to a hospital.[5,6] A successful transplant model consists of a network of TPM coordinators placed on the H-OPU.

This chapter aims at describing the profile and main functions of the TPM coordinator, not only as a healthcare professional specialized in organ donation, but also as a manager of a hospital service with the main purpose of obtaining the highest number of quality organs for transplant.

Functions of the TPM coordinator

The TPM coordinators' responsibilities comprise clinical and nonclinical duties essential for the success of the donation process. Clinical duties are directly related to converting deceased patients into donors for transplant recipients. The clinical duties also extend to living donation, where the main focus is on protecting the donor's rights.

The non-clinical duties involve training hospital staff, managing staff affiliated to the H-OPU, collaborating with research to improve organ, tissue and cell donation, organ and tissue biovigilance, and developing and implementing quality assurance programmes.

Both sets of duties have, as their purpose, the recruitment of as many donors as possible, followed by the fair distribution of procured organs and tissues to the most appropriate recipients.

Clinical duties

The TPM coordinator must analyse all the possibilities for facilitating transplants and coordinate all the aspects that make it possible. The coordinator works around all types of donors including brain death (DBD), circulatory death (DCD), and living donors (Figure 64.1). They detect possible donors and monitor them for evolution to brain

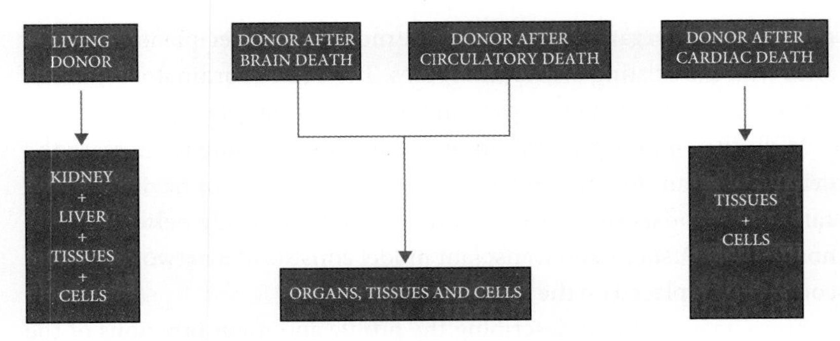

Figure 64.1. Types of Donors

Box 64.1 TPM coordinator's clinical tasks

1. Early detection, referral, and assessment of possible donors
2. Facilitating the diagnosis of brain death
3. Donor management, organ, and tissue viability studies
4. Family Interview for organ donation
5. Organizing the recovery and distribution of organs and tissues
6. Supporting living donor process
7. Konwledge about perfusion techniques after circulatory death
8. Knowledge about Organ Preservation Techniques

death or circulatory arrest (for obtaining organs, and also tissues). The TPM coordinator will also convert cardiac death patients into multi-tissue donors.

The fundamental clinical duties carried out by the TPM coordinator for donor procurement are listed in Box 64.1.

Early detection, referral, and assessment of possible donors

The TPM coordinator knows the donation potentiality of the area of activity and ways to maximize that potentiality. Also, the TPM coordinator is responsible for early and proactive identification and referral of possible donors through daily visits to the main target hospital areas for donors. When there is an electronical medical record system implemented in the hospital, the TPM coordinator performs a daily review of the ICU patients' admissions. Other target unit for donor detection is the emergency rooms; in Spain more than 50% of the possible donors are detected in emergency areas.[7] The TPM coordinator should liaise with emergency unit´s staff in order to avoid losing potential donors. Finally, the evaluation and assessment of the donor to confirm the donor suitability will be an essential duty of the coordinator in order to ensure that no disease is transmitted from the donor to recipient.

Facilitating the diagnosis of death

The TPM coordinator should facilitate death diagnosis by improving knowledge of this in the setting and making the necessary resources available to diagnose brain death at any time and in most likely of places (ICU, Reanimation, Emergency Room, etc.). Also, they could initiate donation manoeuvres in donors after circulatory death once the patient death has been confirmed, initiating perfusion techniques and the preservation of organs and tissues.[8]

Donor management, organ, and tissue viability studies

The TPM coordinator should participate actively in all the donor management aspects, with emphasis on organ and tissue suitability studies in order to take decisions on organ and tissue transplantation viability. Furthermore, the TPM coordinator should work actively to maintain good tissue perfusion and facilitate the necessary treatment and studies to ensure good organ functionality for transplantation and to decide upon clinical use and limitations.[8]

Family interview for organ donation

The TPM coordinator should inform the donor's family about the donation possibility. Donor family care and donation interview are perhaps some of the most important roles of the coordinator; training and experience will be essential to do so. According to the legislative model, opt-in or opt-out, the family should provide authorization and consent for donation. Furthermore, all the necessary administrative and legal steps must be taken, including legal authorization.

Organizing the recovery and distribution of organs and tissues

The TPM coordinator should organize multiorgan and tissue recovery as well as coordinate the necessary and existing resources for surgical procedures, operating room, anaesthesia, nursing wards, surgical teams, etc., and subsequent distribution and transport to the destination.

Supporting living donor process

TPM coordinators work independently from the transplantation teams to manage, evaluate, and record the details of living donation procedures to meet ethical requirements, notably the transparency and legality of the donation. The voluntary nature of living donation must be verified, and it is the TPM coordinator who is finally responsible for protecting the individual from possible coercion. The coordinator speaks to the possible living donors, disclosing all relevant information in a way they can understand, assesses the possibility of socioeconomic vulnerability, and verifies the relationship between donor and recipient. Euro Living Donor (EULID), Euro Living Donor Psychological Follow-up (ELIPSY), and Living Donor Observatory (LIDOBS) are European projects recommending the creation of living donor registries to monitor the psychological and social status and quality of life after donation.[9]

Perfusion techniques after circulatory death

The TPM coordinator should know to reverse ischemic damage after circulatory death, through normothermic regional perfusion. The coordinator must restore organ and tissue metabolism by means of perfusion and other organ preservation techniques.

Non-clinical duties

All the other tasks developed by the TPM coordinator related to the clinical duties will enhance the outcomes of the donation process. Non-clinical task will require specific resources and different skills related to management and communication that the TPM coordinator should account for.

Training and education

Training and education must be of great concern to the TPM coordinator. Fundamentally, they should educate all healthcare professionals and hospital staff (physicians, nurses, auxiliary staff, social workers, hospital administrative workers, etc.) and in particular those working in intensive care and emergency units, neurosurgery, neurology departments, and operating theatres about organ donation and transplantation. Sometimes professionals from transplant units are also in need of education about the organ donation process. A positive attitude towards donation and depth of knowledge among the hospital staff has been associated with a good deceased donation rate.(10)

A European experience in healthcare professional training for organ donation was implemented in the framework of ETPOD Project (European Training Program in Organ Donation) from 2007 to 2009. During this period, seventeen European countries selected a Target Area and performed, among other actions, short EOD (Essentials in Organ Donations) seminars within the hospitals addressed to healthcare professionals. The result of these actions was a 27% increase in the organ donation rates.(11)

The TPM coordinator should also organize educational sessions addressed to the community in collaboration with all the sectors and groups in the society that are in a position to spread knowledge, including opinion and religious leaders. Finally, the TPM coordinator could develop training programmes to assist in the training of other future coordinators.(12)

Research and hospital development

The aim of the research and hospital development of a TPM coordinator is to increase the number and quality of organs and tissues for transplant, along with maximizing the donation potentiality.(13) Potential areas of research in the donation side include the assessment of the donation potentiality, working on the use of expanded criteria donors, donors after circulatory death (DCD) and hepatic and cardiac domino donors among others. Research opportunities from the transplant side comprise ischemia-reperfusion, cardiac transplant from DCD,(14) double renal transplants, partial hepatic transplants from living donors, and combined transplants from different organs or adult-paediatric transplants. The

TPM coordinator shall lead or participate together with other hospital units in research projects that contribute to evolve the organ donation and transplant science.

Tissue and cells transplantation is another area where the TPM coordinator could contribute from the research point of view. Cell viability and transplantation, bioengineering, cryobiology programmes, pancreatic islets, and hepatocyte islets for implants or hepatic bioreactors and vascular tissue for culture could be assisted by the TPM coordinator to generate tissues for research.[15]

Hospital development refers to the actions to build the whole hospital culture in organ donation. The promotion of the concept of organ donation within the hospital is essential to increase the organ donation rates. A systematic approach to create alliances with the hospital staff, ensuring that each possible donor is identified and evaluated, and maximizing conversion rate will ensure the sustainability of the donation and transplant program. Large university hospitals should assist small hospitals in their area of influence in developing the whole organ donation hospital culture.

Organ and tissue biovigilance

Organ and tissues recovered for transplant have the risk related to the transmission of infectious diseases, and further side-effects. Biovigilance system application is a basic requirement for ensuring the quality and safety of organs and tissues intended for transplantation or human use. The TPM Coordinator is responsible for the biovigilance of the organs and tissues recovered in the hospital. It is mandatory to guarantee the safeness of the organs and tissues, and the absence or low risk of disease transmission. Furthermore, in case of any donor-recipient disease transmission, the TPM coordinator should lead the investigation process and the subsequent notification to regulatory offices.

Hospital-based organ procurement unit management

The resource management for the H-OPU and the administrative actions in the donation procedures are another TPM coordinator's responsibility. They should know the requirement of resources for their mission and means to obtain them. The TPM coordinator should analyse all the resources that are necessary to generate a donor, organ, and tissue and determines the costs as well as negotiating the funding.[16]

The H-OPU is a health care service like any other department in a hospital. It is supported by the hospital's infrastructure and has its own budget and resources to perform its assigned tasks. The H-OPUs should have annual plans that define their objectives, should be managed independently from other hospital departments such as ICUs or transplant teams and their budgets should not take into consideration transplantation costs. The manager of an H-OPU is a TPM coordinator who reports directly to the hospital's medical director concerning the team's activities, thereby, circumventing influence from individual transplant teams. The H-OPU management involves registering and analysing data on recruitment and procurement procedures as well as budgeting. In the calculation of the H-OPU's annual budget for organ and tissue donation, it is important to detail the cost of recruiting different organs as well as the costs generated by circulatory-death donors versus brain-death donors, tissue donation and living donation.

Each donation type should have its own cost accounting and hospital reimbursement process. Understanding the management and financial components of the organ donation for transplant process is essential to guarantee the sustainability of the process itself.

Quality assurance in organ donation

The TPM coordinator should always strive for establishing all the necessary mechanisms to guarantee quality in all the phases of the donation and transplantation process. To this end, the TPM coordinator should establish appropriate Standard Operating Procedures, develop a registry of all the activities performed, keep a complete clinical donor record including all required documents and legal procedures, if necessary, and follow up all donor viability studies and laboratory or histological results that could affect the quality of the organ and/or tissue transplanted.

It would be advisable to establish and implement some of the internationally recognized Quality Control Systems for all processes and obtain a quality accreditation for the H-OPU through national and international officially approved societies, organizations, or universities. The Organ Donation European Quality System (ODEQUS) project, developed in Europe from 2011 to 2013, provides a good set of quality criteria, quality indicators, and auditing methodology to help H-OPUs improve their practices.[17]

TPM Coordinator profile

The Organ donation for transplantation is a hospital process with human resources attached to this process; the TPM coordinator is the responsible for the donation duties. The TPM coordinator is a healthcare professional specialized in critical care. In Spain about 80% of TPM coordinators are physicians and 20% nurses. Of the physicians, 80% worked in an ICU or anaesthesiology unit, and the remaining 20% are nephrologists, surgeons, or non-specialists.[1]

The TPM coordinator should have good communication and negotiation skills that help to liaise with other healthcare professionals. The coordinator should be accepted and recognized in the hospital environment and be supported by the medical board. They must also have financial expertise and planning and negotiating skills.

Organ donation process is a teamwork that requires the participation of professionals with different backgrounds. Different professionals could assist the TPM coordinator such as social workers, biologists, or technicians. These professionals will be fundamental for donor family support and follow up, donor recovery logistics, organ distribution arrangements, and other administrative tasks related with the donation process.

The TPM coordinator must be a personnel hired by the hospital, hierarchically reporting to the Medical Director to maintain their independence from the hospital's other departments or units, and placed inside the hospital at the H-OPU next to the donor generating areas such as intensive care and emergency units. This is the case in Spain and some of the donation models in Europe. The in-hospital coordinator figure has proved to have a positive impact in the donation rates.[3,6]

In other models, the coordinators depend on out of hospital organizations rendering integration difficult and costlier. The American model for organ donation account with Organ Procurement Organizations (OPO), where the personnel, most of them being nurses, have a specialized role. Donor detection and referral will be managed by a donation technician; specialists in family authorization will be exclusively dedicated to supporting the family and obtaining donation authorization. An advanced practice coordinator with expertise in critical care and some invasive procedures will be responsible for the donor maintenance. Each step of the donation process will have a technician responsible for it and reports to their OPO.[18]

The TPM coordinator is a specialized job like any other within the hospital; the payment system for coordinators must be mixed, with a fixed part for a day's work, equivalent to other specialists of the centre, and a variable part according to the activity. Depending on the capacity to generate donors, it may be a full-time job, i.e. when more than twelve donors per year are generated, plus tissue donors; and part-time if fewer donors are generated.

Conclusion

Organ donation is a hospital process that requires specialized healthcare professionals dedicated to donation tasks; Transplant Procurement Management coordinators are the specialist for this process. The TPM coordinator guarantees that all possible donors are detected and converted into actual donors. Clinical duties such as donor detection and maximization of conversion rate, and non-clinic duties like training, research, and quality assurance are some of the main obligations of the TPM coordinator. Additionally, organ donation, as a teamwork activity, demands the participation of professionals from different backgrounds such as social workers, biologists, or technicians; nevertheless, the key role will be played by the TPM coordinator.

Highlights

- A hospital-based organ procurement unit should have its own budget and be managed independently from other hospital departments.
- Early detection, referral, and assessment of possible donors are key duties of TPM coordinator.
- TPM Coordinators facilitate the diagnosis of brain death.
- The transplant coordinators participate actively in all donor management aspects, with emphasis on organ and tissue suitability.
- Training and experience are essential to approach the donor family for organ donation.

- Evaluating and recording the details of donation procedures are essential to meet ethical requirements, notably the transparency and legality.

References

1. Manyalich M, Valero R, Paredes D, Paez G. Transplant Procurement Management: Transplant Coordination Organisation Model for the Generation of Donors. In: Transplant Coordination Manual; TPM-Fundacion DTI. Ed. Donation and Transplantation Insitute. Barcelona 2014; 1.9–27.
2. Manyalich M. Trasplantes de órganos y tejidos. In: Farreras-Rozman. Medicina Interna. Ed Elsevier. Barcelona 2004, 2nd Edition: 46–50.
3. Manyalich M, Servicio de coordinación de trasplantes. In: Asenjo MA. Gestión diaria del hospital. Ed Masson, S.A. Barcelona 2006, 3rd Edition, chap. 24: 397–404.
4. Manyalich, M.; Mestres, C.A.; Ballesté, C.; Páez, G.; Valero, R.; Gómez, M.P. Organ Procurement: Spanish Transplant Procurement Management. Asian Cardiovascular & Thoracic Annals, 2011:19; 268–278.
5. Matesanz R, Domı´nguez-Gil B, Coll E, et all. Spanish experience as a leading country: what kind of measures were taken? Transplant International ª 2011 European Society for Organ Transplantation 24 (2011) 333–343.
6. Tocher J, Neades B, Smith GD, Kelly D. The role of specialist nurses for organ donation: A solution for maximising organ donation rates?. J Clin Nurs. 2019 May;28(9–10):2020–2027.
7. R. Matesanz, B. Domınguez-Gil, E. Coll,B. Mahıllo and R. Marazuela. How Spain Reached 40 Deceased Organ Donors per Million Population.American Journal of Transplantation 2017; 17: 1447–1454.
8. Valero R, Cabrer C, Oppenheimer F, Trias E, Sánchez J, de Cabo F, Navarro A, Paredes D, Alcaraz A, Gutiérrez R, Manyalich M. Normothermic recirculation reduces primary graft dysfunction of kidneys obtained from non-heart-beating donors. Transplant International 2000; 13: 303–310.
9. Manyalich M, Ricart A, Martínez I, et al. EULID Project: European Living Donation and Public Health. Transplan Proc 2009; 41(6): 2021–2024.
10. Leo Roels Caroline Spaight Jacqueline Smits Bernard Cohen. Critical Care staffs' attitudes, confidence levels and educational needs correlate with countries' donation rates: data from the Donor Action database. Transplant International Journal compilationª2010 European Society for Organ Transplantation23(2010) 842–850.
11. Manyalich M, Guasch X, Paez G, Valero R, Istrate M ETPOD (European Training Program on Organ Donation): a successful training program to improve organ donation. Transpl Int 2013; 26(4): 373–384.
12. Istrate MG, Harrison TR, Valero R, Morgan SE, Páez G, Zhou Q, Rébék-Nagy G, Manyalich M. Benefits of Transplant Procurement Management (TPM) specialized training on professional competence development and career evolutions of health care workers in organ donation and transplantation. Exp Clin Transplant. 2015 Apr;13 Suppl 1:148–155.

13. Beatriz Domínguez-Gil, Francis L. Delmonico, Faissal A. M. Shaheen, Rafael Matesanz, Kevin O'Connor, Marina Minina, Elmi Muller, Kimberly Young, Marti Manyalich, et al. The critical pathway for deceased donation: reportable uniformity in the approach to deceased donation Transplant International 2011 European Society for Organ Transplantation 24 (2011) 373–378.
14. Iyer A1, Gao L, Doyle A, Rao P, Cropper JR, Soto C, Dinale A, Kumarasinghe G, Jabbour A, Hicks M, Jansz PC, Feneley MP, Harvey RP, Graham RM, Dhital KK, MacDonald PS. Normothermic ex vivo perfusion provides superior organ preservation and enables viability assessment of hearts from DCD donors. Am J Transplant. 2015 Feb;15(2):371–380. doi: 10.1111/ajt.12994.
15. Manyalich, M.; Rüdinger, W.; Gómez, M.P.; Lara, E.; Net, M.; Pinto, H. Non-transplantable liver obtained for cell isolation for therapeutic use. Transplant International, 2009:22(2); 103.
16. Manyalich M., Paredes D., Cabrer C. 2000. Public health issues from European countries. In: Cochat P. (eds) Transplantation and Changing Management of Organ Failure. Transplantation and Clinical Immunology (Symposia Fondation Marcel Mérieux), 2000, vol 32. Springer, Dordrecht. https://doi.org/10.1007/978-94-011-4118-5_2217. Manyalich M, Guasch X, Gomez M, et al. Organ Donation European Quality System: ODEQUS Project Methodology. Transplant Proc 2013; 45(10): 3462–3465.
18. Gunderson S. USA Model for Organ Procurement in Transplant Procurement Management Manual. Ed Donation and Transplantation Institute. Barcelona 2020, 4th Edition, Chap.19-III: 559–567ISBN: 978-84-09-11752-9

65

Role of specialist nurses in organ donation

Lucia Rizzato, Antonino Montemurro

Introduction

The donation and transplantation Coordination Centre's health programmes based on a multidisciplinary approach should necessarily go through the concrete acknowledgement and specific and original contribution of each professional.[1] This, over time, resulted in the creation of the new role of 'donation and transplantation nursing coordinator' who, with specific training, is perfectly able to manage the processes, facilitating the integration, and collaboration between all professionals involved.

On 14 December 2017, in Italy, the Permanent Board for the State, Regions and the Trento and Bolzano Autonomous Provinces relations stated, through the 'National Program to increase organ donation in the 2018–2020 three-year period', that the Hospital Coordination unit of procurement which includes the medical and nursing Local Coordinator shall be thoughtfully selected based on a well-documented aptitude to the task and specific training requirements.[(2)]

Already in March 2002, a State-Regions agreement highlighted the importance of the presence of nursing staff both in Local and Regional Coordination units, anticipating that the complexity of the performed function, together with certified competence, could guarantee a specific career development.[(2)]

In order to train the personnel involved in the donation-transplantation system adequately, many different training courses have been created, such as Transplant Procurement Management (TPM)[3] which is a course promoted by the Italian National Transplant Centre in collaboration with TPM-DTI Foundation, Universitat de Barcelona.

This course is specifically dedicated to the training of coordinator to the processes of donation and organ and tissue retrieval, a training based on national and international experience in the field of donation, retrieval and procurement. Over the years, academic courses for nurses held in different Italian universities have been established which allow, in compliance with Law no. 43 from 1 February 2006, the professionals to be awarded with a first-level master's degree for specialist's functions from the university, thus guaranteeing even higher standards to the 'Italian Transplantation system.[4] In big hospitals, where an elevated number of organ retrievals meet a remarkable potential number of tissue donors, the coordination activity represents an exceptional amount of work and the need for being promptly available. Therefore, a 'coordination office' model composed of physicians and nurses was considered. The model grants the continuity of the service and adequate circulation of tasks and clinical-organizational skills, in addition to the possibility of realizing a thorough and continued training process within the hospital.

By leaving aside those schemes connected to the strict differentiation between medical and nursing tasks, it will be possible to establish a new ability based on knowing to do and knowing to be which allows an efficient and functional integration in performing complex and articulated coordination tasks. Such integration is already an everyday reality for those working in critical fields, with the awareness that the nurse, side by side with the resuscitation specialists, is the first actor of the continuity and quality of the treatment in the intensive care unit (ICU).

As of today, nursing personnel is present at every level of the National Transplant Network, specifically:

- Local Donation Coordination Centre (CL);
- Regional Transplant Coordination Centre (CRT);
- National Transplant Coordination Centre (CNT).

Local Donation Coordination Centre

The State-Regions agreement of March 2002 is the first one to introduce in Italy the presence of nursing staff within regional and local coordination centres and to define the importance of establishing a coordination office made of different professionals, by specifying their functions and responsibilities which can be outlined as follows[5]:

- To prepare the annual programme of the activities to be submitted to the evaluation of the General Director of the Local Healthcare Authority and the Coordinator of the Regional Centre;
- To ensure that the protocol for ascertaining the death of a patient has been activated, in those events foreseen by the Law (L. 578/93—DM 582/94—DM 11/04/2008), through the Medical Directorate, also regardless of organ and tissue donation[6];
- To monitor all brain-damaged patients present in the ICUs of the hospital, in collaboration with the ICU staff everyday;
- To carry out and prepare dedicated courses for the transmission of the material necessary for the typing of the organ and tissue donor to the competent immunology laboratory;
- To ensure the immediate transmission of data related to the donor to the competent CRT for the allocation of organs;
- To coordinate and transmit the administrative acts related to the retrieval surgeries foreseen by the Law;
- To fill, in collaboration with the medical director, the local registry of brain-damaged patients, performed retrievals and the causes of the failure of retrievals, if any;
- To monitor the deaths in order to identify potential donors of corneas, cardiac valves, vascular grafts, osteoarticular segments, skin and to support the resuscitation specialists during the interviews with the donor's family;
- To create programmes for organ and tissue procurement;
- To perform activities on raising awareness and advising the health workers on issues related to donation and transplantation;
- To care for the relationship with the donors' families, both during donation and afterwards;

- To develop organic relations with family medical doctors, in order to raise awareness and correctly inform on the therapeutic possibilities of transplantation and on the social value of donation;
- To develop appropriate relations with local information organizations on the issues related to donation and transplantation, following the indications of the General Director and the Regional Transplant Centre;
- To present to the Medical Director of the Local Healthcare Authority and the coordinator of the Regional Centre an annual report on the activities performed;
- To identify the paths of enhancing hospital logistics of retrieval and transplantation activities, within the programme;
- To organize activities of information, health education and cultural growth within the local community in the field of transplantation, paying attention, in a programmatic manner, to particular targets (schools, religious communities, etc.), together with voluntary associations, following the CRT's guidelines.

In order to better understand the role of the nurse within the local coordination centre, we can summarize the process by streamlining it into four fundamental phases:

1. Identifying the potential donor;
2. Clinical evaluation of the potential donor;
3. Supporting the potential donor family;
4. Training courses and information campaigns on donation and transplantation.

Finding and identifying the potential donor

The resuscitation specialist is the first one to diagnose brain death, assisted by nursing staff who carefully and precociously evaluate such circumstances by identifying some indisputable signs, observed throughout the whole care period. Adequate training and competence of the nurse in-charge of such activity are fundamental elements for reaching a correct diagnosis in a shorter period of time. Undoubtedly, this represents the starting point of the whole process; the identification, within the hospital, of all potential donors through a disclosure management system is fundamental for a good organizational system. The most appropriate modality for the implementation of this systematic approach which puts the nurse on the front line is the daily monitoring of the ICUs. With the support of specific forms for data collection, all potential patients are recorded, monitoring with particular attention, those with severe neurological damage. This activity allows collecting data and information on potential organ and tissue donors, to promptly activate all necessary procedures for ascertaining death.

Creating integration, cooperation, and synergy between medical and nursing staff of ICUs is pivotal to maximize the available resources. The activity that follows consists of elaborating data in order to acquire statistical information on the potential of donation available in one's own reality.

Clinical evaluation of the potential donor

The Local Coordination nurse's care for the donor is one of the most complex and delicate activities since the care of an individual who is brain dead requires highly skilled and prepared staff working in the operational unit in charge. Moreover, other patients in ICUs who need care cannot be ignored; hence, the support from professionals of the Local Coordination Centre becomes essential, not to burden ICUs staff with more work.

The potential donor's clinical assessment undergoes a series of processes which start in the ICU and end in the operating room (OR), during surgery for organ retrieval. This process aims at assessing the donor's suitability for donation and the function of each organ. During this phase, it is crucial to promptly transmit every available data on the potential donor (age, sex, blood type, cause of death, etc.). Simultaneous coordination between the hematochemical and instrumental laboratory tests, the anatomical pathology services indispensable in cases which are difficult to clinically assess and other services which may be useful for the donation process, and finally the on-call OR staff for retrieval are essential. The Local Coordination Centre staff is available in the network for all requests that may be received from the regional centres aiming at producing a thorough organ assessment.

Support to the potential donor's family

During the donation process, emotional and psychological problems include dealing with strong and contradictory feelings such as desperation, loneliness, pain, anguish, anger, and generosity. The interview with the family is one of the most delicate rings of the chain and has to be taken into account, separately.

The Ministerial Decree 739 of 1994 'Regulations concerning the identification of the role and related profile of the nurse' underlines the peculiar relational and educational importance of the nurse. Also the Code of Ethics of nurses states unequivocally the importance of the nurse in the moment of death and through the grieving process.[7] Traditionally, the role of the nurse is perceived by patients and their families as closest to their needs and demands. The type of work they perform and the daily contact with people cared for facilitate the creation of relationships based on communication that is useful and efficient. According to this concept, the interview with the family of the potential donor is carried out in optimal conditions and performed both by a medical doctor and a nurse. The physician has the task to inform on the clinical conditions, on the procedure that is going to be implemented and informs on the death of the relative. The nurse receives the family's reaction, answers to their questions and doubts, and helps them with every need they might have. They build a true relationship based on support, aware of the fact that the relationship with the family often goes beyond the usual communication patterns.

Training and information on donation and transplantation

Another important task of the Local Coordination Centre is the training and information on donation and transplantation. This fundamental activity spreads the culture of donation, acknowledges its importance and its value, and allows every citizen to make a conscious decision on the matter. In every Italian region, nurses employed in schools, churches, and cultural events bring their experience and testimony, in addition to technical knowledge, that are much more effective than words.

Regionale Transplant Coordination Centre

In many CRT centres, the presence of nursing staff is a well-consolidated fact. They work at collecting notifications on potential donors from Local Coordination centres. On hearing about the organ needs from the Italian National Transplant Centre, they offer organs to the transplant centres from their area.

The nurse from the regional coordination centre reads the documentation received, evaluates the presence of potential uncertain elements to be submitted to the medical doctor in charge, and asks for missing data that are necessary for the donor's and organs' suitability assessment. Together with the medical doctor of reference and/or the regional coordinator, they establish the risk level of the donor (notified by their region), in accordance with the national guidelines. This allows the identification of the right recipient for each organ. They also make sure that the necessary immunological tests for the transplant are performed and they take care of every logistical and organizational aspect to reach the final goal—retrieval and transplantation.

The Regional Transplant Centres' functions listed below are reported in comma six of Article 10 of Law number 91/99[8]:

- To coordinate the activities of collection and transmission of data related to the people awaiting transplantation, in accordance with the criteria established by the National Centre;
- To coordinate the activities of retrieval between the resuscitation units present in the territory and the transplant structures;
- To ensure the correct performing of immunological tests necessary for transplantation, with the help of one or more immunology transplantation laboratory;

- To allocate organs by following the criteria established by the National Centre, based on the priorities resulting from the patients' waiting lists;
- To ensure correct performing of immunological compatibility tests in transplant programmes in their territory of competence;
- To coordinate the transportation of biological samples of medical staff and of the organs and tissues in their territory of competence;
- To facilitate the collaboration between healthcare authorities of their territory of competence and the voluntary associations;
- To promote the culture of organ and tissue donation.

When the allocation process is over, the nurse from the Regional Coordination Centre has the task to coordinate the different medical teams involved in the retrieval process. The teams which may be regional or extra-regional; the nurse must make sure that every second-level service is activated, if necessary. They also coordinate the transportation of the medical staff, the organs or the patients, based on the demands of the donation process.

National Operational Transplant Coordination Centre

Since November 2013, the Italian National Transplant Centre is the only national operational representative, interacting directly with the Regional Coordination Centres and ensuring 24/7 support, fundamental for the operational management of the national programmes.[9] The centralization of the management of the allocation process together with that of the waiting list for the national programmes provides the following benefits:

- Smoothens the allocation process through the standardization of processes;
- Provides a univocal interpretation of the rules that currently discipline such programmes and therefore, it makes application more efficient;
- Facilitates immediate communication and resolution;

- Allows a real-time monitoring of donation, allocation streams, and processes' outcomes;
- Translates the work performed into statistical data, updated in real time.

The selection of the personnel and the organization of the work shifts require time and a deep knowledge of the network along with the identification of those features and predispositions of which the selected staff should possess. Considering the above duties, taking as a reference a national average of six donors per day and taking into account the fact that every donor shall be notified to CNTO in order to assess their potential, as far as the national programs are concerned, it has been deemed necessary to create an operational unit made of at least twelve coordination nurses distributed on three shifts and five medical doctors (one shift in the morning, one in the afternoon, and the on-call shifts from 8 p.m.).This structural operational unit represents the indispensable number of people to ensure the service 24/7, 365 days a year.

The nursing staff works at the front office of all national programmes coordination and manages the waiting lists, together with the Transplant IT system. The medical staff play a fundamental role in the assessment of suitability of the donor and as monitoring authority of the whole system.

The National Coordination nurse collects the notifications on all the donors on the national territory and the organ offers coming from other countries establish the operational allocation plan of the organs, and share it with the staff on shift.

As far as the allocation for national programmes is concerned, the nurses read the documentation about the donors, assess the presence of potential pathological clinical elements, doubts and controversies to be submitted to the reference medical doctor and/or CNTO person in charge. The nurses request missing data necessary for the suitability assessment of the donors and/or the organs. The nurses communicate with Regional Coordination Centres involved in the operational allocation plan to make organ offers, according to the established priorities. They share with reference medical doctor and/or CNTO person in charge, potentially critical matters emerging during the allocation procedures, in order to identify resolution strategies. They monitor the correct implementation of the procedures, in case of transportation of the recipients/medical staff for each transplant. They store the documentation of the donors cared for and they write the related reports. They collect the outcomes of the allocation procedures and update in real time, the national programmes' lists managed. The nurses also contribute to the elaboration of new protocols and improvement plans which affect the donation and transplantation processes. They participate in the management of the data collection database and the related elaboration and take part in the discussion on the most complex clinical cases.

Conclusions

We may conclude by stating that the function of the coordination nurses shall be performed by adequately trained personnel. The coordination nurses shall own particular skills and it is necessary to implement the basic knowledge, perfect the cross communicational and relational skills, given that the context in which they operate are well outlined: the end-of-life stage and the donation process. The coordination nurses shall adjust to continuous organizational innovations, and new technical and professional notions which require an immediate response. They shall have the ability to coordinate and support the activities needed for the implementation of clinical/organizational processes, they shall be able to use appropriate communicational forms and adjust their language on the basis of their target in addition to working in an integrated manner with their collaborators. Passion, technical-specialized skills along with communicational, relational, and theoretical skills are the elements which determine the way to face the problems and the ability to solve them, and that allow the creation of the 'Specialist Nurses for Organ Donation'.

Highlights

- The Italian donation and transplantation system sets an example of a good organization;
- Nursing personnel is present at every level of the National Transplant Network;

- The function of the coordination nurses shall be performed by adequately trained personnel;
- The coordination nurses shall adjust to continuous organizational innovations;
- The nurses work in an integrated manner with their collaborators;
- Passion, technical-specialized skills along with communicational, relational, and theoretical skills are the elements which determine the way to face the problems.

References

1. Rizzato L, Venettoni S, Nanni Costa A. The Italian donation and transplantation system: analysis of an integration model of healthcare professionals.Transplants 2007;XI:155–163 (4/2007)
2. State – Regions Conference - Agreement (14.12.2017) Agreement on the 2018 – 2020 National Program for Organ Donation [on line]. Available at: http://www.regioni.it/sanita/2017/12/18/conferenza-stato-regioni-del-14-12-2017-accordo-sul-programma-nazionale-donazione-di-organi-2018-2020-544250/ [consulted in April 2019]
3. Transplant Procurement Management [on line]. 2018. Available at: http://www.trapianti.salute.gov.it/trapianti/dettaglioContenutiCnt.jsp?lingua=italiano&area=cnt&menu=operatori&sottomenu=formazione&id=272 [consulted in April 2019]
4. Law no. 43 from 1 February 2006 Provisions on the nursing, midwifery, rehabilitation, technical-health and prevention health professions and delegation to the Government for the establishment of the related professional associations [on line]. Available at: http://www.parlamento.it/parlam/leggi/06043l.htm [consulted in April 2019]
5. State – Regions Conference—Agreement (21-03-2002) Guidelines for the coordination activities for national organ and tissue procurement for transplantation [on line]. Available at: https://www.gazzettaufficiale.it/eli/gu/2002/06/21/144/sg/pdf [consulted in April 2019]
6. Ministerial Decree 11 April 2008 Aggiornamento del decreto 22 agosto 1994, n. 582 relating to: «Regulations containing the procedures for ascertaining and certifying death » [on line]. Available at: https://www.gazzettaufficiale.it/atto/serie_generale/caricaDettaglioAtto/originario?atto.dataPubblicazioneGazzetta=2008-06-12&atto.codiceRedazionale=08A04067&elenco30giorni=false [consulted in April 2019]
7. Code of Ethics of Nursing Professions. Rome. [on line]. Available at: https://www.fnopi.it/archivio_news/attualita/2629/Il%20testo%20definitivo%20Codice%20Deontologico%20degli%20Ordini%20delle%20%20Professioni%20Infermieristiche%202019.pdf [consulted in April 2019]

8. Law no. 91 from 1 April 1999 Provisions concerning the removal and transplantation of organs and tissues [on line]. Available at: http://www.parlamento.it/parlam/leggi/99091l.htm [consulted in April 2019]
9. PRESS RELEASE N ° 35/2016 Inauguration of the new headquarters of the National Transplant Operative Center [on line]. Available at: http://old.iss.it/pres/?lang=1&id=1703&tipo=1 [consulted in April 2019]

66

Role of education and training programme in organ donation

Alba Coll, Chloë Ballesté, Carmen Blanco, Elisa Vera, Arantxa Quiralte, Ricard Valero, Martí Manyalich

Introduction

Increasing organ donation rates and improving clinical practice must be achieved through a multifactorial approach. Among the main policies to be undertaken, education and training at different social and academic levels and involving all the stakeholders are key to ensure public support and professional practice.

This chapter presents international strategies and projects on successfully implementation of training among healthcare professionals, education in school and university, as well as social awareness towards organ donation.

Educational models

The education model of organ donation and transplantation training includes the following:

- Professional training through the Transplant Procurement Management course,
- University education to medical and health science students with the International Project on Education and Research in Donation at University of Barcelona, and
- School education to create awareness in children.

Professional training—Transplant Procurement Management training courses

Transplant Procurement Management (TPM) is an international educational programme that provides demand-driven, high-quality training to facilitate the transfer of knowledge and development of professional competencies and excellent framework for worldwide networks of donation professionals. Launched in 1991, under the auspice of Universitat de Barcelona (UB), TPM has organized in over 25 years, 304 face-to-face training courses (131 advanced, 93 intermediate, 80 introductory) in 44 countries. The contents are mainly on organ donation, while others are specifically on tissue banking and cell therapies, donation after circulatory death and leadership and quality management. Until 2019, 12,801 participants from 110 countries have been trained in face-to-face courses.

Methodology and contents

To assess the needs, and develop and refine the training programmes according to the participants, TPM applies the ADDIE (Analysis-Design-Development-Implementation-Evaluation) instructional design model. The training programme proposes a student-centred approach tailored to the current profile of the adult learner, with an interactive educational methodology.[(1)]

The blended learning modality allows to implement a training centred in practice. The students initiate the training through access to the support virtual classroom. This is an added value, since it not only allows greater flexibility than a traditional face-to-face course, but also allows more time to invest in activities for practical use of knowledge acquired. This modality also allows students to review part of the course contents before and after the course, for learning reinforcement.

Face-to-face training programmes are delivered at different levels following progression of expertise, aims, and length of awareness courses (8 hours in basic, 40 hours in advanced courses); according to the participants' previous knowledge and experience in the field, adapting the contents and structure of the training for maximizing the learning process. Hence, the blended TPM methodology builds on participants' knowledge based on their previous training and experience in the field through proactive involvement in the learning environment. As proven by Knowles, adult learning is most effective when information is presented in the context of a real-life situation.[2] Thus, TPM combines theoretical lectures with practical simulations and case studies, while promoting participants' engagement and interaction.[3]

The impact of the training is measured in terms of knowledge outcomes before and after the course completion, as well as interaction and active participation. Satisfaction is also assessed in order to contribute to continuous quality improvement.

Reasons for success of TPM

TPM's educational methodology is uncommon, as it offers a blended learning modality (online and face-to-face), also combines theoretical knowledge-transfer with real-life situation exercises. TPM's experience of over twenty-five years in the field of specialized professional training in organ donation represents international recognition and prestige. This reputation distinguishes TPM from any other similar training in organ donation.

In addition to the knowledge acquired and the competencies developed during the course, TPM training allows networking among participants and between faculty and participants, to encourage better practice and experience exchange. After the TPM course completion, the participants may become members of the Donation and Transplantation Institute (DTI) Community, an alumni association that serves as a platform for news on organ donation, additional training opportunities, events, job offers, etc.

The TPM is engaged with the continuous improvement cycle, always pursuing long-life learning and clinical innovation. Hence, although the course structure remains essentially the same, the course materials and contents are constantly updated.

Although Spain, as word leader in organ donation for over two decades, offers several courses for healthcare professionals in organ donation, at the international level, there is no course similar to the TPM in relation to teaching contents, methodology, and use of practical simulations. Figure 66.1 shows 'China's Deceased Donor Evolution and TPM Course participants 2010–2018' and Figure 66.2 shows 'Croatia's Deceased Donor Evolution and TPM Course participants 2010–2018'.[4]

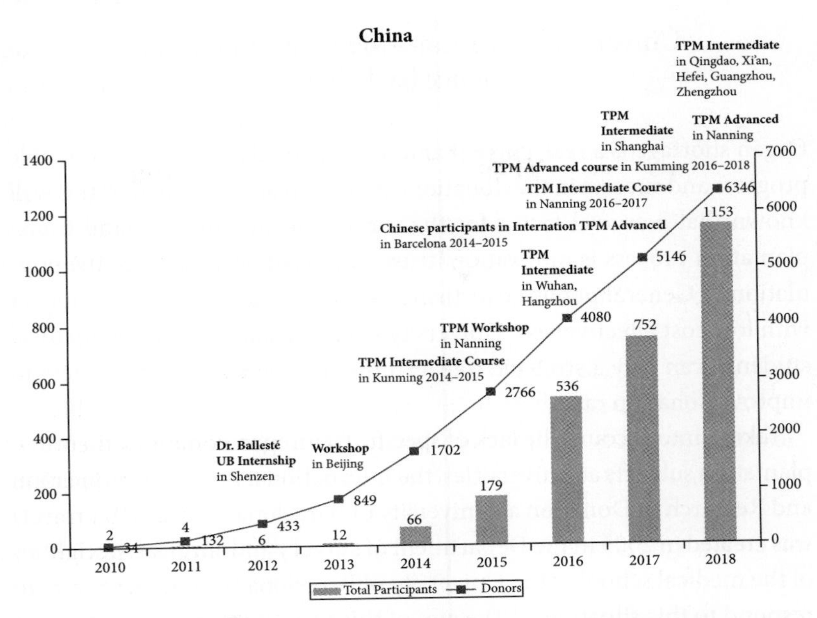

Figure 66.1. China's Deceased Donor Evolution and TPM Course participants 2010–2018

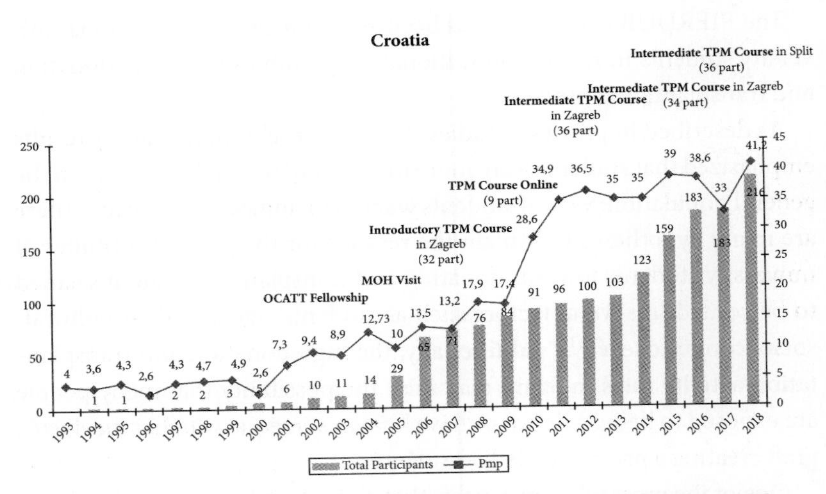

Figure 66.2. The figure shows Croatia's Deceased Donor Evolution and TPM Course participants 2010–2018

University education—Medicine and health science bachelors

Organ shortage is a real, current and international issue despite valuable progress and success in the donation and transplantation field.[5] It is well known that a crucial factor for the success of the donation and transplantation process is motivation, trust, and positive attitude of the population.[6] General public advertising campaigns have short term impact with low cost effectiveness. University students, and specifically medical students, can play a strategic role as future key persons in the society to improve donation rates.[7–13]

Taking into account the lack of specific training in donation and transplantation subjects at Universities, the International Project on Education and Research in Donation at University of Barcelona (PIERDUB project) was created in 2005 in the Department of surgery and surgical specialities of the medical school of the University of Barcelona (UB) with the aim to respond to this situation.[8] The aim of this project was to guarantee that undergraduate students have specific and essential bases in donation and transplantation process during their studies to improve their knowledge and attitudes towards donation.

The PIERDUB experience has been shown great interest among university students in specific educational programmes related to donation and transplantation processes.

As described in previous studies,[8,9,11,13–17] preliminary survey results emphasized that students were more in favour of organ donation than the general population: 97% of students wanted to donate their organs. There are many hypotheses to explain the reasons for the positive attitudes of university students towards donation and transplantation, but it seemed to be related to several factors such as students' age and their cultural/socioeconomic level.[13] Additionally, the high donation and transplantation activity rates in Spain may raise the possibility that many people are exposed to being a donor or have known someone who has received a graft creating a prior knowledge and interest.

One of the most relevant aspects that encourage international training programmes about essential aspects of donation and transplantation was the low degree of knowledge about the concept of brain death. Only half of the answers from the participants' evaluations were correct.[12,16] Previous studies had revealed that university students knew the concept and were well informed.[13]

In conclusion, the PIERDUB experience revealed that the applied strategy is adequate but there is a need for further interventions to ensure well-informed and trained university students, who represent the future key professionals of the society.

Postgraduate education

Postgraduate education is offered by universities around the world to provide advanced training studies that allow participants to achieve a professional specialization or to start a research career.

Since 2004, TPM and the University of Barcelona (UB) offer an official and a specific Masters' programme in donation and transplantation of organs, tissues and cells that gather the up to date efforts carried out by national and international organizations in this field. The programmes use a blended learning methodology that includes online training and face-to-face training with practical simulations. The specific programme also includes a professional internship in different centres around the world, especially in Spain and USA. The main goal of the programme is to bring together the knowledge, skills, and best practices which benefit healthcare professionals working as donor-transplant coordinators, tissue bankers, and advanced cell therapies researchers by developing an updated educational programme.[1] Moreover, the course is designed to increase the knowledge and understanding of donation practices, explore the impact of different ethical frameworks, unique cultural needs, financing models and organizational structures and learn how to inspire health professionals, the community, and nations in donation.

The programme includes four different modules: Organ Procurement, Procurement and Transplantation Management, Organ Transplantation, or Tissue Banking and Advanced Therapies.[20]

Since 2004, 280 participants from thirty-five different nationalities have been trained. So, the strengthening of the online courses in the programme allows and facilitates the training and the interest in Master programmes.[21]

School education

One of the most frequent reasons of familial anxiety and refusal of consent to donation is the uncertainty of a deceased relative's wish in terms of organ donation. Therefore, reducing the number of doubts and stress that arise in this state of emergency and thus decreasing the number of rejections should be one of the main foci in this field.[22] A clue action for increasing society awareness about donation is to identify the optimal population target for campaigns about organ donation. Children are a great means of diffusion since they have a very strong tie with their families. Well educated children will have a personal opinion, will become conscious, and indirectly will educate their relatives.[23] Furthermore, early education may influence decisions in adult life. Modern pedagogical techniques such as gamification, storytelling, and role-playing constitute efficient ways to promote knowledge retention in children.[24,25] It is obtained evidence that the intervention causes an increase in knowledge about transplantation.[26–29] Children are interested in the topic and they share it with their families. Moreover, 11–12 years of age is the best period for children to treat this subject because they study about organs and body functions by mandatory academic guides. If adequate activities could be incorporated into the teaching curriculum, this would ensure a wider and more sustainable approach.

Training programmes in organ donation funded by European Union financing

The EU strategy for education and training focuses on lifelong learning and mobility, quality and efficiency of education, equality, and innovation. Through the strategic framework for education and training, EU countries have identified common objectives, including improving the quality and efficiency of education and training.

The European Commission has strongly supported organ donation programmes of its members, especially through the implementation of effective training programmes for transplant and donors' coordinators, as well as broader projects including training and awareness-raising among other social groups.

Professional and post-graduate training

In recent years, several educational projects have been designed and implemented to establish a specialized organ donation workforce.

European Training Programme on Organ Donation

European Training Programme on Organ Donation (ETPOD) (2007–2009) set the foundation for professional educational projects on organ donation. The ETPOD was a successful initiative addressing three different professional levels in organ donation reaching a high number of European professionals in the field.

1) Essentials in Organ Donation (EOD) Seminar: Basic knowledge of the clinical process of organ donation was addressed to intensive care unit (ICU) and emergency room (ER) professionals to promote donor detection. The seminar was prepared through a 'Training for Trainers' programme, to provide key donation professionals with the knowledge and skills required to replicate the EOD.[30] A total of 51 participants completed the Training for Trainers programme, while the EOD organized training for 3,163 attendees.
2) Professional Training on Organ Donation: This programme aimed to train professionals in charge of the complete donation process at hospital level, and had forty-nine trainees participate in it.
3) Organ Donation Quality Managers Training: Addressed to professionals at national/regional/local or hospital/institutions management level with high organ donation activity, these programmes were conducted to provide the knowledge required to efficiently manage an organ procurement office. About twenty-three participants benefitted from this training.[30]

The ETPOD training programme was specifically addressed to key professionals in donation units (ICU, Postoperative, Recovery, and ER), as well as professionals responsible for the organ donation process' management and donation programme's managers at national, regional, local, and/or hospital level.[1,30]

European-Mediterranean Postgraduate Program on Organ Donation and Transplantation

European-Mediterranean Postgraduate Program on Organ Donation and Transplantation (EMPODaT) (2014–2016) was a TEMPUS project co-funded by the European Commission, designed by four Universities from four different European countries Spain, Germany, France, and Sweden and six Universities from Morocco, Egypt and Lebanon to develop and implement a Postgraduate Program on Organ Donation and Transplantation.[31]

A total of thirteen tutors from Morocco, Egypt, and Lebanon benefitted from the Learn to Teach Training Program (TxT) to become faculty of the Postgraduate Program on Organ Donation and Transplantation. A light increase of knowledge (2.63%) was reported after the course.[31]

The Postgraduate Training (available in English and French) was designed in one academic year of 30 ECTS (European Credit Transfer and Accumulation System) credits (750–900 hours) using blended learning methodology. Pre- and Post-training tests, self-assessing activities, and traineeship activity charts were used to evaluate the students. Around ninety students were trained (fifteen per university), thirty-nine women and fifty-one men, of which seventy-nine were doctors (23% ICU, 22% surgeons), and eleven nurses. Significant differences were found among knowledge improvement between countries and specialization backgrounds. Donation knowledge improved in all countries, but Morocco was the most beneficiated (Mean diff. Morocco 3.71±0.32 > Lebanon 1.83±0.32 >Egypt 1.42±0.32). No significant differences were found between background specialization groups, as can be seen in Figure 66.3. The improvement of transplantation knowledge was no significant among the countries, but the donation background group was significantly more beneficiated (Mean diff. Donation 5.04±0.29> Nursing 4.92±0.49 >Transplantation 4.01±0.23).[31]

Knowledge Transfer and Leadership in Organ Donation from Europe to China

Knowledge Transfer and Leadership in Organ Donation (KeTLOD) (2016–2018) was an Erasmus + project that promoted the development and implementation of a postgraduate programme in organ donation

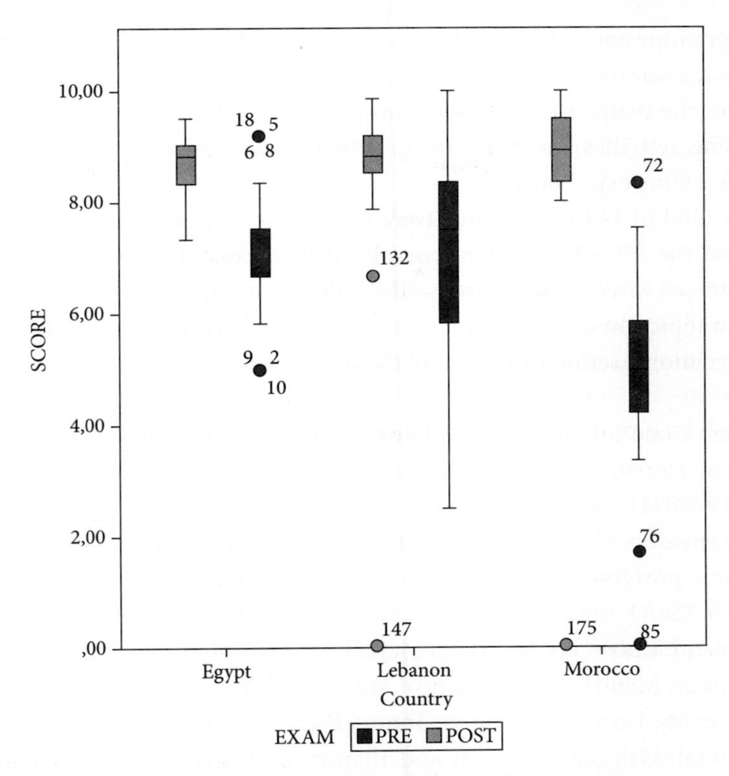

Figure 66.3. Improvement of knowledge between the countries

in seven Chinese universities following the European Space for Higher Education guidelines: Shanghai Jiao Tong University, Hospital Capital Medical University, Kunming University, Wuhan University, Second Military Medical University, Shanghai, Nanchang University, Guangxi University of Chinese Medicine (GUCM)—Transplant institute of medicine Nanning, following successful European models and the experience acquired from the previous EMPODaT project.[32]

The learning strategy was developed in collaboration with three European Universities: University of Barcelona, University Nice Sophia Antipolis, and University of Bologna.

The training was designed in two phases: Train the Trainers (TxT) blended programme (online and face-to-face) and a one-year postgraduate programme (PP) of 25 ECTS credits (625 study hours). The programme applied blended learning methodology with local and international seminars, online training, and traineeships.[32]

For the evaluation of the students pre- and post-training tests, self-assessing activities, and traineeship activity charts were used to enhance the learning experience.

A total of 144 participants were selected on specific criteria and followed the PP; 64% of them completed it successfully. Each university organized three local seminars. The online training, structured in seven main topics on organ donation, was successfully completed by 80% and international seminars by 72% of the students.[32]

Organ Donation Innovative Strategies for Southeast Asia

Organ Donation Innovative Strategies for Southeast Asia (ODISSeA) (2019–2021) is an Erasmus + project funded by the European Commission.[33] The main objective is to design and implement an academic postgraduate programme on organ donation in eight Southeast Asian (SeA) universities from Malaysia, Myanmar, Philippines, and Thailand: University Teknologi Mara, University of Malaya, University of Medicine Mandalay, University of Medicine,[1] Yangon, Ateneo de Davao University, University of Santo Tomas, Faculty of Medicine Ramathibodi Hospital, Mahidol University and Thammasat University, and three universities from European Union (EU): University of Barcelona, University of Bologna, and University of Zagreb School of Medicine.

The training program entails a Train the Trainers (TxT) blended programme (online and face to face) and a postgraduate programme in organ donation (35 participants per institution) of 30 ECTS credits (750 study hours).[33]

The methodology followed involves online training, local, international seminars, informative events, and on-the-job projects. Pre- and post-training questionnaires, self-assessing activities were used to evaluate students.[33]

Public awareness programmes

Training and Social Awareness for Increasing Organ Donation in the European Union and Neighboring Countries (EUDONORGAN) was a service contract awarded by the European Commission, aiming to provide training and increase social awareness in the European Union (EU) and neighbouring countries (NCs) to enhance positive attitude towards organ donation.[34]

The project was divided in two core work packages (WPs), WP1: *Training* and WP2: *Social Awareness*. In WP1, the training programme employed a blended methodology. The beneficiaries included healthcare professionals (HPs) and other key players (OKPs) from the EU and NCs, with a specific e-learning route for each group of beneficiaries. The face to face was practical and promoted best practice exchange. In WP1, 101 participants from 28 countries completed the training: 79 HPs and 22 OKPs. The e-learning registered 25.22% of knowledge improvement among HPs and 29.47% among OKPs. A total of ninety-six participants attended all sessions and were certified.[34]

In WP2, six Member States agreed to organize awareness-raising events, held between September 2018 and April 2019. The events involved EU and NCs and stakeholders: 95 participants in Warsaw from 4 countries, 49 participants in Budapest from 7 countries, 127 participants in Brussels from 33 countries, 95 participants in Stockholm from 9 countries, 96 participants in Athens from 8 countries, and 40 participants in Lisbon from 6 countries, reaching a total of 502 participants.[34]

Conclusion

Training has been proven to be a successful tool to impact positively in the rates of donation of the countries that include these programmes in their regular practice. However, most countries witness a lack of training in organ donation at Higher Education Level, though the efficiency and cost-effectiveness have been demonstrated.

Further efforts to introduce and spread organ donation education in university programmes are key to ensure that this field is considered at the same level to other medical specialities. Moreover, projects funded by public competencies are an additional effective way to reinforce training in areas where the donation rates are low.

Highlights

- Education and training are key factors to improve clinical practice and awareness in organ donation activity.
- Education must be provided at different levels to be successful: school, university, professional training, and social awareness.
- Transplant Procurement Management (TPM) is an international educational programme that provides demand-driven, high-quality training.
- Postgraduate programmes in organ donation use a blended learning methodology that include online training, face-to-face training with practical simulations.
- Several educational projects have been designed and implemented to establish a specialized organ donation workforce.
- The European Commission has strongly supported organ donation programmes through the implementation of effective training programmes for transplant and donors' coordinators.

References

1. Istrate M, Harrison TR, Valero R et al. Benefits of Transplant Procurement Management (TPM) Specialized Training on Professional Competence Development and Career Evolutions of Health Care Workers in Organ Donation and Transplantation. Experimental and Clinical Transplantation (2015) 13 (Suppl 1): 148–155.
2. Knowles MS. The Modern Practice of Adult Education; Andragogy versus Pedagogy. (ERIC Document Reproduction Service No. D043812). 1970. New York, Association Press. ISBN. 0809617560.
3. Kolb DA. Experiential learning: experience as the source of learning and development. Englewood Cliffs, New Jersey: Prentice Hall, 1984.
4. Donation and Transplantation Institute, Annual Report Activity, TPM effect over donation, 2018; 10–11.
5. Organización Nacional de Trasplantes (ONT), Memoria 2008, http://www.ont.es
6. Schaeffner ES, Windisch W, Friedel K, et al. Knowledge and attitudes regarding organ donation among medical students and physicians. Transplantation 2004;77:1714.
7. Corlett S: Professional and system barriers to organ donation. Transplant Proc 1985;17:111.
8. Manyalich, M.; Paredes, D.; Ballesté, C. PIERDUB Project: International project on education and research in donation at University of Barcelona: Training University Students About Donation and Transplantation. Transplant International, volume 22, number 2, 231, 2009

9. Colak M, Ersoy K, Haberal M, et al. A household study to determine attitudes and beliefs related to organ transplantation and donation: a pilot study in Yapracik Village, Ankara, Turkey. Transplant Proc 2008;40:29.
10. Burra P, De Bona M, Canova D, et al. Changing attitude to organ donation and transplantation in university students during the years of medical school in Italy. Transplant Proc 2005;37:547.
11. Garcia CD, Barboza AP, Goldani JC, et al. Educational program of organ donation and transplantation at medical school. Transplant Proc 2008;40:1068.
12. Goz F, Goz M, Erkan M. Knowledge and attitudes of medical, nursing, dentistry and health technician students towards organ donation: a pilot study. J Clin Nurs 2006;15:1371.
13. Feeley TH, Tamburlin J, Vincent DE. An educational intervention on organ and tissue donation for first-year medical students. Prog Transplant 2008;18:103.
14. Canova D, De Bona M, Ruminati R, et al. Understanding of and attitudes to organ donation and transplantation: a survey among Italian university students. Clin Transplant 2006;20:307.
15. Sanavi A, Afshar R, Lotfizadeh AR, et al. Survey of medical students of Shahed University in Iran about attitude and willingness toward organ transplantation. Transplant Proc 2009;41: 1477.
16. Hobeika MJ, Simon R, Malik R, et al. U.S. surgeons and medical student attitudes toward organ donation. J Trauma 2009;67:372.
17. Najafizadeh K, Shiemorteza M, Jamali M, et al. Attitudes of medical students about brain death and organ donation. Transplant Proc 2009;41:2707.
18. Mekahli D, Liutkus A, Fargue S, et al. Survey at first-year medical students to assess their knowledge and attitudes toward organ transplantation and donation. Transplant Proc 2009;41:634–638.
19. Gravoac G, Brkljacic T, Topic I, et al. Attitudes toward organ donation among medical students. Med Teach 2006;28:745.
20. Páez G, Manyalich, M, Valero R. TPM: A Highly Efficient Training Program in Organ and Tissue Donation. Experimental and Clinical Transplantation. MESOT Congress Abstracts, 2012;10(Supple-1).
21. Coll A, Ballesté C, Valero R, Paredes D, Torregrosa V, Diekmann F, Navarro A, Adalia R, Colmenero J, Manyalich M: Modularity and Blended Methodology on Master Education for Donation and Transplantation. Transplantation Proceedings. 2018;50.
22. Guadagnoli E, Christiansen C, DeJong W, McNamara P, Beasley C, Christiansen E, Evanisko M: The Public's willingness to discuss their preference for organ donation with family members. Clinical Transplantation. 1999;13(4): 342–348.
23. McGlade D, Pierscionek B: Can education alter attitudes, behaviour and knowledge about organ donation? A pretest/post-test study. BMJ Open, 2013. Dec 30; 3(12).
24. Durlak JA, Weissberg RP, Dymnicki AB, Shellinger, KB: The Impact of Enhancing Students' Social and Emotional Learning: A Meta-Analysis of School-Based Universal Interventions. Child Development. 2011;82(1): 405–432.
25. Haidet P, Morgan RO, O'Malley K, Moran BJ, Richards BF. A Controlled Trial of Active Versus Passive Learning Strategies in a Large Group Setting. Advances in Health Sciences Education. 2004;9(1): 15–27.

26. Conesa Bernal C, Ríos Zambudio A, Munuera Orenes C: Los escolares de primaria ante la donación de órganos. Encuesta de opinión. Rev. Esp. Trasp; 1996;11: 1–27.
27. Li AH, Rosenblum AM, Nevis IF, Garg AX. Adolescent classroom education on knowledge and attitudes about deceased organ donation: a systematic review. Pediatr Transplant. 2013;17(2): 119–128.
28. Rey JW, Grass V, Galle PR, Werner C, Hoffman A, Kiesslich R, Hammer GP. Education in organ donation among students in Germany—results of an intervention study. Ann Transplant. 2013;18:23–30.4.
29. Muramaki M, Fukuma S, Ikezoe M, Nakamura M, Yamamoto Y, Yamazaki S, Fukuhara S. Effect of an educational program on attitudes towards deceased organ donation. Ann Transplant. 2015;20: 269–278.
30. Manyalich M, Guasch X, Paez G, Valero R, Istrate, M: ETPOD (European Training Program on Organ Donation): a successful training program to improve organ donation; Transpl Int, 2013;26: 373–384.
31. European-Mediterranean Postgraduate Program on Organ Donation and Transplantation, 2014. Accessed from: http://empodat.eu/
32. Knowledge transfer and leadership in Organ Donation. 2018. Accessed from: http://www.ketlod.cn/
33. Organ Donation Innovative Strategies for Southeast Asia. 2019. Accessed from: https://odisseaproject.eu/
34. EUDONORGAN. 2017. Accessed from; http://eudonorgan.eu/

67

The impact of telehealth in management of organ transplantation

Azhar Rafiq, Ding-Yu Fei, Brian Le, Carlo Di Giambattista

Overview of telemedicine and telehealth

The integration of computing technologies into healthcare has become very common with the diagnostic devices or wearable technologies that monitor patients electronically to generate data and the computer systems that store the data for effective record keeping in the digital or electronic format. Such technologies, referred to as Electronic Health (eHealth), are used by partnering healthcare team members. However, the integration of networking capabilities and corresponding technologies for data sharing (interoperability) has become an additional component for distribution of health information collected from patients as well as cross-disciplinary documentation of treatment plans by healthcare teams. These cumulative electronic platforms are the basis for today's healthcare delivery systems globally and are referred to as Information and Communication Technologies (ICTs) by the World Health Organization (WHO).[1] The term to identify such health technology methods has been Telemedicine. The WHO claims that 'Telemedicine … signifies the use of ICT to improve patient outcomes by increasing access to care and medical information.'[1]

As technology continues to evolve with advances in technical capabilities and the use of such tools, the terminology in defining healthcare practices using advanced technology has evolved as well. Telemedicine, the technology used in clinical services for patient care, for example, has gained many perspectives from the types of healthcare services that use technological tools and thus, has varied definitions. The American

Telemedicine Association (ATA) defines Telemedicine as 'the use of medical information exchanged from one site to another via electronic communications to improve a patient's clinical health'.[2] However, with innovative technical progress and advanced computing capacities, the capability to support patients' healthcare with technology has widened to include patient illness diagnosis, care coordination, and education with wider healthcare team members including non-clinical services. The term Telehealth has been used in this wider health care delivery format. The Center for Connected Health Policy (CCHP) has summarized telehealth to include four capabilities of health care management: mobile health or mHealth, remote patient monitoring, store-and-forward care, and live video.[3] Overall, the newly developed and validated telehealth systems have the objective of improving the care of the patients with support from different specialists without their physical presence at the patient's bedside. This technological advancement serves as a precious tool because of its ability to connect patient care teams with additional experts and make knowledge more accessible.

While appreciating that technology can be used by healthcare professionals to support a wider spectrum of patient care, the possibility of managing the complex process of solid organ transplantation using telehealth technologies has been surveyed. The key advantage to the use of telehealth is making healthcare more widely accessible to the patients.[4] In the context of organ transplantation, using telehealth as a viable clinical care delivery method for patient candidates to be matched with organ donors or donation programmes is validated by a series of international programmes.

Phases of solid organ transplantation

Considering the complexity of organ transplantation as a healthcare programme with multiple interdependent phases of patient management, the actual process can be segmented into three main clinical procedural phases: (1) pre-transplant, (2) inpatient, and (3) follow-up care. By identifying these phases of care, it becomes feasible to outline the capacity of successful integration of telehealth to ensure greater patient support and minimal graft rejection. The literature surveys many examples of successful telehealth efforts that encompass a range of patient management techniques and clinical care services to achieve organ transplantation including difficulties of patient identification, organ match alignment, continuing through organ procurement, to the overall surgical procedure, and the long-term follow up of patient wellness. The role of telehealth is noted in these examples to indicate the feasibility of healthcare coordination for the patient management in organ transplantation. The studies cited subsequently are not an exhaustive survey of telemedicine or telehealth literature relative to organ transplant management but a representation of what has been validated and can be adapted widely.

Telehealth in pre-transplant phase

Pre-transplant phase is a period when patients are matched with ideal organ donors, and the patients are actually prepared for the procedure in terms of evaluation. The biggest challenge in organ transplantation is managing the gap between demand for organs and the availability of organs. Additionally, kidney transplant cases can be managed with the coordination among a group of healthcare facilities in managing the overall process of organ transplantation in treatment of end-stage kidney disease.[5] In the Mediterranean Institute for Transplantation and Advanced Specialized Therapies, Italy (ISMETT), participation at the National Transplant Center created a virtual network of hospitals for the sharing of organ donor identification to better manage transplantation from deceased donors.[6] The intention of this effort was to reduce the number of deaths while patients were waiting for organ donation. The National Transplant Center in Italy has created a national programme of protocols and procedures to regulate the management of organs for donation and increasing the number of donors and thus, the transplants.[7] The investigators were also able to demonstrate that telemedicine with videoconferencing in a tele-ICU environment allows early identification of patients who presented with the criteria required to enrol into waiting list. Telehealth is an effective mechanism for immediate management of deceased donors and allows coordination with recipient team management which may be at a distant hospital.[8]

Sigireddi and Carrion have surveyed the use of Extension for Community Healthcare Outcomes (ECHO) telehealth model to conduct pre-liver transplant evaluation of patients.[9] This practice allows for hospital programmes or physicians to seek assistance from experts in the clinical speciality with knowledge and expertise to reach the patients in underserved locales. This has prevented patients from travelling long distances for the initial evaluation as candidacy to receive organ transplantation. Within the United States Department of Veterans Affairs (VA), the Web-based referrals and telehealth programmes are used as part of the National Transplant Program to improve access to healthcare systems for the patients. One Veterans Administration hospital system evaluated the waitlist experience of kidney transplant candidates by incorporating telehealth practices.[10] Clinics used videoconferencing telehealth practices for pre-transplant kidney waitlist evaluation of the patients. This allows the initial evaluation of the patient before the in-patient phase. The outcome with the use of web-based telehealth sessions was that patients could be evaluated sooner with a reduced wait time for initial evaluation; this particularly helped elderly patients.

Additionally, early preventive measures monitored with telehealth practices can reduce complications following the organ transplantation. For example, analysis of liver transplant patients revealed that cardiovascular disease is an aggravating factor for orthotopic liver transplantation. Thus, the benefit of pre-transplant evaluation of cardiac parameters in recipient candidates including electrocardiogram, echocardiography, and exercise stress testing was studied. The outcome was that the investigators were able to profile cardiac risks in liver transplant patients and institute early risk management.[11]

The experience of waiting for transplantation can be a source of psychological impact. Stress management for kidney transplant candidates was evaluated with a mindfulness-based stress reduction programme. Overall, the use of telephone-based teleconference allowed for additional patient engagement sessions from their physical location with mentors and the outcome was noted to be beneficial while preventing long-distance travel.[12]

Role of telehealth in the in-patient phase

The surgical or procedural phase of the transplant process is institution based or within the hospital. In this instance, there can be less motivation to incorporate Telehealth practices. Earlier studies did evaluate the mechanism for sharing the actual surgical field during a surgical procedure.(13) While sharing the surgical field during the procedure was feasible, the concerns for privacy during video transmission and ensuring less distraction of the surgeon during the procedure were of greater concern. One case study did attempt to use telemedicine for paediatric liver transplantation with real-time monitoring and consultation. The consulting team was a Philadelphia, USA, based anaesthesia team connecting to a transplant surgical team in Bangalore, India.(14) Unfortunately, technical challenges made it difficult for successful consultation during the surgery. The consequence was the understanding of the importance of network and computer connections as essential parts of telemedicine and telehealth programmes to be effective.

Telehealth in the follow up or post-transplant phase

In the follow-up phase, there is greater opportunity to integrate telehealth practices in managing patients and ensuring their successful recovery after the organ transplantation. This is especially significant when the transplant patient is viewed to have a similar level of health complexity to those suffering from chronic disease. One arena of follow up care is home monitoring for managing the symptoms that patients experience once they have been discharged from the hospital and preventing possible complications that may result in early readmission or graft failure. The capacity for integrating telehealth technologies within the patient's home is critical.

In cases of long-term care for lung transplant, the success depends on preventing chronic allograft rejection with the continuous monitoring of pulmonary function measurements through the use of daily home spirometry as the best preventive measure. In one study, following lung transplantation, it was possible to collect spirometry data from patients via text message to maintain patient engagement with the care plan and adjust treatments if symptoms are not as expected.[15] The collected data revealed early detection of any unexpected trends in lung performance. In a similar study, wireless transfer was used to collect spirometry data from home monitoring device.[16] Both examples support the hypothesis that home monitoring and data exchange with physicians within a telehealth framework is beneficial to patient recovery. Additionally, feedback messages to lung transplant patients via text messaging from the health care team were found to provide timely decision support to the patients.

A study using wireless technology to collect vital sign data from postoperative patients at home including patient's heart rate, systolic blood pressure, blood glucose, body weight, and temperature data reinforced patient management and successful recovery from surgery. The group of patients fully involved in data exchange had no incidence of readmission within the first thirty days after lung transplant.[17] This finding emphasizes the proactive role of patient-provider interaction in telehealth settings.

Telehealth can also be used to support home monitoring successfully with the use of software in mobile devices as well as questionnaires to monitor patient's well-being following liver transplant in children.[18] Similarly, it is critical for kidney transplant patients to include management of hypertension to prevent premature graft loss. In this study, patients were given blood pressure monitoring devices after surgery for use at home that could transfer their data to the hospital system via the Internet. The study was beneficial as it allowed patient engagement and involvement and the awareness of their symptoms changing over time.[19] Overall, case management with a team of care providers was considered an essential element in being certain that patients are followed regularly for the first post-transplant year using telehealth and revealed reduction in unplanned inpatient acute care.[20] This level of patient engagement reduced nonadherence significantly.

Another variable for the risk of transplant failure is the lack of therapeutic medication compliance by transplant patients. One very important part of the patient's recovery is the adherence to the medication regimen. Thus, the role of a pharmacist is a critical component of the overall care as described by the United Network for Organ Sharing (UNOS). In this context, Jandocitz et al demonstrated that the health centre's pharmacist being in direct contact via telemedicine was an essential part in improving recovery of patients from the transplant procedure.(21) Their dialogue ensured that patients were educated in medication use and were compliant in the treatment. Additional tools for ensuring patients' adherence to medication protocols are mobile technologies. The use of smartphone text messaging with paediatric liver transplant patients was studied and the overall outcome was noted to be an improvement in the level of medication use and a decrease in cellular rejection episodes.(22) Similarly, young adult patients were evaluated to assess if they could benefit more from mobile tools. Such a tool was included in adolescent patient treatment care to ensure compliance with immunosuppressive treatments since they are easy to adapt in using mobile technologies.(23)

The integration of telemedicine in managing organ transplant patients can address some unique challenges in the healthcare systems. For example, the typical backlog of patients waiting in clinics for follow-up visits after transplantation can be managed with telehealth. The use of video conferencing connection between patient and physician was found to be effective in reducing patient wait times for follow up visits.(24) Additionally, the mental state of the patient undergoing organ transplant cannot be overlooked. Understanding that mental shifts such as depressive states can impact treatment outcomes. For example, investigators integrated video conference capabilities and found such a service to be beneficial for the follow up patients.(25)

Review of cost benefits with telehealth integration

Telehealth continues to proliferate in the healthcare industry because of the increased technical evolutions and the ease with which technology is adaptable to engage the patients while they are away from the healthcare facility. In addition to the convenience of access by patients to healthcare teams, the ability to reduce costs is a major driver to integrate telehealth in patient care.(26) Programmes that have integrated videoconferencing as a telehealth practice to manage patients in being evaluated as candidates for organ transplant have analysed the associated costs. Studies on the overall costs for these visits show that associated travel costs for the patients to the clinic and the cost of the clinic for a patient consultation are lowered with telehealth.[27] To manage post kidney transplantation patients, a health system in Germany integrated the telemedicine-based information sharing between transplant centres and nephrologists. The goal was for care management and to sustain lower costs by reducing the rate of hospitalizations and by postponing the need for dialysis.[28] Similarly, the Royal Melbourne Hospital (RMH) in Australia evaluated the management of kidney transplant patients with videoconferencing and the associated impact on costs. While patients in rural areas had no access to local nephrology care, the opportunity for follow up post-transplant care with videoconference meetings allowed for reductions in significant time and expenditure from patients and staff resulting in overall cost savings.[29]

Conclusion

The beneficial opportunities of technologies for the organ transplant patient population in the telehealth arena are endless. This is supported by surveys of patients which have noted that the use of smartphones in monitoring health after organ transplant is an accepted practice.[30] Organ transplant is viewed as being a very complex healthcare event similar to chronic illness management. Innovative nationwide efforts such as the Health Village effort in Finland is seeking to establish digital health practices, or eHealth, to use a common electrical medical record (EMR) tool for sharing records amongst kidney transplant teams and overall nephrological patient care amongst multidisciplinary teams.[31] Coordinating organ transplants from the process of donation to receiving grafts and treatment with follow up can enable more opportunities with telehealth practices that incorporate eHealth tools. Across international borders, there are efforts to explore feasibility for integrated sharing of documents, patient information via effective communication technologies to allow coordination of organ transplant management.[32] Additionally, there are efforts to explore if technical capabilities such as drones can be used to transfer organ donation biological samples to be analysed in reference laboratories. It can be anticipated that such unmanned aerial vehicles can be used in the actual transport of organs from donation sites to receiving facilities. Also, drones can bring life-saving drugs to remote locations for patient management. This is a great benefit for patients that have limited access to transplant case management teams or patients that are not as mobile due to increased age.

Overall, technical advances in computing capacities, electronic medical record sharing, and smartphone software tools are proven to allow for infinite opportunities to integrate telehealth with organ donation. There are ongoing efforts in this evolution to even include the computing capacity of Artificial Intelligence to support clinical image analysis as well as clinical decision support methods. Innovative hardware technologies, software functional tools, and internet connections continue to allow secure and effortless communication between patients and healthcare transplant management teams into more common practice.

Highlights

- The delivery of health care for organ transplant patients is evolving to include computing technologies and Internet-based network access in the form of telehealth.
- Considering that organ transplantation is a complex process in terms of patient management, the use of telehealth facilitates an improved patient engagement.
- Telehealth has demonstrated positive feasibility in monitoring the progress of patients in the transplant process and in being certain that treatment plans are followed by the patient.
- Patient engagement by telehealth allows for patient compliance and reduction in complications following organ transplantation.
- Telehealth has demonstrated potential cost effectiveness for the patients when making follow up visits to hospitals, and for health care facilities in managing the patients at clinics and the volume of visits.

References

1. World Health Organization, editor. Telemedicine: Opportunities and Developments in Member States: Report on the Second Global Survey on EHealth. World Health Organization, 2010.

2. American Telemedicine Association. (2012). What is telemedicine. Retrieved at: http://www.americantelemed.org/about-telemedicine/what-is-telemedicine#.U-b7gIBdWt0.
3. About Telehealth | CCHP Website. Apr 01 2019. https://www.cchpca.org/about/about-telehealth. Accessed 18 Nov. 2019.
4. Mariea Snell Mariea Snell et al. 5 Ways Telehealth Is Taking Modern Healthcare to the Next Level. Technology Solutions That Drive Healthcare, Nov 2012. https://healthtechmagazine.net/article/2019/04/5-ways-telehealth-taking-modern-healthcare-next-level. Accessed 18 Nov. 2019.
5. Blinkhorn T. M. Telehealth in nephrology health care: a review Renal Society of Australasia Journal, 8(3), 132–139.
6. Bonsignore, Pasquale, et al. Crucial Role of Extended Criteria Donors in Deceased Donor Single Kidney Transplantation to Face Chronic Shortage in the Heart of the Mediterranean Basin: A Single-Center Experience. Transplantation Proceedings, vol. 51, no. 9, Nov. 2019, pp. 2868–72.
7. National Transplant Center; http://www.trapianti.salute.gov.it/trapianti Accessed 2 Jan. 2020
8. Gruttadauria, Salvatore, et al. Liver Transplantation for Hemoperitoneum Secondary to Huge Multiple Hemangiomatosis: A Case Report of a Tele-Intensive Care Unit in Deceased-Donor Management. Telemedicine Journal and E-Health, vol. 21, no. 6, June 2015, pp. 499–502.
9. Sigireddi, Rohini R., and Andres F. Carrion. Improving Access to Liver Transplantation through the ECHO Telehealth Model. Texas Heart Institute Journal, vol. 46, no. 1, Feb. 2019, pp. 61–62.
10. Forbes, Rachel C., et al. Implementation of Telehealth Is Associated with Improved Timeliness to Kidney Transplant Waitlist Evaluation. Journal of Telemedicine and Telecare, vol. 24, no. 7, Aug. 2018, pp. 485–91.
11. Główczyńska, Renata, et al. The Pre-Transplant Profile of Cardiovascular Risk Factors and Its Impact on Long-Term Mortality After Liver Transplantation. Annals of Transplantation, vol. 23, Aug. 2018, pp. 591–97.
12. Reilly-Spong, Maryanne, et al. Telephone-Adapted Mindfulness-Based Stress Reduction (TMBSR) for Patients Awaiting Kidney Transplantation: Trial Design, Rationale and Feasibility. Contemporary Clinical Trials, vol. 42, May 2015, pp. 169–84.
13. Rafiq, Azhar, et al. Digital Video Capture and Synchronous Consultation in Open Surgery. Annals of Surgery, vol. 239, no. 4, Apr. 2004, pp. 567–73.
14. Fiadjoe, John, et al. Telemedicine Consultation and Monitoring for Pediatric Liver Transplant. Anesthesia & Analgesia, vol. 108, no. 4, Apr. 2009, p. 1212.
15. Fadaizadeh, Lida, et al. Home Spirometry: Assessment of Patient Compliance and Satisfaction and Its Impact on Early Diagnosis of Pulmonary Symptoms in Post-Lung Transplantation Patients. Journal of Telemedicine and Telecare, vol. 22, no. 2, Mar. 2016, pp. 127–31.
16- Sengpiel, Juliane, et al. Use of Telehealth Technology for Home Spirometry after Lung Transplantation: A Randomized Controlled Trial. Progress in Transplantation (Aliso Viejo, Calif.), vol. 20, no. 4, Dec. 2010, pp. 310–17.

17. Ertel, Audrey E., et al. Use of Video-Based Education and Tele-Health Home Monitoring after Liver Transplantation: Results of a Novel Pilot Study. Surgery, vol. 160, no. 4, Oct. 2016, pp. 869–76.
18. Song, Bianying, et al. Home Monitoring and Decision Support for International Liver Transplant Children. Studies in Health Technology and Informatics, vol. 192, 2013, pp. 268–72.
19. Aberger, Edward W., et al. Enhancing Patient Engagement and Blood Pressure Management for Renal Transplant Recipients via Home Electronic Monitoring and Web-Enabled Collaborative Care. Telemedicine and E-Health, vol. 20, no. 9, July 2014, pp. 850–54.
20. Schmid, A., et al. Telemedically Supported Case Management of Living-Donor Renal Transplant Recipients to Optimize Routine Evidence-Based Aftercare: A Single-Center Randomized Controlled Trial. American Journal of Transplantation, vol. 17, no. 6, June 2017, pp. 1594–605.
21. Jandovitz, Nicholas, et al. Telemedicine Pharmacy Services Implementation in Organ Transplantation at a Metropolitan Academic Medical Center. Digital Health, vol. 4, Dec. 2018, p. 2055207618789322.
22. Miloh, Tamir, et al. Improved Adherence and Outcomes for Pediatric Liver Transplant Recipients by Using Text Messaging. Pediatrics, vol. 124, no. 5, Nov. 2009, pp. e844–50.
23. Reber, S., et al. Mobile Technology Affinity in Renal Transplant Recipients. Transplantation Proceedings, vol. 50, no. 1, Feb. 2018, pp. 92–98.
24. Le, Long B., et al. Patient Satisfaction and Healthcare Utilization Using Telemedicine in Liver Transplant Recipients. Digestive Diseases and Sciences, vol. 64, no. 5, 2019, pp. 1150–57.
25. Shih, F. Jin, et al. Dilemma of Applying Telehealth for Overseas Organ Transplantation: Comparison on Perspectives of Health Professionals and e-Health Information and Communication Technologists in Taiwan. Transplantation Proceedings, vol. 46, no. 4, May 2014, pp. 1019–21.
26. Thompson, Denise A., et al. Assessment of Depressive Symptoms During Post-Transplant Follow-Up Care Performed via Telehealth. Telemedicine and E-Health, vol. 15, no. 7, Aug. 2009, pp. 700–06.
27. Why Telehealth Technology Isn't Enough. 3 Jan 2017. https://www.advisory.com/500?aspxerrorpath=/research/service-line-strategy-advisor/resources/posters/telehealth-technology-isnt-enough. Accessed 19 Jun. 20219
28. Forbes, Rachel C., et al. A Cost Comparison for Telehealth Utilization in the Kidney Transplant Waitlist Evaluation Process. Transplantation, vol. 102, no. 2, 2018, pp. 279–83.
29. Pape, L., et al. The KTx360°-Study: A Multicenter, Multisectoral, Multimodal, Telemedicine-Based Follow-up Care Model to Improve Care and Reduce Health-Care Costs after Kidney Transplantation in Children and Adults. BMC Health Serv Res 2017;17(1):587.
30. Barraclough, K., et al. SAT-073 Travel, Cost and Environmental Savings Resulting from Telehealth follow up of Kidney Transplant Recipients: A Single Centre Experience. Kidney International Reports, vol. 4, no. 7, Supplement, July 2019, pp. S33–34.

31. McGillicuddy, John William, et al. Patient Attitudes toward Mobile Phone-Based Health Monitoring: Questionnaire Study among Kidney Transplant Recipients. Journal of Medical Internet Research, vol. 15, no. 1, Jan. 2013, p. e6.
32. Savikko, J., and V. Rauta. Implementing EHealth in Kidney Transplantation in Finland. Transplantation Proceedings, vol. 51, no. 2, Mar. 2019, pp. 464–65.

68
Communication and organ donation

Alessandro Pacini

Introduction

For centuries it has not been necessary to define death as the common sense identified it with irreversible respiratory arrest together with the appearance of cadaveric phenomena. Important changes have occurred over the last 100 years in the definition and confirmation of death from a clinical and an ethical point of view with subsequent legal implications.

At first, modern scientific knowledge offered means to identify the time of death with the cessation of cardiac activity in addition to respiratory arrest. New therapeutic opportunities such as artificial ventilation and pharmacological and mechanical circulatory support have further modified these concepts, leading to clinical pictures in which the total loss of brain functions is accompanied by cardio-circulatory artificially assisted functions occurring in the Intensive Care Unit (ICU).

There are possibilities of irreversible cessation of entire brain in a patient undergoing intensive resuscitation treatments such as artificial ventilation, or peripheral circulation supported by the residual cardiac activity, either spontaneous or pharmacologically induced, and this condition is called brain death. The Harvard criteria for brain death, 1968, have been codified in the law of every State.

The determination of death with irreversible cessation of the functions of the entire brain has led to an important conceptual change that today is not well understood by the public opinion with residual difficulties even for the professionals.[1–4]

Laws were adapted to this new reality not only for responding to the need of the scientific community but also for the relevant legal effects connected to the transformation of the human being (subject) into a dead body (object). In the meantime, the ethical concept of violation of a dead body as an act contrasting the value of compassion for the deceased was superseded by charity and solidarity when transplant medicine showed the possible use of organs taken from a donor.[5]

Family members of ICU patients

Several emotional aspects connected with death, which represents a universal source of anguish, remain unsolved. When death causes the loss of a family member we keep the image, love, and memory in order to lessen the sense of emptiness. There is active regret for what could have been and had not, the guilt for many little things and many more feelings. This great deal of emotions, the pain, and the tearing conflicts lead, comprehensibly, to refuse a family member's death. The passage of time and the difficult process of mourning will restore the balance.

In addition, the attitudes towards the cadaver are deeper and stronger. Many anthropologists trace the beginning of human history with the respect for the corpse and the burial rites. It is important to highlight that the study of the dead body has been forbidden for centuries and that autopsy arouses fear and resistance.[6]

Between the refusing organ donation and consenting to organ harvesting, there is a wide range of feelings that the family should cope with. The members of the family should accept the loss of a loved one and allow the organ donation with the aim of saving life for one or more unknown human beings. The family should deal with the psychological and ethical dilemma between choosing the sacredness of the body and organ donation.

The modern resuscitation techniques that have determined the appearance of brain death and consequently the need to ascertain death with neurological criteria have revolutionized how death is conceived by operators. Accentuated fears and doubts about the reality of corpse being still warm, with pulse and chest still expanding are worsened by the short time which makes it impossible for the family to cope with the loss and decide within few hours.

It is, therefore, clear that the application of law cannot be a simple notary's deed but it constitutes an important therapeutic act within a wide process that allows the family to cope with the mourning. This process accompanies the family in accepting the violability of the dead body for an ethical, higher goal.

The ICU represents the place where clinical practice, ethical values, and the law concerning death find a unifying moment. In the last decades, due to modern technologies and pharmacological therapies, this ward had to confront the growing need of dealing with the relational aspects of the families with their patients who struggle for life. Often there is a conflict between the healthcare facility and the family's needs when the family members cannot keep an adequate and continuous relationship with their loved ones. In addition, the family has to make a difficult decision that affects a particular relationship and involvement of the staff.[1,7,8]

It is very important to accompany the family during the whole pathway in ICU starting from the hospital admission as the physical distance to patient can cause anxiety, anger, depression, and ideas not related to the reality.

However, this situation does not improve when the family is at the bedside of a dying loved one, as the complex therapeutic equipment they may see and the staff's involvement deprive them of a direct and active participation, causing more anguish.

It is absolutely necessary that the whole ICU staff (doctors and nurses) understands all these aspects for a better reception of the family and the subsequent involvement in the care pathway.

Strategy of communication of brain death

The communication process in ICU requires the involvement of all operators and needs, especially when a brain death occurs in a potential organ donor, the absolute respect of certain roles and a precise strategy that can allow the comprehension of death and the acceptance of a donation. Until the information on the decease, the main actors are the ICU doctors and the nurses.[2,4,7]

In this phase a trained professional (transplant coordinator, doctor, and/or nurse who can work in the same ICU or in another ward) can 'go on stage' meaning inform family about the death and organ donation.

The Spanish specialists have considered this profession as the keystone for a better process that begins with death determination until the procurement of organs and tissues.[2,8–11]

In this phase, this devoted professional will begin to understand the family situation. They get all the necessary details that can be useful, after death determination, to help the family members in a pathway of comprehension and acceptance of death. They support the family in this early mourning phase until gradually requesting for organ and tissues donation.

In the relationship with the family it is important to set goals at the arrival of the patient to ICU.

1) The first aim is at establishing a good therapeutic alliance, mutual understanding, and trust with the family that allow to experience together this pathway of pain. Empathy and human touch expressed with non-verbal communication focusing on little gestures are very important.
   Particular attention is paid to the place where the professional meets the family (it is counterproductive to talk in the corridor). The use of a special room or—if not available—the doctor's lounge is strongly recommended. Genuine attention should be given to listening, because it is therapeutic for the family even if very difficult for the professionals.
2) Another aim is at letting the family understand from the beginning the real clinical situation, its evolution, the meaning of the therapies, and the results that can be achieved, without offering false hopes.

The language must be very easy and not technical as the main aim is at obtaining the full alliance with the family. The family members must be certain that everything possible is being done and it is important that doubts do not arise on the strategies and goals of the professional taking care of the patient. As part of care structure, it is also important to offer the involvement of external specialists to support, if the family wishes it.

When death is about to occur, it is important that the doctor gradually communicates the treatment failure and the poor prognosis. The whole relationship is established from the beginning with the ward and all the professionals play their roles. The relationships among the staff members, grade of efficiency of the structure and communication attitude are all essential for the donation process.

The family members must be aware that every possible effort has been done to let the patient survive and that death diagnosis is based on several factual elements. The diagnosis of death will be confirmed according to the legal criteria established by each nation, in order to avoid any possible uncertainty about this evaluation as the legislation on ascertaining death varies in different countries.

We should keep in mind that for many doctors, it is a thankless task to give information and explanations whenever enquired by the family. Doctors have problems in approaching the family of their patients, particularly when they have to communicate the decease and often dump on the patient family the frustration and anxiety derived from their job.

The resuscitator could begin expressing his/her feelings of pain, for example, 'I am sorry to inform you that the tests carried out', gently introducing the concept of death by expressions that lead to deduce it, for example, 'did not give the desired results'. It is desirable that the family member becomes aware through a personal process of deduction rather than the doctor representing the harsh reality of death.

In this phase, it is important to ask open questions that eases the expression of feelings and actively listen to facilitate a smooth relational process. It is necessary to explain the irreversibility of the situation adapting to the cultural level of the family and trying to give clear and easy answers.

It is important to use expressions that can introduce the family to the concept of death. It is better to use phrases like 'his/her brain does not live any more' than 'his/her brain is dead'; 'this is the final or terminal situation' and wait for the reaction of the family, instead of 'is deceased or is dead'.

In addition, it is important to explain that their loved one is not conscious anymore and breathing with the respirator. The body is artificially kept warm because there is some blood circulation as the heart is still beating due to pharmacological treatment. This will last for a short time because all the organ functions are deteriorating.

The family members often think that a coma is occurring and ask for the confirmation on how a person can come out of a coma. In this case, it must be emphasized that someone who is in a coma is alive while their loved one is in brain death, which means they are dead.

If the family members neither react nor understand the explanation, they will ask further doubts again. They should be offered help and the explanation repeated as much as necessary (much patience and availability of time are needed). Gradually, more painful words are used but with calm and low-pitched voice apologizing for what has to be told to them.

These are moments of great tension; therefore, the ICU professionals involved should reduce the tension with pauses and with the help of listening with interest what the family members say and give a positive evaluation, but returning to the mourning.

For example: 'I know that you are confused. Would you like to ask me any questions?' 'I can understand that in this moment you are not even able to think. Would you like to speak with anybody? A friend, a family member, a priest, etc.'

Questions on burial services or talk of the deceased with the past tense, etc., are indications on the grade of comprehension of the family. It is necessary to keep in mind that during the conversation the family members will try to find the culprits of the occurred death (their guilt, society, the healthcare system, etc.). It is important to let them express their feelings and in case of self-accusation, trying to reduce it without diminishing their feelings. 'I understand that you can feel guilty for . . . , but this could have happened in many other ways.'

The circumstances and destiny must be blamed. Their feelings must be continuously controlled in order to help them from the beginning of mourning.

The role of transplant coordinator

The transplant coordinator must be aware that the subsequent request of donation is largely dependent on the comprehension and trust level that has been reached till then.

During the phase of communication of death, the transplant coordinator, who is introduced by the resuscitator as a doctor delegated by the Medical Direction to help the family in that difficult moment, can assist them in understanding the condition of brain death.[9,10]

During this first contact, the transplant coordinator assesses the family's attitude: calm, hysterical, or angry; and tries to find the most receptive and favourable family member. The coordinator also assesses the necessary approach for the support relationship and whether the family has understood their loved one's death. This last aspect is very important as we cannot proceed with a donation interview if the family has not understood death.

The transplant coordinator, in this role of supporting the potential donor's family, must not be experienced by colleagues in the RTI with frustration as a theft to their role in the RTI. Instead, he must be seen as an expert colleague (doctor or nurse) who, with the help of all RTI professionals, by implementing an effective communication strategy, aims to help the bereaved family and receive consent to the donation.

The Spanish have comprehensively studied the process and have found that to devolve a skilled professional in this phase is the best strategy to help the family in the hard experience and help to obtain the donation consent.[(10)]

This derives from the consideration that for the family, the resuscitator is the doctor who safeguards their loved one's health at all costs. For them, it becomes difficult to see the role of resuscitator changed from attending to their patient's health to attending to the health of possible waiting list patients, after the death of potential donor. When a patient dies, he becomes a potential organ donor. The resuscitator ensures maintenance of good functionality of the deceased' organs and ensures to make them available for transplantation of patients in the waiting list.

For medical team, this can represent redemption from a therapeutic failure; however, this role change can put in crisis the therapeutic alliance which was so important from the beginning for the family.

Devoting a specific professional to perform the subsequent phase and the need to offer an adequate psychological help to the family (in terms of time and competence in this matter) in these initial phases of mourning (support relationship) represent a positive aspect because this role could not be played by the ICU professionals; they are overburdened not only caring for the potential donor but also several other patients in the ward. As we have seen, the communication of death needs much of their time, causing sometimes a crisis in the ward organization.

Brain death in the mass media

The concept of brain death, in case of radio or television interviews, should be treated with high professionalism, clarity, and simplicity. The doubt on brain death represents one of the most forbidden themes, which is better not to deal with, unless it is directly requested by the interviewer or by direct questions on air.

The general principles are: (1) have a prepared answer always; (2) short sentences with structured subjects; (3) clear and credible message, no technicalities; (4) energetic tone and without suspect of doubt.

We should let the audience understand with easy words that brain destruction corresponds to death and in these conditions, with artificial systems located in ICU, blood circulation in the dead body can be maintained until all the necessary acts to certify the death are performed and make the cadaver available for the donation. Otherwise, every artificial treatment will be stopped and the deceased will be transferred to the morgue.

It is important to remember that every patient deceased in the ICU due to brain lesion is a potential organ donor. This donor is a dead body, never a patient, regardless of whether or not his/her organs and tissues will be donated.

Never use the term coma (add the term irreversible instead) as it can cause ambiguity with other situations.

Conclusion

The issue of organ donation, which has developed in recent decades due to modern resuscitation techniques, has led to an improvement in both the relational climate among RTI healthcare workers and among them with the families of patients hospitalized in serious clinical conditions and with poor prognoses. Both the relations are crucial in the reporting and evaluation pathways of potential organ donors with the consequent increase in transplants of patients on the waiting list. Healthcare professionals have made a leap in professional quality, starting to take charge not only of the clinical problems of the patient to be treated, but also of the psycho-relational support of his family and the expectations of possible patients on the waiting list for a transplant that could benefit of a donation. The transplant coordinator (doctor or nurse) is the new professional figure that the Spaniards have experienced over the years in various hospitals. They have contributed to favouring this organizational improvement of the health facilities and of all transplant pathways, supporting these relational and communication aspects in the care pathways.

Highlights

- Death is no longer the end of life, but an opportunity for the continuity of life.
- It is important to take care not only of the patient in RTI but also of his family and patients on the waiting list for an organ transplant.
- The communication strategy is crucial in the care path of the brain-injured patient in RTI to favour the donation of organs and tissues.
- It is essential to provide correct information to the population on the subject of brain death.

References

1. De Bertolini, C, Rupolo GP. La sofferenza psicologica in rianimazione, Paltron Editore, Bologna, 1986, 67–88.
2. Nile, PA, Mattice BJ. The timing factor in the consent process, Journal of the Transplant Coordinator, 1996, 6/2, 84–87.
3. Rupolo GP, Mazzon D, Mascarin S, De Bertoni C, Pozansky C. Il rianimatore e la famiglia del donatore protagonisti di una scelta difficile, Psicologia e psichiatria del trapianto d'organi, Masson Editore.1999
4. Reader TW, Flin R., Cuthbertson BH. Communication skills and error in the intesive care unit, Curr Opin Crit Care, 2007, 13: 732–736.
5. Moore FD. Three Ethical Revolutions: Ancient Assumptiom Remodeled Under Pressure of Transplantation, Transplantation Proceedings, 1988, 1, 1061–1067.
6. Prioreschi P. Determinanti della rinascita della dissezione del corpo umano nel Medioevo, Ipotesi Mediche (2001) (2):56–57.
7. Gardner D, Stewart N. Staff envolvement with families of patients in critical care unit, Heart Lung, 1978, 1, 105.
8. Perez-San Gregorio MA, Blanco-Picaria A. et al. Psychological problems in the family members of gravely traumatised patients admitted into an intensive care unit, Intesive Care Medicine, 1992 a, 18, 279–281.

9. Manialich M, Procaccio F, Gianelli Castiglione A, Nanni Costa A, Manuale Corso Nazionale Coordinatori alla Doanzione a al prelievo, Ed. Compositori (BO), 2012
10. Santiago Guervos C, Gomez Marinero P. Sequenza dell'intervista di donazione, Dispense Corso famiglia e donazione Regione Toscana 2003, 52–60.
11. Trabucco G, Marcanti M, Procaccio F. Dalla criticità al processo, il ruolo delle emozioni nel percorso di donazione, Trapianti, XII, 2009, 135–143.

SECTION 6.

ETHICS AND ORGAN DONATION

69

The consent to organ donation: Opt-in versus opt-out

Deepak Gupta, Anna Teresa Mazzeo, Marco Mazzeo

Introduction

Organ transplantation is indispensable for ensuring the survival of patients with end-stage organ diseases. There is a worldwide shortage of donor organs for transplantation. Although transplant activity has increased globally during recent decades, there remains an insufficient supply of organs to satisfy demand all around the world. While dead persons cannot be harmed by the removal of their organs, the existing sick people and the society, in general, stand to benefit from them (utilitarian and communitarian view).[1] It is estimated that only a small percentage of demand for organs is met while a large percentage of patients die waiting for organ transplants globally.[2] The disparity between supply and demand for organs exists even in countries with an established infrastructure to facilitate transplantation and exhibiting solid results over years. Different strategies have been developed to bridge this gap and ensure that patients do not die waiting for organ transplantation.

The availability of deceased organ donation depends upon the desire or disposition of the person deceased (during life) or the relatives to authorize or veto organ and tissues retrieval.[3]

Different consent models for organ donation

Though only a multifaceted approach can produce significant and lasting results, a topic of special interest in the arena of transplantation is the possibility of adopting different consent models to increase organ donation worldwide. Among fundamental questions in medicine, the appropriate model of consent in transplantation medicine is one of the most debated questions around the world for which a unique approach is far to be reached. In particular, adopting an opt-out system for organ donation (termed 'presumed or deemed consent') versus an opt-in system (termed 'explicit consent') has been proposed to increase organ donor rates, with both positive and negative factors keenly debated.(4,5)

Expressed or presumed consent

Informed consent is crucial in any medical activity and represents the basis for a transparent patient-physician relationship. Trust in healthcare services is essential in this reciprocal alliance and failure to build such a fiduciary relationship will create suspicion, doubts, and eventually result in adverse feelings.

Consent process, whether expressed or presumed, retains a central place in the legal and ethical analysis of transplantation practices.(6) Expressed informed consent alone may not suffice due to multiple reasons including failure of potential donors to sign written directives while alive, possible difficulties in finding the donor cards, failure of hospital personnel to approach families when a donor card is missing.(7) On the other hand, presumed/deemed consent can be misleading because consent is hypothetical and a real positive indication for organ donation after death is lacking.(7,8)

It is often difficult to choose between 'ethics' and 'common good' when it comes to presumed consent in organ donations. Presumed consent has been criticized as a potential violation of the right to choose how one's body will be used after death and potential exploitation of the most vulnerable persons with the risk of not equitable allocation of organs.(7,9) Furthermore, few cultural and religious doctrines emphasize the sacredness of the body, even when the individual has been declared dead.(7,10) Presumed consent laws have also been criticized for taking for granted that organs belong to the society rather than to each person or family.(7) Though presumed consent models may reduce organ shortages, it is important to consider the feelings that society has towards such a change in legislation.

Any chosen system has to balance the value of solidarity with the respect for autonomous choices of the individual in a matter that is rich in ethical, philosophical, religious, and social pressures.

Opt-in versus opt-out consent

Consents, in the context of organ donations, can be either opt-in consent (expressed wish to donate by applicant) or opt-out consent (wherein there is expressed wish not to donate organs) (Box 69.1). In the opt-out system, the willingness to donate is the default option, unless the person explicitly opts not to be an organ donor.

'Opt-in' or 'contracting in' is a system allowing organ donation after death only with appropriate consent.[7] It is estimated that currently 40%

Box 69.1 Opt-in versus opt-out consent model in organ donation

OPT-IN:

Explicit consent

Expressed wish to donate, through organ donor register or organ donor cards

Donor choice is clear and unequivocal.

Relief of family stress during end-of-life discussions and protection against family interference as majority on organ donor register hasn't discussed with family.

OPT-OUT:

Presumed or deemed consent

Expressed wish not to donate

Non selecting opt-out where legislature exists for opt-out, donors are presumed to be consenting for organ donation after death by the state government.

'Soft' opt-out: the family is consulted.

'Hard' opt-out: family is not consulted

of those who opt-in and are in organ donor registers may have not discussed their willingness with family; therefore, without knowing potential donor preferences, the family can't choose with serenity and may refuse organ donation when proposed.[7] In India, opt-in consent model is in practice since the beginning. Lack of widespread awareness programmes and religious and cultural overtones are associated with failure of opt-out system in India.[7]

'Opt-out' or 'contracting out system' of organ donation is the model allowing organ donation unless an express objection is made by the person before the death and is considered to bridge the gap between intention and action. This system could address the possible laziness or apathy or procrastination of those citizens who would have liked to donate. Furthermore, experimental evidence suggests presuming organ donation as the default option for citizens may make them consider that to be a natural choice, whereas presuming the opposite makes the choice special rather than the norm.

In opt-out model, therefore, citizens are automatically deemed to consent for organ donation unless they register an opt-out decision.

There are two types of 'opt-out' systems: a 'soft' opt-out where the family is consulted prior to organ donation to ask their agreement and to honour their wishes, and a 'hard' opt-out where the family is not consulted about the deceased's wishes on organ donation. Regardless of opt-in or opt-out system, it is considered desirable that transplant coordinators and involved teams approach potential donor family to assist them in the most difficult moment of their life. They discuss available options with the ultimate opportunity to offer the family the possibility to express the will of their loved one. This is because it is generally accepted that closest relatives are likely to know what deceased relative wishes would have been, and are most likely to act accordingly.

Opt-out system is assumed to be a civic duty and it may reduce waiting list. It is often a relief at the most stressful time.

Majority of donors who opt-out have fears concerning the validity of brain death criterion as a method of defining irreversible total body death and fear of government control of organs after death. Among critiques to opt-out consent, legislation is the accepting absence of objection as given permission for donation that could undermine the ethical principles of informed consent. On the contrary, the declared choice for individuals in the opt-in system could be a guarantee of their wishes to be honoured, and not overridden by distressed families at the time of death.[11] Deemed consent is advantageous primarily for those who have not actioned intentions to be an organ donor due to laziness and for those with psychological ambivalence towards organ donation as it protects them from making a difficult choice.[11]

Evidences from literature

It is known that proper communication is a critical aspect in the field of organ donation and especially when consent is asked so that individual decisions can be influenced even by minor changes in the terms used and type of language,[12] and this is especially true for topics that are dealt with usual reluctance, such as death. Participation or non-participation of people in a choice is certainly influenced also by the meaning that they individually and collectively attach to the opt-in or opt-out choice in question.[12] Therefore, each country should consider that the way of proposing options relevant to personal and societal decisions will directly influence the meanings that become attached to those decisions, and therefore, will influence the response and the final effect of the proposal.

To overcome the shortage of organ donors globally, several countries have adopted an opt-out donor consent system (France, Greece, Portugal, Spain, Luxemburg, Austria, Belgium, Denmark, Great Britain, and Italy, among others). In some countries, such as Belgium, Spain, and Austria, this resulted in a positive effect on rates of organ donation.[13,8] In other countries, such as Brazil, the opt-out model of consent did not result in the awaited increase of organ donation and transplantation, because it was not accompanied by adequate information and education of citizens.[10] An inadequate divulgation of the rationale of the new consent model at the public level, and also among health professionals and religious leaders were responsible for this failure and for the need to reintroduce opt-in model and family consent.

Several studies addressed the effect of opt-out versus opt-in model to increase organ donor number, with different results. Data analysis on organ donation and transplantation rates registered with the Organization for Economic Co-operation and Development demonstrated no significant difference in deceased donation or solid organ transplantation activity between opt-out versus opt-in countries.[14]

The study findings suggested no significant gain for established opt-in countries considering a switch to opt-out. Some countries observed impressive increase after the introduction of presumed consent, such as Belgium, while others fared badly with either no difference or an actual drop in organ donation rates, including Singapore, Brazil, Chile, Sweden, and more recently, Wales.[15] Wales is the only country within the United Kingdom to be achieving the target 80% family consent rate for deceased donation set by the UK Strategy 'Taking Organ Transplantation to 2020'.[15] Spain with 40 deceased organ donors and 100 transplant procedures per million population considered as a model for a successful deceased organ donation system has no official opt-out register, and family approval is always sought.[16] The learning from the Spanish model of organ transplant is the importance to invest in education, training, and infrastructure for organ transplantation. Presumed consent alone may fail to tackle the apathetic attitude and behaviour among the lay public regarding organ donation.

In the same study,[14] compared to opt-in countries, opt-out countries had fewer living donors per million population (4.8 vs 15.7 respectively) with no significant difference in deceased donors (20.3 vs 15.4 respectively).[14] Overall, no significant difference was observed in rates of kidney (35.2 vs 42.3 respectively), non-renal (28.7 vs 20.9 respectively), or total solid organ transplantation (63.6 vs 61.7 respectively). In a multivariate linear regression model, after adjusting for country-specific variables, an opt-out system was an independent predictor of fewer living donors but was not associated with the number of deceased donors or with transplantation rates.[14] Thus, a simplistic switch to the 'opt-out' model has unintended consequences for living organ donation that does not provide a 'quick fix' to improve donor rates.[14] Furthermore, it should be recognized that models and systems that are successful for some countries may not necessarily work in others.

In a recent systematic review focusing on literature published from 2006 to 2016, reporting data from USA, UK, and Spain, to analyse the effect of opt-out versus opt-in on organ donation and transplantation, an increase in deceased donation rate and deceased transplantation rate was demonstrated.[17] Four studies reported opt-out consent increases deceased donation rate by 21–76% over 5–14 years. Nevertheless, the authors underlined that future research should be focused on public education, awareness, and the role of family consent in the opt-out consent model.(17)

The implication of an opt-out organ transplant policy adoption has also been recently presented by DeRoos et al, in a study simulating the potential implications of a presumed consent policy in the United States.(18) The authors observed that such a policy was associated with modest improvements for waiting lists for all organs, but also emphasized that other factors, such as economic conditions, infrastructure changes, and healthcare system and society characteristics need to be considered when studying the effect of consent model changes.(18)

The positive effect of the implementation of a soft opt-out policy on improved consent rates for deceased organ donation in Wales was described by Noves et al, indicating that even if this cannot be the only strategy, it still represents the starting step of a long journey in this complex scenario.(19) Human Transplantation Act was fully enacted in 2015 in Wales with the primary aim to increase consent rates. In the Welsh soft opt-out system, unless the deceased person has expressed a decision in life (either for or against being an organ donor), it will be assumed that they have no objection to organ donation and their consent can be deemed.(19) In a study analysing data on organ donor registration activity for eighteen months after the introduction of Human Transplantation Act in 2015 in Wales, compared with up to three years pre-implementation, it was observed that the consent rate for all modes of consent was 61%, showing a recovery from the dip to 45.8% in 2014/2015.(19) About 62.4% of cases had registered or expressed their decision to opt-in, 16.5% opted-out, while the number of deceased donors remained relatively static. Authors concluded that further interventions are needed to reach the 2020 target of 80% consent rates.(19)

In a panel study to compare organ donor and transplant rates in forty-eight countries that had either opt-in or opt-out consent, over thirteen years between 2000 and 2012, there were significantly more deceased donors in opt-out than opt-in consent systems.(20) However, there were significantly more living donors in opt-in than opt-out consent systems. Furthermore, the authors observed that the number of living and deceased donors increased over the years. Interestingly, the results were confirmed even after Spain was removed from the analysis.[20] Opt-out consent was also associated with an increase in the total number of livers and kidneys transplanted.

However, as recently highlighted in an editorial article, the implementation of presumed consent alone is unlikely to explain the increased rates of organ donation between countries. Other factors play a significant synergistic role, such as early identification of potential donors from outside the intensive care unit, the use of expanded criteria for organ suitability and the development of donation after circulatory death.[21]

The fact that the introduction of presumed consent may potentially threaten the trust which is an essential component in any doctor-patient alliance, has been considered as a serious drawback related to this shift from opt-in to opt-out model of consent.[21] As for any new system, it is essential that its introduction is gradual, and is accompanied by a corollary of other essential factors to be successful, such as public awareness, among others, as learned from Spanish model.

The main rationale behind opt-out system is that it should bridge the gap between the favour towards organ donation and laziness, thus increasing the pool of potential donors.

A large survey of intentions towards opt-out legislation was conducted in Scotland, England, and Northern Ireland to explore the reasons for participants to plan for opt-in (n = 646), follow deemed consent (n = 205), opt-out (n = 32) and those who were not sure (n = 40). Participants who planned to actively opt-in identified four main reasons: making choices explicitly clear and unequivocal; organs can save lives, the importance of reciprocity (if willing to receive I should be willing to give) and personal experience of donation.[22] Opt-in group organ donors often understand the enormity and emotive nature of the donation decision-making process faced by grieving families.[22] Furthermore, willing to accept an organ in the event of future disease without willing to donate in the event of brain death is certainly not acceptable, so that priming people to consider this fact has led to a positive attitude towards organ donation.[11]

Recently, the Bill for opt-out legislation has been passed in Scotland and England and is planned for implementation in next years.[23] Following the introduction of opt-out consent legislation, if an individual has not registered an active donor choice, consent for organ donation is automatically presumed through deemed consent.[11,24]

While some of the variability in deceased donor rates after adoption of opt-out system might benefit of additional resources and infrastructure to make a deceased donation programme successful,[25] other factors such as the need of education to increase awareness should be considered. A significant lack of knowledge among young university students regarding the presumed post-mortem organ donation law has been recently documented in a study involving first-year students from the University of Porto.[26] The need for more adequate information to make informed end-of-life decisions about organ donation was also demonstrated in polytechnic students in Singapore.[27]

The importance of implementing residency school core curricula on determination of death by neurologic criteria, as a mean to improve awareness on all aspects related to organ donation and transplantation has been recently discussed by our group.[28]

Conclusions

Given that a high percentage of individuals die while waiting for a transplant from select communities, there is an urgent need to increase consent rates and the number of donations all around the world. Only after creating widespread awareness about organ donation and transplantation and addressing the religious, cultural, ethical overtones that are associated with it, this global aim can be reached. Better public awareness on the benefits of transplantation and continuous education of healthcare personnel, together with more dedicated infrastructure is the preferred way to achieve an increase in organ donation.

Finally, a multifaceted scenario, comprehending early identification of the potential organ donor, proper maintenance of the potential organ donor in the intensive care unit, reducing deceased donor solid organ discard rates, increased use of unconventional or high-risk organs, increased public and health system awareness, and better infrastructure dedicated to transplantation, together with the model of consent adequate at each country level, could represent the most successful strategy to adopt, to bridge the gap between supply and demand worldwide.

Highlights

- Opt-in system is one where anyone wishing to donate their organs in the event of death must provide consent by signing up to the organ donor register.
- Opt-out system is presumed consent by default. One is automatically assumed to give consent for the donation of his/her organs in the event of death unless he/she removes him/herself from the organ donor register.
- Family is not consulted in hard opt-out systems, while the family is consulted in soft opt-out organ donation systems.
- Disconnect between the wish for organ transplantation (if ever required) and simultaneous reluctance to be organ donors (if ever possible) is a factor to be addressed in modern society.
- Current evidence suggests that opt-in countries switching to opt-out mechanisms for organ donation do not guarantee an automatic increase in organ donation rates or solid organ transplantation activity if other essential factors are not contextually implemented.

References

1. Prabhu PK. Is presumed consent an ethically acceptable way of obtaining organs for transplant? J Intensive Care Soc. 2019 May;20(2):92–97.
2. Tullius SG, Rabb H. Improving the Supply and Quality of Deceased-Donor Organs for Transplantation. N Engl J Med. 2018;378:1920–1929.
3. MacDonald A. Organ Donation: The Time Has Come to Refocus the Ethical Spotlight. Stan L & Pol'y Rev. 1997;8:177–184.
4. John P. Merrill, Joseph E. Murray, J. Hartwell Harrison, Warren R. Guild. Landmark article Jan 28, 1956: Successful Homotransplantation of the Human Kidney Between Identical Twins. By John P. Merrill, Joseph E. Murray, J. Hartwell Harrison, and Warren R. Guild. JAMA.1984; 251(19):2566–2571.
5. Global Observatory on Donation and Transplantation. Organ Donation and Transplantation Activities: 2016 Activity Report. Global Observatory on Donation and Transplantation WHO-ONT collaboration [Internet]. 2016. Available from: http://www.transplant-observatory.org/download/2016-activity-data-report
6. Price D. Legal and ethical aspects of organ transplantation. Ist Edn. Cambridge University Press; 2000.
7. Kaushik J. Organ transplant and presumed consent: towards an opting out system. Indian J Med Ethics. 2009 Sep;6(3):149–152.

8. Michielsen P. Presumed consent to organ donation: 10 years' experience in Belgium. J R Soc Med. 1996 Dec;89(12):663–666.
9. Rithalia A, McDaid C, Suekarran S, Norman G, Myers L, Sowden A. A systematic review of presumed consent systems for deceased organ donation. Health Technol Assess Winch Engl. 2009 May;13(26):iii, ix–xi, 1–95.
10. Csillag C. Brazil abolishes 'presumed consent' in organ donation. Lancet Lond Engl. 1998 Oct 24;352(9137):1367.
11. Miller J, Currie S, O'Carroll RE. 'If I donate my organs it's a gift, if you take them it's theft': a qualitative study of planned donor decisions under opt-out legislation. BMC Public Health. 2019 Nov 6;19(1):1463.
12. Davidai S, Gilovich T, Ross LD. The meaning of default options for potential organ donors. Proc Natl Acad Sci U S A. 2012 Sep 18;109(38):15201–15205.
13. Matesanz R. Organ procurement in Spain. Lancet Lond Engl. 1992 Sep 19;340(8821):733.
14. Arshad A, Anderson B, Sharif A. Comparison of organ donation and transplantation rates between opt-out and opt-in systems. Kidney Int. 2019 Jun;95(6):1453–1460.
15. NHSBT. Organ Donation and Transplantation Activity Data: WALES [Internet]. 2019. Available from: https://nhsbtdbe.blob.core.windows.net/umbraco-assetscorp/ 15914/nhsbt-wales-summary-report-mar-19.pdf
16. Matesanz R, Domínguez-Gil B, Coll E, Mahíllo B, Marazuela R. How Spain Reached 40 Deceased Organ Donors per Million Population. Am J Transplant Off J Am Soc Transplant Am Soc Transpl Surg. 2017 Jun;17(6):1447–1454.
17. Ahmad MU, Hanna A, Mohamed A-Z, Schlindwein A, Pley C, Bahner I, et al. A Systematic Review of Opt-out Versus Opt-in Consent on Deceased Organ Donation and Transplantation (2006-2016). World J Surg. 2019 Dec;43(12):3161–3171.
18. DeRoos LJ, Marrero WJ, Tapper EB, Sonnenday CJ, Lavieri MS, Hutton DW, et al. Estimated Association Between Organ Availability and Presumed Consent in Solid Organ Transplant. JAMA Netw Open. 2019 Oct 2;2(10):e1912431.
19. Noyes J, McLaughlin L, Morgan K, Walton P, Curtis R, Madden S, et al. Short-term impact of introducing a soft opt-out organ donation system in Wales: before and after study. BMJ Open. 2019 03;9(4):e025159.
20. Shepherd L, O'Carroll RE, Ferguson E. An international comparison of deceased and living organ donation/transplant rates in opt-in and opt-out systems: a panel study. BMC Med. 2014 Sep 24;12:131.
21. The Lancet Gastroenterology Hepatology null. Organ donation: presumed consent is not enough. Lancet Gastroenterol Hepatol. 2018;3(10):655.
22. Miller J, Currie S, O'Carroll RE. 'What if I'm not dead?'—Myth-busting and organ donation. Br J Health Psychol. 2019;24(1):141–158.
23. Opt-out organ donation "in place by 2020" for England. BBC News; 2018.
24. Rosenblum AM, Horvat LD, Siminoff LA, Prakash V, Beitel J, Garg AX. The authority of next-of-kin in explicit and presumed consent systems for deceased organ donation: an analysis of 54 nations. Nephrol Dial Transplant Off Publ Eur Dial Transpl Assoc - Eur Ren Assoc. 2012 Jun;27(6):2533–2546.

25. Tennankore KK, Klarenbach S, Goldberg A. Perspectives on opt-out versus opt-in legislation for deceased organ donation: An opinion piece. Can J Kidney Health Dis. 2021;8:20543581211022151. doi: 10.1177/20543581211022151
26. da Silva Clemente Pinho R, Nogueira da Costa Santos CM, Resende Figueire do Duarte IM. Presumed post-mortem donors: The degree of information among university students. Observational Study. BMC Med Ethics. 2021;22:139.
27. Leung RWS, Ho BSZ, Fong GXY, Boh JJM, Chow YL, Thong DA, Kong SNM, Tan CK. Improving the communication and understanding of the opt-out organ donation law among young adults. Transplant Proc. 2021;53:2095–2104.
28. Mazzeo AT, Gupta D. Implementing residency school core curricula on determination of death by neurologic criteria: A further step toward better uniformity around the world. Transplantation. 2021;105:e48–e49.

70

Spiritualism, ethics in organ transplantation

Ashok K. Mahapatra

Introduction

Following ethical practice in medicine can never be overemphasized. Over the decades, the ethical values have gone down in every sphere of life, and medical profession is no exception. Resorting to unethical practice is not uncommon. Often in the case of organ transplantation, there is high demand for organs because of shortage of available donors, be it living or related, paid living or cadaver donors.[1–4] Due to increased longevity of life and also increased incidence of diabetes, hypertension, and other related kidney damage, the incidence of Chronic Kidney Disease (CKD), renal failure, liver failure, and such other conditions require more and more organ donations for transplantation.[5–7] In such situations, following ethical values have become more imperative than ever before.[1,7,9–12] The ethical and spiritual issues in organ transplantations in general, and Cadaver Organ Transplant in particular[8,9,12] have been highlighted in this chapter.

Unethical practices in organ transplantation

Looking back in the last seventy-five years, ever since organ transplantation started, it has become an obvious, viable alternate to organ failure patients.[1,5] Moreover, with improved care, surgical skill and advances in immunosuppression, it is almost possible for patients to have a normal life following the organ transplantation. For these reasons, the number of people waiting for transplantation has steadily increased, producing imbalance in demand and supply, thus necessitating unethical practices, by exchanging money.[3,7,12]

Unethical practices by donors

As per law organs can be donated by a first-class relative, or a friend in case of relative being unfit for donation. One can sell or purchase organ.[2,3,7,9] It cannot be the monopoly of the Transplant Surgeon to choose the recipient or oblige someone while others are waiting in the list. Almost four decades back, some patient's coma picture was released to show that doctors were killing patients with over dosage of anaesthesia rendering the patients' brain dead and thereafter, harvesting organs. Time and again it has also been reported that when some patient goes for laparotomy for some reason, one of the two kidneys is removed and sold to a recipient for exchange of money.[2,7] These are highly unethical practices and must be prevented.[9–11]

On the other hand, sometimes a living donor is found selling his/her organ to get money, with a false identity of being the patient's blood relation. To prevent these unethical practices in India, authorization committees were formed following the law in 1990s and modified in 2005 and 2014 respectively.[13,14]

Unethical practices by recipient family

In India the live donors outnumber the Cadaver Organ donors due to many reasons. They include lack of awareness in the treating physicians, problems in determining brain death, infection in brain in the dying patients, and more importantly, due to lack of a proper list of prospective recipients waiting to receive transplant. In live donor case, often relatives are unavailable or even if available, are not fit for donating organ. So, the recipient family tries to find out paid donors. Poor people in need for money do sell the organs[2,7,15–17] to such recipients. This used to be rampant, however, due to strict laws, such incidents have decreased across India, and the incidence of paid live donors has significantly reduced. Cadaver donation from brain-dead patients can also have potential scope for money exchange[7,10] which is unethical at any cost. To bust the racket of organ trading, the law has provided significant punishment under Indian organ transplant act. If crime is committed and proved, the paid donor can get five to ten years of imprisonment and 20 Lakh to 1 Crore Indian Rupees as fine[1] as per the Indian 'Human Organ Transplant Act' (THOA) 1994.

Indian Organ Transplant Act and ethical issues

All ethical issues were the highly emphasized guidelines of the Indian organ transplant act[1,5] and the law also had provision of punishment for malpractices. The Act has been modified several times in the last twenty-five years, understanding the limitations and loopholes.[13,14]

a) There are specified doctors who can certify brain death.
b) There are specified hospitals notified by the Government of India to carry out Cadaver organ transplantation.
c) For maintenance of donor, there should be no financial burden on donor family.
d) The transplant surgical team should not interact with donor family.
e) Transplant coordinator is the person who motivates and prepares all the documents as per law once the donor family is ready for organ donation.
f) Proper certification of brain death as per authorized persons prescribed by the Human Organ transplant act is essential.
g) Doctor cannot forcefully or by bribing the relatives to get the consent for organ donation from brain dead patients.
h) Brain death certifying team should not be part of Transplant team.
i) To facilitate post-mortem, the hospital authority should be able to conduct post- mortem at a priority basis, even beyond the official timing. The post-mortem expert must be available at the time of organ retrieval.
j) The organ agreed to be removed in consent form by the relatives can only be removed and not anything extra.

k) The brain death certificate team must meticulously follow brain death criteria certificate as prescribed in the Transplantation of Human Organ Act (THOA, 1994)

Few important criteria as per Euro transplant law

Ethical issues do vary to some extent from one country to another. The ethical issues guidelines followed in Europe are called 'Euro transplant'.[3] Everyone in the society, having realized the shortage of organs available for transplant, should try to maximize the utility of organs. Justice must be done in choosing recipient. It is generally believed to give organ to the sickest patient giving benefit to the worst of patients; however, this action has decreased chances of surgical success. It is also true that defining who among the patients benefit better is a difficult decision and is a major social issue. Thus, large number of factors must be considered to choose the patient for transplant, which include saving life, reducing mortality and morbidity, and relief of suffering caused by the disease. Hence urgency, medical benefit and first or second generation immigrants are few important criteria, as per Euro transplant law or guidelines.[3]

Ethical issues in American organ transplant law

Since 1954, the first human organ transplant was done in the US. The law has been modified several times in the US, considering many issues in any form of Organ Transplantation. An important consideration to take organ from a healthy person for a sick person is that you risk the health of the healthy person. When transplantation was attempted initially, the procedure resulted in varying degrees of success. As early as 1967, ethical issues were discussed by Starzl.[13] In 1966, Ciba Foundation sponsored a conference in London to discuss ethical issues in Transplantations. In 1968, Harvard Medical School appointed an ADHOC committee to find out if brain dead patients can be potential donors for Organ Transplant.[14] The documents produced by the Harvard Committee was widely accepted along with issues between brain death and persistent vegetative state; and being in a Vegetative state, like death, is a serious ethical issue even today.[18,19]

The US president constituted a commission on the request of US Congress[20] to further study brain death from the Organ transplantation point of view. The commission provided more extensive and precise criteria of brain death that was defined as irreversible, cessation of brain stem function.[15] Thus, the deck was cleared to harvest organs from braindead patients. There were also some controversies which were put to rest by the term 'non-beating heart donation'; in these patients, life support was removed prior to harvesting organ.

Over the years, success percentage of transplant has increased as compared to earlier years. Hence, many ethical issues of 1960s and 1970s are no more valid. Selection of subjects and development of skill and technique are two important criteria in ethical consideration; however, the main concern is: 'Do no harm', be it donor or recipient.

Task force recommendations

Ethical issues are more relevant even today due to the fact that there is a scarcity of organs, and it is not possible to provide a transplant to each and every person waiting to receive one. In 1981, the American Nation Organ Transplant Act constituted the task force[19] to go into the details of ethical, social, and financial angles of organ procurement versus transplantation. In that year, 200000 persons were declared brain dead and only 2000 could donate organs, while 50000 potential patients were waiting for various transplantations. This highlights the gap between the need and availability of organs.

Task force recommended two important points:[6]

a) No financial compensation to organ donor family (except medical cost).
b) Organs consented by donor or donor family only to be obtained. It should be purely voluntary.

Hence, the most important ethical issues are suitability from the patient's perspective, and clinical bias from the physician's perspective. Despite limitations and ethical issues, the organ transplantation has evolved over the last sixty years, not only involving patients and physicians but also involving the society and public at large. The awareness of Organ Donation has exponentially increased amongst the people. It is also realized that the organs must be judiciously used to maximize the potential benefit to the recipient.

Chinese organ transplant law

Organ transplant started in China in 1960s. Over the years, there is an increase in the number of transplants. It has been discovered that the people are making China a place of Transplant Tourism. In 2011, important facts emerged that doctors recommended organ harvesting from asylum-seeking persons. In 1984, Chinese law made it legal to remove organs from criminals, being executed. This was considered an important ethical abuse across the world, and also led to corruption. Between 2006 and 2009, 41500 transplants were done. In 2009, it was reported that 65% of organ donations were received from death of prisoners.[8] However, in 2013, Chinese claimed that they followed all ethical issues as per WHO guidelines for Organ Transplantation. Voluntary Organ donation is illegal as per Chinese law.[12,15,21]

Spiritualism and organ transplantation

Spiritualism is the science of study of soul and its connection with God, as believed by various religions. Spiritualism leads to healthy life and less disease and suffering for the human being. Often spiritualism is confused with religiousness. The difference is that religious person are bound by the laws and beliefs of that religion, on the contrary, spiritual person is more open and liberal as he is not bound by strict laws and regulations of any religion. Both have their advantages and limitations. Their laws and faith have tremendous impact and bearing on organ donation, be a live donor or brain-dead patient, and also has limitation of transplantation into recipients. Many health professionals and transplant surgeons may lack knowledge of religious issues involving organ transplantation. One of the reasons for the low rate of donation of organs is due to religious superstitions. These are not confined to any specific religion; these religious beliefs are widespread across the religions, Hindu or Sikh or Islamic or Christianity, even in the far east, amongst Buddhist, Confucianism and Taoism, these factors do operate and influence organ donations.

In a study, Oliver et al[22] reported widespread variations amongst organ donor card holders, which ranged from 42% Buddhist to 97% Muslim in Saudi Arabia. In Iran, 99.5% card holders reported were Muslims. In the US, 76% card holders were Christians. It may not really reflect the truth as the population is not uniform. It is believed in Islam and Buddhism that organ donation is not in line with their laws.

Islamic views

In Islamic view, damaging or cutting human body is not accepted; on the contrary, saving a life is considered highly religious as per the Holy Quran. To facilitate organ donation in the UK, Islamic council made a religious ruling that Organ Transplant is acceptable by Islamic Law.[20] In Iran, Cadaver Kidney Donation and Transplantation started as early as 2008.[23] Many Islamic Schools in Iran, Turkey, Saudi Arabia, and Kuwait have accepted and endorsed organ donation from either live donors or deceased donors.[23–25] However, in 2005 in Turkey, 21% of doctors expressed their religious concern in organ donation. Efforts are constantly made to increase the organ donation among the Islamic countries. In a publication Najafizaden et al[25] reported increased incidence of organ donation in Iran, in the Holy month of Ramadan.

Hindus/Sikhs in relation to organ donation

There are no specific contraindications for organ donation in Hinduism. In fact, kidney transplant started in India as early as 1970s and heart transplantation started in 1994. Indian Human Organ Transplantation act was established in 1994 and several modifications have been made in 2005 and 2014.[26] It is also important that selfless sacrifice and giving are considered as Niyamas (virtual act) in Hinduism. Mythologically,

Lord Siva had transplanted an elephant head in his own son, Lord Ganesh. Similarly, a goat head was transplanted in Dakshya Prajapati, highlighting the principle of extension of life in Hindu mythology from time immemorial. Similarly, Sikhism also believes in good action. There is nothing specific to Sikhism as far as organ donation and transplantation is concerned.[26–28]

Other religious beliefs in organ donation

In Buddhism, there is no view against organ donation. According to some Buddhists, spiritual consciousness is more important than physical consciousness and they believe even after death, spiritual consciousness may remain in the body.[17] Body must not be disturbed for few days until spiritual consciousness departs from the dead body.[17,29–32] In Buddhism, there are confusing concepts and different conclusions. Few of them oppose deceased donation, while few others may allow donation. Sometimes, local scholar of a locality may directly influence followers by their concepts and provide guidance to common man. In a study from Korea, it was obvious that Confucius beliefs are against organ donation.[30] Some other have the just opposite views and approve organ donation. Thus, the large number of religions has different beliefs about the body and the soul, which directly influences organ donation.[30–32]

In Shintoism, organ donation or transplantation is not encouraged. They think after death, body is impure and dangerous.[29,32] A Cardiac Transplant at Sapporo, in 1968, was not accepted well and drew serious criticisms. As the donation and transplantation were not accepted in Japan, the recipients used to go out of the country to receive organ transplantations. In 1997, the law was changed[33] and allowed kidney transplantation from the brain-dead patients; however, 90% of renal transplants are from live donors.[33] It is also true that donor cards are the lowest in Japan as compared to other countries. Nevertheless, cadaver donors' incidence is steadily increasing in Japan.[33]

Overall, it is well understood that religious beliefs and law, across the religions and countries by and large, did not encourage organ donation in the past. Over the last four decades, many countries have changed their laws and spread the awareness to motivate the public for organ donation. As a result, organ donation has increased many folds facilitating transplantation. After the adoption of brain death law, deceased donors have also increased. It is encouraging that deceased donation across religions has been reported. It is also noticed from various countries that Nongovernmental Organizations (NGO) across religions have played important role in motivating public for organ donation. One of the examples is HOPE (Human Organ Procurement and Education) Trust in India, which is working in this field since 2003. There are many Government Organizations like NOTTO and SOTTO in India. This brings out the fact that people have come out from past religious beliefs and started understanding the value of Cadaver Organ donation.

Conclusion

Organ donation and organ transplantation have a large number of social, ethical, and financial issues. Over the last sixty years, these issues have been discussed by various Task Force committee and groups across the world to find out the solutions and to lay down the guidelines. With skill and experience, the result of transplantation has improved multi-fold and complications to the life of donor is minimized. Though there are several issues with cadaver donors, it has gained popularity in the last 3–4 decades. The problems with brain death and organ harvesting from a dying person have been simplified by the laws that have been laid down to minimize unethical practices. However, more practices many things have yet to be done to achieve 100% ethical practice in organ transplantation.

Highlights

- Organ transplantation is a complex process that deals with donor, recipient, and surgeon.
- Transplantation needs social worker, social guides and Transplant co-coordinators to ensure a smooth process.
- The team must be clear about the laws, existing ethical, and financial issues regarding transplantation.

- The spiritual and religious issues must be adequately addressed as different religions have different ways of thinking and practices.

References

1) Institute of Medicine. 2006. Organ donation: Opportunities for action. Washington, DC: The National Academies Press. https://doi.org/10.17226/11643.
2) Goyal M. Mehta RL Schinederman LJ etal. Economic and health consciousness of selling Kidney in India. Journal of American Medical Association 2002;288: 1589–1593.
3) Jame Macarthy " China to tidy up" trade in executed prisoners Organ. The Times 3 December 2005.
4) Reddy KC: In Land W, Dosseta JB (Eds) Organ replacement Therapy. Ethics, Justice and commerce. Newyork. Springer Verlag.1996 page 173.
5) JonsemAR. The ethics of organ transplantation: a brief history. Virtual Mentor. AMA Journal of Ethics 2012;14(3):264–268. doi: 10.1001/virtualmentor.2012.14.3.mhst1-1203
6) Schurtz HS. Bioethical and legal consideration is increasing the supply of transplantable organ. From UAGA to Baby Fac Amer. J Law Med 1985;10:397.437.
7) Delmonico FL, Arnold R, Scheper – Hughess etal. Ethical incentives—not payment, for organ donation. New England Journal of Medicine, 20 June 2002;346(25): 2002–2005.
8) Eooan C McNeio D. Japanese rich buy organ from executed Chinese prisinor. The Indipendent. 21 May 2010. https://www.independent.co.uk/news/world/asia/japan-s-rich-buy-organs-from-executed-chinese-prisoners-5335744.html
9) Matas AJ. Schnitzler M. Payment for living donor. Kidneys: A cost effectiveness analysis. American Journal of Transplantation 2003;4:216:221.
10) Spita A. Donor Benefit is the key to Justifying living Organ donation. Cambridge quarterly of Health Ethics 2004;13:105.109.
11) BBC World Service. Discovery of Chines Organ Transplant, Turism and Transparency—BBC. www. China organtransplant.org. https://www.bbc.co.uk/programmes/w3csxyl4
12) Wikipedia> wiki> Organ – transplantion – in China. Accessed 2020.
13) Starzl TE. Ethical problem in Organ Transplantation a clinicians point and view. Ann Int Med 1967;67:32–35.
14) A definition of irreversible coma. A report of the ADHOC committee at Harvard Medical School to examine the definition of Brain death. JAMA 1968;205:337–340.
15) Dockrill P. Worst fear about Chins Organ Transplant and Prisioner were Just Science Alert, 19 June 2019. https://www.google.com/url?sa=t&rct=j&q=&esrc=s&source=web&cd=&cad=rja&uact=8&ved=2ahUKEwjzwvSly5f0AhUl7rsIHfbvCbAQFnoECAIQAQ&url=https%3A%2F%2Fwww.sciencealert.com%2Four-worst-fears-about-where-china-s-human-organs-come-from-were-just-confirmed&usg=AOvVaw2p-aHFwYhziJDcM8IPqeLm

16) Transplantation of Human Organ and Tissue. The Gazette of Govt of India. 2014. Extra Ordinary Part III Sector 3 March 27 2014
17) Hadacre H. Response of Buddhism and Shinto to the issue of Brain Death and Organ Transplant. Comb Q, Health Ethics 1994;3:584–601.
18) Task force on Organ Transplantation. Organ Transplantation Issues and recommendations. Rockville MD Department of Health and Human Services Xxi. 1986
19) President's commission for study of Ethics in Medicine in Biomedical and Behavioral Research. Defining Death. A report on Medical, Legal and Ethical issue in the Definition of Death. Washington DC US. GoVt. Primary office 1981.
20) Golmakani MM, Niknam MH, Hedayat KM. Transplantation ethics from Islamic point of view. Med. Sci Monitoring 2005;11:105–109.
21) Srivastav A, Mani A, Deceased Organ Donation and Transplantation in India. Promises and challenges. (Guest Common day) Neurology India 2018;66; 316–322.
22) Oliver Michel, Waywood A, Ahmed A et al. Organ donation, Transplantation and religion. Nephrology Dialysis Transplantation. 2011;26:437–444.
23) Einollahi B, Cadaven Z Kidney transplantation in Iran: behind the middle Eastern Countries. Iran J Kidney Dis 2008;2: 55–56.
24) Hassaballah AM. Defination of Death, organ donation interruption of treatment in Islam. Nephrology Dialysis Transplant 1996;11:964–965.
25) Najafizadeth. K, Gorbani F, Hamidinia S etal. Holy month of Ramadan and increased Organ Donation willingness Saudi. J Kidney Dis and Transplant 2010;21:443–446.
26) NHS Blood and Transplant. Hindu Dharma and Organ. WWW. Organ Donation. Nhs.UK. https://www.organdonation.nhs.uk/helping-you-to-decide/your-faith-and-beliefs/hinduism/ Accessed 2020.
27) Excely C, Sim J, Reid N etal. Attitude and beliefs within the Sikh community regarding Organ Donation: a pilot study. Soc Sci Med. 1996;43:23–28.
28) Tai MC. An Asian Perspective of Organ Transplantation. Wien Med Wochensecht, 2009;159:452–456.
29) Namihira E. Shinto concept concerning the dead human body. Transplant Proc, 1990;22:940–941.
30) Kim Jr, Eilliot D, Hyde C. The influence of Socio cultural factors on organ donations and Transplantation in Korea. Finding from key informant interviews J Tran Cult Nurs, 2004;15:147–154.
31) Daar As. The body, the soul and organ donation beliefs of major world religions. Nefrologia, 1994;14:78–81.
32) Danovitch GM. Cultural barriers to kidney transplantation a new frontier. Transplantation 2007;84:462–463.
33) Hanto DW, Ethical Challenges posed by the solicitation of Deceased and living organ donors. NEJM, 2007;356:1062–1066.

71

Conundrums in the definitions of life and death and their ethical implications

Adrian Caceres

> Death commences too early—almost before you're half-acquainted with life—you meet the other.
>
> —Tennessee Williams

Introduction

Throughout the history, man has been confronted with enormous questions such as: Where do we come from? What defines us as human beings? After completing our life cycle, where do we go? These questions are as old as humanity and are a reflection of a need for transcendence beyond our finite earthly presence. Probably nothing generates as much fear and uncertainty as the fact that after death, we envision ourselves devoid of any sensory input, reduced to the insubstantiality of nothingness. It is in this way the need for moral holdings has created, within all human cultures, a system of supernatural, mystical, and dimensionless beliefs that we call religion.

The man being social, by definition, feels a deep fear of solitude that the death poses. Therefore, in the majority of the religions, man postulates other worldly social coexistence. Having fulfilled a finite time on this earth, humans transport to another dimension to continue interacting with other spiritual entities. Before exploring the concept of death, we must be forced to define its counterpart, that is, the concept of life. There is enough evidence that there is no unique, clear framework to define concepts such as time, space, personhood, and life.

Definition of life

Attempting to define life is more complex than defining death. Until relatively recently, multiple examples that surround us throughout the nature are relied upon to explain life; it is defined through its study.

Linus Pauling stated 'with respect to the origin of life, I must say that sometimes it is easier to study an object than to try to define it'.[1] It is obvious to ask the following question: How can we define death when there is no consensus regarding the definition of life? Can the space probes know what they are looking for in the confines of the universe if the meaning of life is not clear on the earth?

Seeking life according to a Platonic/Socratic view according to our perception is an important barrier to understanding the potential diversity of life. Recent discovery about bacteria that do not conform biochemically to the previous defined standards proves that there may be many other potential arrangements not only on earth but in the whole universe. Cleland has stated that it is a mistake to attempt defining the term life rather than defining a general theory of living systems. On the other hand, it is customary among biologists to perform valuable research without a definition.[2,3]

Definitions for the end of life and the beginning of death are not simple. Main dictionaries and encyclopaedias lack satisfactory definitions for both terms. Some of the definitions pointed out by Potter[4] that are accepted as standards of the term 'life' are as follows:

1. The condition that distinguishes animals and plants from inorganic objects and dead organisms, manifested by growth through metabolism, reproduction and the ability to adapt to the environment through changes originating in the medium.
2. An open system of chained organic reactions that are catalysed at low temperatures by specific enzymes that are, in turn, byproducts of the system.

It should be noted that in the former, the concept of homeostasis stands out and in the later, it is the transformation of energy from primary materials that become integrated elements of the system, or waste of these reactions. Life is defined in terms of growth, reproduction, metabolism, movement, and response. However, there are exceptions to these definitions within nature, Fire grows, moves, has metabolism (consumes, transforms, and generates byproducts), and responds to stimuli (i.e. wind). Likewise, computer software can adapt, provide specific responses, consume energy, and duplicate itself but it would be difficult for us to define fire or computer software as a living entity.

Francis Crick included as a basic requirement for life 'the ability of a system to replicate both its own instructions and any machinery necessary in this process'.[5] This concept was further elaborated by Dyson in his double origin theory defining life as the result of the interaction of self-replicating catalytic systems which produce proteins that progressively sophisticated their metabolism eventually generating RNA capable of transmitting genetic information.[6]

Trifonov analysed the vocabulary of published definitions of life, finding 123 terms that could be aggregated in order to generate a 'compact expression' akin to all these definitions—Life is a metabolizing material informational system with ability of self-reproduction with changes (evolution) which requires energy and suitable environment.[7]

The current taxonomy organizing living species includes the domain of Acytota, which is defined as living forms that do not require a cellular structure to exist. Within this category, viruses are the most cited (and disputed) elements. However, this kingdom also includes plasmids, satellites, viroids, and transposable elements all of which, by the way, outnumber any other cell forms.[8]

Within the kingdom of Cytota are bacteria, archaea, chromista, protozoa, plantae fungi, and Animalia.

Recent genome sequencing has enabled to compare genomes of all entities considered alive in search for the last universal common ancestor (LUCA) which is thought to be the single non-extinct ancestor of life.[9,10] Based on this sequencing, scientists consider that this common ancestor existed between 4.2 to 4.5 billion years ago.

Death concepts

> 'Death is not always an enemy, it is often a good medical treatment, it often reaches what medicine cannot solve; it stops suffering.'
> Death must be painless, compassionate and welcomed as an essential part of the process of life.
>
> Christiaan Barnard

The concept of death within primitive cultures was given by the magical-religious context of societies such as druids, Aztecs, and Egyptians among others.[11,12] Death represented a process of transition towards another spiritual dimension. As part of this rite, the shaman or high priest makes his appearance, not only as a healer, but also assisting man in his passage to the unknown dimension. In this union man forms a continuum with his environment, such as the example of the Native American cultures.[13] In contemporary examples such as the Australian aborigines, the acceptance of the death process as an integral part of the social being stands out. The family of the dying person gathers around him, suffering the earthly loss of the individual, but at the same time they congratulate themselves because they are on the way with the destiny.[14] Throughout history, intellectual and technological development has invested man with a false sense of security given by the study and mastery of almost all natural processes that surround him, with one exception, death, which constantly reminds him of his fragile and finite permanence.

Within this desire for existential persistence, religions have generally proposed three options:

1. Division of the soul-body binomial with the transfer of the soul to an outer dimension.
2. Division of the binomial soul body with the reinsertion of the soul into this world through a reincarnation.
3. Division of the binomial soul body with integration with the environment.

This process of division is facilitated by the cremation of the body, a practice that was implemented by the Dorians and is still practised today in the incineration of organisms either in cremation ovens or in pyres, as is customary in several cultures of South Asia. The transcendence of the death rites within the cultural, architectural, and social manifestations takes its greatest exponent in the Egyptians and their architectonic legacies that even marvel us to this day.

The regulation, depersonalization, and ritualization of death occur with the settlement of nomadic tribes. In the early periods of the Christian era, death was conceived as a gradual process, a concept that prevailed until the beginning of this century. After death, the body was involved in a trance, without the evidence of movement or activity, but where hair and nails continued growing. In this state, the soul did not leave the body immediately. Therefore, a vigil was established around the deceased until the appearance of cadaverous signs evidencing the departure of the soul.

Despite the accumulation of science and technology, death is the constant reminder of the inability of man to overcome destiny, the inflexible laws of nature and confronting him with his spiritual creator, to whom he must render an account of his earthly actions. Dying translates the impotence of man against destiny. In the Christian world, the memory of the punishing God of the Old Testament makes death dark, enigmatic, and dreary, implying intrinsic suffering. The conception of hell and paradise appears according to the customs of the Middle Ages.

Due to the idea of the gradual process of death, visualizations appear in the form of spirits, ghosts, and other entities that, in their transition to another dimension, become involved with humans with different purposes. During the Renaissance period, it was customary not to bury the recently deceased in order to avoid errors in the proclamation of death. A classic example of this procedure is seen in Shakespeare's classic 'Romeo and Juliet'. Among the measures customary at that time to prevent the burial of a living stands out the conclamation, an ancient custom consisting of calling the person by his name three times. This rite of conclamation is still carried out when a Pope dies.(15)

In 1740, Wrinslow published his 'Dissertation sur L'incertitude des Signes de la Morte et de l Abus des Enterrements et Embaumements Pricipitis'.(16) In this popular publication, unfounded fears were spread in Western society around the rites of death. The literary appearance of the Frankenstein monster of Mary Shelley and the strange case of M. Valdemar by Allan Poe marked the romantic and phantasmagoric transfiguration of death involving science and postulating the reversibility of this process. This process of death, romantically suspended or even reversible, is at the same time the foundation of stories such as Sleeping Beauty and Snow White.[17]

As a result of these stories deeply rooted in the popular creed, a series of artefacts and devices were arranged near the 'apparent deceased' so that in case of waking up from such an unfortunate situation, one could give notice to his mourners for a 'fast rescue'.

The desecration of tombs for the purpose of anatomical dissection increased the fear of the people, who expressly requested that after the death, their bodies remained without embalming until the signs became evident of cadaveric decomposition which, in addition to protecting against the usurpation of bodies, would protect them from a scientist with resurrectionist aims. According to this custom, it was necessary to create dwellings where several bodies were 'watched'.[18] In this time, the funeral homes or chapels were called vitae dubiae azilia, that is, asylums for life in doubt.

George Washington allegedly requested before dying 'have me decently buried, do not let my body be put into a vault in less than two days after I am dead'.[19]

Even to this day, the purpose of funeral homes is defined by several statements such as to help confirming the reality and finality of death and to provide a declaration that a life has been lived as well that as a sociological statement that death has occurred.

In response to these fears of uncertainty of death, it became necessary to summon a physician to aid with the confirmation of death. The first law that required the participation of the physician in the certification of death was proclaimed in England by William, the Conqueror, in 1836. This law mandated that a doctor who had treated the patient in question during his last days should certify the cause of death.

This law was reviewed in 1874 by the House of Commons and ruled the need to perform an examination of the body in search of unequivocal signs of death.[20] The systematization of the pathological changes associated with the death of the organism was the product of the work of Xavier Bichat & Rudolf Virchow and thus, the forensic science established as criteria the lack of cardiac and respiratory responses.[21] This set of criteria was called cardiorespiratory death which remained unchallenged and up to 1918, there was a law in France that required the need to perform an arteriotomy to demonstrate the lack of blood flow as well as the application of fluorescein to evidence the loss of turgor of the cornea.[22]

The earliest descriptions of the role of the brain in the death process are accounted in the recognition that intracranial disease, manifested by intracranial hypertension, would produce respiratory arrest.[23] Jalland, Horsley, and Duckworth went on to describe how severe respiratory depression could be reversed with measures that alleviated intracranial space conflicts.[24] Harvey Cushing, among his many contributions, described a case in 1902 in which a comatose patient stopped breathing spontaneously and was 'kept alive' through artificial ventilation.[25]

Modern brain death definition criteria

With the introduction of the electroencephalography by Hans Berger in 1929, and the correlation between stoppage of cell function and lack of electrical activity, Oscar Sugar correlated ischemia with a decline in neurological function and eventually death, if the blood flow was not adequately reestablished.[26]

In 1957, Löfstedt and Von Reis demonstrated that patients with a lack of intracranial blood flow would correlate with coma.[27]

By then, Claude Beck had successfully defibrillated a human heart, thus reversing the remainder of the two components of traditional cardiopulmonary death.[24] The correlation of absence of clinical evidence of neurological activity along with no spontaneous breathing when the ventilatory support was withheld marked the definition of brain death and its implications. Curiously, the concept of irreversible state of coma and apnoea, as published by Mollaret and Goulon, who named this clinical picture Le coma depassé in 1959, was not considered at the time as an equivalent to death.[28] An excellent timeline of clinical events and milestones concerning development of medical life-sustaining technology, progress in neurological sciences in the description of disorders of consciousness, and irreversible neurological damage along with the need of an ethical background, especially in the realm of organ donation and transplants, can be found in the papers by De Georgia and Machado.[29,30]

This series of events triggered the need for the Ad Hoc Committee of Harvard Medical School, led by Beecher, Adams, and Sweet, who all in 1968 formulated the criteria for the determination of neurological death.[31] Many criticisms were generated about this pronouncement, alleging that it had been generated in response to the need for a law to obtain organs for transplant, a view that has been challenged by Machado and others.[24]

The criteria formulated to establish brain death by the new Ad Hoc committee definition included:

1. Unresponsiveness.
2. Absence of movement and breathing
3. Absence of brainstem reflexes.
4. An isoelectric EEG was also recommended along with the exclusion of hypothermia or drug intoxication[32].

During the seventies in the United States and Europe, several studies were carried out to validate the conclusions of the Harvard study, notable among them were studied by Mohandas and Chou,[33] Jorgensen et al. of Sweden in 1973,[34] the British report in 1976, the North American Cooperative Study of 1977 and the President's Commission for the Study of Ethical Problems in Medicine and Behavioral Research.

In the classic series of articles written by Christopher Pallis,[35–38] the author mentioned that considering the possibility of a future medical technology that can solve the pathologies that currently require organ transplants, physicians will still be confronted to diagnose patients with brain death. Therefore, Pallis cited the need to establish the definition of brain death to meet several needs as follows:

1. Establish the equivalence of brain death with the death of the patient.
2. Reduce the human stress of both family members and the staff of the intensive care units.
3. Rationalize the use of resources of intensive care units.
4. Collaborate with organ transplant programmes.

After the integration of the concept which, feasibly, demonstrated an irreversibly deteriorated neurological function in an organism that remains with ventilatory and hemodynamic functions replaced by pharmacological and technological means, the extension and location of this neurological lesion that allowed generating the diagnosis of brain death was greatly debated.

The following is a review of the main schools of thought about death and the requirements established by them, as well as the ethical dilemmas they faced. It must be stated that any criteria of brain death should be defensible on biological and philosophical grounds.

Whole brain death and total brain failure postulations

The definition of whole brain death, implying the irreversible destruction of the whole encephalon (cerebral hemispheres, brainstem, and cerebellum) was postulated and defended by James L Bernat et al,[39–44] and later endorsed in 1981 by the study of the President's Commission.[45,46]

This postulation declared that the requisite of living things which is absent in the dead is the body's capacity to organize and regulate itself. Therefore, when the brain completely ceases to function, death is 'the cessation of the functioning of the organism as a whole'.

Additionally, the concept of an inexorable and imminent deterioration of these body's subsystems after the whole brain, as grand integrator, was irreversibly damaged, was an assumption under this postulation.

The resulting Uniform Determination of Death Act stated that death could be determined by:

1. Irreversible cessation of respiratory and circulatory functions.
2. Irreversible cessation of all brain functions of the entire brain, including the brainstem.

While, currently, the concept of death has been firmly established on cardiovascular and neurological criteria, there is still a wide variation of the criteria used to arrive at this diagnosis. On the other hand, this definition has been challenged by Alan Shewmon and others, since patients who meet the criteria of whole brain death exhibit persistent neuron cellular activity, translated through electrical encephalographic activity, evoked auditory responses and through integrity of pituitary hormone systems.[47–49]

The defenders of this theory upheld that all these manifestations of persistent neuronal activity represented extracranial anastomotic blood supply and did not reflect a significant function.[50]

Other detractors from this concept declared that the term brain death could generate the concept of incomplete or double death among lay persons as they could be confused by the anticipatory legal fiction of declaring dead, a patient with a non-functioning brain who would later go on to endure hours, days, months, and, in rare instances, up to fourteen years before experiencing a 'second death'. They concluded in their arguments that a brain-dead patient who is on life support technology but carries out all the other integrative functions (digestion, growth, active combat against infection, fever, and even carrying a foetus to full terminus) cannot be labelled as a corpse.

In 2008, the President's Council on Bioethics rejected the concept of whole brain death given the accumulation of evidence that even in the presence of massive irreversible brain injury, there are areas which will exhibit EEG activity and it is possible to detect neuroendocrine functioning and, in some cases, neuroauditory evoked responses. This council went on to discard the term brain death and replacing it with 'total brain failure' in an attempt to produce a philosophically adequate terminology.[51,52] This report also declared that whenever we are referring to an organism as a whole it does not refer to the whole organism, that is to say to the arithmetical sum of its parts; rather emphasizes that characteristic that turns living organisms into something bigger than a simple addition referring to the mechanism that allows the integration of internal and external stimuli, in such a way that their survival is guaranteed.

Through this definition, the organism can tolerate loss of some of its parts without dying, that is, it can amputate an extremity, a kidney, a lung, etc. But a complete organism with the 'loss of the organism as a whole' is nothing but a set of subsystems lacking interrelation or common purpose.

A novel argument was also the concept that a living organism had the fundamental work of self-preservation. 'This inner need for life is achieved through the organism's need-driven commerce with the surrounding world. This commerce is manifested by the need to breathe and the need of consciousness'; therefore, total brain failure equals death as the organism cannot engage in the essential work that defines living things. These formulations found criticism as it was considered that this rationalization was merely a conclusion that allowed the removal of vital organs without violating the dead donor rule.[53,54]

Truog, Miller, and Halpern stated that it would be more honest to abandon the dead donor rule allowing patients whose death is imminent 'to die in the process of helping others to live' by removal of their vital organs.[55,56] The concern that by following this practice, a patient in critical condition could be electively placed in this pathway where imminent death is rather a decision than an irreversible condition is discussed later in the chapter.[57]

On the other hand, Botkin and Post declared that 'it is our own conviction that the whole brain death standard will probably balance the conflicting needs of our society, despite the confusion it generates, its utility is based on utilitarian considerations.'[58]

Higher brain formulation

The higher brain concept, formulated by Robert Veatch, contemplates the clinical scenario in which a lesion to the brain is capable of producing permanent loss of what constitutes the human essence of a being. Once human powers are lost, death in the moral, social, and legal sense will follow. This injury implies a destruction of the neocortex as well as irreversible loss of consciousness.[59]

Therefore, there are two events which Veatch distinguishes—the death of the personhood, and later, in a variable timeframe, follows the death of the body or organism. Brody and collaborators have refined this concept by articulating it within a mind-body context. For these authors, there is a difference between physical and social existence, where citizenship, rights, and values correspond to the subjective person, not the body. Therefore, once the individual's ability to interact with the society is lost, it is not only permissible to stop the administration of food, fluids, and medicines, but it is also desirable, unless some benefit to others in need can be obtained from it.[60] According to this point of view, it is wrong to treat these bodies as if they were 'living instead of being just alive'.[61]

What is left behind is an artificially sustained living organism which while not biologically dead is morally, legally, and socially dead, and therefore, should be treated as such.[54] Perhaps, we should rephrase these concepts under the sentence: 'Living a life is not equivalent to being alive; in the same way, dying is not the same as being dead.'

One of the criticized points of the higher brain definition is that it does not describe what we call death, and also within this group, we can potentially include patients in persistent vegetative state and those who have never acquired this binomium such as anencephalic patients, where despite not exhibiting any evidence of cognitive or affective activity, certainly we do not consider them as dead.[62]

Brainstem death

The definition of brainstem death was introduced as the backbone of the criteria of the British Committee. Its' main exponent was Christopher Pallis, who refers the need for the coexistence of coma and apnoea as the fundamental criteria of death since both functions have their substratum within the brainstem.[35–38,63,64]

The anatomical substrate of the brainstem provides the organism more than the sum of its parts. The mesencephalon is a prerequisite for the correct functioning of the cortical networks mediating cognitive function. In addition, recent studies have pointed to the relevance of an upper brainstem system that connects the colliculus area of the mesencephalon with the basal diencephalon for the elaboration of conscious contents. Damasio and Edelman also agreed on the integrity of the brainstem for a primary or core consciousness.[65–67] Accumulating evidence that hydranencephalic children can have limited but definitive evidence of conscious activity reinforces the existence of these neural networks.[68]

Some opponents to this approach emphasize that although there is no evidence of the functioning of the brainstem, there is residual activity within the brain. However it is clear that this activity, for practical purposes, does not represent cognitive or affective activity, and therefore, does not correspond to the concept of social, moral, or legal formulation held by Veatch. This definition is probably the most pragmatic, since, as Pallis has shown, this type of patients will unequivocally present asystole in short periods of time. It is important to point out that additionally, by definition, patients in a persistent vegetative state are excluded, who must be treated separately to avoid confusion and committing acts that are unethical.[69]

Return to the concept of cardiorespiratory arrest death

It is clear that death is currently a process that can be 'intervened' with the assistance of vital support technology which prolongs the body's homeostasis, even in the absence of a well-integrated brain capable of fulfilling the concept of personhood. While some authors question that locating human death within the brain is reductionist and does not respect body dignity, it is evident that there is a growing consensus about a unifying medical concept that all human death is located to the brain. De Georgia has defined that for much of the public and to some extent in the medical profession, brain-dead patients are considered practically as good as dead but not really dead.[29]

However, the need for organ procurement in the face of growing waiting lists for transplants has led to the practice of protocols for donation after circulatory determination of death (DCDD). To honour planned decisions to withdraw life support of patients with pathologies beyond medical hope and to assist those in need for an organ, patients who do not fulfil the neurological criteria of brain death are declared dead on the traditional cessation of circulation. This requires witnessing cardiac arrest for a variable period of time, then declaring the patient dead, and immediately proceeding to extract organs (non-beating heart organ donation). It is evident that irreversible damage to the brain follows cessation of breathing and cardiac arrest which eventually leads to secondary brain death, however, this last component is not the premise of this approach.

Therefore, the three components of death after cardiorespiratory arrest are:

1. A clear intention not to attempt cardiopulmonary resuscitation, which would restore circulatory and potentially brain function.

2. An observation period confirming persistent apnoea, absent circulation, and unconsciousness which precludes spontaneous reversal of cardiac function.
3. The prohibition of any intervention that might restore cerebral blood flow.

The steps for establishing the diagnosis of death after cardiorespiratory arrest are similar to the brain death criteria in their evaluation of loss of consciousness (evaluation of pupillary reflexes, absence of corneal reflex, no response to supraorbital noxious stimulus) and that there is a period to observe the persistence of apnoea.(19)

Donation within the framework of non-beating heart includes patients within two categories as described in the Maastricht classification(70):

1. Uncontrolled, which includes those patients brought to the hospital and:
   a. Are declared dead on arrival,
   b. Those who had unsuccessful resuscitation procedures,
   c. Those who present cardiac arrest after brain death.
   d. Those who suffer cardiac arrest as hospital inpatients.
2. Controlled, which include patients in an ICU setting who have non-survivable injuries and had treatment withdrawal, therefore, cardiac arrest is being awaited. If these patients had expressed their will to donate their vital organs, it is possible that the transplant team can be present during the treatment withdrawal, wait for cardiac arrest, observe the no touch period and then proceed to recover the organs in order to ensure their optimal condition for transplant medicine.

There is a variability of this observation or no touch period as in Australia and USA, this time spans between 2 and 5 minutes, in the UK and Canada, it is not less than 5 minutes and Italy requires at least 20 minutes.(19) Devita suggested that the shortest time for DCDD is 65 seconds. However, there is strong criticism if such brief observation periods would violate the dead donor rule as clearly, the heart or the brain could have a recovery potential even within the 5 minute timeframe.(71,72)

The terminology of DCDD was modified in such a way that it would express the cessation of function after cardiocirculatory arrest as 'permanent' which was felt to be unequivocal and contingent with the possibility of restoring the circulation, and at the same time, relies on the clear intention of not attempting resuscitation and prohibiting any action that might restore cerebral blood flow.[19,73]

The fact that these 'recovered' organs continue to function generates another ethical concern. Especially, the heart which initially was excluded from the list of recoverable organs can now be saved by ECMO by restarting the donor heart *in situ*, but only after exclusion of the brain circulation with a balloon.[73]

Legal fictions in the definitions of death

Death should be treated as a legal construct or as a matter of social agreement, however, death as currently defined by all legal standards, has two legal fictions which should be considered:

The status fiction of death is, in essence, to apply similar law considerations to two distinct, but related death definitions.

The concepts of 'whole brain death' and 'total brain death' are not biologically equivalent to death as many patients continue to perform integrative bodily functions in spite of a profound brain damage. These brain-dead patients can host life functions such as homeostasis, hormonal secretion, metabolism and byproduct excretion, fight against infection, physical growth and sexual maturation in the case of children and even continuation of a pregnancy to full term. These functions cannot be found in a corpse, yet these two entities are considered under the law as one. In the words of Shah and cols., 'Whole brain death and total brain failure are used to determine death in an unacknowledged legal fiction which is applied without full recognition of its falsity'.[53]

The next example of legal fiction is commonly applied in order to legally comply with the Uniform Definition of Death Act and it is denominated the anticipatory fiction of death, which requires to consider that something that is about to occur is the same as if it had already happened.

This fallacy has been implied due to the evidence that while most centres who practice DCDD will wait between 2 and 5 minutes, asystole within that period is not unequivocally irreversible.[19] The fact that a procured heart during this practice will reassume its function once transplanted, raises the question of the 'irreversibility' of the donor's circulatory arrest.

Practical approach for the rationale of organ donation within the frameworks of death

This is a modification of the proposal done by Halevy and Brody,[60] which looks for a pragmatical approach to the steps in decision-making whenever conducting transplant medicine in patients under any of the aforementioned definitions of death.

When should we contact the transplant team?

Upon determination of irreversible cessation of conscious functioning in the framework of any of the definitions of brain death.

Whenever there is an imminent cardiac arrest in a patient that has expressed his decision to donate his vital organs.

When a patient ceases to breathe and has unsuccessful cardiac arrest resuscitation.

When can the organs be recovered?

Upon the completion of requirements of the diagnosis of brain death.

After the no touch period has expired in the DCDD patients.

When can the undertaker begin his work?

After asystole in brain death.

After organs have been recovered in the corpse in oxygenation (ECMO)

Conclusion

I shall not wholly die, and a great part of me will escape the grave.

Horace

Medical advances in life support technology, neuromonitoring, and neuroimaging have enabled the challenge of traditional views regarding life and death.

Departing from a cardiorespiratory definition, today, the concept of death rests in the fabric of personhood which is driven by the integrative functions of the brain. While there are schools of thought which on one hand consider the brain cortex as the seat of this function, it is undeniable that none of them can amount to significant activity without the function of the brainstem which provides arousal to integrate and produce consciousness and higher cerebral activities.

The arrival of organ transplantation medicine required new views regarding the biological, philosophical, legal, and ethical implications of defining when a person has ceased to live but can still be able to produce the gift of life through organ donation.

Highlights

- The definitions of life and death rather than marking a single term, describes in both cases, process with either the adequate functioning of a metabolizing material informational system with ability of self-reproduction with changes (evolution) which requires energy and suitable environment or its gradual disintegration and cease of function.
- Progress in medical life support technology along with better medical care led to a common clinical scenario where irreversible cessation of the brain activity can be found in patients whose other physiological functions can be present for variable amounts of time if life support technology can assist breathing and an adequate cardiovascular response.
- The hierarchical order to determine the diagnosis of death should follow the next order: Determining who or what is dead, how death is defined, which criteria are necessary to be fulfilled and which tests are required to reach this conclusion. Also, of paramount importance are the criteria which contraindicate reaching this diagnosis such as hypothermia, shock, or the presence of neurodepressing drugs.
- The higher brain formulation contemplates the clinical scenario in which a lesion to the brain is capable of producing permanent loss of what constitutes the human essence of a being, therefore, it is no longer a human being and should be treated as a corpse on life support technology.

- The brainstem formulation contemplates that irreversible cessation of the activity of the brainstem implies coma and arrest of breathing which are the fundamental components to produce death without the active participation of life support technology.
- The concept of donation after cardiocirculatory determination of death has been attempted with variable success to recover organs from patients who experience cardiorespiratory arrest in either controlled (hospital) or community-based events.

References

1. Pauling L. The origin of life on earth. Oparin A, editor. MacMillan; 1938.
2. Chodasewicz K. Evolution, reproduction and definition of life. Theory Biosci [Internet]. 2014 Mar [cited 2019 Jul 21];133(1):39–45.
3. van Regenmortel MHV. The metaphor that viruses are living is alive and well, but it is no more than a metaphor. Stud Hist Philos Sci Part C Stud Hist Philos Biol Biomed Sci [Internet]. 2016 Oct [cited 2019 Jul 20];59:117–24. Available from: http://www.ncbi.nlm.nih.gov/pubmed/26970895
4. Potter SM. The meaning of life [Internet]. 1986. Available from: https://www.ibiblio.org/jstrout/uploading/potter_life.html
5. Portin P. The birth and development of the DNA theory of inheritance: Sixty years since the discovery of the structure of DNA. J Genet [Internet]. 2014 [cited 2020 Nov 2];93(1):293–302. Available from: https://pubmed.ncbi.nlm.nih.gov/24840850/
6. Dyson FJ. Origins of life. Cambridge University Press; 1999. 100 p.
7. Trifonov EN. Vocabulary of definitions of life suggests a definition. J Biomol Struct Dyn [Internet]. 2011 Oct [cited 2019 Jun 22];29(2):259–66. Available from: http://www.ncbi.nlm.nih.gov/pubmed/21875147
8. Kejnovsky E, Trifonov EN. Horizontal transfer—imperative mission of acellular life forms, *Acytota*. Mob Genet Elements [Internet]. 2016 Mar 3 [cited 2019 Jul 20];6(2):e1154636. Available from: http://www.ncbi.nlm.nih.gov/pubmed/27141324
9. Jain A, Perisa D, Fliedner F, von Haeseler A, Ebersberger I. The evolutionary traceability of a protein. Eyre-Walker A, editor. Genome Biol Evol [Internet]. 2019 Feb 1 [cited 2019 Jul 20];11(2):531–545. Available from: http://www.ncbi.nlm.nih.gov/pubmed/30649284
10. Palacios-Pérez M, José M V. The evolution of proteome: From the primeval to the very dawn of LUCA. Biosystems [Internet]. 2019 Jul [cited 2019 Jul 20];181:1–10. Available from: http://www.ncbi.nlm.nih.gov/pubmed/30995537
11. Aztec Thought and Culture: A Study of the Ancient Nahuatl Mind - Miguel León Portilla—Google Books [Internet]. [cited 2020 Nov 2]. Available from: https://books.google.co.cr/books?hl=en&lr=&id=OI9J7R-R1awC&oi=fnd&pg=

PR7&dq=death+concept+aztecs&ots=qmbYFIBtl_&sig=Ll5ef_qZIWUJoEMPsz73nh7FJ54&redir_esc=y#v=onepage&q=death concept aztecs&f=false
12. Death and Salvation in Ancient Egypt—Jan Assmann—Google Books [Internet]. [cited 2020 Nov 2]. Available from: https://books.google.co.cr/books?hl=en&lr=&id=ATBKDwAAQBAJ&oi=fnd&pg=PR7&dq=death+concept+egypt&ots=2oQengQahZ&sig=NqXrYGrGgTZef8LxqD3YkA--CkQ&redir_esc=y#v=onepage&q=death concept egypt&f=false
13. Schindler S, Greenberg J, Pfattheicher S. An existential perspective on the psychological function of shamans [Internet]. Vol. 41, The Behavioral and brain sciences. NLM (Medline); 2018 [cited 2020 Nov 2]. p. e85. Available from: https://pubmed.ncbi.nlm.nih.gov/31064473/
14. Bohemia, Jack; Mcgregor W. Death practices in the north west of AUSTRALIA on JSTOR. Aborig Hist [Internet]. 1992 [cited 2020 Nov 2];15(No. 1/2):86–106. Available from: https://www.jstor.org/stable/24046404?seq=1
15. A UGR study describes Roman funeral rites—Canal UGR [Internet]. [cited 2020 Nov 2]. Available from: https://canal.ugr.es/prensa-y-comunicacion/science-news-ugr/humanities/a-ugr-study-describes-roman-funeral-rites/
16. Benigne-Winslow MJ. Dissertation sur l'incertitude des signes de la mort et l'abus des enterremens, & embaumemens précipités : par M. Jacques Benigne-Winslow,... traduite, & commentée par Jacques-Jean Bruhier,... - Winslow, Jacques-Bénigne, 1669-1760.... - numelyo - biblioth [Internet]. 1745th ed. A Paris: chez Morel le jeune: Prault, père: Prault, fils: Simon F, editor. Paris; 1742 [cited 2020 Nov 2]. Available from: https://numelyo.bm-lyon.fr/f_view/BML:BML_00GOO0100137001103043795
17. Jean R, Nicks G. Fairy tales and necrophilia: A new cultural context for antebellum American sensationalism. 2006.
18. Kivistö S, Sumiala J, Brattico E, Holmberg EJ, Hämäläinen N, Kennedy J, et al. Cultures of death and dying in medieval and early modern Europe [Internet]. 2015. Available from: www.helsinki.fi/collegium/journal
19. Gardiner D, Shemie S, Manara A, Opdam H. International perspective on the diagnosis of death. Br J Anaesth [Internet]. 2012 Jan [cited 2019 Jun 22];108:i14–28. Available from: http://www.ncbi.nlm.nih.gov/pubmed/22194427
20. Davis GG. Mind your manners Part I: History of death certification and manner of death classification [Internet]. Vol. 18, American Journal of Forensic Medicine and Pathology. Am J Forensic Med Pathol; 1997 [cited 2020 Nov 2]. p. 219–223. Available from: https://pubmed.ncbi.nlm.nih.gov/9290867/
21. Cousins M, Hussain A. Michel Foucault [Internet]. Macmillan Education, Limited; 1984 [cited 2019 Jul 21]. Available from: https://books.google.co.cr/books?id=jEFdDwAAQBAJ&pg=PA166&lpg=PA166&dq=death+concept+bichat&source=bl&ots=1w9_atKgL_&sig=ACfU3U00_t2XXQuH8VQTMub-JEJ4IJ_8rw&hl=en&sa=X&ved=2ahUKEwj3iNnVvsXjAhXKq1kKHdRqCEQQ6AEwDXoECAcQAQ#v=onepage&q=death concept bichat&f=false
22. Orban JC, Ferret E, Jambou P, Ichai C. Confirmation of brain death diagnosis: A study on French practice. Anaesth Crit Care Pain Med [Internet]. 2015 Jun 1 [cited 2020 Nov 2];34(3):145–50. Available from: https://pubmed.ncbi.nlm.nih.gov/26004878/

23. Dinallo S, Waseem M. Cushing reflex [Internet]. StatPearls. 2019 [cited 2020 Nov 2]. Available from: http://www.ncbi.nlm.nih.gov/pubmed/31747208
24. Machado C, Kerein J, Ferrer Y, Portela L, de la C Garcia M, Manero JM. The concept of brain death did not evolve to benefit organ transplants. J Med Ethics [Internet]. 2007 Apr 1 [cited 2019 Jul 20];33(4):197–200. Available from: http://www.ncbi.nlm.nih.gov/pubmed/17400615
25. Machado C. Brain death: a reappraisal. Springer; 2007. 223 p.
26. Cryer PE. Hypoglycemia, functional brain failure, and brain death [Internet]. Vol. 117, Journal of Clinical Investigation. American Society for Clinical Investigation; 2007 [cited 2020 Nov 2]. p. 868–870. Available from: /pmc/articles/PMC1838950/?report=abstract
27. Bergquist E, Bergström K. Angiography in cerebral death. Acta radiol [Internet]. 1972 [cited 2020 Nov 2];12(3):283–288. Available from: https://pubmed.ncbi.nlm.nih.gov/5045423/
28. Mollaret P, Goulon M. [The depassed coma (preliminary memoir)]. Rev Neurol (Paris) [Internet]. 1959 Jul [cited 2019 Jul 20];101:3–15. Available from: http://www.ncbi.nlm.nih.gov/pubmed/14423403
29. De Georgia MA. History of brain death as death: 1968 to the present. J Crit Care [Internet]. 2014 Aug [cited 2019 Jul 20];29(4):673–678. Available from: http://www.ncbi.nlm.nih.gov/pubmed/24930367
30. Machado C, Kerein J, Ferrer Y, Portela L, de la C García M, Manero JM. The concept of brain death did not evolve to benefit organ transplants. J Med Ethics [Internet]. 2007 Apr [cited 2019 Jul 21];33(4):197–200. Available from: http://www.ncbi.nlm.nih.gov/pubmed/17400615
31. Beecher HK, Adams RD, Sweet WH. Procedures for the appropriate management of patients who may have supportive measures withdrawn. JAMA [Internet]. 1969 Jul 21 [cited 2019 Jul 20];209(3):405. Available from: http://www.ncbi.nlm.nih.gov/pubmed/5819439
32. A definition of irreversible coma. Report of the Ad Hoc Committee of the Harvard Medical School to Examine the Definition of Brain Death. JAMA [Internet]. 1968 Aug 5 [cited 2019 Jul 21];205(6):337–340. Available from: http://www.ncbi.nlm.nih.gov/pubmed/5694976
33. Mohandas A, Chou SN. Brain death. J Neurosurg [Internet]. 1971 Aug [cited 2019 Jul 21];35(2):211–218. Available from: http://www.ncbi.nlm.nih.gov/pubmed/5570782
34. Jorgensen EO, Brodersen P. [Criteria of death. The value of cliniconeurologic examination of cerebral circulation for the assessment of brain death]. Nord Med [Internet]. 1971 Dec 23 [cited 2019 Jul 21];86(51):1549–1560. Available from: http://www.ncbi.nlm.nih.gov/pubmed/5134764
35. Pallis CA, Prior PF. Guidelines for the determination of death. Neurology [Internet]. 1983 Feb [cited 2019 Jul 20];33(2):251–252. Available from: http://www.ncbi.nlm.nih.gov/pubmed/6681664
36. Pallis C. ABC of brain stem death. The arguments about the EEG. BMJ [Internet]. 1983 Jan 22 [cited 2019 Jul 20];286(6361):284–287. Available from: http://www.ncbi.nlm.nih.gov/pubmed/6402074

37. Pallis C. ABC of brain stem death. The position in the USA and elsewhere. BMJ [Internet]. 1983 Jan 15 [cited 2019 Jul 20];286(6360):209–210. Available from: http://www.ncbi.nlm.nih.gov/pubmed/6401532
38. Pallis C. ABC of brain stem death. The declaration of death. BMJ [Internet]. 1983 Jan 1 [cited 2019 Jul 20];286(6358):39–39. Available from: http://www.ncbi.nlm.nih.gov/pubmed/6401455
39. Dalle Ave AL, Bernat JL. Inconsistencies between the criterion and tests for brain death. J Intensive Care Med [Internet]. 2018 Jun 21 [cited 2019 Jun 22];088506661878426. Available from: http://www.ncbi.nlm.nih.gov/pubmed/29929410
40. Bernat JL. A defense of the whole-brain concept of death. Hastings Cent Rep [Internet]. [cited 2019 Jun 22];28(2):14–23. Available from: http://www.ncbi.nlm.nih.gov/pubmed/9589289
41. Bernat JL. A conceptual justification for brain death. Hastings Cent Rep [Internet]. 2018 Nov [cited 2019 Jun 22];48:S19–S21. Available from: http://www.ncbi.nlm.nih.gov/pubmed/30584866
42. Bernat J. The definition, criterion, and statute of death. Semin Neurol [Internet]. 1984 Mar 19 [cited 2019 Jul 21];4(01):45–51. Available from: http://www.ncbi.nlm.nih.gov/pubmed/11649667
43. BERNAT JL, Culver CM, Gert B. On the definition and criterion of death. Ann Intern Med [Internet]. 1981 Mar 1 [cited 2019 Jul 21];94(3):389. Available from: http://www.ncbi.nlm.nih.gov/pubmed/7224389
44. Bernat JL. A defense of the whole-brain concept of death. Hastings Cent Rep [Internet]. [cited 2019 Jul 21];28(2):14–23. Available from: http://www.ncbi.nlm.nih.gov/pubmed/9589289
45. Guidelines for the determination of death. Report of the medical consultants on the diagnosis of death to the President's Commission for the Study of Ethical Problems in Medicine and Biomedical and Behavioral Research. JAMA [Internet]. 1981 Nov 13 [cited 2019 Jul 21];246(19):2184–2186. Available from: http://www.ncbi.nlm.nih.gov/pubmed/7289009
46. Sarbey B. Definitions of death: Brain death and what matters in a person. J law Biosci [Internet]. 2016 Dec [cited 2019 Jul 21];3(3):743–752. Available from: http://www.ncbi.nlm.nih.gov/pubmed/28852554
47. Moschella M. Brain death and human organismal integration: A symposium on the definition of death. J Med Philos [Internet]. 2016 Jun [cited 2019 Jun 22];41(3):229–236. Available from: http://www.ncbi.nlm.nih.gov/pubmed/27107428
48. Moschella M. Deconstructing the brain disconnection–brain death analogy and clarifying the rationale for the neurological criterion of death. J Med Philos [Internet]. 2016 Jun [cited 2019 Jun 22];41(3):279–299. Available from: http://www.ncbi.nlm.nih.gov/pubmed/27095749
49. Shewmon DA. Constructing the death elephant: A synthetic paradigm shift for the definition, criteria, and tests for death. J Med Philos [Internet]. 2010 Jun 1 [cited 2019 Jun 22];35(3):256–98. Available from: http://www.ncbi.nlm.nih.gov/pubmed/20439358
50. Baron L, Shemie SD, Teitelbaum J, Doig CJ. Brief review: history, concept and controversies in the neurological determination of death. Can J Anaesth [Internet]. 2006 Jun [cited 2019 Jul 21];53(6):602–608. Available from: http://link.springer.com/10.1007/BF03021852

51. Brugger EC. D. Alan Shewmon and the PCBE's White Paper on brain death: Are brain-dead patients dead? J Med Philos [Internet]. 2013 Apr 4 [cited 2019 Jun 22];38(2):205–218. Available from: https://academic.oup.com/jmp/article-lookup/doi/10.1093/jmp/jht009
52. The President's Council on Bioethics: Controversies in the Determination of Death: A White Paper by the President's Council on Bioethics [Internet]. [cited 2019 Jul 21]. Available from: https://bioethicsarchive.georgetown.edu/pcbe/reports/death/
53. Shah SK, Truog RD, Miller FG. Death and legal fictions. J Med Ethics [Internet]. 2011 Dec 1 [cited 2019 Jul 20];37(12):719–722. Available from: http://www.ncbi.nlm.nih.gov/pubmed/21810923
54. Veatch RM. Killing by organ procurement: Brain-based death and legal fictions. J Med Philos [Internet]. 2015 Jun 1 [cited 2019 Jul 20];40(3):289–311. Available from: http://www.ncbi.nlm.nih.gov/pubmed/25889264
55. Truog RD, Fackler JC. Rethinking brain death. Crit Care Med [Internet]. 1992 Dec [cited 2019 Jun 22];20(12):1705–1713. Available from: http://www.ncbi.nlm.nih.gov/pubmed/1458950
56. Miller FG, Truog RD. The incoherence of determining death by neurological criteria: a commentary on 'Controversies in the determination of death', a White Paper by the President's Council on Bioethics. Kennedy Inst Ethics J [Internet]. 2009 Jun [cited 2019 Jul 21];19(2):185–193. Available from: http://www.ncbi.nlm.nih.gov/pubmed/19623822
57. Dalle Ave AL, Shaw DM. Donation after circulatory determination of death donation after circulatory determination of death: What information to whom? I Introduction [Internet]. [cited 2019 Jul 20]. Available from: http://www.bioethica-forum.ch/docs/16_1/06_Dalle_BF9_1.pdf
58. Botkin JR, Post SG. Confusion in the determination of death: distinguishing philosophy from physiology. Perspect Biol Med [Internet]. 1992 [cited 2019 Jul 21];36(1):129–138. Available from: http://www.ncbi.nlm.nih.gov/pubmed/1475153
59. Veatch R. The death of whole-brain death: The plague of the disaggregators, somaticists, and mentalists. J Med Philos [Internet]. 2005 Aug 1 [cited 2019 Jun 22];30(4):353–378. Available from: http://www.ncbi.nlm.nih.gov/pubmed/16029987
60. Halevy A, Brody B. Brain death: Reconciling definitions, criteria, and tests. Ann Intern Med [Internet]. 1993 Sep 15 [cited 2019 Jul 21];119(6):519. Available from: http://www.ncbi.nlm.nih.gov/pubmed/8357120
61. Kushner T. Having a life versus being alive. J Med Ethics [Internet]. 1984 Mar 1 [cited 2019 Jul 21];10(1):5–8. Available from: http://jme.bmj.com/cgi/doi/10.1136/jme.10.1.5
62. Rothenberg LS. The anencephalic neonate and brain death: An international review of medical, ethical, and legal issues. Transplant Proc [Internet]. 1990 Jun [cited 2019 Jul 21];22(3):1037–1039. Available from: http://www.ncbi.nlm.nih.gov/pubmed/2190370
63. Pallis C. ABC of brain stem death. Prognostic significance of a dead brain stem. BMJ [Internet]. 1983 Jan 8 [cited 2019 Jul 20];286(6359):123–124. Available from: http://www.ncbi.nlm.nih.gov/pubmed/6401485

64. Pallis C. Further thoughts on brainstem death. Anaesth Intensive Care [Internet]. 1995 Feb 22 [cited 2019 Jun 22];23(1):20–23. Available from: http://www.ncbi.nlm.nih.gov/pubmed/7778742
65. Merker B. Consciousness without a cerebral cortex: A challenge for neuroscience and medicine. Behav Brain Sci [Internet]. 2007 Feb 1 [cited 2019 Jul 21];30(1):63–81; discussion 81-134. Available from: https://www.cambridge.org/core/product/identifier/S0140525X07000891/type/journal_article
66. Berlucchi G, Marzi CA. Neuropsychology of consciousness: Some history and a few new trends. Front Psychol [Internet]. 2019 Jan 30 [cited 2019 Jul 21];10:50. Available from: http://www.ncbi.nlm.nih.gov/pubmed/30761035
67. Machado C, Shewmon DA. Brain death and disorders of consciousness. Springer US; 2004. 287 p.
68. Aleman B, Merker B. Consciousness without cortex: A hydranencephaly family survey. Acta Paediatr [Internet]. 2014 Oct [cited 2019 Jul 21];103(10):1057–1065. Available from: http://doi.wiley.com/10.1111/apa.12718
69. Willmott L, White B. Persistent vegetative state and minimally conscious state: Ethical, legal and practical dilemmas [Internet]. Vol. 43, Journal of Medical Ethics. BMJ Publishing Group; 2017 [cited 2020 Nov 2]. p. 425–426. Available from: https://pubmed.ncbi.nlm.nih.gov/28663409/
70. Daemen JW, Kootstra G, Wijnen RM, Yin M HE. Nonheart-beating donors: the Maastricht experience—PubMed [Internet]. Clin Transpl. 1994 [cited 2020 Nov 2]. p. 303–16. Available from: https://pubmed.ncbi.nlm.nih.gov/7547551/
71. DeVita MA. The death watch: certifying death using cardiac criteria. Prog Transplant [Internet]. 2001 Mar [cited 2019 Jul 22];11(1):58–66. Available from: http://www.ncbi.nlm.nih.gov/pubmed/11357558
72. Ozark S, DeVita MA. Non-heartbeating organ donation: ethical controversies and medical considerations. Int Anesthesiol Clin [Internet]. 2001 [cited 2019 Jul 22];39(3):103–16. Available from: http://www.ncbi.nlm.nih.gov/pubmed/11524603
73. McGee A, Gardiner D, Murphy P. Determination of death in donation after circulatory death. Curr Opin Organ Transplant [Internet]. 2018 Feb [cited 2019 Jul 20];23(1):114–119. Available from: http://www.ncbi.nlm.nih.gov/pubmed/29049046

72

Ethics of organ donation in India

Daljit Singh, Rachna Wadhwa, Tanshi Daljit

Introduction

The road to successful organ donation in India is no different from the rest of the world. Organ transplantation is the best treatment option for end-stage organ disease. Organ donation not only helps in mere survival and extending life, but it also confers good quality of life in patients suffering from organ failure. Despite this known fact, the process still needs wide attention, essential knowledge, and public awareness. With improved healthcare facilities, the demand for organ donation and transplantation has increased dramatically. Although transplantation has benefitted thousands of individuals all over the world, the demand for organs still outnumbers the supply. To overcome this crisis, it is mandatory to sensitize the society towards organ donation, identify the potential donors, achieve nationwide organizational support, and implement appropriate laws and rules pertaining to this.

Global and Indian burden on organ donation

India has a population of nearly 1.37 billion, the second largest in the world. It constitutes 17.71% of the world population. According to National Organ Tissue Transplant Organisation (NOTTO) till December 2018, India had performed nearly 10,000 transplants. However, there were about 12758 patients waiting for kidney, 4173 for liver, 425 for heart, and 75 for lung.[1]

There is growing incidence of heart, kidney, lung, and liver diseases and the trends of growing organ failure requiring organ transplant are unimaginable. There are no data that projects the actual ground reality. Nearly 1.4 million people have pledged to donate organs but there are other hindrances beyond the pledge which affect organ donation in India.[1] Guidelines for organ allocation, interstate transfer, information about the donor, and recipient matching process are some of the unique problems. Guidelines for organ allocation, urgency clause, and restriction of donor eligibility pose special threats.

In January 2019, there were 113,000 patients in the waiting list for organs in the USA. The total number of transplantations performed was 36,528. Though 95% of US citizens support organ donation programme, only 58% have actually signed as donors.[2] Around twenty patients die daily waiting for transplantation and one recipient is added to waiting list every 10 minutes. In the UK, there was an 11% increase in the number of deceased donors from the previous figures to 1,574 and the number of donors after brain death increased by 15% to 955, while the number of donors after circulatory death increased by 6% to 619.[3] The number of living donors has also increased by 1% accounting for 40% of total number of organ donors.[3] Organ donation rate is highest in Spain at 46.9 per million, 31.96 per million in USA and in India, it is lowest at 0.86 per million.[4]

In England, Spain, and few other countries, the government has plans to change the law on consent for organ donation. With the introduction of Max's Law, it is presumed that everyone has consent for organ donation unless he or she opts out.[5] In India presumed consent is not yet applicable.

The worlds' estimated population was 7.2 billion with an estimated 57 million deaths per year and only 30,000 cadaveric donors. It amounts to 0.053% donors in deaths and 118,000 transplants. In fact, one million transplants and self-sufficiency can be attained by only 0.5% of cadaveric donors.[6–8]

Mythological evidence of organ donation in India

According to Indian Mythology, the first organ transplant (head transplant) was successfully performed by Lord Shiva for Lord Ganesha. Lord Shiva transplanted the head of an elephant on baby Ganesha after initially decapitating his head. Even in Sushrutasamhita, during the epic war of Gods, Rudra severed the head of Yajna. Ashmani Kumar brothers, who were heavenly surgeons, resutured the head and provided life to Yajna.(9–11)

In the quest of organ donors and recipients, there are several tales of implanting pisces (fishes) on human head. Such a widespread belief has made Indian sub-continent a special geographical zone where organ transplant is a sacred process. We have enriched examples of xenograft in Ganesha and Matsyakanya (human fish hybrid).(12,13)

Though ancient surgeons like Sushruta and Jivika did not find a mention in organ donation, their skills for organ crafting and reshaping laid the foundation of organ transplant today.

Evolution of organ donation in India

In India the first organ transplant was performed in 1965 in Mumbai. Later more centres started performing transplants. In the initial decades of transplant, Indian donors were subjected to kidney racketing. Exploitation of poor patients remained a common process despite voices against it amidst society, doctors, and activists. The Indian subcontinent was slowly becoming a subcentre for organ transplant for sick patients. Though the Government and regulatory bodies like Medical Council India (MCI) exists, there was no concrete law that allowed transparency, licensing, regulation of process, and punishment for any kind of violation errant.

To overcome these deficiencies, Transplant of Human Organ act was enacted in 1994. The same has been later revised to facilitate more kinds of donors for increasing organ donation. This act also defined and conceptualized the criteria of brain death, especially the declaration and various other issues related to organ transplant.(14,15)

The Act of Transplantation of Human Organs laid down the regulations regarding removal, storage, and transplantation of human organs for purely therapeutic purposes. The amendment to the act was passed in 2011 by parliament and subsequent rules were passed and notified in 2014 (THOTA). Various provisions under this act have been adopted from previous publications related to ethics.

There are two types of donors—living and deceased. The living donors include near related donors, spousal donors, and sometimes, other than near related donors. Safety and quality of life of a living donor are important issues apart from ethical concerns. However, motivation of the donor is essential for living organ donation. Ministry of Health and Family Welfare Government of India (MOHFW) have expanded the definition of near relatives under THOTA 1994 clause(i) of section 2 and define 'near relative' as spouse, son, daughter, mother, brother, and sister. Further, the act was amended in 2011 and it also included grandfather, grandmother, grandson, and granddaughter.[16]

Despite this expansion, number of living donors did not increase as grandparents were either too old or had multiple co-morbidities that prohibited their organ donation; grandchildren are also too young to donate. Therefore, the Government of India is yet to expand this list including stepfather, stepmother, stepbrother, stepsister, stepson, stepdaughter, and their spouses.

Various provisions under the act have been summarized to familiarize with the clauses related to regulation of organ donation.[17–19]

The Transplantation of Human Organs and Tissues Act, 1994 (Act No. 42)

It is an Act to regulate the removal, storage, and transplantation of human organs for therapeutic purposes and for the prevention of commercial dealings in human organs and for matters connected therewith or incidental thereto.

Chapter 1 of the act comprises various definitions, precisely, brain death, deceased, donor, human organ, hospital, human organ retrieval centre, minor, near relative, recipient, tissue, tissue bank, transplantation, transplant coordinator, etc. Chapter 2 focuses on the authority for removal of human organs or tissues or both.

1) Any donor, before his death (when alive), can give consent and authorize the removal of any organ or tissue or both from his body for therapeutic purposes.

1A) In case of removal, storage, or transplant, it is the duty of registered medical practitioner of hospital, in coordination with transplant coordinator:
   (i) To check if any person in the ICU has given the authorization for organ donation before his death.
   (ii) If the patient has not given any authorization, they should make that person and his near relative aware about the process of organ donation and give them option for acceptance or declination.
   (iii) The hospital is required to inform in writing to human organ retrieval centre.

1B) The duties of registered medical practitioner mentioned in 1A clauses i and ii have to be carried out, even when hospital is not registered.

2. If donor has authorized for organ and tissue donation in writing, then registered medical practitioner can proceed.
3. If no such authority, but no objection also for organs being therapeutically used, then the person lawfully in possession of that dead body may authorize.
4. The authority as mentioned in 1, 2, and 3 is sufficient for organ and tissue donation but only registered medical practitioner has authority for such removal.
5. It is the duty of registered medical practitioner to confirm before proceeding for organ removal that death has been certified, especially in cases of brain death.
6. In cases of brain death, procedure for removal should begin only after death has been certified by Board of Medical Experts including registered medical practitioner, specialists from panel of names approved by appropriate authority, neurologist, or neurosurgeon from the same panel and the treating physician.
   - Removal of human organ or tissue or both should not be authorized in certain cases, e.g. no authority to remove body parts is granted to a person who has been entrusted with responsibility for intervention, cremation, or other disposal.

In cases of unclaimed bodies in hospital/prison not claimed within 48 hours, the person in charge or management control of hospital or prison has the authority to permit removal of body parts.

- Authority for removal of organ in case of MLC/road traffic accident and preservation of human organ or tissue or both.
- Restriction of removal or transplantation where either donor or recipient being near relative is a foreign national, prior approval of authorization committee shall be received.

Chapter 3 deals in

- Regulation of hospital: No hospital unless registered in the Act shall conduct or associate with removal, storage, or transplantation. Similarly, no medical practitioner unless registered in this Act shall conduct transplant-related activities.

Chapter 4 deals in

- Appropriate authority at either central government or state government level shall grant registration, suspend, or cancel registration, and investigate and inspect the premise.
- Advisory committee can be constructed by state or central government for a term of two years to discharge its function.

Chapters 5 and 6

It defines the guidelines for registration of hospitals, engaged in removal, storage, or transplantation of organs, certificate of registration, supervision of registration (even suo moto) and appeal. It also defines the rules with respect to punishment which may extend up to ten years with fine up to 20 lakhs.

Deceased donation can be carried out after cardiac death or brain death, and have many logistic and important ethical issues. The deceased organ donation can be significantly increased with the implementation of proper guidelines, public awareness, and sensitization. There is an urgent need of establishing infrastructure and education system so as to promote deceased donations.

The provisions in the transplant of human organs and tissues act further define:

a) Living Donor—relatives who can donate without hassles—mother, father, brother, sister, son, daughter, and spouse; first degree relatives require genetic testing and legal formalities. In the absence of authorized donor, appropriate authority can allow permission for transplant of organs based upon clinical and emergent situations.
b) Authorization committee may approve or reject donation from other than the first degree relative. Joint application is made by both donor and recipient in such cases.
c) Appropriate authority which is constituted by state or centre has the responsibility to regulate, license, and appeal. It also inspects places, maintains standards, and separate license is required for each organ.

The act also laid the basis of withdrawal of life support. There has been a widespread concern about vegetative patients who have volunteered for euthanasia and organ donation, yet some of the prevailing laws are insufficient to address the gaps in such issues. Some of the prevailing problems despite the Act are lack of ICU, infrastructure, and skill for transplant.

Limitations of organ transplant process

In an overburdened ICU, the process of brainstem death declaration is considered rather tedious and cumbersome. It has also been perceived that expectation of family members of donors suddenly changes once they agree to donate organs.[20,21] There have been instances when donor family demands financial gain during donation of organs from rather terminal recipient who has otherwise no earning potential for survival.

Motivation for organ donation is lacking in India. There are several reasons for this. There is a common misconception that by donating organs, the soul becomes impure and will not be able to attain *nirvana, moksha,* or salvation.[22,23]

Additionally, removal of organ from unclaimed bodies over 48-hour window has resulted in poor outcome. Often the family traces the body within this period and organ donation is not restricted to the willingness of donor or one of the family members. It requires persuasion and consent of several family members, especially in India as with the social structure of joint family or joint care of family members, their attachment is inherent. Such measures delay and result in crucial time loss to maintain organ survival in the brain dead.

Reward gifting the unrelated donor is also an important ethical issue. Advocates often come into picture in such situations and hamper the process. Financial incentive is a double-edged sword; due to poor socio-economic status of majority of donors and recipients, often it is equated to the principle of business as beg, borrow, or steal. It is better to buy than to die. The enormous market of organ donation generally allows rich to manage early out of the line arrangements than those in the waiting list. In such situations, it is inevitable for the middleman to crop up in the system and exploit it even further.

Cost of transplant: Issue of inequality

Another major reason involving ethics in organ donation in India is the exuberant cost in private sector. In most cases, cost of transplant and its maintenance on immune suppression is quite high and is not affordable by majority of families. There is no system of insurance for transplant, no national programme for transplant and policy to help such cases.

Recently, trends are getting slowly favourable with the help of PM relief fund, AYUSHMAN scheme and help from some NGOs.(24)

The presence of a huge middle-class population in India and mismatch between donor and recipient ratio opens the footpath for inevitable corrupt practices in organ donation. Such mismatch exists all over world, and not only in India. Further mindset of rich people questions paradoxically, like, why donate organ when money is there to purchase it. Therefore, it creates a situation similar to child labour, where labour is available at low cost or prostitution, i.e. paid sexual gratification.(25)

In a study on Economic and Health consequences of selling a kidney in India, 96% had donated kidneys to pay debt. Average amount received was $1070. Nearly 86% of donors had deteriorated after nephrectomy. Therefore, the economic gain as an incentive had only short-lasting benefits. Similar observation had been reported by Lawrence Cohen who reported 'kidney belt region' in south India where females had sold their kidney to cover debt incurred by husband through gambling and addiction.[26,27]

Social and ethical issues of transplantation

The very nature that organ trade market is indiscriminate and promiscuous led to the erosion of social values. Currently, India has over 400 transplant centres. Both government and NGO (Mohan organization, Chennai) are actively involved in encouraging organ donation and transplantation. India has the high potential of organ donation from those who meet fatal accidents or severe subarachnoid haemorrhage. It is estimated that India has over 100,000 fatal deaths every year.[28] Most of these are young adults with otherwise healthy body. Though, it may generate a large pool of potential donors, ethic and emotion attached to sudden loss of family member pose a major obstacle to donation.

India also faces similar problems as the rest of the world. Relevance of cardinal principles of bioethics, i.e. autonomy, beneficence, justice, and non-maleficence are tested more in organ donation.

Autonomy-first cardinal principle where patient has a right to decide for himself is more relevant in clinical trial than organ donation.[29] A diseased person is often not in a mental state to make decisions, unless already consented. Those who had already pledged for organ donation often remain undisclosed and often may not inform other relatives or care giver.[30]

Altruism can be an extension to beneficence as a measure to benefit others by moral duty. Indian mythology also supports such acts. Rishi (sage) Dhadichi had donated his bone to Vajra, a kind of weapon to kill demons. Such tales can be of supportive value in persuasive motivation for donation in India.

Even neuroscience supports sense of gratification as elicited on Functional MRI in midline structure of brain. Subgenual cortex, septal region shows EEG activity of the brain. It may suggest that certain areas of brain are involved in taking altruistic decisions.[31]

Conclusion

The principle of justice in bioethics is often debated in organ donation. Where it may help the recipient, there is always a risk to living donor. Many donors experience pain and morbidity. The risk of surgical complications among living donors is 5–10%. Therefore it may be debated if all the cardinal principles of organ donation be as applicable as in other clinical trials.

All these principles are primarily meant for clinical research and trial during introduction of a new drug or implant. These principles focus on benefit of society at large keeping the ability to choose by an individual. The benefits of trial are largely to a society whereas it is an individual who is benefited in transplant surgery.

Therefore, one may have to evolve different ethical guidelines and principles preventing non-exploitation of potential donor, with informed rather presumed consent that provide justice to society, at large, without malicious gain in the realm of organ donation. India has been the spiritual epicentre of the world and the same spirit can be extended with the support of huge mythological background to enrich the ethics of organ donation without organ broker and transplant tourism.

Highlights

- Indian Mythology claims to have evidence of the first-ever Xenograft for Lord Ganesha.
- In India, Transplant of Human Organ and Tissue Act regulates organ donation.
- India has a high number of potential donors which need to be motivated from school age rather than later years of life.
- Ethical principles should be more people friendly and transparent to facilitate larger utility for patients requiring organ donation.
- There is a need to have more centres which can effectively carry out organ donation programme in India.

References

1. National Organ and Tissue Transplant Organization. Accessed November 2020 from: https://notto.gov.in/
2. Sahay M. Transplantation of human organs and tissues Act—'Simplified'. Indian J Transplant 2018;12:84–89.
3. Smith M. Physiologic changes during brain stem death—lessons for management of the organ donor. J Heart Lung Transplant. 2004;23(9):S217–S222.
4. Pande GK, Patniak PK, Gupta S, Sahni P. Brain death and organ transplantation in India. National Medical Journal of India, New Delhi. 1990.
5. https://www.organdonation.nhs.uk/get-involved/news/max-and-keira-s-law-comes-into-effect-in-england, assessed November 2020
6. The Council of the Transplantation Society: Commercialisation in Transplantation. The problems and some guidelines for practice. Lancet1985;327:715–716.
7. Bakshi A, Nandi P, Guleria S. Cadaveric renal transplants. Our experience with relatives. National Medical Journal of India1994;7:252.
8. Patel CT. Live related donation: a viewpoint. Transplant Proceedings 1988;20:1068–1070.
9. Sanjay Nagral. Ethics of Organ transplant. Medical ethics 1995;3(2):19–22.
10. Reddy KC, Thiagrajan CM, Shunmugasundaram D et al. Unconventional renal transplantation in India: to buy or let die. Transplant Proceedings 1990;22;9 10–11.
11. Salahudeen AK, Woods HF, Pingle A et al. High mortality among recipients of bought living-related donor kidney. Lancet1990;336:725–728.
12. Mani MK. Making an Ass of the Law. Letter from Chennai. Natl Med J India 1997;10:242–243.
13. Kakodkar R, Soin A, Nundy S. Liver transplantation in India: Its evolution, problems and the way forward. Nat Med J India 2007;20:53–56.
14. Goyal M, Mehta RL, Schneiderman LJ, Sehgal AR. Economic and Health Consequences of selling a Kidney in India. Jama 2002;288:1589–1593.
15. The Declaration of Istanbul on Organ Trafficking and Transplant Tourism. International Summit on Transplant Tourism and Oran Trafficking. Clin J Am Soc Nephrol 2008;3:1227–1231.
16. National Organ and Tissue Transplant Organization. Accessed November 2020 from https://notto.gov.in/act-end-rules-of-thoa.htm
17. Organ trafficking and transplant tourism and commercialism: the Declaration of Istanbul. The Lancet 2008:372(9632), 5–6.
18. Rhodes R, Schiano T. Transplant tourism in China: a tale of two transplants. Am J Bioeth 2010; 10: 3–11.
19. Eghtesad B, Jain AB, Fung JJ. Living donor liver transplantation: ethics and safety. Transplant proc 2003; 35: 51–52.
20. Starzl TE, Marchioro TL, porter KA, Brettschneider L. Homotransplantation of the liver. Transplantation 1967; 5: Suppl: 790-uppl:803.

21. Gries CJ, White DB, Truog RD, Dubois J, Cosio CC, Dhanani S, et al. Sharing Statement" ethical and policy considerations in organ donation after circulatory determination of death. Am J Respir Crit Care Med 2013; 188: 103–109.
22. World Health Organization. WHO guiding principles on human cell, tissue and organ transplantation. Transplantation 2010; 90: 229–233.
23. Saunders B. Normative consent and opt-out organ donation. J Med ethics 2010; 36: 84–87.
24. Ayushman Bharat Pradhan Mantri Jan Arogya Yojana. Accessed November 2020 from: https://pmjay.gov.in/
25. Chkhotua A. Incentives for organ donation: pros and cons. Transplant Proc 2012; 44: 1793–1794.
26. Cohen L.R. Where It Hurts: Indian Material for an Ethics of Organ Transplantation. Daedalus 1999;128:135–165.
27. Lavee J. Ethical amendments to the Israeli Organ Transplant Law. Am J Transplant 2013; 13: 1614. doi: 10.1111/ajt.12240.
28. Mortality due to road injuries in the states of India: the Global Burden of Disease Study 1990–2017. Lancet Public Health 2020; 5: e86–98 Published Online December 24, 2019 https://doi.org/10.1016/ S2468-2667(19)30246-4
29. Shroff S. Legal and ethical aspects of Organ donation and transplant. Indian J Urology.2009; 25(3):348–355.
30. Shroff S, Navin S, Abraham G, Rajan PS, Suresh S, Rao S, et al. Cadaver organ donation and transplantation—an Indian prospective. Transplant Proceedings 2003;35:15–17.
31. Shroff S. Working towards ethical organ transplants. Indian J Med Ethics 2007;4:68–69.

73

Family members perspective of organ donation: Concerns and fears

Manikandan Sethuraman

Introduction

Organ donation has saved millions of people with end-stage disease conditions across the world and has become the standard of care in these patients.[1] The donation can be either by deceased or living organ donors. However, the number of patients with end-stage disease is ever-increasing and so is the demand for organs for transplant. The global shortage of availability of organs which is of major concern,[2] the entire demand is not met globally leading to supply-demand imbalance. Millions of people with end-stage disease die while waiting for availability of compatible organs causing a major impact on the healthcare system. Moreover, these patients need repeated hospitalization till the availability of organs for transplantation leading to loss of work, financial constraints as well as demand on the healthcare. Death of the end-stage disease patients before availability of organs will cause severe impact on the family of these patients.

Since the deceased organ donation is a major source of organs, the decision to donate the organ of the dead person entirely depends on the consent of the deceased family members.[3] Many times, the family members have reservations about the organ donation which is a major cause to refusal for donation.[3] A retrospective analysis found family refusal as a cause of failure of organ donation in at least 50% of cases.[4] The family refusal can lead to loss of potential organs that can be transplanted as well as low donation rate in many countries, especially the developing nations. The family concerns can be due to various reasons like illiteracy, inability to take decisions due to bereavement, religious belief, lack of education about organ donation and so on. It is important to understand the factors affecting the organ donation and try to address them. This chapter will provide an overview of family perceptions on organ donation and their concerns.

Factors affecting organ donation by family members

Death of a close kin is one of the most disturbing events for every family member. This is further exaggerated if the death occurs suddenly and due to unnatural causes like accidents, suicide, etc. It is obvious that in such a situation, the family members will be in a state of shock. Most of the deceased organ donations occur from the victims of trauma. Understandably, the family may not be in a situation to take the right decision on organ donation. In addition, various factors may contribute to the refusal/acceptance of family consent for organ donation like lack of knowledge about organ donation, wishes of the deceased, religious and cultural beliefs and obligations, distrust in the healthcare system, fear of disfigurement of the body after organ/tissue donations, etc. Hence, the organ donation/procurement team must understand these issues, and provide appropriate knowledge and support to the families to aid in making the decision on donation.

Having said that the relatives are responsible for consenting, the entire blame on organ refusal must not be on the relatives of the deceased. Sometimes, the hospital management of the deceased, technique, and timing of the approach to relatives of the dead, misinterpretation of the prevailing legal system as well as religious bodies and systems can also be a co-contributor for family refusal.

Healthcare workers and organ donation

Though this chapter deals with family concerns of acceptance of organ donation, the knowledge and attitude of healthcare workers on organ donation process can also influence the family decisions. The rates of organ donation among healthcare workers and their families are also low. In a survey of medical professionals in Argentina, only 82% agreed for their organ donation and 69% agreed for donation of their family members. Almost 94% didn't have adequate information/knowledge about organ donation. Only 20% have registered themselves as organ donor.[5] Moreover, it was found that the medical students do not discuss about organ donation among their family members. In another survey of nursing students, the organ donation willingness and knowledge were found to be low.[6] It is obvious that if the knowledge, attitude, and willingness are low among healthcare workers, then they would not have appropriate knowledge to explain the families of potential donors on the organ donation issues. It is very important to educate the healthcare workers about the medical and social aspects of brain death and organ donation by the way including the same in their curriculum and training them accordingly.[7] This is very important as brain death can occur in smaller hospitals or remote areas in any country or developing nations; the inadequate knowledge and information of treating doctors and nurses on organ transplant process can lead to potential loss of donors even if either the patient had wished to donate before death or family was favouring donation. In a recent large study, it was found that training of emergency personnel in organ donation, an electronic support system to identify and/or refer potential donors, a collaborative care pathway, donation request by a trained professional, and additional family support while patient is in the ICU by a trained nurse were associated with positive response to organ donation emphasizing the importance of training the healthcare professionals.[8]

Organ donation and laws

In order to improve the organ donation rate, different countries have adopted laws to facilitate the organ retrieval. Many families and individuals are not familiar or unaware of the laws present in their country. Some of the laws can have impact on the belief and cultural practices of the family which can lead to refusal of organ donation. It is necessary for the organ procurement team to explain these legal rules to the family so that they feel secure and trust the organ donation process.

Brain death versus biological death and its impact

The first law to be enacted worldwide is the shift in the definition of criteria for death. Over centuries, people in many countries believed and legally defined death as 'cessation of cardiorespiratory functions' of the individual. The concept of brain death came with the understanding that the circulatory and respiratory functions of the individual can be maintained with medical advancement even after cessation of brain functions. With this fact, along with the development of organ transplant programme since 1960s, and the shift of organ procurement from living to cadaveric donors, criteria for brain death have been formulated. Most countries have enacted the definition of brain death as the criteria of somatic death.

People don't accept death when the heart is beating and the patient is kept on ventilatory support.[9] Even though the physicians were aware of the brain death, they were hesitant to declare death and still followed criteria of cardiac death due to apprehension and fear of backlash from the kin of the patient.[10] This is one of the reasons for refusal of organs by the families. Further, this led to unnecessary treatment, bed occupancy especially in the ICUs, and increased the costs. This can lead to inability to provide ICU care to genuine patients due to scarcity of hospital beds. In order to facilitate the health services to improve the organ donation rates, countries like India have enacted laws favouring withdrawal of life support if the patient satisfies the criteria of brain death.[11] Despite the laws, studies have shown that still people are not aware of the concept of brain death and the pathophysiology[12] and organ donation rates were found to be low in many countries. This is due to lack of knowledge and transparency and a part of failure of the healthcare/legal system.[13] The reason was thought to be the inability to take a right decision, religious beliefs, and lack of understanding of the wishes of the deceased, especially in sudden and unexpected death situations.

Laws for consent to organ donation

Obtaining consent of the family is an important prerequisite of organ donation.[14] Despite the best of efforts, the organ donation rate is only 42% in UK.[15] Multiple studies show varying factors contributing to positive and negative consent.[16] Modifiable factors for improving family consent include appropriate timing like when the patient is terminally ill rather than along with declaration of brain death, providing emotional support while explaining the process of brain death and organ donation. In addition, well-trained personnel for obtaining consent have been found to improve donation rates.[17] Considering the above pitfalls in organ donation, countries like England and other European countries have enacted new law stating that all adults will be considered for organ donation when they die (presumed consent) unless specified by the individual against donation or if they fall under exclusion group due to other factors.

There are three types of consent related to organ donation and differ among the countries depending on the law. Majority of the European countries are part of Eurotransplant program wherein 'presumed consent' system exists.[18] In presumed consent, the organ donation is considered automatically in all patients when the diagnosis of brain death is made, unless they have specifically registered their wish not to donate their organs. Countries that have presumed consent include Austria, Germany, Hungary, Slovenia, Croatia, Belgium, and Wales. Netherlands and England have approved presumed consent from 2020 onwards. In the USA, the physician in charge of the deceased donor is expected to speak to the relatives of the victim for organ donation. Nevertheless, in certain states like Texas, there has been a move to go for presumed consent.[19] In a country like India, 'Informed consent' exists where the physician in charge notifies the occurrence of brain death to the state/national agencies (NOTA) who will initiate the process of taking consent for organ donation from the relatives of the patients through the transplant coordinators.[20] Alternate to the above two consent systems is the third one, the 'Conscription system', where the usable organs and tissues are removed posthumously within a short time of death for transplantation regardless of existence of consent or refusal for organ donation.[21,22]

Each of the above systems has advantages and disadvantages. In presumed consent, the state has the right to procure the organs unless opt-out is registered. The rates of organ donation is reported to be 'very low' even in many developed countries in Europe and US as their population are reluctant to consent to donate organs.[23] The fear of presumed donation is that it will increase the people's mistrust on the healthcare system.[24] The autonomy, wishes, and beliefs of the individual and family are violated. Hence, many people would opt out of donation. In some countries like Brazil, the donation rates have come down following presumed donation laws.[25] Moreover, as per the law, presumed consent involves adult patients. Hence, organs from children and others who were disabled before brain death cannot be taken leading to potential loss of donors. In such patients, informed consent is mandatory.

Informed consent maintains the autonomy and self-respect of the individuals. It is also considered more ethical compared to presumed consent. It also helps the individuals to choose their wish of donating which organs/tissues they would like to give. Additionally, the families feel better and proud by voluntarily donating the organs, rather than by force as in presumed consent. Studies have shown that voluntary registering of donors enhances the donation rates. The disadvantage of informed consent is that the grieving families may not be in a right frame of mind to take a decision. Further, even if the deceased has registered willingness to organ donation, families can refuse. The donation rates can be very low based on family beliefs and practices and lack of information.

Wishes of the deceased

Perhaps the most important factor favouring organ donation is the wishes of the deceased. If the deceased had discussed his/her wishes to the family members regarding organ donation, the agreement for organ donation has higher success rate than if the family did not know the wish. The family members have been found to be more satisfied and proud to accomplish the wishes of their close ones. However, if the wishes were unknown, then they are hesitant to agree upon donation. In a questionnaire, factors like body integrity should be preserved after death and that organ donation entails mutilation and disfigurement of their loved ones were found to be of much concern and main reasons for family refusal.[26] Positive attitude to donation of self or family members, level of communication among family members on organ donation, openness to organ donation, registration of a family member as an organ donor all have been associated with improved donation rates. It is also known that if the family members are unaware of the wish to donate before, then the chances of refusal for donation is low.[27] The hospital and organ procurement team must approach the family considering the attitudes of the family to donation. A positive attitude has high success rates. Families who are not keen on donation are less likely to agree. On the other hand, those who neither had positive or negative attitudes nor thoughts about organ donation have been found to consent willingly with extensive and repeated counselling, and improve the success rates of organ donation.[28]

Effects of religion on organ donation

Religious beliefs form an important influence on the organ donation.[29] Almost all the religions followed by people are ancient and the people following are governed by beliefs and traditions that have evolved over centuries. All the religions have their own views on post-death destiny of the deceased and effects of death on human body post-death and its handling.

The concept of organ donation is very new compared to religions. Hence people and their religious leaders have concerns and reservations over donation. The teachings in different religions on after-life, rebirth, destiny, etc. have an impact on the decision-making. Most of the religions like Hinduism, Buddhism, and Christianity considers donation in any form as a good deed, act of selflessness and encourages it. They also consider that relief of human suffering is very important. In some religions like Sikhism, the dead body is not considered important as it gives importance to soul and does not inhibit donation. In Islam, even though violating human body is prohibited, relieving the suffering of individual is considered to be the highest priority. Hence, various Islamic countries encourage organ donation. However, the rates of donation are different in different countries.[30,31]

In Japan, where people practice Shintoism, injuring the body is considered to be harmful even after death. Moreover, interfering with the corpse is considered bad luck.[32] So the rates of organ donation are poor in Japan. Similar concerns exist in people following Taoism and Confucianism. In Jehovah's Witness, transfusion of blood in any form is prohibited; however, with regards to organ donation, no consensus exists and 'to donate or not' depends on the individual concerned.[33]

It is important for the transplant procurement teams to understand the religious beliefs of the families taking it into consideration when counselling for organ donation. This becomes important in countries like USA and UK where people of multiple ethnicity and religions live. Religious concerns of the family may include injuring the body during surgery and disfigurement, rituals like burials or cremation, timing concerns related to taking the body to their place as well as performing the religious rituals and providing information to the near and dear about the death. Some religions like Islam favours burial to be done within 24 hours. The transplant procurement team must be in a position to address the religious concerns through different approaches and include appropriate personnel like various religious organisations. In UK, information booklets are made available to be distributed to people to provide answers to different religious-related concerns on organ donation. People of any particular religion can get sufficient information from the booklets which enhance the acceptability to donation. In some religions, rituals/prayers are usually performed in the presence of Chaplains/Clerics/Priests before death. They play a vital role in helping families of a potential organ donor. Hence if a potential donor is available, personal communication by the healthcare workers with the concerned religious person regarding the possibility of organ donation would be of great help for families in decision process.

Optimal timing of interaction with families

One of the critical and well-recognized factors in organ donation is the optimal timing of 'breaking the bad news' and further progress towards the counselling for organ donation.[34] Premature requests/suggestions for organ donation or a talk about it when the patient is not making progress or deteriorating in the ICU, and not tested for brain death, are not well taken by the relatives.[35] It needs to be ascertained that the relatives know about the concept of brain death. Many people do not know about the brain death. It has been found that the families expect miracles for bringing the patient to life. Hence, in families without prior knowledge, counselling for organ donation without proper information will cause mistrust in the healthcare system and negative attitude towards organ donation, even if the patient has registered willingness to donate organs.

The treating physician plays an important role in identifying the knowledge of the brain death among family members, educating them and continuously informing about the patient's deteriorating conditions. Studies have shown that the relatives consider the information provided by the hospital about the patient's condition was inadequate many times.[36] Studies have shown that for high success rate, the appropriate method and time to explain to relatives would be in two phases. Initially, it involves explanation by the physician to the families about the low chances of recovery, providing information about testing of brain death and the results to make them understand that irreversibility of the condition. In the second phase, counselling for organ donation must be made considering the attitudes of the family members towards the same. It was found that when more number of family members, and friends were present during counselling, the understanding of the situation, acceptance of brain death and willingness for organ donation were higher compared to counselling to a single member. In families who are unable to decide, a second set of counselling would also improve the willingness to donate. Moreover, it was that inadequate and counselling not sensitive to the needs of the relatives was associated with poor organ donation rates.[37] It is important that adequate time is spent with the relatives to clear their apprehensions and their fears regarding organ procurement process.

Tissue versus organ donation

In addition to organs, tissues like skin, bones, heart valves, blood vessels, and musculoskeletal tissues are also being taken from the deceased donors for transplantation. The family consent and response to counselling for tissue donations vary from organ donation.[38] It was found that families may approve organ donations but have concerns for tissue donation and type of tissues retrieved. While it was found that the acceptance for tissues like cornea and heart valves was found to be reasonably constant in a retrospective study in Brazil, the rates of donation for tissues like skin, bone, etc. were low.[39]

This has been attributed to the fact that donation and retrieval of cornea and heart valves are usually done after the heart stops; hence the family acceptability was found to be good. Furthermore, the knowledge about corneal transplant is widespread which could be another reason for high donation rates. Survey shows that the relatives do not want disfigurement of the body after removal and hence, the rates of skin and bone donations were thought to be lower. It is very vital to inform and obtain consent from the relatives of the donor for tissues harvested and organs retrieved as tissue donation is increasingly used in many conditions and the demand is set to increase.

Concerns in paediatric organ donor

Paediatric end-stage disease is one of the major health concerns in children and 7% of transplantations are done in paediatric patients. However, special concerns are availability of donor of suitable size; poor survival in the waiting period for donation contributes to high mortality in paediatric patients. However, once transplanted the survival rates are high compared to adults.(40)

There are key issues and differences in the paediatric organ donor. Foremost is that the paediatric patients cannot first-person consent necessitating the importance of parent's consent. It has been found that parents are far more agreeable for organ donation in paediatric cases. The main concerns of the patients in the donation process were evaluated in a recent study.(41) The key differences between the adult and paediatric deceased donor were that the educational levels of the parents did not influence their decision on donation. Moreover, disfigurement concerns and delays in burial did not influence the decision-making. Fulfilling the expectations of parents regarding the process of organ donation by the critical care physician, nurse, and primary care was found to be a major factor to increase the success rate of paediatric organ donation.(42) With regard to the timing of discussion, parents felt that when the child is critically ill with low chance of survival, the discussion about organ donation must be initiated rather than after declaration of brain death in contrast to adults. The main concern and expectations of the parents were follow-up emotional support which prevented them from regretting about consenting for organ donation.(42)

Concerns of donation after cardiac death

Donation after circulatory determination of death (DCDD) is another method of procuring organs in order to increase the supply of organs for transplant. This method has been projected to increase the organ donation by 10% every year.[43] The DCCD is much more challenging compared to brain death for the organ procurement team and families. Controlled DCDD is the technique employed for the purpose of organ procurement that happens in the critically or terminally ill patients and end of life patients who were otherwise fit to donate organs. The death is declared within two minutes of cessation of circulatory and pulmonary activity. In DCDD, consent for organ donation is obtained if adult from either patients or if they are not fit to give consent from the eligible family members of patients before the declaration of death; whereas in donation after brain death, the family consent must be obtained after diagnosis of brain death. The patients' will is considered to be strong and have more precedence over family wishes regarding organ donation under Uniform Anatomical Gift act.[44] In case of paediatric patients, surrogate consent is needed. However, conflicts can occur for obtaining consent from relatives for doing interventions to maintain organ functions antemortem and post-mortem as well as withdrawal of life support process. The ICU physicians and staff must discuss the details of intervention with the surrogates and obtain consent. The relatives can disagree on this process that can potentially lead to failure to conduct controlled DCDD.[45] The process of DCDD is still not well evolved with only few centres practising it and needs lots of research for further understanding.

Conclusion

Success of the organ donation in a country depends primarily on the caregivers' approach to understand the needs of the bereaving kin of the potential organ donor. They must be provided with adequate information and time to take decisions, and emotional support not only for the donation, but post-donation also and respect their decisions. There must be a combined approach towards family counselling and continuous monitoring of the effective interventions is essential to improve the services.

Highlights

- There is a shortage of supply of organs for donation worldwide and the key factor is refusal of donation by the relatives of the potential organ donor.
- There is lack of knowledge among health care professionals on the organ donation.
- Families' refusal reasons include lack of faith in healthcare system, refusing to accept brain death, and waiting for miracles.
- Other key issues for failure of organ donation include lack of knowledge on organ donation process, poor emotional support, doubts about mutilation of the corpse, and various religious and cultural beliefs.
- The need for transparency, improved overall information, and favourable laws while maintaining family autonomy and ethics will improve the donation rate.

References

1. Directive 2010/53/EU of the European Parliament and of the Council of 7 July 2010 on standards of quality and safety of human organs intended for transplantation. 2010. Available at: http://eurlex.europa.eu/LexUriServ/LexUriServ.do?uri=OJ:L:2010:207:0014: 0029:EN:PDF
2. Siminoff LA, Gordon N, Hewlett J, et al. Factors influencing families' consent for donation of solid organ transplantation. JAMA. 2001;286:71–77.
3. Morgan SE, Miller JK. Beyond the organ donor card: the effect of knowledge, attitudes, and values on willingness to communicate about organ donation to family members. Health Commun.2001;14:121–134.
4. Leblebici M. Prevalence and Potential Correlates of Family Refusal to Organ Donation for Brain-Dead Declared Patients: A 12-Year Retrospective Screening Study. Transplant Proc. 2021;53:548–554.
5. Atamañuk AN, Ortiz Fragola JP, Giorgi M, Berreta J, Lapresa S, Ahuad-Guerrero A, Reyes-Toso CF. Medical Students' Attitude Toward Organ Donation: Understanding Reasons for Refusal in Order to Increase Transplantation Rates. Transplant Proc. 2018;50:2976–2980.
6. Pugliese MR, Degli Esposti D, Venturoli N, et al. Hospital attitude survey on organ donation in the Emilia-Romagna region. Italy. Transpl Int 2001;14:411e9.
7. Fontana F, Massari M, Giovannini L, Alfano G, Cappelli G. Knowledge andAttitudes Toward Organ Donation in Health Care Undergraduate Students in Italy.Transplant Proc. 2017;49:1982–1987.

8. Witjes M, Jansen NE, van der Hoeven JG, Abdo WF. Interventions aimed at healthcare professionals to increase the number of organ donors: a systematic review. Crit Care. 2019 20;23:227.
9. Liu CW, Yeo C, Lu Zhao B, Lai CKY, Thankavelautham S, Ho VK, Liu JCJ. Brain Death in Asia: Do Public Views Still Influence Organ Donation in the 21st Century? Transplantation. 2019;103:755–763.
10. Franz HG, DeJong W, Wolfe SM, Nathan H, Payne D, Reitsma W, Beasley C.Explaining brain death: a critical feature of the donation process. J Transpl Coord. 1997;7:14–21.
11. Lobo Gajiwala A. Regulatory aspects of tissue donation, banking and transplantation in India. Cell Tissue Bank. 2018;19:241–248.
12. Shah SK, Kasper K, Miller FG. A narrative review of the empirical evidence on public attitudes on brain death and vital organ transplantation: the need for better data to inform policy. J Med Ethics. 2015;41:291–296.
13. Gyllström Krekula L, Forinder U, Tibell A. What do people agree to when stating willingness to donate? On the medical interventions enabling organ donation after death. PLoS One. 2018 24;13:e0202544.
14. Chandler JA, Connors M, Holland G, Shemie SD. "Effective" Requesting: A Scoping Review of the Literature on Asking Families to Consent to Organ and Tissue Donation. Transplantation. 2017;101(5S Suppl 1):S1–S16.
15. (Hulme W, Allen J, Manara AR, Murphy PG, Gardiner D, Poppitt E. Factors influencing the family consent rate for organ donation in the UK. Anaesthesia. 2016;71:1053–1063.
16. Brown CV, Foulkrod KH, Dworaczyk S, Thompson K, Elliot E, Cooper H, Coopwood B. Barriers to obtaining family consent for potential organ donors. J Trauma. 2010;68:447–451.
17. Vincent A, Logan L. Consent for organ donation. Br J Anaesth. 2012;108 Suppl 1: i80–i87
18. Samuel U. Regulatory aspects of VCA in Eurotransplant. Transpl Int. 2016;29:686–693.
19. Bruce CR, Koch P. Flawed Assumptions: Ethical Problems With Proposed Presumed Consent Legislation. American Journal of Transplantation 2017; 17: 3262–3263.
20. Mathiharan K. Ethical and legal issues in organ transplantation: Indian scenario. Med Sci Law. 2011;51:134–140.
21. Kaushik J. Organ transplant and presumed consent: towards an 'opting out' system. Indian J Med Ethics. 2009 Jul-Sep;6(3):149–152.
22. Spital A, Taylor JS. Routine recovery of cadaveric organs for transplantation: consistent, fair, and life-saving. Clin J Am Soc Nephrol. 2007 Mar;2(2):300–303.
23. Pfaller L, Hansen SL, Adloff F, Schicktanz S. Saying no to organ donation: An empirical typology of reluctance and rejection. Social Health Illn. 2018;40:1327–1346.
24. Bruce CR, Koch P. Flawed Assumptions: Ethical Problems With Proposed Presumed Consent Legislation. Am J Transplant. 2017;17:3262–3263.
25. Rieu R. The potential impact of an opt-out system for organ donation in the UK. J Med Ethics 2010; 36: 534–538.

26. Holman A, Karner-Huţuleac A, Ioan B. Factors of the willingness to consent to the donation of a deceased family member's organs among the Romanian urban population. Transplant Proc. 2013; 45:3178–3182.
27. L. Murray, A. Miller, C. Dayoub, C. Wakefield, and J. Homewood. Communication and Consent: Discussion and Organ Donation Decisions for Self and Family. Transplantation Proceedings. 2013; 45, 10–12.
28. U.S. Department of Health and Human Services, Health Resources and Services Administration, Healthcare Systems Bureau, 2012 National Survey of Organ Donation Attitudes and Behaviors. Rockville, Maryland: U.S. Department of Health and Human Services, 2013. https://www.organdonor.gov/sites/default/files/organ-donor/professional/grants-research/national-survey-organ-donation-2012.pdf
29. Oliver M, Woywodt A, Ahmed A and Said I. Organ donation, transplantation and religion. Nephrol Dial Transplant 2011; 26: 437–444.
30. Golmakani MM, Niknam MH, Hedayat KM. Transplantation ethics from the Islamic point of view. Med Sci Monit 2005; 11: 105–109.
31. Einollahi B. Cadaveric kidney transplantation in Iran: behind the Middle Eastern countries? Iran J Kidney Dis 2008; 2: 55–56.
32. Namihira E. Shinto concept concerning the dead human body. Transplant Proc 1990; 22: 940–941.
33. Boggi U, Vistoli F, Chiaro MD et al. Kidney and pancreas transplants in Jehovah's Witnesses: ethical and practical implications. Transplant Proc 2004; 36: 601–602.
34. Mihály S, Smudla A, Kovács J. Practices Around Communication About Organ Donation in Hungary. Transplant Proc. 2016;48:2529–2533.
35. Simpkin AL, Robertson LC, Barber VS, Young JD. Modifiable factors influencing relatives' decision to offer organ donation:systematic review. BMJ 2009;338:b991.
36. Blok GA, van Dalen J, Jager KJ, Ryan M, Wijnen RM,Wight C, et al. The European Donor Hospital Education Programme (EDHEP): addressing the training needs of doctors and nurses who break bad news, care for the bereaved, and request donation. Transpl Int 1999;12:161e7.
37. Rodrigue JR, Cornell DL, Howard RJ. Organ donation decision: comparison of donor and nondonor families. Am J Transplant. 2006 Jan;6(1):190–198.
38. Pompeu HP, SilvaSS, RozaBA, BuenoSMV. Factors involved in the refusal to donate bone. Acta Paul Enferm 2014;27:380e4.
39. Dos Santos MJ, Leal de Moraes E, Santini Martins M, Carlos de Almeida E,Borges de Barros E Silva L, Urias V, Silvano Corrêa Pacheco Furtado MC, BritoNunes Á, El Hage S. Trend Analysis of Organ and Tissue Donation forTransplantation. Transplant Proc. 2018;50:391–393.
40. Committee on Hospital Care, Section on Surgery, and Section on Critical Care. Policy statement--pediatric organ donation and transplantation. Pediatrics. 2010;125:822–828.
41. Rodrigue JR, Cornell DL, Howard RJ. Pediatric organ donation: what factors most influence parents' donation decisions? Pediatr Crit Care Med. 2008;9:180–185.
42. Vane DW, Sartorelli KH, Reese J. Emotional considerations and attending involvement ameliorates organ donation in brain dead pediatric trauma victims. J Trauma 2001;51:329–331.

43. Halpern SD, Barnes B, Hasz RD, Abt PL. Estimated supply of organ donors after circulatory determination of death: a population-based cohort study. JAMA 2010;304:2592–2594.
44. Verheijde JL, Rady MY, McGregor JL. The United States Revised Uniform Anatomical Gift Act (2006): New challenges to balancing patient rights and physician responsibilities. Philos Ethics Humanit Med. 2007;2:19.
45. Gries CJ, White DB, Truog RD, Dubois J, Cosio CC, Dhanani S, Chan KM, CorrisP, Dark J, Fulda G, Glazier AK, Higgins R, Love R, Mason DP, Nakagawa TA, ShapiroR, Shemie S, Tracy MF, Travaline JM, Valapour M, West L, Zaas D, Halpern SD. American Thoracic Society Health Policy Committee. An official American Thoracic Society/International Society for Heart and Lung Transplantation/Society of Critical Care Medicine/Association of Organ and Procurement Organizations/United Network of Organ Sharing Statement: ethical and policy considerations in organ donation after circulatory determination of death. Am J Respir Crit Care Med.2013;188:103–109.

74

Contact between organ donor families and their recipients is usually therapeutic for both sides

Reginald Green

Four months after our seven-year-old son, Nicholas, (Photo, Figure 74.1) became an organ donor while we were on a family holiday in Italy, Maggie, my wife, and I went back there and met six of his seven recipients. It was one of the most fulfilling experiences of our lives—and theirs. (The seventh, the heart recipient, had still not fully recovered.)

Nicholas was shot in an attempted carjacking in the extreme south of Italy in 1994, while we were travelling at night on the main divided highway to Sicily. It turned out later that the killers had mistaken our rented car, with its Rome license plates, for one carrying a cargo of jewellery.

I don't think I need to elaborate on the bleakness we felt. I found myself wondering how I could get through the rest of my life without the magical little creature who had brought sunshine into every day and even now the happiest moments come with the thought 'If only Nicholas could see this'. But donating his organs was easy. It was perfectly clear he didn't need that body any more. Others, however, did desperately need what that little body could give.

The results were explosive. Organ donation rates in Italy tripled in the next ten years. An increase of that size must have subsidiary causes but no other country has ever come anywhere close to that rate of increase so it is clear that Italy's generous response to the story of one small boy was predominant. As a result, thousands of people, many of them young, have been saved from an early death.

More widely, the unending flow of articles and interviews round the world in the twenty-seven years since Nicholas was killed has brought

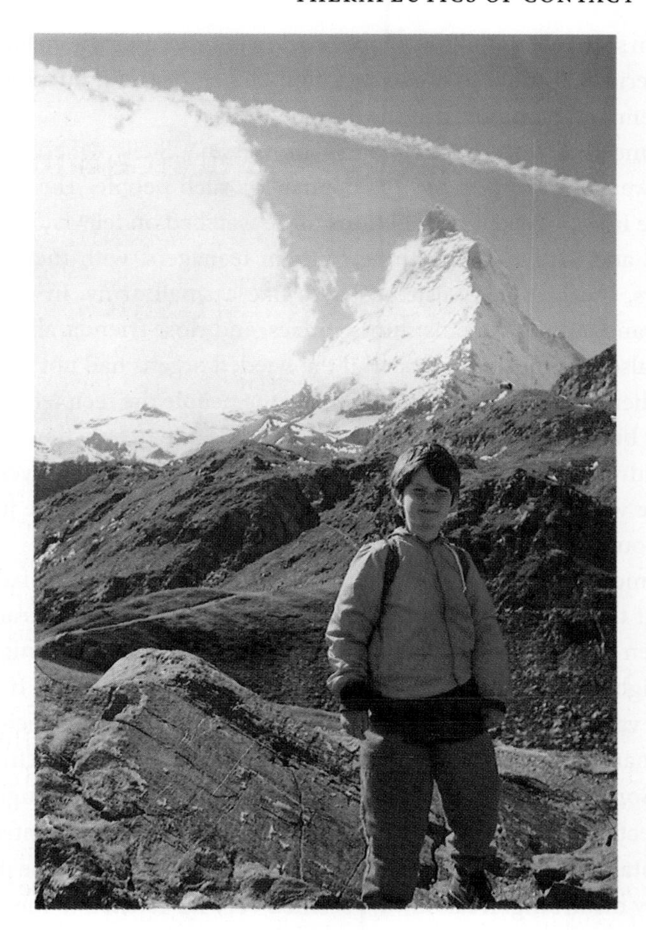

Figure 74.1. Picture of Nicholas at Matterhorn

home to tens of millions of people that if they ever need a new heart or liver or lungs someone else will likely have to die first. More than that, the family of that someone, despite the almost irresistible pressure to turn inward, will have to put their grief aside long enough to help someone in desperate need they never met and can't even visualize.

Lest 'tens of millions' be thought an exaggeration let's consider just one element: the made-for-television movie starring Jamie Lee Curtis, 'Nicholas' Gift' that grew out a book I wrote called 'The Nicholas Effect', has been seen by 100 million people worldwide, many of whom had never given serious thought to organ donation before. I cannot imagine any of them remaining unmoved as the drama unfolds.

The meeting with the recipients—in Messina, Sicily, where Nicholas died—was an unforgettable eye-opener for such people. The large hall we were in was packed and millions more watched on television. A door opened and in they came, three of them teenagers, with their fathers, mothers, brothers, and sisters. It was like a small army. In the wings were grandparents, cousins, aunts, uncles, and close friends, all of whom would also have been devastated if the needed organs had not arrived in time. Then, as in any donation, there are the people the recipients haven't met yet but who will become their best friends, the people they'll marry, the children they'll have. Many more people are affected than ever seems possible when, your mind overwhelmed by the blow you have just suffered, you say 'yes'.

The meeting produced another surprise. I had expected mixed feelings but the sheer life force of the recipients, who before the transplant had been like ghosts, always aware when they went to bed at night that they might not wake up in the morning, drove out the sadness. If we had needed validation for the decision to donate, this would have been it.

Yet many countries place restrictions on the two sides contacting each other. Some make it virtually impossible, including Italy through a law to protect privacy passed in 1999. The authorities in these countries fear any contact, even an unsigned letter expressing thanks, could be psychologically disturbing. It has always seemed very far-fetched to me and the evidence is strongly against it.

Accordingly, with just one helper, an Italian friend, Andrea Scarabelli, and in face of the opposition or indifference of the entire Italian medical establishment I started a media campaign in 2016 to change the law. We felt so alone we called ourselves Don Quixote and Sancho Panza. But the campaign caught fire and the authorities found themselves bombarded by both the media and the public asking, 'If two families with an emotional connection as close as this want to write to each other, or even meet, why should some bureaucrat be able to say no?'

The sudden eruption of public concern about a policy that had been so completely taken for granted that I cannot remember ever hearing it discussed in either medical or political circles opened the way for others to join us. For example, despite his devastation Marco Galbiati of Lecco, whose high-spirited and beloved fifteen-year-old son, Rikky, died in 2017, was also determined to trace the recipients and in a whirlwind campaign collected 50,000 signatures to support changing the law to allow communication.

The whole issue attracted so much popular support that it was referred to the Italian National Bioethics Committee which to everyone's surprise recommended that the two sides should be able to meet under controlled conditions.[1] As I write, a group of Italian legislators has introduced a bill on those lines and the Deputy Minister of Health has issued a statement giving a ringing endorsement for change.[2] My new hope is that, if Italy changes its restrictive policy, other countries will follow suit.

It's true that many families are not interested in contact: they want to put the transplant behind them and make the best of lives that have already had more than their fair share of disturbance. No one would want to challenge that right. Contact should only be possible when both sides want it.

But what better tonic can there be for a donor family than seeing in front of them a lively boy who says he used to have a banged-up old jalopy for a heart—which did not allow him to walk to the door of his apartment without stopping for breath—but after receiving their son's heart now has a Ferrari inside him? Or being hugged by a young woman who had once been on her deathbed but after receiving their son's liver has given birth to a boy to whom she has given the same name as the donor? These are not imaginary examples: they happened to us.

Many recipients also yearn to communicate: they want to know what the donor was like. 'Did he play soccer like I do? What position?' 'Did she have a boyfriend?' More than that, many of them feel guilty that they are alive only because someone else died and they want the family who saved their lives to know they will try to be worthy of the gift. What a relief it is to them to hear that the best thing they can do for the donor family is to have a long and healthy life, because that makes the gift more valuable.

Indeed, if there is psychological damage it seems to me much more likely to be to the families who are denied all knowledge of the people who are living with parts of one of their own members inside them or those who ache to thank the people who rescued them. Many of those people spend the rest of their life feeling something important is missing—as it is—and some of them suffer acutely. What a perverse result of policies that were designed to help them!

Let me give an example that I've told many times of how it works at its best. Inger Jessen has not had an easy life: she has lost both a husband and a son. She herself had a leg amputated because of diabetes and when she was fifty-five her heart was so weak that she could not walk out of her house without help.

But instead of wallowing in self-pity her instincts are to share with others. So, when in 1997 she received a new heart, her overwhelming instinct was to thank the donor family for their generosity and commiserate with them on their loss. Knowing nothing about them, she wrote an unsigned letter through OneLegacy, the organ procurement organization in Southern California.

She received no reply. She was disappointed but understood and put it out of her mind. Years later, however, when she had won two gold medals in swimming at the World Transplant Games—Olympic-style events open only to organ recipients—she decided to write again, thinking that the news would show them in the most vivid way what a difference their donation had meant to her.

But she had no idea how shattered the family had been. The heart had belonged to an eighteen-year-old, Nicole Mason, who had been knocked down by a car while she was walking on a road near home. Nicole's father, Dan remembers how nothing seemed to matter anymore. 'I had no feeling for anything. Sometimes when I was driving I had to pull over to the side of the road to sob', he remembers. 'I had a four-year-old granddaughter and I couldn't even play with her.'

But time passed and for the Masons too thoughts were stirring and, in the end, they decided they would like to know more about this kindly lady with whom they had such an unusual bond. They contacted OneLegacy saying they would like to meet. Inger says that for days after she received the call, she went around in a dream.

On the twentieth anniversary of Nicole's death, a date crammed with memories for all of them, they met and melted into each other's arms, the climax coming when the Masons listened by stethoscope to the strong, regular beat of their daughter's heart, which has worked perfectly from the start. 'I couldn't believe I was listening to Nikki's heart', Dan recalls with awe. 'I think of her every day. She seems so far away. But here she was again.'

For Inger too the meeting had a profound effect. 'Since then', she says, 'I have felt a peace I haven't known in years.'

Luckily, however, we don't have to rely on anecdotes like this to know if communication is therapeutic. Instead, we have statistics. In the United States, where communication has been encouraged for more than twenty-five years, thousands and thousands of transplant families have made contact either by letter or face-to-face, the records show that communication has had positive results for both sides in the overwhelming number of cases. Obviously, things can go wrong—what can't?—but they are the exceptions.

The procedure varies slightly but in most cases a family wanting contact writes an unsigned letter that the OPO (the organ procurement organization) for their area screens. It wants to feel sure, for example, that one side is unlikely to want a more intense relationship than the other would feel comfortable with. If satisfied, it forwards the letter to the other family which is free to decide whether it wants to respond. If not, the process stops and nothing further happens, however persistent the first family is. If, however, the second family is open to the idea it can reply, again anonymously and again through the OPO.

If all goes well, as it usually does, the two sides correspond as they wish, giving whatever information they want. Some write regularly, some infrequently. Or perhaps never again: that first exchange of letters will have given them a trove of information and may be enough. If, however, the relationship warms, the two sides can meet, at first under the supervision of the OPO, then quite freely. Some become close friends, others go to each other's houses for Sunday lunch, console each other when needed: who better?

Like all relationships these wax and wane as moods and interests shift but I can attest, not just from our case but also from watching or reading about others, to the benign strength of the relationship in most cases., The peace of mind Inger Jessen found is repeated over and over again. Nicholas's liver recipient told us that she was dogged by guilt until Maggie said to her, 'Don't cry. If that liver hadn't gone to you, it would have gone to someone else.' Now she thinks of Nicholas guarding her children like an angel. Could there be a more effective cure for recipient guilt?

But if things do come off the rails, the solution is fairly simple: the OPO can tell the offending party that no further contact is allowed. With the whole weight of the health service against them, it would be a brazen family that persisted after that. Nor are these relationships rare: a survey in 2019 by the Association of Organ Procurement Organizations, to which 48 of the 58 American OPOs replied, found that they had reviewed 24,000 letters between recipients and donor families *that year alone* and that excludes not only all letters that went directly between the two families, which they are allowed to send, when their medical advisers agree, but also the increasingly popular emails.[(3)]

Recently I asked the chief executive officers of OPOs in widely differing parts of the United States what their experience has been. Here are their answers:

'For the overwhelming majority, contacts between recipients and donor family members provide comfort to both sides', says Howard Nathan, Gift of Life Donor Program, which covers part of Pennsylvania and Maryland, an area with a population of 11 million.

'The majority of our donor families and recipients that meet go on to create life-long friendships', Suzanne Conrad, Iowa Donor Network, adds.

'Correspondence between donor families and recipients is a tremendously powerful and positive practice. We see many donor families and recipients go on to have incredibly close, family-like relationships, across many years and great distances', says Sue Dunn, Donor Alliance, the organ procurement organization covering Colorado and most of Wyoming.

'OneLegacy, which serves the 20 million residents and 200 hospitals of Southern California, provides every donor family the opportunity to communicate with their loved one's recipients and with mutual agreement meet them. These contacts provide healing to both sides, many have created life-long friendships, and all enable those touched by donation to share their experience, if they wish, with anyone from their closest friends to the world at large—giving anyone who hears them an incentive to become a donor too', Tom Mone comments.

It's a formidable body of experience to argue against, isn't it?

Reg Green (www.nicholasgreen.org)

Highlights

- We donated our seven-year-old son's organs after he had been shot in Italy.
- Italian organ donation rates tripled in the next ten years.
- We met all seven of our son's recipients: that was therapeutic for them and us.
- Many countries put severe restrictions on the two sides being able to communicate either by letter or in person.
- In the United States where contact is encouraged many thousands of donor families have met their recipients and in the overwhelming number of cases the results have been therapeutic for both sides.

References

1) 'Organ donor families should be free to meet their recipients under controlled conditions if both sides wish', say Carlo Petrini, Bioethics Unit, Higher Institute of Health, Rome, and Reg Green, President, Nicholas Green Foundation, La Cañada, CA, USA Annals of the Italian National Institute of Health 2019 | Vol. 55, No. 1: 6–9 http://old.iss.it/binary/publ/cont/ANN_19_01_03_1_.pdf
2) Statement by Dr. PierPaolo Sileri, Italian Deputy Minister of Health, September 23, 2020

'The liberalization of the contacts between recipients and donor families is a deed of humanity and civilization, a right and proper act that must find its rightful position in a modification of the current legislation, the law 91/99. This battle can and must be driven forward, creating a structured system that, beyond the law, can guide recipients and donor families through their grief process. I want to thank once again Nicholas' family who, without their faith in humanity and will to contribute to our emancipation as persons, wouldn't have ever pursued the path of the gift and the campaign for liberalization. It means having your neighbor at heart and waging a battle like Don Quixote, as Reg Green, Nicholas' father, says in his own words. I know very well the battles against the windmills and I want to support in a productive way and through the law, a modification of the 91/99 law—a law that by now is outdated. Together we are stronger and more human, as Nicholas and his family taught us.' (Translation: Andrea Scarabelli)
3) Letters Between Transplant Families (2019 Survey) Association of Organ Procurement Organizations (aopo@aopo.org) 8300 Greensboro Drive, #L1-620, Mclean,Virginia, 22102 (703 556 4242)

75

Perplexities of contact between organ donor families and their recipients

Alicia Pérez Blanco

Introduction

Following the WHO guidelines of 2010,[1] Transplant Organizations and Health Care Systems must guarantee the anonymity of organ donors and recipients as well as the confidentiality surrounding the procedure. All countries, except for the USA and Israel, comply with this recommendation under specific laws[2] aimed at protecting the families with the explicit purpose of shielding them from social media. From the perspective of the individuals involved in the procedure, the purpose is to prevent potential harmful effects such as coercion or stalking. From the point of view of the interest of the community, the goal is to avoid potential abuse that might put the credibility of the transplantation system at risk, compromising the transplantation of patients in need of an organ.

Donation and transplantation activities are part of all modern Health Care Systems, therefore they must comply with the general law that obliges health care professionals (HCP), stakeholders, and institutions to maintain the confidentiality about the identity of patients and their clinical data even after they die.[3]

For the time being, the transplant organizations have successfully managed this commitment with confidentiality and anonymity; however, social media has spread at gigantic proportions and may be used to facilitate disclosure challenging transplant organizations and HCPs. Recipients and family donors willing to contact have a powerful instrument at their disposal and the enforcement of the law that prevents the breach of confidentiality seems much more difficult. Therefore, the controversy emerges as to whether the benefits of disclosure outweigh the harms. Ethicists and psychologists alike discuss vividly whether to move towards a more open policy.[4]

In this chapter, I firstly explain the reasons for sticking to a confidentiality-based policy and the negative consequences of breaking it might be. Secondly, I will put forward the potential benefits for disclosing the identity of the recipient and donor and allowing contact between the donor's family and the recipient. Finally, I shall pose a hypothetical safety scenario for disclosing.

Purpose of maintaining confidentiality

It has been posed that agreed disclosure may be positive for all parties, but it has not been justified. It is well-known that the core of organ donation is generosity, benevolence, and altruism, which are inherently independent of who benefits from it. Indeed, altruism implies not being conditioned by who the recipient is or to what extent they might take advantage of the opportunity of enjoying a new life.

That said, it is also believed that people do not make decisions on organ donation based on ethical reasoning (benevolence and altruism) but based on their wish to resolve a crucial problem of a person in need. According to this experiential view, the necessity to know about the recipient's faring is understandable and perhaps, beneficial.

Negative consequences of disclosure

The available evidence shows the following as to the negative consequences of contacting:

- According to La Spina et al, knowing that some of the donor's organs are living in others may impede the necessary detachment from the deceased loved one making it even harder to develop a healthy grieving process.[5]
- Another concern facing direct contact has to do with the unrealistic expectations from each other.[6] Acknowledging that the recipient's

lifestyle is far from what the family has envisioned may negatively affect their bereavement or even provoke regret. Usually families pursue donation based on what they suppose their loved one would have wanted, not merely what they, themselves, may consider (organ donation as a societal good). Therefore, if the recipient's lifestyle is not in line with the donor's, their family may have to adjust this mismatch adding stress to their bereavement. This may be especially relevant if they have experienced ambivalence when consenting organ donation.[4]

- Contradictory feelings causing additional stress may arise when families directly see the improvement in the recipient's quality of life, in the knowledge that this was made possible by the loss of their loved one.[7]
- Secondary losses will occur if the transplant was unsuccessful or the recipient dies after the transplant. The family who believed that their loved one would still live in others must go through a second bereavement making it harder to gain peace.

The recipient's feeling of being in permanent debt makes him vulnerable, a victim of potential harassment, stalking or coercion from the donor's family.

Psychological problems that may arise are feelings of guilt and responsibility towards the graft. According to Goeztzmann et al[8] 2.7% of recipients experience feelings of guilt knowing that the price for them being alive was the death of the donor and even worse, if the donor was young, which is usually what happens with heart transplantation.[9] Knowing that they are not able to reciprocate may make them feel extraordinarily responsible for the well-being of the graft.[8]

Post-transplant identity problems

The recipient may struggle to assimilate the graft as part of them; according to Kaba et al,[10] 10–20% recipients think that by having a part of another's body, some of their traits are inherited. Direct knowledge of the donor may increase the difficulties of rebuilding a post-transplant identity, potentially inclining the recipient to non-adherence or hiding that they have undergone a transplant.

Potential benefits to uphold recipients and donor's families knowing each other

The most common reasons raised by the donor's family for wanting to know about the recipient are the following: to learn, first-hand, about the positive outcome of the transplant, to reassure them of the goodness of their decision, to conclude the narrative of their tragic loss, and to divulge the donor's personality.[11,12]

Were these expectations met through direct contact? Some authors have reported that donor families who met the recipients had eased their pain by finding a positive meaning from their loss. Feelings of peace arose when the recipients showed their immense gratitude, helping them look to the future, therefore, lessening their grief.[13,10,14]

The recipient's feelings of guilt are alleviated when expressing gratitude to the donor's family.[6] Surveys of transplant recipients reflect their support to any initiative allowing them to contact the donor family, to learn more about the donor and to share their new life with the family. Moreover, they would like to disclose their experience to encourage organ donation amongst others.[15,16,4]

Indeed, paediatric recipients have demonstrated the need for direct contact with donors' families, as has recently occurred in UK.[17,18] Max Johnson's heart transplant and the identity of his donor, Keira Ball, were revealed by the media, breaking all the privacy norms. Moreover, the National Health Service in England published the story, thus, demonstrating support in changing the disclosure policy and showing both the comprehensible need of the family and the benefits of encouraging donation amongst society. This will probably result in crucial shift towards enacting an opt-out law. In the same way, Ashkenazi et al reported that 24% of donor parents were satisfied knowing the outcome, while 60% were interested in direct contact with the recipient.[19]

Hypothetical safety scenario for disclosing

Only USA and Israel bring their donors and recipients the opportunity of legally knowing from each other when there is genuine consent and bilateral agreement. Given this condition and being overseen by psychologists and acknowledged professionals of the transplant organizations, posing the possibility of knowing from each other may be positive to all parties involved, including the societal benefit of promoting donation.

Some HCPs of Canada[20] and bioethicists from Australia[4] have expressed their support for a change in the status quo (prohibition of disclosure) provided both parties consent to it.

There is a general agreement on the following: if regulated and oversighted, disclosure will, at least, prevent from the harm of uncontrolled use of internet and social media. On the other hand, guidance of clinical psychologists and social workers will positively impact the outcome of any kind of contact. For many, correspondence might suffice. Therefore, the positive impact on rebuilding life and coming to terms with a transplant are ended worth taking the risk of disclosure. Donor families' and recipients' capacity to consent at the time of making the decision on organ donation and transplantation should be considered by HCPs and transplant organizations when deciding about their role in deciding about disclosure.[21]

Conclusion

The credibility and sustainability of every Donation and Transplantation System are at stake, all National Health Care Systems struggle to guarantee the confidentiality of all the parties involved. This commitment is considered to be of utmost importance as for its implications on the society, leaving the reasonable desire of disclosure behind.

In order to clarify the implications of disclosure, new studies by bioethicists and involving professionals in donation and transplantation activities should be performed to shed more light on this topic.

Highlights

- Transplantation systems must guarantee anonymity of the donor's families and recipient in order to protect them for coercion or stalking.
- Transplantation systems as part of the Health Care System are committed to maintain the same policies of confidentiality.

- If the parties involved ask for disclosure, this could only be done under the guidance of HCP experienced in confronting these stressful and potentially harmful situations.
- Pilot studies might shed some light on the potential benefits of disclosure; thus transplantation authorities may have proof of concept to attempt any change on the data protection regulation.

References

1 World Health Organization (WHO) 2010. WHO guiding principles in human cell, tissue and organ transplantation. Geneva. Available at: http://www.who.int/transplantation/Guiding_PrinciplesTransplantation_WHA63.22en.pdf?ua¼1.

2 Real Decreto 2070/1999, de 30 de diciembre, por el que se regulan las actividades de obtención y utilización clínica de órganos humanos y la coordinación territorial en materia de donación y trasplante de órganos y tejidos. https://www.boe.es/buscar/doc.php?id=BOE-A-2000-79.(accessed Nov 20, 2019).

3 Ley 41/2002, de 14 de noviembre, básica reguladora de la autonomía del paciente y de derechos y obligaciones en materia de información y documentación clínica. Available at: https://www.boe.es/eli/es/l/2002/11/14/41/con.(accessed Nov 20, 2019).

4 Martin D. Report on the Community Consultative Forum: Contact between donor families and transplant recipients. Australian Government Organ and Tissue Authority 2017. Available at: https://donatelife.gov.au/sites/default/files/Report%20on%20the%20community%20consultative%20forum.pdf.(accessed Nov 20, 2019).

5 La Spina F, Sedda L, Pizzi C et al. Donor families' attitude toward organ donation. The North Italy Transplant Program. Transplantation Proceedings 1993; 25: 1699–1701.

6 Holtkamp S. Wrapped in mourning: the gift of life and organ donor family trauma. In: Brunner-Routledge Eds. New York, 2002.

7 Albert PL. Clinical decision making and ethics in communications between donor families and recipients: How much should they know? Journal of Transplant Coordination 1999; 9: 219–224.

8 Goetzmann L, Irani S, Moser K et al. Psychological processing of transplantation in lung recipients: A quantitative study of organ integration and the relationship to the donor. British Journal of Health Psychology 2009; 14: 667–680.

9 Lewino D, Stocks L, Cole G. Interaction of organ donor families and recipients. Journal of Transplant Coordination 1996; 6: 191–195.

10 Kaba E, Thompson D, Burnard P, Edwards D, Theodosopoulou E. Somebody else's heart inside me: A descriptive study of psychological problems after a heart transplantation. Issues in Ment Health Nurs 2005; 26: 611–625.

11 Albert P. Direct contact between donor families and recipients: crisis or consolation? Journal of Transplant Coordination 1998; 8: 139–144.

12 Merchant SK, Yoshida EM, Lee TK, Richardson P, Karlsbjerg KM, Cheung E. Exploring the psychological effects of deceased organ donation on the families of the organ donors. ClinTransplant 2008; 22:341–347.
13 Kandel I, Merrick J. Organ transplants. Contact between the donor family and recipient. International Journal on Disability and Human Development 2007; 6: 21–27.
14 Clayville L. When donor families and organ recipients meet. Journal of Transplant Coordination 1999; 9: 81–86.
15 Dobbels F, Van Gelder F, Remans K, Verkinderen A, Peeters J, Pirenne J, Nevens F. Should the law on anonymity of organ donation be changed? The perception of liver transplant recipients. ClinTransplant 2009; 23: 375–381.
16 Annema C, Op den Dries S, Van den Berg AP et al. Opinions of Dutch liver transplant recipients on anonymity of organ donation and direct contact with the donors family. Transplantation 2015; 99: 879–884.
17 https://www.organdonation.nhs.uk/helping-you-to-decide/real-life-stories/people-who-have-benefitted-from-receiving-a-transplant/max-heart-transplant-recipient-and-campaigner/.(accessed 20 November 2019).
18 https://www.bbc.co.uk/news/av/health-47373365/organ-donation-law-how-keira-s-heart-saved-max.(accessed 20 November 2019).
19 Ashkenazi T. Do bereaved parents of organ donors want to know about or meet with the recipients? The relationship between parents willingness and 'meaning of life' measures. 2013, 3nd ELPAT Congress on Ethical, Legal and Psychosocial Aspect of Transplantation Global Issues, Local Solutions. page 49.
20 Gewarges M, Poole J, De Luca E, Shildrick M, Abbey S, Mauthner O, Ross H. Canadian Society of Transplantation Members' views on anonymity in organ donation and transplantation. Transplant Proc 2015; 47:2799–2804.
21 Dicks SG, Northam H, van Haren FM, Boer DP. An exploration of the relationship between families of deceased organ donors and transplant recipients: A systematic review and qualitative synthesis. Health Psychol Open. 2018; 5(1):2055102918782172. doi:10.1177/2055102918782172

76

Organ donation: An act of charity

Most Reverend Vincenzo Paglia

Introduction

The relationship between organ donation and charity can be seen clearly in the life of Blessed Don Carlo Gnocchi, who was called by St. John Paul II 'a *Father to children maimed in wartime*. He began his priestly ministry as a teacher, but he later experienced the horrors of the Second World War as a volunteer chaplain, first during the Italian Campaign in Greece and, later, with the mountain troops of the 2nd Alpine Division "Tridentina" in the Battle of Stalingrad. He spent his time with heroic charity for the wounded and dying, and that experience led to his formulation of a wide-ranging plan of care for the poor, orphans, and unfortunates. Fruit of that plan was the *Pro Juventute* Foundation, through which he multiplied social and apostolic initiatives that cared for war orphans and amputee children maimed by exploding ordnance. His generosity lasted beyond his death on 28 February 1956, because he donated his corneas to two blind boys. This was a ground-breaking gesture since there was no legal structure at that time in Italy that regulated organ donation.'(1)

This last act of Father Gnocchi (the donation of his corneas) represented the fulfilment of the life of charity. In the words of Pope Emeritus Benedict XVI, 'Organ donation is a peculiar form of witness to charity. In a period like ours, often marked by various forms of selfishness, it is ever more urgent to understand how the logic of free giving is vital to a correct conception of life ... The act of love which is expressed with the gift of one's vital organs remains a genuine testimony of charity that is able to look beyond death so that life always wins.'(2)

It is not merely a matter of giving something of one's own, but rather giving something of *oneself*, since 'By virtue of its substantial union with a spiritual soul, the human body cannot be considered as a mere complex of tissues, organs and functions, ... rather it is a constitutive part of the person who manifests and expresses himself through it.'[3] 'Accordingly, any procedure which tends to commercialize human organs or to consider them as items of exchange or trade must be considered morally unacceptable, because to use the body as an "object," is to violate the dignity of the human person.'[4]

A gift cannot be reduced to a pure external act, like a simple giving of something that belongs to the giver. Rather, like every gesture of charity, it engages the freedom of the giver as a giver. He offers himself, as a person, and he becomes present in the gift.[5]

Different modalities of organ donation

In the transplant field, there are at least three different ways in which the bond, since a gift, is itself the recognition of a bond, between donor and donee manifests itself. First, if a donor is alive, the donation is made because of a tie, of blood, or other relationship that binds the recipient and the donor. For example, parent to child or wife to husband. The gesture is motivated primarily by the benefit to the loved one, recognizing that it will contribute to improving the life of the recipient, for example, the positive effects of a kidney transplant on the lives of couples and families. Second, there is a kind of donation called *Good Samaritan.* While alive, a person donates an organ without wanting to know who the recipient will be. The recipient is chosen according to criteria established by the scientific community. Third, in the donation of one's body upon death, the donor, if those with vested rights do not object, gives his or her body to the community which, through authorized agencies and following specific guidelines, makes use of the organs of the deceased. The donor does not choose the recipient, does not know who it will be. Just by speaking about these three ways, we can imagine a range of other circumstances. We move from a very strong bond between donor and recipient to the lack of any pre-existing bond at all. How can we reconcile these seemingly diverse approaches? What commonality is there between donations made to known persons and a donation made to a stranger?[6–11]

Gifts are circular

There is an old maxim that says a person who gives a gift forgets having done it, but a person who receives a gift remembers it forever. This seems to make the donor completely autonomous and the recipient completely dependent. It appears to be a one-way street, with no way to express gratitude. But is that really what a gift is? Doesn't a gift reflect a true relationship, one that creates and fosters a bond? A gift, 'is not a one-sided loss of something, a kind of protuberance on one side that simply fits into a cavity on the other. A gift is always a kind of exchange and of correspondence that is not based on wealth or poverty. It is always, in various ways, based on an awareness of the human quality of human relationships. That humanity makes loving and suffering worthwhile, and it makes boundaries acceptable, but it also gives us the courage to overcome limitations, to accept the risk of real human relationships and to appreciate our ability to respect the bonds that make those relationships human'.(12)

Many, many acts of gratuitousness have radically changed those who performed them! Many people who have given their consent to the donation of a loved one's organs have said that this gesture influenced their whole lives, sometimes significantly. Thus, a gift is never one-way; indeed, it creates its own reciprocity. An exchange relationship is both active and passive, and it is so on two sides: the one who is the giver and the one who is the donee but who also reciprocates. The Gospel is instructive here. Luke writes, 'As He was entering a village, ten lepers met Him. They stood at a distance from Him and raised their voice, saying, "Jesus, Master! Have pity on us!" And when He saw them, He said, "Go show yourselves to the priests." As they were going, they were cleansed. And one of them, realizing he had been healed, returned, glorifying God in a loud voice; and he fell at the feet of Jesus and thanked Him. He was a Samaritan. Jesus said in reply, "Ten were cleansed, were they not? Where are the other nine? Has none but this foreigner returned to give thanks to God?" Then He said to him, "Stand up and go; your faith has saved you"' (Lk, 17:12–19).

Gratitude from the foreigner shows that he appreciated and understood the meaning of the gift; gratitude tells the donor that his gesture (as well as he himself) has been recognized and is therefore good. This was not the case with the other nine, even though every person wants his or her most authentic identity be recognized. Paul Ricoeur notes, 'And if, happily, I chance to be recognized, shouldn't I be grateful to all those who, in one way or another, have, by recognizing me, recognized my identity?[13] An authentic gift always brings with it the hope of gratitude; gratitude is expected and welcomed. But in a true gift, gratitude is not demanded. Demanding gratitude for a gift would destroy its meaning.

The gift betrayed

In the light of the connection between gratuitousness and gratitude, that is, of the reciprocal nature of the gift, we must be aware that certain ways of giving rob the gift of what should be its nature. A gift would not be a gift if it were the result of opportunism or constraint, or if it took advantage of the ignorance or weakness of the recipient, blackmailing him more or less subtly. A gift would not be a gift if the recipient were obligated to return it; or if there were not the risk of receiving nothing in return, or if the donor were not giving up something of value, objective or subjective, or indeed if the donor did not openly make it known that the recipient had no obligation to return the gift on demand.

The following story is instructive: 'Three sons were required to share equitably an inheritance seventeen camels, received from their father. The father provided that the first would receive half the camels (8.5), the second would receive a third (5.6) and the last a ninth (1.9). They were not allowed to sell or kill the animals. The boys found themselves entangled in a dispute that threatened to get worse and worse, particularly because each one tried to "round-up" his share to a whole number that favored him. Their heated arguments were finally settled by an elder who gifted one camel to the boys, resulting in a number of camels that is divisible by 2, 3, and 9. Thus, nine camels went the first, six to the second and two to the third, for a total of seventeen, exactly the original number of camels that was impossible to divide using the father's formula. And happily, there was still the additional camel left over, the one the elder had given. After the seventeen camels had been distributed, he was able to get his own camel back! Thus, he settled the dispute without any loss to himself, but only after allowing for the possibility of such a loss.'[14] Still, there is nothing wrong with appropriately hoping to receive a gift as well as giving one, even a gift that is received in return for the one given. Note, however, that if one who gives a gift receives nothing in return, he or she can reasonably conclude that the gift was not appreciated or was even felt to be inappropriate.

The liberating gift

At times it seems some people take a mischievous delight in maintaining a state of mutual indebtedness and unbalanced exchanges. The greater a gift, the more it undermines the freedom of the recipient by imposing on him or her a duty to reciprocate.[15] In the donation of an organ by one living person to another, where there is generally a close relationship, and thus frequent contact, between donor and donee, there is also an imbalance such that the donee feels continuously indebted to the donor. In the mentality of the market, which admits of only quantifiable and monetizable forms of reciprocity, the only way (short of bankruptcy) to get out of debt is to pay it off, either in the same medium or by agreeing on a different medium of equivalent value.[16–21]

In a gift context, the thinking is different. Equivalent value is determined flexibly. As I said above, reciprocity is desired, even expected, but not demanded. The risk of getting nothing in return is recognized, even welcomed. In the experience of giving, a man reaches the height of his possibilities, sacrificing his most precious asset, freedom. For this reason, a gift 'remains an experience linked to love and gratuitousness; it cannot be the child of a legal the command or guaranteed by the fear of possible punishment ... It cannot be the product of a domineering, authoritarian manner that relies on fear rather than on trust and on a sense of responsibility.'[22] The more someone is convinced that the other is not obligated to give back, the more he is freed from this reciprocal obligation, the more his gesture will be free. It will arise out of the strength of the relationship; it will nurture the existing bond and protect it.[23]

Conclusion

I think it is necessary to get beyond a cultural approach that represents gift as a heroic, monodirectional choice, closed in on itself—a sort of excessive altruism, which makes a true gift inevitably impossible,[24–25] unreal, and therefore not attractive, not fruitful. The most altruistic gift 'is one that gives the other the possibility of reciprocity, that restores his or her ability to give in return'.[26] It reminds everyone of 'their filial identity: I would not be alive if I had not received and if I did not continue to receive'.[27] It is not a question of extraordinary gestures or actions, but spinning and strengthening the thread from which all life is woven.

In this optic we understand the connection between, first, giving to someone we know, the donation of an organ from one living person to another; second, a donation to the community, the so-called Good Samaritan donation; and third, a donation of a cadaver upon death. All these donations are recognitions of how much we receive from each other, from others, and the whole community. It is in recognizing basic relationships with others that we open ourselves freely to gift, and in so doing, we make it possible for giving and receiving, gratuitousness and gratitude, activeness and passiveness, to call out to each other and keep each other safe.

Highlights

- Organ donation represents one of the most extraordinary and heroic acts of charity.
- Different bonds are in place between donor and donee: tied of blood or other relationship; without any previous tie (donation to the community, Good Samaritan); after donor's death.
- A true gift must be free from all conditions.
- The gift benefits both the donor and the donee: everybody enriches from it.

References

1. John Paul II. Allocution to the Participants in the Pilgrimage of the 'Don Carlo Gnocchi' Foundation. Saturday, November 30, 2002.

2. Benedict XVI. Allocution to Participants in the International Congress on the Subject: 'A Gift for Life. Considerations of Organ Donation'. Sponsored by the Pontifical Academy for Life. November 7, 2008.
3. Congregation for the Doctrine of the Faith. Donum vitae. 1987; 3.
4. John Paul II. Allocution to the 18th International Congress of the Transplantation Society. August 29, 2000.
5. Benedict XVI. Deus Caritas est. 2005; 34.
6. Thomasma DC. The quest for organ donors: a theological response. Health progress. 1988; 69 (7): 22–4, 28.
7. Gerrand N. The notion of gift-giving and organ donation. Bioethics. 1994; 8 (2): 127–150.
8. Lamb D. Organ transplants and ethics. Aldershot; Brookfield USA: Avebury. 1996.
9. Daar AS. Altruism and reciprocity in organ donation: compatible or not? Transplantation. 2000; 70 (4): 704–705.
10. John Paul II P. Address to the International Congress on Transplants. The National Catholic Bioethics Quarterly. 2001; 1 (1): 89–92.
11. Morrissey P, Dube C, Gohh R et al. Good Samaritan kidney donation. Transplantation. 2005; 80 (10): 1369–1373.
12. Sequeri P. L'uomo alla prova. Soggetto, identità, limite. Milano: Vita e Pensiero. 2002. 129.
13. Ricoeur P. Percorsi del riconoscimento. Milano: Cortina. 2005; 5.
14. Pietroni D, Rumiati R. Il mediatore. Una nuova figura professionale per spegnere i conflitti. Bologna: Il Mulino. 2012; 29.
15. Mauss M. Saggio sul dono. Forma e motivo dello scambio nelle società arcaiche. In: Mauss M. Teoria generale della magia e altri saggi. Torino: Einaudi. 1965; 153–292.
16. Manga P. A commercial market of organs? Or not. Bioethics. 1987; 1 (4): 321–338.
17. Delmonico FL et al. Ethical incentives—not payment—for organ donation. NEJM. 2002; 346 (25): 2002–5.
18. Council of Europe. Convention for the Protection of Human Rights and the dignity of the human being with regard to the application of biology and medicine. Convention on Human Rights and Biomedicine. Strasbourg: Council of Europe. 2003.
19. International Summit on Transplant Tourism and Organ Trafficking. The Declaration of Istanbul on Organ Trafficking and Transplant Tourism. Istanbul: The Transplantation Society and International Society of Nephrology. 2008.
20. Directorate General of Human Rights and Legal Affairs. Trafficking in organs, tissues and cells and trafficking in human beings for the purpose of the removal of organs. France: Joint Council of Europe/United Nations Study. 2009.
21. Sixty-Third World Health Assembly. WHO guiding principles on human cell, tissue and organ transplantation, WHA63.22, Geneva: World Health Organization. 2010.
22. Cucci G. Altruismo e gratuità. I due polmoni della vita. Assisi: Cittadella. 2014; 197–198.
23. Capron AM. More blessed to give than to receive? Transplantation proceedings. 1992; 24 (5): 2185–2187.

24. Derrida J. Donare il tempo. Milano, Cortina. 1996.
25. Derrida J. Donare la morte. Milano, Jaca Book. 2002.
26. Rastoin M. Si è più beati nel dare che nel ricevere. La Civiltà Cattolica. 2013; IV, 313–326, 325.
27. Pagazzi GC. La carne. Cinisello Balsamo: San Paolo. 2018; 27–28.

77

My transplant story

Anita Siletto

Everyone who has had a transplant knows that their rebirth is linked to a gift of love and generosity.

My name is Anita Siletto, I live in Turin with my family, and I am an extremely fortunate woman.

Thanks to the gift of a liver transplant, nine years ago I started living again.

The transplant experience has been a long and arduous climb, full of difficulties, and obstacles, a test that above all forced me to overcome my fear, find courage, and keep hope alive every day. The important steps on my journey towards the transplant were characterized by feelings, states of mind, and extraordinarily strong emotions. First fear, then hope, suspense, and finally rebirth and gratitude.

My journey took four years, starting from a sudden hospitalization, during which I was diagnosed with an incurable disease and the only way to survive was a transplant.

Today, some years on, I can say that there is a cure which can beat my illness. I got through the transplant and I am better. Another blessing in my life!

The illness and the need for a transplant imposed great change on my life. Everything happened very quickly, making me face the truth that I could not avoid and that frightened me.

There were so many questions to which I did not have an answer: 'Will I make it? Will the doctors be able to look after me while I am waiting for a new organ? Will it arrive in time?'

I often lived daily life uncertain of timings, results, and waiting, fearing that these had worsened.

Sometimes I was afraid that I would not be able to control or face any of this. I felt that my body was abandoning me, and my mind was not always clear enough to react.

At that time, I was also very worried about my delicate family situation. My daughter was my constant thought, she was at that delicate age of adolescence and, because of my worsening health, I could not always take enough care of her. My biggest worry was that I would not be able to support her in future years as I did not know if I would have any more to come. To this were added the sadness and pain for the loss of my father who had been seriously sick for years and the worry of being a burden on my mother, who was then eighty, fragile, and exhausted, with my state of health.

My whole family had been subjected to limitations on their own lives due to my poor physical conditions and this added to my unease and frustration.

My husband never left me alone, my tender daughter, and my mother, who had taught me never to give up, were all my anchors who, every time I became discouraged or sad, gave me the strength to hope and keep on trying to see the light at the end of the tunnel.

My serious health conditions forced me to leave my job as a nursery schoolteacher and 'my' school. For a long time, I hoped that I would be able to resume my job, but it was not so. It was hard to leave my job for good after twenty-seven years. Teaching had given me so much satisfaction and the children had been a source of joy and cheerfulness.

Giving up my job, I felt even more isolated and left more room for fear. Also, for this reason, my life was changing, and I was not ready for it.

Despite the treatment for my illness, my conditions were gradually getting worse: I could not do the shopping or the housework, sometimes not even getting dressed or walking. Often, I needed someone to help me do all these things and I was admitted to hospital many times before my transplant operation.

I was incredibly angry with the disease and the whole world. At the same time, I realized that I could not let fear in, it would have overpowered me and taken away my will to live and fight. I was forty-eight years old and I still had so much will to live and do so many things.

The solitude in which I sometimes hid, allowed me, little by little, to become fully aware of my illness and, in part, accept it.

In those years I kept hope alive, I needed it in order to stay connected to life. I tried to accumulate positive energy and strength to prepare myself for the transplant, only in this way could I face the operation better. I changed my priorities, grasping the beautiful things that helped me smile and give me strength. Just one phone call, a visit, or a smile was enough to help me go on. I intensified my prayers and I found comfort in them.

In the two years following my admission to hospital, the doctors were able to keep my illness under control. After which, there was a long phase of tests in order to be put on the transplant waiting list. They were tiring and persistent tests that put my body and mind to the test. I was afraid that the tests would bring up problems that would impede the possibility of a transplant.

After numerous tests, I got onto the waiting list and from that moment I realized that I was starting a journey of no return. Getting onto the waiting list was almost like overcoming an important step on my journey but the fear of taking that unknown path remained. On the other hand, I had a lot of faith and hope in the new life that I would acquire.

The six months which passed after getting onto the list was like a period of 'suspension', where everything stopped but anything could happen. It is a period of preparation, waiting for 'the phone call', I prepared a bag like expectant mothers, I tried to leave everything tidy. You never know—I told myself—if after the phone call I would never return home if it goes badly.

In the early afternoon on that long-awaited day, I received the phone call that all transplant patients wait for anxiously, apprehensively, and expectantly because our lives hang by that phone call. With that gift you know that you can start living, dreaming, and making plans again. The coordinator of the Transplant Centre kindly and calmly told me 'there is a liver for you, can you come to the hospital quickly?' Firstly, I told my husband, then my mother, and then my daughter who had just left that morning for camp. Then I set off hurriedly to the hospital.

So many contrasting emotions invaded my mind: fear, joy, a thought for the donor—someone that was no longer there, so generous, giving me a chance to be reborn. Those moments were full of uncertainty because, on the one hand, I knew that a family was suffering the loss of their dear loved one, and on the other, I wanted to live. So, I grasped at that thought and quietly to myself thanked that person and their family for the great gift they had given me.

The operation went well, despite some complications which made my progress longer than normal.

The day of my return home was unforgettable, the joyous welcome of my family and the emotion of my first trip out a few months after my transplant: it was as if I was discovering the sea, the sun, and the sky for the very first time!

Life had restarted and I soon felt full of energy and strength!

A few months after the transplant, I felt the need to go back to school to revisit the place I loved, my colleagues, and the children, and to give them some of my time.

The idea of becoming a volunteer grew inside me because I wanted to give back to life the best of what the transplant experience had given me.

So, I decided to become a volunteer for the Italian Liver Transplant Association (AITF). My job is to meet the patients who have to get onto the transplant waiting list, telling them about my experience, encouraging them, supporting them, and accompanying them on this journey of waiting, being sympathetic and compassionate of their fears, reassuring them, and helping them never to lose faith and hope. It is wonderful meeting them after their transplant, seeing them joyfully returning to life!

Doing that allowed me to feel that I can give something back and, more specifically, show my immense gratitude to science, humanity, and the Turin medical community. Another job of mine as a volunteer is to go into schools and speak about organ donations along with the doctors of the Regional Coordination for Organ and Tissue Donation. It is an immense pleasure being with young people, they are new life, hope, and our future. It is important that young people are informed about donations, that they speak about it together and with their families, so that, when it is time, they have clear ideas and can make an informed choice. I hope that they live their lives to the best, remembering how precious it is, asking them to stop every now and then to think about living it well so as to become consistent and responsible in their choices.

I celebrate two birthdays. The day I was born, thanks to my parents, and the day I was reborn, thanks to the generosity of someone who saw life after death. For the latter, I don't want presents, the best gift is being here every day, living again, being with my family, enjoying my daughter, and seeing her grow, seeing my eighty-eight-year-old mother, who supported me and helped me not to give up, being with my husband and continuing many years of life together.

I feel the deepest gratitude and respect towards my donor, their family, blood donors, doctors, nurses, friends, relatives, and everyone who made it possible for me to receive the miracle of a new life.

Every day I thank my donor, they allowed me and my family to resume a normal life, start dreaming again, making plans, hoping for a future again. I received a 'baton' from them, like in a relay race, and I feel I have an obligation to honour this gift daily, carrying it with me in my life to the best of my abilities. There is a special tie to my donor which unites us, many times when I manage to do something wonderful or important, I lightly touch my stomach and I tell them 'look, we managed to do it, we did it together!'

Every day I thank all the blood donors without whom transplants could not happen. I will always remember my first transfusion, I was weak, frightened and while I watched the many drops of blood dripping down, I thought about how many people, with this gesture of love, give life, and hope to strangers in difficulty.

I thank the families of the donors that have the strength and the courage to transform their rage and pain into Life and Rebirth for other people. A friend of mine, the wife of a donor, says that the choice of donating is a victory over death. That which death has taken from her and her two daughters have been gifted to the life of other people. During these years I have met a few donor families and I feel they are part of my family. Meeting them and getting to know them has given me strength, has enriched my life even more. In the warmth of their embrace, every time that I meet them, I feel I can hug and thank my donor and his loved ones.

My sincere thanks and profound gratitude are extended to the scientists who, with their research, made the advancement of organ transplantation possible. My thanks and gratitude are also extended to the countries that were able to create laws to improve and legalize the entire process, to the hospitals, and to the doctors and nurses who are highly dedicated to their work in achieving success in this field.

This letter is a testimonial of my organ transplant experience, a celebration of donor generosity and of the serious commitment of the communities who help and support patients who need organ transplants, without whom this miracle of life could not happen. It is appropriate then, that nations, regions, states, and cities continue the network created so far, and expand knowledge and support further, so that organ donation is neither a taboo nor a religious or cultural choice. It should be a way of embracing our responsibility for the lives of others and can be the gift of being reborn for a second time. Miracles exist!

78

Global impact of SARS-CoV2 pandemic on organ donation and transplantation

Anna Teresa Mazzeo, Deepak Gupta

Introduction

In March 2020, the World Health Organization (WHO) declared Severe Acute Respiratory Syndrome Coronavirus type 2 (SARS-CoV-2) as a global pandemic. The disease has already spread around the world and its dramatic effects are visible not only on healthcare systems but also on the life of each of us.(1)

Emergence of new viruses (West Nile, Ebola, H1N1 influenza, Zika, SARS-CoV, MERS-CoV, etc.) is not a rare event faced by the transplantation system. Nevertheless COVID-19 pandemic has been showing its negative effects on the transplantation rates all over the world, therefore presenting a big challenge to an already challenging arena.(2)

While scientific community is working hard to explore intensely about this previously unknown disease, several questions have aroused in the transplant programmes at this time. The commonest is the risk of transmission of SARS-CoV-2 from donor to recipient by organ transplantation, the degree and duration of viremia, the uncertainty regarding the outcome of COVID-19 infection in immunosuppressed recipients, and the best way to avoid post-transplant infections. Whether or not COVID-19 is a risk to the procurement team remains a concern.

Major lessons from previous epidemic outbreaks prompted the development of operative protocols and recommendations. These include plans for recipient evaluation in the case of temporary inactivity of a specific transplant centre, or identification of alternative centres where candidates can be listed when the epidemic is affecting a specific geographic location.[2] Recommendations for the evaluation and testing of deceased organ donors with regards to SARS-CoV-2 and the operative plans for the entire transplantation process have been issued at national level.[3–6] Recommendations and policies to mitigate the impact of the COVID-19 pandemic on specific population, such as patients with liver disease[7] or for the organization and management of kidney transplantation under current pandemic situation[8] have been published. As for any evolving disease, reviews and updates of the newly released procedures are expected.

As there is a rather wide degree of medical urgency among solid organ transplants (SOT), transplant organizations have been instructed to set priorities. Centres in the less affected areas continue to do their best to keep actual standards, while centres most affected by the epidemiological hit limit their activity to pursuing donation only from ideal donors to providing transplantation to critically ill patients or other specific and urgent situations. A phased approach to decreasing transplant activity from a 25%, 50%, to 75% trigger for activity reduction depending on risk tolerance, hospital capacity, and degree of virus activity in the jurisdiction has been proposed in the early phase of pandemic.[9]

Ethical principles which guide transplant programmes are applied during the COVID-19 era as well. Clearly, the pre-pandemic availability of resources in each country, and the position on the COVID incidence curve will have a significant effect on the threshold for transplantation.[10]

Impact of COVID-19 pandemic on transplantation rates

Spain, the most active country in the world in the field of organ donation and transplantation, has also been one of the most affected countries in the world by this pandemic. In a challenging and unprecedented scenario, which is severely striking the healthcare system at all levels, sustaining a deceased donation programme has become highly complex.[11] In 2019, Spain reached a historical maximum in the rates of organ donation (2302 deceased donors, 49 per million population) and organ transplantation (5449 transplant procedures, 116 per million population). A dramatic decrease in the numbers of organ donation and transplantation has been registered since the beginning of the pandemic alarm. The effects on patients in the waiting lists are still difficult to measure and could become an indirect effect of the pandemic.(11) Potential donor losses could be due to multiple factors including the overwhelmed healthcare system, unavailability of intensive care unit (ICU) beds even for neurocritical patients, consequent decrease in potential donor referral to local coordination teams combined with logistic factors such as reduced mobility, reduced resources, or prolonged times needed for SARS-CoV-2 testing, especially in the early phases of pandemic.(11)

In a study to quantify the contemporary effects of the COVID-19 pandemic on organ donation and transplantation in France and the USA, a strong association between the increase in COVID-19 infections and a dramatic reduction in overall solid-organ transplantation procedures was demonstrated. The overall reduction in deceased donor transplantations was 90.6% in France and 51.1% in the USA, respectively, mostly driven by kidney transplantation, but with significant effect on other organ transplantation as well.(12)

In a questionnaire survey by Ahmed et al. distributed to nineteen selected organ procurement organizations (OPOs) throughout the US to compare two specific ninety-day periods from March–May 2019 and March–May 2020, the total number of organs transplanted fell by 18% ($n = 2580$ vs $n = 3148$ organs, $p = 0.0001$) in 2020 when compared to the year 2019.(13) The greatest differences were reported in heart and lung transplantation. There was an 11% decrease in organ authorization by donor families in 2020 when compared to the same ninety-day period in 2019. Interestingly, COVID-19 testing was initially performed in only 49% of potential organ donors in March 2020 but was extended to all potential donors by May 2020.(13)

In the UK, the comparison between donor and transplantation activity during the COVID-19 lockdown period 23 March to 10 May 2020, and the same time period in 2019 showed that the number of deceased donors reduced by 66% and the number of deceased donor transplants decreased by 68%, also referrals of potential donors decreased by 39%.(14)

Preliminary Italian data demonstrated that in the first four weeks of COVID-19 pandemic, a 25% reduction of procured organs occurred.[15] Therefore, transplant physicians are compelled to use even more stringent prioritization criteria to select transplant candidates in this new scenario.[15]

Even countries, such as Australia, which experienced a lower incidence of COVID-19 infections, had a significant negative impact on organ donation and transplantation. Kidney transplantation was 27% less compared to 2019, liver 8%, and lung 12% less respectively. Conversely, heart and pancreas transplant activity has increased by 26% and 32%, respectively.[16]

Few countries like India have converted their trauma centres into COVID centres and hence organ harvest rates have dropped to zero figures post COVID-19 pandemic. The entire health infrastructure is currently involved in the care of prevention and treatment of COVID-19 suspects/positive cases, therefore severely compromising the availability/commitment of team for organ transplantations.

The early effects of the first few months of the pandemic on organ transplantation in the Middle East have also been reported.[17]

The impact of COVID-19 on organ donation, procurement, and liver transplantation has been specifically addressed. The importance of improved communication and telehealth in the field of transplant setting has been recognized.[18]

Recently, a large study of the Scientific Registry of Transplant Recipients in the US reported a considerable increase in the waitlist deaths in the states with the highest COVID-19 incidence during the earliest wave of the pandemic. Interestingly, early period of the pandemic saw major changes in transplant practices in the COVID-affected areas. However, in the later part of the pandemic, the newly COVID-affected areas did not seem to be affected to the same extent, due to adaptability of the transplant programmes.[19]

Furthermore, a very recent report from the Spanish experience demonstrated that recommendations to guide centres to optimize donation and transplantation programmes in relation to the dynamic and heterogeneous epidemiological challenges are starting to give good results and the programme has recovered and is now rebuilding in the context of COVID-19.[20]

Impact of COVID-19 pandemic on SOT recipients

There is insufficient data regarding SOT recipients suffering from COVID-19 and viral transmission of SARS-CoV-2 from organ donors to recipients at this time. In a single centre in Netherlands, twenty-three organ recipients who were diagnosed with COVID-19 were studied and nineteen out of twenty-three were hospitalized. All hospitalized patients had chest radiographs consistent with viral pneumonia. Five patients (22%) died from COVID-19.[(21)]

In a larger multi-centre cohort study of SOT recipients with laboratory-confirmed COVID-19, 482 SOT recipients from >50 transplant centres were included. Among them, 78% were hospitalized, 31% required mechanical ventilation, and 20.5% died by twenty-eight days after diagnosis.[(22)] In this study, mortality was mainly related to underlying medical comorbidities and certain clinical features at presentation, rather than surrogate measures of immunosuppression intensity.[(22)]

A very high early mortality among kidney-transplant recipients with Covid-19, 28% at three weeks, was reported in a group of thirty-six consecutive adult kidney-transplant recipients, between 16 March and 1 April 2020. Of the thirty-six kidney recipients, 94% had hypertension, 69% had diabetes mellitus, 36% had a history of smoking tobacco or were current smokers, and 17% had heart disease. In this series, 78% were admitted to the hospital and 96% of the hospitalized patients had radiographic evidence of viral pneumonia, 39% requiring mechanical ventilation.[(23)]

Another study of ninety SOT recipients with COVID-19 at two large academic centres during the initial three weeks of the epidemic in New York City revealed 18% patients died (sixteen patients), 24% were hospitalized, 52% were ICU patients, and 54% (thirty-seven patients) were discharged. Average time from transplant to infection in this cohort was almost six years.[(24)]

A case-fatality rate of 27.8% (5/18) was reported in another preliminary single-centre analysis including SOT recipients diagnosed with COVID-19 from 5 March to 23 March 2020, in Spain.[(25)]

Conversely, a study to compare outcomes in SOT versus non-SOT COVID-19 patients admitted in the ICU throughout the US, from 4 March to 8 May 2020 demonstrated that twenty-eight-day mortality in

SOT COVID-19 patients was similar to non-SOT COVID-19 patients. Furthermore, no difference in the ICU length of stay, risk of acute respiratory distress syndrome (ARDS), secondary infection, thromboembolic events, vasopressor use, or receipt or duration of invasive mechanical ventilation was reported between the two groups, while a 30% higher risk of acute kidney injury requiring renal replacement therapy was documented in SOT COVID-19 patients.[26]

In a case series from a single, large academic heart transplant programme in New York, between 1 March and 24 April 2020, twenty-eight recipients of heart transplant were infected with COVID-19. Overall, seven patients (25%) died; among twenty-two patients (79%) who were admitted, 50% were discharged home, 18% remained hospitalized at the end of the study, and 32% died during hospital stay.[27]

In a recently reported large experience by the Spanish Group from the Study of COVID-19 in Transplant Recipients, the incidence of COVID-19 in SOT recipients was 11.9/1,000 persons at risk (two-fold higher compared to the Spanish general population).[28] No donor-derived COVID-19 was suspected. Infection was hospital-acquired in 13% of cases, with a reported median interval from transplantation of twenty months for this group of recipients, and of sixty-five months for community-acquired cases. About 3% of patients acquired SARS-CoV-2 infection in the first month after transplantation. Overall, 27% patients died and the cause of death was considered to be COVID-19 in 93% of cases. The course of infection was described as worse in lung transplant recipients.[28]

Lung transplantation as a rescue therapy in COVID-19 pneumonia refractory to maximal medical therapy

On the other side of this multifaceted relation between the actual pandemic and transplantation system, one should also consider the potential need of transplantation for patients affected by COVID-19. Lung transplantation as a rescue therapy for end-stage pulmonary fibrosis related to acute respiratory distress syndrome induced by SARS-Cov2 infection has been reported.[29,30] A series of three cases of lung transplantation for

COVID-19 patients who could not be weaned off ECMO support was published. Bilateral lung transplant was taken into consideration as the primary choice of treatment. Three critical points have been recommended in order to evaluate lung transplant candidacy: confirmed irreversibility of respiratory failure refractory to maximal medical support; confirmed positive-turned-negative virology status by repeated consecutive nucleic acid tests with samples derived from multiple sites; and absence of other organ dysfunction contraindicating transplantation.(29) More recently, Cypel and Keshavjee listed ten considerations that should be carefully weighed when assessing a patient with COVID-19-associated ARDS regarding potential candidacy for lung transplantation.(31)

Conclusion

In the critically challenging arena of organ donation and transplantation, the ongoing strike of the dramatic COVID-19 pandemic is seriously affecting donation and transplantation rates all over the world.

In this rapidly evolving circumstance, individualized decision-making regarding transplantation, balancing risk of death on waiting list, risk of infection transmission, actual lack of specific therapies for SARS-CoV-2, and the potential serious effects of severe COVID-19 disease in SOT recipients should be carefully considered. Nevertheless, unjustified fears and misinformation should be contained, in order to avoid the real risk of deaths indirectly related to COVID-19 pandemic on patients requiring organ transplantation. Clinical practice recommendations that address the priorities of organ donation and transplantation activity during the actual pandemic have been recently published, guiding decisions around deceased donation evaluation and the management of SOT recipients and patients in the waiting list.(32)

Highlights

- SARS-CoV-2 pandemic has profoundly affected healthcare systems and will have a long-lasting impact on the organ donation and transplantation systems all over the world.

- Maximum precautions are applied with international guidance on the evaluation and screening of donors for SARS-CoV-2 infection.
- Dramatic decrease in organ donation and transplantation rates during the pandemic has been documented during the early phase of pandemic.
- Overwhelmed healthcare system, unavailability of intensive care unit beds, reduced mobility, reduced resources, prolonged times needed for SARS-CoV-2 testing are among the factors responsible for this decreased activity.
- The impact of immunosuppression on the burden of the disease is still uncertain; on one side there is potentially greater infection risk, and on the other side potential protective effect from cytokine storm.
- Despite a dramatic decrease of organ donation and transplantation during the early phase of the pandemic, a recovery of the program has been described, which will hopefully return to pre-pandemic levels soon.

References

1. Mazzeo AT. Vitruvian Man Redesigned in the COVID-19 Era. Neurol India 2020;68:955–956.
2. Michaels MG, La Hoz RM, Danziger-Isakov L, et al. Coronavirus disease 2019: Implications of emerging infections for transplantation. J Transplant. 2020;20:1768–1772.
3. Summary of Spanish recommendations regarding organ donation and transplantation in relation to the COVID-19 outbreak. http://www.ont.es/infesp/RecomendacionesParaProfesionales/Spanish%20Recommendations%20on%20Organ%20Donation%20and%20Transplantation%20COVID-19%20ONT.pdf. Accessed April 13, 2020
4. Trapianti CN. 28 Febbraio 2020 Prot. 482/CNT 2020.; 2020
5. https://optn.transplant.hrsa.gov/news/information-for-transplant-programs-andopos-regarding-2019-novel-coronavirus/
6. Ritschl PV, Nevermann N, Wiering L, et al. Solid organ transplantation programs facing lack of empiric evidence in the COVID-19 pandemic: A By-proxy Society Recommendation Consensus approach. Am J Transplant. 2020;00:1–12.
7. Fix OK, Hameed B, Fontana RJ, et al. Best Practice Advice for Hepatology and Liver Transplant Providers During the COVID-19 Pandemic: AASLD Expert Panel Consensus Statement. Hepatology. 2020. PMID: 32298473 doi:10.1002/HEP.31281
8. Vistoli F, Furian L, Maggiore U, et al. COVID-19 and kidney transplantation: an Italian Survey and Consensus. Journal of Nephrology 2020; https://doi.org/10.1007/s40620-020-00755-8

9. Kumar D, Manuel O, Natori Y, et al. COVID-19: A global transplant perspective on successfully navigating a pandemic. Am J Transplant. 2020;00:1–7.
10. Stock PG, Wall A, Gardner J. Ethical Issues in the COVID Era: Doing the Right Thing Depends on Location, Resources, and Disease Burden. Transplantation 2020; 104:1316–1320.
11. Dominguez-Gil B, Coll E, Fernandez-Ruiz M, et al. COVID-19 in Spain: Transplantation in the midst of the pandemic. Am J Transplant. 2020;00:1–6.
12. Loupy A, Aubert O, Reese PP, et al. Organ procurement and transplantation during the COVID-19 pandemic. The Lancet 2020; 395: 295–296.
13. Ahmed O, Brockmeier D, Lee K, Chapman WC, Doyle M. Organ donation during the COVID-19 pandemic. Am J Transplant. 2020;00:1–8. DOI: 10.1111/ajt.16199
14. Manara AR, Mumford L, Callaghan CJ, Ravanan R, Gardiner D. Donation and transplantation activity in the UK during the COVID-19 lockdown. The Lancet 2020;396: 465–466.
15. Angelico R, Trapani S, Manzia TM et al. The COVID-19 outbreak in Italy: Initial implications for organ transplantation programs. Am J Transplant. 2020;20:1780–1784.
16. Chadban SJ, McDonald M, Wyburn K, Opdam H, Barry L, Coates PT. Significant impact of COVID-19 on organ donation and transplantation in a low-prevalence country: Australia., Kidney International 2020; doi: https://doi.org/10.1016/j.kint.2020.10.007
17. Zidan A, Alabbad S, Ali T, et al. Position Statement of Transplant Activity in the Middle East in Era of COVID-19 Pandemic. Transplantation 2020; 104: 2205–2207.
18. Merola J, Schilsky ML, Mulligan, DC. The Impact of COVID-19 on Organ Donation, Procurement and Liver Transplantation in the United States. Hepatol Commun. 2020 Sep 29: 10.1002/hep4.1620. doi: 10.1002/hep4.1620
19. Strauss AT, Boyarsky BJ, Garonzik Wang JM, et al: Liver transplantation in the United States during the COVID-19 pandemic: national and center-level Responses. Am Journ Tranplant 2020, in press, doi: 10.1111/AJT.16373
20. Dominguez-Gil B, Fernandez-Ruiz M, Hernandez D, et al. ORGAN DONATION AND TRANSPLANTATION DURING THE COVID-19 PANDEMIC: A SUMMARY OF THE SPANISH EXPERIENCE. Transplantation, Publish Ahead of Print DOI: 10.1097/TP.0000000000003528
21. Hoeck RAS, Manintveld OC, Betjes MGH, et al. COVID-19 in solid organ transplant recipients: a single-center experience. Transpl Int. 2020 May 27;10.1111/tri.13662. doi: 10.1111/tri.13662
22. Kates OS, Haydel BM, Florman SS, et al. COVID-19 in solid organ transplant: A multi-center cohort study. Clin Infect Dis. 2020 Aug 7: ciaa1097. Published online 2020 Aug 7. doi: 10.1093/cid/ciaa1097
23. Akalin E, Azzi Y, Bartash R et al. Covid-19 and Kidney Transplantation. N Engl J Med 2020;382:2475–2477.
24. Pereira MR, Mohan S, Cohen DJ, et al. COVID-19 in solid organ transplant recipients: Initial report from the US epicenter. Am J Transplant. 2020;00:1–9.
25. Fernandez-Ruiz M, Andres A, Loinaz C, et al. COVID-19 in solid organ transplant recipients: A single-center case series from Spain. Am J Transplant. 2020;20:1849–1858.

26. Molnar MZ, Bhalla A, Azhar A, et al. Outcomes of critically ill solid organ transplant patients with COVID-19 in the United States. Am J Transplant. 2020;20:3061–3071.
27. Latif F, Farr MA, Clerkin KJ, et al. Characteristics and Outcomes of Recipients of Heart Transplant With Coronavirus Disease 2019. JAMA Cardiol. 2020;5(10):1165–1169.
28. Coll E, Fernandez-Ruiz M, Sanchez-Alvarez JE, et al: COVID-19 in transplant recipients: The Spanish experience. Am J Transplant 2020, doi: 10.1111/AJT.16369, in press.
29. Chen JY, Qiao K, Liu F, et al. Lung transplantation as therapeutic option in acute respiratory distress syndrome for coronavirus disease 2019-related pulmonary fibrosis. Chin Med J 2020;133(12):1390–1396
30. Luo WR, Yu H, Gou JZ et al. Histopathologic Findings in the Explant Lungs of a Patient With COVID-19 Treated With Bilateral Orthotopic Lung Transplant. Transplantation: November 2020;104(11): e329–e331.
31. Cypel M, Keshavjee S. When to consider lung transplantation for COVID-19. Lancet Respir Med 2020;8:944–946.
32. Weiss MJ, Homby L, Foroutan F, Belga S, Bernier S, et al. Clinical practice guideline for solid organ donation and transplantation during the COVID-19 pandemic. Transplant Direct. 2021 Oct; 7(10): e755. doi: 10.1097/TXD.0000000000001199.

Index

Tables and figures are indicated by t and f following the page number